G000123454

Textbook and Color Atlas
of Traumatic Injuries to the Teeth

A. T. Hyatt.

J. O. ANDREASEN AND F. M. ANDREASEN

Textbook and Color Atlas of Traumatic Injuries to the Teeth

THIRD EDITION

MUNKSGAARD · COPENHAGEN

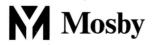

St. Louis Baltimore Boston Chicago London Madrid Philadelphia Sydney Toronto

Munksgaard

TEXTBOOK AND COLOR ATLAS OF TRAUMATIC INJURIES TO THE TEETH

3RD EDITION, 1ST PRINTING 1994

COPYRIGHT © 1981, 1994 BY MUNKSGAARD, COPENHAGEN, DENMARK

ALL RIGHTS RESERVED

ISBN 87-16-10637-7

LAYOUT, GRAPHIC DESIGN, DIAGRAMS: LARS THORSEN

COVER-LAYOUT: MUNKSGAARDS TEGNESTUE

COVER ILLUSTRATION: HENNING DAHLHOF

COLOR DRAWINGS: HENNING DAHLHOF

REPRODUCTION: HIGH TECH REPRO A/S, COPENHAGEN

PRINTER: PROOST INTERNATIONAL BOOK PRODUCTION, BELGIUM

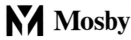

Dedicated to Publishing Excellence

DISTRIBUTED IN NORTH AND SOUTH AMERICA BY MOSBY YEAR-BOOK, INC.

11830 WESTLINE INDUSTRIAL DRIVE ST. LOUIS, MISSOURI 63146

ISBN 0-8151-0127-9

NO PART OF THIS PUBLICATION MAY BE REPRODUCED, STORED IN A RETRIEVAL SYSTEM, OR TRANSMITTED IN ANY FORM OR BY ANY MEANS, ELECTRONIC, MECHANICAL PHOTOCOPYING, RECORDING OR OTHERWISE WITHOUT PRIOR PERMISSION BY THE COPYRIGHT OWNER.

Preface

"Seeing implies making ourselves free of prejudices, becoming aware of our being manipulated by old frames of references, acquiring new ones through the collection of knowledge, giving truth priority over the way we would like things to be, interpreting imaginatively so that development forward becomes visible"
BRÄNNSTRÖM 1981

While these remarks were true in the early 1980's when Martin Brännström presented his revolutionary concepts of the role of bacteria in pulpal response to restorative materials, they are certainly as relevant now in our views of pulpal and periodontal healing after trauma. The past decade since the publication of the 2nd edition of *Traumatic Injuries of the Teeth* has witnessed advances in our understanding of wound healing after injury, developments in restorative dental materials - not the least of which is the evolution of dentin and universal bonding agents - and knowledge about pulpal responses to these materials. About a century ago, G.V. Black developed his ideas of cavity preparation, based on the materials available at that time: gold foil and silver amalgam. Composite resin restorations weren't even imagined. The acid etch technique and composite resin restorations demanded rethinking on the part of the profession and led to the concept of very conservative preventive resin restorations, tunnel preparations and the like to preserve tooth structure. Recent and ongoing research into dentin bonding agents and pulpal responses to a bacteria-tight seal under dental restorations once again force us to re-think treatment strategy in order to save tooth structure and maintain pulp vitality.

Recent advances in the understanding of wound healing related to dental trauma, tooth and bone transplantation and implantation have opened up new treatment avenues which for the first time make it possible to fully restore even the most severely traumatized dentition. The sad reality, however, is that these sophisticated treatment alternatives are inaccessible for most patients due to their cost. The challenge, therefore, is to simplify these procedures and thereby bring them within the grasp of the general public.

A significant portion of the first part of this 3rd edition is devoted to wound healing principles in general, and as they relate to healing after acute dental trauma. The deeper one delves into healing principles, the more one becomes aware of the role infection plays in the development of healing complications.

Since the publication of the 1st edition in 1972, progress has been dramatic. The increase in the size of the volumes reflects this. In 1972, the 1st edition comprised 334 pages, in 1981, 450 pages, now, more than 760 pages.

The goal of this 3rd edition, *Textbook of Traumatic Injuries to the Teeth* is to tell the reader of the vast treatment potential now available for tooth preserving, tooth restoring and tooth replacement. The latter includes the use of autotransplantation and implantation. Apart from these innovative treatment procedures, long-term clinical investigations, as well as experimental studies in various aspects of dental traumatology, have been instrumental in developing a biological treatment foundation based on the science of wound healing in the dental pulp and periodontium after injury. This has permitted the development of a sometimes very conservative treatment strategy.

It is on this biological basis and the development of new treatment modalities that it is now possible to save more teeth and restore the esthetics and function to the traumatized dentition. It is our wish that this progress will be to the benefit of that significant part of the population which has suffered dental injury.

Finally, we would like to express our gratitude to the administration and our colleagues in the dental department at the University Hospital and Departments of Pediatric Dentistry and Oral and Maxillofacial Surgery at the Dental School, Copenhagen, for providing the working environments in which this text could be written. Thanks, too, to photographers Leise Ellegaard and Tove Rasmussen for their professional assistance.

Gratitude is expressed to Drs. Torsten Reumert and Stig Bolund of the Plastic Surgery Unit, University Hospital, Copenhagen, for their critical review of the section on soft tissue wounds. Thanks, too, to the librarians at the University Library, and the libraries of the Dental Schools, Copenhagen and Århus University, for their painstaking efforts in the literature review necessary in the production of each chapter.

Particular thanks are extended to Drs. Jette Daugaard-Jensen and E. Christian Munksgaard for their strong personal and professional support and collaboration.

Also personal thanks to international colleagues for their advice and recommendations particularly in the realm of pulpal responses, dentin bonding agents and composite resin restorations, which has helped raise the art of restorative dentistry to the science that it is today. These include: Dr. Gunnar Bergenholtz (Gothenburg, Sweden), Dr. David Pashley (Augusta, Georgia), Dr. John Gwinnett (Stony Brook, New York), Dr. Charles Cox (Birmingham, Alabama), and Dr. Erik Asmussen (Copenhagen, Denmark). Of course the spirit of the research initiated by Dr. Martin Brännström has pervaded this arena.

Finally, a special thanks to Lene Due Andreasen for her painstaking typing of the manuscript for this 3rd edition.

J.O. Andreasen and F.M. Andreasen
Copenhagen, October 1993

List of Contributors

P.K. ANDERSEN, Cand.Stat., PhD
Statistical Research Unit
University of Copenhagen
Copenhagen
Denmark

J.O. ANDREASEN, DDS,
Odont Dr. HC, F.R.C.S,
Department of Oral and Maxillo-
facial Surgery
University Hospital
Copenhagen
Denmark

F.M. ANDREASEN, DDS, LDS
Department of Oral and Maxillo-
facial Surgery
Department of Pedodontics
Dental School
Copenhagen
Denmark

N.H.J. CREUGERS, DDS, Odont Dr.
Department of Oral Function and
Prosthetic Dentistry
Dental School
Nijmegen
The Netherlands

M. CVEK, DDS, Odont Dr.
Department of Pedodontics
Eastman Dental Institute
Stockholm
Sweden

C. DAHLIN, DDS, Odont Dr.
Department of Oral and Maxillo-
facial Surgery
Norra Älvsborg County Hospital
Trollhatan
Sweden

R.D. FINKELMAN, DDS, PhD
Hard Tissue Research Laboratory
Institute of Molecular Biology
Worcester
Massachusetts
USA

L. GOLDSON, DDS
Department of Orthodontics
Eastman Dental Institute
Stockholm
Sweden

F. GOTTRUP, MD., D.M.Sci.
Copenhagen Wound Healing Center
Hvidovre and Bispebjerg Hospital
and Rigshospitalet
Copenhagen
Denmark

J. JENSEN, DDS
Department of Oral and Maxillo-
facial Surgery
Aarhus University Hospital
Aarhus
Denmark

R.E. JORDAN, DDS, MSD, F.I.C.D
Faculty of Dentistry
University of Manitoba
Winnipeg
Manitoba
Canada

L. KRISTERSON, DDS, Odont Dr.
Department of Oral and Maxillo-
facial Surgery
Malmö General Hospital
Malmö
Sweden

7

B. MALMGREN, DDS
Department of Pedodontics
Eastman Dental Institute
Stockholm
Sweden

O. MALMGREN, DDS, Odont Dr.
Department of Orthodontics
Eastman Dental Institute
Stockholm
Sweden

H. NILSON, DDS, LDS
Department of Prosthetic Dentistry
University of Umeå
Umeå
Sweden

P. PALACCI, DDS
10 Rue Fargès
Marseille
France

B. SCHEER, BDS, LDS
Department of Paediatric Dentistry
Kings College School of Medicine
and Dentistry
London
England

O. SCHWARTZ, DDS, PhD
Department of Oral and
Maxillofacial Surgery
Bispebjerg Hospital
Copenhagen
Denmark

M. TORABINEJAD, DMD, MSD
Department of Endodontics
School of Dentistry
Loma Linda
California
USA

M. TSUKIBOSHI, DDS
5-14 Genji
Kanie-cho, Amagun
Aichi 497
Japan

R.R. WELBURY, MD, BS, PhD,
FDSRCS (Eng)
Department of Child Dental Health
Dental Hospital and School
University of Newcastle-upon-Tyne
Newcastle-upon-Tyne
England

R.R. WINTHER, DDS
Department of Fixed Prosthodontics
Marquette University
Milwaukee
Wisconsin
USA

Contents

19. Autotransplantation of Teeth to the Anterior Region

J.O. ANDREASEN, L. KRISTERSON,
M. TSUKIBOSHI & F.M. ANDREASEN

20. Implants in the Anterior Region

J.O. ANDREASEN, L. KRISTERSON,
H. NILSON, K. DAHLIN,
O. SCHWARTZ, P. PALACCI &
J. JENSEN

21. Prevention of Dental and Oral Injuries

B. SCHEER

22. Prognosis of Traumatic Dental Injuries

P. K. ANDERSEN, F.M. ANDREASEN
& J.O. ANDREASEN

CHAPTER 1

Wound Healing Subsequent to Injury

F. GOTTRUP & J.O. ANDREASEN

Traumatic dental injuries usually imply wound-healing processes in the periodontium, the pulp and sometimes associated soft tissue. The outcome of these determines the final healing result (Fig. 1.1).

The general response of soft and mineralized tissues to surgical and traumatic injuries is a sensitive process, where even minor changes in the treatment procedure may have an impact upon the rate and quality of healing.

In order to design suitable treatment procedures for a traumatized dentition, it is necessary to consider the cellular and humoral elements in wound healing. In this respect considerable progress has been made in understanding of the role of different cells involved.

In this chapter the general response of soft tissues to injury is described, as well as the various factors influencing the wound healing processes. For progress to be made in the treatment of traumatic dental injuries it is necessary to begin with general wound-healing principles. The aim of the present chapter is to give a general survey of wound healing as it appears from recent research. For more detailed information about the various topics the reader should consult recent textbooks devoted to wound healing (1-13,172, 542-544, 549).

Nature of a Traumatic Injury

Whenever injury disrupts tissue, a sequence of events is initiated whose ultimate goal is to heal the damaged tissue. The sequence of events after wounding is control of bleeding; establishing a line of defense against infection; cleansing the wound site of eventual necrotic tissue elements, bacteria or foreign bodies, closing the wound gap with newly-formed connective tissue and epithelium; and finally modifying the primary wound tissue to a more functionally suitable tissue.

This healing process is basically the same in all tissues, but may vary clinically according to the tissues involved. Thus wound healing after dental trauma is complicated by the multiplicity of cellular systems involved (Fig. 1.1).

During the last two decades, significant advances have been made in the understanding of the biology behind wound healing in general and new details concerning the regulating mechanisms have be discovered.

While a vast body of knowledge exists concerning the healing of cutaneous wounds, relatively sparse information exists concerning healing of oral mucosa and odontogenic tissues. This chapter describes the general features of wound healing, and the present knowledge of the cellular systems involved. Wound healing as it applies to the specific odontogenic tissues will be described in Chapter 2.

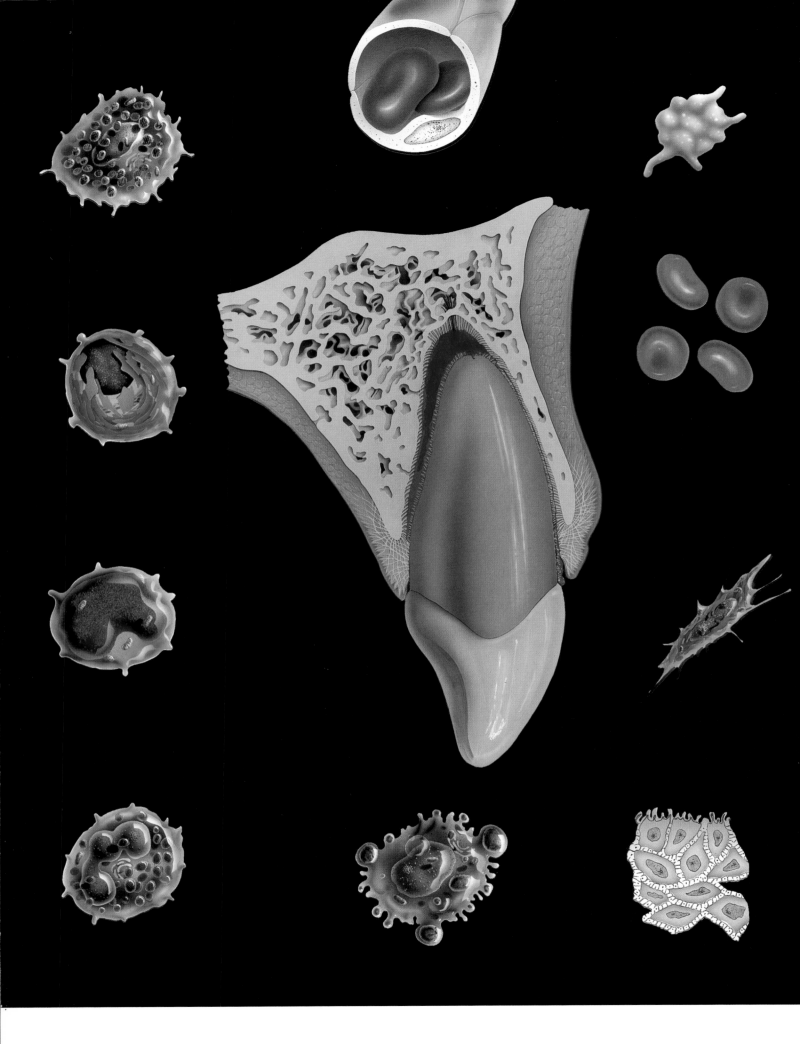

←
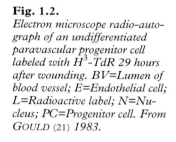

Fig. 1.1. Cells involved in the healing events after a tooth luxation. Clockwise from top left:
Endothelial cells
Thrombocyte (platelet)
Erythrocytes
Fibroblast
Epithelial cells
Macrophage
Neutrophil
Lymphocyte
Plasma cell
Mast cell

Repair versus Regeneration

The goal of the wound-healing process after injury is to restore the continuity between wound edges and to reestablish tissue function. In relation to wound healing, it is appropriate to define various terms, such as *repair* and *regeneration*. In this context, it has been suggested that the term *regeneration* should be used for a biologic process by which the structure and function of the disrupted or lost tissue is completely restored, whereas *repair* is a biologic process whereby the continuity of the disrupted or lost tissue is regained by new tissue which does not restore structure and function (14). Throughout the text, these terms will be used according to the above definitions. The implication of repair and regeneration as they relate to oral tissues is discussed in Chapter 2, p. 77.

Cell Differentiation

Cell differentiation is a process whereby an embryonic non-functional cell matures and changes into a tissue-specific cell, performing one or more functions characteristic of that cell population. Examples of this are the *mesenchymal perivascular cells*

in the periodontal ligament and the pulp, and the *basal cells* of the epithelium. A problem arises as to whether already functioning odontogenic cells can revert to a more primitive cell type. Although this is known to take place in cutaneous wounds (15), it is unsettled with respect to dental tissues (see Chapter 2, p.77). With regard to cell differentiation, it appears that extracellular matrix compounds, such as proteoglycans, have a significant influence on cell differentiation in wound healing (16).

Progenitor Cells (Stem Cells)

Among the various cell populations in oral and other tissues, a small fraction are *progenitor cells*. These cells are self-perpetuating, nonspecialized cells, which are the source of new differentiating cells during normal tissue turnover and healing after injury (17-19).

The typical morphologic features of progenitor cells are that they have retained an embryonic appearance, i.e. small size, scarcity of intracellular organelles and a high nuclear/cytoplasmatic ratio (20, 21).

The progenitor cells are predominantly placed around blood vessels close to the basement membrane of the vasculature

Fig. 1.2.
Electron microscope radio-autograph of an undifferentiated paravascular progenitor cell labeled with H^3-TdR 29 hours after wounding. BV=Lumen of blood vessel; E=Endothelial cell; L=Radioactive label; N=Nucleus; PC=Progenitor cell. From GOULD (21) 1983.

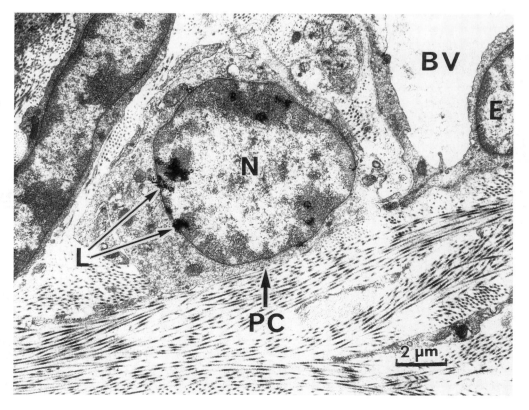

(Fig. 1.2). In contrast to differentiated cells, progenitor cells appear to be rather resistant to even extended periods of ischemia (22, 23). In this context the preferential paravascular location appears to be optimal for nutrition of the progenitor cells during trauma events, such as a compromized vascularity following injury, as well as during revascularization in the form of end-to-end anastomoses (see p. 48). In both instances the paravascular position implies that the progenitor cell will be the last cell to suffer during vascular shut-down and the first to benefit from eventual revascularization.

Progenitor cell activation after wounding has been studied in various oral tissues such as *gingiva* (24, 25), *pulp* (26-34), *periodontal ligament* (PDL) (21, 31, 35-37), *bone* (20, 31, 37), *skin* (38), *mucosa* (39), and *muscle* (40).

In surgical periodontal wounds in monkeys the paravascularly placed progenitor cells within the nearest 200 μm of the wound defect have been found to respond with mitosis after one day (41). It is anticipated, but not yet proven, that one of the daughter cells then starts to migrate towards the wound area (35). During this migration further cell divisions take place which continue as the cells move into the wound site (41).

Signals for initial progenitor cell mitosis and the later amplifying divisions of the newly generated progenitor offspring could be initiated from the wound edge, where significant changes in pO_2, pCO_2, lactate and pH are found (42) (See p. 55).

The continued division of migrating cells thus allows a small population of progenitor cells to provide the cells necessary for restoring the damaged tissue with phenotypic cells able to regenerate the PDL wound. The question is then whether different progenitor cells exist for the regeneration of bone, PDL fibers and cementum or whether all three components derive from *one* type of progenitor cell offspring which will differentiate into the appropriate PDL cell (osteoblasts, fibroblasts or cementoblasts) according to local matrix signals. Recent studies indicate that at least two progenitor cell populations exist in the PDL, one population close to bone probably giving rise to bone-committed cells and a cell population near the root surface possibly responsible for cementum and periodontal ligament regeneration (35).

In the pulp, similar healing responses have been found (31). Thus progenitor cell proliferation is seen 2 days after injury and differentiation into odontoblasts and pulp cells is seen within 4 days (31).

An unsettled question is whether the progenitor cell response elicited by wounding represents a pool of resting undifferentiated cells or already differentiated cells which, as a response to injury, dedifferentiate and proliferate and then redifferentiate into osteoblasts, cementoblasts and odontoblasts after contact with the respective tissue matrices (31). Presently, the concept of the matrix modulating the phenotype of the repopulating cells into prospective cementoblasts, osteoblasts or odontoblasts appears doubtful as recent wound-healing studies have shown that repopulating cells in contact with dentin may form not only dentin but also cementum and bone (22). Likewise, exposed cementum matrix may elicit both cementogenesis and osteogenesis (43), apparently suggesting that the phenotype of the tissue formed after injury is related primarily to the origin of repopulating cells (i.e. whether of pulp, periodontal or bone marrow origin). This implies that attempts at guided tissue regeneration (i.e. determining the source of cells invading a wound area) should be based upon knowledge of the type, location and speed of tissue proliferation (22,41,44) (see Chapter 2 p. 77).

Cell Cycle

Prior to mitosis, DNA must duplicate and, RNA be synthesized. Since materials needed for cell division occupy more than half the cell, a cell that is performing functional synthesis (e.g. a fibroblast producing collagen, an odontoblast producing dentin or an epithelial cell producing keratin) does not have the resources to undergo mitosis. Conversely, a cell preparing for or undergoing mitosis has insufficient resources to undertake its functional chores. This may explain why it is usually the least differentiated cells that undergo proliferation in a damaged tissue, and why differentiated cells do not often divide (15).

The interval between consecutive mitoses has been termed the *cell cycle* which represents an ordered sequence of events

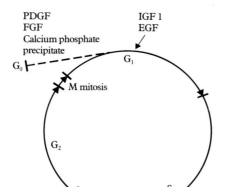

Fig. 1.3. Cell cycle.
G_0 = *resting phase*
G_1 = *time before onset of DNA synthesis*
S = *replication of DNA*
G_2 = *time between DNA replication and mitosis*
M = *mitosis*

that are necessary before the next mitosis (Fig. 1.3). The cell cycle has been subdivided into phases such as G_1, the time before the onset of DNA synthesis. In the S phase the DNA content is replicated, G_2 is the time between the S phase and mitosis, and M the time of mitosis (Fig. 1.3). The cumulative length of S, G_2 and M is relatively constant at 10-12 hours, whereas differences occur among cell types in the duration of G_1 [45].

Cells that have become growth-arrested enter a resting phase, G_0, which lies outside the cell cycle. The G_0 state is reversible and cells can remain viable in G_0 for extended periods.

In vivo, cells can be classified as continuously dividing (e.g. epithelial cells, fibroblasts), non-dividing post-mitotic (e.g. ameloblasts) and cells reversibly growth-arrested in G_0 that can be induced to reenter the proliferative cycle.

Factors leading to fibroblast proliferation have been studied in the fibroblast system. Resting cells are made *competent* to proliferate (i.e. entry of G_0 cells into early G_1 stage) by so-called *competence factors* (i.e. platelet-derived growth factor (PDGF), fibroblast growth factor (FGF) and calcium phosphate precipitates). However, there is no progression beyond G_1 until the appearance of progression factors such as insulin-like growth factor-1 (IGF-1), epidermal growth factor (EGF) and other plasma factors [45] (Fig. 1.3).

Cell Migration

Optimal wound repair is dependent upon an orderly influx of cells into the wound area. Directed cell motion requires polarization of cells and formation of both a leading edge that attaches to the matrix and a trailing edge that is pulled along. The stimulus for directional cell migration can be a soluble attractant (*chemotaxis*), a substratum-bound gradient of a particular matrix constituent (*haptotaxis*) or the three-dimensional array of extracellular matrix within the tissue (*contact guidance*). Finally there is a *free edge effect* which occurs in epithelial wound healing (see p. 53) [46, 47].

Typical examples of cells responding to *chemotaxis* are circulating neutrophils and monocytes (see p. 34). The chemoattractant is regulated by diffusion of the attractant from its source into an attraction-poor medium.

Cells migrating by *haptotaxis* extend lamellipodia more or less randomly and each of these protruding lamellipodiae competes for a matrix component to adhere to, whereby a leading edge will be created on one side of the cell and a new membrane inserted into the leading edge [48]. In that context, fibronectin and laminin seem to be important for adhesion [46].

Contact guidance occurs as the cell is forced along paths of least resistance through the extracellular matrix. Thus, migrating cells align themselves according to the matrix configuration, a phenomenon that can be seen in the extended fibrin strands in retracting blood clots (see p. 23), as well as in the orientation of fibroblasts in granulation tissue [49]. In this context it should be mentioned that mechanisms also exist whereby spaces are opened within the extracellular area when cells migrate. Thus both fibroblasts and macrophages use enzymes such as plasmin, plasminogen and collagenases for this purpose [50].

During wound repair, a given parenchymal cell may migrate into the wound space by multiple mechanisms occurring concurrently or in succession. Factors related to cell migration in wound healing are described later for each particular cell type.

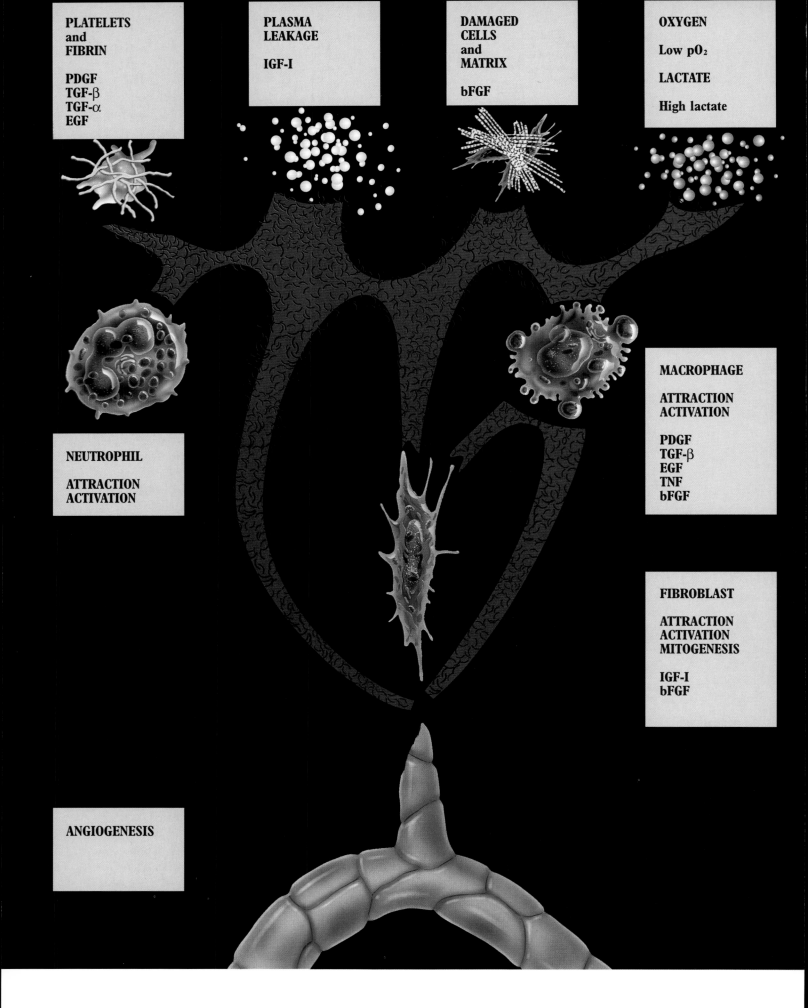

PLATELETS
and
FIBRIN

PDGF
TGF-β
TGF-α
EGF

PLASMA
LEAKAGE

IGF-I

DAMAGED
CELLS
and
MATRIX

bFGF

OXYGEN

Low pO₂

LACTATE

High lactate

MACROPHAGE

ATTRACTION
ACTIVATION

PDGF
TGF-β
EGF
TNF
bFGF

NEUTROPHIL

ATTRACTION
ACTIVATION

FIBROBLAST

ATTRACTION
ACTIVATION
MITOGENESIS

IGF-I
bFGF

ANGIOGENESIS

←
**Fig. 1.4. Cellular compo-
nents and mediators in the
wound-healing module**
*Signals for wound healing are re-
leased by platelets, fibrin, plasma
leakage, damaged cells and matrix. Furthermore low oxygen tension and a high lactate concentration in the injury site contribute
an important stimulus for healing.*

Dynamics of Wound Repair:

Wound-Healing Phases and Wound Types

Classically the events taking place after wounding can be divided into three phases, namely the *inflammation, prolifera-tion* and the *remodelling phases*. The inflammation phase may, however, be subdivided into a *hemostasis phase* and an *inflammatory phase*. But, it should be remembered that wound healing is a continuous process where the beginning and end of each phase cannot be clearly determined and phases do overlap.

Hemostasis Phase

The trauma event usually results in rupture of the vasculature, resulting in bleeding. This event is controlled by combined vasoconstriction, platelet aggregation and activation, and the enzymatic activation of the clotting, complement and kinin cascades, and plasminogen activation.

Activation of platelets and the formation of a fibrin clot release a number of substances which provoke a vascular and cellular response, incorporating mast cells, endothelial cells, neutrophils, lymphocytes, macrophages and fibroblasts whereby the next phases are initiated.

Inflammatory Phase

Neutrophils, lymphocytes and macrophages are the first cells to arrive at the site of injury. Their major role is to guard against the threat of infection, as well as to cleanse the wound site of cellular matrix debris and foreign bodies. The macrophages appear to direct the concerted action of the wound-cell team. Numerous growth factors are released by macrophages and lymphocytes which cause a further influx of neutrophils and initiate the third phase in wound healing (Fig. 1.4).

Proliferative Phase (Fibroplasia)

Stimulated by growth factors and other signals, fibroblasts and endothelial cells divide, and cause a capillary network to move into the wound site which is characterized by ischemic damaged tissue or a coagulum. The increasing numbers of cells in the wound area induce hypoxia, hypercapnia and lactacidosis, due to the increased need for oxygen in an area with decreased oxygen delivery because of the tissue injury (51, 52). Simultaneously, the basal cells in the epithelium divide and move into the injury site, thereby closing the defect. Along with revascularization, new collagen is formed which, after 3-5 days, adds strength to the wound. The high rate of collagen production continues for 10-12 days, resulting in strengthening of the wound. At this time healing tissue is dominated by capillaries and immature collagen.

The arrangement of cells in the proliferative phase has been examined in rabbits using ear chambers where wounds heal between closely approximated, optically clear membranes (52, 53). It appears from these experiments that macrophages infiltrate the tissue in the dead space, followed by immature fibroblasts. New vessels are formed next to these fibroblasts which synthesize collagen. This arrangement of cells, which has been termed the *wound-healing module*, continues to migrate until the tissue defect is obliterated. The factors controlling the growth of the wound healing module are described on p. 55.

Remodelling Phase

In the remodelling phase, the vascularity decreases and a reorganization of the collagen lattice takes place, together with a contraction of the wound.

The extent of the *remodelling phase* is unknown but it is believed to last a year or longer, depending primarily upon the type of tissue involved. During this phase, pronounced changes in the form, bulk and strength of the scar take place. The scar tissue now consists of dense connective tissue dominated by collagen fibers. The turnover rate of collagen is still higher than normal but less rapid than during the proliferative phase. The phase is characterized by remodelling with a further strengthening of the wound, albeit less rapidly than during the proliferation phase.

Types of Wounds after Injury

From a clinical point of view, wounds can be divided into different types, according to healing and associated wound-closure methods (54, 55, 551) (Fig. 1.5). This distinction is based on practical treatment regimens while the basic biological wound-healing sequences are similar for all wound types.

Primary healing, or healing by *first intention*, occurs when wound edges are primarily and anatomically accurately opposed and healing proceeds without complication. This type of wound heals with a good cosmetic and functional result and with a minimal amount of scar tissue. These wounds, however, are sensitive to complications, such as infection.

Secondary healing, or healing by *second intention*, occurs in wounds associated with tissue loss or when wound edges are not accurately opposed. This type of healing is usually the natural biological process that occurs in the absence of surgical intervention. The defect is gradually filled by granulation tissue and a considerable amount of scar tissue will be formed despite an active contraction process. The resulting scar is less functional and often sensitive to thermal and mechanical injury. Furthermore, this form of healing requires considerable time for epithelial coverage and scar formation, but is rather resistant to infection, at least when granulation tissue has developed.

Surgical closure procedures have combined the advantages of the two types of healing. This has led to a technique of *delayed primary closure*, where the wound is left open for a few days but closure is completed before granulation tissue becomes visible (usually a week after wounding) and the wound is then healed by a process similar to primary healing (56, 57). The resulting wound is more resistant to healing complications (primarily infection) and is functionally and cosmetically improved. If visible granulation tissue has developed before either wound closure or wound contraction has spontaneously approximated the defect, it is called *secondary closure*. This wound is healed by a process similar to secondary healing and scar formation is more pronounced than after delayed primary closure. The different closure techniques are shown in Fig. 1.5.

The following section describes the sequential changes in tissue components and their interactions seen during the wound-healing process.

Hemostasis Phase

Coagulation Cascade

An injury that severs the vasculature leads to extravasion of plasma, platelets, erythrocytes and leukocytes. This initiates the coagulation cascade that produces a blood clot usually after a few minutes and which, together with the already induced vascular contraction, limits further blood loss (Fig. 1.6). The tissue injury disrupts the endothelial integrity of the vessels, and exposes the subendothelial structures and various connective tissue components. Especially exposure of type IV and V collagen in the subendothelium promotes binding and aggregation of platelets and their structural proteins (58, 59). Exposure of collagen and other activating agents provokes endothelial cells and platelets to secrete several substances, such as fibronectin, serotonin, platelet-derived growth factor (PDGF), adenosine diphosphate (ADP), thromboxane A and others. Following this activation, platelets aggregate and platelet clot formation begins within a few minutes. The clot formed is impermeable to plasma and serves as a seal for ruptured vasculature as well as to prevent bacterial invasion (59). In addition to platelet aggregation and activation, the coagulation cascade is initiated (Fig. 1.6).

The crucial step in coagulation is the conversion of fibrinogen to fibrin which will create a threadlike network to entrap plasma fractions and formed elements. This fibrin blood clot is formed both intra- and extravascularly and supports the initial platelet clot (Fig. 1.6). Extrinsic and intrinsic clotting mechanisms are activated, each giving rise to cascades that will convert prothrombin to thrombin, and in turn cleave fibrinogen to fibrin which then polymerizes to form a clot (60).

The *extrinsic* coagulation pathway is initiated by tissue thromboplastin and coagulation Factor VII, whereas the initiator of the *intrinsic* coagulation cascade consists of Hageman factor (Factor XII), prekallikrein and HMW-kinogen. The *extrinsic* coagulation pathway is the primary

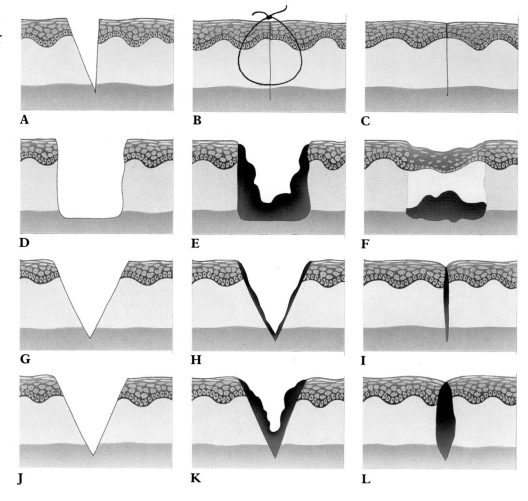

Fig. 1.5. Wound-healing events related to the type of wound and subsequent treatment
A - C: Incisional wound with primary closure.
D - F: Open and non sutured wound.
G - I: Delayed primary closure.
J - L: Secondary closure.
From GOTTRUP (54) 1991.

A   B   C

D   E   F

G   H   I

J   K   L

source of clotting, while the *intrinsic* coagulation pathway is probably most important in producing bradykinin, a vasoactive mediator that increases vascular permeability (61).

Products of the coagulation cascade regulate the cells in the wound area. Thus *intact thrombin* serves as a potent growth stimulator for fibroblasts and endothelial cells (62, 63) whereas *degraded thrombin* fragments stimulate monocytes and platelets (64, 65). Likewise *plasmin* acts as a growth factor for parenchymal cells (66). *Fibrin* acts as a chemoattractant for monocytes (67) and induces angiogenesis (61). Other mediators created by blood coagulation for wound healing include *kallikrein*, *bradykinin*, and *C3a* and *C5a* through a spillover activation of the complement cascade and most of these factors act as chemoattractants for circulating leukocytes. Thus apart from ensuring hemostasis, the clot also initiates healing (Fig. 1.4).

If the blood clot is exposed to air it will dry and form a scab which serves as a temporary wound dressing. A vast network of fibrin strands extends throughout the clot in all directions (Fig. 1.6). These strands subsequently undergo contraction and become reoriented primarily in a plane parallel to the wound edges (68, 69). As the fibrin strands contract, they exert tensional forces on the wound edges whereby serum is extruded from the clot and the distance between wound edges is decreased. Contraction and reorientation of the fibrin strands later serve as pathways for migrating cells (see p. 23).

If proper adaptation of the wound edges has occurred the extravascular clot forms a thin gel filling the narrow space between the wound edges and gluing the wound edges together with fibrin.

If hemostasis is not achieved, blood will continue to leak into the tissue, leading to a hematoma and a coagulum which consists of serum plasma fraction, formed elements and fibrin fragments. The presence of such a hematoma will delay the wound healing and increase the risk of infection.

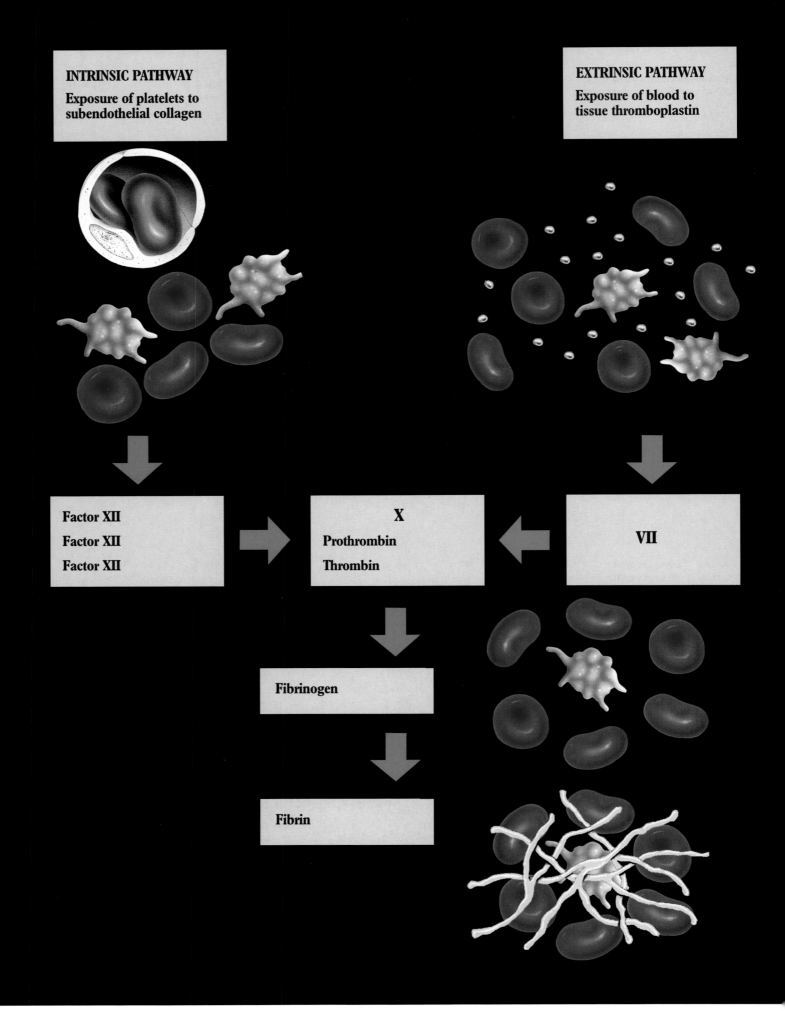

INTRINSIC PATHWAY

Exposure of platelets to
subendothelial collagen

EXTRINSIC PATHWAY

Exposure of blood to
tissue thromboplastin

Factor XII
Factor XII
Factor XII

X
Prothrombin
Thrombin

VII

Fibrinogen

Fibrin

Coagulation

More extensive blood clot formation is undesirable in most wounds as the clots present barriers between tissue surfaces and force wounds that might have healed primarily without a clot to heal by secondary intention. In oral wounds such as extraction sockets, blood clots are exposed to heavy bacterial colonization from the saliva (70). In this location neutrophil leukocytes form a dense layer on the exposed blood clot and the most superficial neutrophils contain many phagocytosed bacteria (71).

The breakdown of coagulated blood in the wound releases ferric ions into the tissue which have been shown to decrease the nonspecific host response to infection (72). Furthermore, the presence of a hematoma in the tissue may increase the chance of infection (73).

Clot adhesion to the root surface appears to be important for periodontal ligament healing. Thus an experiment has shown that heparin impregnated root surfaces, which prevented clot formation, re-sulted in significantly less connective tissue repair and an increase in downgrowth of pocket epithelium after gingival flap surgery (74).

Fibrin

During the coagulation process, fibrinogen is converted to fibrin which via a fishnet arrangement with entrapped erythrocytes, stabilizes the blood clot (Fig. 1.6).

In the early acute inflammatory period extravasation of a serous fluid from the leaking vasculature accummulates as an edema in the tissue spaces. This transudate contains fibrinogen which forms fibrin when acted upon by thrombin. Fibrin plugs then seal damaged lymphatics and thereby confine the inflammatory reaction to an area immediately surrounding the wound.

Fibrin has recently been found to play a significant role in wound healing by its capacity to bind to fibronectin (60). Thus fibronectin present in the clot will link to both fibrin and to itself (75, 76).

Fig. 1.7.
Schematic illustration of the presence of fibrin *in experimental skin wounds in guinea-pigs. The scale is semiquantitative, graded from 0 to 3. From* ROSS *&* BENDIT *1961* (85).

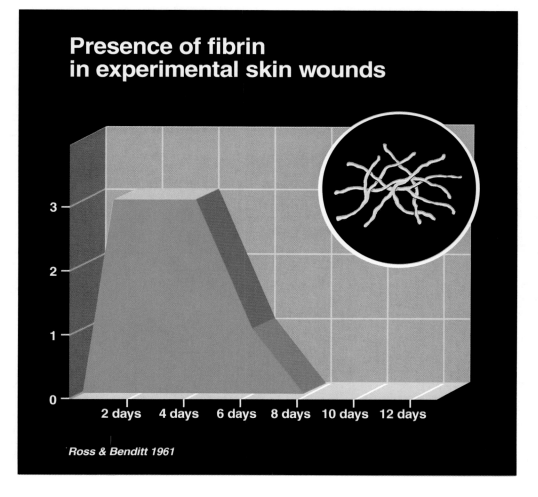

Presence of fibrin in experimental skin wounds

Ross & Benditt 1961

Fibrin clots and fibrinopeptides are weak stimulators of fibroblasts (77), an effect which is prevented by depletion of fibronectin (78). It has also been proposed that an interaction may take place between hyaluronic acid and fibrin which creates an initial scaffold on which cells may migrate into the wound (79).

The extravascular fibrin forms a hygroscopic gel that facilitates migration of neutrophils and macrophages, an effect which possibly reflects a positive interaction between the macrophage surface and the fibrin matrix (80). Fibrin has also been shown to elicit fibroblast migration and angiogenesis, both of which initiate an early cellular invasion of the clot (60, 61, 80-82).

Fibrin clots are continuously degraded over a one to three weeks period (83-85). This occurs during the fibrinolysis cascade which is activated by the plasminogen present in damaged endothelial cells and activated granulocytes and macrophages (83, 84, 86).

In experimental replantation of teeth in monkeys it has been found that collagen fiber attachment to the root surface was preceded by fibrin leakage, and that this leakage was an initial event in the wound-healing response (87).

In summary, the blood clot, apart from being responsible for hemostasis, also serves the purpose of initiating wound healing including functioning as a matrix for migrating connective cells.

Fibronectin

Fibronectin is a complex glycoprotein, which can be present as *soluble plasma fibronectin*, produced by hepatocytes, or *stromal fibronectin*, found in basal laminas and loose connective tissue matrices where it is produced by fibroblasts, macrophages and epithelial cells (88, 89). During wound healing, fibronectin is also produced locally by fibroblasts (90), macrophages in regions where epidermal cell migration occurs (89), endothelial cells (91, 92), and by epidermal cells (93).

Fibronectin plays many roles in wound healing, including platelet aggregation, promotion of reepithelialization, cell migration, matrix deposition and wound contraction (89, 94).

In wound healing, fibronectin is the first protein to be deposited in the wound (95) and therefore, together with fibrin, serves as a preliminary scaffold and matrix for migrating cells (96) (see p. 56). Thus plasma fibronectin is linked to fibrin which has been spilled from damaged vessels or from highly permeable undamaged vessels (see p. 23) (83, 97). The fibrin-fibronectin complex forms an extensive meshwork throughout the wound bed which facilitates fibroblast attachment and migration into the clot (76, 98-100). Furthermore, soluble fibronectin fragments are chemotactic for fibroblasts and monocytes (101).

Fibronectin appears also to guide the orderly deposition of collagen within the granulation tissue. Thus fibronectin serves as the scaffold for deposition of types III and I collagen (102-106) as well as collagen type VI (106). As dermal wounds age, bundles of type I collagen become more prominent at the expense of type III collagen fibronectin (103). Finally, fibronectin seems to represent a necessary link between collagen and fibroblasts which makes it possible to generate the forces in wound contraction (89, 107)

In endothelium during wound healing, fibronectin is found in the basement membrane and reaches a maximum at approximately the same time as the peak in endothelial cell mitosis occurs, indicating a possible role of fibronectin in endothelial cell migration (548).

In epithelialization, it has been found that fibronectin is implicated in epidermal cell adhesion, migration and differentiation (93, 108-111). Thus migrating epithelial cells are supported by an irregular band of fibrin-fibronectin matrix which provides attachment and a matrix for prompt migration (83, 105).

Clinically, fibronectin has been used with a certain effect to promote attachment of connective tissue to the exposed root and surfaces, and thereby limiting epithelial downgrowth (112, 563, 541). Furthermore fibronectin has been shown to accelerate healing of periodontal ligament fibers after tooth replantation (113). This effect has also been shown to occur in experimental marginal periodontal defects in animals (114, 115) as well as in humans (116).

Complement System

The complement system consists of a

group of proteins that play a central role in the inflammatory response. One of the activated factors, C 5a, has the ability to cleave its C-terminal arginil residue by a serum carboxypeptidase to form C5a-des-arg which is a potent chemotactic factor for attracting neutrophils to the site of injury (117, 118).

Necrotic Cells

Dead and dying cells release a variety of substances that may be important for wound healing such as tissue factor, lactic acid, lactate dehydrogenase, calcium lysosomal enzymes and fibroblast growth factor (FGF) (119).

Matrix

PROTEOGLYCANS AND HYALURONIC ACID

All connective tissues contain proteoglycans. In some tissues, such as cartilage, proteoglycans are the major constituent and add typical physical characteristics to the matrix (120).

CHONDROITIN SULFATE PROTEOGLYCANS

Chondrocytes, fibroblasts and smooth muscle cells are all able to produce these proteoglycans. Chondroitin sulfate impairs the adhesion of cells to fibronectin and collagen and thereby promotes cell mobility. Skin contains proteoglycans, termed dermatan sulfates, which are involved in collagen formation.

HEPARIN AND HEPARAN SULFATE PROTEOGLYCANS

Heparins are a subtype with an anticoagulant activity. Heparan sulfates are produced by mast cells and adhere to cell surfaces and basement membranes.

Keratan sulfates are limited to the cornea, sclera and cartilage. Their role in wound healing is unknown.

Hyaluronic acid is a ubiquitous connective tissue component and plays a major role in the structure and organization of the extracellular matrix. Hyaluronic acid has been implicated in the detachment process of cells that allows cells to move. Furthermore hyaluronic acid inhibits cell differentiation. Because of its highly charged nature, hyaluronic acid can absorb a large volume of water (121).

The role of proteoglycans during wound healing is not fully understood (122). *Heparin* may play a role in the control of clotting at the site of tissue damage. Proteoglycans are also suspected of playing an important role in the early stages of healing when cell migration occurs. Thus *hyaluronic acid* may be involved in detachment of cells so that they can move (123). Furthermore, proteoglycans may provide an open hydrated environment that promotes cell migration (122, 124-126).

The proliferative phase of healing involves cell duplication, differentiation and synthesis of extracellular matrix components. Thus hyaluronidate has been found to keep cells in an undifferentiated state which is compatible with proliferation and migration (122). At this stage *chondroitin* and *heparan sulfate*s are apparently important in collagen fibrillogenesis (122) and mast cell *heparin* promotes capillary endothelial proliferation and migration (127). Furthermore, when endothelium is damaged, a depletion of growth-suppressing heparan sulfate may allow PDGF or other stimuli to *stimulate* angiogenesis (128) (see p. 45).

In conclusion the combined action of substances released from platelets, blood coagulation and tissue degradation results in hemostasis, initiation of the vasculatory response and release of signals for cell activation, proliferation and migration.

Inflammatory Phase

The sequence of the inflammatory process is directed by different types of chemical mediators which are responsible for vascular changes and migration of cells into the wound area (Fig 1.6.).

Mediators Responsible for Vascular Changes

Inflammatory mediators such as histamine, kinins and serotonin cause vasodilatation unless autonomic stimulation overrules them.

The effect of these mediators is constriction of smooth muscles. This influences endothelial and periendothelial cells, pro-

Table 1.1. Mediators of vascular response in inflammation. Modified from VENGE (556) 1985

	Mediator	Originating cells
Humoral	Complement	
	Kallikrein - Kinin system	
	Fibrin	
Cellular		
	Histamine	Thrombocytes
		Mast cells
		Basophils
	Serotonin	Thrombocytes
		Mast cells
	Prostaglandins	Inflammatory cells
	Thromboxane A$_2$	Thrombocytes
		Neutrophils
	Leukotrienes	Mast cells
		Basophils
		Eosinophils
		Macrophages
	Cationic Peptides	Neutrophils
	Oxygen Radicals	Neutrophils
		Eosinophils
		Macrophages

viding reversible opening of junctions between cells and permitting a passage of plasma solutes across the vascular barrier. These mediators are released primarily during the process of platelet aggregation and clotting. The best-known mediators related to the vascular response are shown in Table 1.1.

HISTAMINE

The main sources of histamine in the wound appear to be platelets, mast cells, and basophil leukocytes. The histamine release causes a short-lived dilation of the microvasculature (129, 130) and increased permeability of the small venules. The endothelial cells swell and separations occur between the individual cells. This is followed by plasma leaking through the venules and the emigration of polymorphonuclear leukocytes (131-134).

The role of the anticoagulant heparin is to temporarily prevent coagulation of the excess tissue fluid and blood components during the early phase of the inflammatory response.

SEROTONIN

Serotonin (5-hydroxytryptamine) is generated in the wound by platelets and mast cells. Serotonin appears to increase the permeability of blood vessels, similarly to histamine, but appears to be more potent (132, 133). Apart from causing *contraction* of arterial and venous smooth muscles and *dilation* of arterioles, the net hemodynamic effect of serotonin is determined by the balance between dilation and contraction (129, 130, 135).

PROSTAGLANDINS

Other mediators involved in the vascular response are prostaglandins (PG). These substances are metabolites of arachidonic acid and are part of a major group called eicosanoids, which are also considered primary mediators in wound healing (136). Prostaglandins are the best known substances in this group and are released by cells via arachidonic acid following injury to the cell membrane. These include PGD$_2$, PGE$_2$, PGF$_2$, thromboxane A$_2$ and prostacycline (PGI$_2$). These components have an important influence on vascular changes and platelet aggregation in the inflammatory response and some of the effects are antagonistic. Under normal circumstances, a balance of effects is necessary. In case of tissue injury, the balance will shift towards excess thromboxane A2, leading to a shut-down of the microvasculature (136).

New research suggests that prostaglandins, and especially PGF2, could be endogenous agents that are able to initiate repair or reconstitute the damaged tissue (137). Thus biosynthesis of PGF2 has been shown to have an important effect on fibroblast reparative processes (138), for which reason this prostaglandin may also have an important influence on later phases of the wound-healing process. The effect of prostaglandins on the associated inflammatory response elicited subsequent to infection is further discussed in Chapter 2, p. 120.

BRADYKININ

Bradykinin released via the coagulation cascade relaxes vascular smooth muscles and increases capillary permeability leading to plasma leakage and swelling of the injured area.

NEUROTRANSMITTERS (NOREPINEPHRINE, EPINEPHRINE AND ACETYLCHOLINE)

The walls of arteries and arterioles contain adrenergic and cholinergic nerve fibers. In some tissue the sympathetic adrenergic nerve fibers may extend down to the capillary level. Tissue injury will stimulate the release of neurotransmitters which results in vasoconstriction.

Mediators with Chemotactic Effects

These mediators promote migration of cells to the area of injury and are thus responsible for the recruitment of the various cells which are involved in the different phases of wound healing (Fig. 1.4).

The first cells to arrive in the area are the leukocytes. The chemotactic effects are mediated through specific receptors on the surface of these cells. Complement activated products like C5a, C5a-des-arg, and others cause the leukocytes to migrate between the endothelial cells into the in-flammatory area. This migration is facilitated by the increased capillary permeability that follows the release of the earlier mentioned mediators. Further leukocyte chemoattractants include kallikrein and plasminogen activator, PDGF and platelet factor 4.

Other types of chemotactic receptors are involved when leukocytes recognize immunoglobulin (Ig) and complement proteins such as C3b and C3bi. The mechanism appears to be that B lymphocytes, when activated, secrete immunoglobulin which again triggers the activation of the complement system resulting in production of chemoattractants such as C5a-des-arg (139).

Other mediators involved in chemoattraction will be mentioned in relation to the cell types involved in the wound healing process.

Growth Factors and Interleukins

Migration and proliferation of cells in response to tissue injury is important for the healing process (Fig 1.4). These events are in large part controlled and directed by specific growth and chemoattractive factors leading to proliferation and migration of cells active in the wound-healing process (140-142, 558). These cell mediators are sometimes categorized as secondary mediators, based on their function which more resembles that of regulators or modulators. These mediators can be produced by different types of cells. If produced by mononuclear phagocytes, they are called *monokines*. If produced by lymphocytes, they are termed *lymphokines*. Collectively, they may be classified as *cytokines* since they modulate inflammatory and immunological responses. In wound-healing research, however, it is more convenient to divide these substances into *growth factors* and *cytokines*.

Growth factors can be defined as signaling peptides, acting via specific cell surface receptors and exerting endochrine, paracrine and/or autocrine stimulation of cell proliferation and migration. Recently, it has also been shown that growth factors may enhance cell motility (143).

The most notable of these growth factors are shown in Fig. 1.4 and in Table 1.2. Generally the effects of growth factors and interleukins are modulation of inflamma-

Table 1.2. The most notable growth factors in wound healing

	Originating cells	Responding cells
Platelet-Derived Growth Factor (PDGF)	Platelets Macrophages Smooth muscle cells Endothelial cells	Epidermal cells Fibroblasts Smooth muscle cells Chondrocytes Glial cells
Transforming Growth Factor α and β (TGF-α and TGF-β)	Platelets Macrophages Lymphocytes Fibroblasts Chondrocytes Osteoblasts Tumor cells	Epidermal cells Endothelial cells Fibroblasts (Most other cells)
Epidermal Growth Factor (EGF)	Platelets Macrophages Salivary gland cells Duodenal gland cells Liver cells	Epidermal cells Endothelial cells Fibroblasts Odontogenic cells
Fibroblast Growth Factor (aFGF and bFGF)	Keratinocytes Macrophages Fibroblasts Chondrocytes Osteoblasts	Epidermal cells Endothelial cells Fibroblasts Smooth muscle cells Peripheral nerve cells Chondrocytes
Insulin-like Growth Factor (1-2) (IGF-1 and IGF-2)	Endothelial cells Macrophages Fibroblasts Smooth Muscle cells	Epithelial cells Fibroblasts Mesenchymal cells
Tumor Necrosis Factor α and β (TNF -α and TNF-β)	Macrophages Mast cells Lymphocytes	Fibroblasts
Keratinocyte Growth Factor (KGF)	Fibroblasts	Epithelial cells

tion, participation in debridement, microbicidal events and regulation of various cellular events in the healing process.

PLATELET-DERIVED GROWTH FACTOR

As the name implies, platelet-derived growth factor (PDGF) is released from platelets activated by thrombin or fibrillar collagen (144-149) (Fig. 1.4). Recent studies have shown that PDGF can also be released by other cells such as endothelial cells, vascular smooth muscle cells and activated blood monocytes (150-152).

PDGF is a strong promotor of healing and, since it is released by platelets, is one of the first growth factors to reach the wound site. An important effect of the PDGF release by activated platelets is chemoattraction and activation of monocytes and neutrophils (153-158). Thus, attracted and activated neutrophils will release lysosomal enzymes and neutral proteases to remove damaged tissues and superoxide to kill microorganisms (157).

PDGF released by platelets, activated macrophages, smooth muscle cells and endothelial cells is important for fibroblast activation and proliferation as well as for angiogenesis (152, 159, 160) (Fig. 1.4). Furthermore the orderly migration of neutrophils, macrophages and then fibroblasts correlates with the concentration of PDGF required for maximum chemotaxis (156).

Clinically the administration of PDGF has been shown to accelerate the healing of incisional wounds in rats (161, 162). An important feature is that PDGF also appears to work synergestically with other growth factors such as IGF-1 and FGF, an effect which has been found to lead to accelerated healing of incision wounds (see p. 30).

In summary, PDGF acts as an important mediator regulating migration, proliferation and/or matrix synthesis of a variety of cells.

TRANSFORMING GROWTH FACTOR (TGF)

This factor has been divided into α and ß subtypes, where the latter is the most important for the wound-healing process (163). Platelets are a major source of TGF-ß, which is released together with PDGF to effect platelet and T-lymphocyte activation (164-167).

TGF-ß is a potent chemoattractant for monocytes. When these cells enter the wound area they are exposed to increasing concentrations of TGF-ß and other cytokines and become activated to other growth factors and mediators (168) (see p. 30). *In vivo* experiments have shown that exogenously applied TGF-ß results in fibroblast infiltration in the wound and increased collagen deposition (168-170), as well as angiogenesis and mucopolysaccharide synthesis (170, 171). This results in an accelerated healing of incisional wounds (172, 173). Furthermore, it has been shown that the effect of TGF-ß can be potentiated by the presence of PDGF and epidermal growth factor (EGF) (169, 174, 175). Since all three growth factors are present in human platelets, the concerted action of these during initiation of the wound-healing response is evident (Fig.1.4).

In conclusion the effect of TGF-ß in the wound-healing process appears to be a direct stimulation of the synthesis of connective tissue by fibroblasts and an indirect stimulation of fibroblasts proliferation mediated by PDGF. Furthermore, recent studies seem to imply that TGF-ß is intimately related to scar formation. Thus the elimination of TGF-ß from incisional wounds in rats (by neutralizing antibody) is able to prevent scar tissue formation (176).

EPIDERMAL GROWTH FACTOR (EGF)

This was the first growth factor isolated. It is produced by platelets, salivary glands and duodenal glands, and is also found in urine. The receptor for EGF is expressed in almost all cells but is most dense in epithelial cells, fibroblasts and endothelial cells (177).

In the oral cavity, receptors for EGF have been found in oral epithelium, enamel organ, periodontal ligament fibroblasts and preosteoblasts (178). Stimulation of the EGF receptor causes the cells to become less differentiated and to divide and grow rapidly. In wounds, EGF has been found to encourage cells to continue through the cell cycle. Such a cell proliferative effect has been demonstrated in epithelial cells (179) endothelial cells and periosteal fibroblasts (180, 181). EGF has also been shown to be chemotactic for epithelial cells (182) and to stimulate fibroblast collagenase production (183). In oral tissues it has been shown that EGF controls the proliferation of odontogenic cells (184) and accelerates tooth eruption (185).

In experimental skin wounds in animals an acceleration of both connective tissue and epithelial healing was found after topical application of EGF (186-189, 545, 553). However, topical application of EGF turned out to have no effect on reepithelialization of experimental wounds in humans (190).

An interesting observation in mice has been that saliva rinsing of skin wounds (by communal licking) both enhances coagulation (191) and leads to acceleration of wound healing (189, 192-194). Due to the high concentration of EGF found in saliva (195) this effect has been suggested to be caused by EGF. Later experiments with induced tongue wounds in mice have shown that EGF (and possibly also TGF-ß) is involved in healing of wounds of the oral mucosa (196, 197) (Fig. 1.4).

FIBROBLAST GROWTH FACTOR (FGF)

This growth factor is present in an acidic and a basic form, with the basic growth factor (bFGF) being more than 10 times as potent as the acidic form (aFGF) (198).

bFGF is a potent mitogen for fibroblasts, endothelial cells (119, 199), smooth muscle cells and peripheral nerve cells (198, 200-202) and stimulates epithelialization (203).

Recently a number of growth factors

with mesodermal mitogenic effects have been isolated from various tissues that share the common property of binding to heparin (198). It is anticipated that bFGF is present in the tissues bound to heparin or heparan sulfate residues in the extracellular matrix. Because of this extracellular storage it can be used whenever necessary (201, 204). Thus, an injury causing platelet release of heparin-degrading enzymes may release bFGF and start the angiogenic cascade (205-207, 547) (see p. 45).

The net effect of bFGF action upon fibroblasts and endothelial cells appears to be an acceleration in the formation of granulation tissue (159, 160, 208) (Fig. 1.4).

Clinically, topical application of bFGF has been found to accelerate wound-healing in incisional wounds (209). In oral tissues, dentin-bound bFGF has been found to positively influence the adhesion, migration and proliferation of human endothelial cells (202, 210) and periodontal ligament cells (211). The clinical effect of this has yet to be demonstrated.

INSULIN-LIKE GROWTH FACTOR (IGF)

This growth factor is found in two versions IGF-1 and IGF-2. IGF-1 especially is related to wound-healing. IGF-1 is an aminoacid peptide with the ability to facilitate DNA synthesis in multiple cell types (212). The major source of IGF-1 is the liver. Synthesis and secretion is regulated by growth hormone (213-215). IGF-1 is of major importance in expressing the growth-promoting effect of growth hormone (GH) during postnatal life (560). In oral tissues a recent study has shown that IGF-1 can stimulate DNA synthesis of PDL fibroblasts, probably via binding to high-affinity cell surface receptors (215).

Receptors for IGF-1 are expressed in a variety of tissues and are structurally similar to the receptor for insulin.

Administration of IGF-1 in skin wounds has no influence upon fibroblast proliferation or activity, or upon epithelialization (130, 216-218). However, if IGF-1 is administered together with PDGF or FGF, a marked fibroblast proliferation and collagen production can be observed as well as enhanced epithelialization (217, 218) (Fig. 1.4).

IGF-1 appears also to be a progression factor when cells have been made competent by PDGF or FGF (see p. 17) (140, 219, 220).

GROWTH HORMONE (GH)

Growth hormone, or somatotropin, is not a local growth factor but a hormone secreted from the anterior pituitary gland. GH probably promotes growth both by a direct action on target cells, as well as by stimulating the hepatic production of IGF-1. GH has an anabolic action in the stimulation of protein synthesis and, additionally, affects the metabolism of carbohydrates, lipids, minerals and fluid. From a wound healing point of view, increased protein synthesis and an anabolic state may be of importance in improved healing, as well as in decreased healing time. The presence of GH receptors has been found on epithelial cells as well as fibroblasts (221).

Systemic GH treatment in rats has shown increased mechanical strength in incisional wounds after 4 days of healing (222, 223, 559). Furthermore, local injection of growth hormone significantly increased the amount of granulation tissue and IGF-1 gene expression in subcutaneously placed wound chambers in rats (224).

SYNERGISTIC EFFECT OF GROWTH FACTORS

Recent experimental studies have shown that the application of single growth factors such as PDGF, IGF-1, EGF and FGF had little or no effect on the healing of connective tissue or epithelium in standardized skin wounds in pigs (216-218, 225). However, a combination of PDGF and IGF-1 produced a dramatic synergistic increase in both epithelium and connective tissues (140, 169, 216, 217). Likewise, PDGF and TGF–β promote synergistic fibroblast proliferation and collagen synthesis but have no effect on epithelialization.

Clinically, the combination of PDGF and IGF-1 has also been shown to promote bone healing around titanium implants (174) and promote periodontal ligament healing in marginal periodontal defects (225). Thus cementum, bone and periodontal ligament healing were found to be enhanced (175, 226), indicating that PDGF and IGF may be potent chemotactic agents and mitogens for both cementoblasts, fibroblasts and osteoblasts (174, 225, 227, 228, 549).

Fig. 1.8. Activated platelet (Thrombocyte)

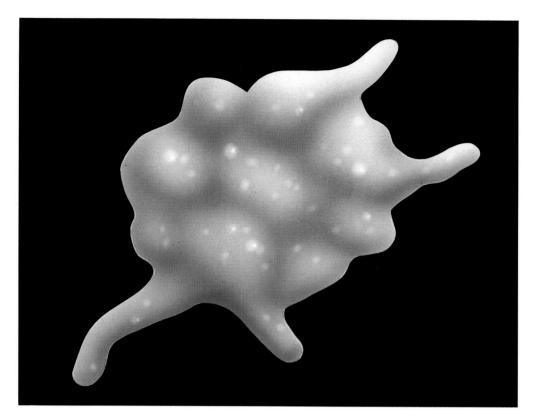

OTHER GROWTH FACTORS

Other factors have been found to be involved in the wound-healing process but their relations are most often not fully understood and will therefore not be discussed.

Cells in Wound Healing

PLATELETS

Platelets (thrombocytes) are anucleate discoid fragments with a diameter of 2 μm (Fig. 1.8). They are formed in the bone marrow as fragments of cytoplasmatic buddings of megakaryocytes and have a life span of 7-10 days in the blood (229). Platelets contain various types of granules which, after release, have a number of effects upon hemostasis and initiation of wound-healing processes (152, 213, 230) (Fig 1.4).

The capacity of the platelets to adhere to exposed tissue surfaces as well as to each other after vessel injury is decisive for their hemostatic capacity. Adhesion and activation of platelets occurs when they contact collagen and microfibrils of the subendothelial matrix and locally generated factors such as thrombin, ADP, fibrinogen, fibronectin, thrombospondin and von Willebrand factor VIII.

Platelet activation results in degranulation and release of adenosine diphosphate (ADP), serotonin, thromboxane, prosta-glandins and fibrinogen. The release of these substances initiates binding of other platelets to the first adherent platelets whereby blood loss is limited during formation of a hemostatic platelet plug (231). The blood loss is further reduced by the vasoconstrictor effect of thromboxane and serotonin.

The inflammatory response is initiated by activation of platelets due to liberation of serotonin, kinins and prostaglandins which leads to increased vessel permeability.

The platelet release of cytokines such as platelet derived growth factor (PDGF), platelet derived angiogenesis factor (PDAF), transforming growth factor α and ß (TGF-α, TGF-ß) and platelet factor 4 leads to an initiation of the wound-healing process (Fig. 1.9). Thus PDGF has been shown to have a chemotactic and activating effect upon neutrophils, monocytes and fibroblasts as well as a mitogenic effect upon fibroblasts and smooth muscle cells (156, 230). The release of TGF-ß has been found to induce angiogenesis and collagen deposition (165, 166). Platelet-derived angiogenesis factor (PDAF) has been shown to cause new capillary formation from the existing microvasculature (232-234). Finally, platelet factor 4 has been found to be a chemoattractant for neutrophils (235).

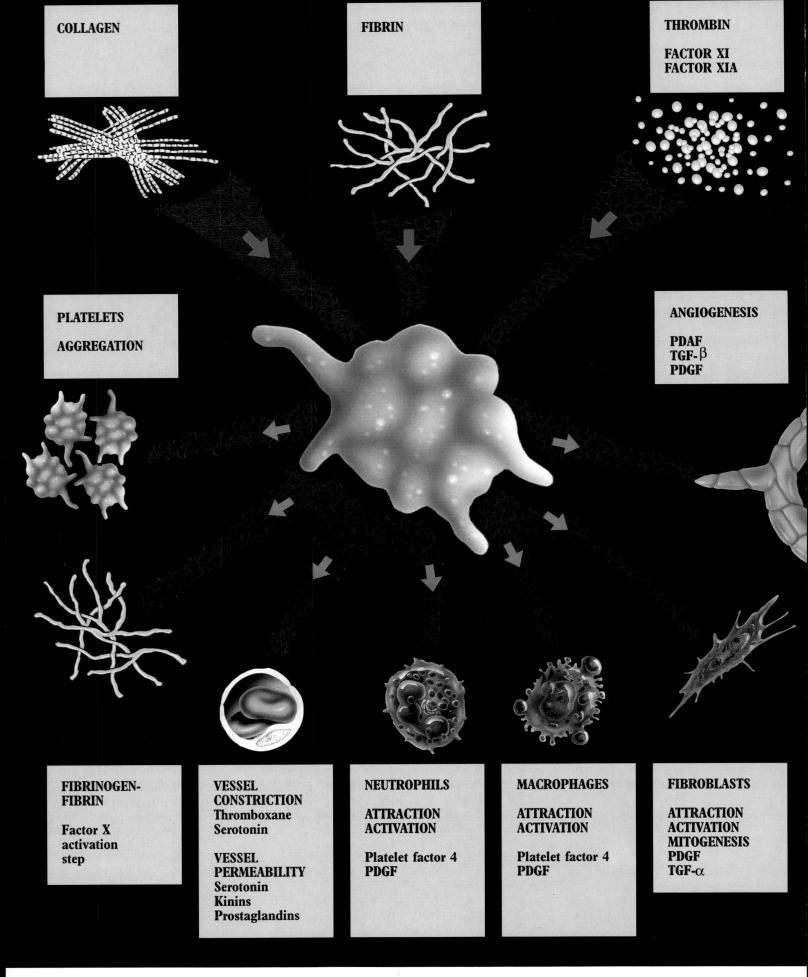

COLLAGEN

FIBRIN

THROMBIN

FACTOR XI
FACTOR XIA

PLATELETS

AGGREGATION

ANGIOGENESIS

PDAF
TGF-β
PDGF

FIBRINOGEN-
FIBRIN

Factor X
activation
step

VESSEL
CONSTRICTION
Thromboxane
Serotonin

VESSEL
PERMEABILITY
Serotonin
Kinins
Prostaglandins

NEUTROPHILS

ATTRACTION
ACTIVATION

Platelet factor 4
PDGF

MACROPHAGES

ATTRACTION
ACTIVATION

Platelet factor 4
PDGF

FIBROBLASTS

ATTRACTION
ACTIVATION
MITOGENESIS
PDGF
TGF-α

Fig. 1.9.
Exposure of platelets to collagen, fibrin, thrombin, factor XI and factor XI-A results in activation and degranulation. This then results in the release of a series of mediators influencing coagulation, vessel tone and permeability. Furthermore the initial cellular response of neutrophils, macrophages, fibroblasts and endothelial cells is established.

In summary, the platelets are the first cells brought to the site of injury. Apart from their role in *hemostasis*, they exert an effect upon the *initiation* of the vascular response and *attraction* and *activation* of neutrophils, macrophages, fibroblasts and endothelial cells. As wound healing progresses, the latter tasks are gradually assumed by macrophages.

ERYTHROCYTES

The influence of erythrocytes upon wound healing is not adequately documented. In one study it was found that neovascularization was stimulated in areas with erythrocyte debris (236). Another effect of the breakdown of erythrocytes is the liberation of hemoglobin, which has been found to enhance infection (237-240). In addition, the heme part of hemoglobin may contribute to the production of oxygen free radicals that can produce direct cell damage (241).

MAST CELLS

Masts cells, distinguished by their large cytoplasmatic granules, are located in a perivenular position at portals of entry of noxious substances and are especially prominent within the body surfaces that are subject to traumatic injury, such as mucosa and skin (242, 243) (Fig. 1.10).

The mast cell participates in the initial inflammatory response after injury via a series of chemical mediators such as histamine, heparin, serotonin, hyaluronic acid, prostaglandins and chemotactic mediators for neutrophils.

The release of mast cell mediators may occur as a direct result of trauma inflicted on the cell. Another means of activation after trauma appears to be when coagulation generates the mast cell activator bradykinin. An alternative means of mast cell activation appears to be the release of endotoxin during infection and the generation of C3a, C5a and cationic neutrophil protein during the inflammatory response (242).

Fig. 1.10. Mast cell in perivenular position

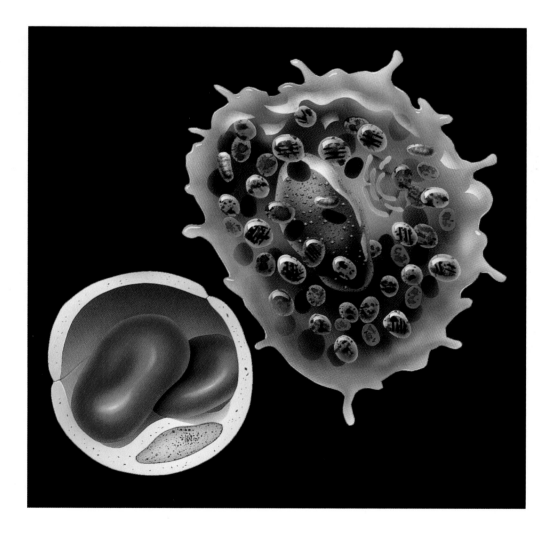

WOUND HEALING SUBSEQUENT TO INJURY

Fig. 1.11. Neutrophil leuko-cyte

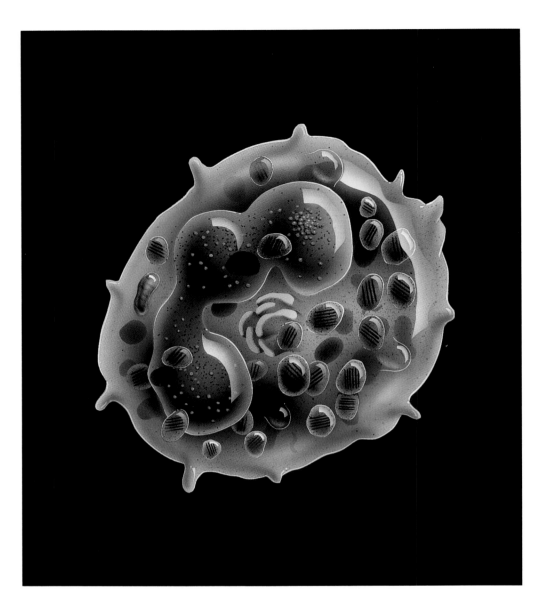

The release of the mast cell mediators such as histamin, heparin, serotonin and slow-reacting substance of anaphylaxis (SRS-A) results in active vasodilation of the small venules, which allows for the entrance of water, electrolyte and plasma proteins into the microenvironment. The maintenance of an open channel for this influx is promoted by the anticoagulant activity of heparin and by the proteolytic enzymes such as chymase. Histamine and heparin may also potentiate the angiogenesis when other angiogenic factors are present (244) (see p. 45).

The liberation of a neutrophil chemotactic factor and a lipid chemotactic factor from activated mast cells both result in attraction of neutrophils and the release of a platelet-activating factor results in degranulation and aggregation of platelets.

Finally, hyaluronic acid promotes cell movement and may be crucial for cell division, which is essential in this phase of wound healing (9).

In summary the mast cell plays a role, together with platelets, in being the initiator of the inflammatory response. However, experiments with corneal wounds have shown that healing can proceed in the absence of mast cells (245).

NEUTROPHILS

The first wave of cells entering the wound site are the neutrophil leukocytes which migrate from the microvasculature (Figs. 1.11 and 1.12). The primary function of neutrophils is to phagocytize and kill microorganisms present within the wound (246, 247). They then degrade tissue macromolecules such as collagen, elastin, fibrin and fibronectin by liberation of digestive enzymes (Table 1.3). Finally, neutrophils

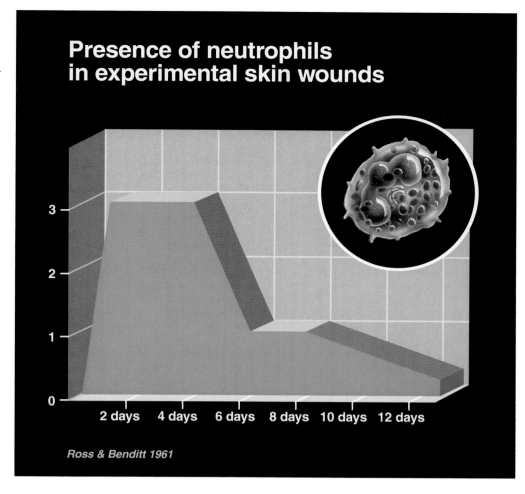

Table 1.3. Neutrophil produced degrading products

Primary Granules (unspecific, azurophilic)

Cathepsin A, G
Elastase
Collagenase (unspecific)
Myeloperoxidase
Lyzozyme

Secondary Granules (specific)

Lactoferrin
Collagenase (specific)
B_{12}-binding protein
Lyzozyme

Other Products

Gelatinase
Kininogenase
Oxygen radicals

Table 1.4. Some chemotactic and chemokinetic agents. Modified from VENGE (556) 1985

Humoral

Chemotactic	C3 and C5 fragments
	Fibrin degradation products
	Kallikrein
	Plasminogen activator
	Fibronectin
	Casein
Chemokinetic	C3 and C5 fragments
	Acute phase proteins
	(Orosomucoid α_1, $_1$-antitrypsin)
	α_2-macroglobulin
	Hyaluronic acid

Cellular

Chemotactic	Leukotriene B_4 (precursors and derivatives)
	Platelet-activating factor (PAF)
	Transforming Growth Factor- β (TGF-β)
	Lymphokines
	NCFs (neutrophil chemotactic factors)
	ECFs (eosinophil chemotactic factors)
	MCFs (monocyte chemotactic factors)
	Formylated tri-peptides (e.g. FMLP)
Chemokinetic	Cathepsin G

release a series of inflammatory mediators which serve as chemotactic or chemokinetic agents (Fig. 1.4 and Table 1.4).

Upon exposure to chemoattractants from the clot, such as platelet factor 4, platelet-derived growth factor (PDGF) kallekrein, C5a, leukotriene B_4 (153, 154) and bacterial endotoxins (248, 249, 257), the granulocytes start to adhere locally to the endothelium of the venular part of the microvasculature next to the injury zone (250). Neutrophils begin to penetrate the endothelium between endothelial cells, possibly by active participation of the endothelium 2-3 hours after injury (251-254), and migrate into the wound area (252-254). Once a neutrophil has passed between endothelial cells, other leukocytes and erythrocytes follow the path (254, 255).

After the neutrophil has passed between the endothelial cells it traverses the basement membrane by a degradation process and then moves into the interstitial tissue in the direction of the chemoattractant. This movement may be facilitated by proteolytic activity and enhanced by contact guidance. Thus neutrophils move preferentially along fiber alignments, suggesting that tissue architecture may be a significant determinant of the efficacy of cellular mobilization.

At this point the wound contains a network of fibrin, leukocytes and a few fibroblasts. By the end of the 2nd day most of the neutrophils have lost their ameboid properties and have released their granula into the surrounding tissue. This event apparently triggers a second migration where plasma, erythrocytes and neutrophils again leave the venules (256). In the case of uncomplicated non-infected healing, the numbers of neutrophils decrease after 3-5 days (Fig. 1.12).

When the neutrophils have reached the site of injury they form a primary line of defence against infection by the phagocytosis and intracellular killing of microorganisms (257). In this process each phagocyte may harbor as many as 30 or more bacteria (258).

Phagocytosis of bacteria by neutrophils induces a respiratory burst that produces toxic oxygen metabolites. These products include hypohalides, superoxide anion

Fig. 1.13. Macrophage

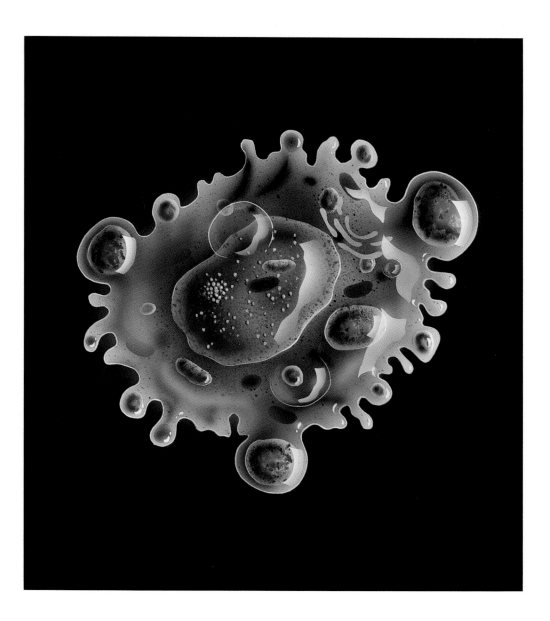

and hydroxyl radicals (257). Furthermore, they can generate chloramine formed by the reaction of hypochlorite with ammonia or amines (259). As a result of stimulation, phagocytosis or lysis, the neutrophils may release the content of their granules into the extracellular space. These granules contain oxygen radicals and neutral proteases, such as cathepsin G, elastase, collagenases, gelatinase and cationic proteins (257). All these products result in tissue damage and breakdown at an acid pH (260). A decrease or elimination of these products provided by experimental neutropenia have prevented the normally found decrease in wound strength in early intestinal anastomosis (261).

Despite these effects upon the wound the presence of neutrophils is not essential for the wound-healing process itself. Thus wound healing has been found to proceed normally as scheduled in uncontaminated wounds in the absence of neutrophils (247, 262). A recent study, however, demonstrating neutrophil expression of cytokines and TGF-ß may indicate a positive influence on wound healing (263).

In summary, the main role of neutrophils in wound healing appears to be limited to elimination of bacteria within the wound area.

MACROPHAGES

Following the initial trauma and neutrophil accumulation, monocytes become evident in the wound area (Fig. 1.13). These cells arise from the bone marrow and circulate in blood (264, 265). In response to release of chemoattractants monocytes leave the bloodstream in the same way as neutrophils. These cells are a heterogenous group of cells which can express an almost

Fig. 1.14.
Schematic illustration of the presence of <u>macrophages</u> *in experimental skin wounds in guinea-pigs. The scale is semiquantitative, graded from 0 to 3. From* ROSS & BENDIT (85) *1961* .

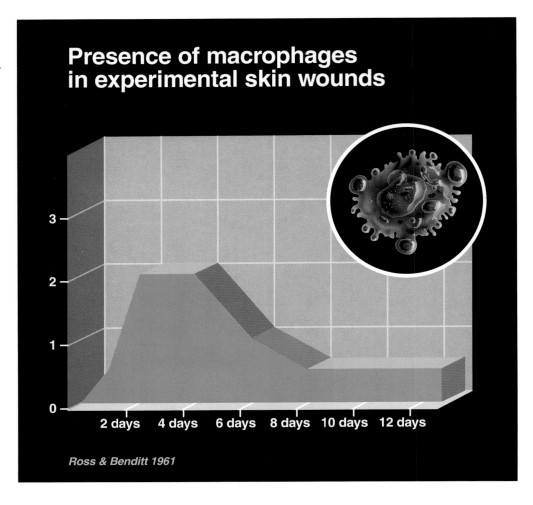

infinite variability of phenotypes in response to changes (270-272).

Monocytes appear in the wound after 24 hours, reach a peak after 2-4 days, and remain in the wound until healing is complete (85) (Fig. 1.14). When monocytes invade the wound area, they undergo a phenotypic metamorphosis to macrophages (266, 267). It should be mentioned that tissue macrophages can proliferate locally (266-269) and possibly play a significant role in the initial inflammatory response.

The arrival of macrophages in the wound area is a response to various chemoattractants released from injured tissue, platelets, neutrophils, lymphocytes and bacteria (Fig. 1.4). In Table 1.4 series of chemotactic factors are listed which have been shown to be chemotactic for macrophages. In this context, it should be mentioned that monocytes express multiple receptors for different chemotactic factors (269). As shown in Table 1.4

connective tissue fragments appear to be *chemotactic* for macrophages, i.e. forming gradients enabling directional movements, and *chemokinetic*, i.e. alter the rate of cell movements. These tissue fragments are possibly generated by neutrophils which precede the appearance of monocytes (see p. 34). It has been shown that neutrophils contain enzymes such as elastase, collagenase and cathepsin which may degrade collagen and elastin, and fibronectin, (Table 1.3) and thereby attract monocytes (269).

In contrast to neutrophils, depletion of circulating blood monocytes and tissue macrophages results in a severe retardation of tissue debridement and a marked delay in fibroblast proliferation and subsequent wound fibrosis (264). Macrophages therefore seem to have an important regulatory role in the repair process.

After migration from the vasculature into the tissue, the monocyte rapidly differentiates to an inflammatory macrophage, the mechanism of which is largely unknown. However, the binding of monocytes to connective tissue fibronectin has been found to drive the differentiation of monocytes into inflammatory macrophages (273, 274).

The regulatory and secretory properties of macrophages seem to vary depending on the state of activity: *At rest, intermediate* or in an *activated* state. Macrophage activation can be achieved by the already mentioned chemoattractants in higher concentrations. Further activation can be achieved through the products released from the phagocytotic processes described. These various stimuli induce the macrophages to release a number of biologically active molecules with potential as chemical messengers for inflammation and wound repair (275) (Tables 1.1 and 1.2).

At the inflammatory site the macrophages undertake functions similar to neutrophils, i.e. bacterial phagocytosis and killing and secretion of lysozomal enzymes and oxygen radicals O_2^-, H_2O_2, $\cdot OH$ (59). Activated inflammatory macrophages have been found to be responsible for the degradation and removal of damaged tissue structures such as elastin, collagen, proteoglycans and glycoproteins by the use of secreted enzymes such as elastase, collagenase, plasminogen activator and cathepsin B and D. Both extra- and intracellular tissue debridement can occur (269).

Macrophages have been shown to release growth factors such as PDGF, TNF and TGF-ß which stimulate cell proliferation in wound healing (276-278) (Fig. 1.4). These growth factors are collectively known as macrophage-derived growth factors (MDGF). The level of MDGF can be significantly increased following stimulation of macrophages with agents such as fibronectin and bacterial endotoxin (279, 280).

Activation of macrophages has been found to lead to fibroblast proliferation (276, 281), increased collagen synthesis (277) and neovascularization (282-285).

Macrophages release their angiogenic mediator only in presence of low oxygen tension in the injured tissue (i.e. 2-30 mm Hg) (232, 233). However, as macrophages have been found to release lactate even while they are well-oxygenated, the stimulus to collagen synthesis remains even during hyperoxygenation (286, 287), a finding which is of importance in the use of hyperbaric oxygen therapy (see p.58).

Finally, it should be mentioned that macrophages can release a polypeptide, interleukin-1, that can function as a messenger for lymphocytes The role of macrophages in the immune response is further discussed on p. 40.

In summary, the macrophage seems to be the key cell in the inflammatory and proliferative phase of wound-healing by secreting factors which stimulate proliferation of fibroblasts and secretion of collagen, as well as stimulation of neovascularization (Fig 1.4). The macrophages also act as scavengers in the wound area and remove traumatized tissue and bacteria and neutralize foreign bodies by forming giant cells which engulf or surround the foreign matter. Moreover, signals released by traumatized bone or tooth substances cause some monocytes to fuse and form osteoclasts which will subsequently resorb damaged hard tissue (see Chapter 2, p. 112). Finally, macrophages play a important role in the immune response to infection (see p. 59 and Chapter 2 p. 112).

Fig. 1.15. Lymphocyte

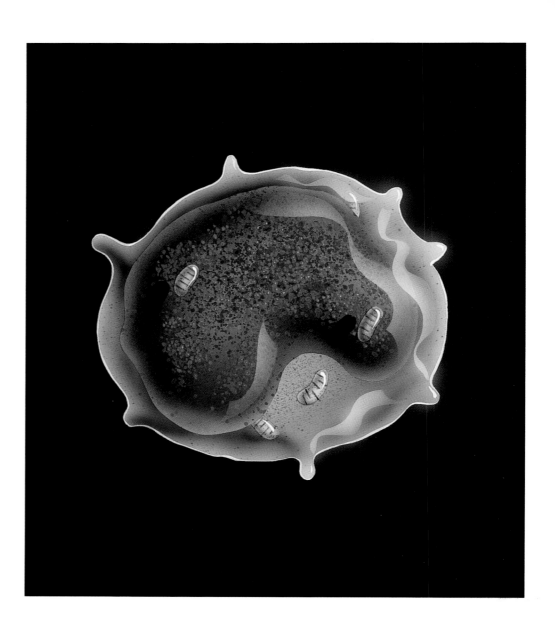

LYMPHOCYTES

Lymphocytes emigrating from the bloodstream into the injury site become apparent after 1 day and reach a maximum after 6 days (85) (Figs. 1.15 and 1.16). The role of these lymphocytes in the wound-healing process has for many years been questioned as earlier investigations have pointed out that lymphocytes like neutrophils were not necessary for normal progression of healing in non-infected wounds (262). However, recent research has demonstrated that lymphocytes together with macrophages may modulate the wound healing process (288-290) (Fig. 1.17).

Lymphocytes can be divided into *T lymphocytes* (thymus-derived lymphocytes) and *B lymphocytes* (bone marrow-derived lymphocytes). Both types are attracted to the wound area, probably by activated complement on the surface of macrophages and neutrophils.

Lymphocyte infiltration in wounds is a dynamic process where both T-helper/effector and T-suppressor/cytotoxic lymphocytes are present in the wound after 1 week (291). These activated lymphocytes produce a variety of lymphokines of which interferon (IFN-α) and TGF-ß have been shown to have a significant effect on endothelial cells and thereby may have an effect on angiogenesis. This effect may be secondary to other effects such as macrophage stimulation and activation (292). TGF-ß is also a potent fibroblast chemotactic molecule and, in addition, induces monocyte chemotaxis and secretion of fibroblast growth factor and activating factors (293).

Fig. 1.16.
Schematic illustration of the presence of lymphocytes in experimental skin wounds in guinea-pigs. The scale is semiquantitative, graded from 0 to 3. From ROSS & BENDIT (85) *1961.*

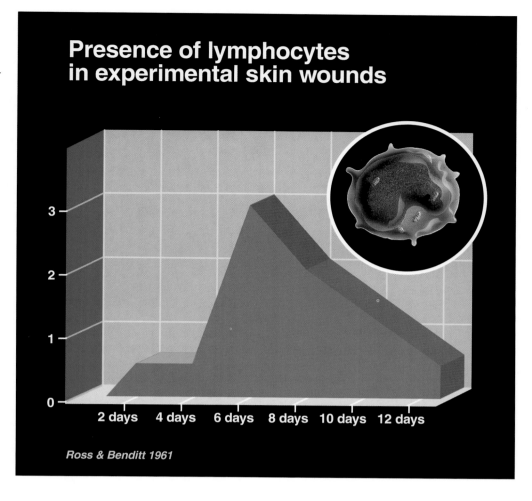

Fig. 1.16.
Schematic illustration of the presence of lymphocytes in experimental skin wounds in guinea-pigs. The scale is semiquantitative, graded from 0 to 3. From ROSS & BENDIT (85) *1961.*

Recent studies have indicated that there are at least two populations of T cells involved in wound healing. One population bearing the all-T-cell marker appears to be required for successful healing, as shown by the impairment in healing caused by their depletion. The T-supressor/cytotoxic subset appears to have a counterregulatory effect on wound healing, as their depletion enhances wound rupture strength and collagen synthesis (288-290, 292).

Based on present evidence, *BARBUL* and coworkers have postulated the following theory: Macrophages exert a direct stimulatory effect on endothelial cells and fibroblasts (Fig. 1.17). A T-cell marker-positive subset (T$^+$), which is not yet fully characterized, has a direct action on endothelial cells and fibroblasts and acts indirectly by stimulating macrophages. T-supressor/cytotoxic cells (Ts/c) down-regulate wound healing by direct action on macrophages and T cells (292, 293) (Fig. 1.17).

There is presently no evidence to suggest that the humoral immune system (B lymphocytes) participates in the wound healing process. The influence of lymphocytes therefore seems primarily to be through T lymphocytes.

In summary, lymphocytes appear indirectly to influence the balance between the stimulatory and inhibitory signals to fibroblasts and endothelial cells via the macrophages.

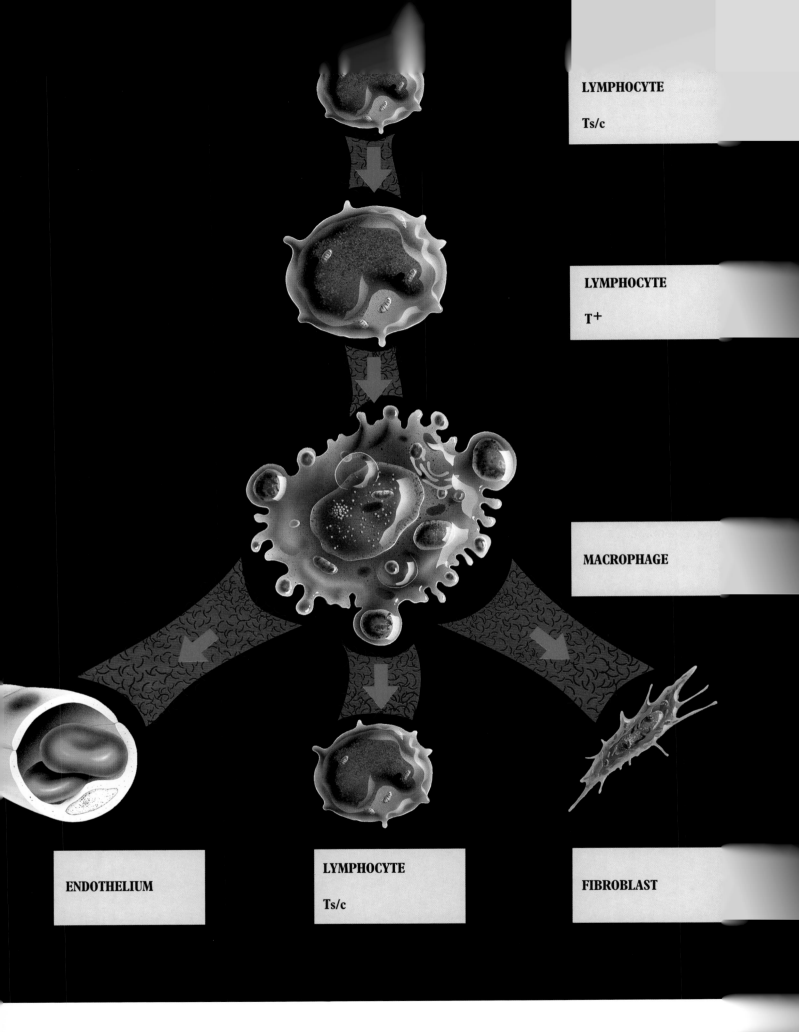

LYMPHOCYTE

Ts/c

LYMPHOCYTE

T+

MACROPHAGE

ENDOTHELIUM

LYMPHOCYTE

Ts/c

FIBROBLAST

CHA

←

**Fig. 1.17. Role of lympho-
cytes in wound healing**
*Macrophages exert a direct stimu-
latory effect on endothelial cells
and fibroblasts. A T-cell marker-
positive subset (T⁺), which is
not fully characterized, has direct
action on endothelial cells and fibroblasts and acts indirectly by
stimulating macrophages. T-sup-
pressor/cytotoxic cells (Ts/c)
down regulate wound healing by
direct action on macrophages
and T cells. From* BARBUL (292)
1992 .

FIBROBLASTS

The fibroblast is a pleomorphic cell. In the
resting, non-functional state it is called a
fibrocyte. The cytoplasm is scanty and
often difficult to identify in ordinary histologic sections. In the activated, mature
form the cell becomes stellate or spindle-
shaped and is now termed a *fibroblast*. The
most characteristic feature is now the extensive development of a dilated endoplasmic reticulum, the site of protein synthesis (294) (Fig. 1.18).

In the wound the fibroblast will produce
collagen, elastin and proteoglycans (295).

After wounding, fibroblasts start to invade the area after 3 days stimulated by
platelets and macrophage products and
they become the dominating cell 6 to 7
days after injury, being present in considerable concentration until the maturation
phase of the healing process (85) (Fig.
1.19).

Several studies have suggested that new
fibroblasts arise from the connective tissue
adjacent to the wound, principally from
the perivascular undifferentiated mesenchymal cells (stem cells) (296-301) (see p.
15) and not from hematogenous precursors (301).

Once fibroblast precursors receive the
proper signal they begin to reproduce and
a mitotic burst is seen between the 2nd
and 5th day after injury (302). Proliferating
fibroblasts develop through cell divisions
every 18 to 20 hours and remain in the
mitotic phase for 30 minutes to 1 hour.
The primary function of the activated fibroblast in the wound area is to produce
collagen, elastin and proteoglycans. However, during the mitotic phase, the fibroblast does not synthesize or excrete external components. Progression factors are
necessary to stimulate the fibroblast to
undergo replication. Before this can happen the fibroblast must be made *competent*
(see p. 17). Factors which induce this
competence are platelet-derived growth
factor (PDGF), fibroblast growth factor
(FGF) and calcium phosphate precipitates (45). PDGF-induced competence requires only transient exposure of cells to
the factor. When competent, the fibro-

Fig. 1.18. Active fibroblast

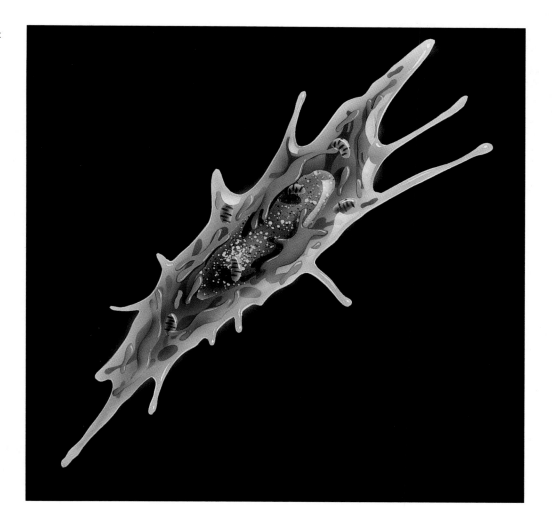

Fig. 1.19.
Schmatic illustration of the presence of <u>fibroblasts</u> *in experimental skin wounds in guinea-pigs. The scale is semiquantitative, graded from 0 to 3. From* ROSS & BENDIT (85) *1961.*

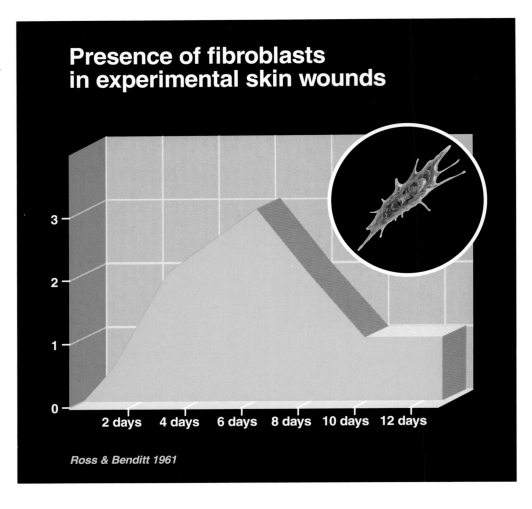

blast can replicate after stimulation by progression factors such as insulin-like growth factor-1 (IGF-1), epidermal growth factor (EGF) and other plasma factors (45). This dual control of fibroblast proliferation explains why fibroblasts can remain in a reversible quiescent state in the presence of progression factor. The transition to a proliferative stage then awaits the release of competence factors by activated cells, such as platelets, macrophages and lymphocytes (see p. 17).

PDGF is released in response to injury by platelets and production is continued by activated macrophages, which can induce migration into the wound and proliferation of fibroblasts over an extended period of time (Fig. 1.4).

TGF-ß is a growth stimulator for mesenchymal cells and has been found to accelerate wound healing in rats (168, 303) by direct stimulation of connective tissue synthesis by fibroblasts and indirect stimulation of fibroblast proliferation by PDGF (161, 162). Other factors which may

be involved in fibroblast proliferation include tumor-necrosis factors (TNF-α and TNF-ß) (45).

The best-characterized inhibitor of fibroblast proliferation is ß-fibroblast interferon (IFN-ß). It has been suggested that IFN-ß inhibits events involved in fibroblast competence and induction of competence of fibroblasts and by PDGF inhibition (304, 305).

Regulatory systems of fibroblast activity may operate through activation of macrophages, which generate an endogenous stimulus to fibroblast proliferation. Alternatively, a fibroblast proliferation might be slowed by either inhibition of the release and activation of PDGF and TGF-ß or by stimulation of inhibitory substances, such as IFN-ß. Clinically this may suggest a specific stimulation of fibroblast proliferation by treatment with exogenous growth factors such as PDGF and TGF-ß or by their activation (45).

Once fibroblasts have migrated into the wound, they produce and deposit large quantities of fibronectin, types I and III collagen and hyaluronidate. TGF-ß is presently considered to be the most important stimulator of extracellular matrix production (306, 307).

Multiplication and differentiation of fibroblasts and synthesis of collagen fibers require oxygen as well as amino acids, carbohydrates, lipids, minerals and water. Collagen cannot be made in the mature fibroblast layer without oxygen (310-314). Consequently the nutritional demands of the wound are greater than that of non-wounded connective tissue (308) and the demand is greatest at a time when the local circulation is least capable of complying with that demand (309).

After collagen molecules are secreted into the extracellular space, they are polymerized in a series of steps in which the hydroxylysine groups of adjacent molecules are condensed to form covalent crosslinks. This step is rate-dependent on oxygen tension and gives collagen its strength (310, 315).

Fibroblasts have been shown to have chemotactic attraction to types I, II, III collagen as well as collagen-derived peptides, with binding of these peptides directly to fibroblasts (316, 317).

Fibroblasts have been known for many years to be involved in wound *contraction*. In relation to this phenomenon, a specific type of fibroblast has been identified which has the characteristics of both fibroblasts and smooth muscle cells for which reason they have been termed *myofibroblasts*. These cells are richly supplied with microfilament bundles that are arranged along the long axis of the cells and are associated with dense bodies for attachment to the surrounding extracellular matrix (318, 319). Besides numerous cytoplasmic microfilaments, large amounts of endoplasmic reticulum are also seen. In this respect these cells have characteristics of fibroblasts.

The myofibroblast has contractive properties and has been demonstrated in many tissues that form contracted and/or nodular scars (320). Myofibroblasts are present throughout granulation tissue and along wound edges at the time when active contraction occurs (321). For this reason the most generally accepted theory of wound contraction has involved the contribution by myofibroblasts (320).

Recently, *EHRLICH* and coworkers have presented a new theory for the phenomenon of wound contraction (322). In this *fibroblast theory* it is suggested that fibroblast locomotion is the mechanism that generates the contractive forces in wound contraction and that the connective tissue matrix is important in controlling these forces. It is suggested that the histological existence of myofibroblasts is a transitional state of the fibroblast in granulation tissue.

In summary, the fibroblasts are late-comers in the inflammation phase of wound healing. Their main function is to synthesize and excrete the major components of connective tissue: collagen, elastin and proteoglycans. The fibroblast is also involved in wound-contraction through a specific cell called the *myofibroblast* which has characteristics of both fibroblasts and smooth muscle cells.

Angiogenesis

Between 2 and 4 days after wounding, proliferation of capillaries and fibroblasts begins at the border of the lesion. However, studies have shown that blood cells and plasma perfuse the wound tissue several hours before the space is invaded by sprouting capillaries (256, 323). At first the blood cells move around randomly in the meshes of the fibrinous network but gradually preferential channels are formed in the wound through which cells pass more or less regularly. This phenomenon has been termed *open circulation* and it is suggested that the blood cells at this time are transported in a simple tube system which has not yet acquired an endothelial lining (256, 323, 324).

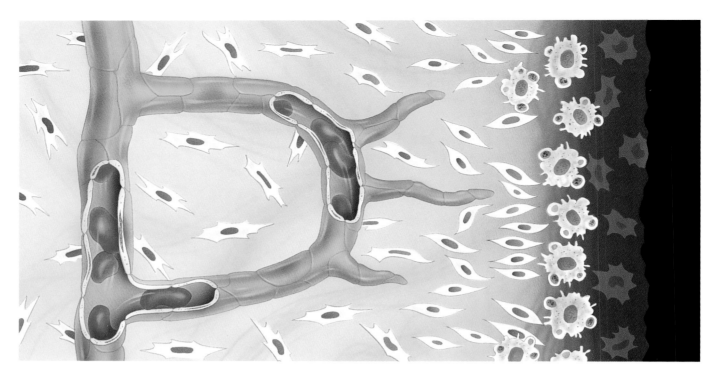

Fig. 1.20.
New capillaries start as outgrowths of endothelial cells lining existing venules. Subsequent arcading sprouts unite and tubulization allows circulation to be established.

Angiogenesis is the process of formation of new blood vessels by directed endothelial migration, proliferation and lumen formation (213, 325-330). (Fig. 1.20). In wound healing, angiogenesis is crucial for oxygen delivery to ischemic or newly-formed tissue. New vessels arise in most cases as capillaries from existing vessels and only from venules (330, 331) (Fig. 1.21). In early granulation tissue, after the wound-healing module is assembled, capillary sprouts move just behind the advancing front of macrophages. Collagen-secreting fibroblasts are placed between these sprouts and are nourished by the new capillaries (Fig. 1.26, p. 56).

Variants in healing of the vascular network are found according to the type of tissue involved and the extent of the injury. In skin or mucosal lacerations, primarily closed, existing vessels may anastomose spontaneously and thereby reestablish circulation. In wounds with tissue defects or in non-closed wounds, a new vascular network has to be created via granulation tissue. The third variant in vascular healing is the revascularization of ischemic tissue as seen after skin grafting, tooth luxation, tooth replantation and transplantation. In these situations angiogenesis takes place in existing ischemic or necrotic tissue. The healing in these cases usually occurs as a mixture of gradual ingrowth of new vasculature combined with occasional end-to-end anastomosis between existing and in-growing vessels (see p. 45).

Angiogenesis in wounds has been examined in different *in vivo* assays such as the *rabbit ear chamber* (233, 332), the *Algire chamber* where a transparent plastic window is placed in the dorsal subcutaneous tissue of a mouse (333) or the *hamster cheek pouch* (334, 335). Furthermore, angiogenesis has been tested in *corneal pockets* (233, 336, 337), and *chicken chorioallantoic membrane* (338). These assays have been used to describe the dynamic process of angiogenesis together with the influence of different types of external factors on vascular proliferation.

Our current knowledge of the biochemi-

Fig. 1.21. Capillary

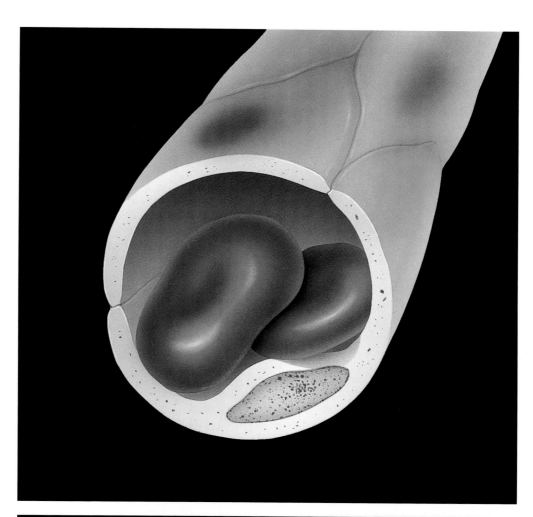

Fig. 1.22.
Schematic illustration of the presence of new <u>capillaries</u> in experimental skin wounds in guinea-pigs. The scale is semiquantitative graded from 0 to 3. From ROSS & BENDIT (85) *1961.*

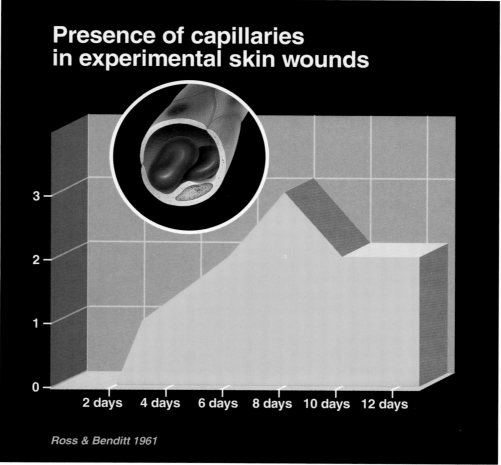

Presence of capillaries in experimental skin wounds

Ross & Benditt 1961

cal nature of the signals that induce angiogenesis has been derived primarily from *in vitro* observations using cultured vascular endothelial cells. *In vitro* assays have been used extensively in the identification and the purification of angiogenetic factors. In this context, as angiogenesis is considered to be a process of capillary growth, cultured capillary endothelial cells seem to be optimal for testing angiogenesis (339).

CELLULAR EVENTS IN ANGIOGENESIS

New capillaries usually start as outgrowths of endothelial cells lining existing venules. After exposure to an angiogenic stimulus, endothelial cells of the venules begin to produce enzymes that degrade the vascular basement membrane on the side facing the stimulus (330). After 24 hours the endothelial cells migrate through the degraded membrane in the direction of the angiogenic stimulus (Fig. 1.20). Behind the tip of the migrating wound edges, trailing endothelial cells divide and differentiate to form a lumen. The sprouts or buds can either connect with other sprouts to form vascular loops or can continue migrating. Capillary bud formation is found after 48 hours and these buds arise solely from venules (331).

When endothelial migration tips join to form capillary loops or join across a wound edge, blood flow begins within the formed lumen. As vessels mature, extracellular matrix components are laid down to form a new basement membrane (325, 330). Recent studies have shown that angiogenesis is closely related to fibroblast activity. Thus it appears that new vessels cannot grow beyond their collagenous support (310, 340).

The speed of neovascularization has been investigated in ear chambers and been found to range from 0.12 to 0.24 mm per day (236, 256, 341, 342). In dental pulps which become revascularized after replantation or transplantation, the speed is approximately twice this rate (see Chapter 2 p. 104).

In raised and repositioned skin flaps, angiogenesis along the cut margins is rapid and capillary sprouts advance across the wound space from the host bed. In rats, new vascular channels across the wound margin can be demonstrated within 3 days; and in pigs, normal blood flow has been observed within 2 to 3 days (343-346).

After tissue grafting, specific vascular healing processes take place. Thus it has been shown in skin transplants that after an initial contraction of the vessels a so-called plasmatic circulation takes place in the zone next to the graft bed (347-354). This supply of fluids serves to prevent drying of the graft before blood supply has been restored (352). The role of the plasmatic circulation as a source of nourishment is, however, debatable (352).

Vascularization of skin transplants, although initially sluggish, takes place after 3 to 5 days (355-364). The role of already existing graft vessels is unsettled. Thus, in some studies, it has been shown that the original vessels act only as non-viable conduits for ingrowth of new vessels (342), and that revascularization takes place primarily from invading new vessels (362, 365). In other experiments, however, it has been shown that, depending upon the degree of damage to the grafted tissues and on local hemodynamic factors, the original graft vessels may be incorporated in the established new vascular network (363-367).

Teeth have a vascular system which in some situations is dissimilar to skin. In replantation and transplantation procedures of immature incisors, the severed periodontal ligament and the pulp can be expected to become revascularized. The process of revascularization of the periodontal ligament seems to follow the pattern of skin grafts (see Chapter 2 p. 95). On the contrary, there is very limited diffusion of nutrients from the graft bed to the dental pulp due to its hard tissue confinement and extended length, which again leads to specific vascular healing events (see Chapter 2 p. 104).

In a primarily closed skin wound, circulation bridging the wound edges can be established as early as the 2nd or the 3rd day and appears to be at a maximum after 8 days (85) (Fig. 1.22). The the new vascular network is then remodelled. Some vessels differentiate into arteries and veins while others recede. The mechanism regulating this process is largely unknown. Active blood flow within the lumen may be a factor, as capillaries with decreased blood flow typically recede while those with active flow are usually maintained or expand into larger vessels (332, 368).

Factors determining angiogenesis represent a series of cellular and humoral events which lead to the initiation, progression and termination of angiogenesis (Figs. 1.4 and 1.23). Initiation of angiogenesis appears to be related to signals released from activated platelets and fibrin at the site of vascular rupture (82, 146, 154, 369). During platelet activation, enzymes are released that degrade heparin and heparan sulfate components from the vascular basement membranes, whereby stored bFGF is liberated (204-207, 370). This liberation of FGF has been shown to induce angiogenetic activity (371). Other bFGF signals are released from injured cells and matrix (330). This growth factor is partly responsible for angiogenesis through initiating a cascade of events (372). Thus bFGF stimulates endothelial cells to secrete procollagenase, plasmin and plasminogen. Plasmin, as well as plasminogen, activates procollagenase to collagenase. Together, these enzymes can digest the blood vessel basement membrane. Subsequently endothelial chemoattractants, such as fibronectin fragments generated from extracellular matrix degradation and heparin released from mast cells, draw endothelial cells through the disrupted basement membrane to form a nascent capillary bud (127).

Recruited and activated macrophages soon also promote angiogenesis (373) by liberating potent direct-acting angiogenic factors such as tumor-necrosis factor alpha (TNF-α), wound angiogenesis factor (WAF) and fibroblast growth factor (FGF). The macrophage signal seems to diminish as angiogenesis proceeds (232, 233, 310, 315, 374-377). Recent studies indicate that the effect of hypoxia within the wound upon angiogenesis is possibly mediated via stimulated macrophages (232, 378, 379) (see p. 55).

OTHER FACTORS CONTROLLING ANGIOGENESIS

Recently, a number of angiogenetic factors have been isolated which either have a *direct* effect on endothelial cell migration/proliferation or have an *indirect* effect via other cells. The exact mechanisms behind indirect angiogenetic activity are not yet known; but it is possible that they cause accumulation of other types of cells, e.g. platelets or macrophages, that release direct-acting factors (330, 380).

Once new blood vessels form, they acquire a layer of pericytes and the composition of their basement membrane changes. Pericytes inhibit the growth of adjacent endothelial cells and thereby direct growth toward the site of attraction (381).

Finally, it should be mentioned that angiogenesis is dependent upon the composition of the extracellular matrix (382). Thus, fibrin appears to promote angiogenesis (61) and the fibrin-fibronectin extravascular clot serves as a provisional stroma providing a matrix for macrophages, fibroblasts and new capillary migration. In this way, the fibrin-fibronectin gel is transformed to granulation tissue.

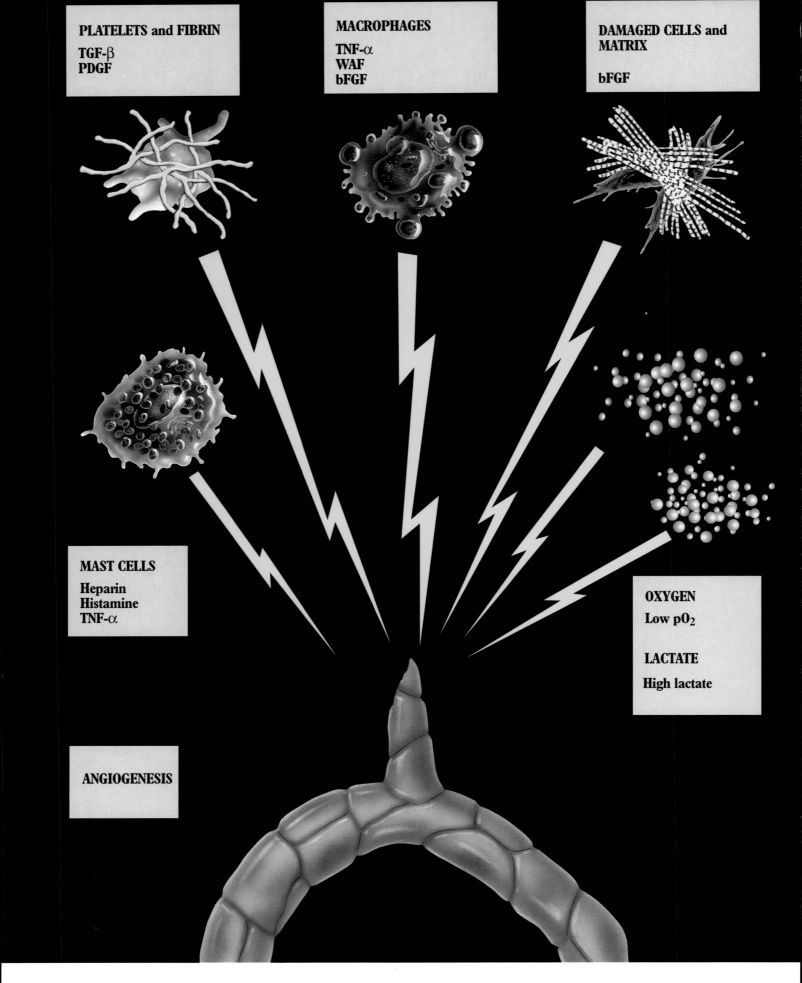

PLATELETS and FIBRIN

TGF-β
PDGF

MACROPHAGES

TNF-α
WAF
bFGF

DAMAGED CELLS and MATRIX

bFGF

MAST CELLS

Heparin
Histamine
TNF-α

OXYGEN

Low pO_2

LACTATE

High lactate

ANGIOGENESIS

←
Fig. 1.23. Cellular and humoral events leading to angiogenesis

Platelets, fibrin, mast cells, macrophages, injured cells and matrix all release angiogenic signals. Low oxygen tension and a high lactate concentration in the wound space represent also an important stimulation to angiogenesis.

Collagen Biochemistry and Mechanical Strength

The tensile strength of a wound is, from a functional point of view, the most important property in wound healing. The strength of a healing wound is related to the amount of collagen deposited and, later, to crosslinking and organization of existing collagen fibers (383-386) (Fig. 1.24). Moreover, not only does wound strength vary considerably according to time after injury, but also according to the type of tissue injured (Fig. 1.25).

Collagen constitutes the principal structural protein of the body and is the main constituent of extracellular matrix in all species. At least 13 types of collagen have been identified. Despite their differences, all collagen molecules consist of a triple helix matrix protein which gives the tissues their strength (15, 387-392). Current literature on wound-healing and collagen contains only sparse information about the different types of collagens (387).

Type I collagen is the major structural components of skin, mucosa, tendons and bone (390).

Type II collagen is located almost exclusively in hyaline cartilage.

Type III collagen, also called reticular fibers (393), is found in association with Type I collagen although the ratio varies in different tissues (390).

In a rat model, type III collagen could be demonstrated 10 hours after the start of wound healing in skin (39), and after 3 days in healing PDL wounds (395, 396). The early appearance of type III collagen has been found associated with the deposition of fibronectin (see p. 24), indicating that type III collagen together with fibronectin may provide the initial scaffolding for subsequent healing events (397, 398).

In children, type III collagen can be detected between 24 and 48 hours in skin wounds, whereas no type I collagen is found in this type of wound (399). From 72 hours and onwards a substantial increase in type I collagen is found, together with

Fig. 1.24.
Schematic illustration of the presence of <u>collagen</u> in experimental skin wounds in guinea-pigs. The scale is semiquantitative graded from 0 to 3. From Ross & Benditt (85) *1961.*

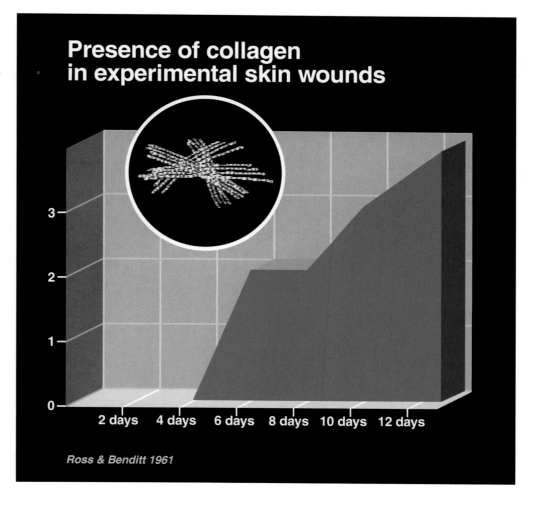

Fig. 1.25.
Relative healing rates for linear incisional wounds in different tissues in rats and rabbits; the tensile strength being calculated in percent of that of the respective intact tissues (taken as 100%). From VIIDIK & GOTTRUP (410) 1986.

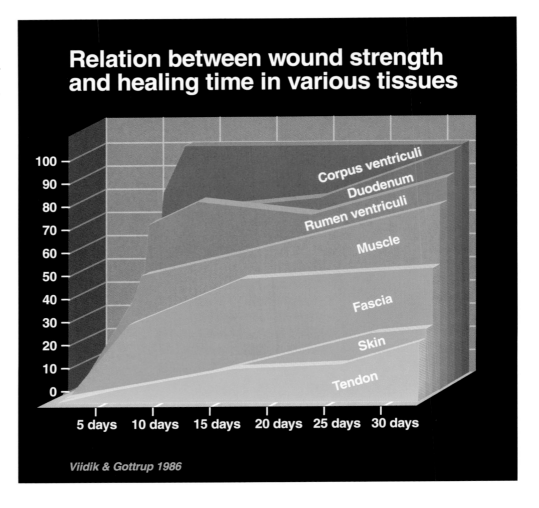

Relation between wound strength and healing time in various tissues

Viidik & Gottrup 1986

the appearance of mature fibroblasts (399).

Type IV collagen together with other components, including heparan sulfate, proteoglycans and laminin, makes up the basement membranes in both epidermis and endothelium.

In dermal wound healing, type IV collagen synthesis by epidermis is connected with the reformation of the basement membrane and is a relatively late event in the wound-healing process (400-402).

Type V collagen is found in almost all types of tissue and has been proposed to be involved in migration of capillary endothelial cells during angiogenesis (391). Type V collagen is synthesized while epidermal cells migrate; however, the regeneration of the basement membrane is delayed until the wound defect is covered and the epidermal cells are no longer in a migrating phase (401).

Type VII collagen has been found to be an anchoring fibril that attaches the base-ment membrane to underlying connective tissue (403-406).

The remaining types of collagen are less known in relation to the wound-healing process and are therefore not discussed.

Collagen represents a key component in wound healing. Thus, immediately after injury the exposure of collagen fibers to blood results in platelet aggregation and activation with resultant coagulation and the release of chemotactic factors from platelets that initiate healing (e.g. PDGF, platelet factor IV, IGF-1 TGF-ß and an unidentified chemoattractant to endothelial cells) (see p. 31). Collagen fragments are then degraded by the attracted neutrophils and leukocytes, which leads to attraction of fibroblasts.

Synthesis of new collagen in a wound starts with fibroblast proliferation and invasion and the deposition of a collagen-based extracellular matrix. This event takes place after 3-5 days and persists for

CHAPTER 1

10-12 days. During this period of time, there is a rapid synthesis primarily of type III and later of type I collagen, resulting in an increase in the tensile strength of the wound which is primarily dependent on the build-up of type I collagen (399, 407-409).

Remodelling Phase

Remodelling of the extracellular matrix is a continuous process which starts early in the wound-healing process. Thus most fibronectin is eliminated within 1 or 2 weeks after granulation tissue is established. Hyaluronidate is replaced or supplemented with heparan sulfate proteoglycans in basement membrane regions and with dermatan chondroitin sulfate proteoglycans in the interstitium (58).

Type III collagen fibers are gradually replaced by type I collagen which becomes arranged in large, partly irregular, collagen bundles. These fiber bundles become oriented according to lines of stress and provide a slower increase in the tensile strength of the healing wound than found during the proliferation phase (409). In most tissues, this remodelling phase ultimately leads to formation of a scar (see p. 45).

The functional properties of the scar tissue vary considerably depending on the content of collagen in the intact original tissue. The healing rate, measured as the mechanical strength of the wound compared to adjacent intact tissue, therefore varies from one tissue type to another. In tissue with a low collagen content before injury (e.g. gastrointestinal tract (565) and other intra-abdominal organ systems), the primarily closed wound shows a rapid increase in relative strength (strength of wounded tissue compared to intact tissue) (410). As shown in Fig. 1.25 tensile strength close to the level of intact tissue levels of tensile strength is reached after 10-20 days of healing in tissues with a low collagen content before injury. In tissues with a high collagen content (e.g. tendon and skin) the increase in relative strength is much slower; and more than 100 days of healing are needed to achieve half the strength of intact tissue. In the wounded PDL, a very rapid increase in tensile strength has been found after severance of Sharpey's fibers (see Chapter 2 p. 95)

Investigations of wounds closed 3-6 days after injury (delayed primary closure) has shown that this type of wound was significantly stronger than primarily closed wounds after 20 days of healing. After 60 days of healing, delayed primarily closed wounds were almost twice as strong as primarily closed wounds; and this difference persisted after 120 days (56, 57, 411). The mechanisms behind the different wound strength in primarily and delayed primarily closed wounds are probably related to an increase in tissue perfusion and oxygenation due to increased angiogenesis and oxygen delivery to the tissues (412).

Epithelial Cells

Epithelium covers all surfaces of the body, including the internal surfaces of the gastrointestinal, respiratory and genitourinary tract. The major function of epithelium is to provide a selective barrier between the body and the environment. The epithelial barrier is the primary defense against threats from the environment and is also a major factor in maintaining internal homeostasis. Physical and chemical injury of the epithelial layer must therefore be repaired quickly by cell proliferation.

After injury to the epidermis, wound protection is provided in two steps: within minutes there is a temporary coverage of the wound by coagulated blood which serves as a barrier to arrest the loss of body fluids. The second step is the movement of adjacent epithelium beneath the clot and over the underlying dermis to complete wound closure. Re-epithelialization of an injured surface is achieved either by movement or growth of epithelial cells over the wound area (413, 414, 552). In early phases of wound healing the most important process is cell migration which is independent of cell division (415-417).

In deep wounds the new epithelial cover arises from the wound periphery; whereas shallow wounds usually heal from residual pilosebaceous or eccrine structures (359, 418-420).

The cellular response of epithelial cells to an injury can be divided into four basic steps: *mobilization* (freeing of cells from their attachment; *migration* (movement of cells); *proliferation* (replacement of cells by mitosis of preexisting cells) and *differentiation* (restoration of cellular function, e.g. keratinization).

The first response of the epithelium after injury is *mobilization*, which starts after 12-24 hours. This involves detachment of the individual cells in preparation for migration. Epithelial cells lose hemidesmosomal junctions; the tonofilaments withdraw from the cell periphery; and the basal membrane becomes less well-defined (15, 413, 421, 422). In addition, the cells of the leading edge become phagocytic, engulfing tissue debris and erythrocytes. Epithelialization occurs most rapidly in superficial wounds where the basal membrane is intact. Short tongues of epithelial cells grow out from the residual epithelial structures. By the 2nd or 3rd day, most of the wound base is covered with a thin epithelial layer; and, by the 4th day, by layered keratinocytes (403, 423, 424).

Migration of epithelial cells occurs as movement of clusters or sheets of cells. This movement of epithelial cells has been proposed to take place in a "leap-frog" fashion of epidermal sheet movement (425). This model suggests that cells in the migrating front adhere to the tissue only to be replaced at the front successively by cells coming from behind and moving over the newly adherent basal cell in a "leap-frog" fashion. Fibronectin in connection with fibrin seems to make a provisional matrix for cellular anchorage and self-propelling traction of the epithelial cell for migration. A speculative mechanism has been that fibronectin is produced in front of the wound edge by epidermal cells and these then slide over the deposited fibronectin matrix and finally break down this matrix at a distance of some cell diameters behind the wound edge (426, 427). It seems that the motile cells use secreted fibronectin as a temporary basal membrane and use collagenase and plasminogen activators to facilitate passage through reparative connective tissue (561).

The specific signals or stimuli for epithelialization are unknown. Migration of epithelial cells takes place in a random fashion; however, orientation of the substrate on which the cells move, as well as the presence of other cells of the same type are determinants of the extent and direction of cell movement. Furthermore, cell migration appears to be at least in part initiated by a negative feed-back mechanism from other epithelial cells in the free edge of the wound (5). Substances in the substrate which are important for direction of the migration seem to be collagen fibers, fibrin and fibronectin, as earlier described. Fibronectin appears to be a substrate for cell movement and to have a binding capacity for epithelial cells as well as monocytes, fibroblasts, and endothelial cells (98, 427-429).

Proliferation of epidermal cells starts after 1 to 2 days in the cells immediately behind the migrating edge, thereby generating a new pool of cells to cover the wound (417, 429). Mitosis in epidermal epithelium has a diurnal rhythm, being greatest during rest and inactivity. In normal epidermis, very few basal cells are in mitosis at any given time. Epidermal wounds, however, result in a change of the diurnal mitotic rhythm in cells adjacent to the wound, resulting in an absolute increase in mitotic activity and an increase in the size of epidermal cells (403). The maximal mitotic activity is found on the 3rd day and continues until epithelialization is complete and epithelial cells have reverted to their normal phenotype and reassumed their intercellular and basement membrane contacts by *differentiation* (553).

A number of stimuli for epidermal cell growth and thereby wound closure have been indentified, such as calcium in low concentration, interleukin-1, basic fibroblast growth factor (bFGF), epidermal growth factor (EGF), platelet-derived growth factor (PDGF) and transforming growth factor-alpha (TGF-α) (413, 427). The only factor known to block epithelial growth is TFG-ß (423, 430). Most of these molecules are released from cells within the wound environment such as platelets, inflammatory cells, endothelial cells and smooth muscle cells (Fig. 1.4).

Another factor which influences epithelialization is oxygen tension. Thus a high pO_2 has been found to increase epithelialization (431, 432).

Epithelial repair differs temporally in different types of wound. In *incisional wounds*, mobilization and migration of epithelial cells is a rapid response compared to other events of the wound-healing process. Already after 24 to 48 hours the epithelial cells have bridged the gap in clean incisional and sutured wounds (136). In small *excised and non-sutured wounds* which heal by secondary intention the surface is initially covered by a blood clot. Migrating epithelium does not move through the clot, but rather beneath it in direct contact with the original wound bed. Epithelial cells appear to secrete a proteolytic enzyme that dissolves the base of the clot and permits unimpeded cell migration.

In *large excised wounds*, all stages of epithelial repair may be seen simultaneously. In such wounds epithelialization will not be complete before granulation tissue has developed. Epithelial cells will use this bed for subsequent migration. Depending upon the size of wound the surface will subsequently be covered by a *scar epithelium* which is thin, and lacks strong attachment to the underlying dermis as well as lacking Langerhans cells and melanocytes.

One factor which has a strong influence upon epithelial healing is the depth of the wound. In superficial wounds the regeneration from hair follicles coincides with epithelialization from the wound edges. In deeper wounds, all epidermal regrowth occurs from the wound edge.

Finally, it should be mentioned that re-epithelialization is significantly enhanced if the wound is kept moist (426).

In the oral cavity the morphological changes seen during epithelialization of the rat molar extraction socket appear to be similar to wounds that involve oral mucosa (70, 433-437). Thus the epithelium migrates down into and across the wound with either fibrin-fibronectin or granulation tissue-fibronectin below it and the superficial wound contents (i.e. neutrophil leukocytes, tissue debris, food elements and bacteria) above it. This layer is subsequently lost in the form of a scab following reepithelialization (435).

Microenvironment in Wounds

Microenvironments in wounds are the sum of the single processes mentioned earlier. Of particular interest for the wound-healing process is the influence of the wound microenvironment as an *initiator*, *supporter* and *terminator* of the wound-healing processes (438).

Cellular activity in the wound has already been discussed in detail, but can be described as three waves of cells invading the wound area. Apart from their role in hemostasis, *platelets* serve as the initiators of wound healing by their release of substances such as growth factors (e.g. PDGF platelet factor IV, IGF-1, TGF-ß and an uncharacterized chemoattractant of endothelial cells at the moment of injury (Fig. 1.4)). As the access of platelets to the wound area is limited by the coagulation process the supply of these factors is limited.

The second set of cells, *polymorphonuclear leukocytes*, migrate into the wound after a few hours largely under the direction of complement factors. Their role in the wound-healing process appears mainly to be the control of infection.

The third type of cell invading the wound area are the *monocytes*, which are attracted to the injury site by platelet factors, complement and fibrinopeptides. After entering the wound, these cells are transformed to macrophages and take over the control of healing processes. It would appear that macrophages have the capacity to detect and interpret changes in the wound environment and thereby initiate appropriate healing responses.

In the early wound, cells float around in the tissue fluid of the wound and their function and movement are directed by different growth factors (e.g. TGF-ß, IL-6, IGF-1 and insulin produced by platelets and/or macrophages).

The amino acid content of wound fluids reflects to some extent the metabolic events. Amino acid concentrations are initially close to those of serum. Later, they approach that of inflammatory cells. After some time particularly glutamine and glutamate rise well over that of serum, whereas arginine concentration falls to low levels due to conversion to ornithin and citrullin (438). Arginine has been shown to be active in influencing the wound-healing process and seems to activate macrophages (439, 440).

It would seem that the wound fluid, with its mixture of growth factors, amino acids and other components, is conducive to cell proliferation. Thus, it has been found experimentally that cell growth was optimized in the presence of wound fluid compared to cell growth in serum (282).

Wound microenvironments have been studied in rabbit ear chambers in which healing tissues can be visualized between closely-approximated, optically clear membranes mounted under a microscope

Fig. 1.26. Cellular build-up, oxygen tension and lactate concentration in a rabbit ear chamber

The center of the wound is to the right on the drawing. At this location where macrophages operate there is very low oxygen tension and a high lactate concentration. It appears that oxygen tension is closely related to the location of the vasculature. Replication of fibroblasts takes place ahead of the regenerating vessels, whereas fibroblasts begin collagen production when the neovascular front reaches the proliferating fibroblasts. From HUNT & VAN WINKLE (557) 1976.

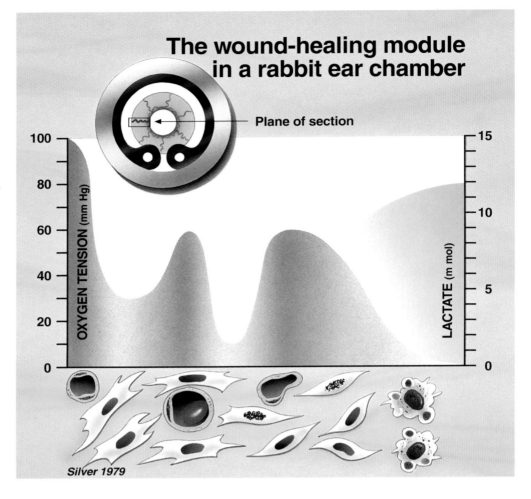

The wound-healing module in a rabbit ear chamber

Plane of section

OXYGEN TENSION (mm Hg)

LACTATE (m mol)

Silver 1979

(Fig. 1.26). This narrow space, as thin as 50 μm, forces healing cells to travel in coherent order, so that one or two cells pass at one time (53). In this model, influence of oxygen tension and lactate concentration could be measured by microprobes and has been characterized (53). An oxygen gradient from the central wound space in the chamber to the peripheral normal tissue has been described. While oxygen tension along the edges of the wound is very low, with hypoxia close to 0 mm Hg, the oxygen tension at the periphery of the wound is up to 100 mm Hg. This oxygen tension gradient seems to be important in the initiation of the wound-healing process. Concurrently, lactate concentration in the wound space is 10-20 times that of venous blood, resulting in a fall in pH to 7.25 (441).

Wound-Healing Module

After the first phase of the inflammatory process has taken place, a characteristic cell build-up is found after 3 to 4 days. At the edge of a wound is a vanguard of scavenging cells, the majority of which in the non-infected wound are macrophages. If the wound is infected, these macrophages are accompanied by large numbers of neutrophilic leukocytes.

Beneath the phagocytes is a layer of immature fibroblasts, floating in a gelatinous, non-fibrillar matrix, which are unable to divide because of local hypoxia. Beneath this layer of fibroblasts is a group of dividing fibroblasts which are associated with the most distal perfused arcaded capillaries, and behind the first perfused capillary loops are more dividing fibroblasts which provide cells to form the new tissue.

Distal to this zone, blood vessels increase in size and become less dense, probably as a result of enlargement or coalescence of a few vessels, as the other channels recede from the pattern of vascular flow. Between these vessels lie mature fibroblasts and new fibrillar collagen. This arrangement of cells creates an environment that is favorable to angiogenesis and collagen deposition and has been termed the *wound-healing module.*

Fibroblasts in mitosis are always found just ahead of the regenerating vessels, where the tissue oxygen tension is optimal for replication (i.e. about 40 mm Hg). It is assumed that these fibroblasts behave as growth centers and that new fibroblasts remain at this location until reached by the neovascular zone, whereafter they initiate collagen production (442). The hyperemic neovascular front has a higher pO_2 (Fig. 1.26) which is optimal for collagen synthesis. Thus the fibroblasts *replicate* and *produce* collagen in different wound environments.

It has been found that hypoxia or exposure to a high lactate concentration increases the capacity of fibroblasts to synthesize collagen when they are subsequently placed in an oxygenated environment (443, 444). It has been suggested that lactate stimulates collagen synthesis, (438). Thus lactate has been shown to induce an increase in procollagen mRNA. Lactate concentration in test wounds is greatest in the central space and persists well into the zone of collagen synthesis (Fig. 1.26). It is therefore suggested that new vessels overtake the immature fibroblasts and change their environment from high lactate and low oxygen tension to high lactate and high oxygen tension and thereby increase both their collagen synthesis and their deposition. When the wound cavity is totally filled with granulation tissue, the hypoxia and high lactate concentration gradually diminish as does macrophage stimulation, whereupon the wound-healing process will stop.

Oxygen tension in the wound has been shown to be important for collagen deposition and the development of the tensile strength of the wound (431, 445), for regulation of angiogenesis (233) and for the epithelialization of wounds (417). Oxygen in the wound's extracellular environment also has an important role in the intracellular killing of bacteria by granulocytes (446).

Neutrophil *migration*, *attachment* and *ingestion* of bacteria apparently are independent of oxygen; however, the *killing* of the most important wound pathogens is achieved by mechanisms that require molecular oxygen (447). These mechanisms are introduced through reducing extracellular molecular oxygen to superoxide which is then inserted into phagosomes. Here the superoxide is converted to high-energy bactericidal oxygen radicals for optimal bacterial killing (448).

Several studies in normal volemic animals have shown that they clear bacteria from wounds in proportion to the fraction of oxygen in the inspired gas. Infection was less invasive or failed to develop in hyperoxygenated guinea pigs when bacteria were injected into skin (448). Furthermore, infected skin lesions in dogs became invasive in tissues with extracellular fluid oxygen tension under 60 mm Hg; however, they remained localized if the tissue was better oxygenated, as in the case of higher inspiratory oxygen concentration (449). Experience in human subjects tends to support these findings; but no trial has yet been performed supporting these observations.

Factors Affecting the Wound-Healing Process

Blood Circulation and Oxygenation of the Wound

Oxygen has, as already described, a very significant effect in the initiation, continuation and termination of the wound-healing process (431, 445, 450-452). Blood supply and oxygen delivery provide energy and nutrition to the cells within the wound. Healing is not possible without adequate local circulation. A fundamental factor in the healing process therefore is the restoration of microcirculation and oxygen delivery by angiogenesis.

Tissue perfusion is determined by a variety of general and local factors. Peripheral tissue perfusion is influenced by multiple cardiovascular regulatory mechanisms. In response to hemorrhage, these mechanisms maintain blood flow to vital organs, such as heart and brain, while blood flow to other tissues is decreased (453, 550). Circulatory adjustments are effected by local as well as systemic mechanisms that change the caliber of the arterioles and alter hydrostatic pressure in the capillaries. Detection of poor tissue perfusion, and especially tissue oxygenation, is crucial in the postinjury and care periods.

If wound edges show signs of ischemia, there is a risk of impaired wound healing with development of wound leakage and infection. From the knowledge of healing wounds of the oral cavity and the anus, it is obvious that perfusion is the major factor in resistance to infection. Despite contamination of both types of wound with bacteria, they almost always heal without infection if patients have a normally functioning immune system. The difference between these and other wounds (e.g. extremities) is not related to local immunity, but to differences in perfusion and oxygenation.

Increased oxygen tension improves resistance to infection through local leukocyte function (454). Thus, experimental data have shown that the killing capacity of granulocytes is normal only to the extent to which molecular oxygen is available (446, 455-460). Bacteria killing involves two major components. The first is degranulation of neutrophils in which bacteria located within the phagosome are exposed to various antimicrobial compounds from the granules. The effect of this system is unrelated to the environment of the leukocytes. The second system is the so-called *oxidative killing* and depends upon molecular oxygen absorbed by the leukocytes and converted to high-energy radicals such as superoxide, hydroxyl radical, peroxides, aldehydes, hypochlorite, and hypoiodite, all substances which to varying degrees are toxic to bacteria. In this regard it is important to consider that the efficacy of oxidative bacteria killing is directly proportional to local oxygen tension (461).

The clinical relevance of blood flow and oxygen supply to healing and infection has been shown experimentally in skin flaps in dogs (51, 346, 349). In flaps with a high perfusion and tissue oxygen tension, no infection was found after injection of bacteria; whereas invasive, necrotizing infections were found in flap areas in which oxygen tension was less than 40 mm Hg. When oxygen tension in inspired gas and arterial blood was raised or lowered, the infection rate corresponded to tissue oxygen tension, but not to oxygen carrying capacity.

With respect to healing of dental tissues, the oxygen tension may have a significant effect. Thus, several *in vivo* tissue culture studies have shown that low oxygen tension (e.g. a 5% oxygen atmosphere) results in reduced collagen and bone formation. A concentration of 35% O_2 was found to be optimal for collagen and bone formation, while a high oxygen concentration (95%) resulted in depression of collagen and bone formation as well as osteoclastic resorption of bone and cartilage (462-464). This *in vitro* relation between high oxygen concentration and osteoclastic activity may have an *in vivo* counterpart in the so-called vanishing bone disease (*Gorhams disease* or *vanishing facial bone*) (465, 466) as well as the *internal surface resorption* phenomena seen in revascularization of the pulps of luxated or root-fractured teeth (43). In both instances active local hyperemia and increased oxygen supply may be related to osteoclastic activity.

Among local factors which can control blood supply and tissue perfusion to the injured tissue, tension caused by splints or sutures may seriously jeopardize local circulation. Thus, splinting types exerting pressure on the periodontium may disturb or prevent uneventful PDL or pulp healing and lead to disturbances, such as root resorption, ankylosis and pulp necrosis (see Chapter 2, p. 95). Furthermore, tension of sutured soft tissue wounds may lead to ischemia with subsequent risk of wound infection (see Chapter 13, p. 499).

Hyperbaric Oxygenation (HBO)

Recently hyperbaric oxygen (HBO) has been introduced in treatment of various oral conditions such as problem wounds subsequent to irradiation as well as in cases of grafting procedures where vascularization appears compromised (467).

HBO is administered in pressurized tanks where the patients inhale 100% oxygen at a pressure of 2 atmospheres. The interaction of HBO to hypoxic tissue has a range of effects (7). The most significant effect of HBO is that it augments the oxygen gradient within the wound-healing site, thus leading to increased fibroblast

Fig. 1.27. Importance of the decisive period
The period of active tissue anti-bacterial activity (decisive period) relates well to the establishing of the inflammatory response, as reflected by increased vascular permeability and leukocyte migration into the wound site. From LEAK ET AL (478) 1974.

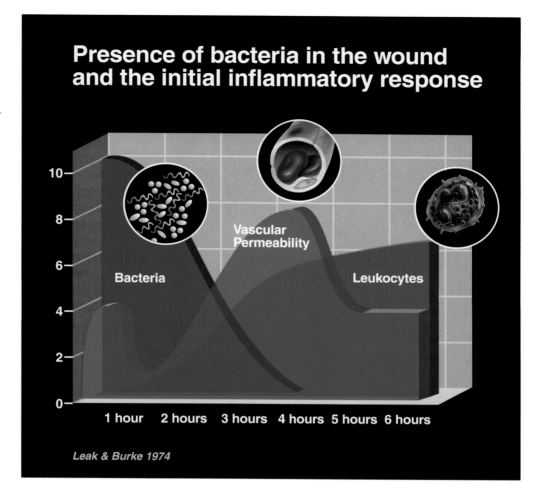

and endothelial activity (233, 468-471) as well as increased epithelialization (432). HBO may also suppress growth of certain bacteria (454).

In experimental gingival wounds in rats, it has been found that HBO augments gingival connective tissue healing during the first 2 weeks, whereafter no difference was seen in comparison to wounds healed at normal atmosphere (472). In more extensive wounds in rats, where mandibular ramus osteotomy wounds severed the neurovascular supply in the mandibular canal, it was found that HBO reduced or prevented the ischemic damage to pulp cells, ameloblastema and adjacent bone on a short-term basis (i.e. after 10 days). With an observation period of 30 days, HBO was found to stimulate osteodentin and bone formation in the zones of injury (473).

This beneficial effect of HBO on bone healing after injury is supported by a human study where acceleration of bone healing after osteotomy could be demonstrated after the use of hyperbaric oxygen (474).

Infection

Infection is the most common complication which can disturb wound-healing (277). Development of infection is determined by the number and type of contaminating organisms, host defense capability and local environment (475).

When bacteria invade a wound, the final outcome of this event is related to the success of the inital phase of the inflammatory response in establishing an antibacterial defense (Fig. 1.27). Timing is critical and the fate of the contaminating bacteria appears to be determined within the first 3 to 4 hours after injury. During this period, the early inflammatory process is established and will usually result in the elimination of bacteria (476-478).

The risk of infection appears to be directly related to the number of bacteria initially present in the wound (479). If the bacteria are not eliminated during these first critical hours, a series of events which will effect wound-healing will occur. Thus the formation of fibroblasts will be disturbed in several ways and fibroblast proliferation is generally inhibited; but stimulation may occur in certain circumstances (480-484, 554, 555). Liberation of toxins, enzymes and waste products from bacteria decrease or inhibit collagen synthesis (485) and increase the synthesis of collagenase, resulting in lysis of collagen (486). Furthermore, some bacteria decrease the amount of oxygen available in the infected tissue (487, 488) whereby healing processes suffer. Collagen formation is reduced, cell migration is delayed or arrested, cellular necrosis and microvascular thrombosis may result (489). Wounds have been classified as:

Clean wounds, which are uninfected operative wounds in which no inflammation is encountered.

Potentially contaminated wounds, in which the respiratory, alimentary or genitourinary tracts are entered under controlled condition during surgery.

Contaminated wounds where acute inflammation (without pus) is encountered or where there is a gross spillage from a hollow viscus during surgery.

Dirty wounds and infected wounds which are old traumatic wounds and operating wounds in the presence of pus or those involving clinical infection of perforated viscera (477).

The level of aerobic and anaerobic contamination expressed as bacteria in the wound (i.e. colony forming units per unit area) is for *clean wounds* 2.2, for *potentially contaminated wounds* 2.4×10^1, for *contaminated wounds* 1.1×10^3 and for *dirty wounds* 3.7×10^3 (490).

Oral wounds are associated with a high risk of contamination as saliva contains 10^{8-9} bacteria per milliliter (491).

The infective dose of bacteria which results in a *microscopic* infection has been found to be 10^5 bacteria per gram of tissue (492). A correlation has been found in different types of wounds between pre-closure bacterial density of aerobic and anaerobic bacteria and post-surgical wound infections (490). It is recognized that both aerobic and anaerobic organisms are implicated in most wound infections.

The use of antibiotics to supplement the natural host resistance (i.e. the early inflammatory response) has been found to be additive and sometimes even synergistic in bacteria killing. However, if antibiotics are given with more than a 3-hour delay, animal experiments have shown that the effect of antibiotics such as penicillin, erythromycin, chloramphenicol and tetracyclin was eliminated (493). The timing of antibiotics therefore seems to be of utmost importance.

Many factors are described as contributing to impaired wound-healing as well as increased risk of infection. Some of these factors may have a direct influence on the healing process while others factors have an indirect influence by changing circulation and thereby oxygenation.

Foreign Bodies

The presence of foreign bodies can contribute to delayed healing, but is normally not by itself sufficient to prevent healing. Foreign bodies provide a focus for bacterial growth, and consequently a smaller amount of bacteria is needed to cause infection in the wound area. More than 30 years ago it was observed that just a single silk suture present in the wound area increased the susceptibility to bacteria (staphylococcus) by a factor of x 10,000 (494, 495). Other types of foreign materials, such as soil, clothing and drains have also been shown to increase the risk of postoperative infection and impaired wound-healing (496-498). Recently it has been found that bacteria may be camouflaged on artificial surfaces by producing an extracellular carbohydrate film (499). This film seriously affects the host response by inhibiting chemotaxis, bacterial engulfment and the oxidation response of the phagocytes.

Foreign bodies in oral and other soft tissue wounds consist mainly of soil and its contaminants (496), but also tooth fragments can be found. Soil has four major components: inorganic minerals, organic matter, water and air. The coarser components of soil are stone, gravel and sand. The smallest inorganic particle found in soil is clay. Not only does soil carry bacterial contamination into the wound, but the mere presence of inorganic and organic particles has been shown to lead to impairment of leukocyte ability to ingest and kill bacteria (496). Therefore very few bacteria are able to elicit purulent infections in the presence of foreign bodies. As there is no way of neutralizing the effect of soil, therapeutic efforts should be directed towards removing it from the wound area (see Chapter 13 p. 498).

In traumatic wounds, foreign bodies can usually be removed, improving wound healing and decreasing the risk of infection. In surgical wounds, however, this may not always be the case. The most common foreign bodies in surgical wounds are sutures, drains and biological materials such as hematomas.

Sutures

The ideal suture can be described as free of infection, non-irritating to tissues, achieving its purpose and disappearing when the work is finished (500). Such ideal sutures are still not available; but by choosing the best material, the complication rate provided by the suture material itself can be decreased. Bulky and braided suture materials are generally more likely to cause trouble than fine monofilament sutures (501, 566) (see Chapter 13, p. 499).

In non-infected multifilamentous sutures, fibroblasts and giant cells appear early and the suture strands remain tightly bound in comparison to infected sutures where bacteria are entrapped within the braids, leading to pus formation (502).

The reaction around a monofilament suture is minimal and a fibrous capsule appears after 10 days, even in the presence of infection. Apart from the knots, there is no space for bacteria to lodge (502). The ideal suture is therefore a monofilament type of suture with sufficient strength to hold the wound edges together until significant healing has occurred, even in delayed healing. The use of absorbable and non-absorbable sutures in relation to wound healing and infection is still controversial (503-505). The use of sutures in soft tissue wounds is further discussed in Chapter 13, p. 499.

Distant Wound Response

For decades it has been known that a wound preceded by a previous injury heals faster than a primary wound. Thus from a mechanical point of view (wound strength) a second wound heals faster than the first (506). The explanation for this phenomenon is still uncertain. Another distant wound response is found when two wounds occur simultaneously in distant parts of the body. In these cases impaired blood circulation may be found in the wounds leading to impaired healing (507).

Age

FETAL WOUND HEALING

Healing of experimental oral wounds in a mammalian fetus differs greatly from similar wounds in adults (508-512). Thus accelerated healing without scarring is found in fetal wounds, even in defect wounds. The wound response appears to be without acute inflammation and with minimal fibroblast and endothelial cell proliferation (513). Furthermore the extracellular matrix appears collagen-poor and rich in hyaluronic acid.

Hyaluronic acid is laid down early in the matrix of both fetal and adult wounds; but sustained deposition of hyaluronic acid is unique to fetal wound healing (514). Hyaluronic acid is presently thought to play a decisive role in the regenerative process, as it provides a permissive environment for cell proliferation and mobility (508, 509, 513, 515) and suppresses macrophage-effected post-natal repair (515). Lately it has been shown that the elimination of transforming growth factor ß (TGF-ß) from healing wounds in adult rats reversed the typical fibrous scar formation to a stage of fetal wound healing without scar tissue (176). This implies that the control of selected cytokines may be a future approach to control scarring.

ADULT WOUND HEALING

The relationship between age and healing of *skin wounds* in respect to speed of healing has been studied experimentally in *rats* (516-523), *rabbits* (524, 525) and in *humans* (526, 527). Experiments examining the role of the age factor upon wounding of *oral mucosa* and *gingiva* has been performed in *rats* (528-532) *mice* (533) and *humans* (534-536). In the most comprehensive studies using experimental skin wounds in rats and gingival wounds in humans, it was found that healing of gingival defects is slower and regeneration more incomplete in old than in young individuals. Furthermore, wound strength develops more slowly in old rats than in young rats, a finding which was related to the better functional arrangement of collagen fibers in the young animals (537). In the gastro-intestinal tract, however, aging seems not to have an adverse influence on wound healing (538).

Wound infection is also strongly related to age (539, 540). Thus, in a prospective study on wound infection subsequent to surgical wounds, a wound infection rate of 0.6% was found in children aged 1-14 years and this rate rose to a maximum of 3.8% in patients over 66 years of age (539).

Optimizing Oral Wound Healing

An important principle to consider in this context is that the mode of action of both normal wound healing and the response to infection seem to follow a general pattern which is sometimes in conflict with the *regeneration* of injured organs. This is apparent in skin wounds where the need for rapid wound closure (in order to prevent infection from invading microorganisms) usually results in the formation of a scar. In the dental organ, an effective response against bacteria takes priority with activation of the neutrophils, lymphocytes macrophages and osteoclasts leading to frequent bone and tooth loss due to hard tissue resorption (see Chapter 2 , p. 112).

Presently, the most likely avenue whereby healing problems can be avoided appears to be careful tissue handling whereby tissue perfusion is reestablished or stabilized and wound contaminants (e.g. foreign bodies and microbes) are reduced or eliminated.

To achieve this goal, various steps are necessary in the diffent phases of wound healing. In the coagulation phase, assistance in achieving hemostasis may be necessary. In performing this, it is important not to use excessive cautery, which results in tissue necrosis, or topical hemostatic agents (e.g. Surgicel ®, Oxycel ®, Gelfoam ®) that may have a potentiating effect for infection (240). Instead, firm pressure exerted with a gauze sponge for several minutes usually results in hemostasis.

In handling oral wounds, a local anesthetic is usually necessary. In this regard it should be borne in mind that the vasoconstriction of the anesthetic solution increases the risk of infection of the wound due to interference with the inflammatory response in the critical first hours after injury (496, 562). Regional block anesthesia rather than local infiltration of the anesthetic solution is therefore to be recommended.

Wound debridement should be limited to removal of foreign bodies and obviously damaged tissue which cannot be anticipated to survive or become revascularized (see Chapter 13, p. 496).

The elimination and/or reduction in the size of the blood clot should be attempted in order to facilitate wound healing, including revascularization. This applies to soft tissues as well as tooth and bone repositioning.

The value of complete immobilization of the wound edges is presently under debate so only a few treatment principles can be suggested:

In soft tissue wounds any sutures used to immobilize the wound edges must be regarded as foreign bodies which increases the risk of infection (240, 496). Thus a minimal number of sutures should be used, and a suture type should be chosen which elicits minimal side effects (see Chapter 13, p. 499).

In regard to hard tissue healing, splinting should generally be performed. These splints should not augment the risk of infection, whereby the application and the design of the splints becomes crucial (see Chapter 9, p. 347).

The value of antibiotics in oral wound healing is presently unsettled (see Chapters 11 and 13). If indicated, antibiotics should be administered as early as possible and preferably not later than in the first 3 to 4 hours after trauma and only maintained for a short period of time (475) (see Chapters 11 and 13).

Acceleration of oral wound healing by the use of growth factors is in its initial stage and has the potential to be an essential part of trauma treatment (143). The fascinating perspective in the use of growth factors is the achievement of an orchestrated healing response whereby certain parts of the cellular response are promoted (e.g. angiogenesis, fibrillogenesis, dentinogenesis, osteogenesis and epithelialization). The initial attempts at such an approach to oral wound healing appear very promising (225).

Essentials

Regeneration is a process whereby the original architecture and function of disrupted or lost tissue is completely restored.

Repair is a process whereby the continuity of disrupted or lost tissue is restored by new tissue, but which does not reproduce the original structure and function.

THE GENERAL STEPS IN WOUND HEALING INCLUDE

Control of bleeding by the combined action of vaso-constriction and coagulation.

Inflammatory response, whereby leukocytes migrate into the wound in order to protect the area against infection and perform cleansing of the wound site.

Connective and epithelial tissue migration and proliferation, which obturate the wound defect and add mechanical strength to the wound.

Reorganization of the tissue by a remodelling process which results in more functionally oriented collagen fibers which increase the strength of the wound.

THE MAIN ROLES OF THE INDIVIDUAL TISSUE CELLS INCLUDE

Platelets, apart from their role in initial hemostasis and their activation of the coagulation cascade, serve as initiators of the wound-healing process.

Polymorphonuclear leukocytes prevent bacterial infection within the wound site.

Macrophages are scavengers of tissue remnants and foreign bodies including bacteria and the key cells in coordinating the cellular events in wound healing.

Fibroblasts produce collagen and ground substance which fills out the wound defect and adds mechanical strength to the wound.

Endothelial cells in the venules are the key cells in angiogenesis. By coordinated endothelial cell proliferation and migration, a new vascular network is formed at the wound site.

Epithelial cells close the gap against the external environment by cell migration and proliferation.

The coordinated action of the above-mentioned cells is found in the *wound-healing module* created a few days after injury where leading macrophages clear damaged tissue, foreign bodies and bacteria with trailing fibroblasts and newly formed capillaries.

Significant stimuli for the invasive growth of new formed connective tissue and also termination of the wound-healing module appear to be growth factors as well as oxygen tension and lactate concentration in the injury zone ahead of the wound-healing module.

Of many factors known to disturb wound healing, the following are the most likely candidates in wound healing affecting mucosa, skin, as well as the periodontium and the pulp of traumatized teeth:

Low oxygen delivery to the wound site due to the initial trauma and/or improper tissue handling technique (e.g. suturing, splinting or lack of repositioning of tissues).

Infection due to contamination of the injury site.

Foreign bodies including inappropriate use of sutures and drains.

Bibliography

1. SUNDEL B, ed. *Symposium on wound healing: plastic surgical and dermatological aspects.* Espoo 1979.

2. HUNT TK, ed. *Wound healing and wound infection: theory and surgical practice.* New York: Appelton-Century-Crofts, 1980.

3. DINEEN P, HILDIC-SMITH G, eds. *The surgical wound.* Philadelphia: Lea & Febiger, 1981.

4. HUNT TK, HEPPENSTALL RB, PINES E, ROVEE D, eds. *Soft and hard tissue repair: biological and clinical aspects.* New York: Praeger, 1984.

5. PEACOCK JR EE. *Wound repair.* 3rd edn. Philadelphia: WB Saunders Company, 1984.

6. WOO SLY, BUCKWALTER JA, eds. *Injury and repair of the musculoskeletal soft tissues.* Illinois: American Academy of Orthopedic Surgeons, 1988.

7. DAVIS JC, HUNT TK, eds. *Problem wounds: the role of oxygen.* New York: Elsevier, 1988.

8. CLOWES JR GHA, ed. *Trauma, sepsis, and shock: the physiological basis of therapy.* New York: Mercel Dekker, 1988.

9. CLARK RAF, HENSON PM, eds. *The molecular and cellular biology of wound repair.* New York: Plenum Press, 1988.

10. LUNDBORG G. *Nerve injury and repair.* Edinburgh: Churchill Livingstone, 1988.

11. KLOTH LC, MCCULLOCH JM, FEEDAR JA, eds. *Wound healing: alternatives in management.* Philadelphia: FA Davis Company, 1990

12. JANSSEN H, ROOMAN R, ROBERTSON JIS, eds. *Wound healing.* Petersfield: Wrightson Biomedical Publishing Ltd, 1991.

13. COHEN IK, DIEGELMANN RF, LINDBLAD WJ, eds. *Wound healing: biochemical and clinical aspects.* Philadelphia: WB Saunders Company,1992.

14. GILLMAN T. Tissue Regeneration. In: BOURNE GH, ed. *Structural aspects of ageing.* London: Pitman, 1961:144-176.

15. FEINBERG SE, LARSEN PE. Healing of traumatic injuries. In: FONSECA RJ, WALKER RV, eds. *Oral and maxillofacial trauma.* Philadelphia: WB Saunders, 1991:13-56.

16. BERNFIELD M, BANERJEE SD, KODA JE, RAPRAEGER AC. Remodelling of the basement membrane: morphogenesis and maturation. In: *Basement membranes and cell movement.* London: Pitman (Ciba Foundation symposium 108),1984: 179-196.

17. POTTEN CS. *Stem cells: Their identification and characterization.* New York: Churchill Livingstone, 1983.

18. CAIRNIE AB, LAMERTON LF, STEEL GG. Cell proliferation studies in the intestinal epithelium of the rat. I. and II *Exp Cell Res* 1965;**39**:528-538.

19. LEBLOND CP, CHENG H. Identification of stem cells in the small intestine of the mouse. In: CAIRNIE AB, LAla PK, OSMOND DG, eds. *Stem Cells of Renewing Populations.* New York: Academic Press, 1976:7-31.

20. ROBERTS WE, MOZSARY PG, KLINGLER E. Nuclear size as a cell-kinetic marker for osteoblast differentiation. *Am J Anat* 1982;**165**:373-384.

21. GOULD TRL. Ultrastructural characteristics of progenitor cell populations in the periodontal ligament. *J Dent Res* 1983;**62**:873-876.

22. ANDREASEN JO, ANDREASEN FM. Cellular changes during pulpal revascularization after experimental tooth replantation in monkeys. In preparation 1993.

23. SNOW MH. Myogenic cell formation in regenerating rat skeletal muscle injured by mincing: II. An autoradiographic study. *Anat Rec* 1977;**188**:200-218.

24. RAMFJORD SP, ENGLER WO, HINIKER JJ. A radiographic study of healing following simple gingivectomy.II. The connective tissue. *J Periodontol* 1966;**37**:179-189.

25. TONNA E, STAHL SS. A (3H)-thymidine autoradiographic study of cell proliferative activity of injured periodontal tissues of 5-week old mice. *Arch Oral Biol* 1973;**18**:617-627.

26. SVEEN OB, HAWES RR. Differentiation of new odontoblasts and dentine bridge formation in rat molar teeth after tooth grinding. *Arch Oral Biol* 1968;**13**:1399-1412.

27. ZACH L, TOPAL R, COHEN G. Pulpal repair following operative procedures. Radioautographic demonstration with tritiated thymidine. *Oral Surg Oral Med Oral Pathol* 1968;**28**:587-597.

28. FEIT J, METELOVA M, SINDELKA Z. Incorporation of 3H-thymidine into damaged pulp of rat incisors. *J Dent Res* 1970;**49**:783-786.

29. LUOSTARINEN V. Dental pulp response to trauma. An experimental study in the rat. *Proc Finn Dent Soc* 1971;**67**:1-51.

30. FITZGERALD M. Cellular mechanics of dentinal bridge repair using 3H-thymidine. *J Dent Res* 1979;**58**:2198-2206.

31. YAMAMURA T, SHIMONO M, KOIKE H, et al. Differentiation and induction of undifferentiated mesenchymal cells in tooth and periodontal tissue during wound healing and regeneration. *Bull Tokyo Dent Coll* 1980;**21**:181-221.

32. YAMAMURA T. Differentiation of pulpal cells and inductive influences of various matrices. *J Dent Res* 1985;**64**:530-540.

33. SENZAKI H. A histological study of reparative dentinogenesis in the rat incisor after colchicine administration. *Arch Oral Biol* 1980;**25**:737-743.

34. RUCH JV. Odontoblast differentiation and the formation of the odontoblast layer. *J Dent Res* 1985;**64**:489-498.

35. GOULD TRL, MELCHER AH, BRUNETTE DM. Migration and division of progenitor cell populations in periodontal ligament after wounding. *J Periodont Res* 1980;**15**:20-42.

36. MCCULLOCH CAG. Progenitor cell populations in the periodontal ligament of mice. *Anat Rec* 1985;**211**:258-262.

37. TONNA EA, CRONKITE EP. Cellular response to fracture studied with tritiated thymidine. *J Bone Joint Surg* 1961;**43A**:352-362.

38. POTTEN CS. Stem cells in epidermis from the back of the mouse. In: POTTEN CS, ed. *Stem Cells: Their identification and characterisation.* New York: Churchill Livingstone, 1983: 200-232.

39. HUME WJ. Stem cells in oral epithelia. In: POTTEN CS, ed. *Stem cells. Their identification and characterization.* New York: Churchill Livingstone, 1983:233-270.

40. SNOW MH. Myogenic cell formation in regenerating rat skeletal muscle injured by mincing: I. A fine structural study. *Anat Rec* 1977;**188**:181-200.

41. IGLHAUT J, AUKHIL I, SIMPSON DM, JOHNSTON MC, KOCK G. Progenitor cell kinetics during guided tissue regeneration in experimental wounds. *J Periodont Res* 1987;**23**:107-117.

42. SILVER IA. Local and systemic factors which affect the proliferation of fibroblasts. In: KALONEN E, PIKARAINEN J, eds. *Biology of the fibroblasts.* New York: Academic Press,1973;507.

43. ANDREASEN JO, ANDREASEN FM. Root resorption following traumatic dental injuries. *Proc Finn Dent Soc* 1992;**88**(Suppl 1):95-114.

44. HANCOCK EB. Regeneration procedures. In: NEVINS M, BECKER W, KORNMAN K, eds. *Proceedings of the world workshop in clinical Periodontics.* Princeton: America Academy of Periodontology, 1989: VI.1-20.

45. MORGAN CJ, PLEDGER WJ. Fibroblast proleferation. In: COHEN IK, DIEGELMANN RF, LINDBLAD WJ, eds. *Wound healing: biochemical and clinical aspects.* Philadelphia: WB Saunders, 1992:63-78.

46. MCCARTY JB, SAS DF, FURCHT LT. Mechanisms of parenchymal cell migration into wounds. In: CLARK RAF, HENSON PM, eds. *The molecular and cellular biology of wound repair.* New York: Plenum Press, 1988:281-319.

47. SINGER SJ, KUPFER A. The directed migration of eukaryotic cells. *Ann Rev Biol* 1986;**2**:337-365.

48. BERGMANN JE, KUPFER A, SINGER SJ. Membrane insertion at the leading edge of motile fibroblasts. *Proc Natl Acad Sci USA* 1983;**80**:1367-1371.

49. BRYANT WM. *Wound healing*. Ciba Clin Symp 1977;**29**:1-36.

50. REICH E, RIFKIN DB, SHAW E, eds. *Proteases and biological control*. Cold Spring Harbor: Cold Spring Harbor conference on cell proliferation. 1976.

51. GOTTRUP F, FIRMIN R, HUNT TK, MATHES S. The dynamic properties of tissue oxygen in healing flaps. *Surgery* 1984;**95**:527-537.

52. HUNT TK. Physiology of wound healing. In: CLOWES GHA, ed. *Trauma, sepsis, and shock*. New York: Marcel Dekker, 1988:443-471.

53. SILVER IA. The physiology of wound healing. In: HUNT TK, ed. *Wound healing and wound infection: theory and surgical practice*. New York: Appelton-Century-Crofts, 1980:11-31.

54. GOTTRUP F. Acute wound healing - aspects of wound closure. In: LEAPER DJ, ed. *International symposium on wound management*. Bussum, the Netherlands: Medicom Europe, 1991:11-18.

55. GOTTRUP F. Advances in the biology of wound healing. In: HARDING KG, LEAPER DL, TURNER TD, eds. *Proceedings of 1st european conference on advances in wound management*. London: MacMillan, 1992:7-10.

56. GOTTRUP F, FOGDESTAM I, HUNT TK. Delayed primary closure: an experimental and clinical review. *J Clin Surg* 1982;**1**:113-124.

57. GOTTRUP F. Delayed primary closure of wounds. *Infect Surg* 1985;**4**:171-178.

58. CLARK RAF. Cutaneous wound repair: a review with emphasis on integrin receptor expression. In: JANSSEN H, ROOMAN R, ROBERTSON JIS, eds. *Wound healing*.Petersfield: Wrightson Biomedical Publishing Ltd, 1991:7-17.

59. WAHL LM, WAHL SM. Inflammation. In: COHEN IK, DIEGELMANN RF, LINDBLAD WJ, eds. *Wound healing: biochemical and clinical aspects*. Philadelphia: WB Saunders, 1992:40-62.

60. DVORAK HF, KAPLAN AP, CLARK RAF. Potential functions of the clotting system in wound repair. In: CLARK RAF, HENSON PM, eds. *The molecular and cellular biology of wound repair*. New York: Plenum Press, 1988:57-85.

61. DVORAK HF, HARVEY VS, ESTRELLA P, et al. Fibrin containing gels induce angiogenesis. Implications for tumor stroma generation and wound healing. *Lab Invest* 1987;**57**:673-686.

62. CHEN LB, BUCHANAN JM. Mitogenic activity of blood components. I. Thrombin and prothrombin. *Proc Natl Acad Sci USA* 1975;**72**:131-135.

63. WESLER BB, LEY CW, JAFFE EA. Stimulation of endothelial cell prostacycline production by thrombin, trypsin, and ionophore A23187. *J Clin Invest* 1978;**62**:923-930.

64. BAR- SHIVAT R, WILNER GD. Biologic activities of nonenzymatic thrombin: Elucidation of a macrophage interactive domain. *Sem Throm Hem* 1986;**12**:244-249.

65. BAR- SHIVAT R, KAHN AJ, MANN KG, et al. Identification of a thrombin sequence with growth factor activity on macrophages. *Proc Natl Acad Sci USA* 1986;**83**:976-980.

66. CARNEY DH, CUNNINGHAM DD. Role of specific cell surface receptors in thrombin-stimulated cell division. *Cell* 1978;**15**:1341-1349.

67. GRAY AJ, REEVES JT, HARRISON NK, et al. Growth factors for human fibroblasts in the solute remaining after clot formation. *J Cell Sci* 1990;**96**:271-274.

68. MAJNO G, BOUVIER CA, GABBIANI G, RYAN GB, STAIKOV P. Kymographic recording of clot retraction: Effects of papaverine, theophylline and cytochalasin B. *Thromb Diath Haemorrh* 1972;**28**:49-53.

69. ORDMAN LN, GILLMAN T. Studies in the healing of cutaneous wounds. Part III. A critical comparison in the pig of the healing of surgical incisions closed with sutures or adhesive tape based on tensile strength and clinical and histologic criteria. *Arch Surg* 1966;**93**:911-928.

70. MCMILLAN MD. An ultrastructural study of the relationship of oral bacteria to the epithelium of healing tooth extraction wounds. *Arch Oral Biol* 1975;**20**:815-822.

71. MCMILLAN MD. The healing of oral wounds. *N Zealand Dent J* 1986;**82**:112-116.

72. POLK HC JR, MILES AA. Enhancement of bacterial infection by ferric ion: kinetics, mechanisms and surgical significance. *Surgery* 1971;**70**:71-77.

73. POLK HC JR, FRY DE, FLINT LM. Dissemination and causes of infection. *Surg Clin North Am* 1976;**56**:817-829.

74. WIKESJÖ UME, CLAFFEY N, EGELBERG J. Periodontal repair in dogs: effect of heparin treatment of the root surface. *J Clin Periodontol* 1991;**18**:60-64.

75. GRINNELL F, BENNETT MH. Fibroblast adhesion on collagen substrata in the presence and absence of plasma fibronectin. *J Cell Sci* 1981;**48**:19-34.

76. MOSHER DF, JOHNSON RB. Specificity of fibronectin-fibrin cross-linking. *Ann NY Acad Sci* 1983;**408**:583-594.

77. KITTLICK PD. Fibrin in fibroblast cultures: A metabolic study as a contribution of inflammation and tissue repair. *Exp Pathol (Jena)* 1979;**17**:312-326.

78. KNOX P, CROOKS S, RIMMER CS. Role of fibrinectin in the migration of fibroblasts into plasma clots. *J Cell Biol* 1986;**102**:2318-2323.

79. WEIGEL PH, FULLER GM, LEBOEUF RD. A model for the role of hyaluronic acid and fibrin in the early events during the inflammatory response and wound healing. *J Theor Biol* 1986;**119**:219-234.

80. CIANO P, COLVIN R, DVORAK A, et al. Macrophage migration in fibrin gel matrices. *Lab Invest* 1986;**54**:62-70.

81. RICHARDSON DL, PEPPER DS, KAY AB. Chemotaxis for human monocytes by fibrinogen-derived peptides. *Br J Haematol* 1976;**32**:507-513.

82. KNIGHTON DR, HUNT TK, THAKRAL KK, et al. Role of platelets and fibrin and the healing sequence: An in vivo study of angiogenesis and collagen synthesis. *Ann Surg* 1982;**196**:379-388.

83. CLARK RAF, LANIGAN JM, DELLAPELLE P, et al. Fibronectin and fibrin provide a provisional matrix for epidermal cell migration during wound re-epithelialization. *J Invest Dermatol* 1982;**79**:264-269.

84. KURKINEN M, VAHERI A, ROBERTS PJ, et al. Sequential appearance of fibronectin and collagen in experimental granulation tissue. *Lab Invest* 1980;**43**:47-51.

85. ROSS R, BENDITT EP. Wound healing and collagen formation. I. Sequential changes in components of guinea pig skin wounds observed in the electron microscope. *J Biophys Biochem Cytol* 1961;**11**:677-700.

86. ALLEN RA, PEPPER DC. Isolation and properties of human vascular plasminogen activator. *Thromb Haemost* 1981;**45**:43-50.

87. POLSON AM, PROYE MP. Fibrin linkage: a precursor for new attachment. *J Periodont* 1983;**54**:141-147.

88. MCDONALD JA. FIBRONECTIN. A primitive matrix. In: CLARK RAF, HENSON PM, eds. *The molecular and cellular biology of wound repair*. New York: Plenum Press, 1988:405-435.

89. WATER VAN DE L, BROWN L, DUBIN D, LAVIGNE L, MURPHY T. *Macrophages regulate their fibronectin splicing pattern during wound healing*. Submitted, 1991.

90. WILLIAMS IF, MCCULLAGH KG, SILVER IA. The distribution of types I and III collagen and fibronectin in the healing equine tendon. *Connect Tissue Res* 1984;**12**:211-227.

91. MCAUSLAN B, HANNAN G, REILLY W, STEWART F. Variant endothelial cells: fibronectin as a transducer of signals for migration and neovascularization. *J Cell Physiol* 1980;**104**:177-186.

92. MCAUSLAN B, HANNAN G, REILLY W. Signals causing change in morphological phenotype, growth mode, and gene expression of vascular endothelial cells. *J Cell Physiol* 1982;**112**:96-106.

93. KUBO M, NORRIS DA, HOWELL SE, RYAN SR, CLARK RA. Human keratinocytes synthesize, secrete, and deposit fibronectin in the pericellular matrix. *J Dermatol* 1984;**82**:580-586.

94. LIVINGSTON, WATER VAN DE, CONSTANT C, BROWN L. Fibronectin expression during cutaneous wound healing. In: ADZICK NS, LONGAKER MT, eds. *Fetal wound healing.* New York: Elsevier, 1992:281-301.

95. KLEINMAN HK. Interactions between connctive tissue matrix macromolecules. *Connective Tissue Res* 1982;**10**:61-72.

96. REPESH LA, FITZGERALD TJ, FURCHT LT. Fibronectin involvement in granulation tissue and wound healing in rabbits. *J Histochem Cytochem* 1982;**30**:351-358.

97. CLARK RA, WINN HJ, DVORAK HF, COLVIN RB. Fibronectin beneath reepithelializing epidermis in vivo: sources and significance. *J Invest Dermatol* 1982;**77**:26-30.

98. GRINNELL F, FELD MK. Initial adhesion of human fibroblasts in serum free medium: possible role of secreted fibronectin. *Cell* 1979;**17**:117-129.

99. GUSTAFSON GT. Ecology of wound healing in the oral cavity. *Scand J Haematol* 1984;**33**(suppl 40):393-409.

100. IRISH PS, HASTY DL. Immunocytochemical localization of fibronectin in human cultures using a cell surface replica technique. *J Histochem Cytochem* 1983;**31**:69-77.

101. POSTLETHWAITE A, KESKI-OJA J, BALIAN G, et al. Induction of fibroblast chemotaxis by fibronectin. Localization of the chemotactic region to a 140,000 molecular weight non-gelatin-binding fragment. *J Exp Med* 1981;**153**:494-499.

102. MCDONALD JA, KELLEY DG, BROEKELMANN TJ. Role of fibronectin in collagen deposition: Fab' to the gelatin-binding domain of fibronectin inhibits both fibronectin and collage organization in fibroblast extracellular matrix. *J Cell Biol* 1982;**92**:485-492.

103. GRINNEL F, BILLINGHAM RE, BURGES L. Distribution of fibronectin during wound healing *in vivo. J Invest Dermatol* 1981;**76**:181-189.

104. HØLUND B, CLEMMENSEN I, JUNKER P, LYON H. Fibronectin in experimental granulation tissue. *Acta Pathol Microbiol Immunol Scand (A)* 1982;**90**:159-165.

105. DVORAK HF, FORM DM, MANSEAU EJ, SMITH BD. Pathogenesis of desmoplasia. I. Immunofluoreecence identification and localization of some structural proteins of line 1 and line 10 guinea pig tumors and of healing wounds. *J Natl Cancer Inst* 1984;**73**:1195-1205.

106. CARTER WG. The role of intermolecular disulfide bonding in deposition of GP140 in the extracellular matrix. *J Cell Biol* 1984;**99**:105-114.

107. BAUR JR. PS, PARKS DH. The myofibroblast anchoring strand: the fibronectin connection in wound healing and the possible loci of collagen fibril assembly. *J Trauma* 1983;**23**:853-862.

108. TAKASHIMA A, GRINNELL F. Human keratinocyte adhesion and phagocytosis promoted by fibroblast. *J Invest Dermatol* 1984;**83**:352-358.

109. TAKASHIMA A, GRINNELL F. Fibronectin-mediated keratinocyte migration and initiation of fibronectin receptor function in vitro. *J Invest Dermatol* 1985;**85**:304-308.

110. CLARK RAF, FOLKVORD JM, WERTZ RL. Fibronectin as well as other extracellular matrix proteins, mediate human keratinocyte adherance. *J Invest Dermatol* 1985;**84**:378-383.

111. O'KEEFE EJ, PAYNE RE, JR, RUSSELL N, WOODLEY DT. Spreading and enhanced motility of human keratinocytes on fibronectin. *J Invest Dermatol* 1985;**85**:125-130.

112. FERNYHOUGH W, PAGE RC. Attachment, growth and synthesis by human gingival fibroblasts on demineralized or fibronectin-treated normal and diseased tooth roots. *J Periodontol* 1983;**54**:133-140.

113. NASJLETI C, CAFFESSE RG. Effect of fibronectin on healing of replanted teeth in monkeys: a histological and autoradiographic study. *Oral Surg Oral Med Oral Pathol* 1987;**63**:291-299.

114. CAFFESSE RG, HOLDEN MJ, KON S, et al. The effect of citric acid and fibronectin application on healing following surgical treatment of naturally occurring periodontal disease in beagle dogs. *J Clin Periodont* 1985;**12**:578-590.

115. RYAN PC, WARING GJ, SEYMOUR GJ. Periodontal healing with citric acid and fibronectin treatment in cats. *Aust Dent J* 1987;**32**:99-103.

116. THOMPSON EW, SEYMOUR GJ, WHYTE GJ. The preparation of autologous fibronectin for use in periodontal surgery. *Aust Dent J* 1987;**32**:34-38.

117. FERNANDEZ HN, HENSON PM, OTANI A, HUGLI TE. Chemotactic response to human C3a and C5a anaphylatoxins. I. Evaluation of C3a and C5a leukotaxis *in vitro* and under stimulated *in vivo* conditions. *J Immunol* 1978;**120**:109-115.

118. FERNANDEZ HN, HUGLI TE. Primary structural analysis of the polypeptide portion of human C5a anaphylatoxin. *J Biol Chem* 1978;**253**:6955-6964.

119. FOLKMAN J, KLAGSBRUN M. Angiogenesic factors. *Science* 1987;**235**:442-447.

120. WEITZHANDLER M, BERNFIELD MR. Proteoglycan glycoconjungates. In: COHEN K, DIEGELMANN RF, LINDBLAD WJ, eds. *Wound healing: biochemical and clinical aspects.* Philadelphia: WB Saunders Company, 1992:195-208.

121. STERN MG, LONGAKER MT, STERN R. Hyaluronic acid and its modulation in fetal and adult wounds. In: ADZICK NS, LONGAKER MT, eds. *Fetal wound healing.* New York: Elsevier, 1992:189-198.

122. COUCHMAN JR, HÖÖK M. Proteoglycans and wound repair. In: CLARK RAF, HENSON PM, eds. *The molecular and cellular biology of wound repair.* New York: Plenum Press, 1988:437-470.

123. LATERRA J, ANSBACHER R, CULP LA. Glycosaminoglycans that bind cold-insoluble globulin in cell-substratum adhesion sites of murine fibroblasts. *Proc Natl Acad Sci USA* 1980;**77**:6662-6666.

124. TOOLE BP, GROSS J. The extracellular matrix of the regenerating newt limb: synthesis and removal of hyaluronate prior to differentiation. *Dev Biol* 1971;**25**:57-77.

125. ALEXANDER SA, DONOFF RB. The glycosaminoglycans of open wounds. *J Surg Res* 1980;**29**:422-429.

126. GRIMES NL. The role of hyaluronate and hyaluronidase in cell migration during the rabbit ear regenerative healing response. *Anat Rec* 1981;**199**:100.

127. AZIZKHAN RG, AZIZKHAN JC, ZETTER BR, FOLKMAN J. Mast cell heparin stimulates migration of capillary endothelial cells *in vitro. J Exp Med* 1980;**152**:931-944.

128. ROSS R, GLOMSET JA. The pathogenesis of atherosclerosis. *N Engl J Med* 1976;**295**:369-377.

129. CLEMENTI F, PALADE GE. Intestinal capillaries. II. Structural effects of EDTA and histamine. *J Cell Biol* 1969;**42**:706-714.

130. MAJNO G, GILMORE V, LEVENTHAL M. On the mechanism of vascular leakage caused by histamine-type mediators. *Circ Res* 1967;**21**:833-847

131. KAHLSON G, NILSSON K, ROSENGREN E, ZEDERFELDT B. Histamine: Wound healing as dependent on rate of histamine formation. *Lancet* 1960;**2**:230-234.

132. MAJNO G, PALADE GE. Studies on inflammation. I. The effect of histamine and serotonin on vascular permeability: An electron microscopic study. *J Biol Phys Biochem Cytol* 1961;**11**:571-605.

133. MAJNO G, SCHOEFL GI, PALADE G. Studies on inflammation. II. The site of action of histamine and serotonine on the vascular tree: A topographic study. *J Biophys Biochem Cytol* 1961;**11**:607-626.

134. MAJNO G, SHEA SM, LEVENTHAL M. Endothelial contraction induced by histamine-type mediators. An electron microscopic study. *J Cell Biol* 1969;**42**:647-672.

135. PARRAT JR, WEST GB. Release of 5-hydroxytryptamine and histamine from tissues of the rat. *J Physiol* 1957;**137**:179.

CHAPTER 1

136. ROBSON MC, HEGGERS JP. Eicosanoids, cytokines, and free radicals. In: COHEN IK, DIEGELMANN RF, LINDBLAD WJ, eds. *Wound healing: biochemical and clinical aspects.* Philadelphia: WB Saunders, 1992:292-304.

137. HEGGERS JP, ROBSON MC. Eicosanoids in wound healing. In: WATKINS WD, ed. *Prostaglandins in clinical practice.* New York: Raven Press, 1989:183-194.

138. PENNEY NS. Prostaglandins in skin. In: KALAMAZOO: *Current Concept/ Scope Publication* Upjohn, 1980.

139. FRANK MM. *Complement.* KALAMAZOO In: *Current Concept/Scope Publication* Upjohn, 1975.

140. LYNCH SE. Interactions of growth factors in tissue repair. In: BARBUL A, CALDWELL MD, EAGLESTEIN WH, et al, eds. *Clinical and experimental approaches to dermal and epidermal repair. Normal and chronical wounds.* New York: Wiley-Liss, 1991:341-357.

141. DAVIDSON JM, BROADLEY KN. The response of experimental wounds to endogenous and exogenous growth factors. In: JANSSEN H, ROOMAN R, ROBERTSON JIS, eds. *Wound healing.* Petersfield, England: Wrightson Biomedical Publishing, 1991:81-90.

142. FALANGA V. Growth factors: Status and expectations. In: LEAPER DJ, ed. *International symposium on wound management.* Bussum, The Netherlands: Medicom Europe, 1991: 87-94.

143. STEENFOS HH. *Growth factors and formation of granulation tissue.* Departments of Plastic Surgery and Physiology, University of Göteborg, 1992 Vasastadens Bokbinderi AB, Sweden.

144. ROSS R, VOGEL A. The platelet-derivied growth factor. *Cell* 1978;14:203-210.

145. ROSS R, GLOMSET JA, KARTYA B, HARKER L. A platelet-dependent serum factor that stimulates the proliferation of arterial smooth muscle cells *in vitro. Proc Natl Acad Sci USA* 1974;71:1207-1210.

146. ROSS R, RAINES EW, BOWEN-POPE DF. The biology of platelet-derived growth factor. *Cell* 1986;46:155-169.

147. WITTE LD, KAPLAN KL, NOSSEL HL, et al. Studies of the release from human platelets of the growth factor for cultured human arterial smooth muscle cells. *Circ Res* 1978;42: 402-409.

148. KAPLAN DR, CHAO FC, STILES CD, et al. Platelet-alpha granules contain a growth factor for fibroblasts. *Blood* 1979;53:1043-1052.

149. KAPLAN KL, BROEKMAN MJ, CHERNOFF A, et al. Platelet-alpha granule proteins: studies on release and subcellular localization. *Blood* 1979;53:604-616.

150. GROTENDORST GR, CHANG T, SEPPA HEJ, et al. Platelet-derived growth factor is a chemoattractant for vascular smooth muscle cells. *J Cell Physiol* 1982;113:261-266.

151. SENIOR RM, GRIFFIN GL, HUANG JS, WALZ DA, DEUEL TF. Chemotactic activity of platelet alpha granule proteins for fibroblasts. *J Cell Biol* 1983;96:382-385.

152. HUANG JS, OLSEN TJ, HUANG SS. The role of growth factors in tissue repair I.: Platelet-derived growth factor. In: CLARK RAF, HENSON PM, eds. *The molecular and cellular biology of wound repair.* New York: Plenum Press, 1988:243-251.

153. DEUEL TF, SENIOR RM, CHANG D, et al. Platelet factor 4 is chemotactic for neutrophils and monocytes. *Proc Natl Acad Sci USA* 1981;78:4584-4587.

154. DEUEL TF, SENIOR RM, HUANG JS, GRIFFIN GL. Chemotaxis of monocytes and neutrophils to platelet-derived growth factor. *J Clin Invest* 1982;69:1046-1049.

155. DEUEL TF, HUANG JS. Platelet-derived growth factor: Purification, properties, and biological activities. *Prog Haematol* 1983;13:201-221.

156. DEUEL TF, HUANG JS. Platelet-derived growth factor: Structure, function, and roles in normal and transformed cells. *J Clin Invest* 1984;74:669-676.

157. TZENG DY, DEUEL TF, HUANG JS, SENIOR RM, BOXER LA, BAEHNER RL. Platelet-derived growth factor promotes polymorphonuclear leukocyte activation. *Blood* 1984;64:1123-1128.

158. TZENG DY, DEUEL TF, HUANG JS, BAEHNER RL. Platelet-derived growth factor promotes human peripheral monocyte activation. *Blood* 1985;66:179-183.

159. STEENFOS HH, HUNT TK, SCHEUENSTUHL H, GOODSON WH. Selective effects of tumor necrosis factor-alpha on wound healing in rats. *Surgery* 1989;106:171-176.

160. STEENFOS HH, LOSSING C, HANSSON H-A. Immunohistochemical demonstration of endogeneous growth factors in wound healing. *Wounds* 1990;2:218-226.

161. PIERCE GF, MUSTOE TA, SENIOR RM, et al. In vivo incision wound healing augmented by platelet-derived growth factor and recombinant c-sis gene homodimeric proteins. *J Exp Med* 1988;167:974-987.

162. PIERCE GF, MUSTOE TA, LINGELBACH J, et al. Platelet-derived growth factor and transforming growth factor-beta enhance tissue repair activities by unique mechanisms. *J Cell Biol* 1989;109:429-440.

163. ASSOIAN RK. The role of growth factors in tissue repair IV.: Type beta-transforming growth factor and stimulation of fibrosis. In: CLARK RAF, HENSON PM, eds. *The molecular and cellular biology of wound repair.* New York: Plenum Press, 1988:273-280.

164. ASSOIAN RK, KOMORIYA A, MEYERS CA, MILLER DM, SPORN MB. Transforming growth factor-beta in human platelets: identification of a major storage site, purification, and characterization. *J Biol Chem* 1983;258:7155-7160.

165. ASSOIAN RK, SPORN MB. Type beta transforming factor in human pletelets: release during platelet degranulation and action on vascular smooth muscle cells. *J Cell Biol* 1986;102:1217-1223.

166. ASSOIAN RK, SPORN MB. Anchorage-independent growth of primary rat embryo cells is induced by platelet-derived growth factor and inhibited by type-beta transforming growth factor. *J Cell Physiol* 1986;126:312-318.

167. PIRCHER R, JULLIEN P, LAWRENCE DA. Beta-transforming growth factor is stored in human blood platelets as a latent high molecular weight complex. *Biochem Biophys Res Commun* 1986;136:30-37.

168. SPORN MB, ROBERTS AB, SHULL JH, et al. Polypeptide transforming growth factor beta isolated from bovine sources and used for wound healing *in vivo. Science* 1983; 219:1329-1331.

169. LAWRENCE WT, SPORN MB, GORSCHBOTH C, NORTON JA, GROTENDORST GR. The reversal of an adriamycin induced healing impairment with chemoattractants and growth factors. *Ann Surg* 1986;203:142-147.

170. ROBERTS AB, SPORN MB, ASSOIAN RK, et al. Transforming growth factor type beta: rapid induction of fibrosis and angiogenesis in vivo and stimulation of collagen formation in vivo. *Proc Natl Acad Sci USA* 1986;83:4167-4171.

171. OGAWA Y, SAWAMURA SJ, KSANDER GA, et al. Transforming growth factors-b1 and b2 induce synthesis and accumulation of hyaluronate and chondroitin sulfate in vivo. *Growth Factors* 1990;3:53-62.

172. MUSTOE TA, PIERCE GF, THOMASON A, et al. Accelerated healing of incisional wounds in rats induced by transforming growth factor-beta. *Science* 1987;237:1333-1336.

173. BROWN GL, CURTSINGER LJ, WHITE M, et al. Acceleration of tensile strength of incisions treated with EGF and TGF-β. *Ann Surg* 1988;208:788-794.

174. LYNCH SE, BUSER D, HERNANDEZ RA, et al. Effects of the platelet-derived growth factor/insulin-like growth factor-I combination on bone regeneration around titanium dental implants. Results of a pilot study in beagle dogs. *J Periodontol* 1991;62:710-716.

175. LYNCH SE, RUIZ DE CASTILLA G, WILLIAMS RC, et al. The effect of short-term application of platelet-derived and insulin-like growth factors on periodontal wound healing. *J Periodontol* 1991;**62**:458-467.

176. SHAH M, FOREMAN DM, FERGUSON MWJ. Control of scarring in adult wounds by neutralising antibody to transforming growth factor. *Lancet* 1992;**339**:213-214.

177. BANKS AR. The role of growth factors in tissue repair II: Epidermal growth factor. In: CLARK RAF, HENSON PM, eds. *The molecular and cellular biology of wound repair*. New York: Plenum Press, 1988:253-263.

178. CHO M, LEE YL, GARANT PR. Radioautographic demonstration of receptors for epidermal growth factor in various cells of the oral cavity. *Anat Rec* 1988;**222**:191-200.

179. GROVE RI, PRATT RM, Influence of epidermal growth factor and cyclic AMP on growth and differentiation of palatal epithelial cells in culture. *Dev Biol* 1984;**106**:427-437.

180. CANALIS E, RAISZ LG. Effect of epidermal growth factor on bone formation in vitro. *Endocrinology* 1979;**104**:862-869.

181. NAKAGAWA S, YOSHIDA S, HIRAO Y, et al. Biological effects of biosynthetic human EGF on the growth of mammalian cells in vitro. *Differentiation* 1985;**29**:284-288.

182. BLAY J, BROWN KD. Epidermal growth factor promotes the chemotactic migration of cultured rat intestinal cells. *J Cell Physiol* 1985;**124**:107-112.

183. CHUA CC, GEIMAN DE, KELLER GH, et al. Induction of collagenase secretion in human fibroblast cultures by growth promoting factors. *J Biol Chem* 1985;**260**:5213-5216.

184. STEIDLER NE, READE PC. Epidermal growth factor and proliferation of odontogenic cells in culture. *J Dent Res* 1981;**60**:1977-1982.

185. COHEN S. Isolation of a mouse submaxillary gland protein accelerating incisor eruption and eyelid opening on newborn animal. *J Biol Chem* 1962;**237**:1555-1562.

186. FRANKLIN JD, LYNCH JB. Effects of topical applications of epidermal growth factor on wound healing: experimental study on rabbit ears. *Plast Reconst Surg* 1979;**64**:766-770.

187. BROWN GL, CURTSINGER L, BRIGHTWELL JR, et al. Enhancement of epidermal regeneration by biosynthetic epidermal growth factor. *J Exp Med* 1986;**163**:1319-1324.

188. BROWN GL, NANNEY LB, GRIFFEN L, et al. Enhancement of wound healing by topical treatment with epidermal growth factor. *N Engl J Med* 1989;**321**:76-79.

189. NIALL M, RYAN GB, O'BRIEN BM. The effect of epidermal growth factor on wound healing in mice. *J Surg Res* 1982;**33**:164-169.

190. GREAVES MW. Lack of effect of topically applied epidermal growth factor (EGF) on epidermal growth in man *in vivo*. *Clin Exp Dermatol* 1980;**5**:101-103.

191. VOLKER JF. The effect of saliva on blood coagulation. *Am J Orthodont* 1939;**25**:277-281.

192. HUTSON J, NIALL M, EVANS D, FOWLER R. The effect of salivary glands on wound contraction in mice. *Nature (London)* 1979;**279**:793-795.

193. BODNER L, KNYSZYNSKI A, ADLER-KUNIN S, DANON D. The effect of selective desalivation on wound healing in mice. *Exp Gerontol* 1991;**26**:357-363.

194. LI AK, KOROLY MJ, SCHATTENKERK ME, MALT RA, YOUNG M. Nerve growth factor: Acceleration of the rate of wound healing in mice. *Proc Natl Acad Sci USA* 1980;**77**:4379-4381.

195. BYYNY RL, ORTH DN, DOYNE ES. Epidermal growth factor: effects of androgens and adrenergic agents. *Endocrinology* 1974;**95**:776-782.

196. NOGUCHI S, OHBA Y, OKA T. Effect of epidermal growth factor on wound healing of tongue in mice. *Am J Physiol* 1991;**260**:E620-5.

197. YEH YC, GUH JY, YEH J, YEH HW. Transforming growth factor type alpha in normal human adult saliva. *Mol Cell Endocrinol* 1989;**67**:247-254.

198. FOX GM. The role of growth factors in tissue repair III. Fibroblast growth factor. In: CLARK RAF, HENSON PM, eds. *The molecular and cellular biology of wound repair*. New York: Plenum Press, 1988:265-271.

199. KNIGHTON DR, PHILLIPS GD, FIEGEL VD. Wound healing angiogenesis: indirect stimulation by basic fibroblast growth factor. *J Trauma* 1990;**30**(suppl 12):134-144.

200. GOSPODAROWICZ D, BIALECKI H. The effect of epidermal and fibroblast growth factors on the replicative lifespan of cultured bovine granulosa cells. *Endocrinology* 1978;**103**:854-858.

201. BAIRD A, GONZALEZ AM, BUSCAGLIA M, LAPPI DA. *Growth factors in health and disease: basic and clinical aspects*. Amsterdam: Exerpta Medica, 1990.

202. TWEDEN KS, SPADONE DP, TERRANOVA VP. Neovascularisation of surface demineralized dentin. *J Periodontol* 1989;**60**:460-466.

203. FOURTANIER A, COURTY J, MULLER E, et al. Eye-derived growth factor isolated from bovine retina and used for epidermal wound healing in vivo. *J Invest Dermatol* 1986;**87**:76-80.

204. VLODASKY I, FOLKMAN J, SULLIVAN R, et al. Endothelial cell-derived basic fibroblast growth factor synthesis and deposition into subendothelial extracellular matrix. *Proc Natl Acad Sci USA* 1987;**84**:2292-2296.

205. OOSTA GM, FAVREAU LV, BEELER DL, et al. Purification and properties of human platelet heparitinase. *J Biol Chem* 1982;**257**:11248-11255.

206. BUNTROCK P, JENTZSCH KD, HEDER G. Stimulation of wound healing, using brain extract with fibroblast growth (FGF) activity.I. Quantitative and biochemical studies into formation of granulation tissue. *Exp Pathol* 1982;**21**:46-53.

207. BROADLEY KN, AQUINO AM, WOODWARD SC, et al. Monospecific antibodies implicate basic fibroblast growth factor in normal wound repair. *Lab Invest* 1989;**61**:571-575.

208. SPRUGEL KH, McPHERSON JM, CLOWES AW, ROSS R. Effects of growth factors in vivo: cell ingrowth into porous subcutaneous chambers. *Am J Pathol* 1987;**129**:601-613.

209. McGEE G, DAVIDSON JM, BUCKLEY A, et al. Recombinant fibroblast growth factor accelerates wound healing. *J Surg Res* 1988;**45**:145-153.

210. TERRANOVA VP, ODZIEMIEC C, TWEDEN KS, SPADONE DP. Repopulation of dentin surfaces by periodontal ligament cells and endothelial cells: effect of basic fibroblast growth factor. *J Periodontol* 1989;**60**:293-301.

211. TERRANOVA VP, WIKESJÖ UME. Extracellular matrices and polypeptide growth factors as mediators of functions of cells of the periodotium. A review. *J Periodont* 1987;**58**:371-380.

212. HUMBEL RE. Insulin-like growth factors I and II. *Eur J Biochem* 1990;**190**:445-462.

213. JENNINGS RW, HUNT TK. Overview of postnatal wound healing. In: ADZICK NS, LONGAKER MT, eds. *Fetal wound healing*. New York: Elsevier, 1992:25-52.

214. CLEMMONS DR. Structural and functional analysis of insulin-like growth factors. *Br Med Bull* 1989;**45**:465-480.

215. BLOM S, HOLMSTRUP P, DABELSTEEN E. The effect of insulin-like growth factor-I and human growth hormone on periodontal ligament fibroblast morphology, growth pattern, DNA synthesis, and receptor binding. *J Periodontol* 1992;**63**:960-968.

216. LYNCH SE, NIXON JC, COLVIN RB, ANTONIADES HN. Role of platelet-derived growth factor in wound healing: synergistic effects with other growth factors. *Proc Natl Acad Sci USA* 1987;**84**:7696-7700.

217. LYNCH SE, COLVIN RB, ANTONIADES HN. Growth factors in wound healing: single and synergistic effects on partial thickness porcine skin wounds. *J Clin Invest* 1989;**84**:640-646.

218. LYNCH SE, COLVIN RB, KIRISTY CP, ANTONIADES HN. Comparative effects of growth factors on soft tissue repair. *J Dent Res* 1989;**68**(Spec. Issue):326(Abstr. 1153).

219. COLVIN RB, ANTONAIDES HN. Role of platelet-derived growth factor in wound healing: synergistic effects with other growth factors. *Proc Natl Acad Sci USA* 1987;**84**:7696-7700.

220. STILES CD, CAPONE GT, SCHER CD, et al. Dual control of cell growth by somatomedin and platelet derived growth factor. *Proc Natl Acad Sci USA* 1979;**76**:1279-1283.

221. LOBIE PE, BREIPOHL W, LINCOLN DT, GARCIA - ARAGON J, WATERS MJ. Localization of the growth hormone receptor binding protein in skin. *J Endocrinol* 1990;**126**:467-472.

222. ZAIZEN Y, FORD EG, COSTIN G, ATKINSON JB. The effect of perioperative exogeneous growth hormone on wound bursting strength in normal and malnourished rats. *J Pediatr Surg* 1990;**25**:70-74.

223. ZAIZEN Y, FORD EG, COSTIN G, ATKINSON JB. Stimulation of wound bursting strength during protein malnutrition. *J Surg Res* 1990;**49**:333-336.

224. STEENFOS HH, JANSSON J-O. Growth hormone stimulates granulation tissue formation and insulin-like growth factor-I gene expression in wound chambers in the rat. *J Endocrinol* 1992;**132**:293-298.

225. LYNCH SE, WILLIAMS RC, POLSON RC, HOWELL TH, REDDY MS, ZAPA UE, ANTONAIDES HN. A Combination of platelet-derived and insulin-like growth factors enhances peridontal regeneration. *J Clin Periodontal* 1989;**16**:545-548.

226. RUTHERFORD RB, NIEKRASH CE, KENNEDY JE, CHARETTE MF. Platelet-derived and insuline-like growth factors stimulate regeneration of periodontal attachment in monkeys. *J Periodont Res* 1992;**27**:285-290.

227. CANALIS E, McCARTHY TL, CENTRELLA M. Effects of platelet-derived growth factor on bone formation in vitro. *J Cell Physiol* 1989;**140**:530-537.

228. PICHE JE, CARNES JR. DL, GRAVES DT. Initial characterization of cells derived from human periodontia. *J Dent Res* 1989;**68**:761-767.

229. HARKER LA, FINCH CA. Thrombokinetics in man. *J Clin Invest* 1969;**48**:963-974.

230. TERKELTAUB RA, GINSBERG MH. Platelets and response to injury. In: CLARK RAF, HENSON PM, eds. *The molecular and cellular biology of wound repair.* New York: Plenum Press, 1988:35-55.

231. MARR J, BARBORIAC JJ, JOHNSON SA. Relationship of appearance of adenosine diphosphate, fibrin formation, and platelet aggregation in the haemostatic plug *in vivo. Nature(London);***205**:259-262.

232. KNIGHTON DR, HUNT TK, SCHEUENSTUHL H, HALLIDAY BJ, WERB Z, BANDA MJ. Oxygen tension regulates the expression of angiogenesis factor by macrophages. *Science* 1983;**221**:1283-1285.

233. KNIGHTON DR, SILVER IA, HUNT TK. Regulation of wound healing angiogenesis: effect of oxygen gradients and inspired oxygen concentrations. *Surgery* 1981;**90**:262-270.

234. KNIGHTON DR, OREDSSON S, BANDA M, HUNT TK. Regulation of repair: hypoxic control of macrophage mediated angiogenesis. In: HUNT TK, HEPPENSTALL RB, PINES E, ROVEE D, eds. *Soft and hard tissue repair.* New York: Praeger, 1984:41-49.

235. HITI-HARPER J, WOHL H, HARPER E. Platelet factor 4: an inhibitor of collagenase. *Science* 1987;**199**:991-992.

236. ZAWICKI DF, JAIN RK, SCHMID - SHOENBEIN GW, CHIEN S. Dynamics of neovascularization in normal tissue. *Microvasc Res* 1981;**21**:27-47.

237. DAVIS JH, YULL AB. A toxic factor in abdominal injury. II. The role of the red cell component. *J Trauma* 1964;**4**:84-90.

238. KRIZEK TJ, DAVIS JH. The role of the red cell in subcutaneous infection. *J Trauma* 1965;**5**:85-95.

239. PRUETT TL, ROTSTEIN OD, FIEGEL VD, et al. Mechanism of the adjuvant effect of hemoglobin in experimental peritonitis. VIII. A leukotoxin is produced by *escherichia coli* metabolism in hemoglobin. *Surgery* 1984;**96**:375-383.

240. EDLICH RF, RODEHEAVER GT, THACKER JG. Surgical devices in wound healing management. In: COHEN IK, DIEGELMANN RF, LINDBLAD WJ, eds. *Wound healing: biochemical and clinical aspects.* Philadelphia: WB Saunders, 1992:581-600.

241. ANGEL MF, NARAYANAN K, SWARTZ WM, et al. The etiologic role of free radicals in hematoma-induced flap necrosis. *Plast Reconstr Surg* 1986;**77**:795-801.

242. YURT RW. Role of mast cells in trauma. In: DINEEN P, HILDRICK-SMITH G, eds. *The surgical wound.* Philadelphia: Lea & Febiger, 1981:37-62.

243. ZACHRISSON BU. *Histochemical studies on the mast cell of the human gingiva in health and inflammation.* Oslo: Universitetsforlaget,1968:135.

244. CLARK RAF. Cutaneous tissue repair: Basic biologic considerations. *J Am Acad Dermatol* 1985;**13**:701-725.

245. HEROUX O. Mast cells in the skin of the ear of the rat exposed to cold. *Can J Biochem and Physiol* 1961;**39**:1871-1878.

246. SIMPSON DM, ROSS R. Effects of heterologous antineutrophil serum in guinea pigs: hematologic and ultrastructural observations. *Am J Pathol* 1971;**65**:79-96.

247. SIMPSON DM, ROSS R. The neutrophilic leukocyte in wound repair: a study with antineutrophil serum. *J Clin Invest* 1972;**51**:2009-2023.

248. BERGENHOLTZ G, WARFVINGE J. Migration of leucocytes in dental pulp in response to plaque bacteria. *Scand J Dent Res* 1982;**90**:354-362.

249. SAGLIE R, NEWMAN MG, CARRANZA JR FA. A scanning electron microscopic study of leukocytes and their interaction with bacteria in human periodontitis. *J Periodont* 1982;**53**:752-761.

250. WILKINSON PC. *Chemotaxis and inflammation,* 2nd edn. New York: Churchill Livingstone, 1982.

251. SHAW JO. Leukocytes in chemotactic-fragment-induced lung inflammation. *Am J Pathol* 1980;**101**:283-291.

252. JANOFF A, SCHAEFER S, SHERER J, et al. Mediators in inflammation in leucocyte lysozymes. II Mechanisms of action of lysosomal cationic protein upon vascular permeability in the rat. *J Exp Med* 1965;**122**:841-851.

253. TEPLITZ C. The pathology and ultrastructure of cellular injury and inflammation in the progression and outcome of trauma, sepsis, and shock. In: CLOWES JR GHA, ed. *Trauma, sepsis, and shock: the physiological basis of therapy.* New York: Marcek Dekker Inc, 1988.

254. MARCHESI VT. Some electron microscopic observations on interactions between leucocytes, platelets,and endothelial cells in acute inflammation. *Ann NY Acad Sci* 1964;**116**: 774-788.

255. JOHNSTON DE. Wound healing in skin. *Vet Clin North Am* 1990;**20**:1-25.

256. LINDHE J, BRÅNEMARK P-I. Observations on vascular proliferation in a granulation tissue. *J Periodont Res* 1970;**5**:276-292.

257. TONNESEN MG, WORTHEN GS, JOHNSTON JR. RB. Neutrophil emigration, activation, and tissue damage.In: CLARK RAF, HENSON PM, eds. *The molecular and cellular biology of wound repair.* New York: Plenum Press,1988:149-183.

258. BEASLEY JD, GROSS A, CUTRIGHT DE. Comparison of histological stained sections with culturing techniques in the evaluation of contaminated wounds. *J Dent Res* 1972;**51**:1624-1631.

259. THOMAS EL. Myeloperoxidase, hydrogen peroxide, chloride antimicrobial system: Nitrogen-chlorine derivatives of bactericidal action against *Escherichia coli. Infect Immun* 1979;**23**:522-531.

260. RAUSCHENBERGER CR, TURNER DW, KAMINSKI EJ, OSETEK EM. Human polymorphonuclear granule components: relative level detected by a modified enzyme-linked immunosorbent assay in normal and inflamed dental pulps. *J Endodont* 1991;**17**:531-536.

261. HÖGSTRÖM H, HAGLUND K. Neutropenia prevents decrease in strength of rat intestinal anastomoses: partial effect of oxygen free radicals scavengers and allopurinol. *Surgery* 1986;**99**:716-720.

262. STEIN JM, LEVENSON SM. Effect of the inflammatory reaction on subsequent wound healing. *Surg Forum* 1966;**17**:484-485.

263. GROTENDORST GR, SMALE G, PENCEV D. Production of transforming growth factor beta by human peripheral blood monocytes and neutrophils. *J Cell Physiol* 1989;**140**:396-402.

264. LEIBOVICH SJ, ROSS R. The role of the macrophages in wound repair. A study with hydrocortisone and antimacrophage serum. *Am J Pathol* 1975;**78**:71-100.

265. STEWARD RJ, DULEY JA, DEWDNEY J, ALLARDYCE RA, BEARD MEJ, FIZGERALD PH. The wound fibroblast and macrophage. II. Their origin studied in a human after bone marrow transplantation. *Br J Surg* 1981;**68**:129-131.

266. VAN FURTH R, COHEN ZA. The origin and kinetics of mononuclear phagocytes. *J Exp Med* 1968;**128**:415-435.

267. VAN FURTH R, DIESSELHOFF - DEN DULK MMC, MATTIE H. Quantitative study on the production and kinetics of mononuclear phagocytes during an acute inflammatory reaction. *J Exp Med* 1973;**138**:1314-1330.

268. VAN FURTH R, NIBBERIN PH, DISSEL VAN JT, DIESSELHOFF-DEN DULK MMC. The characterization, origin and kinetics of skin machrophages during inflammation. *J Invest Dermatol* 1985;**85**:398-402.

269. RICHES DWH. The multiple roles of macrophages in wound repair. In: CLARK RAF, HENSON PM, eds. *Muscular and cellular biology of wound repair*. New York: Plenum Press, 1988:213-239.

270. COHN ZA. The activation of mononuclear phagocytes: fact, fancy, and future. *J Immunol* 1978;**121**:813-816.

271. VAN FURTH R. Current view of the mononuclear phagocyte system. *Immunbiol* 1982;**161**:178-185.

272. WERB Z. How the macrophage regulates its extracellular environment. *Am J Anat* 1983;**166**:237-256.

273. HOSEIN B, BIANCO C. Monocyte receptors for fibronectin characterized by a monoclonal antibody that interferes with receptor activity. *J Exp Med* 1985;**162**:157-170.

274. HOSEIN B, MOSESSEN MW, BIANCO C. Monocyte receptors for fibronectin. In: VAN FURTH R, ed. *Mononuclear phagocytes: characteristics, physiology, and function*. Dordrecht: Martinus Nijhoff, 1985:723-730.

275. BOUCEK RJ. Factors affecting wound healing. *Otolaryngol Clin North Amer* 1984;**17**:243-264.

276. LEIBOVICH S, ROSS R. A macrophage-dependent factor that stimulates the proliferation of fibroblasts in vitro. *Am J Pathol* 1976;**84**:501-514.

277. HUNT TK, KNIGHTON DR, THAKRAL KK, GOODSON WH, ANDREWS WS. Studies on inflammation and wound healing: angeniogenesis and collagen synthesis stimulated *in vivo* by resident and activated wound macrophages. *Surgery* 1984;**96**:48-54.

278. MILLER B, MILLER H, PATTERSON R, RYAN SJ. Retinal wound healing. Cellular activity at the vitreoretinal interface. *Arch Ophthalmol* 1986;**104**:281-285.

279. GLENN KC. ROSS R. Human monocyte-derived growth factor(s) for mesenchymal cells: activation of secretion by endotoxin and concanavalin A. *Cell* 1981;**25**:603-615.

280. MARTIN BM, GIMBRONE MA, UNANUE ER, COTRAN RS. Stimulation of nonlymphoid mesenchymal cell proliferation by a macrophage-derived growth factor. *J Immunol* 1981;**126**:1510-1515.

281. LEIBOVICH SJ. Production of macrophage-dependent fibroblast-stimulation activity(M-FSA) by murine macrophages. *Exp Cell Res* 1978;**113**:47-56.

282. GREENBERG GB, HUNT TK. The proliferative response in vitro of vascular endothelial and smooth muscle cells exposed to wound fluid and macrophages. *J Cell Physiol* 1978;**97**:353-360.

283. THAKRAL KK, GOODSON WH, HUNT TK. Stimulation of wound blood vessel growth by wound macrophages. *J Surg Res* 1979;**26**:430-436.

284. POLVERINI PJ, COTRAN RS, GIMBRONE MA, UNANUE ER. Activated macrophages induce vascular proliferation. *Nature (London)* 1977;**269**:804-806.

285. POLVIRINI PJ, LEIBOVICH SJ. Induction of neovascularization in vivo and endothelial proliferation in vitro by tumor associated macrophages. *Lab Invest* 1984;**51**:635-642.

286. HUNT TK, ANDREWS WS, HALLIDAY B, et al. Coagulation and macrophage stimulation of angiogenesis and wound healing. In: DINEEN P, HILDICK-SMITH G, eds. *The surgical wound*. Philadelphia: Lea & Febiger, 1981:1-18.

287. JENSEN JA, HUNT TK, SCHEUENSTUHL H, BANDA MJ. Effect of lactate, pyruvate and pH on secretion of angiogenesis and mitogenesis factors by macrophages. *Lab Invest* 1986;**54**:574-578.

288. PETERSON JM, BARBUL A, BRESLIN RJ, et al. Significance of T lymphocytes in wound healing. *Surgery* 1987;**102**:300-305.

289. BRESLIN RJ, BARBUL A, WOODYARD JP, et al. T-lymphocytes are required for wound healing. *Surg Forum* 1989;**40**:634-636.

290. BARBUL A, BRESLIN RJ, WOODYARD JP, et al. The effect of *in vivo* T helper and T suppressor lymphocyte depletion on wound healing. *Ann Surg* 1989;**209**:479-483.

291. FISHEL RS, BARBUL A, BESCHORNER WE, et al. Lymphocyte participation in wound healing. Morphological assesment using monoclonal antibodies. *Ann Surg* 1987;**206**:25-29.

292. BARBUL A. Role of immune system. In: COHEN IK, DIEGELMANN RF, LINDBLAD WJ, eds. *Wound healing: biochemical and clinical aspects*. Philadelphia: WB Saunders, 1992:282-291.

293. REGAN MC, BARBUL A, Regulation of wound healing by the T cell-dependent immune system. In: JANSSEN H, ROOMAN R, ROBERTSON JIS, eds. *Wound healing*. Petersfield, England: Wrightson Biomedical Publishing, 1991:21-31.

294. GABBIANI G, RUNGGER - BRÄNDLE E. The fibroblast. In: GLYNN LE, ed. *Handbook of inflammation: Tissue repair and regeneration*. Amsterdam: Elsevier/ North Holland Biomedical Press, 1981:1-50.

295. ROSS R. The fibroblasts and wound repair. *Biol Rev* 1968;**43**:51-96.

296. MCDONALD RA. Origin of fibroblasts in experimental healing wounds: autoradiographic studies using tritiated thymidine. *Surgery* 1959;**46**:376-382.

297. GRILLO HC. Origin of fibroblasts in wound healing: an autoradiographic study of inhibition of cellular proliferation by local X-irradiation. *Ann Surg* 1963;**157**:453-467.

298. GLÜCKSMANN A. Cell turnover in the dermis. In: MONTAGNA W, BILLINGHAM RE, eds. *Advances in biology of skin*. Wound healing (vol 5). Oxford: Pergamon Press, 1964: 76-94.

299. ROSS R, LILLYWHITE JW. The fate of buffy coat cells grown in subcutaneously implanted diffusion chambers. A light and electron microscopic study. *Lab Invest* 1965;**14**:1568-1585.

300. SPECTOR WG. Inflammation. In: DUNPHY JE, VAN WINKLE HW, eds. *Repair and regeneration*. New York: McGraw-Hill Book Company, 1969:3-12.

301. ROSS R, EVERETT NB, TYLER R. Wound healing and collagen formation. VI. The origin of the wound fibroblast studied in parabiosis. *J Cell Biol* 1970;**44**:645-654.

302. HUNT TK. Disorders of repair and their management. In: HUNT TK, DUNPHY JE, eds. *Fundamentals of wound management*. New York: Appelton-Century-Crofts, 1979:68-118.

303. SHIPLEY GD, TUCKER RF, MOSES HL. Type beta-transforming growth factor/growth inhibitor stimulate entry of monolayer culture of AKR-2B cells into S phase after prolonged prereplicative interval. *Proc Natl Acad Sci USA* 1985;**82**:4147-4151

304. PLEDGER WJ, HART CA, LOCATELL KL, et al. Platelet-derived growth factor-modulated proteins: constitutive synthesis by a transformed cell line. *Proc Natl Acad Sci USA* 1981;**78**:4358-4362.

CHAPTER 1

305. LIN SL, KIKUSKI T, PLEDGER WJ, et al. Interferon inhibits the establishment of competence in G0/S phase transition. *Science* 1986;**233**:356-359.

306. SPORN MB, ROBERTS AB, WAKEFIELD LM, DE CROMBRUGGHE B. Some recent advances in the chemistry and biology of transforming growth factor-beta. *J Cell Biol* 1987;**105**:1039-1045.

307. WELCH MP, ODLAND GF, CLARK RAF. Temporal relationships of f-actin bundle formation, fibronectin and collagen assembly, fibronectin receptor expression to wound concentration. *J Cell Biol* 1990;**110**:133-145.

308. SCARPELLI DG, KNOUFF RA, ANGERER CA. Cortisone on oxygen consumption of granulation tissue from the rabbit. *Proc Soc Exp Biol* (N.Y.) 1953;**84**:94-96.

309. HUNT TK, ZEDERFELDT B. Nutritional and environmental aspects of wound healing. In: DUNPHY JE, van WINKLE HW, eds. *Repair and regeneration.* New York: McGraw-Hill Book Company, 1969:217-228.

310. HUNT TK, PAI MP. Effect of varying ambient oxygen tension on wound metabolism and collagen synthesis. *Surg Gynecol Obstet* 1972;**135**:561-567.

311. HUNT TK. Disorders of repair and their management. In: HUNT TK, DUNPHY JE, eds. *Fundamentals of wound management in surgery.* New York: Appelton-Century-Crofts, 1979:68-169.

312. NIINIKOSKI J, PENTTINEN R, KULONEN E. Effects of oxygen supply on the tensile strength healing wound and of granulation tissue. *Acta Physiol Scand* (Suppl) 1966;**277**:146.

313. LEVENSON S, SEIFTER E, van WINKLE E JR. Nutrition. In: HUNT TK, DUNPHY JE, eds. *Fundamentals of wound Management.* New York: Appelton-Century-Crofts, 1979:286-363.

314. DOUGLAS NJ, TWOMEY P, HUNT TK, DUNPHY JE. Effects of exposure to 94% oxygen on the metabolism of wounds. *Bull Soc Int Chir* 1973;**32**:178-185.

315. NIINIKOSKI J. Effect of oxygen supply on wound healing and formation of experimental granulation tissue. *Acta Physiol Scand* 1969 (Suppl 78);**334**:1-72.

316. POSTLETHWAITE AE, SEYER JM, KANG AH. Chemotactic attraction of human fibroblasts to type I, II and III collagens and collagen-derived peptides. *Proc Natl Acad Sci USA* 1978;**75**:871-875.

317. CHIANG TM, POSTLETHWAITE AE, BEACHEY EH, et al. Binding of chemotactic collagen-derived peptides to fibroblasts: the relationship to fibroblast chemotaxis. *J Clin Invest* 1978;**62**:916.

318. GABBIANI G, HIRSCHEL BJ, RYAN GB, et al. Granulation tissue as a contractile organ. A study of structure and function. *J Exp Med* 1972;**135**:719-734.

319. RUDOLPH R, GRUBER S, SUZUKI M, et al. The life cycle of the myofibroblast. *Surg Gynecol Obstet* 1977;**145**:389-394.

320. RUDOLPH R, BERG JV, EHRLICH HP. Wound contraction and scar contracture. In: COHEN IK, DIEGELMANN RF, LINDBLAD WJ, eds. *Wound healing: biochemical and clinical aspects.* Philadelphia: WB Saunders, 1992:96-114.

321. MANGO G, GABBIANI G, HIRSCHEL BJ, et al. Contraction of granulation tissue in vitro: similarity to smooth muscle. *Science* 1971;**173**:548-550.

322. ERHLICH HP. The modulation of contraction of fibroblast populated collagen lattices by type I, II and III collagen. *Tiss Cell* 1988;**20**:47-50.

323. BRÅNEMARK P-I. Capillary form and function. The microcirculation of granulation tissue. *Bibl Anat* 1965;**7**:9-28.

324. BRÅNEMARK P-I, BREINE U, JOSHI M, et al. Microvascular pathophysiology of burned tissue. *Ann NY Acad Sci* 1968;**150**:474-494.

325. AUSPRUNK DH, FOLKMAN J. Migration and proliferation of endothelial cells in performing and newly formed blood vessels during tumor angiogenesis. *Microvasc Res* 1977;**14**:53-63.

326. CLARK ER, CLARK EL. Observations on changes in blood vascular endothelium in the living animal. *Am J Anat* 1935;**57**:385-438.

327. CLARK ER, CLARK EL. Microscopic observations on the growth of blood capillaries in the living mammal. *Am J Anat* 1939;**64**:251-301.

328. HUNT TK, CONOLLY WB, ARONSON SB. Anaerobic metabolism and wound healing. An hypothesis for the initiation and cessation of collagen synthesis in wounds. *Am J Surg* 1978;**135**:328-332.

329. MADRI JA, PRATT BM. Angiogenesis. In: CLARK RAF, HENSON PM, eds. *The molecular and cellular biology of wound repair.* New York: Plenum Press, 1988:337-358.

330. WHALAN GF, ZETTER BR. Angiogenesis. In: COHEN IK, DIEGELMANN RF, LINDBLAD WJ, eds. *Wound healing: biochemical and clinical aspects.* Philadelphia: WB Saunders, 1992:77-95.

331. PHILLIPS GD, WHITHEAD RA, KNIGHTON DR. Initiation and pattern of angiogenesis in wound healing in rats. *Am J Anat* 1991;**192**:257-262.

332. SANDISON JC. Observations on the growth of blood vessels as seen in the transparent chamber introduced in the rabbits ear. *Am J Anat* 1928;**41**:475-496.

333. ALGIRE GH, LEGALLAIS FY. Recent developments in transparant-chamber technique as adapted to mouse. *J Natl Cancer Inst* 1949;**10**:225-253.

334. SANDERS AG, SHUBIK P. A transparent window for use in the Syrian hamster. *Israel J Exp Med* 1964;**11**:118a.

335. GOODALL CM, SANDERS AG, SHUBIK P. Studies of vascular patterns in living tumors with a transparent chamber inserted in a hamster cheek pouch. *J Natl Cancer Inst* 1965;**35**:497-521.

336. LANGHAM ME. Observations on the growth of blood vessels into the cornea. Application of a new experimental technique. *Br J Ophthalmol* 1953;**37**:210-222.

337. GIMBRONE MA, COTRAN RS, LEAPMAN SB, et al. Tumor growth and neovascularization: an experimental model using the rabbit cornea. *J Natl Cancer Inst* 1974;**52**:413-427.

338. AUERBACH R, KUBAI L, KNIGHTON D, et al. A simple procedure for the long term cultivation of chicken embryos. *Dev Biol* 1974;**41**:391-394.

339. ZETTER BR. Endothelial heterogeneity: influence of vessel size, organ location and species specifity on the properties of cultured endothelial cell. In: RYAN U, ed. *Endothelial cells.* Orlando FL: CRC Press, 1988:63-80.

340. MCGRATH MH, EMERY JM. The effect of inhibition of angiogenesis in granulation tissue on wound healing and the fibroblast. *Ann Plast Surg* 1985;**15**:105-122.

341. CLIFF WJ. Kinetics of wound healing in rabbit ear chambers: a time lapse cinemicroscopic study. *Quart J Exp Physiol Cog Med Sci* 1965;**50**:79-89.

342. ZAREM HA, ZWEIFACH BW, MCGEHEE JM. Development of microcirculation in full thickness autogeneous skin grafts in mice. *Am J Physiol* 1967;**212**:1081-1085.

343. TSUR H, DANNILER A, STRAUCH B. Neovascularization of the skin flap: route and timing. *Plast Reconstr Surg* 1980;**66**:85-93.

344. NAKAJIMA T. How soon do venous drainage channels develop at the periphery of a free flap? A study on rats. *Br J Plast Surg* 1978;**31**:300-308.

345. GATTI JE, LAROSSA D, BROUSSEAU DA, et al. Assessment of neovascularization and timing of flap division. *Plast Reconstr Surg* 1984;**73**:396-402.

346. GOTTRUP F, OREDSON S, PRICE DC, MATHES SJ, HOHN D. A comparative study of skin blood flow in musculocutaneous and random pattern flaps. *J Surg Res* 1984;**37**:443-447.

347. MIR Y, MIR L. Biology of the skin graft. *Plast Reconstr Surg* 1951;**8**:378-389.

348. HYNES W. The early circulation in skin grafts with a consideration of methods to encourage their survival. *Br J Plast Surg* 1954;**6**:257-263.

WOUND HEALING SUBSEQUENT TO INJURY

349. CONVERSE JM, BALLANTYNE DL, ROGERS BO, RAISBECK AP. "Plasmatic circulation" in skin grafts. *Transplant Bull* 1957;4:154.

350. CLEMMESEN T. The early circulation in split skin grafts. *Acta Chir Scand* 1962;124:11-18.

351. CLEMMESEN T. The early circulation in split-skin grafts. Restoration of blood supply to split-skin autografts. *Acta Chir Scand* 1964;127:1-8.

352. CLEMMESEN T. Experimental studies on the healing of free skin autografts. *Dan Med Bull* 1967;14(Suppl.2):1-74.

353. PSILLAKIS JM, DE JORGE FB, VILLARDO R, DE M ALBANO A, MARTINS M, SPINA V. Water and electrolyte changes in autogeneus skin grafts. Discussion of the so-called "Plasmatic circulation". *Plast Reconstr Surg* 1969;43:500-503.

354. TEICH-ALASIA S, MASERA N, MASSAIOLI N, MASSÉ C. The disulphine blue colouration in the study of humoral exchanges in skin grafts. *Br J Plast Surg* 1961;14:308-314.

355. SCOTHORNE RJ, MCGREGOR IA. The vascularisation of autografts and homografts of rabbit skin. *J Anat* 1953;87:379-386.

356. MARKMANN A. Autologous skin grafts in the rat: vital microscopic studies of the microcirculation. *Angiology* 1966;17:475-482.

357. OHMORI S, KURATA K. Experimental studies on the blood supply to various types of skin grafts in rabbit using isotope P^{32}. *Plast Reconstr Surg* 1960;25:547-555.

358. PIHL B, WEIBER A. Studies of the vascularization of free full-thickness skin grafts with radioisotope technique. *Acta Chir Scand* 1963;125:19-31.

359. HINSHAW JR, MILLER ER. Histology of healing split-thickness, full thickness autogenous skin grafts and donor site. *Arch Surg* 1965;91:658-670.

360. HENRY L, DAVID C, MARSHALL C, FRIEDMAN A, GOLDSTEIN DP, DAMMIN GJ. A histologic study of the human skin autograft. *Am J Pathol* 1961;39:317-332.

361. CONVERSE JM, RAPAPORT FT. The Vascularization of skin autografts and homografts. An experimental study in man. *Ann Surg* 1956;143:306-315.

362. CONVERSE JM, FILLER M, BALLANTYNE DL. Vascularization of split-thickness skin autografts in the rat. *Transplantation* 1965;3:22-27.

363. HALLER JA, BILLINGHAM RE. Studies of the origin of the vasculature in free skin grafts. *Ann Surg* 1967;166:896-901.

364. SMAHEL J, GANZONI N. Contribution to the origin of the vasculature in free skin autografts. *Br J Plast Surg* 1970;23:322-325.

365. CONVERSE JM, BALLANTYNE DL, ROGERS BO, RAISBECK AP. A study of viable and non-viable skin grafts transplanted to the chorio-allantoic membrane of the chick embryo. *Transplantation* 1958;5:108-120.

366. MERWIN RM, ALGIRE GH. The role of graft and host vessel in the vascularization of grafts of normal and neoplastic tissue. *J Natl Cancer Inst* 1956;17:23-33.

367. LAMBERT PM. Vascularization of skin grafts. *Nature* 1971;232:279-280.

368. SCHOEFL GT. Electron microscopic obsrvations on the reactions of blood vessels after injury. *Ann NY Acad Sci* 1964;116:789-802.

369. KNIGHTON DR, CIRESI KF, FIEGEL VD, et al. Classification and treatment of chronic non-healing wounds. Successful treatment with autologous platelet derived wound healing factors. *Ann Surg* 1986;104:322-330.

370. BAIRD A, LING N. Fibroblast growth factors are present in the extracellular matrix produced by endothelial cells in vitro: implications for a role of heparinase-like enzymes in the neovascular response. *Biochem Biophys Res Commun* 1987;142:428-435.

371. SHING Y, FOLKMANN J, SULLIVAN R, BUTTERFIELD C, MURRAY J, KLAGSBRUN M. Heparin affinity: purification of a tumor-derived capillary endothelial cell growth factor. *Science* 1984;223:1296-1299.

372. MIGNATTI P, TSUBOI R, ROBBINS E, RIFKIN DB. *In vitro* angiogenesis on the human amniotic membrane: requirement for basic fibroblast growth factor-induced proteinases. *J Cell Biol* 1989;108:671-682.

373. POLVERINI PJ, COTRAN RS, GIMBRONE MA, et al. Activated macrophages induce vascular proliferation. *Nature* 1977;269:804-806.

374. HOCKEL M, BECK T, WISSLER JH. Neomorphogenesis of blood vessels in rabbit skin produced by a highly purified monocyte-derived polypeptide (monocyto-angiotropin) and associated tissue reactions. *Intl J Tiss Reac* 1984;6:323-331.

375. MELTZER T, MEYERS B. The effect of hyperbaric oxygen on the bursting strength and rate of vascularization of skin wounds in the rat. *Am J Surg* 1986;52:659-662.

376. SILVER IA. The measurement of oxygen tension in healing tissue. *Prog Resp Res* 1969;3:124-135.

377. HUNT TK, CONOLLY WB, ARONSON SB, et al. Anaerobic metabolism and wound healing: An hypothesis for the initiation and cessation of collagen synthesis in wounds. *Am J Surg* 1978;135:328-332.

378. BANDA MJ, KNIGHTON DR, HUNT TK, et al. Isolation of a non-mitogenic angiogenesis factor from wound fluid. *Proc Natl Acad Sci USA* 1982;79:7773-7777.

379. HUNT TK, HALLIDAY B, KNIGHTON DR, et al. Impairment of microbicidal function in wounds: correction with oxygen. In: HUNT TK, HEPPENSTALL RB, PINES E, et al, eds. *Soft tissue repair*. Biological and clinical aspects. Surgical Science Series, vol 2. New York: Praeger,1984:455-468.

380. D'AMORE P, BRAUNHUT SJ. Stimulatory and inhibitory factors in vascular growth control. In: RYAN U, ed. *The endothelial cell*. Boca Raton FL: CRC Press, 1988:13-36.

381. ORLIDGE A, D'AMORE P. Inhibition of capillary-endothelial cell growth by pericytes and smooth muscle cells. *J Cell Biol* 1987;105:1455-1461.

382. HAY ED. *Cell biology of the extracellular matrix*. New York, Plenum Press: 1981.

383. DUNPHY JE, UDUPA KN. Chemical and histochemical sequences in the normal healing of wounds. *New Engl J Med* 1955;253:847-851.

384. PEACOCK EE. Some aspects of fibrinogenesis during the healing of primary and secondary wounds. *Surgery Gynec Obstet* 1962;115:408-414.

385. SANDBERG N, ZEDERFELDT B. The tensile strength of healing wounds and collagen formation in rats and rabbits. *Acta Chir Scand* 1963;126:187-196.

386. VILJANTO J. Biochemical basis of tensile strength in wound healing: an experimental study with viscose cellulose sponges on rats. *Acta Chir Scand* 1964 (Suppl 333).

387. MCPHERSON JM, PIEZ KA. Collagen in dermal wound repair. In: CLARK RAF, HENSON PM, eds. *The molecular and cellular biology of wound repair*. New York: Plenum Press, 1988:471-496.

388. PHILLIPS C, WENSTRUP RJ. Biosynthetic and genetic disorders of collagen. In: COHEN IK, DIEGELMANN RF, LINDBLAD WJ, eds. *Wound healing: biochemical and clinical aspects*. Philadelphia: WB Saunders, 1992:152-176.

389. MILLER EJ. Chemistry of collagens and their distribution. In: PIEZ KA, REDDI AH, eds. *Extracellular matrix biochemistry*. New York: Elsevier, 1984:41-78.

390. MARTIN GR, TIMPL R, MULLER PK, KUHN K. The genetically distinct collagens. *Trans Int Biol Soc* 1985;115:285-287.

391. MILLER EJ, GAY S. Collagen structure and function.In: COHEN IK, DIEGELMANN RF, LINDBLAD WJ, eds. *Wound healing: biochemical and clinical aspects*. Philadelphia: WB Saunders, 1992:130-151.

392. VIIDIK A, VUUST J, eds. *Biology of collagen*. London: Academic Press, 1980.

CHAPTER 1

393. Kang AH. Connective tissue: collagen and elastin. In: Kelley WN, Harris Jr ED, Ruddy S, Sledge CB, eds. *Textbook of rheumatology*. Philadelphia: W B Saunders,1981: 221-238.

394. Clore JN, Cohen IK, Diegelmann RF. Quantitation of collagen types I and III during wound healing in rat skin. *Proc Soc Exp Biol Med* 1979;**161**:337-340.

395. Andreasen JO. Histometric study of healing of periodontal tissues in rats after surgical injury. *Odont Rev* 1976;**27**:115-130.

396. Andreasen JO. Histometric study of healing of periodontal tissues in rats after surgical injury. *Odont Rev* 1976;**27**:131-144.

397. Kurkinen M, Vaheri A, Roberts PJ, et al. Sequential appearance of fibronectin and collagen in experimental granulation tissue. *Lab Invest* 1980;**43**:43-47.

398. Grinnell F, Billingham RE, Burgess L. Distribution of fibronectin during wound healing in vivo. *J Invest Dermatol* 1981;**76**:181.

399. Gay S, Viljanto J, Raekallio J, Pettinen R. Collagen types in early phase of wound healing in children. *Acta Chir Scand* 1978;**144**:205-211.

400. Fine JD. Antigenic features and structural correlates of basement membranes. *Arch Dermatol*. 1988;**124**:713.

401. Stenn KS, Madri JA, Roll JF. Migrating epidermis produces AB2 collagen and requires continued collagen synthesis for movement. *Nature(London)* 1979;**277**:229-232.

402. Stanley JR, Alvarez OM, Bere EW JR, et al. Detection of basement membrane zone antigens during epidermal wound healing in pigs. *J Invest Dermatol* 1981;**77**:240.

403. Odland G, Ross R. Human wound repair. I. Epidermal regeneration. *J Cell Biol* 1968;**39**:135-151.

404. Sakai LY, Keene DR, Morris NP, et al. Type VII collagen is a major structural component of anchoring fibrils. *J Cell Biol* 1986;**103**:2499-2509.

405. Bentz H, Morris NP, Murray LW, Sakai LY, Hollister DW, Burgeson RE. Isolation and partial characterization of a new human collagen with an extended triple-helical structural domain. *Proc Natl Acad Sci USA* 1983;**80**:3168-3172.

406. Gipson IK, Spurr-Michaud SJ, Tisdale SJ. Hemidesmosomes and anchoring fibril collagen appear synchronous during development and wound healing. *Develop Biol* 1988;**126**:253-262.

407. Ross R, Benditt EP. Wound healing and collagen formation.I. Sequental changes in components of guinea pig skin wounds observed in the electron microscope. *J Biophys Biochem Cytol* 1961;**11**:677-700.

408. Madden JW, Peacock EE. Studies on the biology of collagen during wound healing. I. Rate of collagen synthesis and deposition in cutaneous wounds of the rat. *Surgery* 1968;**64**:288-294.

409. Heughan C, Hunt T. Some aspects of wound healing research: a review. *Can J Surg* 1975;**18**:118-126.

410. Viidik A, Gottrup F. Mechanics of healing soft tissue wounds. In: Schmid-Schonbein GW, Woo SLY, Zweifach BW, eds. *Frontiers in biomechanics*. New York: Springer, 1986:263-279.

411. Fogdestam I. A biomechanical study of healing rat skin incisions after delayed primary closure. *Surg Gynecol Obstet* 1981;**153**:191-199.

412. Fogdestam I. *Delayed Primary Closure. An experimental study on the healing of skin incisions*. Doctoral Thesis University of Gothenburg, Sweden, 1980.

413. Stenn KS, Malhotra R. Epitheliazation. In: Cohen IK, Diegelmann RF, Lindblad WJ, eds. *Wound healing: biochemical and clinical aspects*. Philadelphia: WB Saunders, 1992:115-127.

414. Stenn KS, Depalma L. Re-epitheliazation. In: Clark RAF, Henson PM, eds. *The molecular and cellular biology of wound repair*. New York: Plenum Press, 1988:321-335.

415. Arey LB. Wound healing. *Physiol Rev* 1936;**16**:327-406.

416. Kuwabara T, Perkins DG, Cogan DG. Sliding of the epithelium in experimental corneal wounds. *Invest Ophthalmol* 1976;**15**:4-14.

417. Winter GD. Epidermal regeneration studied in the domestic pig. In: Maibach HI, Rovee DT, eds. *Epidermal wound healing*. Chicago: Year Book Med Publ. Inc, 1972:71-112.

418. Pang SC, Daniels WH, Buck RC. Epidermal migration during the healing of suction blisters in rat skin: a scanning and transmission electron microscopic study. *Am J Anat* 1978;**153**:177-191.

419. Gillman T, Penn J, Brooks D, et al. Reactions of healing wounds and granulation tissue in man to autothiersch, autodermal and homodermal grafts. *Br J Plast Surg* 1963;**6**:153-223.

420. Miller TA. The healing of partial thickness skin injuries. In: Hunt TK, ed. *Wound healing and wound infection*. New York: Appelton-Century-Crofts, 1980:81-96.

421. Andersen L, Fejerskov O. Ultrastructure of initial epithelial cell migration in palatel wounds of guinea pigs. *J Ultrastruc Res* 1974;**48**:313-324.

422. Gabbiani G, Ryan GB. Developments of contractile apparatus in epithelial cells during epidermal and liver regeneration. *J Submicr Cytol* 1974;**6**:143-157.

423. Mansbridge JN, Hanawalt PC. Role of transforming growth factor beta in maturation of human epidermal keratinocytes. *J Invest Dermatol* 1988;**90**:336-341.

424. Fejerskov O. Excision wounds in palatal epithelium in guinea pigs. *Scand J Dent Res* 1972;**80**:139-154.

425. Winter GD. Movement of epidermal cells over the wound surface. *Dev Bil Skin* 1964;**5**:113-127.

426. Jonkman MF. *Epidermal wound healing between moist and dry*. Thesis, Groningen 1990.

427. Clark RAF. Fibronectin matrix deposition and fibronectin receptor expression in healing and normal skin. *J Invest Dermatol* 1990;**94**:128-134S.

428. Clark RAF, Folkvord JM, Wertz RL. Fibronectin as well as other extracellular matrix proteins, mediates keratinocytes adherence. *J Invest Dermatol* 1985;**84**:378-383.

429. Horsburg CR, Clark RAF, Kirkpatrick CH. Lymphokines and platelets promote human monocytes adherence to fibrinogen and fibronectin in vitro. *J Leuk Biol* 1987;**4**:14-24.

430. Moses HL, Coffey RJ, Leof EB, et al. Transforming growth factor beta regulation of cell proleferation. *J Cell Physiol* 1987;(Suppl)**5**:1-7.

431. Pai MP, Hunt TK. Effect of varying ambient oxygen tensions on wound metabolism and collagen synthesis. *Surg Gynecol Obst* 1972;**135**:561-567.

432. Winter GD, Perrins JD. Effects of hyperbaric oxygen treatment on epidermal regeneration. In: Wada J, Iwa T, eds. *Proceedings of the fourth international congress on hyperbaric medicine*. Tokyo: Igaku Shoin, 1970:363-368.

433. McMillan MD. Oral changes following tooth extraction in normal and alloxan diabetic rats. Part II, microscopic observations. *N Z Dent J* 1971;**67**:23-31.

434. McMillan MD. Effects of histamine-releasing agent (compound 48-80) on extraction healing in rats. *N Z Dent J* 1973;**69**:101-108.

435. McMillan MD. *The healing tooth socket and normal oral mucosa of the rat*. PhD Thesis, University of Otago, 1978.

436. McMillan MD. Transmission and scanning electron microscope studies on the surface coat of oral mucosa in the rat. *J Periodont Res* 1980;**15**:288-296.

437. McMillan MD. Intracellular desmosome-like structures in differentiating wound epithelium of the healing tooth socket in the rat. *Arch Oral Biol* 1981;**26**:259-261.

438. Hunt TK, Hussain Z. Wound microenvironment. In: Cohen IK, Diegelmann RF, Lindblad WJ, eds. *Wound healing: biochemical and clinical aspects*. Philadelphia: WB Saunders, 1992:274-281.

439. BARBUL A, LAZAROU SA, EFRON DT, et al. Arginine enhances wound healing and lymphocyte immune responses in humans. *Surgery* 1990;**108**:331-337.

440. ALBINA JE, CALDWELL MD, HENRY WL, et al. Regulation of macrophage functions by L-arginine. *J Trauma* 1989;**29**:842-846.

441. HUNT TK, BANDA MJ, SILVER IA. Cell interactions in post-traumatic fibrosis. In: EVERED D, WELAND J, eds. *Fibrosis.* Ciba Foundation Symposium 114, London: Pitman, 1985:127-129.

442. HUNT TK, ZEDERFELDT B, GOLDSTICK TK. Oxygen and healing. *Am J Surg* 1969;**118**:521-525.

443. GREEN H, GOLDBERG B. Collagen and cell protein synthesis by an established mammalian fibroblast line. *Nature* 1964;**204**:347-349.

444. COMSTOCK JP, UDENFRIEND S. Effect of lactate on collagen proline hydroxylase activity in cultured L-929 fibroblasts. *Proc Natl Acad Sci USA* 1970;**66**:552-557.

445. STEPHENS FO, HUNT TK. Effects of changes in inspired oxygen and carbon dioxide tensions on wound tensile strength. *Ann Surg* 1971;**173**:515-519.

446. HOHN DC, MACKAY RD, HALLIDAY B, HUNT TK. The effect of O_2 tension on the microbicidal function of leucocytes in wounds and *in vitro. Surg Forum* 1976;**27**:18.

447. AUSPRUNK DH, FALTERMAN K, FOLKMAN J. The sequence of events in the regression of corneal capillaries. *Lab Invest* 1978; **38**:284-294.

448. KNIGHTON DR, HALLIDAY B, HUNT TK. Oxygen as an antibiotic: the effect of inspired oxygen on infection. *Arch Surg* 1984;**119**:199-204.

449. JONSSON K, HUNT TK, MATHES SJ. Effect of environmental oxygen on bacterial induced tissue necrosis in flaps. *Surg Forum* 1984;**35**:589-591.

450. NIINIKOSKI J, GOTTRUP F, HUNT TK. The role of oxygen in wound repair. In: JANSSEN H, ROOMAN R, ROBERTSON JIS, eds. *Wound healing.* Petersfield, England: Wrightson Biomedical Publishing, 1991:165-174.

451. JONSSON K, HUNT TK, MATHES SJ. Oxygen as an isolated variable influences resistance to infection. *Ann Surg* 1988;**208**:783-787.

452. SCHANDALL A, LOWDER R, YOUNG HL. Colonic anastomotic healing and oxygen tension. *Br J Surg* 1986;**72**:606-609.

453. GOTTRUP F. Measurement and evaluation of tissue perfusion in surgery (to optimize wound healing and resistance to infection). In: LEAPER DJ, BRANICKI FJ, eds. *International surgical practice.* Oxford: Oxford University Press, 1992:15-39.

454. RABKIN JM, HUNT TK. Infection and oxygen. In: DAVIS JC, ed. *Problem wounds: the role of oxygen.* New York: Elsevier, 1988:9-16.

455. BEAMAN L, BEAMAN BL. The role of oxygen and its derivatives in microbial pathogenesis and host defence. *Ann Rev Microbiol* 1984;**38**:27-48.

456. HOHN DC. Host resistance of infection: established and emergin concepts. In: HUNT TK, ed. *Wound healing and wound infection: theory and surgical practice.* New York: Appelton-Century-Crofts, 1980:264-280.

457. HOHN DC. Oxygen and leucocyte microbial killing. In: DAVIS JC, HUNT TK, eds. *Hyperbaric oxygen therapy.* Bethesda: Undersea Medical Society, 1977:101-110.

458. HUNT TK, HALLIDAY B, KNIGHTON DR, et al. Oxygen in prevention and treatment of infection. In: ROOT RK, TRUNKEY DD, SANDE MA, eds. *Contemporary issues in infectious diseases,* vol 6. New York: Churchill Livingstone, 1986.

459. KLEBANOFF S. Oxygen metabolism and the toxic properties of phagocytes. *Ann Intern Med* 1980;**93**:480-489.

460. MANDELL G. Bactericidal activity of aerobic and anaerobic polymorphonuclear neutrophils. *Infect Immun* 1974;**9**:337-341.

461. JONSSON K, HUNT TK, MATHES SJ. Effect of environmental oxygen on bacterial induced tissue necrosis in flaps. *Surg Forum* 1984;**35**:589-591.

462. GOLDHABER P. The effect of hyperoxia on bone resorption in tissue culture. *Arch Pathol* 1958;**66**:635-641.

463. SHAW JL, BASSETT CAL. The effects of varying oxygen concentrations on osteogenesis and embryonic cartilage *in vitro. J Bone and Joint Surg* 1967;**49**:73-80.

464. BASSETT CAL, HERRMANN I. Histology: influence of oxygen concentration and mechanical factors on differentiation of connective tissues *in vitro. Nature* 1961;**190**:460-461.

465. GORHAM LW, STOUT AP. Massive osteolysis (Acute spontaneous absorption of bone, phantome bone, disappearing bone). Its relation to hemangiomatosis. *J Bone and Joint Surg* 1955;**37-A**:985-1004.

466. FREDERIKSEN NL, WESLEY RK, SCIUBBA JJ, HELFRICK J. Massive osteolysis of the maxillofacial skeleton: a clinical, radiographic, histologic, and ultrastructural study. *Oral Surg Oral Med Oral Pathol* 1983;**55**:470-480.

467. MARX RE, JOHNSON RP. Problem wounds in oral and maxillofacial surgery: the role of hyperbaric oxygen. In: DAVIS JC, HUNT TK, eds. *Problem wounds: the role of oxygen.* New York: Elsevier, 1988:123.

468. UDENFRIEND S. Formation of hydroxyproline in collagen. *Science* 1966;**152**:1335-40.

469. NIINIKOSKI PB, RAJAMAKI A KULONEN E. Healing of open wounds: effects of oxgen, distributed blood supply and hyperemia by infrared radiation. *Acta Chir Scand* 1971;**137**:399-401.

470. KETCHUM SA, THOMAS AN, HALL AD. Angiographic studies of the effect of hyperbaric oxygen on burn wound revascularization. In: WADA J, IWA T, eds. *Proceedings of the fourth international congress on hyperbaric medicine.* Tokyo: Igaku Shain, 1970:388.

471. SILVER IA. Oxygen and tissue repair, an environment for healing: the role of occlusion. *Int Cong Symp Ser/Roy Soc Med* 1987;**88**:15.

472. SHANNON MD, HALLMON WW, MILLS MP, NEWELL DH. Periodontal wound healing responses to varying oxygen concentrations and atmospheric pressures. *J Clin Periodontol* 1988;**15**:222-226.

473. NILSSON LP, GRANSTRÖM G, RÖCKERT HOE. Effects of dextrans, heparin and hyperbaric oxygen on mandibular tissue damage after osteotomy in an experimental system. *Int J Oral Maxillofacial Surg* 1987;**16**:77-89.

474. WILCOX JW, KOLODNY SC. Acceleration of healing of maxillary and mandibular osteotomies by use of hyperbaric oxygen (a preliminary report). *Oral Surg Oral Med Oral Pathol* 1976;**11**;423-429.

475. BURKE JF. Infection. In: HUNT TK, DUNPHY JE, eds. *Fundamentals of wound management.* New York: Appelton-Century-Crofts, 1979:170-240.

476. BURKE JF. Effects of inflammation on wound repair. *J Dent Res* 1971;**50**:296-303.

477. BURKE JF. Infection. In: HUNT TK, DUNPHY JE, eds. *Fundamentals of wound management.* New York: Appelton-Century-Crofts, 1979:170-241.

478. LEAK LV, BURKE JF. In: ZWEIFACH BW, GRANT L, McCLUSKEY RR, eds. *The inflammatory process,* vol.III 2nd edn. New York: Academic Press, 1974:207

479. MORRIS PJ, BARNES BA, BURKE JF. The nature of "irreducible minimum" rate of incisional sepsis. *Arch Surg* 1966;**92**:367-370.

480. LEVENSON SM, KAN-GRUBER D, GRUBER C, MOLNAR J, SEIFTER E. Wound healing accelerated by *Staphylococcus aureus. Arch Surg* 1983;**118**:310-320.

481. KAN-GRUBER D, GRUBER C, MOLNAR J, et al. Acceleration of wound healing by a strain of *Staphylococcus aureus.* I. *Surg Forum* 1980;**31**:232-234.

482. KAN-GRUBER D, GRUBER C, SEIFTER E, et al. Acceleration of wound healing by *Staphylococcus aureus.* II. *Surg Forum* 1981;**32**:76-79.

483. TENORIO A, JINDRAK K, WEINER M, et al. Accelerated healing in infected wounds. *Surg Gynecol Obstet* 1976;**142**:537-544.

484. OLOUMI M, JINDRAK K, WEINER M, et al. The time at which infected postoperative wounds demonstrate increased strength. *Surg Gynecol Obstet* 1977;**145**:702-704.

485. NIINIKOSKI J. *Oxygen and trauma: studies on pulmonary oxygen poisoning and the role of oxygen in repair processes.* London: European Research Office United States Army, 1973:59.

486. LARJAVA H. Fibroblasts: bacteria interactions. *Proc Finn Dent Soc* 1987;**83**:85-93.

487. SMITH IM, WILSON AP, HAZARD EG, et al. Death from staphylococci in mice. *Infect Dis* 1960;**107**:369-78.

488. BULLEN JJ, CUSHNIE GH, STONER HB. Oxygen uptake by *Clostridium welchi* type A: its possible role in experimental infections in passively immunized animals. *Br J Exp Pathol* 1966;**47**:488.

489. IRVIN TT. Wound infection. In: IRVIN TT, ed. *Wound healing: principles and practice.* London: Chapman and Hall, 1981:64.

490. RAAHAVE D. Wound contamination and post-operative infection. In: TAYLOR EW, ed. *Infection in surgical practice.* Oxford: Oxford University Press, 1992:49-55.

491. BECKER GD. Identification and management of the patient at high risk for wound infection. *Head Neck Surg* 1986;**8**:205-210.

492. ROBSON MC, HEGGERS JP. Delayed wound closure based on bacterial counts. *J Surg Oncol* 1970;**2**:379-383.

493. BURKE JF. The effective period of preventive antibiotic action in experimental incisions and dermal lesions. *Surgery* 1961;**50**:161-168.

494. ELEK SD. Experimental staphylococcal infections in skin of man. *Ann NY Acad Sci* 1956;**65**:85-90.

495. ELEK SD, CONEN PE. The virulence of *Staphylococcus Pyogens* for man. A study of the problems of wound infection. *Br J Exp Pathol* 1957;**38**:573-586.

496. EDLICH RF, RODEHEAVER G, THACKER JG, EDGERTON MT. Technical factors in wound management. In: HUNT TK, DUNPHY JE, eds. *Fundamentals of wound management.* New York: Appelton-Century-Crofts, 1979:364-454.

497. DOUGHERTY SH, SIMMONS RL. Infections in bionic man: the pathobiology of infections in prosthetic devices- Part II. *Curr Prob Surg* 1982;**19**:265-312.

498. TAYLOR EW. General principles of antibiotic prophylaxis. In: TAYLOR EW, ed. *Infection in surgical practice.* Oxford: Oxford University Press, 1992:76-81.

499. COSTERTON JW, CHENG KJ, GEESEY GG, et al. Bacterial biofilms in nature and disease. *Ann Rev Microbiol* 1987;**41**:435-464.

500. MOYNIHAM BJA. The ritual of surgical operations. *Br J Surg* 1920;**8**:27-35.

501. BUCKNALL TE. Factors affecting healing. In: BUCKNALL TE, ELLIS H, eds. *Wound healing.* London: Bailliere Tindall, 1984:42-74.

502. CAPPERAULD I, BUCKNALL TE. Sutures and dressings. In BUCKNALL TE, ELLIS H, eds. *Wound healing for surgeons.* London: Bailliere Tindall, 1984:73-93.

503. BUCKNALL TE, ELLIS H. Abdominal wound closure, a comparison of monofilament nylon and polyglycolic acid. *Surgery* 1981; **89**:672-677.

504. SAVOLAINEN H, RISTKARI S, MOKKA R. Early laparotomy wound dehiscence: a randomized comparison of three suture materials and two methods of fascial closure. *Ann Chir Gynecol* 1988;**77**:111-113.

505. LARSEN PN, NIELSEN K, SCHULTZ A, MEJDAHL S, LARSEN T, MOESGAARD F. Closure of the abdominal fascia after clean and clean-contaminated laparotomy. *Acta Chir Scand* 1989;**155**:461-464.

506. VIIDIK A, HOLM-PEDERSEN P, RUNDGREN Å. Some observations on the distant collagen response to wound healing. *J Plast Reconstr Surg* 1972;**6**:114-122.

507. ZEDERFELDT B. Factors influencing wound healing. In: VIIDIK A, VUUST S, eds. *Biology of collagen.* London: Academic Press, 1980:347-362.

508. ADZICK NS, LONGAKER MT. Characteristics of fetal tissue repair. In: ADZICK NS, LONGAKER MT, eds. *Fetal Wound healing.* New York: Elsevier, 1992:53-70.

509. ADZICK NS, LONGAKER MT. Scarless fetal healing: therapeutic implications. In: ADZICK NS, LONGAKER MT, eds. *Fetal wound healing.* New York: Elsevier, 1992:317-324.

510. LONGAKER MT, KABAN LB. Fetal models for craniofacial surgery: cleft lip/palate and craniosynostosis. In: ADZICK NS, LONGAKER MT, eds. *Fetal wound healing.* New York: Elsevier, 1992:83-94.

511. FERGUSON MWJ, HOWARTH GF. Marsupial models of scarless fetal wound healing. In: ADZICK NS, LONGAKER MT, eds. *Fetal wound healing.* New York: Elsevier, 1992:95-124.

512. ADZICK NS. Fetal animal and wound implant models. In: ADZICK NS, LONGAKER MT, eds. *Fetal wound healing.* New York: Elsevier, 1992:71-82.

513. MAST BA, KRUMMEL TM. Acute inflammation in fetal wound healing. In: ADZICK NS, LONGAKER MT, eds. *Fetal wound healing.* New York: Elsevier, 1992:227-240.

514. CHIU E, LONGAKER MT, ADZICK NS, et al. Hyaluronic acid patterns in fetal and adult wound fluid. *Surg Forum* 1990;**41**:636-639.

515. BURD DAR, SIEBERT J, GARG H. Hyaluronan-protein interactions. In: ADZICK NS, LONGAKER MT, eds. *Fetal wound healing.* New York: Elsevier, 1992:199-214.

516. PAUL HE, PAUL MF, TAYLOR JD, MARSTERS RW. Biochemistry of wound healing. II. Water and protein content of healing tissue of skin wounds. *Arch Biochem* 1948;**17**:269-274.

517. BOURLIÈRE F, GOURÉVITCH M. Age et vitesse de réparation des plaies expérimentales chez le rat. *C R Soc Biol (Paris)* 1950;**144**:377-379.

518. CUTHBERTSON AM. Concentration of full thickness skin wounds in the rat. *Surg Gynec Obstet* 1959;**108**:421-432.

519. ENGELHARDT GH, STRUCK H. Effect of aging on wound healing. *Scand J Clin Lab Invest* 1972;**29** (Suppl 123).

520. HOLM-PEDERSEN P, ZEDERFELDT B. Strength development of skin incisions in young and old rats. *Scand J Plast Reconstr Surg* 1971;**5**:7-12.

521. HOLM-PEDERSEN P, VIIDIK A. Maturation of collagen in healing wounds in young and old rats. *Scand J Plast Reconstr Surg* 1972;**6**:16-23.

522. HOLM-PEDERSEN P, NILSSON K, BRÅNEMARK P-I. The microvascular system of healing wounds in young and old rats. *Advanc Microcirc* 1973;**5**:80-106.

523. HOLM-PEDERSEN P, VIIDIK A. Tensile properties and morphology of healing wounds in young and old rats. *Scand J Plast Reconstr Surg* 1972;**6**:24-35.

524. BILLINGHAM RE, RUSSEL PS. Studies on wound healing, with special refference to the phenomenon of contracture in experimental wounds in rabbits skin. *Ann Surg* 1956;**144**:961-981.

525. LÖFSTRÖM B, ZEDERFELDT B. Wound healing after induced hypothermia. III. Effect of age. *Acta Chir Scand* 1957;**114**:245-251.

526. SANDBLOM P, PETERSEN P, MUREN A. Determination of the tensile strength of the healing wound as a clinical test. *Acta Chir Scand* 1953;**105**:252-257.

527. OLSSON A. Sårläkning hos homo. *Nord Med* 1955;**53**:128.

528. FORSCHER BK, CECIL HC. Some effect of age on the biochemistry of acute inflammation. *Gerontologia (Basel)* 1958;**2**:174-182.

529. STAHL SS. The healing of gingival wounds in male rats of various ages. *J Dent Med* 1961;**16**:100-103.

530. STAHL SS. Soft tissue healing following experimental gingival wounding in female rats of various ages. *Periodontics* 1963;**1**:142-146.

531. BUTCHER EO, KLINGSBERG J. Age, gonadectomy, and wound healing in the palatal mucosa of the rat. *Oral Surg Oral Med Oral Pathol* 1963;**16**:484-493.

532. BUTCHER EO, KLINGSBERG J. Age changes and wound healing in the oral tissues. *Ann Dent (Baltimore)* 1964;**23**:84-95.

533. ROVIN S, GORDON HA. The influence of aging on wound healing in germfree and conventional mice. *Gerontologia (Basel)* 1968;**14**:87-96.

534. HOLM-PEDERSEN P, LÖE H. Wound healing in the gingiva of young and old individuals. *Scand J Dent Res* 1971;**79**:40-53.

535. STAHL SS, WITKIN GJ, CANTOR M, BROWN R. Gingival healing.II. Clinical and histologic repair sequences following gingivectomy. *J Periodont* 1968;**39**:109-118.

536. GROVE GL. Age-related differences in healing of superficial skin wounds in humans. *Arch Dermatol Res* 1982;**272**: 381-385.

537. HOLM-PEDERSEN P. *Studies on healing capacity in young and old individuals. Clinical, biophysical and microvascular aspects of connective tissue repair with special reference to tissue function in man and rat.* Copenhagen: Munksgaard, 1973.

538. GOTTRUP F. Healing of incisional wounds in stomach and duodenum. The influence of aging. *Acta Chir Scand* 1981;**147**:363-369.

539. CRUSE PJE, FOORD R. A five-year prospective study of 23,649 surgical wounds. *Arch Surg* 1973;**107**:206-210.

540. DAVIDSON AIG, CLARK C, SMITH G. Postoperative wound infection: a computer analysis. *Br J Surg* 1971;**58**:333-337.

541. CATON JG, POLSON AM, PINI PG, BARTOLUCCI EG, CLAUSER C. Healing after application of tissue-adhesive material to denuded and citric-treated root surfaces. *J Periodontol* 1986;**157**:385-390.

542. BARBUL A, CALDWELL MD, EAGLESTEIN WH, eds. *Clinical and experimental approaches to dermal and epidermal repair.* New York: Wiley-Liss, 1991.

543. BUCKNALL TE, ELLIS H. *Wound healing for surgeons.* London: Bailliere Tindall, 1984.

544. HARTING G, ed. *Advanced wound healing resource theory.* Copenhagen: Coloplast, 1992.

545. BORNSIDE GH. Bactericidal effect of hyperbaric oxygen determined by direct exposure. *Proc Soc Exp Biol Med* 1969;**130**:1165-1167.

546. BUCKLEY A, DAVIDSON JM, KAMERATH CD, et al. Epidermal growth factor increases granulation tissue formation dose dependently. *J Surg Res* 1987;**43** 322-328.

547. BUNTROCK P, JENTZSCH KD, HEDER G. Stimulation and wound healing, using brain extract with fibroblast growth factor (FGF) activity. II. Histological and morphometric examination of cells and capillaries. *Exp Pathol* 1982;**21**:62-67.

548. CLARK RAF, DELLAPELLA P, MANSEAU E, LANIGAN JM, DVORAK HF, COLVIN RB. Blood vessel fibronectin increases in conjunction with endothelial cell proliferation and capillary ingrowth during wound healing. *J Invest Dermatol* 1982;**79**:269-276.

549. PICHE JE, GRAVES DT. Study of growth factor requirements of human bone-derived cells: a comparison with human fibroblasts. *Bone* 1989;**10**:131-138.

550. GOTTRUP F, NIINIKOSKI J, HUNT TK. Measurements of tissue oxygen tension in wound repair. In: JANSSEN H, ROOMAN R, ROBERTSON JIS, eds. *Wound healing.* Petersfield, England: Wrightson Biomedical Publishing, 1991:155-164.

551. GOTTRUP F. Surgical wounds - Healing types and physiology. In: HARTING K, ed. *Advanced wound healing resource theory.* Copenhagen: Coloplast,1992, Chapter X:1-17.

552. KRAWCZYK WS. A pattern of epidermal cell migration during wound healing. *J Cell Biol* 1971;**49**:247-263.

553. LAATO M, NIINIKOSKI J, GERDIN B, et al. Stimulation of wounds healing by epidermal growth factor: a dose dependent effect. *Ann Surg* 1986;**203**:379-381.

554. RAJU R, JINDRAK K, WEINER M, et al. A study of the critical bacterial inoculum to cause a stimulus to wound healing. *Surg Gynecol Obstst* 1977;**144**:347-350.

555. LEVENSON SM, GRUBER DK, GRUBER C, et al. Wound healing accelerated by Staphylococcus aureus. *Arch Surg* 1983;**118**:310-319.

556. VENGE P. What is inflammation?. In: VENGE P, LINDBLOM A, eds. *Inflammation.* Stockholm: Almquist & Wiksell International, 1985:1-8.

557. HUNT TK, VAN WINKLE W JR. Wound healing: disorders of repair. In: DUNPHY JE, ed. *Fundamentals of wound management in surgery.* South Plainfield: Chirurgecom, 1976:37

558. ROTHE M, FALANGA V. Growth factors: their biology and promise in dermatologic diseases and tissue repair. *Arch Dermatol* 1989;**125**:1390-1398.

559. JØRGENSEN PH, ANDREASSEN TT. Influence of biosynthetic human growth hormone on biomechanical properties of rat skin incisional wounds. *Acta Chir Scand* 1988;**154**:623-626.

560. ISAKSSON OGP, LINDAHL A, NILSSON A, ISGAARD J. Mechanism of the stimulatory effect of growth hormone on longitudinal bone growth. *Endocrine Rev* 1987;**8**:426-438.

561. GRØNDAHL-HANSEN J, LUND LR, RALFKIER E, et al. Urokinase and tissue-type plasmin activators in keratinocytes during wound re-epithelization in vivo. *J Invest Dermatol* 1988;**90**:790-795.

562. STEVENSON TR, RODEHEAVER GT, GOLDEN GT, et al. Damage to tissue defenses by vasoconstrictors. *J Am Coll Emerg Phys* 1975;**4**:532

563. RIPAMONTI U, PETIT J-C, LEMMER J, AUSTIN JC. Regeneration of the connective tissue attachment on surgically exposed roots using a fibrin-fibronectin adhesive system. An experimental study on the baboon (Papio ursinus). *J Periodont Res* 1987;**22**:320-326.

564. MANSBRIDGE JN, KNAPP AM. Changes in keratinocyte maturation during wound healing. *J Invest Dermatol* 1987;**89**:253-263.

565. GOTTRUP F. Healing of intestinal wounds in the stomach and duodenum. An experimental study. *Danish Med Bull* 1984,**31**:31-48.

566. OSTHER PJ, GJØDE P, MORTENSEN BB, BARTHOLIN J, GOTTRUP F. Abdominal fascia clossure. A randomized comparision of glycolic and polyglyconate sutures on wound complications in patients with suspected impaired wound healing. Submitted 1993.

CHAPTER 1

Response of Oral Tissues to Trauma

J. O. ANDREASEN

and

Inflammation and Mediators of Hard Tissue Resorption

M. TORABINEJAD & R. D. FINKELMAN

Repair and Regeneration of Oral Tissues

An injury can be defined as an interruption in the continuity of tissues, and healing as the reestablishment of that continuity. The result of this process can either be *tissue repair,* where the continuity is restored but the healed tissue differs in anatomy and function, or *tissue regeneration,* where both anatomy and function are restored.

In lower vertebrates, the regeneration of appendages such as limbs, tails and fins is common. In mammals, this healing capacity has generally been lost, although it has been reported that, in humans, digits amputated distal to the distal interphalangeal joint can regenerate in children (1). The explanation for this general loss of healing capacity in mammals is presently under investigation. However, the rapid epidermal healing response in mammals, which optimizes wound closure and thereby limits the risk of infection, is currently believed to present an obstacle to tissue regeneration (2).

Healing of most wounds in humans, whether caused by trauma or surgery, includes repair with more or less fibrous scar tissue formation which subsequently leads to problems in function of the particular organ affected. In the oral region, skin wounds and to a lesser degree the oral mucosa are repaired with scar formation (see Chapter 13, p. 496).

Dental tissues are unique in comparison to most other tissues in the body due to their marked capacity for regeneration. Thus tooth germs split by trauma or surgery may completely regenerate (see p. 85). Similarly injured dentin, cementum, bone, and gingiva often will regenerate (see later).

Injuries to the pulp and the periodontal ligament may regenerate or show repair with scar tissue or bone after wounding.

Understanding the circumstances leading to repair and regeneration in oral tissues has been a formidable challenge (3). In this regard, wounding releases a variety of signals that induce neighboring cell populations to respond by the alteration of a number of cell functions including proliferation, migration, or differentiation. The first prerequisite for tissue regeneration is that a tissue-specific cell population is present after wounding (e.g. pulp or PDL progenitor cells). If these cells are not present, repair rather than regeneration will take place. A typical example of

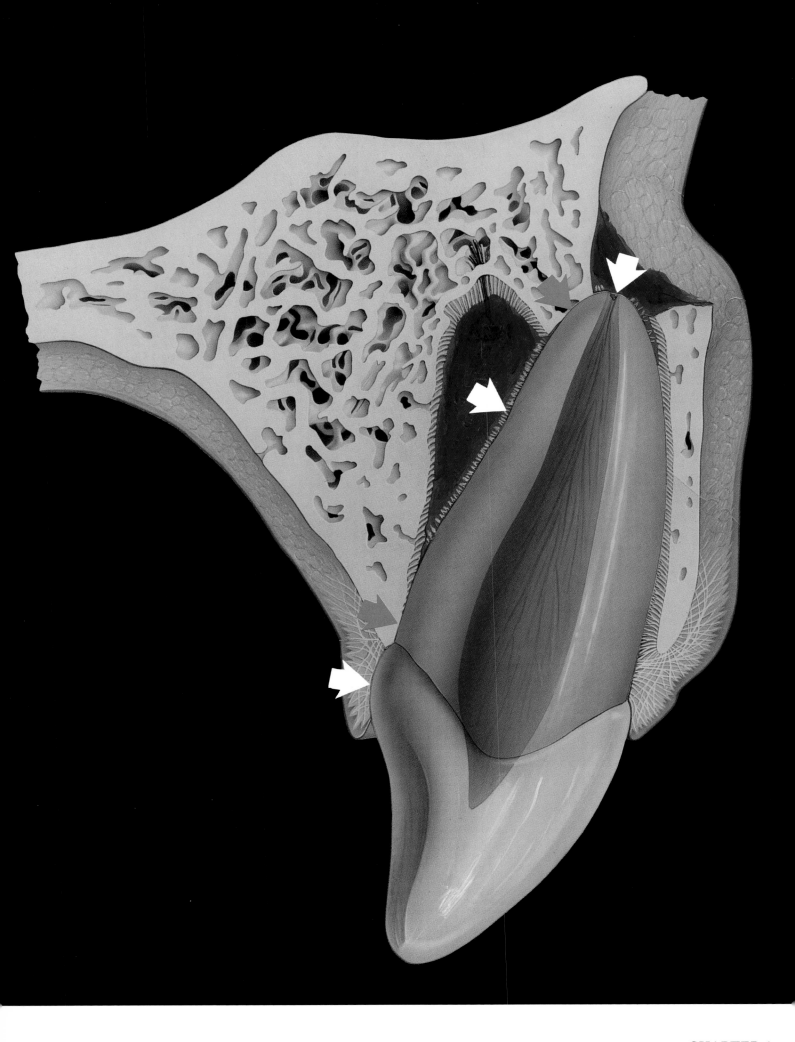

←

Fig. 2.1. Injury zones after tooth luxation
A lateral luxation implies trauma to multiple cell systems in the periodontium and the pulp, as rupture (white arrows) or compression (blue arrows) or ischemia damage these cellular compartments. The outcome of the healing processes is entirely dependent upon the healing capacity of the different cellular systems involved. From AN-DREASEN & ANDREASEN (3) 1992.

this concept is the healing by ankylosis of teeth replanted with an avital periodontal ligament(see p. 100).

A second prerequisite for regeneration is that conditions exist that are conducive to migration of tissue-specific cells into the wound site. Thus, incomplete repositioning of a luxated tooth may lead to damage to the epithelial root sheath and ingrowth of PDL-derived cells and bone into the pulp canal. Another situation in which the topographic conditions of the wound may determine whether repair or regeneration take place is related to loss of periodontal attachment on a root or implant. In this situation the insertion of a membrane may direct bone cells into the wound site (see Chapter 20, p. 698).

A third factor that may determine tissue repair or regeneration in oral wounds is the presence of contaminating foreign bodies and/or bacteria. Inflammation related to a contaminated wound has been found to lead to repair rather than regeneration, possibly because contamination leads to formation of a non-tissue-specific, inflamed granulation tissue at the expense of the proliferation and migration of tissue-specific cells.

When assessing wound healing after trauma, it is not enough to understand the healing capacity of individual cell types, one must also consider the various tissue compartments, each consisting of different cellular systems. Differences in healing capacity and rates of healing can lead to competitive situations and thereby to variations in wound healing. Ischemia or the total destruction of cell layers may occur (1) (Fig. 2.1). This chapter will present a brief description of the anatomy and function of cell compartments typically involved following a traumatic event. In the description of these compartments, anatomical borders have been chosen which are typically the result of separation lines or contusion subsequent to trauma. Using this approach, the following anatomical zones evolve in relation to teeth with completed root development: *gingival- and periosteal complex*; *cemento-perio-dontal ligament complex; alveolar bone complex* and *dentino-pulpal complex*.

In developing teeth, the following structures should be added: *dental follicle;, enamel* and *enamel-forming organ*; and *Hertwig's epithelial root sheath*.

For each tissue compartment, a description will be given of its anatomy and healing responses to trauma and infection.

Developing Teeth
Dental Follicle

The dental follicle (dental sac) has traditionally been considered the formative organ of the periodontium (Fig. 2.2). This concept has been supported by experimental studies of transplanted tooth germs which indicate that the innermost layer (dental follicle proper, which is in contact with the tooth germ) can give rise to all of the components of the periodontium (4-6). Based on these findings, it has been suggested that the term *dental follicle* should be reserved for the innermost layer of connective tissue separating the tooth germ from its crypt (7). The remaining peripheral tissue would therefore be designated as the perifollicular mesenchyme (2,5,8). However, until further research has definitely ruled out the possibility of perifollicular mesenchymal participation in the formation of the periodontal attachment, it appears justified to use the term *dental follicle* for all the mesenchymal tissue interposed between the tooth germ and alveolar bone.

In addition to the role of the dental follicle in the formation of cementum and periodontal ligament fibers, it also has a significant osteogenic capacity. Thus, in several experiments it has been shown that heterotopic transplantation of tooth germs, including their follicles, to soft tissue sites results in formation of a complete periodontium including cementum, periodontal ligament fibers and an adjacent shell of bone (alveolar bone proper) (3,5,8-15).

A number of events have been suggested

Fig. 2.2. Anatomy of a dental follicle of a monkey maxillary central tooth germ
Note the close proximity between the primary tooth and the permanent successor as well as the loose structure of the follicle. x 12.

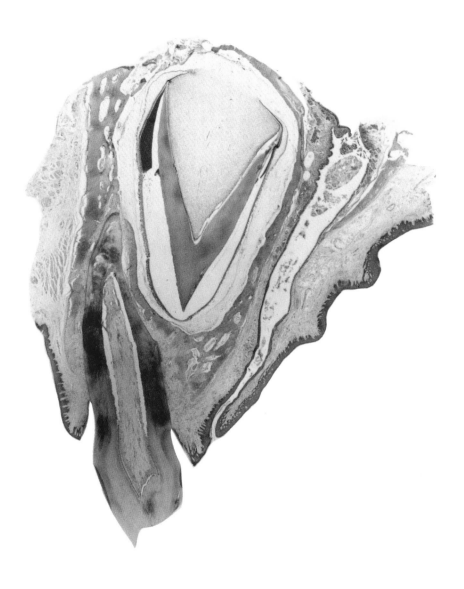

as being responsible for tooth eruption, including root growth, dentin formation, pulp growth and changes in the dental follicle and the periodontal ligament (16-22). However, recent experiments in dogs and monkeys have demonstrated that changes in the dental follicle (including the reduced enamel epithelium) are possibly responsible for the coordinated en-largement of the eruption pathway and movement of the tooth germ in the initial phases of eruption (23-26). These findings, together with the established relationship between the dental follicle and distinct areas of bone resorption and bone forma-tion, suggest that the dental follicle and/or the reduced enamel epithelium coordinate these processes during eruption (21,22-30)

CHAPTER 2

Fig. 2.3. Eruption of a permanent maxillary central monkey incisor
Note bone apposition apically, while active bone and tooth resorption takes place coronally. x 12.

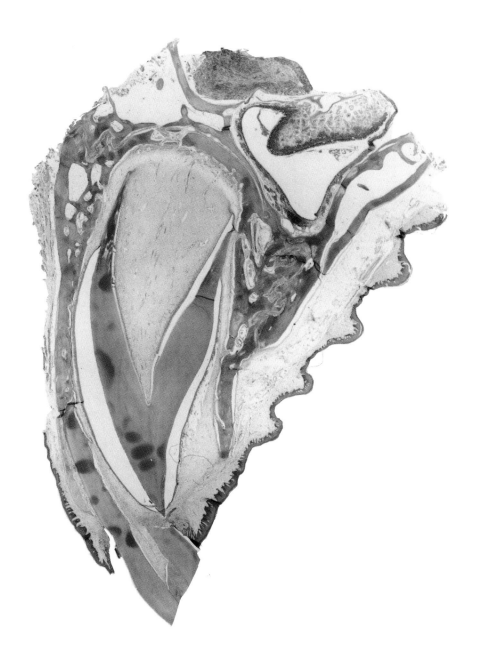

(Fig. 2.3). Consequently, severe disturbances in eruption can be anticipated if there is damage to the follicle due to trauma or infection.

RESPONSE TO TRAUMA
Histologic studies have revealed a very close relationship between the primary teeth and the permanent dentition, especially in the initial phases of development (31,32) (Figs. 2.2 and 2.3). Traumatic injuries can therefore be transmitted easily from the primary to the permanent dentition (34).

While there is abundant clinical evidence to show that the dental follicle has a remarkable healing capacity after injury,

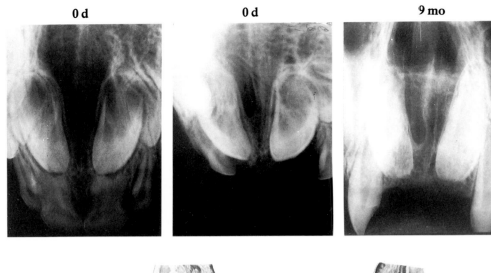

Fig. 2.4. Replantation of maxillary monkey tooth germs with damaged follicles
Preoperative and postoperative radiographs and the condition after 9 months. No eruption has taken place. Low power view of both central incisors. Note the lack of eruption despite almost complete root formation. Furthermore note the ankylosis sites affecting the crowns of both teeth (arrows). From KRISTERSON & ANDREASEN (25) 1984.

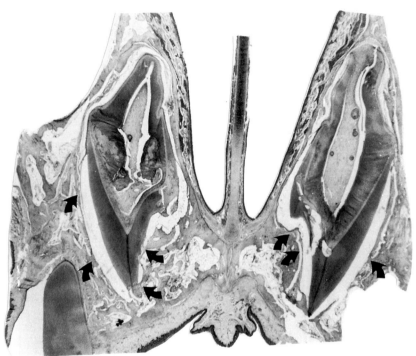

certain limitations do exist. Thus, it has been shown that, when larger parts of the dental follicle are removed, an ankylosis is formed between the tooth surface and the crypt and eruption is arrested (23,25) (Fig. 2.4). The extent to which a follicle can be damaged without leading to this complication is not known.

RESPONSE TO INFECTION
Very little information exists on the reaction of the dental follicle to infection. In monkeys, it was found that follicles of permanent incisor tooth germs were resistant to short-term chronic periapical infection originating from the root canals of primary incisors (Fig. 2.5), and no influence could be demonstrated on the permanent successors with respect to enamel mineralization (33). In rare instances, acute infection has been found to spread to the entire follicle and to lead to sequestration of the tooth germ (34). Such events have been reported after traumatic injuries to the primary dentition, in jaw fractures where the line of fracture involves a tooth germ, or in cases of osteomyelitis which

Fig. 2.5. Follicular changes
after pulp necrosis of a
maxillary monkey central
primary incisor

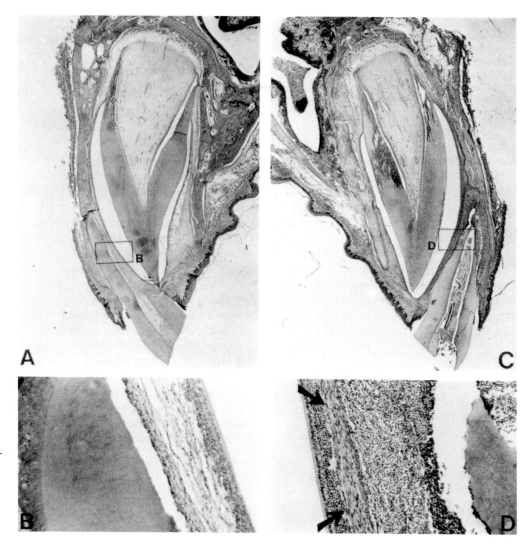

**Fig. 2.5. Follicular changes
after pulp necrosis of a
maxillary monkey central
primary incisor**
*Late stages of tooth development
of permanent tooth germs. Low
power view of control tooth (A)
and experimental tooth (C). x 7.*

Changes in the follicle
*Normal reduced enamel epithe-
lium in control tooth. In the experimental tooth there is intense
periapical inflammation demarcated from reduced enamel epithelium by a thin layer of fibrous
tissue (arrows). x 75. From AN-
DREASEN & RIIS (33) 1978.*

affect the bony regions containing dental follicles (34). Apart from these rare occurrences, the dental follicle appears to be rather resistant to infection.

Enamel-Forming Organ

The formation and maturation of enamel in the permanent dentition is often disturbed or arrested by trauma transmitted from primary teeth after displacement and/or periapical inflammation resulting from infection. The outcome of such events depends primarily upon the stage of enamel formation at the time of the injury.

The usual stage at which primary tooth injuries interfere with odontogenesis of the permanent dentition is the beginning of mineralization of the incisal portion of the crown. At this stage of development, the enamel-forming organ consists of the cervical loop placed apically to the site of active enamel and dentin formation. Coronally, the enamel epithelium is divided into the inner and outer enamel epithelium with an intervening stratum intermedium and stellate reticulum between them. The reduced enamel epithelium is found more coronally, where the full ena-

Fig. 2.6. Immediate changes after intrusion of a primary monkey incisor

A. Low power view of specimen. x 8. B. Dislocation between mineralized tissues and cervical loop. x 75. C. Rupture and bleeding in stellate reticulum. x 75. D. Destruction of reduced enamel epithelium. x 75. E. Separation of reduced enamel epithelium from connective tissue. x 75. From AN-DREASEN (37) 1976.

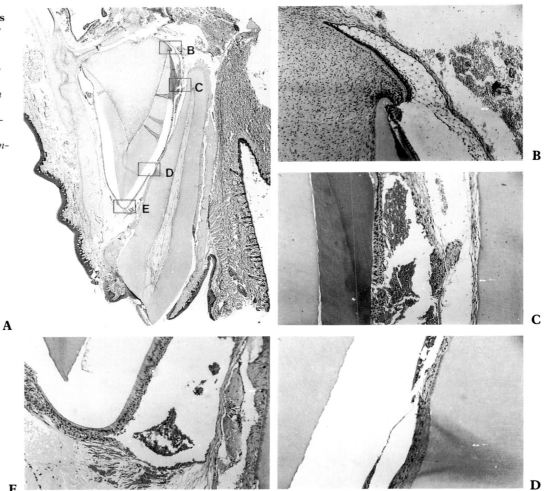

mel thickness has been formed and mineralization completed. In the following, a synopsis of the anatomy and function of these structures will be presented, as well their response to trauma and infection.

Cervical Loop

At the free border of the enamel organ, the inner and outer enamel epithelial layers are continuous and form the cervical loop (35,36). Progression of tooth development is entirely dependent upon the growth and action of this structure.

RESPONSE TO TRAUMA

The cervical loop is highly resistant to trauma. Simple separation of the cervical enamel and dentin matrix does not prevent further enamel or dentin formation (37,38) (Figs. 2.6 and 2.7). However, pro-

found contusion of this structure, as after intrusion of a primary incisor into the developing successor, may result in total arrest of further odontogenesis.

RESPONSE TO INFECTION

The response of the cervical loop to infection has not yet been studied.

Inner Enamel Epithelium

According to function, the inner enamel epithelium (ameloblasts) evolves through a number of functional stages (39-41) (Fig. 2.8). The first is the *morphogenetic stage* whereby the future outline of the crown is determined. This stage is followed by an *organizing stage*, with initiation of dentin formation. *The formative stage* is then reached, where enamel matrix formation as well as initial mineralization take place. The *maturation stage* follows enamel mat-

Fig. 2.7. Late changes after intrusion of primary incisors in a monkey
Low power view of specimen (A), where the intruded tooth is preserved and the contralateral side where the intruded tooth was extracted (D). x 8.

Changes in enamel and dentin
Morphologic changes in enamel matrix and dentin (B). x 20. Destruction of enamel epithelium and abnormal matrix formation (C). x 75. Partial arrest of enamel matrix formation (E). x 30. Metaplasia of enamel epithelium and abnormal matrix formation (F). x 75. From ANDREASEN (37) 1976.

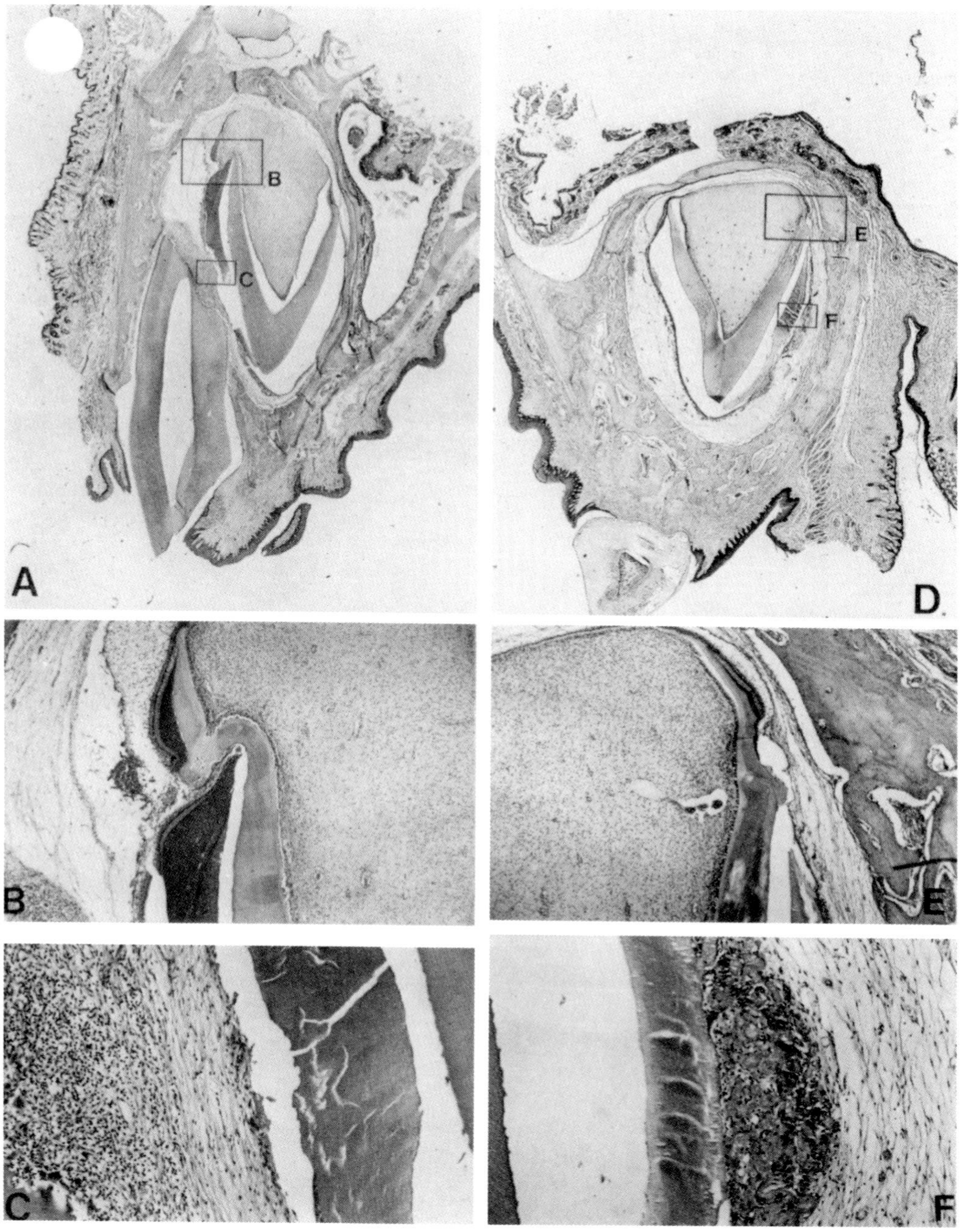

rix formation. During this stage, there is partial removal of the organic enamel matrix accompanied by a complex mineralization process proceeding from the region immediately adjacent to dentin and progressing outward (42). These are followed by the *protective* and *desmolytic* stages, which will be described later. During these two stages, the tissue layer is now designated the *reduced enamel epithelium*.

RESPONSE TO TRAUMA
To date, only limited knowledge exists concerning the response of the inner enamel epithelium to trauma (37,38,43-46). In the case of total loss of ameloblasts in the

secretory phase, no regenerative potential exists (44). In the case of partial damage, the ameloblasts in the *secretory* stage may survive and continue enamel matrix formation, and later maturation may occur (42,45-47) (Figs. 2.6 and 2.7).

If there is total loss of the ameloblasts during the *maturation* stage, a hypomineralized area of enamel will develop. If partial damage occurs, the ameloblasts may recover and the result may be only a limited zone of hypomineralization (42).

RESPONSE TO INFECTION
When chronic periapical inflammation develops due to the necrosis of an infected

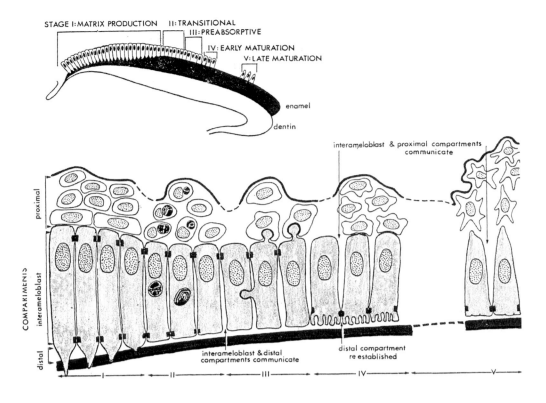

STAGE I: MATRIX PRODUCTION II: TRANSITIONAL
III: PREABSORPTIVE
IV: EARLY MATURATION
V: LATE MATURATION

enamel
dentin

interameloblast & proximal compartments communicate

proximal

COMPARTMENTS

interameloblast

distal

interameloblast & distal compartments communicate

distal compartment re established

I   II   III   IV   V

pulp in primary teeth, the effect upon permanent successors is very limited, at least over a short time (i.e. months) (33) (Fig. 2.5). When infection persists over longer periods (i.e. years), however, experimental and clinical studies have shown that enamel formation and maturation may be affected (48-50).

The response to acute infection is similar to the response to trauma and may lead to localized arrest of enamel formation (51-58). At the site of injury, a cementum-like tissue may later be deposited (59,60). In this situation, the cementoblasts are most probably recruited from the follicle, shown to have cementogenic potential (426).

Reduced Enamel Epithelium

When enamel matrix formation is complete and enamel maturation begun, the ameloblasts become compact and the stellate reticulum disappears, whereby a multilayered epithelium is formed of cuboidal or sometimes flattened cells. The following functions are currently linked to the reduced enamel epithelium: Protection of the enamel against the follicle until the tooth erupts (61), regulation of osteo-

clastic activity in the follicle preparatory to eruption (61), and participation in the breakdown of the connective tissue overlying the crown (62-65). In addition, the reduced enamel epithelium may play an active part in fusion with the oral epithelium as the tooth emerges into the oral cavity (63).

RESPONSE TO TRAUMA
Minor injury to the reduced enamel epithelium is repaired with a thin squamous epithelium (37) (Fig. 2.9). The influence of this event upon eruption is presently unknown, but with larger areas of destruction of the reduced enamel epithelium, ankylosis and tooth retention have been demonstrated (66) (Fig. 2.4).

RESPONSE TO INFECTION
The short-term effect (i.e. months) of chronic inflammation on primary teeth appears to be negligible (33) (Fig. 2.5), while the long-term effect appears to be ectopic or accelerated eruption (50).

Enamel and Enamel Matrix

Mature enamel has the highest mineral content of any tissue in the body (i.e.

Fig. 2.9. Late changes after intrusion in monkey

Low power view of specimen (A) where the intruded primary tooth was preserved and the contralateral side where the intruded tooth was extracted (D). Arrows indicate length of disturbed reduced enamel epithelium. x 8.

Changes in follicle and hard tissues

B. Periapical inflammation and disturbed enamel epithelium (arrows). x 75. C. Amorphous eosinopilic substance deposited upon enamel (arrows). E. Area with temporary arrest of enamel matrix formation. x 75. F. Metaplastic reduced enamel epithelium. From ANDREASEN (37)1976.

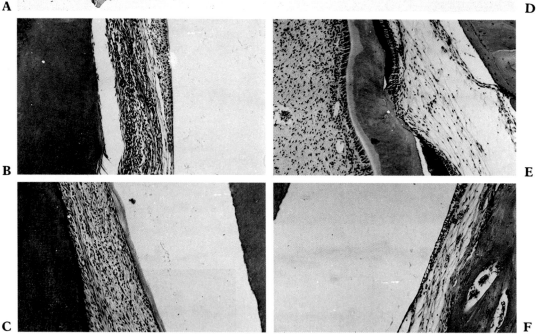

A   D

B   E

C   F

96-98%), whereas enamel matrix is considerably less mineralized. Thus, if maturation is interrupted due to infection or trauma, enamel hypomineralization will result. One may see problems clinically with increased caries or perhaps with difficulties regarding acid-etch restorative techniques. This problem is further discussed in Chapter 12, p. 483.

RESPONSE TO TRAUMA

Trauma to a primary tooth may cause contusion of the permanent enamel matrix (37,38). The ameloblasts will also be destroyed, thereby arresting enamel maturation and resulting in a permanent hypomineralized enamel defect (see Chapter 12, p. 466). In mature enamel, the result of a direct impact will be enamel infraction, i.e. a split along the enamel rods usually ending at the dentino-enamel junction (see Chapter 6, p. 224), or a fracture, whereby part of the crown is lost.

RESPONSE TO INFECTION

The response of enamel matrix or enamel to infection has been discussed earlier.

Fig. 2.10. Hertwig's epithelial root sheath
The root sheath consists of 2 to 3 layers of epithelial cells.

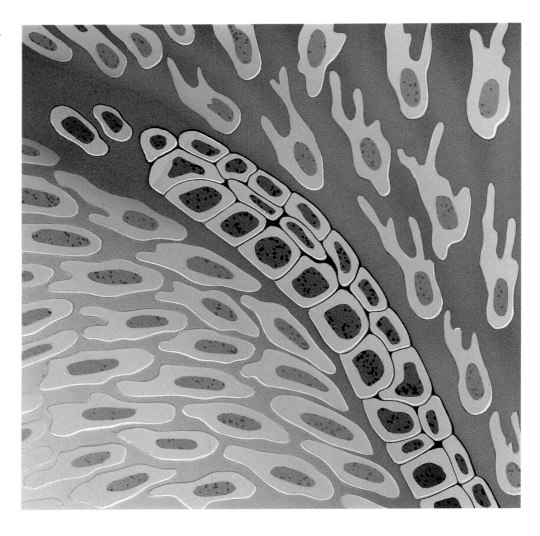

Hertwig's Epithelial Root Sheath (HERS)

HERS is a continuous sleeve of epithelial cells which separates the pulp from the dental follicle. In all primates it consists of an inner layer of cuboidal cells and an outer layer of more flattened cells (67). (Fig. 2.10). Occasionally, there is an intermediate layer of elongated cells (68).

HERS completely encloses the dental papilla except for an opening in its base, the *primary apical foramen*, through which the pulp receives its neurovascular supply. *Root formation* is determined by the activity of HERS (69-73), and root growth is dependent upon a continuous proliferation of epithelium (74,75). More incisally, dentin and cementum develop synchronously,

ensuring a relatively constant sheath length throughout root formation up to the final phases of root development, when the root sheath becomes considerably shorter.

The width of the primary apical foramen as well as the number of vessels entering it appears to be relatively constant until final root length has been achieved (73). Thus, in a luxation, a replantation or a transplantation situation the chances of revascularization through the primary apical foramen should theoretically be the same throughout the early stages of root development, until apical constriction starts. Such a relationship has in fact been found for luxated (218) and replanted incisors (427) as well as for autotransplanted human premolars (428).

Fig. 2.11. Epithelial island of Mallassez

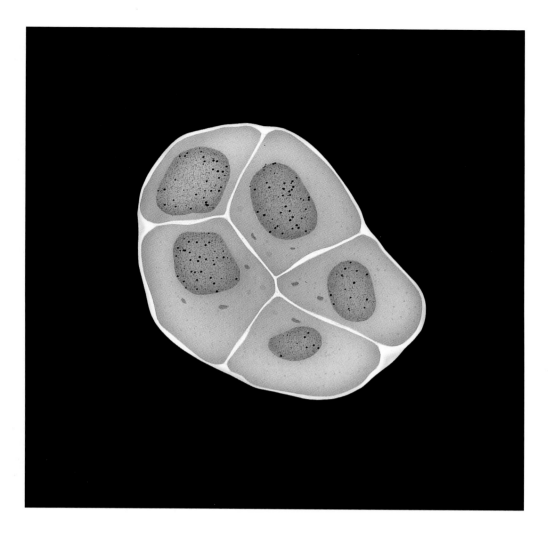

In the following, a closer look will be taken at the role of HERS in *dentin* and *cementum formation*. Odontoblastic differentiation takes place adjacent to the basal aspect of HERS, after which the first dentin matrix is deposited (*mantle dentin*). At this time, the innermost layer of cells in the root sheath secretes a material which combines with the mantle dentin to form the so-called *intermediate cementum layer*. This layer has been found to contain enamel matrix protein and later becomes hypercalcified (76-78). The intermediate cementum layer has recently attracted interest. It has been found to be an effective barrier against the penetration of noxious elements placed in the root canal to the periodontal ligament via the dentinal tubules and possibly also to toxins produced by bacteria within the root canal (79).

After odontoblast induction and formation of intermediate cementum, the root sheath degenerates and the epithelial cells migrate away from the root surface to form the epithelial rests of Mallassez (Fig. 2.11). At the same time, cells from the periodontal ligament migrate towards the root surface and become cementoblasts. These cells then synthesize collagen and other organic constituents of cementum. The role of the epithelial root sheath in the induction of cementoblasts, however, has recently been questioned (74,80-82).

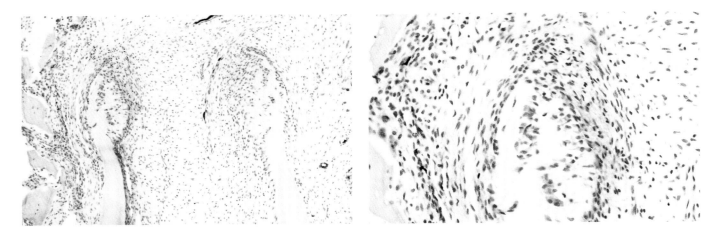

Fig. 2.12.
Hyperactivity og HERS with excessive production of dentin after replantation of a permanent maxillary lateral incisor. x 25 and x 75. Observation time: 1 week.

RESPONSE TO TRAUMA

Chronic trauma to the Hertwig's epithelial root sheath, such as orthodontic intrusion of immature teeth, often leads to its fragmentation. In these cases the epithelial fragments displaced into the pulp canal can induce true denticle formation (i.e. dentin-containing pulp stones) (83-87).

An injury close to the root sheath (e.g. a laceration in the PDL) may result in temporary hyperactivity of the root sheath which can initiate rapid production of both dentin and cementum in the apical area (Fig. 2.12). However, activity of the root sheath will later return to normal (see Chapter 10, p. 415).

An *acute* trauma to the epithelial root sheath, transmitted *indirectly*, for example by the intrusion of a primary tooth, or *directly* by forceful displacement of imma-

ture permanent teeth, can damage HERS and lead to partial or complete arrest of root development (88-91) (Fig. 2.13).

During replantation, the root sheath may be injured either during avulsion, during extraoral storage, or by the repositioning procedure. Following such injury, further root growth will be partially or totally arrested; and bone and PDL-derived tissue from the base of the socket may invade the root canal to form intraradicular bone which is separated from the canal wall by an *internal periodontal ligament* (92) (Fig. 2.14) (see also Chapter 10, p. 415). A similar bony invasion into the pulp of immature teeth is found when the epithelial root sheath is resected *in situ* (93-95), or when the root sheath is injured chemically, as with devitalization procedures that employ formaldehyde (96,97).

Fig. 2.13.
Damage to the cervical diaphragm or the HERS subsequent to replantation of permanent lateral monkey incisors. Observation period: 1 week. A. Displacement of cervical diaphragm. x 25. B. Fragmentation of the root sheath. x 75.

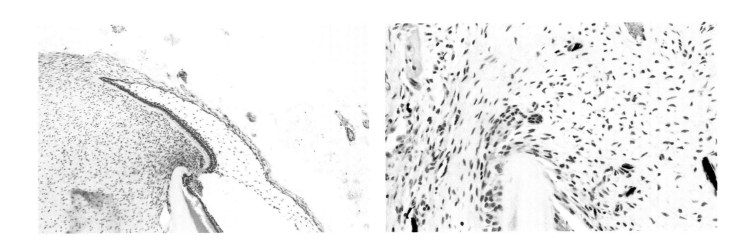

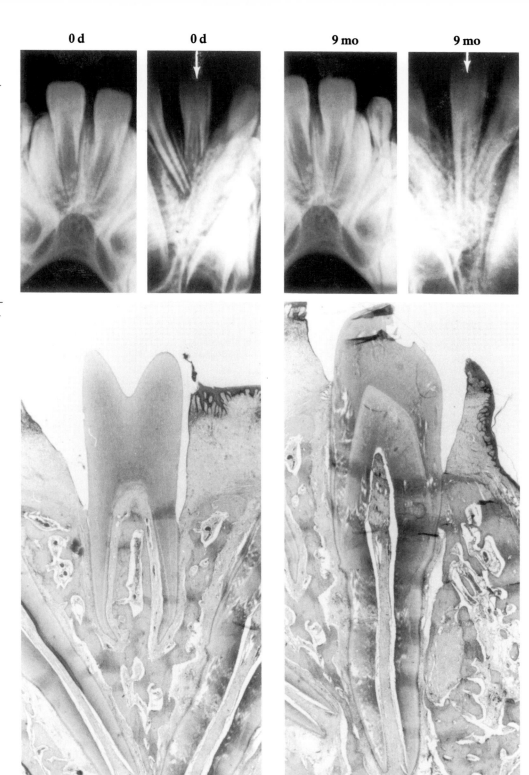

Fig. 2.14. Effect of trauma to HERS upon root growth
The right permanent central incisor in a monkey was extracted and the HERS was traumatized by pressing the apex against the socket wall before repositioning. The left central incisor was extracted and repositioned as a control.

Condition 9 months after surgery in a monkey
Root development has stopped and bone has entered the root canal in the right central incisor. The left central incisor shows normal root development. From AN-DREASEN ET AL. (93) 1988

0 d   0 d   9 mo   9 mo

RESPONSE TO INFECTION

Hertwig's epithelial root sheath is rather resistant to inflammation in connection with partial pulp necrosis. Although sometimes restricted, root formation has been found to occur in most cases of partial pulp necrosis irrespective of whether endodontic therapy has been instituted or not (see also Chapter 10, p. 415). This would seem to imply that HERS can continue to function despite inflammation (93,98-104). In this context, there appears to be a critical distance between the root sheath and pathological changes in the pulp. If that distance is too short, inflammation will destroy the root sheath and

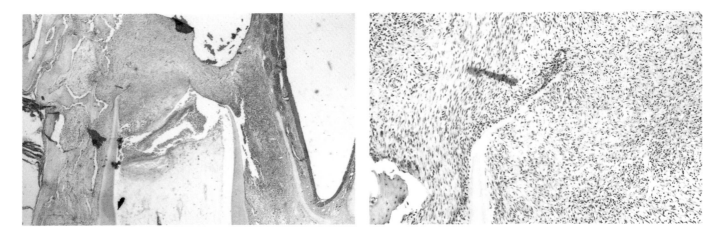

Fig. 2.15.
Critical distance between pulp necrosis and survival of HERS. The permanent central maxillary incisor was autotransplanted to the contralateral side in a monkey 1 week previously. x 25. Pulp necrosis extending to the apex mesially whereas the pulp necrosis zone is 1 mm short of the distal aspect of the apex. The HERS has survived and some root formation has occurred. x 75. From AN-DREASEN ET AL. (93) *1988.*

root formation will be arrested (93) (Fig. 2.15). The fact that the epithelial root sheath can continue to function despite inflammation elicited by a partial pulp necrosis demonstrates that continued root development and apical closure as such cannot be taken as criteria for pulpal vitality (see Chapter 14, p. 542).

Teeth with Developed Roots

Gingival and Periosteal Complex

The gingiva is usually involved during crown-root and root fractures, luxation injuries and always during tooth avulsion. In addition, the periosteum is always involved during lateral luxation and alveolar bone fractures. In the following, the anatomy and function of the gingiva and periosteum will be described, as will their response to trauma and infection.

Gingiva

Gingiva is defined from an anatomic point of view as either *free* or *attached*. The *free gingiva* comprises the vestibular and oral gingival tissue as well as the interdental papillae. Clinically, the apical border of the free gingiva is usually circumscribed by the *free gingival groove* (Fig. 2.16).

The *attached gingiva* is circumscribed coronally by the free gingival groove and apically by the mucogingival junction. The attached gingiva is firmly bound to the periosteum by collagenous fibers and is resistant to elevation.

The *alveolar mucosa* borders the attached gingiva and is loosely bound to periosteum, thereby offering minimal resistance to the formation of a subperiosteal hematoma which can develop after lateral luxation, alveolar fracture, or rupture from traction due to an impact parallel to the labial surface of the mandible or maxilla.

The function of the *free gingiva* is to seal, maintain and defend the critical area where the tooth penetrates its connective tissue bed and enters the oral cavity.

The gingival epithelium immediately adjacent to the tooth and *junctional epithelium* is designed to seal the periodontium from the oral cavity (Fig. 2.16).

Gingival epithelium displays a specific anatomy, being narrow and consisting of a few cell layers without rete pegs. The development of the junctional epithelium is closely related to tooth eruption. Thus, the junctional epithelium shows cell division originating in the basal layers, with cells being ultimately exfoliated into the gingival sulcus. Two zones can be recognized by transmission electron microscopy between the superficial cells of the junctional epithelium and the enamel; namely, the *lamina densa* and the *lamina lucida*, together called the *internal basement lamina*. Hemidesmosomes are formed by the epithelium adjacent to the lamina lu-

Fig. 2.16. Anatomy of the gingiva and periosteal complex
1. *Sharpey's fibers*
2. *Dentoperiosteal fibers*
3. *Alveologingival fibers*
4. *Dentogingival fibers*
5. *Junctional epithelium*
6. *Gingival epithelium*
7. *Sulcular Epithelium*
8. *Periosteogingival fibers*
9. *Intergingival fibers*
10. *Circular fibers*

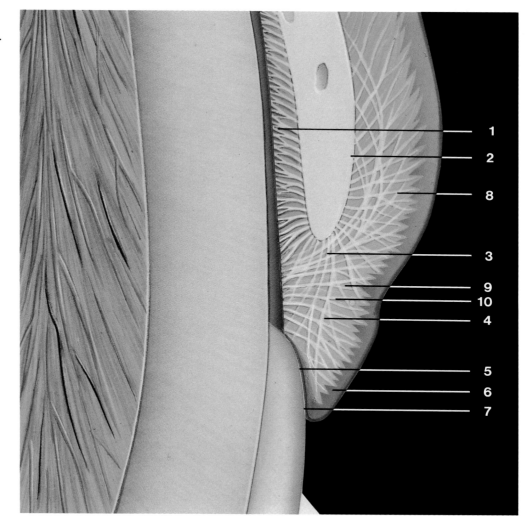

cida, and these create an interphase with the enamel analogous to that with the subepithelial connective tissue (105).

Dental cuticle and sometimes a layer of fibrillar cementum can be seen interposed between this epithelium and the enamel. The *sulcular epithelium* faces the tooth without being in direct contact with it (Fig. 2.16). This epithelium is thicker than the junctional epithelium and has abundant rete pegs.

The *fibrillar system* of the gingiva is complex, comprising groups of collagen fibers with different sites of insertion (106-112) (Fig. 2.16):

The *dentinogingival fibers* originate in cementum and insert in the free gingiva. The *dentoperiosteal fibers* start at the same site, but insert into the attached gingiva. The *transseptal fibers* extend from cementum in the supra-alveolar region and insert into the supra-alveolar cementum of the adjacent tooth. The *circular fibers* encircle the tooth in a ring-like, supra-alveolar course. These fibers are responsible for the very rapid initial closure of an extraction wound (see p. 102), as well as the rapid adaptation of the gingiva around luxated or replanted teeth (see p. 95). Finally, *alveolo-gingival fibers* emanate from the top of the alveolar crest and fan out into the attached gingiva.

The blood supply to the gingiva originates from three sources: The *periodontal ligament*, the *crestal bone* and the *supra-periosteal blood vessels* (see p. 97). This ensures survival of the marginal gingiva even after severe laceration or contusion (see Chapter 13, p. 50).

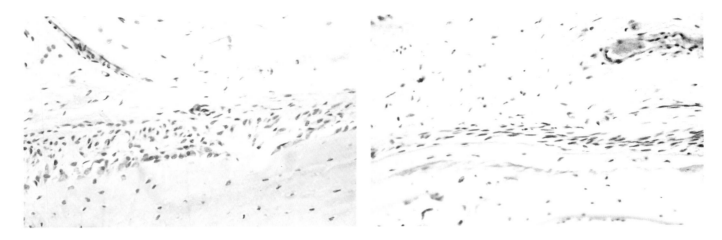

Fig. 2.17.
A. Cellular alveolar periosteum in a young *monkey (root development of permanent incisors incomplete). O= osteoblasts. P=precursor cells. F=fibroblasts. x 75. B. Periosteum in an* old *monkey. Note the difference in the configuration of periosteum. x 75.*

Periosteum

The *alveolar periosteum* covers the alveolar process. In *young* individuals, at the time of active bone growth, it consists of an inner layer of *angular* osteoblasts followed by spindle-shaped precursor cells supported by loosely arranged collagen fibers (Fig. 2.17). In *older* individuals, where growth has ceased, the inner layer consists of *flattened* osteoblasts followed by an outer fibrous layer of inactive osteoprogenitor cells which however, still maintain their potential for cell division (113-115) (Fig. 2.17).

The periosteum serves an important function in appositional growth, remodelling and bone repair after injury. Furthermore, it anchors muscles and carries blood vessels, lymphatic vessels and nerves.

RESPONSE TO TRAUMA
The gingival attachment is often torn during luxation injuries and always during avulsions. In an experimental replantation study in monkeys, the junctional epithelium showed increased autoradiographic labelling of cells as early as after 1 day, and reached a peak after 3 days. After 7 days, a new junctional epithelium was formed (116). In the connective tissue, the ruptured gingival and transseptal collagen fibers were united in the majority of cases after 1 week (117-119) (see also p. 99).

The response of periosteum to trauma is not very well described. Displacement of the attached gingiva or the alveolar mucosa involves injury to the periosteum and the underlying bone (120-157). Thus, the surface of bone is affected in several ways. Firstly, the cortical bone plate loses an important part of its vascular supply. Secondly, the cellular cover of bone provided by the innermost layer of periosteum is partially or totally removed. These two events invite an initial resorption of the bony surface which, however, is then followed by bony deposition to repair the initial loss.

In addition to bone loss due to displacement of gingiva or alveolar mucosa, bone may also be lost directly due to trauma. In such cases, an important factor related to healing is the osteogenic potential of the periosteum, which is strongly influenced by age (148-150). Thus, when a periosteal flap is raised in *adult* animals, the osteogenic layer is usually disrupted and periosteal osteogenesis can only take place from the periphery of the wound where progenitor cells have not been disturbed (151-154), implying that bony repair will be limited and fibrous scar tissue will often form in its place (158,159).

Conversely, in young animals, cells in the cambium layer of elevated flaps exhibit osteogenic potential and the bone contour is often fully repaired. In humans, surgical removal of large portions of the mandible, but with intentional preservation of the periosteum, has been seen to result in extensive new bone formation (156,157).

RESPONSE TO INFECTION
The general reaction of gingiva to infection has been the subject of numerous studies related to plaque-induced gingi-

vitis and is beyond the scope of this text. The significance of infection will be discussed only as it relates to the gingival attachment after traumatic or surgical injury. In monkeys, it has been shown that incisional wounds from the gingival sulcus to the alveolar crest lead to epithelial growth through most of the supracrestal area when gingival inflammation is induced (160).

The role of bacteria in gingival healing after surgical injury has been assessed only indirectly through the effect of antibiotic therapy. The use of antibiotics (tetracycline) in rats after injuries to pulpal, gingival and root tissues was shown to promote gingival and periodontal reattachment (161-163). In humans, it was demonstrated that the administration of erythromycin for 4 days after gingivectomy led to completed epithelialization after 1 week, in contrast to only two-thirds of the specimens when no antibiotic coverage was given (163). In conclusion, there is some evidence that bacteria-induced gingival inflammation has a negative influence upon wound healing after trauma and surgical injury.

If an odontogenic infection spreads from bone marrow to the periosteal layer and an abscess is formed between periosteum and cortical bone, the blood supply to the immediately underlying cortical bone can be compromised. The cortical bone can then undergo ischemic necrosis, resulting in an undermining resorption (164).

Periodontal Ligament-Cementum Complex

The anatomical border for the periodontal ligament (PDL) is the most cervically located of the principal fibers (Sharpey's fibers) that insert into both cementum and alveolar bone (Fig. 2.18). In this context, only the anatomy and function of the more important cellular and fibrillar structures of the periodontal ligament will be considered.

Cementoblasts

Cementoblasts are spindle or polyhedral shaped cells whose long axes are usually oriented parallel to the root surface. The cytoplasm is basophilic and the nuclei are round or ovoid (Fig. 2.19). These cells are said to be active or resting according to the relative amount of cytoplasm. Resting cells contain less cytoplasm than active cementoblasts (165). Cementoblasts produce the organic matrix of cementum (i.e. intrinsic collagen fibers and ground substance), while the extrinsic fibers (i.e. Sharpey's fibers) are formed by fibroblasts from the PDL (166). If the cementoblast becomes incorporated into the mineralizing front, cellular cementum is formed. The deposition of cementum appears to occur rhythmically throughout life, at a speed of approximately 3 μm per year (167). Periods of activity alternate with periods of quiescence, thereby giving rise to incremental lines (168).

Periodontal Fibroblasts

These cells are spindle-shaped, with several points of contact with adjacent cells. The nuclei are oval, containing one or more prominent nucleoli (Fig. 2.18). In sections parallel to Sharpey's fibers, fibroblasts appear as spindle-shaped cells with only occasional contact with other fibroblasts (Fig. 2.18). In transverse sections, however, they are seen as stellate cells whose processes envelope the principal periodontal fiber bundles and connect with many other fibroblasts to form a cellular network (169). This intricate relationship between fibroblasts and Sharpey's fibers after injury may be important in the rapid degradation or reformation of Sharpey's fibers (171,172). Recent anatomical (170) and *in vitro* studies (173) suggest that different fibroblast populations exist in the PDL (174).

Fibroblasts are responsible for the formation, maintenance and remodelling of PDL fibers and their associated ground substance. By using tritiated thymidine labelling, it has been found that fibroblasts comprise a very active cell renewal system. In mice, for example, a cell turnover rate of 30% was seen when continuous labelling was used over a period of 25 days (174,175). Furthermore, cell renewal took place as a clonal paravascular proliferation of cells. Together with simultaneous cell death in the PDL, a steady state was created in the cellular content of the periodontal ligament (175-177).

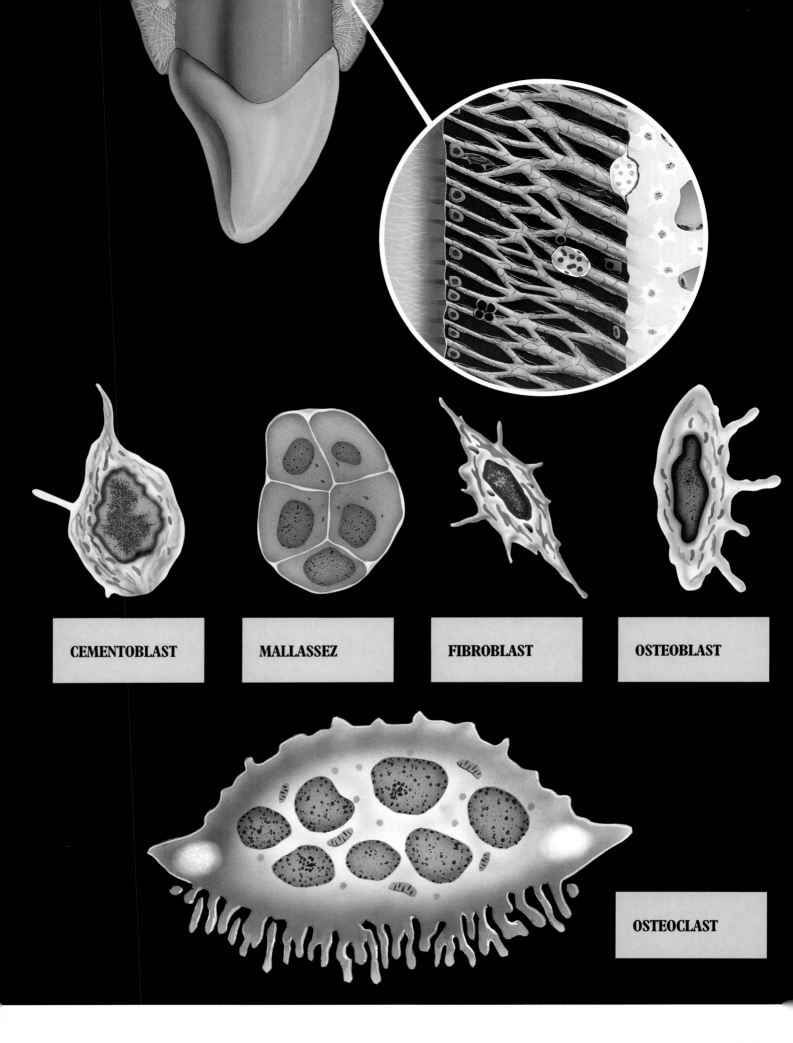

CEMENTOBLAST

MALLASSEZ

FIBROBLAST

OSTEOBLAST

OSTEOCLAST

Fig. 2.18. Anatomy of the periodontal ligament
Sharpey's fibers
Cementoblast
Mallassez epithelial island
Fibroblast
Osteoblast
Osteoclast

Another important function of fibroblasts in the PDL is the maintenance of periodontal fibers. This function is manifested by very rapid collagen synthesis and degradation (turnover)(178-182), occurring primarily in the middle zone of the PDL (183). Thus, it has been shown that the half-life of collagen in the PDL of rats is about 6-9 days (184,185). Moreover, collagen turnover is considerably more rapid in PDL collagen than in that of gingiva, pulp or other connective tissues in the body (186,187). This very rapid turnover in the PDL is in agreement with findings from studies in PDL wound healing, where very rapid healing of the periodontium has been demonstrated after surgical injury (see p. 98).

Finally, for the sake of completeness, it should be mentioned that periodontal fibroblasts are also responsible for synthesis and maintenance of other fibers, such as elastin and oxytalan.

Osteoblasts

The osteoblast is slightly larger than the cementoblast and has a circular or ovoid nucleus which is usually located eccentrically. The cytoplasm is abundant and very basophilic during osteogenesis (Fig. 2.18). Like the cementoblast, the osteoblast is found in an active or resting form, as revealed by less cytoplasm in the latter form.

Epithelial Rests of Mallassez

A network of epithelial cells is found in the PDL positioned close to the root surface (Fig. 2.18). These cells originate from the successive breakdown of the Hertwig's epithelial root sheath during root formation(see p. 88).

These epithelial cells have been proposed as playing a role in the homeostasis of the PDL (439, 440). However, recent experimental studies do not support this theory (441,442,443). On the other hand, these cells represent an important part of the defense system of the PDL against invading bacteria from the root canal. Bacterial invasion of both the main and lateral canals leads to proliferation and adherence of the epithelial cells to the root canal openings to the PDL to form an epithelial barrier against the invaders (444).

Periodontal Ligament Fibers

The vast majority of collagen fibers in the PDL are arranged in bundles, the so-called principal fibers (Sharpey's fibers) (Fig. 2.18). These fibers are embedded in both cementum and bone. In their course from cementum to alveolar bone, they are often wavy at their midpoint, giving the impression of an intermediate plexus, with interdigitation of fibers. However, recent scanning electron microscopic studies seem to indicate that the majority of the principal fibers span the entire PDL space, although they usually branch and join adjacent fibers to create a ladder-like architecture in the PDL (188-202) (Fig. 2.18). The principal fibers extending from cementum to bone can be classified according to their direction and location into horizontal, oblique and apical fibers. In the gingiva, the supraalveolar (gingival) fibers can be classified into dento-gingival fibers, dentoperiosteal fibers, interdental fibers and circular fibers (Fig. 2.16)(see p. 93).

The main function of the PDL is to support the tooth in its alveolus during function. Whenever functional demands are changed, corresponding adjustments take place in the architecture of the PDL, such that the orientation, amount and insertion pattern of the principal fibers are altered.

Periodontal Vasculature

The blood supply to the PDL at the *midportion* of the root appears to arise from branches of the superior or inferior alveolar arteries. Before theses arteries enter the apical foramen, they give off branches to the interdental bone. On their way to the alveolar crest, they give off multiple branches which perforate the socket wall and form a plexus which surrounds the root surface (203-208)(Fig. 2.19). This plexus is located in the interstitial spaces between Sharpey's fibers. In primates, the majority of these vessels are located close to the bone surface (207) (Fig. 2.19). *Apically*, the blood supply to the PDL originates from branches of the dental arteries which are released as they cross the PDL and enter the pulp. *Cervically*, however, anastomoses are formed with gingival vessels (Fig. 2.19).

The blood supply to the *gingiva* appears

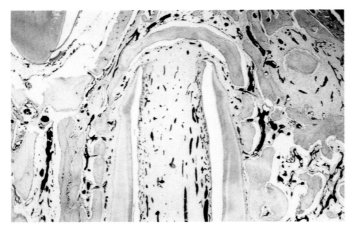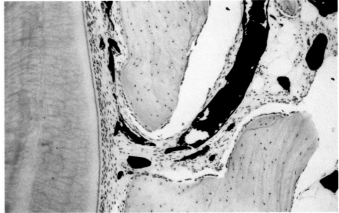

Fig. 2.19.
Vascular supply to the PDL in a longitudinally sectioned permanent maxillary central incisor in a monkey shown by indian ink perfusion. x 10. The interdental arteries give off multiple branches to the midportion of the PDL. x 100.

to arise primarily from the supraperiosteal blood vessels, which anastomose in the gingiva with vessels from the PDL and branches of the interdental arteries and which perforate the crestal bone margin or the labial or lingual bone plate.

Periodontal Innervation

The PDL has receptors for pain, touch, pressure and proprioception, which all belong to the somatic nervous system. Autonomic nerves are also present, which innervate the blood vessels. In general, periodontal innervation follows the same pathways as the blood supply.

Homeostatic Mechanism of PDL

PDL appears to exist throughout life with minimal variations in width (209). This dimension is primarily controlled by age and function, but it is also affected by pathology (505).

The decisive structure for preserving homeostasis appears to reside within the innermost layer of the PDL (i.e. possibly cementoblasts and immediately adjacent cells) (209).

RESPONSE TO TRAUMA
Following a severe dental injury (e.g. lateral luxation or intrusion) the PDL must respond to a variety of insults. These can include temporary compressive, tensile or shearing stresses, which result in hemorrhage and edema, rupture or contusion of the PDL. Each of these injuries can induce varying wound-healing signals.

The cellular kinetics of healing in the PDL associated with a surgical wound have been examined using tritiated thymidine labelling of proliferating cells. Thus, in mice, paravascular cells were labelled within 100 μm of the margin of the injured PDL. Some of these cells moved into the injury zone 3-5 days after injury and divided (211). It would appear that in the PDL there is a population of paravascular cells which exhibits a high nuclear/cytoplasmic ratio and which remains stable throughout wound healing, but provides a front of new cells that migrate into the wound and then divide (210,214) (Fig. 2.20). The identity of these progenitor cells is only partially known at present. It is possible that progenitor cells placed in the middle of the PDL supply the fibroblast population (211, 214), while progenitor cells close to the alveolar bone develop into osteoblasts (211-216). Cementoblasts precursors have not yet been identified; however, there is some indication that the progenitors for this cell population are located away from blood vessels (214,216).

Bleeding and Edema
Very little is known about healing events after bleeding or edema in the PDL sub-

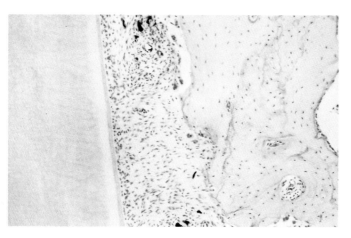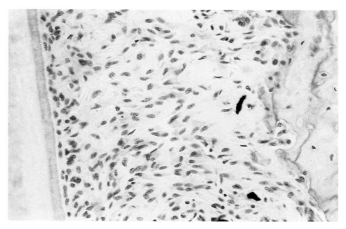

Fig. 2.20.
A. Healing of the periodontal ligament after replantation of a permanent monkey incisor. The monkey was perfused with indian ink at sacrifice 1 week after replantation. x 25. B. The PDL is very cellular and has lost its typical parallel arrangement of the fibroblasts. In a few places Sharpey's fibers appear united. x 100.

sequent to minor trauma (e.g. concussion or subluxation). However, in a clinical luxation study, a higher frequency of surface resorption was seen following concussion injury than after subluxation (217), suggesting that pressure from bleeding into the PDL after a mild injury might elicit minor areas of damage to the root surface. In the case of subluxations, where the impact is great enough to cause tooth loosening, this pressure can be relieved; however when no loosening results (i.e. concussion), pressure will be reflected in subsequent surface resorption.

Rupture of the PDL
There has been little investigation into the healing of a ruptured PDL. The few available studies are either of extrusive luxation (215,219-221) or of extraction and subsequent replantation (116-118,222).

In monkeys, it appears that rupture of the fibers after extrusion or extraction usually occurs midway between the alveolar bone and the root surface. However, rupture can also be seen close to either the alveolar wall or the root surface. After 1 week, the split in the periodontal ligament is occupied by proliferating fibroblasts and blood vessels. In isolated areas, union of

Fig. 2.21. Healing with minor injury to the periodontal ligament
The injury site is resorbed by macrophages and osteoclasts. Subsequent repair takes place by the formation of new cementum and Sharpey's fibers.

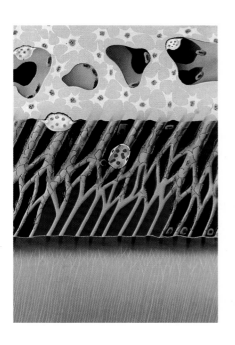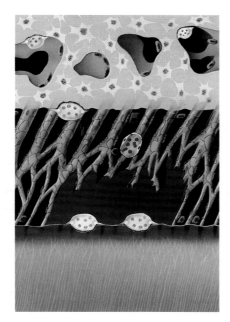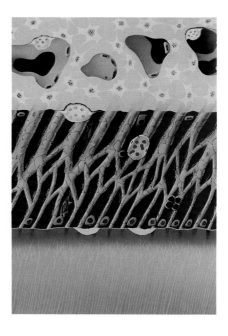

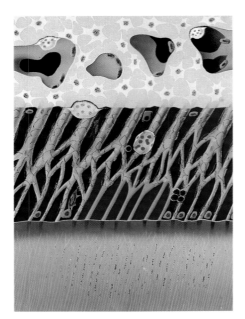 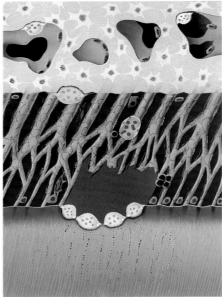 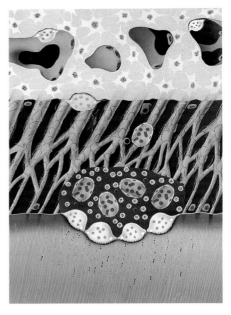

Fig. 2.22. Healing with moderate injury to the periodontal ligament and associated infection in the pulp and/or dentinal tubules

The initial injury to the root surface triggers a macrophage and osteoclast attack on the root surface. If the resorption cavity exposes infected dentinal tubules which can transmit bacterial toxins, the resorption process is accelerated and granulation tissue ultimately invades the root canal.

Fig. 2.23. Healing after extensive injury to the periodontal ligament

Ankylosis is formed because healing occurs almost exclusively by cells from the alveolar wall.

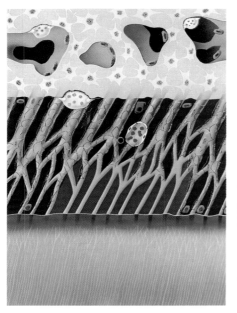 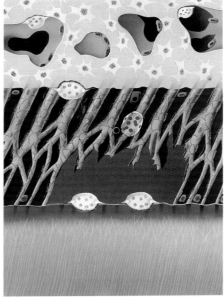 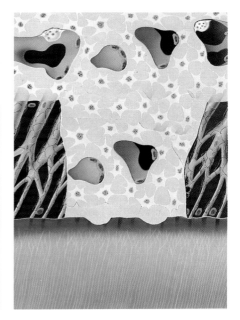

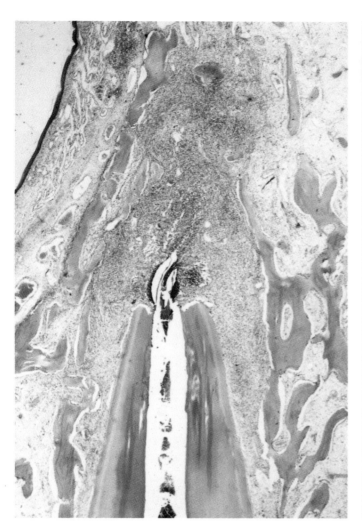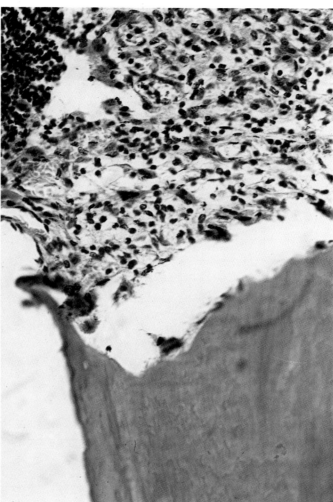

Fig. 2.24.
Periapical inflammation and apical root resorption subsequent to pulp necrosis in a replanted permanent monkey incisor. x 10 and x 100.

the principal fibers has already taken place (Fig. 2.20). After 2 weeks, a substantial number of principal fibers have healed (118). At that time, the mechanical properties of the injured PDL are about 50-60% of that of an uninjured PDL (219). With longer observation periods, an increased number of healed principal fibers can be seen. After 8 weeks, the injured PDL cannot be distinguished histologically from an uninjured control (219).

Contusion Injuries of the PDL
During intrusion, lateral luxation or avulsion with subsequent replantation, contusion of the PDL is a common occurrence. Wound healing is subsequently initiated when damaged tissue is removed by macrophage or osteoclast activity (see p. 112). During these events, not only are necrotic PDL tissue remnants removed, but sometimes also bone and cementum. The latter can lead to either surface or inflammatory resorption, depending upon the age of the patient, the stage of root development and

pulp status (Figs. 2.21 and 2.22) (209,223). When large areas of the PDL are traumatized, competitive wound healing processes begin between bone marrow-derived cells destined to form bone and PDL-derived cells which are programmed to form PDL fibers and cementum (209,223) resulting in either a transient or permanent ankylosis (Fig. 2.23).

RESPONSE TO INFECTION
Progression of gingival infection or spread of infection from the root canal through the apical foramen, accessory canals or dentinal tubules are the most common routes of infection of the PDL. Accordingly, the following discussion will emphasize PDL reactions due to infection in the root canal.

Cellular kinetics of the PDL due to pulpal infection have been examined in rats using tritiated thymidine. It was shown that after 1 hour there was increased labelling of fibroblasts, osteoblasts and cementoblasts which reached a peak after 2 to 3 days. The increase in cellular activity continued in osteoblasts and fibroblasts for 30 days (the end of the experiment) while the cementoblast layer returned to its normal level after 25 days (224,225).

Moderate or intense periapical inflammation has been found to lead to a breakdown of PDL fibers and resorption of the root apex and bone, resulting in an expansion of the PDL space or a periapical rarefaction (226-233) (Fig. 2.24). This resorption response has been found to be related to the presence of bacteria and their toxins in the root canal (234-243). The stimulus for osteoclastic activity affecting the root surface and alveolar bone appears to be a combination of a direct influence of bacteria and their toxins and an indirect influence on the osteoclast in response to inflammatory changes (209,223,244,245).(Fig 2.24)(see p. 112). The cell population in the PDL, however, appears to be rather resistant to infection in the sense that, when infection has been eliminated, the PDL usually returns to normal. This phenomenon has been found in the marginal periodontium (246,247), in the apical periodontium (248,249) and in situations involving the entire PDL, such as after osteomyelitis (250). However, if the infection is not completely eradicated, chronic inflammation will develop and allow only minimal cementum and PDL repair (225,251).

Alveolar Bone and Marrow Complex

The alveolar process may be defined as the tooth-supporting region of the mandible or maxilla (Fig. 2.25). It is made up of three components: (1) the *alveolar bone proper*, consisting of a thin plate of bone which provides attachment for either the dental follicle or the principal fibers of the PDL (252), (2) the *cortical bone plates* which form the outer and inner plates of the alveolar process, and (3) the *cancellous bone* and *bone marrow* which occupy the area between the cortical bone plates and the alveolar bone proper.

The *alveolar bone proper* consists of a thin, perforated bone plate which appears radiographically as a radiopaque lining around the radiolucent PDL space (i.e. lamina dura). The perforations in the socket wall function as gateways for vascular channels that supply the periodontal ligament (253) (see p. 98).

The *cortical bone plates* form the lateral borders of the alveolar process and are usually much thinner in the maxilla than in the mandible. In the incisor and canine regions, there is usually no cancellous bone or bone marrow to separate the lamina dura from the cortical plates, and this results in a fusion of these structures. For this reason, lateral luxation of maxillary incisors produces a combined fracture of the lamina dura and the cortical bone plate.

The *cancellous bone* consists of thin bone trabeculae which encircle the bone marrow. These trabeculae are lined with a delicate layer of connective tissue cells, the *endosteum*. The *bone marrow* consists of a reticulate tissue in which cells representing different stages of hematogenesis occupy the mesh (*red bone marrow*). If the hematopoietic cells disappear, the reticulate tissue is replaced either by adipose tissue (*yellow bone marrow*) or, as in some areas in the alveolar process, by fibrous tissue (*fibrous bone marrow*) (254). The exact topographical distribution of the various types of bone marrow in humans has not yet been documented.

As previously mentioned, the primary function of the *alveolar process* is to protect and support the dentition. More specifically, the *alveolar bone proper* protects the developing tooth and later provides an anchorage for the fibers of the PDL (255). Apart from its hemopoietic function, the *bone marrow* plays an important role in osteogenesis. Thus, the reticular cells of the bone marrow stroma can manifest osteogenic activity when stimulated by trauma (256). Furthermore, bone marrow plays an important role in the defense against infection (243).

RESPONSE TO TRAUMA
The most common traumatic injury to the alveolar bone complex is the extraction/avulsion or luxation wound with displacement. Furthermore, the bone becomes involved after alveolar and bone fractures (see Chapter 11 p. 436).

Extensive studies have been conducted regarding socket healing after extraction whereas none has yet been performed relating to tooth luxation. The following is a synopsis of what is presently known about human extraction wounds.

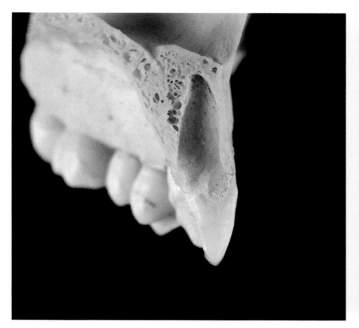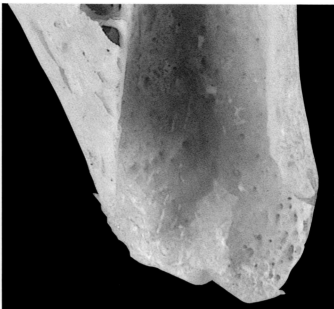

Fig. 2.25. Anatomy of the alveolar bone.
Section through the central incisor region in a human jaw. Note the fused alveolar bone proper and cortical bone plate labially whereas both structures can be recognized palatally. Furthermore, multiple vascular canals perforate the lamina dura.

Histologic Evidence of Socket Healing

The following *overlapping* stages have been found histologically, based on biopsies from healing of normal extraction wounds in human patients (257-269).

Stage I. A *coagulum* is formed once hemostasis has been established. It consists of erythrocytes and leukocytes, in the same ratio as in circulating blood, entrapped in a mesh of precipitated fibrin.

Stage II. Granulation tissue is formed along the socket walls 2-3 days postoperatively and is characterized by proliferating endothelial cells, capillaries and many leukocytes. Within 7 days, granulation tissue has usually replaced the coagulum.

Stage III. Connective tissue formation begins peripherally and, within 20 days postoperatively, replaces granulation tissue. This newly-formed connective tissue comprises cells, collagen and reticular fibers dispersed in a metachromatic ground substance.

Stage IV. Bone development begins 7 days postoperatively. It starts peripherally, at the base of the alveolus. The major contributors to alveolar healing appear to be cancellous bone and bone marrow while the remaining PDL apparently plays an insignificant role (270,271). By 38 days, the socket is almost completely occupied by immature bone. Within 2-3 months, this bone is mature and forms trabeculae; after 3-4 months, maturation is complete (268).

Stage V. Epithelial repair begins closing the wound 4 days after extraction and is usually complete after 24 days.

Finally, it should be mentioned that socket healing has been found to be significantly influenced by the *age* of the individual (259,269). Thus, histological alveolar socket repair is more active 10 days postoperatively in individuals in the 2nd decade of life, while the same stage of activity is seen about 20 days postoperatively in individuals in the 6th decade or more. However, after 30 days, the healing sequence levels out and becomes identical in the two age groups (269).

RESPONSE TO INFECTION

The most common situations in which the alveolar bone becomes involved in infection is during marginal or periapical periodontitis (272,273). As the most frequent complication after replantation procedures and certain luxation types is infection of necrotic pulp tissue, emphasis will be placed on the reaction of the alveolar bone to periapical infection.

Infected necrotic pulp tissue can elicit chronic or acute periapical inflammation. *Acute inflammation* in the form of a periapical abscess is the response to invasion by virulent bacteria or immune complexes in the periapex (274). Histologically, there

is an accumulation periapically of polymorphonuclear leukocytes and disintegration of the PDL. More peripherally, there
is intense osteoclastic activity to remove
periapical bone in order to provide space
for the granulation tissue required to com-
bat infection (275).

The result of a low-grade periapical infection is *chronic inflammation* in the formation of a periapical granuloma. In this
situation, the bacterial front is either in the
root canal or just outside the apical foramen (276-278). Lymphocytes appear to be
the dominant cells in the immediate
periapical region, accompanied by polymorphonuclear leukocytes, macrophages and fibroblasts (277-286,445-447).
This cell population is identical to that
of the infiltrate found in advanced marginal periodontitis (273,286-289). In the
capsule surrounding the periapical inflammatory zone, the dominant cell is
the PDL fibroblast. This can be regarded as an extension of the PDL (286).

The osteoclastic activity responsible for
resorption of periapical bone and subsequent expansion of the developing granuloma is most likely the result of the combined action of breakdown products of
arachidonic acids (i.e. prostaglandins,
thromboxanes, leukotrines and lipoxines)
from phospholipids of cell membranes
from leukocytes, macrophages and platelets (282,290-299,310). Cytokines released
by activated lymphocytes and plasma cells
(294-302) include immunecomplexes released by B lymphocytes (291), and bacterial toxins (e.g. lipopolysaccaride (LPS),
muramyl dipeptide (MDP) and, lipotei-
choic acid (LTA) (303-309,448), (Fig. 2.27)).
These events are described in more detail
in the section on hard tissue resorption
(see p. 113).

Periapically, the long-term effect of
chronic infection is a change in the bone
marrow from predominantly fatty to predominantly fibrous (313,314). An occasional
finding is periapical osteosclerosis, whereby
bone marrow is replaced by thickened spon-
giosa, resulting in a radiodense area (315,316).
The latter reaction is assumed to be the
response to a low-grade irritant (infection ?)
in the area. Supporting this hypothesis is the
finding that osteosclerotic lesions often disappear when proper endodontic therapy is instituted (317,318).

In jaw fractures, *acute* infection in the
line of the fracture has been found to be
related to a number of different factors,
which are described in Chapter 11.

Dentin-Pulp Complex
Dentin

Dentin consists of a mineralized organic
matrix dominated by an intricate collagen
lattice skeleton and traversed by dentinal
tubules.

Rɛsponse to trauma
Any deviation in the composition of the
organic structure of dentin may lead to
fracture. Thus, teeth in patients suffering
from dentinogenesis imperfecta, with its
inherent defects in the collagen matrix,
have a high risk of tooth fracture (319-321).
Furthermore, exposure of dentinal tubules during trauma leads to bacterial invasion with a resultant permanent or tran-
sitory inflammatory reaction in the pulp
(322,323). Finally, a weakening of the dentin
under physical loads may occur due to
early pulpectomy in immature teeth
(324,325). This may be intensified if inflammatory resorption weakens the root structure, especially in the cervical region (325).

Pulp

The pulp is a highly specialized loose connective tissue with a specific response to
surgical and traumatic injuries, as well as
to bacterial insults (Fig. 2.26). The predominant cells in the pulp are the fibroblasts, which appear as spindle-shaped or
stellate cells with oval nuclei and are dispersed uniformly throughout the pulp, except in the subodontoblastic layer. Undifferentiated mesenchymal cells are located
paravascularly and can be recognized by
their stunted or rounded form and their
few, short processes. These cells probably
play an important role in pulpal repair (326)
(see p. 106). Pericytes and macrophages
are also found in the same location (Fig.
2.26).

Odontoblasts are elongated cells subjacent to the dentin. They have a distally
oriented nucleus and processes which extend some distance into the dentinal tubules (327,328) (Fig. 2.26). Their appearance varies from the coronal to the apical
aspect of the pulp, being columnar coronally and flattened apically. Moreover,

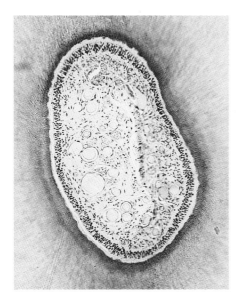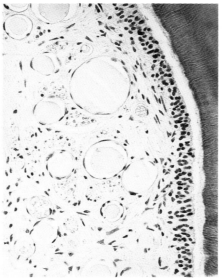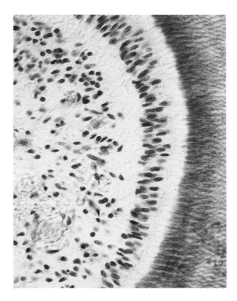

Fig. 2.26.
A. Horizontal section of a pulp from a maxillary permanent monkey incisor. Root development is complete. Note the distribution of the larger vessels and nerves x 10. B and C. The odontoblast layer and the subodontoblastic cell free zone. x 40 and x 100

their appearance is also related to their functional stage (i.e. preodontoblasts, secretory, transitional or aged (329)). Odontoblasts have many junctions, suggestive of communication between cells (330).

In the crown, a cell-free layer (i.e. the subodontoblastic layer or zone of Weil) exists that contains a network of nerve endings and vessels which, to a lesser degree, is also found in other parts of the pulp.

The cellular activities of odontoblasts are very complex. Beyond elaboration of the organic matrix of predentin and control of calcium and phosphate ion transfer, the odontoblast plays a major role in degradative processes of components of the organic matrix (330). The average production of primary human dentin appears to be 3 μm per day during tooth formation and eruption (331). When eruption is complete, dentin formation decreases in the pulp chamber. In the root, production continues unchanged until root formation is complete, at which time dentin production is decreased to an extent that is not measurable over a 3-week period. Dentinogenesis, however, can be reactivated by external stimuli, such as dental caries, attrition and dentin fracture and luxation injuries. The production of new dentin can then rise to a level of that of primary dentin (331,332).

Pulpal Vasculature

The vascular supply to the immature human dental pulp consists of multiple thin-walled arterioles, venules and veins passing through the apical foramen (333-335). In the mature tooth, vessels can also enter the tooth through lateral canals. The arterioles and venules run parallel to the canal walls up to the pulp horns (Fig. 2.27). En route, they give off branches to form a dense peripheral capillary plexus in the subodontoblastic layer. A few loops are also found between the odontoblasts (333-335) (Fig. 2.27).

Within the pulp, especially apically, there are many arterio-venous connections (shunts) which facilitate and regulate blood flow (336-339). These shunts are important in the control of tissue pressure due to inflammation when, during the initial inflammatory reaction, several vasoactive agents are released (see p. 120). These agents cause edema and an increase in tissue pressure. When this pressure exceeds that of the venules, a decrease in blood flow results. The arterio-venous anastomoses in the apical part of the pulp dilate in this situation and carry the blood away from the injury zone (337).

The number of vessels entering the apical foramen appears to a certain degree to be related to the maturity of the tooth. However, the density of the vessels is not in direct proportion to the constriction of the pulpo-periodontal interphase.

The pulpal nerves generally follow the course of the blood vessels (Fig. 2.26). Two types of nerves are found, the *nonmyelinated nerves* which are responsible for vasoconstriction and dilation, and the *myelinated nerves* which respond to pain stimuli. The number of myelinated fibers increases with tooth maturity and, at the

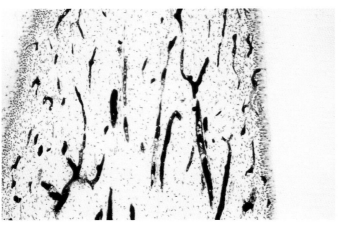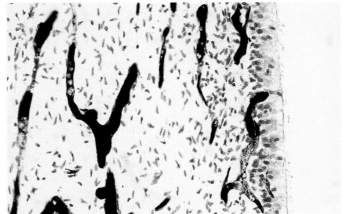

Fig. 2.27.
Vascular pattern in the pulp of a permanent monkey incisor as revealed by indian ink perfusion.
x 40. B. Note the dense network of capillaries next to the odontoblastic layer. x 100.

same time, the threshold for electometric pulp stimulation is lowered (340-343).

The function of the dentin-pulp complex is multiple. First, together with Hertwig's epithelial root sheath, root formation is accomplished. Later, the function becomes a protective and reparative one against noxious stimuli, such as dentin exposure due to attrition, the progression of caries, cavity preparation, or trauma.

RESPONSE TO TRAUMA

The pulp must respond to a spectrum of traumatic events, such as exposed dentin due to fracture with subsequent bacterial invasion into the tubules (332,323). Furthermore, the pulp can be directly exposed to bacterial contamination from saliva following a complicated enamel-dentin fracture. Another, and usually sterile, exposure occurs during root fracture, when the pulp is exposed to the periodontal ligament via the fracture line. Finally, the pulp may become partly or totally severed and sometimes crushed at the apical foramen or at the level of a root fracture during luxation injuries. These different traumatic insults, all of which interfere with the neurovascular supply to the pulp, give rise to various healing and defense responses ranging from localized or generalized secondary dentin formation to pulpal inflammation, internal resorption, and bone metaplasia, as well as pulp necrosis with and without infection (344).

Two basic responses determine the healing result; namely, a *pulpal wound healing response*, whereby damaged pulp tissue is replaced with newly differentiated

tissue, and a *defense response*, aimed at neutralizing, or controlling, microbial invasion. The stimuli for a pulpal wound healing response have not yet been adequately defined, whereas bacterial toxins are known to elicit a defense response (245).

The general feature of the pulpal wound healing response is replacement of damaged tissue with newly formed pulp tissue. This can occur along the pulpo-dentin border if localized damage has been inflicted on the odontoblast layer (e.g. after dentin exposure), along an amputation zone in the coronal part of the pulp, or as a replacement of the major parts of the pulp if it has become necrotic because of ischemia (e.g. after a luxation injury). A common denominator of these different events is *replacement of pulp tissue* by the invasion of macrophages, new vessels, and pulpal progenitor cells in the injury zone, whereby the traumatized pulp tissue is gradually replaced by new pulp tissue. The exact nature of this process is only partly understood at present (344).

The character of the pulpal wound healing response varies according to the origin of the progenitor cells involved. Thus, in the case of PDL-derived progenitor cells, PDL tissue will be formed with associated cementum deposition along the root canal walls. Moreover, if there is a patent apical foramen, bone may invade the root canal accompanied by inserting Sharpey's fibers. It has been found that if an *accidental exposure* of the pulp is left untreated, even over a period of 1 week, inflammation is superficial and limited to a depth of 2 mm. It can be seen at that time that the pulp tissue

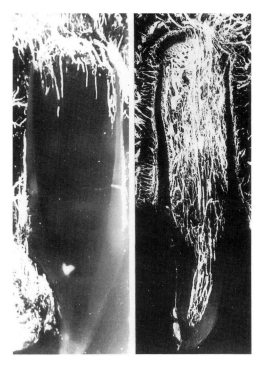

Fig. 2.28.
Ingrowth of vessels in the pulp after immediate replantation of an immature tooth in a dog demonstrated by a microangiographic technique. A. After 4 days, revascularization has begun in the apical portion of the pulp. B. After 3 weeks, revascularization is complete. From SKOGLUND ET AL. (356) 1978.

has proliferated through the exposure site (345,346) (see also Chapter 14, p. 521). In cases where the entrance to the exposure site is covered with a suitable capping material (i.e. which limits or prevents bacterial contamination), a hard tissue barrier

is normally established (347,348). The cells responsible for the formation of this dentin bridge are apparently not odontoblasts, but more probably are the mesenchymal cells located paravascularly that subsequently differentiate into odontoblasts (327,349-354). This has been shown very convincingly in a recent study where the odontoblast population was eliminated in rats by colchicine administration. After 3-5 days, revascularization and cell proliferation into the necrotic cell layer adjacent to the predentin were observed. New odontoblasts seemed to develop from paravascular cells and, after initial formation of a non-mineralized collagenous matrix, tubular dentin was formed (355).

Luxation injuries often imply severance of the neurovascular supply. The ensuing ischemia affects all cells in the pulp. Healing processes begin apically, move coronally and are highly dependent upon the size of the pulpo-periodontal interface (i.e. stage of root development). The outcome of pulpal rupture will be either pulpal revascularization (Fig. 2.28) or the development of partial or total pulp necrosis, usually determined by the presence or absence of bacteria in the injury zone.

In some cases of successful revascularization, an intact odontoblast layer will be found with an apparent continuity of the odontoblastic processes (Fig. 2.29). The mechanism of this is speculative, but end-to-end anastomoses in the ruptured apical vascular supply is a possibility (356,357). The

Fig. 2.29.
Continued dentin formation in a replanted maxillary permanent central incisor in a monkey. Observation period 8 weeks. Note continued dentinogenesis after replantation. Only a slight change in the direction of the dentinal tubules indicates the time of replantation. An average daily production of 2 μm of dentin was formed in the observation period. x 25 and x 50.

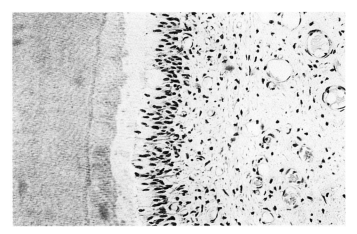 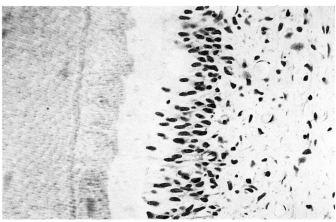

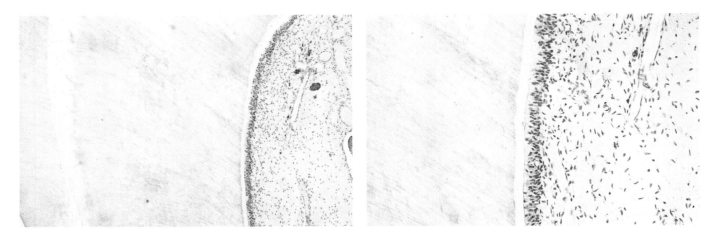

Fig. 2.30.
A. Extensive dentin production after autotransplantation of a permanent maxillary central incisor in a monkey. Observation period: 9 months. x 10. B. An intact odontoblast layer is seen forming tubular dentin. The dentin formed immediately after transplantation is acellular. The average dentin production after transplantaion is 4 μm. daily x 40.

source of the repopulating endothelial cells is not known (358). In most cases, osteo-dentin, bone or cementum-like tissue is formed on the canal walls as a response to the pulpal injury. The reasons for these varying responses have not yet been investigated.

Dentin formation after revascularization is usually very extensive and soon leads to total pulp canal obliteration. In replanted or transplanted monkey incisors observed for 9 months, it was found that the average daily dentin production was 4 μm (25) (Fig. 2.30). The explanation for this accelerated dentin production is presumably a loss of autonomic and/or sensory nervous control of the odontoblast (359-371).

An untreated dentin fracture is a common pathway for pulpal infection following bacterial invasion of the dentinal tubules. Pulpal reactions to crown fracture will be further described in (Chapters 6 and 14). If the vascular supply to the pulp is intact and the bacterial insult moderate, the event will result in secondary dentin formation and the pulp will survive (322,323). However, if bacteria gain access to the pulp via dentin tubules, as in the case of dental caries or crown fracture, or if pulpal vascularity is in any way compromised, as after a luxation injury, pulpal healing will not take place (372,373). This is probably due to diminished or absent immunological defense and/or a loss of the pulpal hydrostatic pressure that presents a powerful barrier to bacterial invasion (374,375). An alternative route is through the apical foramen via a severed PDL (372,373,384). Finally, a hematogenous route (anachoresis) cannot be excluded (376-381). The explanation for this transmission of bacteria appears to be an increased vascular leakage in the tissue bordering the traumatized pulp tissue (382,383).

An interesting finding is that necrotic but sterile pulpal tissue can persist over a prolonged period (years) without becoming infected (274,385-387).

If the pulp becomes infected in its ischemic state, revascularization is apparently permanently arrested and a leukocyte zone is formed which separates infected necrotic tissue from the ingrowing apical connective tissue (79) (Fig. 2.31). In these cases, bacteria are found in the necrotic pulp as well as in the leukocyte zone, but seldom in the adjacent vital connective tissue.

The pulpal response to infection differs from the general response to infection by the end-organ character of the tissue, implying limitations in the initial inflammatory response to infection (i.e. swelling) and a restricted access of the defense system to privileged sites for bacteria, such as the dentinal tubules, lateral canals and vascular inclusions in dentin. These anatomical obstructions usually make complete microbial kill impossible. The best compromise is usually the creation of a barrier against microorganisms, either by granulation tissue, hard tissue such as secondary dentin or cementum or proliferation of epithelium (230,388-390). Obviously, this type of defense system is not absolute and, with a change in the number of bac-

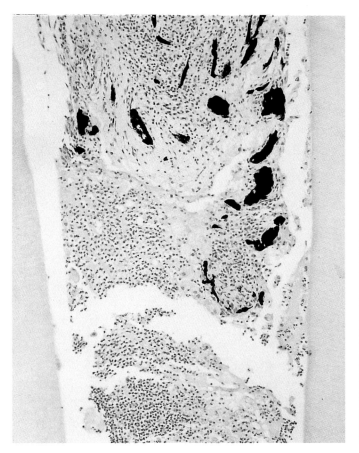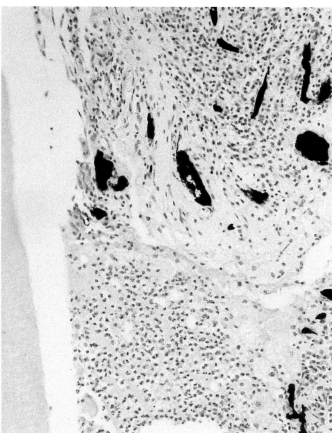

Fig. 2.31.
Infection in the pulp has caused arrest of pulpal revascularization. Status of a replanted permanent lateral incisor in a monkey. A. Low power view. There is autolysis and infection in the coronal part of the pulp. x 40. B. A leukocyte zone separating the infected part of the pulp from the revascularized part. x 100.

teria, their virulence, or the level of resistance of the patient, an exacerbation of the infection may occur.

A specific response may be encountered during revascularization of an ischemic pulp if bacteria have invaded dentinal tubules, as with an untreated dentin fracture. Resorption may then occur in relation to infected dentinal tubules.

The response of Hertwig's epithelial root sheath to infection is also a part of the pulpal response. This response has already been described (see p. 88).

Oral Mucosa and Skin

The lips comprise a complex unit of highly vascularized connective tissue, musculature, salivary glands and hair follicles (Fig. 2.32). This anatomy implies an injury that can affect a number of different anatomical structures whereby wound healing disturbances may arise.

RESPONSE TO INJURY
The main injuries affecting alveolar mucosa and lips are abrasions and lacerations. A combination of laceration and contusion is seen in the penetrating lip wound, where teeth have been forced through the tissues. In this type of lesion, tissue is lacerated and contused and contaminated by foreign bodies and bacteria.

The wound healing response in both oral mucosa and skin has been researched after incision injury (391-399) or excision injury (400-414). An excellent review on the healing events in oral mucoperiosteal wound healing has recently been published (415).

Within 4 to 24 hours after injury, epithelial cells begin their migration from the basal cell layer peripherally to the base of the coagulum. A thin epithelial cover is thereby able to close a simple wound within 24 hours (401,402). This event is seen earlier in mucosa than in cutis and is possibly related to the moist environment found in the oral cavity (393). By mitotic activity this epithelium will eventually achieve normal thickness.

In the connective tissue, a number of wound-healing processes will be initiated. Thus after 2 days, proliferation of endothelium can be observed. A wound-healing module is created whereby macrophages, fibroblasts and capillaries, originating from existing venules, invade the injury zone (409). This process will close the wound with young mature connective

**Fig. 2.32. Anatomy of
human lip.**
1. *Hair follicles*
2. *Sebaceous glands*
3. *Musculature*
4. *Connective tissue*

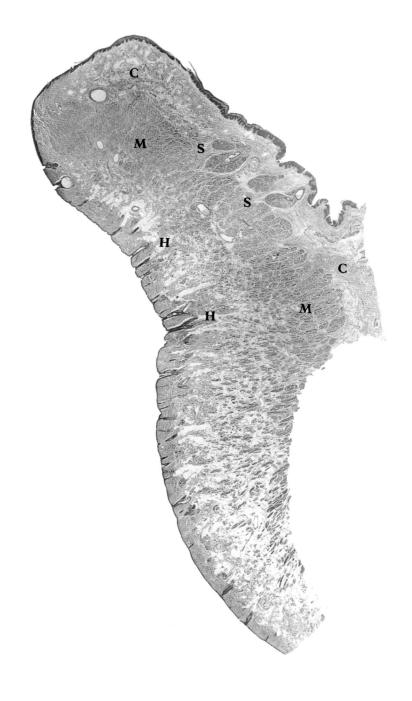

**Fig. 2.33. Healing compli-
cations after a penetrating
lip lesion**

*Scarring in a lower lip due to per-
sistence of foreign bodies. The patient has suffered a penetrating
lip lesion 6 months previously. In-
duration is felt in the lower lip
and a radiographic examination
shows foreign bodies.*

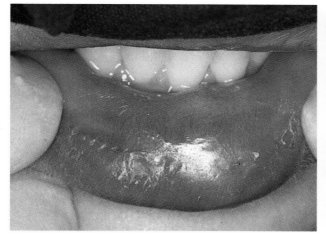
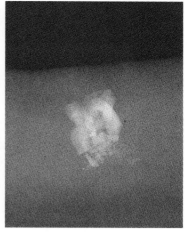

Removed tissue

*The indurated tissue was
removed and a histologic examination showed that it consisted of
fibrous tissue and multiple
foreign bodies, most likely enamel
and dentin fragments x 10 and
x 40.*

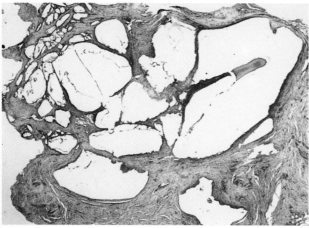
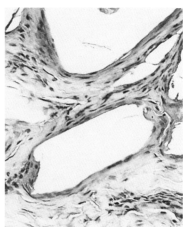

tissue within 5-10 days. These events are described in detail in Chapter 1.

In general, wound healing processes are facilitated by a good vascular supply, as is seen in the lips; a fact which may explain the relatively rare occurrence of serious complications such as tissue necrosis in this region.

In an experimental study in monkeys, it was found that a penetration wound caused by an impact forcing the incisors through the lower lip resulted in crushing of musculature and salivary gland tissue, as well as occasional entrapment of foreign bodies (plaque, calculus, tooth fragments and remnants from the impacting object) (416). These events imply a complex pattern of healing in the oral mucosa, salivary gland tissue, muscular tissue and skin, simultaneously. The regenerative potential of each of these tissue components, as well as their response to infection, varies significantly. For example, oral mucosa lesions – in contrast to skin lesions – generally heal without scarring, an observation which is presently based only on clinical documentation.

Healing of damaged salivary gland

tissue is presently not very well researched. However, considering that these cells are highly differentiated, only limited or no regenerative potential can be expected.

Muscle can regenerate (418-425), but this process is often complicated by competition from connective tissue, frequently leading to formation of scar tissue in the lips.

The incorporation of foreign bodies during wound healing implies a risk of infection by their mere presence, as well as possible bacterial contamination. Furthermore, even sterile foreign bodies usually invoke a foreign body reaction and formation of fibrous scar tissue (see Chapter 1, p. 60). A longstanding chronic foreign body reaction and/or infection may lead to fibrosis which encapsulates the foreign body by a concentration of macrophages or giant cells (Fig. 2.33).

A common foreign body in the lips appears to be enamel fragments. The reaction to these appears to be fibrous encapsulation and a macrophage/giant cell response, whereas resorption by osteoclasts (recruited from the bloodstream) is sometimes found.

RESPONSE OF ORAL TISSUES TO TRAUMA

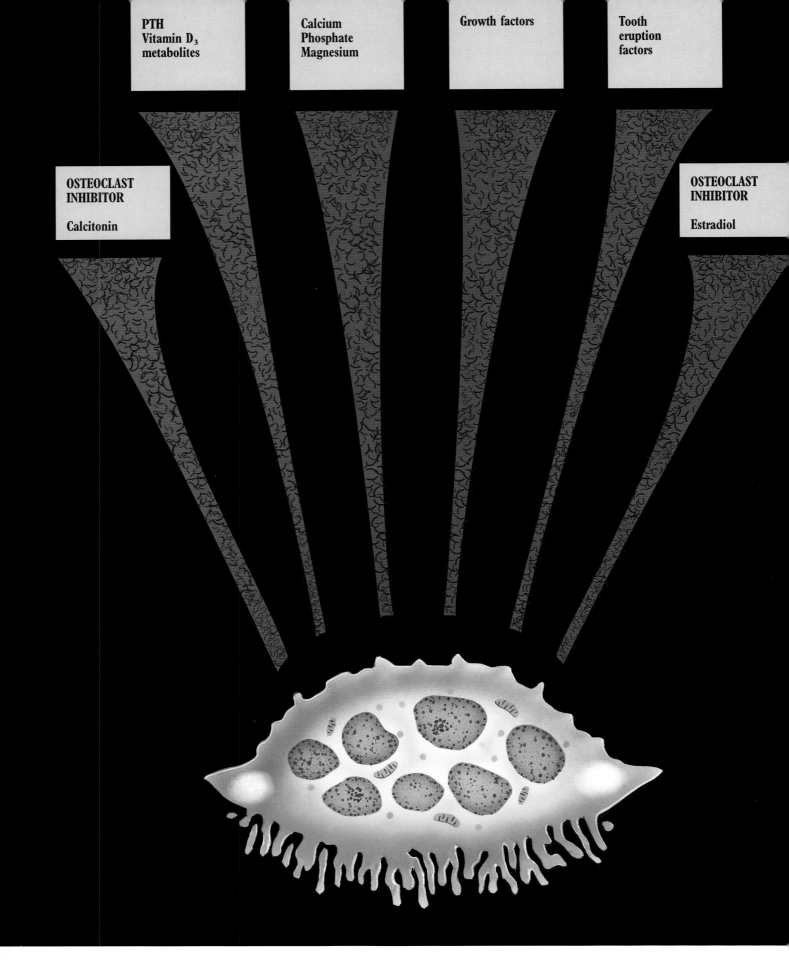

OSTEOCLAST INHIBITOR

Calcitonin

PTH
Vitamin D$_3$
metabolites

Calcium
Phosphate
Magnesium

Growth factors

Tooth
eruption
factors

OSTEOCLAST INHIBITOR

Estradiol

Inflammation and Mediators of Hard Tissue Resorption

Osteoclast Activation

The osteoclast, the main bone-resorbing cell, plays an important role in the normal healing events after trauma to bone as well as in the defense system established in response to infection (439-452). Consequently, marked osteoclastic activity may be the explanation for a number of radiographic phenomena including transient or permanent apical and marginal breakdown of the bony socket as well as external and internal root resorption (451), (see Chapter 9, p, 366).

Under normal physiologic conditions, osteoclast activity is regulated by a combination of direct and indirect osteoclast *activators* (e.g. parathyroid hormone (PTH), vitamin D metabolites, plasma calcium concentration, neurotransmitters, growth factors and cytokines (453), and osteoclast *inhibitors* (e.g. calcitonin and estrogen) (451), (Fig. 2.34)). The sum of osteoblast/osteoclast activity (i.e. net bone balance) can be seen in normal tooth eruption, growth and maintenance of the jaws, as well as homeostasis of plasma calcium and phosphate.

Hard tissues may be injured following trauma either directly (e.g., crushing injuries) or indirectly, (e.g. ischemic injuries). In both instances, an inflammatory response is elicited which results in the liberation of cytokines and the promotion of hard tissue resorption (Figs. 2.35 and 2.36). The purpose of this response is to remove the damaged hard tissue prior to healing. In this regard, the integrity of the cementoblast and odontoblast layers that cover cementum and dentin, respectively, is of paramount importance. If the traumatic event results in an irreparable injury to these cell layers, the hard tissue surface may succumb to resorption due to the intense osteoclastic activity that results from the liberation of a series of osteoclast-activating factors (452), (Figs. 2.35 and 2.36).

In the case of bacterial contamination of dentin and pulp, this response is a necessary step in the fight against invading bacteria (Fig. 2.36). Resorption of dentin serves to eliminate bacteria residing in dentinal tubules and the pulp canal while periapical bone resorption and the development of an apical granuloma builds up an area of defense against the bacteria residing in the pulp canal (449).

With respect to wound healing in hard tissues, the osteoclast can be considered analogous to the macrophage system operating in soft tissue wounds in its response to trauma and/or infection (447,454). The following is a summary of current knowledge concerning mediators for osteoclast activity, as well as the origin and function of osteoclasts.

There are three hard tissues in the oral cavity that are subject to resorption subsequent to trauma, *alveolar bone, dentin* and *cementum.* Alveolar bone is itself highly vascular, while dentin and cementum are adjacent to the vascular tissues of the dental pulp and periodontal ligament (PDL), respectively. Thus, all three of these hard tissues are readily accessible to blood-derived inflammatory cells and serum proteins and can be resorbed as a result of inflammatory reactions.

Regardless of whether the source of the injury is bacterial, mechanical or chemical, tissue injury leads to the host response of inflammation. The inflammatory reaction is characterized by the movement of fluid, proteins and white blood cells from the intravascular compartment into the extravascular space (see Chapter 1, p. 19). The inflammatory reaction can also initiate a resorptive process, the net result of which is a loss of hard tissue volume. In the following, the cells and chemical mediators involved in inflammation and hard tissue resorption will be described.

Cells of Inflammation

Although the inflammatory response is not completely understood, the precipitating event in any inflammatory process is

←
Fig. 2.34.
Activators and inhibitors regulating osteoclast activation during growth and maintenance of bone.

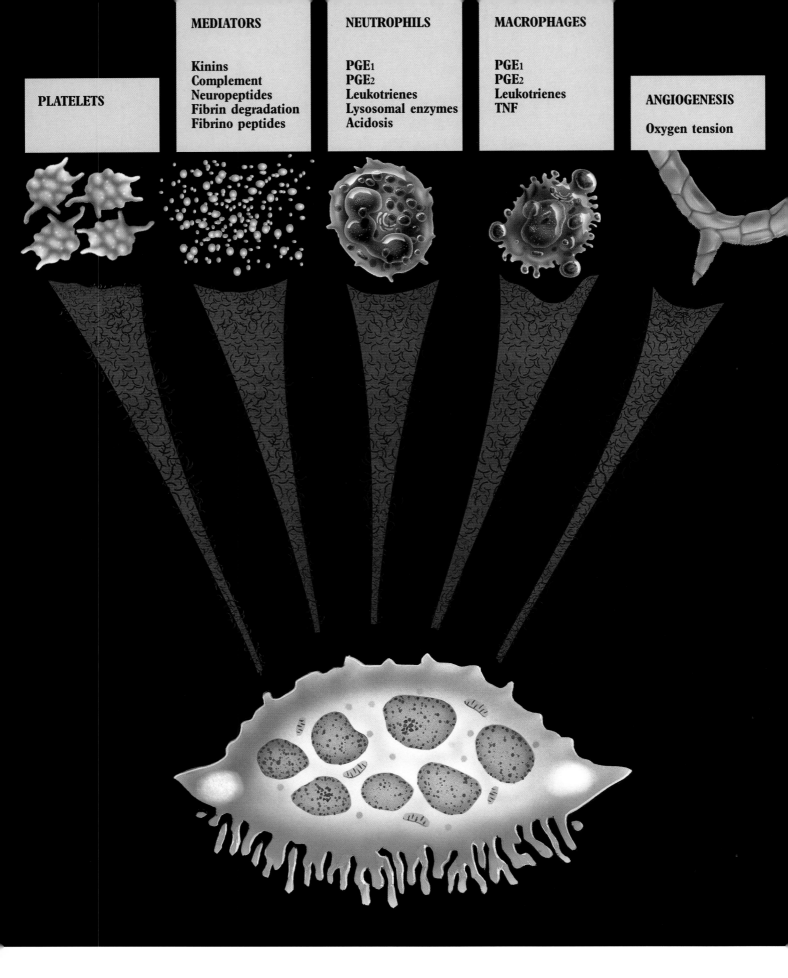

PLATELETS

MEDIATORS

Kinins
Complement
Neuropeptides
Fibrin degradation
Fibrino peptides

NEUTROPHILS

PGE1
PGE2
Leukotrienes
Lysosomal enzymes
Acidosis

MACROPHAGES

PGE1
PGE2
Leukotrienes
TNF

ANGIOGENESIS

Oxygen tension

tissue injury. Such injury is quickly followed by a vascular response that includes vasodilation, vascular stasis and increased vascular permeability, which then results in the extravasation of fluid and soluble components into the surrounding tissues (455-457). These vascular changes lead to the redness, heat, swelling and pain that are the cardinal signs of inflammation. The vascular response also includes margination of leukocytes, pavementing of these cells and, finally, their egress from the vascular space. The immune system consists of a number of inflammatory cell types that can control and direct the activities of other cells via secreted factors. Inflammatory cells involved in the various stages of tissue injury and repair include platelets, polymorphonuclear (PMN) leukocytes, mast cells, basophils, eosinophils, macrophages and lymphocytes.

The response of these cells to injury has already been described in detail in Chapter 1.

Chemical Mediators of Inflammation

Immune cells, along with other cells associated with local tissue injury and inflammation, produce a number of soluble factors that further accentuate the inflammatory response and may elicit osteoclastic activity (Figs. 2.35 to 2.38). These endogenous chemical mediators of inflammation include neuropeptides, fibrinolytic peptides, kinins, complement components, vasoactive amines, lysosomal enzymes, arachidonic acid metabolites and other mediators of immune reactions.

NEUROPEPTIDES

Neuropeptides are proteins generated from somatosensory and autonomic nerve fibers following tissue injury. A number of neuropeptides have been characterized, including substance P (SP), calcitonin gene-related peptide (CGRP), dopamine-β-hydrolase (DβH), neuropeptide Y (NPY), originating from sympathetic nerve fibers, and vasoactive intestinal polypeptides (VIP), generated from parasympathetic nerve fibers (458). Physiological and pharmacological studies have shown that these substances have both vasodilatory and vasoconstrictive effects.

Substance P, (SP) and *calcitonin gene-related peptide* (CGRP). SP is a neuropeptide present both in the peripheral and central nervous systems. The release of SP can cause vasodilation, increased vascular permeability and increased blood flow during inflammation. In addition, it can cause the release of histamine from mast cells and potentiate inflammatory responses. SP may play an important role in the pathogenesis of rheumatoid arthritis (459-461).

CGRP, another neuropeptide, which contains 37 amino acid residues, has been localized in small to medium sensory nerve fibers of several organs of experimental animals.

Both SP and CGRP have been found associated with dental tissues. SP was the first neuropeptide to be detected in dental pulp (462), and the presence of CGRP in dental pulp was demonstrated almost ten years later (463-465). Sectioning of the inferior alveolar nerve resulted in the complete disappearance of SP- and CGRP-containing granules from nerve fibers, suggesting that these substances originate from the sensory fibers of the trigeminal ganglion (463-467). *DAVIDOVITCH* and co-workers found intense staining for SP in PDL tension sites in cats 1 hour after orthodontic tooth movement (468). Intraarterial infusion with SP and CGRP produces vasodilation in feline dental pulps as measured by laser Doppler flowmetry and ^{125}I clearance techniques (469). Other investigators have also demonstrated the presence of CGRP in the pulp and PDL of rats 5 days following orthodontic movement of maxillary molars in tension sites (471).

Other peptides. VIP, a 28-amino acid residual peptide originally extracted from porcine duodenum, appears to be a stimulator of bone resorption. *HOHMANN* and associates have shown that VIP stimulates bone resorption by a prostaglandin (PG)-E$_2$-independent mechanism (472). Furthermore, they showed the presence of functional receptors for VIP on human osteosarcoma cells (473). VIP has been reported to be present in the dental pulp (458). Sectioning of the inferior alveolar nerve or sympathectomy did not result in the dis-

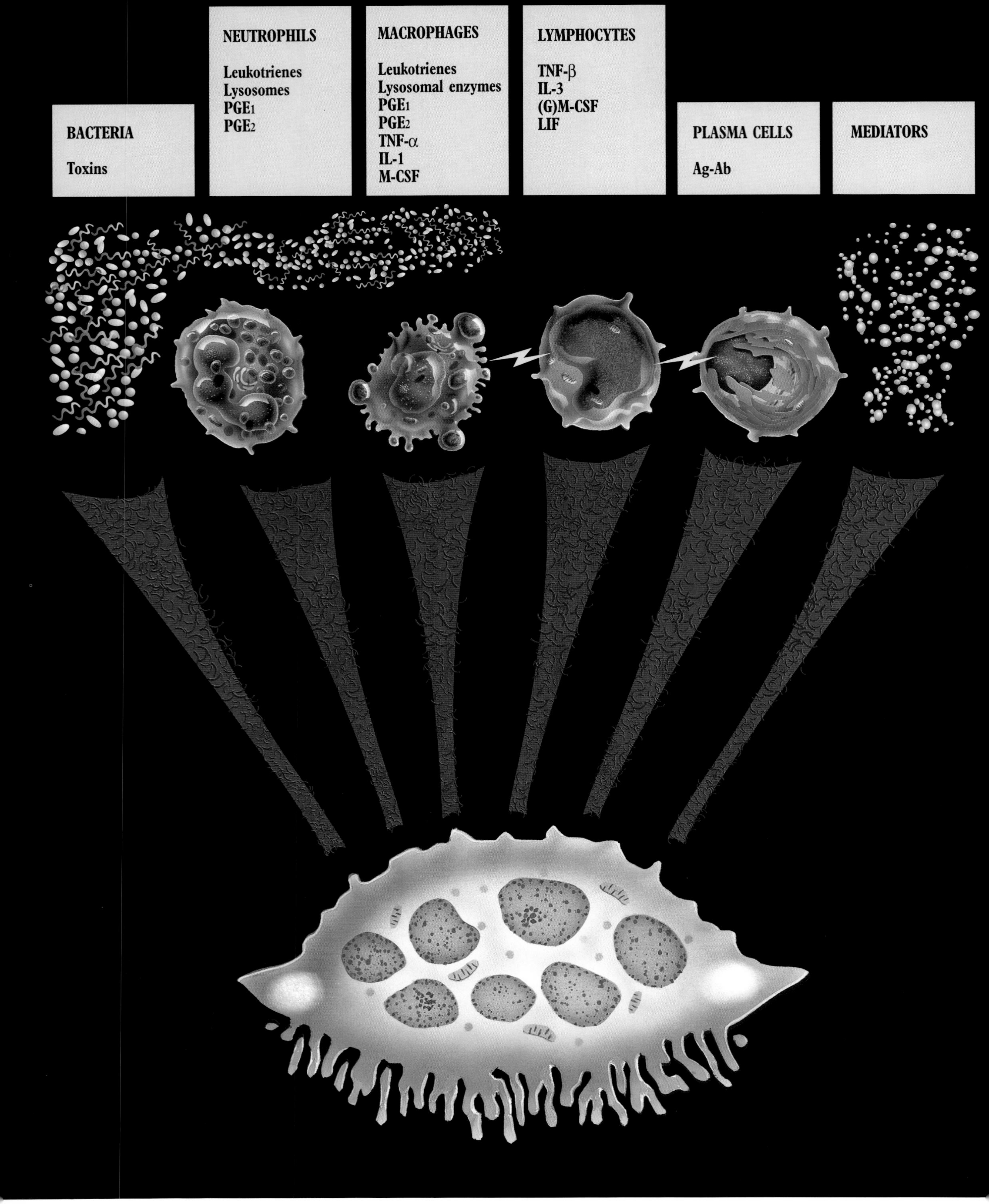

BACTERIA

Toxins

NEUTROPHILS

Leukotrienes
Lysosomes
PGE1
PGE2

MACROPHAGES

Leukotrienes
Lysosomal enzymes
PGE1
PGE2
TNF-α
IL-1
M-CSF

LYMPHOCYTES

TNF-β
IL-3
(G)M-CSF
LIF

PLASMA CELLS

Ag-Ab

MEDIATORS

Fig. 2.37.
Concentrations of kinins in chronic (yellow) and acute (red) human periapical lesions as well as uninflammed negative control connective tissue (green), mg/g of tissue weight. From TORABINE-JAD ET AL. (478) *1968.*

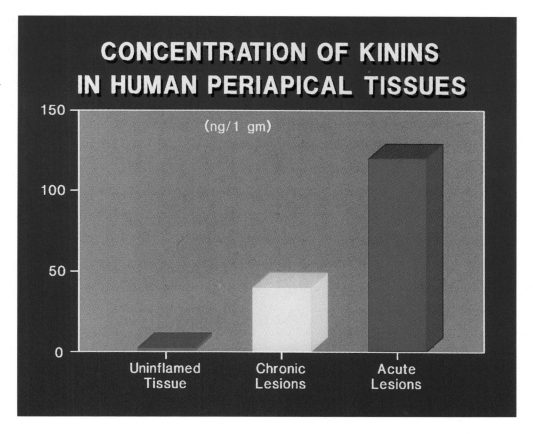

Fig. 2.37.
Concentrations of kinins in chronic (yellow) and acute (red) human periapical lesions as well as uninflammed negative control connective tissue (green), mg/g of tissue weight. From TORABINE-JAD ET AL. (478) *1968.*

appearance of VIP-containing granules from nerve fibers, indicating that VIP is of parasympathetic origin (458).

Lastly, two other neuropeptides that have been only briefly characterized, DβH and NPY, have been localized in dental pulp (458). In this case, removal of the superior cervical ganglion resulted in the complete disappearance of NPY from nerve fibers, indicating that the origin of NPY in fibers is sympathetic in nature.

The presence of these neuropeptides has been clearly demonstrated in pulpal tissues; however, their role in the pathogenesis of periapical pathology following pulpal necrosis has not been completely elucidated.

FIBRINOLYTIC PEPTIDES

Activation of the *Hageman factor* (blood clotting factor XII) results in the stimulation of the clotting cascade and the fibrinolytic, kinin and complement systems (Fig. 2.38). Major activators of the *Hageman factor* include glass, kaolin, collagen, basement membrane, cartilage, sodium urate crystals, trypsin, kallikrein, plasmin, clotting factor XI and bacterial lipopolysaccharides (474). Proper hemostasis depends on the coordinated activity of blood vessels, platelets and plasma proteins.

Following tissue injury, circulating platelets immediately adhere to the subendothelial collagen and form a primary platelet plug. This initial hemostasis is followed by the coagulation cascade which involves both an intrinsic pathway and exposure of coagulation factor XII to negatively charged collagen and an extrinsic pathway and activation of factor VII. After a complex sequence of reactions, both pathways jointly convert prothrombin into thrombin which in turn cleaves fibrinogen to fibrin (see Chapter 1, p. 23).

Even as hemostasis is still occurring, however, a fibrinolytic system is activated which will subsequently dissolve the newly formed blood clot. Circulating plasminogen is activated to plasmin (fibrinolysin) by the action of factor XIIa or by a tissue factor (474). Plasmin digests the clot and forms fibrin and fibrinogen degradation products. Fibrinopeptides and fibrin degradation products are themselves promoters of inflammation and cause increased vascular permeability and chemotaxis of leukocytes to the site of injury (474).

Severance of the blood vessels in the PDL or bone during root canal instrumentation can activate intrinsic and extrinsic coagulation pathways. Contact of the *Hageman factor* with the collagen of base-

←
Fig. 2.36.
Osteoclast activators released by bacteria and the associated inflammatory response.

CLOTTING

FIBRINO PEPTIDES

KININS

INJURY

INFECTION

PHAGO-CYTOSIS

LYSOSOMAL ENZYMES

TYPE II, III IMMUNE REACTIONS

TYPE IV IMMUNE REACTIONS

ARACHIDONIC ACID METABOLITES

VASOACTIVE AMINES

CYTO-KINES

BACTERIA TOXINS

COMPLEMENT SYSTEM

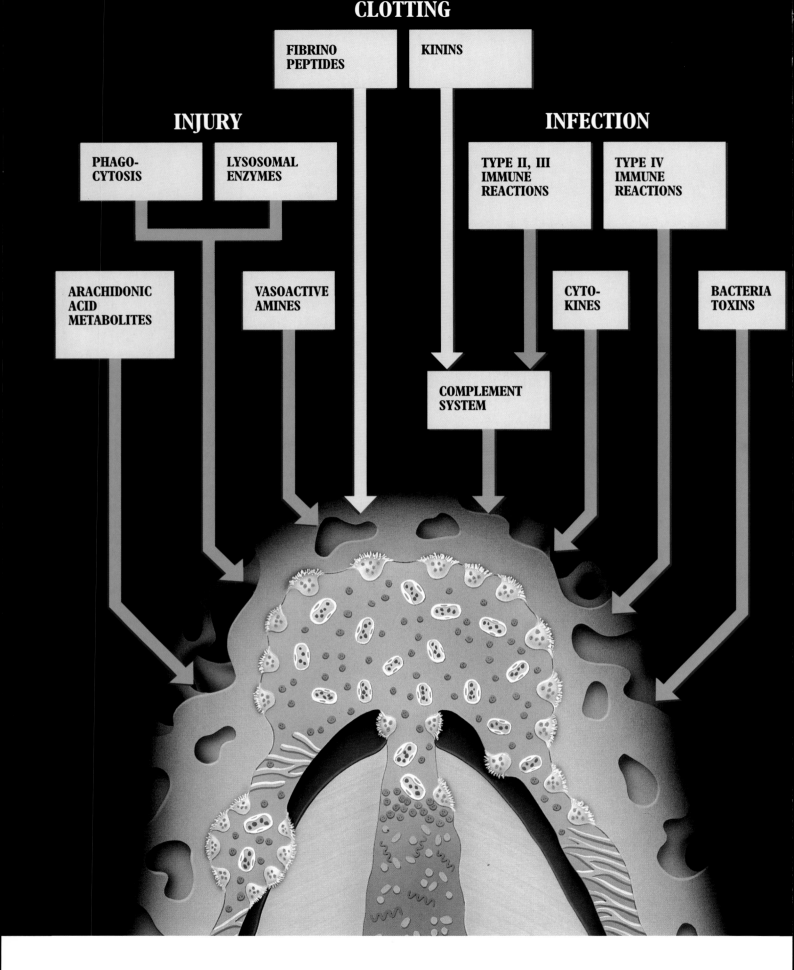

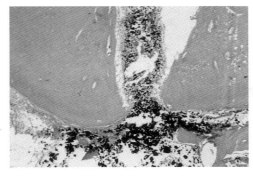 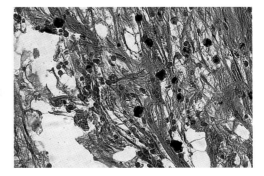

Fig. 2.39.
Egress of vitreous carbon particles from the root canal of a canine tooth into the periodontal ligament. x 20. B. Phagocytosis of carbon particles by macrophages present in the periodontal ligament. x 200.

ment membranes, with enzymes such as kallikrein or plasmin or even with endotoxins from infected root canals can all activate the clotting cascade and the fibrinolytic system. Fibrinopeptides released from fibrinogen molecules and fibrin degradation products released during the proteolysis of fibrin by plasmin can also contribute to the inflammatory process.

KININS

The kinins are able to produce many of the characteristic signs of inflammation (475). They can cause chemotaxis of inflammatory cells, contraction of smooth muscles, dilation of peripheral arterioles and increased capillary permeability. They are also able to cause pain by direct action on the nerve fibers. The kinins are produced by proteolytic cleavage of kininogen by trypsin-like serine proteases, the kallikreins. The kinins are subsequently inactivated by removal of the last one or two C-terminal amino acids by the action of peptidase (476). The kallikreins are also able to react with other systems, such as the complement and coagulation systems, to generate other trypsin-like serine proteases (477). Elevated levels of kinins have been detected in human periapical lesions (478), with acute periradicular lesions containing higher concentrations than chronic ones (Fig. 2.37).

COMPLEMENT SYSTEM

The complement system consists of at least 26 distinct plasma proteins capable of interacting with each other and with other systems to produce a variety of effects (479). Complement is able to cause

both cell lysis if activated on the cell membrane and to enhance phagocytosis through interaction with complement receptors on the surface of phagocytic cells. Complement can also increase vascular permeability and act as a chemotactic factor for granulocytes and macrophages. The complement system is a complex cascade that has two separate activation pathways that converge to a single protein (C3) and complete the cascade in a final, common sequence. Complement can be activated through the classical pathway by antigen-antibody complexes or through the alternate pathway by directly interacting with complex carbohydrates on bacterial and fungal cell walls or with substances such as plasmin (Figs. 2.36 and 2.38).

Several investigators have found C3 complement components in human periradicular lesions (480-482). Activators of the classical and alternative pathways of the complement system include IgM, IgG, bacteria and their by-products, lysosomal enzymes from PMN leukocytes and clotting factors. Most of these activators are present in periradicular lesions. Activation of the complement system in these lesions can contribute to bone resorption either by destruction of already existing bone or by inhibition of new bone formation via the production of prostaglandins (PGs). Addition of complement to organ cultures of fetal rat long bones *in vitro* stimulates the release of previously incorporated ^{45}Ca to a greater extent than heat-inactivated complement (483,484).

The activated complement system can stimulate phospholipid metabolism (485) and cause the release of lipids from cell

←
Fig 2.38.
Mediators for inflammation and tooth and bone resorption released by a mechanical, chemical or bacterial injury to the pulp or periodontium.

membranes (486-488). Consequently, the activated complement system may provide a source for the precursor of PGs, arachidonic acid (see below).

VASOACTIVE AMINES

The two major vasoactive amines involved in inflammatory reactions are histamine and serotonin. Both exist preformed in a variety of cells, most notably in mast cells, basophils and platelets. These two factors lead to increased capillary permeability and dilation and can cause smooth muscle contraction. In humans, histamine is the most important of the two species (489). Histamine is present in preformed granules in mast cells and is released by a number of stimuli including physical and chemical injury (490), complement activation products (491), activated T lymphocytes (492) and bridging of membrane-bound IgE by allergens (493). These stimuli initiate a transmembrane signal in the mast cell that eventually culminates in the release of histamine and perhaps other more minor vasoactive amines (474).

Numerous mast cells have been detected in human periradicular lesions (494,495). Physical or chemical injury of periradicular tissues during cleaning, shaping or obturation of the root canal system with antigenic substances can cause mast cell degranulation. Mast cells discharging vasoactive amines into the periradicular tissues can in turn initiate an inflammatory response or aggravate an existing inflammatory process.

LYSOSOMAL ENZYMES

Lysosomal enzymes are potent proteolytic enzymes that are stored in small, membrane-bound bodies termed lysosomes within the cytoplasm of inflammatory cells such as neutrophils, macrophages and platelets (496). Major enzymes released from lysosomes include acid and alkaline phosphatases, lysozyme, peroxidase, cathepsins and collagenase. Lysosomal enzymes are released via two principal mechanisms: 1) cytotoxic release during cell lysis (as in gout or silicosis); and 2) secretory release, often during phagocytosis.

The effects of lysosomal enzyme release have been well demonstrated in the Arthus reaction (496). After injection of an antigen, it can precipitate with its corresponding antibody to form an immune complex. These complexes bind complement, resulting in the release of anaphylatoxins which, in turn, cause histamine release and neutrophil infiltration. Neutrophils then ingest the immune complexes and release their lysosomal enzymes, leading to local tissue damage. The importance of lysosomal enzymes in this process has been demonstrated experimentally. The complete elimination of neutrophils (by nitrogen mustard treatment) will block the Arthus reaction (496). Depending on their physiological pH activities, the lysosomal enzymes have been subdivided into acid, basic and neutral proteases. Because the inflammatory site typically has an acidic pH, the acidic proteases may have the greatest activity in these locations. Factors that could help to determine the extent of tissue damage after the release of lysosomal enzymes might include the nature of the stimulus, the type of tissue or the absence of appropriate control mechanisms. For example, one group of patients with pulmonary emphysema was shown to exhibit a deficiency of α_1-antitrypsin, a potent inhibitor of neutral protease activity (496).

Release of lysosomal enzymes can also result in increased vascular permeability and further chemotaxis of leukocytes and macrophages. In addition, lysosomal enzymes can cause cleavage of C5 and generation of C5a, a potent chemotactic component, and liberate active bradykinin from plasma kininogen (496).

Lysosomal enzyme release can also occur following endodontic manipulation. Extrusion of filling materials into the periradicular tissues can result in phagocytosis and release of lysosomal enzymes (242) (Fig. 2.39). Thus, root canal obturating materials themselves, if improperly used, can be potent sources of inflammation.

ARACHIDONIC ACID METABOLITES

Arachidonic acid is a naturally occurring acid that is incorporated into phospholipids of the cell membrane. Oxidation of arachidonic acid leads to the generation of a group of biologically important products including prostaglandins (PGs), thromboxanes and leukotrienes. Products of the arachidonic acid cascade are not preformed and stored within intracellular granules but instead are synthesized from cell membrane components as a result of cell membrane injury (497). There

Fig. 2.40. Pathways of arachidonic acid metabolism.

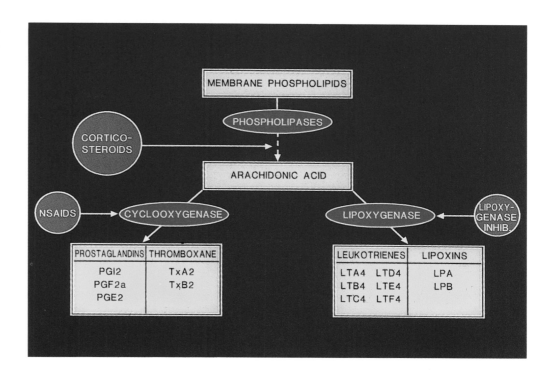

are several pathways by which arachidonic acid is metabolized (Fig. 2.40).

Prostaglandins (PGs). PGs are produced from arachidonic acid via the cyclooxygenase pathway. The PGs, particularly PGE_2 and PGI_2, have been shown to be associated with vascular permeability and pain in conjunction with the action of other chemical mediators of acute inflammation, such as histamine and kinins (474).

PGs have been implicated in pathological changes associated with human pulpal and periradicular diseases (498). The role of PGs in periradicular bone resorption was investigated by TORABINEJAD ET AL. (499) who demonstrated that the formation of periradicular lesions in cats was inhibited by systemic administration of indomethacin (Fig. 2.41). Recently

MCNICHOLS ET AL. (500) showed the presence of high levels of PGE_2 in acute periradicular abscesses. The mechanisms by which PGs are involved in bone resorption will be discussed in greater detail later in this chapter.

Leukotrienes. The leukotrienes are produced from arachidonic acid via the lipo-oxygenase pathway. The biological activities of leukotrienes include chemotactic effects for neutrophils, eosinophils and macrophages, increased vascular permeability, and release of lysosomal enzymes from PMN leukocytes and macrophages (501). High concentrations of leukotriene B4, a potent chemotactic agent, have been found in periradicular lesions (502). In addition, a positive correlation was found between the concentra-

Fig. 2.41.
A horizontal 5 µm section of periradicular tissue of a feline tooth after 6 weeks of exposure to the oral flora, stained histochemically for PGE_2. Note: dark staining for the presence of PGE_2 on the surface of alveolar bone, x 500. No staining is noted in the periradicular tissues of the contralateral tooth not exposed to the oral flora. From TORABINEJAD ET AL (499) 1979.

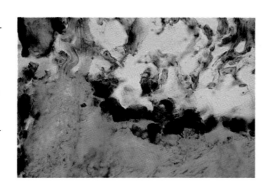 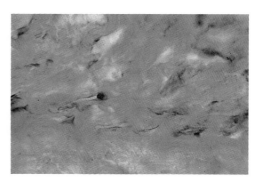

tion of this substance and the number of PMN leukocytes. The actions of these mediators can be further enhanced by the vasoactive amines and kinins.

Immunological Reactions

Immunological reactions can be divided into antibody- and cell-mediated reactions. The role of IgE-mediated reactions in hard tissue resorption was described earlier under vasoactive amines. In addition to immediate hypersensitivity reactions, immune complex reactions as well as cell- mediated reactions can also participate in inflammation and hard tissue reactions.

Antigen-antibody complex reactions

Immune complexes in periradicular tissues can be formed when extrinsic antigens such as bacteria or their by-products interact with either IgG or IgM antibodies. The resultant complexes bind to platelets, leading to the release of vasoactive amines and to increased vascular permeability and PMN leukocyte chemotaxis. The binding of immune complexes in periradicular lesions has been demonstrated in experimental animals. Simulated immune complexes placed in feline root canals led to the rapid formation of periradicular lesions, notably characterized by bone loss and the accumulation of numerous PMN leukocytes and osteoclasts [499] (Fig. 2.42). This finding was confirmed by TORABINEJAD & KIGER [503] who immunized cats with subcutaneous

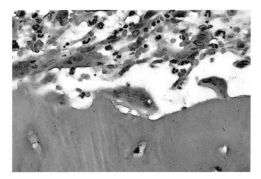

Fig. 2.42.
Accumulation of PMN leukocytes and osteoclasts in periradicular tissues of a feline tooth after the deposition of immune complexes in the root canal. x 200. From TORABINEJAD ET AL. [499] 1979.

injections of keyhole limpet hemocyanin until the presence of circulating antibody to this antigen was detected. Challenge doses of the same antigen were then administered via the root canals. Radiographic and histological observations suggested the development of periradicular lesions consistent with characteristics of an Arthus-type reaction.

Immune complexes in periradicular tissues in humans have been studied as well. TORABINEJAD & KETTERING [504], using the anticomplement immunofluorescence technique, presented evidence to support the localization of immune complexes in human periradicular specimens (Fig. 2.43). Furthermore, in two separate investigations, TORABINEJAD and associates quantitated the serum concentrations of circulating immune complexes, various classes of immunoglobulins and a C3 complement component in patients with chronic and acute periradicular lesions [505,506]. The results indicated that immune complexes formed in chronic periradicular lesions are either minimal or are confined within the lesions and do not enter into the systemic circulation. In contrast, when the serum concentrations of circulating immune complexes in patients with acute abscesses were compared with those of individuals without these lesions, a significant difference was found between the two groups. Complexes were present in the circulation of patients with lesions, but they were undetectable in the blood of unaffected controls.

Although immune complex formation can often be considered a protective mechanism for the neutralization and elimination of antigens, the data from studies on experimental animals and from patients with periradicular lesions suggest that this complex formation in the periapical space can lead to periradicular lesions that can include hard tissue resorption.

Cell-mediated immune reactions

The presence and relative concentration of B and T lymphocytes and their subpopulations were determined in human periradicular lesions by the indirect immunoperoxidase method [507]. Many B cells, T suppressor (S) cells and T helper (H) cells were detected in these lesions; but the T cells outnumbered the B cells

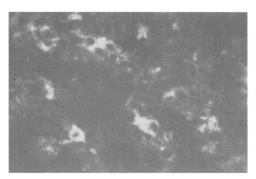

Fig. 2.43.
Detection of immune complexes in phagocytic cells of a human periapical lesion using anti-complement immunofluorescence technique. x 200. From TORABINEJAD & KETTERING (504) *1979.*

significantly (Fig. 2.44). Other investigators found approximately equal numbers of T-cell subsets in chronic lesions (TH/TS ratio) (508-511). Further immune cell specificity in developing lesions was shown by *STASHENKO* and associates (510), who demonstrated in rats that TH cells outnumber TS cells during the acute phase of lesion expansion, whereas TS cells predominate at later time periods when lesions are stabilized. Based on these results it appears that TH cells may participate in the development of periradicular lesions, whereas TS cells may decrease excessive immune reactivity, leading to cessation of lesion growth.

The specific role of T lymphocytes in the pathogenesis of periradicular lesions has recently been studied by a number of investigators. *WALLSTRÖM* (512) exposed the pulps of mandibular molars of athymic and conventional rats and left them open to the oral flora for 2, 4 or 8 weeks. Tissue sections were quantified by percentages of surface areas of bone, connective tissue,

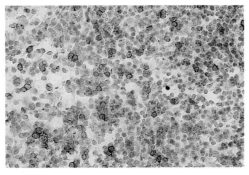

Fig. 2.44.
Presence of numerous T lymphocytes (red cell membrane) in a human periradicular lesion. From TORABINEJAD & KETTERING (507)*1985.*

bone marrow, intrabony spaces, periradicular lesions and numbers of osteoclasts. Statistical analysis showed no significant difference between periradicular tissue responses of the two treated groups. Finally, WATERMAN (513) compared periradicular lesion formation in immunosuppressed rats with that in normal rats and found no significant histologic differences between the two groups. These findings suggest that the pathogenesis of periradicular lesions is a multifactorial phenomenon and is not totally dependent on the presence of circulating lymphocytes.

Cells of Hard Tissue Resorption

Osteoclasts: Origin, Structure and Ultrastructure

The process of bone resorption requires the controlled removal of both the organic and inorganic components of bone by specific bone-resorbing cells, the osteoclasts. At the light microscopic level, osteoclasts are large, multinucleated, tartrate-resistant acid phosphatase (TRAP)-positive cells which normally reside on the bone surface (514,515), although the specificity of multinuclearity or TRAP as osteoclastic markers has not been conclusively established (516). Osteoclasts cause the erosion of the adjacent bone and/or tooth surface and can typically be found in resorption cavities or Howship's lacunae.

At the ultrastructural level, osteoclasts contain abundant mitochondria, free polysomes and rough endoplasmic reticula, circumnuclear Golgi and multiple vacuoles and dense granules. Most osteoclasts may contain 20-30 nuclei, although some may contain as many as 100 or more. The most striking feature of the osteoclast is the presence of a brush or ruffled border, a specialized area of the plasma membrane adjacent to the bone surface (for review see 517-519). The ruffled border is a complex system of folds in the cell membrane that results in the creation of a large array of finger-like projections of cytoplasm. As in the intestine, these projections serve to increase greatly the surface area of cell membrane. Adjacent to the ruffled border is an area of cytoplasm, termed the clear

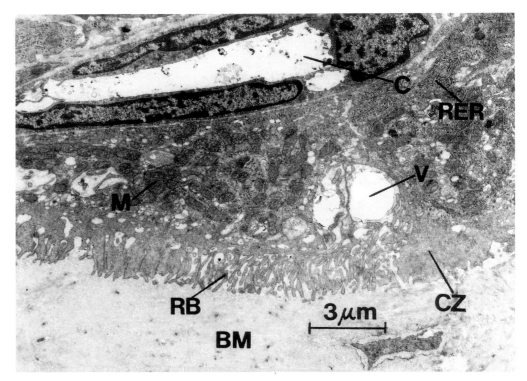

Fig. 2.45.
Electron microscopic section of an osteoclast. BM, bone matrix; C, capillary; CZ, clear zone; M, mitochondria; RER, rough endoplasmic reticulum; RB, ruffled border; V, vacuole. x 6,500. Courtesy of Dr. P.J. McMILLAN, Loma Linda University.

zone, which is completely devoid of cellular organelles and contains a system of microfilaments (Fig. 2.45).

The origin of the osteoclast has remained obscure for quite some time. Studies with parabiotic animals (520-522) and quail-chick chimeras (523,524) have demonstrated that the osteoclast is derived from blood and not from bone. The available data have indicated that the osteoclast is derived from hematopoietic stem cell precursors in the bone marrow, but its lineage has not been clearly defined. It was first thought that osteoclasts derive from cells of the mononuclear phagocyte system (523,525-530). Indeed, monocytes and macrophages may directly cause bone resorption independently of osteoclastic activity (531). However, a clear distinction between the two cell types has evolved, and more recent evidence suggests that the osteoclast may derive from an even more primitive precursor cell (532-535). The formation of functional osteoclasts requires contact with bone marrow stromal cells (536-538).

It appears that osteoclasts are derived from a multilineage precursor and that complete osteoclastic differentiation requires osteoclastic precursors or multilineage colonies in contact with bone marrow stromal cells, including the activity of an as yet unidentified osteoclast-inductive signal produced by these stromal cells (539). Hormones and cytokines may play a role in the induction of functionally mature bone resorbing cells (see below).

Mechanisms of Osteoclastic Bone Resorption

The process of bone resorption is a complex one that must involve sequentially regulated actions of acidic mineral dissolution and organic matrix degradation by both collagenolytic and noncollagenolytic enzymatic activity. Thus, acid and enzymes must be delivered by bone-resorbing cells in a spatially and temporally directed manner to the bone-resorbing surface. Osteoclasts have the ability to degrade both bone mineral and matrix (for reviews, see 451,518,540). Isolated osteoclasts have been demonstrated to resorb both components of bone (541). It is generally agreed that this resorption occurs adjacent to the cell's ruffled border.

It appears that the critical initial event

facilitating bone resorption is the establishment of a segregated extracellular space subjacent to the ruffled border of the osteoclast and adjacent to the resorbing bone surface. This space is established by the attachment of the clear zone of the osteoclast to the bone, a binding that may be mediated by specific noncollagenous bone proteins, most notably osteopontin, that contain a unique arginine-glycine-aspartic acid (RGD) attachment sequence (542-544). The osteoclast then acidifies this microenvironment to promote the dissolution of bone mineral. It has long been proposed that osteoclasts secrete organic acids during bone resorption (545-547), and large extracellular acidic microcompartments were found associated with osteoclasts in situ (548). Experiments using a pH microprobe conclusively demonstrated the acidic nature of the subosteoclastic compartment (549), acidified by the osteoclast itself (548).

The acidification of the subosteoclastic space requires that osteoclasts possess a mechanism for the generation and delivery of H^+ ions. A proton-ATPase pump has been demonstrated in the osteoclast ruffled border (550-552), and the large base-equivalent burden that results from this proton flux is eliminated by passive chloride-bicarbonate exchange at the basolateral membrane (553). Indeed, the proton pump of the osteoclast membrane is charge-coupled to a passive Cl^- permeability in the same membrane (554).

Although a number of organic acids have been considered in the mechanism of subosteoclastic acidification, it is currently thought that carbonic acid may play a major role in this process (555,556). Carbonic anhydrase, the enzyme that reversibly catalyzes the production of carbonic acid from CO_2, has been localized to osteoclasts from chicks (545,557-559), mice (563), rats (560,561) and humans (562). A potent inhibitor of carbonic anhydrase was shown to cause a significant reduction in bone resorbing activity of isolated chick osteoclasts (564). Similarly to observations of osteoclasts (565) or gastric mucosa (566) treated with acetazolamide, this inhibition was only partial, suggesting that enzymatic carbonic anhydrase activity is not the complete mechanism of osteoclast-mediated acid formation.

Following acid dissolution of mineral, the next step in bone resorption requires enzymatic digestion of the organic matrix. Demineralization exposes the matrix to enzymatic proteolytic activity. Osteoclasts are enriched in lysosomal enzymes, resulting from high biosynthetic activity and not phagocytosis (548,567,568). Numerous enzymes have been localized in the lumen of endoplasmic reticula and Golgi complexes and in the many vesicles and vacuoles near the ruffled border (548,567).

It seems that, after synthesis, osteoclastic enzymes proceed through the Golgi and are transported to the ruffled border in coated vesicles. These vesicles then fuse with the plasma membrane, and the enzymes are released into the bone-resorbing compartment (548,567). The enzymes that degrade bone matrix most likely belong to two major classes, matrix metalloproteinases and cysteine-proteinases (569). Collagenase and lysosomal cathepsins are thought to be the most important of these.

Since bone matrix is mostly collagen, the majority of the initial degradation must involve collagenolytic activity. Collagenase has been demonstrated in bone (570-575), and selective inhibition of collagenase activity almost completely inhibits bone resorption (575-577). Somewhat controversial is the active site and source of collagenolytic activity during bone resorption. Fibroblasts and osteoblasts may also be a source of neutral collagenase (578,579), and other enzymes including acid hydrolases may degrade collagen, especially in an acidified microenvironment (580). The inhibition of cysteine-proteinases, but not of collagenase, was also shown to inhibit resorptive activity of isolated osteoclasts on devitalized dentin (581). Lysosomal enzymes might act in concert with collagenase in the degradation of the collagenous matrix of bone during resorption. The most recently available data suggest that multiple enzymes are necessary for the removal of bone matrix after the solubilization of the bone mineral at the resorbing surface (569). The cellular source of collagenolytic activity in bone resorption, however, remains to be determined.

Osteoclast Regulation: Osteoclast / Osteoblast Interactions

Multiple factors, including hormonal and paracrine agents, exist to regulate osteoclast activity. Perhaps one of the most exciting findings of recent research is the observation that many factors which affect osteoclast function do not act on osteoclasts directly but instead function by binding to bone-forming cells, the osteoblasts, which in turn act on osteoclasts. Thus osteoblast-osteoclast interactions play a significant role in osteoclast formation and the regulation of bone resorption. However, these factors may not operate in dental tissues (432,452).

Several systemic hormones have important effects on osteoclastic bone resorption (Fig. 2.37) *Parathyroid hormone* (PTH) has long been known acutely to stimulate bone resorption (582,583) and to inhibit bone formation (584,585). Chronic daily injections of low doses of PTH, however, result in increased bone formation in animals (586-589) and in humans (590,591), suggesting direct effects of PTH on bone-forming cells. Indeed, direct stimulation of osteoblast-like cell growth by PTH has been shown in several species (592-595). To induce bone resorption, however, PTH does not act directly on osteoclasts. Osteoclasts may not even possess detectable PTH receptors (596,597). Rather, PTH binds to receptors on osteoblasts which then communicate this hormonal signal to osteoclasts (598,599). PTH also acutely inhibits matrix synthesis by osteoblasts (600).

The active metabolite of vitamin D3, *1,25-dihydroxyvitamin D3(1,25(OH)2D3)*, is a potent stimulator of bone resorption, 1,000 times more potent than other vitamin D3 metabolites (601), (Fig. 2.34). 1,25(OH)2D3 also seems to exert its effect on osteoclastic resorption via an osteoblast-like cell intermediary (598). As with PTH, 1,25(OH)2D3 acutely inhibits osteoblastic synthesis of bone matrix collagen (602). The bone resorption stimulated by vitamin D3 appears to be mediated by an effect whereby 1,25(OH)2D3 stimulates osteoclast formation from precursor cells (599,603,604). As indicated earlier, this effect requires accessory stromal or osteoblast-like (599,605) cells.

The major hormone that acts directly on osteoclasts is *calcitonin*. Osteoclasts are known to possess calcitonin receptors (606), and calcitonin acutely causes contraction of osteoclasts and inhibits their activity (607-609) (Fig. 2.37). Since bone formation and bone resorption are constantly occurring in the normal processes of bone remodelling and turnover, the net effect of calcitonin is to promote mineral gain in bone (610,611).

Sex steroids may also have a role in osteoclast regulation. Estrogen receptors have been detected on osteoclasts (612,613), (Fig. 2.37). *Estradiol* causes a dose-dependent inhibition of bone resorption (613), perhaps by reducing local synthesis of cytokines such as interleukins (ILs) (614,615) or by stimulating secretion of local bone growth factors such as transforming growth factor β (TGF-β) (616,617). Such changes are likely to play an important role in mediating the well-known reduction of bone mass that accompanies estrogen deficiency.

The observation that accessory cells are necessary for the development of mature osteoclasts and for the action of several *calciotropic* agents led to research regarding the local factors that could be released by these cells which then act on the osteoclast lineage. Presently, a large slate of factors known to stimulate osteoclast activity are produced by osteoblast-like cells. These local factors will be discussed later in this chapter. In addition, it appears probable that other soluble factors produced by osteoblastic cells that are relatively uncharacterized also mediate this activity (618).

Finally, environmental conditions may affect osteoclast activity. For example, *acidosis* stimulates bone mineral release and hypercalcuria in humans (619,620) and bone resorption in animals (621,622). *In vitro* studies have demonstrated the stimulation of ^{45}Ca release from prelabeled bone in response to a reduced pH of the medium, an effect thought to be due merely to the physicochemical dissolution of bone mineral (623,624). Others had suggested that increased cell-mediated release also contributes (625), and it now seems clear that low pH will directly stimulate osteoclast-mediated bone resorption (626). This finding has important implications for inflammation (Fig. 2.37). Bone resorption may be increased in inflammatory disease simply because the local environment often has a reduced pH.

Assays of Hard Tissue Resorption

Some of the uncertainty regarding osteoclastic activity has resulted from the difficulty of developing unambiguous models of bone resorption. It must be realized that any data regarding bone resorption depends on the assay system used and varying assays may respond differently to the same factor. Some assay systems may possess different percentages of mature osteoclasts or perhaps contain osteoclasts that exist at different stages along the developmental pathway. These differences will may directly impact on the interpretation of the results.

IN VITRO ASSAYS

When it was first realized in the early 1970's that inflammatory cells can release an agent (first called osteoclast activating factor or OAF) that stimulates bone resorption (627), there essentially existed only two assays for bone resorption, organ cultures of either fetal rat long bones or neonatal mouse calvariae. In both assays bone was prelabeled *in vivo* with ^{45}Ca or with a radiolabeled amino acid, and the liberation of radiolabel *in vitro* in response to varying factors was then measured. These assays contain all of the cellular events leading to bone resorption including the differentiation and formation of new osteoclasts and the activity of mature, preexisting cells.

Differences do exist, however. Mouse calvariae contain more mature osteoclasts than fetal rat long bones (628). Thus the mouse calvarial assay may respond in a more pronounced fashion to those agents which may act on more mature osteoclasts, while the fetal rat assay may respond preferentially to those factors that act on cells that exist earlier in the osteoclastic pathway. These assays have the advantage of keeping all cells *in situ*; but they do not allow the isolation of effects on particular cells due to the heterogeneity of cell types present.

Other assays have been developed using marrow mononuclear cell cultures from a number of species including human (516,599,629-634). These assays have offered the advantage of allowing for the study of the osteoclast lineage and development, and for studying the effects of different factors at different points along the developmental pathway.

The final type of *in vitro* resorption assay that has been used to study bone resorption is the assay in which isolated osteoclasts are studied on mineralized surfaces (541,610,627, 635,636). The mineralized tissue can be prelabeled with radioisotope, but more commonly, resorption is quantitated by measuring the number, area or volume of resorption lacunae formed on the surface of the mineralized slices. These assays have the advantage of being able to determine the effects of added factors on specific cells, but suffer from the disadvantage of the osteoclasts not being in communication with other local cells which may affect their activity. Indeed, resorption lacunae are generally not formed when osteoclast preparations are highly purified, further suggesting that nonosteoclast-like accessory cells are necessary for normal bone resorption (637). The technical measurement of resorption lacunae may suffer from methodological difficulties, further complicating data interpretation (638).

IN VIVO ASSAYS

Recently, bone resorption has been studied *in vivo* following the injection of various factors in rodents. The ability to produce adequate amounts of cytokines or other agents has allowed for these types of assays. Effects have included the development of severe hypercalcemia (639) and increased bone resorption as assessed by bone histomorphometry (639-641).

Finally, *in vivo* bone resorptive activity has been assessed using Chinese hamster ovarian (CHO) cells transfected with the gene for specific factors. Nude mice bearing CHO cells thus transfected with inflammatory cytokines developed hypercalcemia and a marked increase in bone resorption (642,643).

Chemical Mediators of Hard Tissue Resorption: Cytokines and Local Factors

The discovery of the so-called osteoclast-activating factor (OAF) sparked an abundance of interest in local factors or cytokines that regulate osteoclast function. These cytokines can be derived from bone marrow mononuclear cells or from bone cells directly. Cytokines might also be incorporated into bone matrix to be released in a biologically active form during bone resorption. These cytokines may play a role not only in physiological bone remod-

Table 2.1. Local factors that may affect osteoclasts

Effect on osteoclasts			
Factor	kDa	Osteoclast precursor growth or differentiation	Function of mature osteoclasts
IL-1	17.4	↑	↑
IL-3	28	↑	-
IL-6	23-30	↑	-
TNFs	17-18.8	↑	↑
CSFs	14-35	↑	-
PGs	0.35	↑	↓
1,25(OH)$_2$D$_3$	0.42	-	↑
LIF	45-58	↑	↑
TGF-β★	25	↓	↓

IL, interleukin; TNF, tumor necrosis factor; CSF, colony-stimulating factor; PG, prostaglandin; 1,25(OH)$_2$D$_3$, 1,25-dihydroxyvitamin D$_3$; LIF, leukemia inhibitory factor; TGF-β, transforming growth factor β.
Signatures: ↑ increases; ↓ decreases; - effects not shown.
★TGF-β stimulates PG production by mouse calvariae, causing increased bone resorption in the neonatal mouse calvarial assay.

elling but also in inflammatory and bone remodelling diseases. These cytokines may, in fact, be the major local regulators of osteoclasts (628).

An abundant list of cytokines and other factors that have effects on osteoclasts has developed (Fig. 2.37 and Table 2.1). Some of these factors are stimulatory while others are inhibitory. Interactions among the cytokines may be important as well. The availability of assays to study bone resorption has allowed for the determination of the effects of these factors both *in vitro* and *in vivo*.

INTERLEUKIN-1 (IL-1)
The cytokine most widely studied for its effects on bone resorption is IL-1. IL-1 is produced primarily by monocytes and macrophages (644,645), and human monocytes produce at least two IL-1 species, IL-1α and IL-1β (646). IL-1β is the major form secreted by human monocytes. The chief component of OAF was purified and found to be identical to IL-1β (647). IL-1β is the most active of the cytokines in stimulating bone resorption *in vitro* (half-maximal activity at 4.5 x 10^{-11} M), 15-fold more potent than IL-1α and 1,000-fold more potent than the tumor necrosis-factors (TNFs) (648). The genes for IL-1 have been cloned, and IL-α and IL-β are related molecules of nearly identical

molecular weight (17.4 kDa), but sharing only 35% sequence homology (646).

The effects of IL-1 on bone resorption have been widely studied. IL-1 strongly stimulates bone resorption (649) and inhibits bone formation (650). IL-1 stimulates the growth of osteoclast precursor cells, the differentiation of committed osteoclast precursors and the activity of mature osteoclasts (651,652). As is the case with other bone resorptive agents, the actions of IL-1 on osteoclasts are mediated through osteoblasts (652). IL-1β is also produced by osteoblasts and hence may serve as a messenger to communicate bone-resorptive signals to osteoclasts (653).

IL-1 has been associated with increased bone resorption *in vivo* in several disease conditions. For example, IL-1 is produced by tumor cells in several malignancies associated with increased bone resorption and hypercalcemia (654-657). In addition, since IL-1 may be produced by activated macrophages or inflammatory cells and has been identified in human dental pulp (658), IL-1 has been implicated in the bone resorption of several chronic inflammatory diseases including periodontal disease (659) and periradicular lesions (660-663).

INTERLEUKIN-3 (IL-3)
IL-3 is a T lymphocyte-derived, 28 kDa glycoprotein which supports growth and

differentiation of hematopoietic progenitor cells (664,665). In bone marrow, IL-3 will induce the differentiation of precursors to osteoclast-like cells, an effect that was independent of $1,25(OH)_2D_3$ and inhibited by an anti-IL-3 inhibitory antibody (666,667). IL-3 has also been implicated in the bone resorption that occurs in chronic inflammatory diseases, such as rheumatoid arthritis or periodontitis (666,668).

INTERLEUKIN-6 (IL-6)

IL-6 is a glycoprotein produced by a large number of cells and with a wide range of cell targets (671). It is produced by osteoblasts, but in response to other bone resorptive agents including PTH, IL-1 and $1,25(OH)_2D_3$ (672). IL-6 has been reported to be a potent stimulator of osteoclast-like cell formation in human bone marrow cultures (673), although it did not stimulate resorption in neonatal mouse calvariae (674). It does stimulate resorption, however, in an organ culture system that contains more primitive osteoclastic precursors (675).

IL-6 is produced during immune responses and may play a role in human disease. For example, IL-6 may be an important mediator of the increased number of osteoclasts in Paget's disease (676), implicating IL-6 in the pathogenesis of diseases of increased osteoclast formation. Nude mice carrying CHO tumors overexpressing IL-6 develop hypercalcemia (643), and IL-6 may be involved in the hypercalcemia and bone lesions associated with other malignancies. Lastly, IL-6 may play a role in the bone resorption observed with inflammatory diseases. Thus IL-6 has been isolated from diseased tissues associated with adult periodontitis (677) and rheumatoid arthritis (678).

TUMOR NECROSIS FACTORS (TNFs)

The monocyte-macrophage- derived TNF-α and the lymphocyte-derived TNF-β (previously called lymphotoxin) have effects on bone resorption that are similar to IL-1. Both stimulate resorption and inhibit formation of bone in organ culture (648), and the TNFs stimulate both the growth of osteoclast progenitor cells and the differentiation of committed precursors (651). Their effects on osteoclasts are also indirect and are mediated through osteoblasts (679). The ability of TNF-α to stimulate bone resorption is dependent on prostaglandin (PG) synthesis (680).

TNFs may be associated with bone resorption in vivo in a number of diseases. Although TNF has not been shown to be produced directly by solid tumor cells, many such tumors cause host defense cells to produce excess TNFs, leading to increased resorption and hypercalcemia of malignancy (632,681,682). Direct injections in vivo of TNF-α in intact mice cause hypercalcemia (226). TNF has been implicated in the hypercalcemia and bone resorption with multiple myeloma as well (683). Finally, the TNFs, produced by activated immune cells, may be associated with bone resorption resulting from chronic inflammatory disease. For example, TNFs were detected in all samples of gingival and periradicular tissues associated with disease but were scarcely detectable in sites associated with health (659,663).

COLONY-STIMULATING FACTORS (CSFs)

The CSFs are a broad class of hematopoietic growth factors that support the growth and differentiation of a wide lineage of hematopoietic cells. The following discussion will focus on those that may be involved in the regulation of bone resorbing cells.

This factor, also known as CSF-1, whose effect is restricted to cells of the mononuclear phagocyte system (685), may be critically important for osteoclast development. M-CSF directly stimulates proliferation of osteoclast precursors (232), perhaps in concert with IL-1 or IL-3 (687), although M-CSF may inhibit osteoclast formation in some models (667). M-CSF is produced by osteoblasts themselves and thus could serve to communicate bone resorptive signals from osteoblasts to osteoclasts (688-692). M-CSF production by osteoblasts is enhanced by other bone resorbing cytokines such as IL-1 and TNF (689,691,692).

Compelling evidence for a role for M-CSF in osteoclast development came from the study of the murine mutation osteopetrosis, a phenotype of impaired bone resorption due to a lack of functional osteoclasts. The osteoclast deficiency results from a lack of M-CSF and a defect in the M-CSF gene (693,694). Replacement of M-CSF into the op/op osteopetrotic mouse in vivo corrects the bone resorption deficit and induces the appearance of resorbing osteoclasts and resident bone marrow macrophages (695). In addition, M-CSF administration reduced osteopetrosis, induced large numbers of osteoclasts in bones and macrophages in the peritoneal cavity and bone marrow and permitted tooth eruption in the toothless (*tl/tl*) rat mutation *in vivo* (696).

Granulocyte (G) M-CSF is a T lymphocyte-derived, 22 kDa glycoprotein that affects a multitude of functions of mature granulocytes, monocytes and some mesenchymal cells. GM-CSF stimulates the formation of osteoclast-like cells in long-term marrow cultures (631), but it will also stimulate the growth of osteoblast-like cells (697). Osteoblast-like cells produce GM-CSF (698,699), and the production of GM-CSF is stimulated by osteotropic agents such as PTH or the bacterial component lipopolysaccharide (699). GM-CSF may act in concert with other cytokines such as IL-6 (700), and GM-CSF may both increase the production of other cytokines and be stimulated itself by other cytokines (701-703). Thus, GM-CSF may also be associated with bone resorption in the process of inflammation, and it may also be involved in the mechanism of hypercalcemia of malignancy (704).

PGs, products of arachidonic acid metabolism as described earlier, have long been implicated in bone resorption. PGE$_1$ and PGE$_2$ were first reported to stimulate ^{45}Ca release from fetal rat bone *in vitro* in 1970 (705). The stimulatory effect of PGEs on bone resorption has been confirmed by many groups (706-709). Paradoxically, CHAMBERS and coworkers reported that PGE$_2$ had a direct inhibitory effect on bone resorption by isolated osteoclasts (710) and inhibited osteoclast motility (711), suggesting that the stimulation of bone resorption by PGs in organ culture is due to indirect effects of PGs on cells other than osteoclasts. This suggestion was further strengthened by the finding that PGE$_2$ initially inhibited and then stimulated bone resorption in isolated rabbit osteoclast cultures, consistent with the idea that the stimulated resorption was due to late, indirect effects mediated by marrow stromal cells (712). It appears that PGs induce osteoclastic differentiation

from precursor cells but inhibit the activity of mature osteoclasts (713).

PGs have been implicated in both the local bone resorption of chronic inflammation and in systemic resorption as well. PGE$_2$ is elevated in inflamed, periodontally diseased sites and in symptomatic pulpal tissue compared to control sites (714-717). The importance of PGs in periodontal disease progression was further suggested by the finding that an inhibitor of PGs, flurbiprofen, decreased naturally occurring periodontal disease destruction in beagle dogs (718). Synovial tissue from patients with rheumatoid arthritis produced PGE$_2$ and caused bone resorption *in vitro*, an effect inhibited by indomethacin (719). Tumor cells producing large amounts of PGE$_2$ lead to extensive bone resorption and hypercalcemia, effects also blocked by indomethacin (720,721). Similarly to PTH, however, infusions of PGE$_2$ *in vivo* actually increase bone formation (722), and PG inhibitors decrease fracture repair (723).

PGs may interact with other local cytokines. IL-1 (724,725) and TNF-α (680) increase PGE$_2$ production. PGE$_2$ has been reported to inhibit IL-1 production, perhaps acting as a negative feedback system (726). PTH-related protein will also stimulate PGE$_2$ from human osteoblast-like cells, suggesting that PGs also may communicate bone resorptive signals locally (727).

LIF, a glycoprotein derived from activated T lymphocytes which stimulates differentiation of myeloma cells to mature monocytes (728), is identical in activity to a glycoprotein shown to stimulate bone resorption *in vitro* called differentiation-inducing factor (DIF, 729). It also stimulates osteoclast-like cell formation in marrow cultures (730).

Local Inhibitors of Resorption

Three local inhibitors of osteoclastic bone resorption have been described. *Transforming growth factor-β* (TGF-β) is one of several growth factors that are abundant in bone and known to stimulate bone cell growth. TGF-β is a powerful stimulator of bone cell growth and function and has been shown to stimulate bone formation in a number of *in vivo* models (731-734). TGF-β also affects bone resorption, but its effects vary depending on the model system studied. For example, in human marrow cultures, TGF-β inhibits the formation of osteoclast-like cells (735). In the neonatal mouse calvarial assay, however, TGF-β treatment leads to an increase in bone resorption secondarily due to an increased production of PGs (610,736).

Another agent shown to inhibit osteoclastic bone resorption is γ-*interferon*. γ-interferon completely abolished the resorption stimulated by IL-1, TNF-α and TNF-β, but that stimulated by PTH and 1,25(OH)$_2$D$_3$ was not significantly affected (737). In addition, γ-interferon also inhibited the bone resorption induced by bradykinin, only partially through a PG-mediated mechanism (738).

The most recently described local inhibitor of osteoclastic bone resorption is the *IL-1 receptor antagonist (IL-1ra)* (739-742). *IL-1ra* is a cytokine that is related to the IL-1 family and specifically inhibits the bone-resorptive effects of IL-1α and IL-1β, but not that of PTH or 1,25(OH)$_2$D$_3$

(743,744). It also inhibits the bone resorption and hypercalcemia caused by IL-1 injections *in vivo*.

As summarized in Fig. 2.37, present studies indicate that multiple mechanisms are involved in the pathological changes that are associated with hard tissue resorption. Mechanical injury to the periodontium or periradicular tissues is likely to initiate the release of nonspecific mediators of inflammation and activate several pathways of inflammation. Continuous egress of irritants, antigens or toxic bacterial materials, as from a pathologically involved root canal, can result in one or more immunological reactions. Present data indicate that a number of these reactions can lead to hard tissue resorption at both the periradicular and periodontal sites. Because of complex interactions between the various components of these systems, the dominance of any one pathway or substance may be difficult to establish. Much research is still needed to characterize the specific roles of mediators of inflammation in pathogenesis of hard tissue resorption

Essentials

Dental follicle

The dental follicle has some regenerative potential. Severe damage leads to ankylosis and/or disturbances in tooth eruption.

Cervical loop

This structure has a great regenerative potential, after trauma whereby crown and later root formation can usually be completed.

Ameloblasts

These cells are very sensitive to trauma and infection. Both events usually lead to partial or total arrest of enamel formation and secondary mineralization.

Reduced enamel epithelium

It has limited, if any, regenerative potential. Trauma and infection may therefore lead to defects in secondary mineralization.

Enamel organ

The enamel organ is sensitive to trauma and infection; injuries lead to disturbances in mineralization and enamel matrix formation. Short-term chronic inflammation (i.e. months) has very little or no effect whereas persisting inflammation (years) results in disturbances in enamel matrix formation and mineralization.

Hertwig's epithelial root sheath

This structure can be damaged directly during a luxation injury or indirectly by delayed revascularization due to incomplete repositioning. It has a certain regenerative potential and, depending on the extent of injury partial or total arrest of root development may occur. It appears to be rather resistant to even prolonged pulpal infection.

Gingiva and periosteal complex

Regeneration of gingival anatomy usually takes place 1-2 weeks after wounding.

Periodontal ligament-cementum complex

Traumatic injury to the periodontal ligament can lead to various types of resorption (i.e. surface resorption, inflammatory resorption and replacement resorption), depending upon the extent of the PDL injury, pulpal condition and the age of the patient. The periodontal ligament-cementum complex is resistant to chronic infection. However, acute infection leads to degradation of PDL fibers. Resorption of the root surface can occur subsequent to chronic or acute infection.

Alveolar bone and marrow complex

The response to fracture or contusion is resorption of necrotic bone and subsequent osteogenesis. The reaction of bone to chronic infection is bone resorption and formation of granulation tissue which delimits the focus of infection. In acute infection, bacteria spread to the bone and bone marrow where they elicit severe inflammatory changes.

Dentin-pulp complex

The pulp exhibits a regenerative potential after traumatic injury as long as infection is avoided. This applies to accidental exposure of the coronal part of the pulp, where a hard tissue barrier usually walls off the exposure. In case of severance of the vascular supply to the pulp due to luxation or root fracture, the width of the pulp-periodontal interface is decisive for successful revascularization. If infection occurs in the pulp in its ischemic phase after luxation or replantation, the revascularization process becomes permanently arrested.

Oral mucosa and skin

The lips have, due to their vascularity, an excellent healing capacity. Scar tissue formation is frequent in skin but rare in mucosa. Acute or chronic infection usually results from penetrating lip wounds due to contamination with foreign bodies.

Bibliography

1. ILLINGWORTH CM. Trapped fingers and amputated fingertips in children. *J Pediatr Surg* 1974;**9**:853-8.

2. GOSS RJ. Regeneration versus repair. In: COHEN IK, DIEGELMANN RF, LINDBLAD JW, eds. *Wound healing: biochemical and clinical aspects.* Philadelphia: W.B. Saunders Company, 1992:20-39.

3. ANDREASEN JO, ANDREASEN FM. Biology of traumatic dental injuries. *Tandlægebladet* 1989;93:385-92.

4. TEN CATE AR. Formation of supporting bone in association with periodontal ligament. *Arch Oral Biol* 1975;**20**:137-8.

5. TEN CATE AR, MILLS C, SOLOMON G. The development of the periodontium. A transplantation and autoradiographic study. *Anat Rec* 1971;**170**:365-80.

6. PALMER RM, LUMSDEN AGS. Development of periodontal ligament and alveolar bone in homografted recombinations of enamel organs and papillary, pulpal and follicular mesenchyme in the mouse. *Arch Oral Biol* 1987;**32**:281-9.

7. SCHROEDER HE. *The periodontium.* Springer-Verlag, Berlin Heidelberg, 1986:12-22.

8. FREEMAN E, TEN CATE AR, Development of the periodontium: an electron microscopic study. *J Periodont* 1971;**42**:387-95.

9. HOFFMAN RL. Formation of periodontal tissues around subcutaneously transplanted hamster molars. *J Dent Res* 1960;**39**:781-98.

10. HOFFMAN RL. Bone formation and resorption around developing teeth transplanted into the femur. *Am J Anat* 1960;**118**:91-102.

11. HOFFMAN RL. Tissue alterations in intramuscularly transplanted developing molars. *Arch Oral Biol* 1967;**12**:713-20.

12. BARTON JM, KEENAN RM. The formation of Sharpeys fibres in the hamster under nonfunctional conditions. *Arch Oral Biol* 1967;**12**:1331-36.

13. FREEMAN E, TEN CATE AR, DICKINSON J. Development of a gomphosis by tooth germ implants in the parietal bone of the mouse. *Arch Oral Biol* 1975;**20**:139-40.

14. YOSHIKAWA DK, KOLLAR EJ. Recombination experiments on the odontogenic roles of mouse dental papilla and dental sac tissues in ocular grafts. *Arch Oral Biol* 1981;**26**:303-7.

15. BARRETT P, READE PC. The relationship between degree of development of tooth isografts and the subsequent formation of bone and periodontal ligament. *J Periodont Res* 1981;**16**:456-65.

16. FREUND G. Über die Zahnleisten Kanäle und ihre Bedeutung für die Ätiologie der Follikularzysten und der Zahnretention. *Acta Anat* 1954;**21**:141-54.

17. CAROLLO DA, HOFFMAN RL, BRODIE AG. Histology and function of the dental gubernacular cord. *Angle Orthod* 1971;**41**:300-407.

18. MAGNUSSON B. *Tissue changes during molar tooth eruption. Histologic and autoradiographic studies in monkeys and rats with special reference to dental epithelium, oral mucosa, periodontium, apical pulp and periapical tissue.* Trans Royal Dent Sch Stockholm, Umeå 1968;**13**.

19. BERKOVITZ BKB. Theories of tooth eruption. In: POOLE DFG, STACK MV, eds. *The eruption and occlusion of teeth.* London: Butterworths, 1976:193-204.

20. JENKINS GN. Eruption and resorption. In: JENKINS GN, ed. *The physiology and biochemistry of the mouth.* 4th edn. Oxford, London, Edinburgh, Melbourne: Blackwell Scientific Publications, 1978:197-214.

21. CAHILL DR, MARKS SC, WISE GE, GORSKI JP. A review and comparison of tooth eruption systems used in experimentation - a new proposal on tooth eruption. In: DAVIDOVITCH Z, ed. *The Biological Mechanisms of Tooth Eruption and Root Resorption.* Birmingham: EBSCO Media, 1988:1-7.

22. MARKS SC, GORSKI JP, CAHILL DR, WISE GE. Tooth eruption - a synthesis of experimental observations. In: DAVIDOVITCH Z, ed. *The Biological Mechanisms of Tooth Eruption and Root Resorption.* Birmingham: EBSCO Media, 1988:161-9.

23. CAHILL DR, MARKS SC JR. Tooth eruption: evidence for the central role of the dental follicle. *J Oral Pathol* 1980;**9**:189-200.

24. CAHILL DR, MARKS SC JR. Cronology and histology of exfoliation and eruption of mandibular premolars in dogs. *J Morphol* 1982;**171**:213-8.

25. KRISTERSON L, ANDREASEN JO. Autotransplantation and replantation of tooth germs in monkeys. Effect of damage to the dental follicle and position of transplant in the alveolus. *Int J Oral Surg* 1984;**13**:324-33.

26. BARFOED CO, NIELSEN LH, ANDREASEN JO. Injury to developing canines as a complication of intranasal antrostomy. *Int J Oral Surg* 1984;**13**:445-7.

27. CAHILL DR. Histological changes in the bony crypt and gubernacular canal of erupting permanent premolars during deciduous premolar exfoliation in beagles. *J Dent Res* 1974;**53**:786-91.

28. MARKS SC JR, CAHILL DR, WISE GE. The cytology of the dental follicle and adjacent alveolar bone during tooth eruption in the dog. *Am J Anat* 1983;**168**:277-89.

29. MARKS SC JR, CAHILL DR. Experimental study in the dog of the non-active role of the tooth in the eruptive process. *Arch Oral Biol* 1984;**29**:311-22.

30. WISE GE, MARKS SC JR, CAHILL DR. Ultrastructural features of the dental follicle associated with formation of the tooth eruption pathway in the dog. *J Oral Pathol* 1985;**14**:15-26.

31. OOË T. On the early development on human dental lamina. *Folia Anat Jap* 1957;**30**:198-210.

32. OOË T. Changes of position and development of human anterior tooth germs after birth. *Folia Anat Jap* 1968;**45**:71-81.

33. ANDREASEN JO, RIIS I. Influence of pulp necrosis and periapical inflammation of primary teeth on their permanent successors. Combined macroscopic and histological study in monkeys. *Int J Oral Surg* 1978;**7**:178-87.

34. ANDREASEN JO. *Traumatic injuries of the teeth.* 2nd edn. Copenhagen: Munksgaard, 1981:304.

35. DIAMOND M, APPLEBAUM E. The epithelial sheath: Histogenesis and function. *J Dent Res* 1942;**21**:403-11.

36. SCHOUR I. *Noyes' Oral Histology and Embryology,* 8th edn. Philadelphia: Lea & Febiger, 1962.

37. ANDREASEN JO. The influence of traumatic intrusion of primary teeth on their permanent successors. A radiographic and histologic study in monkeys. *Int J Oral Surg* 1976;**5**:207-19.

38. THYLSTRUP A, ANDREASEN JO. The influence of traumatic intrusion of primary teeth on their permanent successors in monkeys. A macroscopic, polarized light and scanning electron microscopic study. *J Oral Pathol* 1977;**6**:296-306.

39. REITH EJ. The stages of amelogenesis as observed in molar teeth of young rats. *J Ultrastruct Res* 1970;**30**:111-151.

40. REITH EJ, COTTY VF. The absorptive activity of ameloblasts during maturation of enamel. *Anat Rec* 1967;**157**:577-88.

41. YEAGER JA. Enamel. In: BHASKAR N, ed. *Orban's Oral histology and embryology.* Saint Louis: The CV Mosby Company, 1976:45.

42. SUGA S. Enamel hypomineralization viewed from the pattern of progressive mineralization of human and monkey developing enamel. *Adv Dent Res* 1989;**3**:188-98.

43. SUCKLING GW, CUTRESS TW. Traumatically induced defects of enamel in permanent teeth in sheep. *J Dent Res* 1977;**56**:1429.

44. MCKEE MD, WARSHAWSKY H. Response of the rat incisor dental tissues to penetration of the labial alveolar bone in preparation of a surgical window. *J Biol Buccale* 1986;**14**:39-51.

45. SUCKLING GW, PURDELL - LEWIS DJ. The pattern of mineralization of traumatically-induced developmental defects of sheep enamel assessed by microhardness and microradiography. *J Dent Res* 1982;**61**:1211-6.

46. SUCKLING GW. Developmental defects of enamel - historical and present-day perspectives of their pathogenesis. *Adv Dent Res* 1989;**3**:87-94.

47. SUCKLING GW, NELSON DGA, PATEL MJ. Macroscopic and scanning electron microscopic appearance and hardness values of developmental defects in human permanent tooth enamel. *Adv Dent Res* 1989;**3**:219-33.

48. VALDERHAUG J. Periapical inflammation in primary teeth and its effect on the permanent successors. *Int J Oral Surg* 1974;**3**:171-82.

49. ANDO S, SANKO Y, NAKASHIMA T, et al. Studies on the consecutive survey of succedaneous and permanent dentition in Japanese children. Part III. Effects of periapical osteitis in the deciduous predecessors on the surface malformation of their permanent successors. *J Nihon Univ Sch Dent* 1966;**8**:233-41.

50. MCCORMICK J, FILOSTRAT PJ. Injury to the teeth of succession by abscess of the temporary teeth. *ASDC J Dent Child* 1967;**34**:501-4.

51. RADKOVEC F. Les dents de Turner. *8 congrés dentaire international.* Paris 1931, 210-21.

52. MORNINGSTAR CH. Effect of infection of the deciduous molar on the permanent tooth germ. *J Am Dent Assoc* 1937;**24**:786-91.

53. BAUER W. Effect of periapical processes of deciduous teeth on the buds of permanent teeth. Pathological-clinical study. *Am J Orthod* 1946;**32**:232-41.

54. TAATZ H, TAATZ H. Feingewebliche Studien an permanenten Frontzähnen nach traumatischer Schädigung während der Keimentwicklung. *Dtsch Zahnärztl Z* 1961;**16**:995-1002.

55. HITCHIN AD, NAYLOR MN. Acute maxillitis of infancy. Late sequelae of three cases, including a rhinolith containing a tooth and a compound composite odontome. *Oral Surg Oral Med Oral Pathol* 1964;**18**:423-31.

56. BINNS WH, ESCOBAR A. Defect in permanent teeth following pulp exposure of primary teeth. *ASDC J Dent Child* 1967;**34**:4-14.

57. KAPLAN NL, ZACH L, GOLDSMITH ED. Effects of pulpal exposure in the primary dentition of the succedaneous teeth. *ASDC J Dent Child* 1967;**34**:237-42.

58. MATSUMIYA S. Experimental pathological study on the effect of treatment of infected root canals in the deciduous tooth on growth of the permanent tooth germ. *Int Dent J* 1968;**18**:546-59.

59. TURNER JG. Two cases of hypoplasia of enamel. *Br Dent Sci* 1912;**55**:227-8.

60. HALS E, ORLOW M. Turner teeth. *Odont T* 1958;**66**:199-212.

61. WEINMANN JP, SVOBODA JF, WOODS RW. Hereditary disturbances of enamel formation and calcification. *J Am Dent Assoc* 1945;**32**:397-418.

62. MCHUGH WD. The development of the gingival epithelium in the monkey. *Dent Pract Dent Rec* 1961;**11**:314-24.

63. TOTO PD, SICHER H. Eruption of teeth through the oral mucosa. *Periodontics* 1966;**4**:29-32.

64. MELCHER AH. Changes in connective tissue covering erupting teeth. In: ANDERSON DJ, EASTOE JE, MELCHER AH, PICTON DCA, eds. *The mechanism of tooth support.* Bristol: Wright, 1967:94-7.

65. TEN CATE AR. Physiological resorption of connective tissue associated with tooth eruption. *J Periodont Res* 1971;**6**:168-81.

66. KRISTERSON L, ANDREASEN JO. Autotransplantation and replantation of tooth germs in monkeys. Effect of damage to the dental follicle and position of transplant in the alveolus. *Int J Oral Surg* 1984;**13**:324-33.

67. NOBLE HW, CARMICHAEL AF, RANKINE DM. Electron microscopy of human developing dentine. *Arch Oral Biol* 1962;**7**:395-9.

68. OOË T. *Human tooth and dental arch development.* Tokyo: Ishiyaku Publishers, Inc 1981:86-94.

69. DIAMOND M, APPLEBAUM E. The epithelial sheath: histogenesis and function. *J Dent Res* 1942;**21**:403-11.

70. GRANT D, BERNICK S. Morphodifferentiation and structure of Hertwig's root sheath in the cat. *J Dent Res* 1971;**50**:1580-8.

71. OWENS PDA. A light microscopic study of the development of the roots of premolar teeth in dogs. *Arch Oral Biol* 1974;**20**:525-38.

72. OWENS PDA. Ultrastructure of Hertwig's epithelial root sheath during early root development in premolar teeth in dogs. *Arch Oral Biol* 1978;**23**:91-104.

73. ANDREASEN FM, ANDREASEN JO. *The relationship in monkeys between the fuctional, histological and radiographic diameter of the apical foramen and blood supply to the pulp.* In preparation 1993.

74. DIAB MA, STALLARD RE. A study of the relationship between epithelial root sheath and root development. *Periodontics* 1965;**3**:10-7.

75. SHIBATA F, STERN IB. Hertwig's sheath in the rat incisors. II. Autoradiographic study. *J Periodont Res* 1968;**2**:111-20.

76. LINDSKOG S. Formation of intermediate cementum I: early mineralization of aprismatic enamel and intermediate cementum in monkey. *J Craniofac Genet Dev Biol* 1982;**7**:142-60.

77. LINDSKOG S. Formation of intermediate cementum II: a scanning electron microscopic study of the epithelial root sheath of Hertwig in monkey. *J Craniofac Genet Dev Biol* 1982;**2**:161-9.

78. LINDSKOG S, HAMMARSTRÖM L. Formation of intermediate cementum III: 3 H-tryptophan and 3 H-proline uptake into the epithelial root sheath of Hertwig in vitro. *J Craniofac Genet Dev Biol* 1982;**2**:171-7.

79. ANDREASEN JO. Relationship between surface and inflammatory resorption and changes in the pulp after replantation of permanent incisors in monkeys. *J Endod* 1981;**7**:294-301.

80. KENNEY EB, RAMFJORD SP. Cellular dynamics in root formation of teeth in rhesus monkeys. *J Dent Res* 1969;**48**:114-9.

81. LESTER KS. The unusual nature of formation in molar teeth of the laboratory rat. *J Ultrastruct Res* 1968;**28**:481-506.

82. THOMAS HF, KOLLAR EJ. Tissue interactions in normal murine root development. In: DAVIDOVITCH Z, ed. *The Biological Mechanisms of Tooth Eruption and Root Resorption.* Birmingham: EBSCO Media, 1988:145-51.

83. STENVIK A. Pulp and dentine reactions to experimental tooth intrusion. (A histologic study - long-term effects). *Trans Eur Orthod Soc* 1970;**45**:449-64.

84. STENVIK A. The effect of extrusive orthodontic forces on human pulp and dentin. *Scand J Dent Res* 1971;**79**:430-5.

85. STENVIK A, MJÖR IA. Epithelial remnants and denticle formation in the human dental pulp. *Acta Odontol Scand* 1970;**28**:721-8.

86. STENVIK A, MJÖR IA. Pulp and dentine reactions to experimental tooth intrusion. A histologic study of the initial changes. *Am J Orthod* 1970;**57**:370-85.

87. STENVIK A, MJÖR IA. The effect of experimental tooth intrusion on pulp and dentine. *Oral Surg Oral Med Oral Pathol* 1971;**32**:639-48.

88. ANDREASEN JO, SUNDSTRÖM B, RAVN JJ. The effect of traumatic injuries to primary teeth on their permanent successors. I. A clinical and histologic study of 117 injured permanent teeth. *Scand J Dent Res* 1971;**79**:219-83.

89. ANDREASEN JO, RAVN JJ. The effect of tramatic injuries to primary teeth on their permanent scuccessors. II. A clinical and radiographic follow-up study of 213 teeth. *Scand J Dent Res* 1971;**79**:284-94.

90. ANDREASEN JO. The influence of traumatic intrusion of primary teeth on their permanent successors. A radiographic and histologic study in monkeys. *Int J Oral Surg* 1976;5:207-19.

91. ANDREASEN JO. *Traumatic injuries of the teeth.*2nd edn. Copenhagen: Munksgaard, 1981:302-4.

92. ANDERSON AW, MASSLER M. Periapical tissue reactions following root amputation in immediate tooth replants. *Isr J Dent Med* 1970;19:1-8.

93. ANDREASEN JO, KRISTERSON L, ANDREASEN FM. Damage to the Hertwig's epithelial root sheath: effect upon growth after autotransplantation of teeth in monkeys. *Endod Dent Traumatol* 1988;44:145-51.

94. WALDHART E, LINARES HA. Ist die Zahnpulpa zur Knochenbildung befähigt? *Dtsch Zahnärztl Z* 1972;27:52-55.

95. ANDREASEN JO, BORUM M, ANDREASEN FM. Replantation of 400 avulsed permanent incisors. III. Factors related to root growth. *Endod Dent Traumatol*: To be submitted.

96. CVEK M, RÜDHMER M, GRANATH L-E, HOLLENDER L. First permanent molars subjected to mortal amputation before maturation of roots. I. Roentgenographic periradicular changes and peripheral root resorption after four years' observation. *Odont Revy* 1969;20:119-22.

97. GRANATH L-E, HOLLENDER L, CVEK M, RÜDHMER M. First permanent molars subjected to mortal amputation before maturation of roots. II. Roentgenologic and histologic study of ingrowth of vital tissue into devitalized, fixed pulp tissue. *Odont Revy* 1970;21:319-30.

98. STEWART DJ. Traumatised incisors. An unusual type of response. *Br Dent J* 1960;108:396-9.

99. RULE DC, WINTER GB. Root growth and apical repair subsequent to pulpal necrosis in children. *Br Dent J* 1966;120:586-90.

100. BARKER BCW, MAYNE JR. Some unusual cases of apexification subsequent to trauma. *Oral Surg Oral Med Oral Pathol* 1975;39:144-50.

101. TORNECK CD, SMITH J. Biologic effects of endodontic procedures on developing incisor teeth. I. Effect of partial and total pulp removal. *Oral Surg Oral Med Oral Pathol* 1970;30:258-66.

102. TORNECH CD. Effects and clinical significance of trauma to the developing permanent dentition. *Dent Clin North Am* 1982;26:481-504.

103. LIEBERMAN J, TROWBRIDGE H. Apical closure of nonvital permanent incisor teeth where no treatment was performed: case report. *J Endod* 1983;9:257-60.

104. HOLLAND R, DE SOUZA V. Ability of a new calcium hydroxide root canal filling material to induce hard tissue formation. *J Endod* 1985;11:535-43.

105. SCHROEDER HE, LISTGARTEN MA. Fine structure of the developing epithelial attachment of human teeth. *Monographs In Developmental Biology* 1971;2:1-134.

106. GOLDMAN HM. The topography and role of the gingival fibers. *J Dent Res* 1951;30:331-6.

107. ARNIM SS, HAGERMAN DA. The connective tissue fibers of the marginal gingiva. *J Am Dent Assoc* 1953;47:271-81.

108. MELCHER AH. The interpapillary ligament. *Dent Practit* 1962;12:461-2.

109. SMUKLER H, DREYER CJ. Principal fibres of the periodontium. *J Periodont Res* 1969;4:19-25.

110. PAGE RC, AMMONS WF, SCHECTMAN LR, DILLINGHAM LA. Collagen fibre bundles of the normal marginal gingiva in the marmoset. *Arch Oral Biol* 1974;19:1039-43.

111. ATKINSON ME. The development of transalveolar ligament fibres in the mouse. *J Dent Res* 1978;57:151(abstract).

112. GARNICK JJ, WALTON RE. Fiber system of the facial gingiva. *J Periodont Res* 1984;19:419-23.

113. TONNA EA, CRONKITE EP. The periosteum: Autoradiographic studies of cellular proliferation and tranformation utilizing tritiated thymidine. *Clin Orthop* 1963;30:218-33.

114. TONNA EA. Electron microscopy of aging skeletal cells. III. The periosteum. *Lab Invest* 1974;31:609-32.

115. TONNA EA. Response of the cellular phase of the skeleton to trauma. *Periodontics* 1966;4:105-14.

116. NASJLETI CE, CAFESSE RG, CASTELLI WA, HOKE JA. Healing after tooth reimplantation in monkeys. A radioautographic study. *Oral Surg Oral Med Oral Pathol* 1975;39:361-75.

117. HURST RW. Regeneration of periodontal and transseptal fibres after autografts in Rhesus monkeys. A qualitative approach. *J Dent Res* 1972;51:1183-92.

118. ANDREASEN JO. A time-related study of periodontal healing and root resorption activity after replantation of mature permanent incisors in monkeys. *Swed Dent J* 1980;4:101-10.

119. PROYE MP, POLSON AM. Repair in different zones of the periodontium after tooth reimplantation. *J Periodontol* 1982;53:379-89.

120. BORDEN SM. Histological study of healing following detachment of tissue as is commonly carried out in the vertical incision for the surgical removal of teeth. *Can Dent Assoc* 1948;14:510-5.

121. DEDOLPH TH, CLARK HB. A histological study of mucoperiosteal flap healing. *J Oral Surg* 1958;16:367-76.

122. KOHLER CA, RAMFJORD SP. Healing of gingival mucoperiosteal flaps. *Oral Surg Oral Med Oral Pathol* 1960;13:89-103.

123. TAYLER AS, CAMBELL MM. Reattachment of gingival epithelium to the tooth. *J Periodontol* 1972;43:281-94.

124. GRUNG B. Healing of gingival mucoperiosteal flaps after marginal incision in apicoectomy procedures. *Int J Oral Surg* 1973;2:20-5.

125. TONNA EA, STAHL SS, ASIEDU S. A study of the reformation of severed gingival fibers in aging mice using ^{3}H-proline autoradiography. *J Periodont Res* 1980;15:43-52.

126. ENGLER WD, RAMFJORD SP, HINIKER JJ. Healing following simple gingivectomy. A tritiated thymidine radioautographic study. I. Epithelialization. *J Periodontol* 1966;37:298-308.

127. RAMFJORD SP, ENGLER WO, HINIKER JJ. A radiographic study of healing following simple gingivectomy. II. The connective tissue. *J Periodontol* 1966;37:179-89.

128. LISTGARTEN MA. Electron microscopic features of the newly formed epithelial attachment after gingival surgery. *J Periodontol* 1966;2:46-52.

129. HENNING FR. Healing of gingivectomy wounds in the rat: Reestablishment of the epithelial seal. *J Periodontol* 1968;39:265-9.

130. STAHL SS, WITKIN GJ, DICEASARE A, BROWN R. Gingival healing I. Description of the gingivectomy sample. *J Periodontol* 1968;39:106-8.

131. STAHL SS, WITKIN GJ, CANTOR M, BROWN R. Gingival healing II. Clinical and histologic repair sequences following gingivectomy. *J Periodontol* 1968;39:109-18.

132. STAHL SS, TONNA EA. Comparison of gingival repair following chemical or surgical injury. *Periodontics* 1968;6:26-9.

133. STAHL SS, TONNA EA, WEISS R. Autoradiographic evaluation of gingival response to injury - I. Surgical trauma in young adult rats. *Arch Oral Biol* 1968;31:71-86.

134. TONNA EA, STAHL SS, WEISS R. Autoradiographic evaluation of gingival response to injury - II. Surgical trauma in young rats. *Arch Oral Biol* 1969;14:19-34.

135. INNES PB. An electron microscopy study of the regeneration of gingival epithelium following gingivectomy in the dog. *J Periodont Res* 1970;5:196-204.

136. HOLM-PEDERSEN P, LÖE H. Wound healing in the gingiva of young and old individuals. *Scand J Dent Res* 1970;79:40-53.

137. LISTGARTEN MA. Normal development, structure, physiology and repair of gingival epithelium. *Oral Sci Rev* 1972;1:63-8.

138. TONNA EA. A routine mouse gingivectomy procedure for periodontal research in aging. *J Periodontol* 1972;7:261-5.

139. TONNA EA, STAHL SS. A (^{3}H)-thymidine autoradiographic study of cell proliferative activity of injured parodontal tissues of 5-week-old mice. *Arch Oral Biol* 1973;18:617-27.

140. BRAGAAM, SQUIER CA. Ultractructure of regenerating junctional epithelium in the monkey. *J Periodontol* 1980;51:386-92.

141. WIRTHLIN MR, YEAGER JE, HANCOCK EB, GAUGLER RW. The healing of gigival wounds in miniature swine. *J Periodontol* 1980;51:318-27.

142. WIRTHLIN MR, HANCOCK EB, GAUGLER RW. The healing of atraumatic and traumatic incisions in the gingivae of monkeys. *J Periodontol* 1984;55:103-13.

143. LISTGARTEN MA, ROSENBERG S, LERNER S. Progressive replacement of epithelial attachment by a connective tissue junction after experimental periodontal surgery in rats. *J Periodontol* 1982;53:659-79.

144. WENNSTRÖM J. Regeneration of gingiva following surgical excision. A clinical study. *J Clin Periodontol* 1983;10:287-97.

145. SABAG N, MERY C, GARCÍA M, VASQUEZ V, CUETO V. Epithelial reattachment after gingivectomy in the rat. *J Periodontol* 1984;55:135-40.

146. HENNING FR. Epithelial mitotic activity after gingivectomy - Relationship to reattachment. *J Periodontol* 1969;4:319-24.

147. MONEFELDT I, ZACHRISSON BU. Adjustment of clinical crown height by gingivectomy following orthodontic space closure. *Angle Orthod* 1977;47:256-64.

148. HOLM-PEDERSEN P, LÖE H. Wound healing in the gingiva of young and old individuals. *Scand J Dent Res* 1971;79:40-53.

149. HOLM-PEDERSEN P. *Studies on healing capacity in young and old individuals. Clinical, biophysical and microvascular aspects of connective tissue repair with special reference to tissue function in man and the rat* (Thesis). Copenhagen: Munksgaard, 1973.

150. LINDHE J, SOCRANSKY S, NYMAN S, WESTFELT E, HAFFAJEE A. Effect of age on healing following periodontal therapy. *J Clin Periodontol* 1985;12:774-87.

151. MELCHER AH. Role of the periosteum in repair of wounds of the parietal bone of the rat. *Arch Oral Biol* 1969;14:1101-9.

152. MELCHER AH. Wound healing in monkey (Macaca irus) mandible: Effect of elevating periosteum on formation of subperiosteal callus. *Arch Oral Biol* 1971;16:461-4.

153. MELCHER AH, ACCURSI GE. Osteogenic capacity of periosteal and osteoperiosteal flaps elevated from the parietal bone of the rat. *Arch Oral Biol* 1971;16:573-80.

154. HJØRTING-HANSEN E, ANDREASEN JO. Incomplete bone healing of experimental cavities in dog mandibles. *Br J Oral Surg* 1971;9:33-40.

155. MASCRÈS C, MARCHAND JF. Experimental apical scars in rats. *Oral Surg Oral Med Oral Pathol* 1980;50:164-74.

156. NWOKU AL. Unusually rapid bone regeneration following mandibular resection. *J Maxillofac Surg* 1980;8:309-15.

157. SHUKER S. Spontaneous regeneration of the mandible in a child. A sequel to partial avulsion as a result of a war injury. *J Maxillofac Surg* 1985;13:70-3.

158. DAHLIN C, LINDE A, GOTTLOW J, NYMAN S. Healing of bone defects by guided tissue regeneration. *Plast Reconstr Surg* 1988;81.672-76.

159. DAHLIN C, GOTTLOW, LINDE A, NYMAN S. Healing of maxillary and mandibular bone defects using a membrane technique. *Scand J Plast Reconstr Hand Surg* 1990;24:13-9.

160. YUMET JA, POLSON AM. Gingival wound healing in the presence of plaque-induced inflammation. *J Periodontol* 1985;56:107-19.

161. STAHL SS. The influence of antibiotics on the healing of gingival wounds in rats. II. Reattachment potential of soft and calcified tissues. *J Periodontol* 1963;34:166-74.

162. STAHL SS. The influence of antibiotics on the healing of gingival wounds in rats. III. The influence of pulpal necrosis on gingival reattachment potential. *J Periodontol* 1963;34:371-4.

163. STAHL SS, SOBERMAN A, DE CESARE A. Gingiva healing. V. The effects of antibiotics administered during the early stages of repair. *J Periodontol* 1969;40:521-3.

164. KILLEY HC, KAY LW, WRIGHT HC. Subperiosteal osteomyslitis of the mandible. *Oral Surg Oral Med Oral Pathol* 1970;29:576-89.

165. YAMASAKI A, ROSE GG, PINERO GJ, MAHAN CJ. Ultrastructural and morphometric analyses of human cementoblasts and periodontal fibroblasts. *J Periodontol* 1987;58:192-201.

166. SELVIG KA. The fine structure of human cementum. *Acta Odontol Scand* 1965;23:423-41.

167. ZANDER HA, HÜRZELER B. Continuous cementum apposition. *J Dent Res* 1958;37:1035-44.

168. STOOT GG, SIS RF, LEVY BM. Cemental annulation as an age criterion in forensic dentistry. *J Dent Res* 1982;61:814-7.

169. ROBERTS WE, CHAMBERLAIN JG. Scanning electron microscopy of the cellular elements of rat periodontal ligament. *Arch Oral Biol* 1978;23:587-9.

170. BEERTSEN W, EVERTS V. Junction between fibroblasts in mouse periodontal ligament. *J Periodont Res* 1980;15:655-68.

171. GARANT PR. Collagen resorption by fibroblasts. A theory of fibroblastic maintenance of the periodontal ligament. *J Periodontol* 1976;47:380-90.

172. DEPORTER DA, TEN CATE AR. Collagen resorption by periodontal ligament fibroblasts at the hard tissue-ligament interfaces of the mouse periodontum. *J Periodontol* 1980;51:429-32.

173. BORDIN S, NARAYANAN AS, REDDY J, CLEVELAND D, PAGE RC. Fibroblast subtypes in the periodontium. A possible role in connective tissue regeneration and periodontal reattachment. *J Periodont Res* 1984;19:642-44.

174. McCULLOCH CAG, BORDIN S. Role of fibroblast subpopulations in periodontal physiology and pathology. *J Periodont Res* 1991;26:144-54.

175. GOULD TRL, BRUNETTE DM, DOREY J. Cell turnover in the periodontium in health and periodontal disease. *J Periodont Res* 1983;18:353-61.

176. McCULLOCH CAG, MELCHER AH. Continuos labelling of the periodontal ligament of mice. *J Periodont Res* 1983;18:231-41.

177. McCULLOCH CAG, MELCHER AH. Cell density and cell generation in the periodontal ligament of mice. *Am J Anat* 1983;167:43-58.

178. LISTGARTEN MA. Intracellular collagen fibrils in the periodontal ligament of the mouse, rat, hamster, guinea pig and rabbit. *J Periodont Res* 1973;8:335-42.

179. TEN CATE AR, DEPORTER DA. The degradative role of the fibroblast in the remodelling and turnover of collagen in soft connective tissues. *Anat Rec* 1974;182:1-14.

180. CRUMLEY PJ. Collagen formation in the normal and stressed periodontium. *Periodontics* 1964;2:53-61.

181. GARANT PR. Collagen resorption by fibroblasts. A theory of fibroblastic maintenance of the periodontal ligament. *J Periodontol* 1976;47:380-90.

182. IMBERMAN M, RAMAMURTHY N, GOLUB L, SCHNEIR M. A reassessment of collagen half-life in rat periodontal tissues: application of the pool-expansion approach. *J Periodont Res* 1986;21:396-402.

183. BEERTSEN W, EVERTS V. The site of remodelling of collagen in the periodontal ligament of the mouse incisor. *Anat Rec* 1977;189:479-98.

184. RIPPIN JW. Collagen turnover in the periodontal ligament under normal and altered functional forces. I. Young rat molars. *J Periodont Res* 1976;11:101-07.

185. ORLOWSKI WA. Biochemical study of collagen turnover in rat incisor periodontal ligament. *Arch Oral Biol* 1978;23:1163-5.

CHAPTER 2

186. SKOUGAARD MR, LEVY BM, SIMPSON J. Collagen metabolism in skin and periodontal membrane of the marmoset. *Scand J Dent Res* 1970;**78**:256-62.

187. KAMEYAMA Y. Autoradiographic study of H 3 -proline incorporation by rat periodontal ligament, gingival connective tissue and dental pulp. *J Periodont Res* 1975;**10**:98-102.

188. BOYDE A, JONES SJ. Scanning electron microscopy of cementum and Sharpeys fibre bone. *Z Zellforsch* 1968;**92**:536-48.

189. SHACKLEFORD JM, ZUNIGA MA. Scanning electron microscopic studies of calcified and noncalcified dental tissues. *Proc Cambridge Sterioscan Colloquium* 1970; 113-19.

190. SHACKLEFORD JM. Scanning electron microscopy of the dog periodontium. *J Periodont Res* 1971;**6**:45-54.

191. SHACKLEFORD JM. The indifferent fiber plexus and its relationship to principal fibers of the periodontium. *Am J Anat* 1971;**131**:427-42.

192. SVEJDA J, KREJSA O. Die Oberflächenstruktur des Alveolarknochens, des extrahierten Zahnes und des Periodontiums im Rastereelektronenmikroskop (REM). *Schweiz Monatsschr Zahnheilk* 1972;**82**:763-76.

193. SVEJDA J, SKACH M. The periodontium of the human tooth in the scaning electron microscope (Stereoscan). *J Periodontol* 1973;**44**:478-84.

194. KVAM E. Scanning electron microscopy of organic structures on the root surface of human teeth. *Scand J Dent Res* 1972;**80**:297-306.

195. BERKOVITZ BKB, MOXHAM BJ. The development of the periodontal ligament with special reference to collagen fibre ontogeny. *J Biol Buccale* 1990;**18**:227-36.

196. YAMAMOTO T, WAKITA M. The development and structure of principal fibers and cellular cementum in rat molars. *J Periodont Res* 1991;**26**:129-37.

197. KVAM E. Topography of principal fibers. *Scand J Dent Res* 1973;**81**:553-7.

198. SHACKLEFORD JM. Ultrastructural and microradiographic characteristics of Sharpey's fibers in dog alveolar bone. *Ala J Med Sci* 1973;**10**:11-20.

199. SLOAN P, SHELLIS RP, BEKOVITZ BKB. Effect of specimen preparation on the apperance of the rat periodontal ligament in the scanning electron microscope. *Arch Oral Biol* 1976;**21**:633-5.

200. BERKOVITZ BKB, HOLLAND GR, MOXHAM BJ. *A colour atlas and textbook of oral anatomy, histology and embryology.* London: Wolfe Medical Publications Ltd, 1992.

201. SLOAN P. Scanning electron microscopy of the collagen fibre architecture of the rabbit incisor periodontium. *Arch Oral Biol* 1978;**23**:567-72.

202. SLOAN P. Collagen fibre architecture in the periodontal ligament. *J Roy Soc Med* 1979;**72**:188-91.

203. KINDLOVA M. The blood supply of the marginal periodontium in Macacus Rhesus. *Arch Oral Biol* 1965;**10**:869.

204. FOLKE LEA, STALLARD RE. Periodontal microcirculation as revealed by plastic microspheres. *J Periodont Res* 1967;**2**:53-63.

205. LENZ P. Zur Gefässstruktur des Parodontiums. Untersuchungen an Korrosionspräparaten von Affenkiefern. *Dtsch Zahnärztl Z* 1968;**23**:357-61.

206. EDWALL LGA. The vasculature of the periodontal ligament. In: BERKOVITZ BKB, MOXHAM BJ, NEWMAN HN, eds. *The periodontal ligament in health and disease.* Oxford, New York, Toronto, Sydney, Paris, Frankfurt: Pergamon Press, 1982:151-71.

207. LINDHE J, KARRING T. The anatomy of the periodontium. In: LINDHE J. *Textbook of clinical periodontology.* Copenhagen: Munksgaard, 1983:19-66.

208. KVAM E. Topography of principal fibers. *Scand J Dent Res* 1973;**81**:553-7.

209. ANDREASEN JO. Review of root resorption systems and models. Etiology of root resorption and the homeostatic mechanisms of the periodontal ligament. In: DAVIDOVITCH D, ed. *The Biological Mechanisms of Tooth Eruption and Root Resorption.* Birmingham: EBSCO Media:9-21.

210. COOLIDGE ED. The thickness of the human periodontal membrane. *Am Dent Cosmos* 1937;**24**:1260-70.

211. GOULD TRL, MELCHER AH, BRUNETTE DM. Location of progenitor cells in periodontal ligament of mouse molar stimulated by wounding. *Anat Rec* 1977;**188**:133-42.

212. YEE JA, KIMMEL DB, JEE WSS. Periodontal ligament cell kinetics following orthodontic tooth movement. *Cell Tissue Kinet* 1976;**9**:293-302.

213. ROBERT WE, CHASE DC. Kinetics of cell proliferation and migration associated with orthodontically induced osteogenesis. *J Dent Res* 1982;**60**:174-81.

214. GOULD TRL. Ultrastructural characteristics of progenitor cell population in the periodontal ligament. *J Dent Res* 1983;**62**:873-6.

215. BURKLAND GA, HEELEY JD, IRVING JT. A histological study of regeneration of the completely disrupted periodontal ligament in the rat. *Arch Oral Biol* 1967;**21**:349-54.

216. McCULLOCH CAG, BORDIN S. Role of fibroblast subpopulations in periodontal physiology and pathology. *J Periodont Res* 1991;**26**:144-54.

217. ANDREASEN FM, VESTERGAARD PEDERSEN B. Prognosis of luxated permanent teeth - the development of pulp necrosis. *Endod Dent Traumatol* 1985;**1**:207-20.

218. ANDREASEN FM, YU Z, THOMSEN BL. The relationship between pulpal dimensions and the development of pulp necrosis after luxation injuries in the permanent dentition. *Endod Dent Traumatol* 1986;**2**:90-8.

219. MANDEL U, VIIDIK A. Effect of splinting on the mechanical and histological properties of the healing periodontal ligament after experimental extrusive luxation in the monkey. *Arch Oral Biol* 1989;**34**:209-17.

220. MIYASHIN M, KATO J, TAKAGI Y. Experimental luxation injuries in immature rat teeth. *Endod Dent Traumatol* 1990;**6**:121-8.

221. MIYASHIN M, KATO J, TAKAGI Y. Tissue reactions after experimental luxation injuries in immature rat teeth. *Endod Dent Traumatol* 1991;**7**:26-35.

222. ACETOZE PA,L SABBAG YS, RAMALHO AC. Luxacao dental. Estudo das alteracoes teciduais em dentes de crescimento continuo. *Rev Fac Farm Odont Araraquara* 1970;**4**:125-45.

223. ANDREASEN JO, ANDREASEN FM. Root resorption following traumatic dental injuries. *Proc Finn Dent Soc* 1991;**88**:95-114.

224. STAHL SS, WEISS R, TONNA EA. Autoradiographic evaluation of periapical responses to pulpal injury. I. Young rats. *Oral Surg Oral Med Oral Pathol* 1969;**28**:249-58.

225. STAHL SS, TONNA EA, WEISS R. Autoradiographic evaluation of periapical responses to pulpal injury. II. Mature rats. *Oral Surg Oral Med Oral Pathol* 1970;**29**:270-4.

226. COOLIDGE ED. The reaction of cementum in the presence of injury and infection. *J Am Dent Assoc* 1931;**18**:499-25.

227. TAGGER M. Behaviour of cementum of rat molars in experimental lesions. *J Dent Res* 1964;**43**:777-8.

228. SINAI I, SELTZER S, SOLTANOFF W, GOLDENBERG A, BENDER IB. Biologic aspects of endodontics. Part II. Periapical tissue reactions to pulp extirpation. *Oral Surg Oral Med Oral Pathol* 1967;**23**:664-79.

229. TORNECK CD, TULANANDA N. Reaction of alveolar bone and cementum to experimental abscess formation in the dog. *Oral Surg Oral Med Oral Pathol* 1969;**28**:404-16.

230. NAIR PNR, SCHROEDER HE. Pathogenese periapikaler Läsionen (eine Literaturübersicht). *Schweiz Monatsschr Zahnheilk* 1983;**93**:935-52.

231. BLOCK RM, BUSHELL A, RODRIGUES H, LANGELAND K. A histopathologic, histobacteriologic, and radiographic study of periapical endodontic surgical specimens. *Oral Surg Oral Med Oral Pathol* 1976;**42**:656-78.

232. WALTON RE, GARNICK JJ. The histology of periapical inflammatory lesions in permanent molars in monkeys. *J Endod* 1986;**12**:49-53.

RESPONSE OF ORAL TISSUE TO TRAUMA

233. TAGGER M, MASSLER M. Periapical tissue reactions after pulp exposure in rat molars. *Oral Surg Oral Med Oral Patol* 1975;**39**:304-17.

234. VAN MULLEM PJ, SIMON M, LAMERS AC, DE JONGE J, DE KOK JJ, LAMERS BW. Hard-tissue resorption and deposition after endodontic instrumentation. *Oral Surg Oral Med Oral Pathol* 1980;**49**:544-8.

235. MÖLLER ÅJR, FABRICIUS L, DAHLÉN G, ÖHMAN AE, HEYDEN G. Influence on periapical tissues of indigenous oral bacteria and necrotic pulp tissue in monkeys. *Scand J Dent Res* 1981;**89**:475-84.

236. PITT FORD TR. The effects on the periapical tissues of bacterial contamination of the filled root canal. *Int Endod J* 1982;**15**:16-22.

237. SIMON M, VAN MULLEM PJ, LAMERS AC, et al. Hard tissue resorption and deposition after preparation and disinfection of the root canal. *Oral Surg Oral Med Oral Pathol* 1983;**56**:421-4.

238. DWYER TG, TORABINEJAD M. Radiographic and histologic evaluation of the effect of endotoxin of the periapical tissues of the cat. *J Endod* 1981;**7**:31-5.

239. PITTS DL, WILLIAMS BL, MORTON TH. Investigation of the role of endotoxin in periapical inflammation. *J Endod* 1982;**8**:10-8.

240. SCHONFELD SE, GREENING AB, GLICK DH, FRANK AL, SIMON JH, HERLES SM. Endotoxin activity in periapical lesions. *Oral Surg Oral Med Oral Pathol* 1982;**53**:82-7.

241. JOHNSON NW, LINO Y, HOPPS RM. Bone resorption in periodontal diseases: role of bacterial factors. *Int Endod J* 1985;**18**:152-7.

242. MATTISON GD, HADDIX JE, KEHOE JC, PROGULSKE-FOX A. The effect of Eikenella corrodens endotoxin on periapical bone. *J Endod* 1987;**13**:559-65.

243. WANNFORS K, HAMMARSTRÖM L. A proliferative inflammation in the mandible caused by implantation of an infected dental root. A possible experimental model for chronic osteomyelitis. *Int J Oral Maxillofac Surg* 1989;**18**:179-83.

244. PIERCE AM. Experimental basis for the management of dental resorption. *Endod Dent Traumatol* 1989;**5**:255-65.

245. STASHENKO P. The role of immune cytokines in the pathogenesis of periapical lesions. *Endod Dent Traumatol* 1990;**6**:89-96.

246. KANTOR M, POLSON AM, ZANDER HA. Alveolar bone regeneration after removal of inflammatory and traumatic factors. *J Periodontol* 1976;**47**:687-95.

247. POLSON AM, MEITNER SW, ZANDER HA. Trauma and progression of marginal periodontitis in squirrel monkeys. IV. Reversibility of bone loss due to trauma alone and trauma superimposed upon periodontitis. *J Periodont Res* 1976;**11**:290-8.

248. JORDAN RE, SUZUKI M, SKINNER DH. Indirect pulp-capping of carious teeth with periapical lesions. *J Am Dent Assoc* 1978;**97**:37-43.

249. MALOOLEY JR. J, PATTERSON SS, KAFRAWY A. Response of periapical pathosis to endodontic treatment in monkeys. *Oral Surg Oral Med Oral Pathol* 1979;**47**:545-54.

250. MOSKOW BS, WASSERMAN BH, HIRSCHFELD LS, MORRIS ML. Repair of periodontal tissues following acute localized osteomyelitis. *Periodontics* 1967;**5**:29-36.

251. MERTE K, GÄNGLER P, HOFFMAN T. Morphophysiologische Untersuchungen der Zahnbildungs- und funktionsabhängigen Variationsmünster der periodontalen Regeneration. *Zahn Mund Kieferheilk* 1983;**71**:566-74.

252. BHASKAR SN. Maxilla and mandible (alveolar process). In: BHASKAR SN, ed. *Orban's Oral histology and embryology.* St. Louis: The CV Mosby Company, 1976:234-53.

253. BIRN H. The vascular supply of the periodontal membrane. An investigation of the number and size of perforations in the alveolar wall. *J Periodont Res* 1966;**1**:51-68.

254. WEINMANN JP, SICHER H. *Bone and bones. Fundamentals of bone biology.* St Louis: The CV Mosby Company, 1955:51-2.

255. SCOTT J. The development, structure and function of alveolar bone. *Dent Practit* 1968;**19**:19-22.

256. MCLEAN FC, URIST MR. Bone. *An introduction to the physiology of skeletal tissue.* 2nd edn. Chicago: The University of Chicago Press, 1961.

257. AMLER MH, JOHNSON PL, SALMAN I. Histological and histochemical investigation of human alveolar socket healing in undisturbed extraction wounds. *J Am Dent Assoc* 1960;**61**:32-44.

258. AMLER MH, SALMAN I, BUNGENER H. Reticular and collagen fiber characteristics in human bone healing. *Oral Surg Oral Med Oral Pathol* 1964;**17**:785-96.

259. AMLER MH. The time sequence of tissue regeneration in human extraction wounds. *Oral Surg Oral Med Oral Pathol* 1969;**27**:309-18.

260. AMLER MH. Pathogenesis of disturbed extraction wounds. *J Oral Surg* 1973;**31**:666-74.

261. AMLER MH. The age factor in human extraction wound healing. *J Oral Surg* 1977;**35**:193-7.

262. AMLER MH. The interrelationship of dry socket sequelae. *NY J Dent* 1980;**50**:211-7.

263. SYRJÄNEN SM, SYRJÄNEN KJ. Influence of Alvogyl on the healing of extraction wound in man. *Int J Oral Surg* 1979;**8**:22-30.

264. BOYNE PJ. Osseous repair of the postextraction alveolus in man. *Oral Surg Oral Med Oral Pathol* 1966;**21**:805-13.

265. YOSHIKI S, LANGELAND K. Alkaline phosphatase activity in the osteoid matrix of healing alveolar socket. *Oral Surg Oral Med Oral Pathol* 1968;**26**:381-9.

266. SYRJÄNEN SM, SYRJÄNEN KJ. Mast cells in the healing process of the extraction wound in man. *Proc Finn Dent Soc* 1977;**73**:220-4.

267. SYRJÄNEN SM, SYRJÄNEN KJ. Prevention and treatment of post-extraction complications. A comparison of the effects of Alvogyl and a new drug combination on wound healing. *Proc Finn Dent Soc* 1981;**77**:305-11.

268. EVIAN CI, ROSENBERG ES, COSLET JG, CORN H. The osteogenic activity of bone removed from healing extraction sockets in humans. *J Periodontol* 1982;**53**:81-5.

269. PEREA PAZ MB. Caraterísticas histologicas del epitelio neoformado durante la reparacion alveolar post-extraccior en diferentes edades. *Estomatologia Peruana* 1983;**37**:9-17.

270. GERGELY E, BARTHA N. Die Wirkung der in der Extractionswunde gebliebenen Wurzelhautreste auf den Heilungsverlauf. *Dtsch Stomatol* 1961;**11**:494-8.

271. SIMPSON HE. The healing of extraction wounds. *Br Dent J* 1969;**126**:555-7.

272. GUGGENHEIM B, SCHROEDER HE. Reactions in the periodontium to continuous antigenic stimulation in sensitized gnotobiotic rats. *Infec Immun* 1974;**10**:565-77.

273. PAGE RC, SCHROEDER HE. Pathogenesis of inflammatory periodontal disease. *Lab Invest* 1976;**33**:235-49.

274. SUNDQVIST G. *Bacteriological studies of necrotic dental pulps.* Thesis. Umeå: Umeå University-Odontological Faculty, 1976.

275. FISH EW. Bone Infection. *J Am Dent Assoc* 1939;**26**:691-712.

276. MÖLLER ÅJR. Microbiological examination of root canals and periapical tissues of human teeth. Thesis. *Odontologisk Tidsskrift* (Special Issue) 1966;**74**:1-380.

277. ANDREASEN JO, RUD J. A histobacteriologic study of dental and periapical structures after endodontic surgery. *Int J Oral Surg* 1972;**1**:272-81.

278. WALTON RE. Histological evaluation of the presence of bacteria in induced periapical lesions in monkeys. *J Endod* 1992;**18**:216-21.

279. LANGELAND K, BLOCK RM, GROSSMAN LI. A histopathologic and histobacteriologic study of 35 periapical endodontic surgical specimens. *J Endod* 1977;**3**:8-23.

280. TORABINEJAD M, KIGER RD. Experimentally induced alterations in periapical tissues of the cat. *J Dent Res* 1980;**59**:87-96.

281. TORABINEJAD M, KETTERING JD. Identification and relative concentration B and T lymphocytes in human chronic periapical lesions. *J Endod* 1985;**11**:479-88.

282. TORABINEJAD M, EBY WC, NAIDORF IJ. Inflammatory and immunological aspects of the pathogenesis of human periapical lesions. *J Endod* 1985;**11**:479-88.

283. STERN H, MACKLER BF, DREIZEN S. A quantitative analysis of cellular composition of human periapical granuloma. *J Endod* 1981;**7**:70-4.

284. STERN H, DREIZEN S, MACKLER BF, SELBST AG, LEVY BM. Quantitative analysis of cellular composition of human periapical granuloma. *J Endod* 1981;**7**:117-22.

285. STERN H, DREIZEN S, MACKLER BF, LEVY BM. Isolation and characterization of inflammatory cell from the human periapical granuloma. *J Dent Res* 1982;**61**:1408-12.

286. BERGENHOLTZ G, LEKHOLM U, LILJENBERG B, LINDHE J. Morphometric analysis of chronic inflammatory periapical lesions in root-filled teeth. *Oral Surg Oral Med Oral Pathol* 1983;**55**:295-301.

287. LINDHE J, LILJENBERG B, LISTGARTEN M. Some microbiological and histopathological features of periodontal disease in man. *J Periodontol* 1980;**51**:264-9.

288. YANAGISAWA S. Pathologic study of periapical lesions. I. Periapical granulomas: clinical, histopathologic and immunohistopathologic studies. *J Oral Pathol* 1980;**9**:288-300.

289. CYMERMAN JJ, CYMERMAN DH, WALTERS J, NEVINS AJ. Human T lymphocyte subpopulations in chronic periapical lesions. *J Endod* 1984;**10**:9-11.

290. KLEIN DC, RAISZ LG. Prostaglandins: Stimulation of bone resorption in tissue culture. *Endocrinology* 1970;**86**:1436-40.

291. RAISZ LG, SANDBERG AL. GOODSON JM, SIMMONS HA, MERGENHAGEN SE. Complement-dependent stimulation of prostaglandin synthesis and bone resorption. *Science* 1974,**185**:789-91.

292. TORABINEJAD M, CLAGETT J, ENGEL D. A cat model for the evaluation of mechanisms of bone resorption: induction of bone loss by simulated immune complexes and inhibition by indomethacin. *Calcif Tissue Int* 1979;**29**:209-14.

293. MATEJKA M, PORTEDER H, KLEINERT W, ULRICH W, WARZEK G, SINZINGER H. Evidence that PGI-generation in human dental cysts is stimulated by leucotrienes C and D . *J Maxillofac Surg* 1985;**13**:93-6.

294. HORTON JE, RAISZ G, SIMMONS HA, OPPENHEIM JJ, MERGENHAGEN SE. Bone resorbing activity in supernatant fluid from cultured human peripheral blood leucocytes. *Science* 1972;**177**:793-5.

295. LUBEN RA, MUNDY GR, TRUMMEL CL, RAISZ LG. Partial purification of osteoclast-activating factor from phytohemagglutinin-stimulated human leukocytes. *J Clin Invest* 1974;**53**:1473-80.

296. DIETRICH JW, GOODSON JM, RAISZ LG. Stimulation of bone resorption by variuos prostaglandins in organ culture. *Prostaglandins* 1975;**10**:231-40.

297. HORTON JE, WEZEMAN FH, KUETTNER KE. Regulation of osteoclast-activating factor (OAF)-stimulated bone resorption *in vitro* with an inhibitor of collagenase. In: HORTON JE, TARPLEY TM, DAVIS WF, eds. *Mechanisms of localized bone loss.* Arlington: Information Retrieval Inc, 1978:127-50.

298. HORTON JE, KOOPMAN WJ, FARRAR JJ, FULLER-BONAR J, MERGENHAGEN SE. Partial purification of a bone-resorbing factor elaborated from human allogeneic cultures. *Cell Immunol* 1979;**43**:1-10.

299. HOLTROP ME, RAISZ LG. Comparison of effects of 1,25-dihydroxycholecalciferol, prostaglandin E , and osteoclast-activating factor with parathyroid hormone on the ultrastructure of osteoclasts in cultures long bones of fetal rats. *Calcif Tissue Int* 1979;**29**:201-5.

300. LUBEN RA, MOHLER MA, NEDWIN GE. Production of hybridomas secreting monclonal antibodies agains the lymphokine osteoclast activating factor. *J Clin Invest* 1979;**64**:337-41.

301. DEWHIRST FE, MOSS DE, OFFENBACHER S, GOODSON JM. Levels of prostaglandin E , thrombozane, and prostacyclin in periodontal tissues. *J Periodont Res* 1983;**18**:156-63.

302. TORABINEJAD M, LUBEN RA. Presence of osteoclast activating factor in human periapical lesions. *J Endod* 1985;**10**:145.

303. HAUSMANN E, RAISZ LG, MILLER WA. Endotoxin stimulation of bone resorption in tissue culture. *Science* 1970;**168**:862-4.

304. RAISZ LG, ALANDER C, EILON G, WHITEHEAD SP, NUKI K. Effects of two bacterial products, muramyl dipeptide endotoxin on bone resorption in organ culture. *Calcif Tissue Int* 1982;**34**:365-9.

305. CHAMBERS TJ. The cellular basis of bone resorption. *Clin Orthop* 1980;**151**:283-93.

306. RAISZ LG, NUKI K, ALANDER CB, CRAIG RG. Interactions between bacterial endotoxin and other stimulators of bone resorption in organ culture. *J Periodont Res* 1981;**16**:1-7.

307. NAIR BC, MAYBERRY WR, DZIAK R, CHEN PB, LEVINE MJ, HAUSMANN E. Biological effects of a purified lipopolysaccharide from Bacteroides gingivalis. *J Periodont Res* 1983;**18**:40-9.

308. JOHNSON NW, IINO Y, HOPPS RM. Bone resorption in periodontal diseases: role of bacterial factors. *Int Endod J* 1985;**18**:152-7.

309. MILLAR SJ, GOLDSTEIN EG, LEVINE MJ, HAUSMANN E. Lipoprotein: a Gram-negative cell wall component that stimulates bone resorption. *J Periodont Res* 1986;**21**:256-9.

310. YONEDA T, MUNDY GR. Monocytes regulate osteoclast-activating factor production by releasing prostaglandins. *J Exp Med* 1979;**149**:338-50.

311. YONEDA T, MUNDY GR. Prostaglandins are necessary for osteoclast-activating factor production by activated peripheral blood leukocytes. *J Exp Med* 1979;**149**:279-83.

312. BOCKMAN RS, REPO MA. Lymphokine-mediated bone resorption requires endogenous prostaglandin synthesis. *J Exp Med* 1981;**154**:529-34.

313. ANDREASEN JO, RUD J. Modes of healing histologically after endodontic surgery in 70 cases. *Int J Oral Surg* 1972;**1**:148-60.

314. BRYNOLF I. A histological and roentgenological study of the periapical region of human upper incisors. *Odontologisk Revy* 1967;**18**:Suppl 11:1-176.

315. BOYLE PE. *Kronfeld's histopathology of the teeth and their surrounding structures.* 4th edn. Philadelphia: Lea & Fibiger, 1955:17-9.

316. BENDER IB, MORI K. The radiopaque lesion: A diagnostic consideration. *Endod Dent Traumatol* 1985;**1**:2-12.

317. MOSCOW BS, WASSERMAN BH, HIRSCHFELD LS, MORRIS ML. Repair of periodontal tissues following acute localized osteomyelitis. *J Am Soc Periodont* 1967;**5**:29-36.

318. HEDIN M, POLHAGEN L. Follow-up study of periradicular bone condensation. *Scand J Dent Res* 1971;**79**:436-40.

319. WILSON GW, STEINBRECHER M. Heriditary hypoplasia of the dentin *J Am Dent Ass* 1929;**16**:866-86.

320. HODGE HC. Correlated clinical and structural study of hereditary opalescent dentin. *J Dent Res* 1936;**15**:316-7.

321. OVERVAD H. Et tilfælde af osteogenesis imperfecta med dentinogenesis imperfecta. *Tandlægebladet* 1969;**73**:840-50.

322. BRÄNNSTRÖM M. Observations on exposed dentine and the corresponding pulp tissue. A preliminary study with replica and routine histology. *Odont Revy* 1962;**13**:235-45.

323. BRÄNNSTROÖM M, ÅSTRÖM A. A study on the mechanism of pain elicited from the dentin. *J Dent Res* 1964;**43**:619-25.

324. FUSAYAMA T, MAEDA T. Effect of pulpectomy on dentin hardness. *J Dent Res* 1969;**48**:452-60.

325. CVEK M. Prognosis of luxated non-vital maxillary incisors treated with calcium hydroxide and filled with guttapercha. A retrospective clinical study. *Endod Dent Traumatol* 1992;**8**:45-55.

326. BAUME LJ. The biology of pulp and dentine. A historic, terminologic-taxonomic, histologic-biochemical, embryonic and clinical survey. *Monographs in Oral Science* 1980;**8**:1-220.

327. RUCH JV. Odontoblast differentiation and the formation of the odontoblast layer. *J Dent Res* 1945;**64**:489-98.

328. HOLLAND GR. The odontoblast process: form and function. *J Dent Res* 1985;**64**:499-514.

329. COUVE E. Ultrastructural changes during the life cycle of human odontoblasts. *Arch Oral Biol* 1986;**31**:643-51.

330. FRANK RM, NALBANDIAN J. Development of dentine and pulp. In: BERKOVITZ BKB, BOYDE A, FRANK RM, et al., eds. *Teeth*. Berlin: Springer-Verlag, 1989:73-171.

331. MELSEN B, MELSEN F, RÖLLING I. Dentin formation rate in human teeth. *Calcif Tissue Res* 1977;**24**:Suppl:Abstr no 62.

332. STANLEY HR, WHITE CL, MCCRAY L. The rate of tertiary (reparative) dentine formation in the human tooth. *Oral Surg Oral Med Oral Pathol* 1966;**21**:180-9.

333. KRAMER IHR, RUSSELL LH. Observations on the vascular architecture of the dental pulp. *J Dent Res* 1956;**35**:957.

334. KRAMER IRH. The vascular architecture of the human dental pulp. *Arch Oral Biol* 1960;**2**:177-89.

335. SAUNDERS RL. X-ray microscopy of the periodontal and dental pulp vessels in the monkey and in man. *Oral Surg Oral Med Oral Pathol* 1966;**22**:503-18.

336. TAKAHASHI K, KISHI Y, KIM S. Scanning electron microscope study of the blood vessels of dog pulp using corrosion resin casts. *J Endod* 1982;**8**:131-5.

337. KIM S. Microcirculation of the dental pulp in health and disease. *J Endod* 1985;**11**:465-71.

338. KIM S. Regulation of pulpal blood flow. *J Dent Res* 1985;**64**:590-6.

339. HEYERAAS KJ. Pulpal, microvascular, and tissue pressure. *J Dent Res* 1985;**64**:585-9.

340. BERNICK S. Differences in nerve distribution between erupted and non-erupted human teeth. *J Dent Res* 1964;**43**:406-11.

341. FULLING H-J, ANDREASEN JO. Influence of maturation status and tooth type of permanent teeth upon electrometric and thermal pulp testing. *Scand J Dent Res* 1976;**84**:286-90.

342. JOHNSEN DJ, HARSHBARGER J, RYMER HD. Quantitative assessment of neural development in human premolars. *Anat Rec* 1983;**205**:421-9.

343. JOHNSEN DJ. Innervation of teeth: qualitative, quantitative, and developmental assessment. *J Dent Res* 1985;**64**(Special Issue):555-63.

344. ANDREASEN JO, KRISTERSON L, ANDREASEN FM. Relation between damage to the Hertwig's epithelial root sheath and type of pulp repair after autotransplantation of teeth in monkeys. *Endod Dent Traumatol*, In preparation.

345. CVEK M, CLEATON-JONES PE, AUSTIN JC, ANDREASEN JO. Pulp reactions to exposure after experimental crown fractures of grinding in adult monkeys. *J Endod* 1982;**9**:391-7.

346. HEIDE S, MJÖR IA. Pulp reactions to experimental exposures in young permanent monkey teeth. *Int Endod J* 1983;**16**:11-9.

347. WATTS A, PATERSON RC. Cellular responses in the dental pulp: a review. *Int Endod J* 1981;**14**:10-21.

348. CVEK M. Endodontic treatment of traumatized teeth. In: ANDREASEN JO. *Traumatic injures of the teeth*. Copenhagen: Munksgaard, 1981:321-83.

349. SVEEN OB, HAWES RR. Differentiation of new odontoblasts and dentine bridge formation in rat molar teeth after tooth grinding. *Arch Oral Biol* 1968;**13**:1399-412.

350. ZACH L, TOPAL R, COHEN G. Pulpal repair following operative procedures. Radioautographic demonstration with tritiated thymidine. *Oral Surg Oral Med Oral Pathol* 1969;**28**:587-97.

351. FEIT J, METELOVA M, SINDELKA Z. Incorporation of ^{3}H-thymidine into damaged pulp of rat incisors. *J Dent Res* 1970;**49**:783-6.

352. LUOSTARINEN V. Dental pulp response to trauma. An experimental study in the rat. *Proc Finn Dent Soc* 1971;**67**:1-51.

353. FITZGERALD M. Cellular mechanics of dentinal bridge repair using ^{3}H-thymidine. *J Dent Res* 1979;**58**:2198-206.

354. YAMAMURA T. Differentation of pulpal cells and inductive influences of various matrices. *J Dent Res* 1985;**64**:530-40.

355. SENZAKI H. A histological study of reparative dentinogenesis in the rat incisor after colchicine administration. *Arch Oral Biol* 1980;**25**:737-43.

356. SKOGLUND A, TRONSTAD L, WALLENIUS K. A micorangiographic study of vascular changes in replanted and autotransplanted teeth of young dogs. *Oral Surg Oral Med Oral Pathol* 1978;**45**:17-28.

357. SKOGLUND A. Vascular changes in replanted and autotransplanted apicoectomized mature teeth of dogs. *Int J Oral Surg* 1981;**10**:100-10.

358. BARRETT AP, READE PC. Revascularization of mouse tooth isografts and allografts using autoradiography and carbon-perfusion. *Arch Oral Biol* 1981;**26**:541-5.

359. AVERY JK, STRACHAN DS, CORPRON RE, COX CF. Morphological studies of the altered pulps of the New Zealand white rabbit after resection of the inferior alveolar nerve and/or superior cervical ganglion. *Anat Rec* 1971;**171**:495-508.

360. AVERY JK, COX CF, CORPRON RE. The effects of combined nerve resection and cavity preparation and restoration on response dentin formation in rabbit incisors. *Arch Oral Biol* 1974;**19**:539-48.

361. AVERY JK, COX CF, CHIEGO DJ JR. Presence and location of adrenergic nerve endings in the dental pulps of mouse molars. *Anat Rec* 1980;**198**:59-71.

362. CHIEGO DJ JR, SINGH IJ. Evaluation of the effects of sensory deervation on osteoblasts by ^{3}H-proline autoradiography. *Cell Tissue Res* 1981;**217**:569-76.

363. CHIEGO DJ JR, KLEIN RM, AVERY JK. Tritiated thymidine autoradiographic study of the effect of inferior alveolar nerve resection of the proliferative compartments of the mouse incisor formative tissue. *Arch Oral Biol* 1981;**26**:83-9.

364. CHIEGO DJ JR, FISHER MA, AVERY JK, KLEIN RM. Effects of denervation of ^{3}H-fucose incorporation by odontoblasts in the mouse incisor. *Cell Tissue Res* 1983;**230**:197-203.

365. CHIEGO DJ JR, KLEIN RM, AVERY JK, GRUHL IM. Denervation induced changes in cell proliferation in the rat molar after wounding. *Anat Rec* 1986;**214**:348-52.

366. CHIEGO DJ JR, AVERY JK, KLEIN RM. Neuroregulation of protein synthesis in odontoblasts of the first molar of the rat after wounding. *Cell Tissue Res* 1987;**248**:119-23.

367. KLEIN RM, CHIEGO DJ JR, AVERY JK. Effect of chemical sympathectomy on cell proliferation in the progenitive compartments of the neonatal mouse incisor. *Arch Oral Biol* 1981;**26**:319-25.

368. KUBOTA K, YONAGA T, HOSAKA K, KATAYAMA T, NAGAE K, SHIBANAI S, SATO Y, TAKADA K. Experimental morphological studies on the functional role of pulpal nerves in dentinogenesis. *Anat Anz* (Jena)1985;**158**:323-36.

369. ANDREASEN FM. Pulpal healing after luxation injuries and root fracture in the permanent dentition. *Endod Dent Traumatol* 1989;**5**:111-31.

370. ANDREASEN FM, JUHL M, ANDREASEN JO. Pulp reaction to replantation of teeth with incomplete root development. *Endod Dent Traumatol* 1993. To be submitted.

371. INOUE H, KUROSAKA Y, ABE K. Autonomic nerve endings in the odontoblast/predentin border and predentin of the canine teeth of dogs. *J Endod* 1992;**18**:149-51.

372. CVEK M, CLEATON-JONES P, AUSTIN J, KLING M, LOWNIE J, FATTI P. Pulp revascularization in reimplanted immature monkey incisors - predictability and the effect of antibiotic systemic prophylaxis. *Endod Dent Traumatol* 1990;**6**:157-9.

373. CVEK M, CLEATON-JONES P, AUSTIN J, LOWNIE J, KLING M, FATTI P. Effect of topical application of doxycycline on pulp revascularization and periodontal healing in reimplanted monkey incisors. *Endod Dent Traumatol* 1990;**6**:170-6.

374. OLGART L, BRÄNNSTRÖM M, JOHNSON G. Invasion of bacteria into dentinal tubules. Experiments in vivo and in vitro. *Acta Odontol Scand* 1974;**32**:61-70.

375. VONGSAVAN N, MATTEWS B. Fluid flow through cat dentine in vivo. *Arch Oral Biol* 1992;**37**:175-85.

376. ROBINSON HBG, BOLING LR. The anachoretic effect in pulpitis. I. Bacteriologic studies. *J Am Dent Assoc* 1941;**28**:268-82.

377. BOLING LR, ROBINSON HBG. Anachoretic effect in pulpitis. II. Histologic studies. *Arch Pathol* 1942;**33**:477-86.

378. BURKE GW, KNIGHTON HT. The localization of microorganisms in inflamed dental pulps of rats following bacteremia. *J Dent Res* 1960;**39**:205-14.

379. GIER RE, MITCHELL DF. Anachoretic effect of pulpitis. *J Dent Res* 1968;**47**:564-70.

380. SMITH LS, TAPPE GD. Experimental pulpitis in rats. *J Dent Res* 1962;**41**:17-22.

381. CSERNYEI J. Anachoresis and anachoric effect of chronic periapical inflammations. *J Dent Res* 1939;**18**:527-31.

382. ALLARD U, STRÖMBERG T. Inflammatory reaction in the apical area of pulpectomized and sterile root canals in dogs. *Oral Surg Oral Med Oral Pathol* 1979;**48**:463-6.

383. ALLARD U, NORD C-E, SJÖBERG L, STRÖMBERG T. Experimental infections with staphylococcus aureus, streptococcus sanguis, pseudomonas aeruginosa, and bacteroides fragilis in the jaws of dogs. *Oral Surg Oral Med Oral Pathol* 1979;**48**:454-62.

384. GROSSMAN LI. Origin of migroorganisms in traumatized, pulpless, sound teeth. *J Dent Res* 1967;**46**:551-3.

385. BERGENHOLTZ G. Microorganisms from necrotic pulp of traumatized teeth. *Odont Revy* 1974;**25**:347-58.

386. MÖLLER ÅJR, FABRICIUS L, DAHLÉN G, ÖHMAN AE, HEYDEN G. Influence on periapical tissues of indigenous oral bacteria and necrotic pulp tissue in monkeys. *Scand J Dent Res* 1981;**89**:475-84.

387. DELIVANIS PD, SNOWDEN RB, DOYLE RJ. Localization of blood-borne bacteria in instrumented unfilled root canals. *Oral Surg Oral Med Oral Pathol* 1981;**52**:430-2.

388. SONNABEND E, OH CS. Zur Frage des Epithels im apikalen Granulationsgewebe (Granulom) menschlicher Zähne. *Dtsch Zahnärztl Z* 1966;**21**:627-43.

389. NAIR PNR. Light and electron microscopic studies of root canal flora and periapical lesions. *J Endod* 1987;**13**:29-39.

390. NAIR PNR, SCHROEDER HE. Epithelial attachment at diseased human tooth-apex. *J Periodont Res* 1985;**20**:293-300.

391. ROSS R. Wound healing. *Sci Am* 1969;**220**:40-8.

392. ROSS R, ODLAND G. Human wound repair. II. Inflammatory cells. Epithelial-menechymal interrelations, and fibrinogenesis. *J Cell Biol* 1968;**39**:152-68.

393. SCIUBBA JJ, WATERHOUSE JP, MEYER J. A fine structural comparison of the healing of incisional wounds of mucosa and skin. *J Oral Pathol* 1978;**7**:214-27.

394. FEJERSKOV O, PHILIPSEN HP. Incisional wounds in palatal epithelium in guinea pigs. *Scand J Dent Res* 1972;**80**:47-62.

395. FEJERSKOV O. Excision wounds in palatal epithelium in guinea pigs. *Scand J Dent Res* 1972;**80**:139-54.

396. LUOMANEN M. A comparative stydy of healing of laser and scalpel incision wound in rat oral mucosa. *Scand J Dent Res* 1987;**95**:65-73.

397. LUOMANEN M, VIRTANEN I. Healing of laser and scalpel incision wound of rat tongue mucosa as studied with cytokeratin antibodies. *J Oral Pathol* 1987;**16**:139-44.

398. LUOMANEN M, MEURMAN JH, LEHTO V-P. Extracellular matrix in healing CO laser incision wound. *J Oral Pathol* 1987;**16**:322-31.

399. LUOMANEN M, LEHTO V-P, MEURMAN JH. Myofibroblasts in healing laser wounds of rat tongue mucosa. *Arch Oral Biol* 1988;**33**:17-3.

400. ROVIN S, COSTICH ER, FLEMING JE, GORDON HA. Healing of tongue wounds in germfree and conventional mice. *Arch Pathol* 1965;**79**:641-3.

401. FEJERSKOV O. Excision wounds in palatal epithelium in guinea pigs. *Scand J Dent Res* 1972;**80**:139-54.

402. FEJERSKOV O, PHILLIPSEN HP. Incisional wounds in palatal epithelium in guinea pigs. *Scand J Dent Res* 1972;**80**:47-62.

403. DABELSTEEN E, MACKENZIE I. Selective loss of blood group antigens during wound healing. *Acta Pathol Microbiol Scand* 1974;**84**:445-50. Sect A.

404. ANDERSEN L, FEJERSKOV O. Ultrastructure of initial epithelial cell migration in palatal wounds of guinea pigs. *J Ultrastruct Res* 1974;**48**:113-24.

405. ANDERSEN L, FEJERSKOV O. Ultrastructural localisation of acid phosphatase in oral mucosal wounds. In: BIERRING E, ed. *Proc 9th Congress Nord Soc Cell Biol*. Odense: Odense University Press, 1976:89-99.

406. ANDERSEN L. Quantitative analysis of epithelial changes during wound healing in palatal mucosa of guinea pigs. *Cell Tissue Res* 1978;**193**:231-46.

407. ANDERSEN L. Cell junctions in squamous epithelium during wound healing in palatal mucosa of guinea pigs. *Scand J Dent Res* 1980;**88**:328-339.

408. ANDERSEN L. Ultrastructure of squamous epithelium during wound healing in palatal mucosa of guinea pigs. *Scand J Dent Res* 1980;**88**:418-29.

409. NOBUTO T, TOKIOKA T, IMAI H, SUWA F, OHTA Y, YAMAOKA A. Microvascularization of gingival wound healing using corrosion casts. *J Periodontol* 1987;**58**:240-6.

410. WIJDEVELD MGMM, GRUPPING EM, KUIJPERS-JAGTMAN AM, MALTHA JC. Wound healing of the palatal mucoperiosteum in beagle dogs after surgery at different ages. *J Craniomaxillofac Surg* 1987;**15**:51-7.

411. KAHNBERG K-E, THILANDER H. Healing of experimental excisional wounds in the rat palate. I. Histological study of the interphase in wound healing after sharp dissection. *Int J Oral Surg* 1982;**11**:44-51.

412. HEDNER E, VAHLNE A, HIRSCH J-M. Herpes simplex virus (type 1) delays healing of oral excisional and extraction wounds in the rat. *J Oral Pathol Med* 1990;**19**:471-6.

413. HARRISON JW, JUROSKY KA. Wound healing in the tissues of the periodontium following periradicular surgery. I. The incisional wound. *J Endod* 1991;**17**:425-35.

414. HARRISON JW, JUROSKY KA. Wound healing in the tissues of the periodontium following periradicular surgery. II. The dissectional wound. *J Endod* 1991;**17**:544-52.

415. HARRISON JW. Healing of surgical wounds in oral mucoperiosteal tissue. *J Endod* 1991;**17**:401-8.

416. ANDREASEN JO. Histologic aspects of penetrating lip wounds. 1993. In preparation.

417. ALLBROOK D, BAKER W DE C, KIRKALDY-WILLIS WH. Muscle regeneration in experimental animals and in man. The cycle of tissue change that follows trauma in the injured limb syndrome. *J Bone Joint Surg* 1966;**48**:153-69.

418. BETZEH, FIRKET H, REZNIK M. Some aspects of muscle regeneration. In: BOURNE GH, DANIELLI JF, eds. *International Review of Cytology*. New York London: Academic Press, 1966; Ch.19, pp.203-25.

419. CHURCH JCT, NORONHA RFX, ALLBROOK DB. Satellite cells and skeletal muscle regeneration. *Br J Surg* 1966;**53**:638-42.

420. JÄRVINEN M, SORVARI T. Healing of a crush injury in rat striated muscle. I. Description and testing of a new method of inducing a standard injury to the calf muscles. *Acta Pathol Microbiol Scand* 1975;**83**:259-65.

421. JÄRVINEN M. Healing of a crush injury in rat striated muscle. II. A histological study of the effect of early mobilization and immobilization of the repair processes. *Acta Pathol Microbiol Scand* 1975;**83**:269-82.

422. ROWSELL AR. The intra-uterine healing of foetal muscle wounds: experimental study in the rat. *Br J Plast Surg* 1984;**37**:635-42.

423. GARRETT WE JR, SEABER AV, BOSWICK J, URBANIAK JR, GOLDNER JL. Recovery of skeletal muscle after laceration and repair. *J Hand Surg* 1984;**9**:683-92.

424. LEHTO M, ALANEN A. Healing of a muscle trauma. Correlation of sonographical and histological findings in an experimental study in rats. *J Ultrasound Med* 1987;**6**:425-9.

425. HURME, T KALIMO H, LEHTO M, JÄRVINEN M. Healing of skeletal muscle injury: an ultrastructural and immunohistochemical study. *Med Sci Sports Exerc* 1991;**23**:801-10.

426. SILNESS J, GUSTAVSEN F, FEJERSKOV O, KARRING T, LÖE H. Cellular, afibrillar coronal cementum in human teeth. *J Periodontal Res* 1976;**11**:331-8.

427. ANDREASEN JO, BORUM M, JACOBSEN HL, ANDREASEN FM. Replantation of 400 avulsed permanent incisors. II. Factors related to pulp healing. *Endod Dent Traumatol* 1993: To be submittid.

428. ANDREASEN JO, PAULSEN HU, YU Z, BAYER T, SCHWARTZ O. A long-term study of 370 autotransplanted premolars. Part II. Tooth survival and pulp healing subsequent to transplantation. *Eur J Orthod* 1990;**12**:14-24.

429. LÖE H, WAERHAUG J. Experimental replantation of teeth in dogs and monkeys. *Arch Oral Biol* 1961;**3**:176-83.

430. LINDSKOG S, BLOMLÖF L, HAMMARSTRÖM L. Evidence for a role of odontogenic epithelium in maintaining the periodontal space. *J Clin Periodontol* 1988;**15**:371-3.

431. WESSELINK PR. *Disturbances in the homeostatis of the periodontal ligament: dento-alveolar ankylosis and root resorption.* Amsterdam: Joko Offset, 1992:100.

432. ANDREASEN JO. Review of root resorption systems and models. Etiology of root resorption and the homeostatic mechanisms of the periodontal ligament. In: DAVIDOVITCH Z, ed. *The biological mechanisms of tooth eruption and root resorption.* Birmingham: EBSCO Media, 1988:9-21.

433. ANDREASEN JO. Summary of root resorption. In: DAVIDOVITCH Z, ed. *Proceedings of the international conference on the biological mechanisms of tooth eruption and tooth resorption.* Birmingham: EBSCO Media, 1988:399-400.

434. ANDREASEN JO, ANDREASEN FM. Root resorption following traumatic dental injuries. *Proc Finn Dent Soc* 1992;**88**:95-114.

435. NAIR PNR, SCHROEDER HE. Epithelial attachment at diseased human tooth-apex. *J Periodont Res* 1985;**20**:293-300.

436. YU SM, STASHENKO P. Identification of inflammatory cells in developing rat periapical lesions. *J Endodont* 1987;**13**:535-40.

437. SCIUBBA JJ. In situ characterization of mononuclear cells in human dental periapical inflammatory lesions using monoclonal antibodies. *Oral Surg Oral Med Oral Pathol* 1984;**58**:160-65.

438. STASHENKO P, YU SM, WANG C-Y. Kinetics of immune cell and bone resorptive respons to endodontic infections. *J Endodont* 1992;**18**:422-26.

439. ISHIHARA Y, NISHIHARA T, MAKI E, NOGUCHI T, KOGA T. Role of interleukin-1 and prostaglandin in *in vitro* bone resorption induced by *Actinomycetemcomitans* lipopolysaccharide. *J Periodont Res* 1991;**26**:155-60.

440. TORABINEJAD M, BAKLAND LK. Prostaglandins: their possible role in the pathogenesis of pulpal and periapical diseases, part 1. *J Endodont* 1980;**6**:733-39.

441. TORABINEJAD M, BAKLAND LK. Prostaglandins: their possible role in the pathogenesis of pulpal and periapical diseases, part 2. *J Endodont* 1980;**6**:769-75.

442. TORABINEJAD M, EBY WC, NEIDORF IJ. Inflammatory and immunological aspects of the pathogenesis of human periapical lesions. *J Endodont* 1985;**11**:479-87.

443. STERRETT JD. The osteoclast and periodontitis. *J Clin Periodontol* 1986;**13**:258-69.

444. ANDREASEN JO. External root resorption: its implication in dental traumatology, paedodontics, periodontics, orthodontics and endodontics. *Int Endodont J* 1985;**18**:109-18.

445. HAMMARSTRÖM L, LINDSKOG S. General morphological aspects of resorption of teeth and alveolar bone. *Int Endodont J* 1985;**18**:93-08.

446. ANDREASEN JO. Experimental dental traumatology: development of a model for external root resorption. *Endodont Dent Traumatol* 1987;**3**:269-87.

447. ANDREASEN FM, ANDREASEN JO. Resorption and mineralization prosesses following root fracture of permanent incisors. *Endod Dent Traumatol* 1988;**4**:202-14.

448. PIERCE AM. Experimental basis for the management of dental resorption. *Endod Dent Traumatol* 1989;**5**:255-65.

449. STASHENKO P. The role of immune cytokines in the pathogenesis of periapical lesions. *Endod Dent Traumatol* 1990;**6**:89-96.

450. TORABINEJAD M, GOTTI E, LESSARD G. Leukotrienes: their possible role in pulpal and periapical diseases. *Endod Dent Traumatol* 1991;**7**:233-41.

451. PIERCE AM, LINDSKOG S, HAMMARSTRÖM L. Osteoclasts: structure and function. *Electron Microsc Rev* 1991;**4**:1-45.

452. ANDREASEN JO, ANDREASEN FM. Root resorption following traumatic dental injuries. *Proc Finn Dent Soc* 1992;**88**(Suppl.1):95-14.

453. CAHILL DR, MARKS JR SC, WISE GE, GORSKI JP. A review and comparison of tooth eruption systems used in experimentation- a new proposal on tooth eruption. In: DAVIDOVITCH Z, ed. *The biological mechanisms of tooth eruption and root resorption.* Birmingham: EBSCO Media, 1988:1-7.

454. HEPPENSTALL RB. Fracture healing. In: HUNT TK, HEPPENSTALL RB, PINES E, ROVEE D, eds. *Soft and hard tissue repair.* New York: Praeger, 1984:101-42.

455. FANTONE JC, WARD PA. Inflammation. In: RUBIN E, FARBER JL, eds. *Pathology.* Philadelphia: JB Lippincott, 1988:34-64.

456. TROWBRIDGE HO, EMLING RC, *Inflammation: a review of the process* Bristol, Pennsylvania: 2nd edn. Comsource Distribution Systems Inc. 1983.

457. SELTZER S. *Inflammation: an update.* The Research and Education Foundation of the American Association of Endodontists, 1990.

458. WAKISAKA S. Neuropeptides in the dental pulps: distribution, origin, and correlation. *J Endodont* 1990:67-69.

459. LOTZ M, CARSON DA, VAUGHAN JH. Substance P activation of rheumatoid synoviocytes: neural pathway in pathogenesis of arthritis. *Science* 1987;**235**:893-95.

460. YOKOYAMA MM, FUJIMOTO K. Role of lymphocytes activation by substance P in rheumatoid arthritis. *Int J Tissue React* 1990;**12**:1-9.

461. O'BRYNE EM, BLANCUZZI VJ, WILSON DE, WONG MM, PEPPARD J, SIMKE JP, JENG AY. Increased intra-articular substance P and prostaglandin E_2 following injection of interleukin-1 in rabbits. *Int J Tissue React* 1990;**12**:11-14.

462. OLGART L, HOCKFELT T, NILSSON G, PERNOW B. Localization of substance P-like immunoreactivity in nerves of the tooth pulp. *Pain* 1977;**4**:153-59.

463. UDDMAN R, GRUNDITZ T, SUNDLER F. Calcitonin gene-related peptide: a sensory transmitter in dental pulp. *Scand J Dent Res* 1986;**94**:219-24.

464. WAKISAKA S, ICHIKAWA H, NISHIKAWA S, MATSUO S, TAKANO Y, AKAI M. The distribution and origin of calcitonin gene-related peptide-containing nerve fibers in feline dental pulp: relationship with substance-P containing nerve fibers. *Histochemistry* 1987;**86**:585-89.

465. SILVERMAN JD, KRUGER L. An interpretation of dental innervation based upon the pattern of calcitonin gene-related (CGRP)-immunoreactive thin sensory axons. *Somatosens Res* 1987;**5**:157-75.

466. WAKISAKA S, ICHIKAWA H, NISHIMOTO T, et al. Substance P-like immunoreactivity in the pulp-dentine zone of human molar teeth demonstrated by indirect immunofluorescence. *Arch Oral Biol* 1984;**29**:73-75.

467. WAKISAKA S, NISHIKAWA S, ICHIKAWA H, MATSUO S, TAKANO Y, AKAI M. The distribution and origin of substance P-like immunoreactivity in rat molar pulp and periodontal tissues. *Arch Oral Biol* 1985;**30**:813-18.

468. DAVIDOVITCH Z, NICOLAY OF, NGAN PW, SHANFELD JL. Neurotransmitters, cytokines, and the control of alveolar bone remodeling in orthodontics. *Dent Clin N Am* 1988;**31**:411-35.

469. GAZELIUS B, EDWALL B, OLGART L, LUNDBERG JM, HÖKFELT T, FISCHER JA. Vasodilatory effects and coexistence of calcitonin gene-related peptide (CGRP) and substance P in sensory nerves of cat dental pulp. *Acta Physiol Scand* 1987;**130**:33-40.

470. TAKAHASHI O, TRAUB RJ, RUDA MA. Demonstration of calcitonin gene-related peptide immunoreactive axons containing dynorphin A (1-8) immunoreactive spinal neurons in a rat model of peripheral inflammation and hyperalgesia. *Brain Res* 1988;**475**:168-72.

471. KVINNSLAND I, KVINNSLAND S. Changes in CGRP-immunoreactive nerve fibers during experimental tooth movements in rats. *Eur J Orthodont* 1990;**12**:320-29.

472. HOHMANN E, LEVINE L, TASHJIAN AH JR. Vasoactive intestinal peptide stimulates bone resorption via a cyclic adenosine 3', 5'-monophosphate-dependent mechanism. *Endocrinology* 1983;**112**:1233-39.

473. HOHMANN E, TASHJIAN AH JR. Functional receptors for vasoactive intestinal peptide of human osteosarcoma cells. *Endocrinology* 1984;**114**:1321-27.

474. TORABINEJAD M, EBY WC, NAIDORF IJ. Inflammatory and immunological aspects of the pathogenesis of human periapical lesions. *J Endodon* 1985;**11**:479-88.

475. MARCEAU F, LUSSIER A, REGOLI D, GIROUD JP. Pharmacology of kinins: their relevance to tissue injury and inflammation. *Gen Pharmacol* 1983;**14**:209-29.

476. PLUMMER TH, ERODOS EG. Human plasma carboxypeptidase. *Methods Enzymol* 1981;**80**(part c):442-49.

477. KAPLAN AP, SILVERBERG M, DUNN JT, GHEBREHIWET B. Interaction of the clotting, kinin-forming, complement and fibrinolytic pathways in inflammation. C-reactive protein and the plasma protein response to tissue injury. *Ann NY Acad Sci* 1982;**389**:23-38.

478. TORABINEJAD M, MIDROU T, BAKLAND L. Detection of kinins in human periapical lesions. *J Dent Res* 1968;**68**:201 (Abs 156).

479. MULLER-EBERHARD HJ. Chemistry and reaction mechanisms of complement. *Adv Immunol* 1968;**8**:1-80.

480. MALMSTROM M. Immunoglobulin classes of IgG, IgM, IgA, and complement components C3 in dental periapical lesions of patients with rheumatoid disease. *Scand J Rheumatol* 1975;**4**:57-64.

481. KUNTZ DD, GENCO RJ, GUTTUSO J, NATIELLA JR. Localization of immunoglobulins and the third component of complement in dental periapical lesions. *J Endodon* 1977;**3**:68-73.

482. PULVER WH, TAUBMAN MA, SMITH DJ. Immune components in human dental periapical lesions. *Arch Oral Biol* 1978;**23**:435-43.

483. RAISZ LG, SANDBERG AL, GOODSON JM, SIMMONS HA, MERGENHAGEN SE. Complement dependent stimulation of prostaglandin synthesis and bone resorption. *Science* 1974;**185**:789-91.

484. SANDBERG AL, RAISZ LG, GOODSON JM, SIMMONS HA, MERGENHAGEN SE. Initiation of bone resorption by the classical and alternative C pathways and its mediation by prostaglandins. *J Immunol* 1977;**119**:1378-81.

485. KALINER M, AUSTEN KF. CYCLIC AMP, ATP, and reversed anaphylactic histamine release from rat mast cells. *J Immunol* 1974;**112**:664-74.

486. GUTTLER F. Phospholipid synthesis in HeLa cells exposed to immunoglobulin G and complement. *Biochem J* 1972;**128**:953-60.

487. INOUE K, KINOSHITA T, OKADA M, AKIYAMA Y. Release of phospholipids from complement-mediated lesions on the surface structure of Escherichia coli. *J Immunol* 1977;**119**:65-72.

488. SCHLAGER SI, OHANIAN SH, BORSOS T. Stimulation of the synthesis and release of lipids in tumor cells under attack of antibody and complement. *J Immunol* 1978;**120**:895-901.

489. OWEN DAA, WOODWARD DF. Histamine and histamine H1- and H2- receptor antagonists in acute inflammation. *Biochem Soc Trans* 1980;**8**:150-55.

490. WILHELM DL. The mediation of increased vascular permeability in inflammation. *Pharmacol Rev* 1962;**14**:251-80.

491. WILLOUBY DA, DIEPPE P. Anti-inflammatory models in animals. *Agents Actions* 1976;**6**:306-12.

492. van LOVEREN H, KRAEUTER-KOPS S, ASKEMASE PW. Different mechanisms of release of vasoactive amines by mast cells occur in T cell-dependent compared to IgE-dependent cutaneous hypersensitivity responses. *Eur J Immunol* 1984;**14**:40-47.

493. ISHIZAKA K, ISHIZAKA T. Immune mechanisms of reversed type reaginic hypersensitivity. *J Immunol* 1973;**103**:588-95.

494. MATHIESEN A. Preservation and demonstration of mast cells in human apical granulomas and radicular cysts. *Scand J Dent Res* 1973;**81**:218-29.

495. PERRINI N, FONZI L. Mast cells in human periapical lesions: ultrastructural aspects and their possible physiopathological implications. *J Endodon* 1985;**11**:197-202.

496. RYAN GB, MAJNO G. *Inflammation*. Kalamazoo, MI: The Upjohn Company, 1980:52-55.

497. TORABINEJAD M, BAKLAND LK. Prostaglandins: their possible role in the pathogenesis of pulpal and periapical diseases. Part 1. *J Endodon* 1980;**6**:733-39.

498. TORABINEJAD M, BAKLAND LK. Prostaglandins: their possible role in the pathogenesis of pulpal and periapical diseases. Part 2. *J Endodon* 1980;**6**:769-76.

499. TORABINEJAD M, CLAGETT J, ENGEL D. A cat model for evaluation of mechanism of bone resorption: induction of bone loss by simulated immune complexes and inhibition by indomethacin. *Calcif Tissue Int* 1979;**29**:207-14.

500. MCNICHOLAS S, TORABINEJAD M, BLANKENSHIP J, BAKLAND LK. The concentration of prostaglandin E2 in human periradicular lesions. *J Endodon* 1991;**17**:97-100.

501. NACCACHE PH, SHAAFI RI. Arachidonic acid, leukotriene B4, and neutrophil activation. *Ann NY Acad Sci* 1983;**14**:125-39.

502. TORABINEJAD M, COTTI E, JUNG T. The concentration of leukotriene B4 in symptomatic and asymptomatic lesions. *J Endodon* 1992;**18**:205-08.

503. TORABINEJAD M, KIGER RD. Experimentally induced alterations in periapical tissues of the cat. *J Dent Res* 1980;**59**:87-96.

504. TORABINEJAD M, KETTERING JD. Detection of immune complexes in human periapical lesions by anticomplement immunofluorescence technique. *Oral Surg Oral Med Oral Pathol* 1979;**48**:256-61.

505. TORABINEJAD M, THEOFILOPOULOS AN, KETTERING JD, BAKLAND LK. Quantitation of circulating immune complexes, immunoglobulins G and M, and C3 complement in patients with large periapical lesions. *Oral Surg Oral Med Oral Pathol* 1983;**55**:186-90.

506. KETTERING JD, TORABINEJAD M. Concentration of immune complexes, IgG, IgM, IgE, and C3 in patients with acute apical abscesses. *J Endodon* 1984;**10**:417-21.

RESPONSE OF ORAL TISSUE TO TRAUMA

507. TORABINEJAD M, KETTERING JD. Identification and relative concentration of B and T lymphocytes in human chronic periapical lesions. *J Endodon* 1985;**11**:122-25.

508. BABAL P, SOLER P, BROZMAN M, JAKUBOVSKY J, BEYLY M, BASSET F. *In situ* characterization of cells in periapical granulomas by monoclonal antibodies. *Oral Surg* 1987;**64**:548-52.

509. CYMERMAN JJ, CYMERMAN DH, WALTERS J, NEVINS AJ. Human T lymphocyte subpopulations in chronic periapical lesions. *J Endodon* 1984;**10**:9-11.

510. STASHENKO P, YU SM. T helper and T suppressor cells reversal during the development of induced rat periapical lesions. *J Dent Res* 1989;**68**:830-34.

511. BARKHORDAR RA, RESOUZA YG. Human T lymphocyte subpopulations in periapical lesions. *Oral Surg Oral Med Oral Pathol* 1988;**65**:763-66.

512. WALLSTRÖM J. *Surgical exposure of pulp tissues in conventional and nude rats.* Thesis, Loma Linda University, 1990.

513. WATERMAN PA. *Development of periapical lesions in immunosuppressed rats.* Thesis, Loma Linda University, 1992.

514. KALLIO DM, GARANT PR, MINKIN C. Ultrastructural effects of calcitonin on osteoclasts in tissue culture. *J Ultrastruct Res* 1972;**39**:205-16.

515. MINKIN C. Bone acid phosphatase: tartrate-resistant acid phosphatase as a marker of osteoclast function. *Calcif Tissue Int* 1982;**34**:285-90.

516. HATTERSLEY G, CHAMBERS TJ. Generation of osteoclastic function in mouse bone marrow cultures: multinuclearity and tartrate-resistant acid phosphatase are unreliable markers for osteoclastic differentiation. *Endocrinology* 1989;**124**:1689-96.

517. MUNDY GR, ROODMAN GD. Osteoclast ontogeny and function. In: PECK WA, ed. *Bone and Mineral Research* Annual 5. New York: Elsevier, 1987:209-79.

518. VAES G. Cellular biology and biochemical mechanism of bone resorption. A review of recent developments on the formation, activation, and mode of action of osteoclasts. *Clin Orthop* 1988;**231**:239-71.

519. MARKS SC JR, POPOFF SN. Bone cell biology: the regulation of development, structure and function in the skeleton. *Am J Anat* 1988;**183**:1-44.

520. WALKER DG. Congenital osteopetrosis in mice cured by parabiotic union with normal siblings. *Endocrinology* 1972;**91**:916-20.

521. WALKER DG. Osteopetrosis cured by temporary parabiosis. *Science* 1973;**180**:875.

522. GÖTHLIN G, ERICSSON JL. On the histogenesis of the cells in fracture callus. Electron microscopic autoradiographic observations in parabiotic rats and studies on labeled monocytes. *Virchows Arch B Cell Pathol* 1973;**12**:318-29.

523. KAHN AJ, SIMMONS DJ. Investigation of cell lineage in bone using a chimaera of chick and quail embryonic tissue. *Nature* 1975;**258**:325-27.

524. JOTEREAU FV, LE DOUARIN NM. The developmental relationship between osteocyte and osteoclasts: a study using the quail-chick nuclear marker in endochondral ossification. *Dev Biol* 1978;**63**:253-65.

525. LOUTIT JF, NISBET NW. Resorption of bone. *Lancet* 1979;**ii**:26-27.

526. CHAMBERS TJ. The cellular basis of bone resorption. *Clin Orthop* 1980;**151**:283-93.

527. MARKS SC JR. The origin of the osteoclast. *J Oral Pathol* 1983;**12**:226-56.

528. KO JS, BERNARD GW. Osteoclast formation in vitro from bone marrow mononuclear cells in osteoclast-free bone. *Am J Anat* 1981;**161**:415-25.

529. BONUCCI E. New knowledge on the origin, function and fate of osteoclasts. *Clin Orthop* 1981;**158**:252-69.

530. KAHN AJ, STEWART CC, TEITELBAUM SL. Contact-mediated bone resorption by human monocytes in vitro. *Science* 1978;**199**:988-90.

531. MUNDY GR, ALTMAN AJ, GONDEK MD, BANDELIN JG. Direct resorption of bone by human monocytes. *Science* 1977;**196**:1109-11.

532. LOUTIT JF, NISBET NW. The origin of osteoclasts. *Immunobiology* 1982;**161**:193-203.

533. CHAMBERS TJ, HORTON MA. Failure of cells of the mononuclear phagocyte series to resorb bone. *Calcif Tissue Int* 1984;**36**:556-58.

534. BURGER EH, VAN DER MEER JWM, NIJWEIDE PJ. Osteoclast formation from mononuclear phagocytes: role of bone-forming cells. *J Cell Biol* 1984;**99**:1901-06.

535. SCHEVEN BAA, VISSER JWM, NIJWEIDE PH. *In vitro* osteoclast generation from different bone marrow fractions, including a highly enriched haematopoietic stem cell population. *Nature* 1986;**321**:79-81.

536. UDAGAW N, TAKAHASHI N, AKATSU TT, et al. The bone marrow-derived stromal cell lines MC3T3-G2/PA6 and ST2 support osteoclast-like cell differentiation in cocultures with mouse spleen cells. *Endocrinology* 1989;**125**:1805-13.

537. HATTERSLEY G, CHAMBERS TJ. Generation of osteoclasts from hemopoietic cells and a multipotential cell line in vitro. *J Cell Physiol* 1989;**140**:478-82.

538. HATTERSLEY G, CHAMBERS TJ. The role of bone marrow stroma in induction of osteoclastic differentiation. In: COHN DV, GLORIEUX FH, MARTIN TJ, eds. *Calcium Regulation and Bone Metabolism.* Amsterdam: Excerpta Medica, 1990: Ch. 10, pp. 439-42.

539. HATTERSLEY G, KERBY JA, CHAMBERS TJ. Identification of osteoclast precursors in multilineage hemopoietic colonies. *Endocrinology* 1991;**128**:259-62.

540. BARON R. Molecular mechanisms of bone resorption by the osteoclast. *Anat Rec* 1989;**224**:317-24.

541. BLAIR HC, KAHN AJ, CROUCH EC, JEFFREY JJ, TEITELBAUM SL. Isolated osteoclasts resorb the organic and inorganic components of bone. *J Cell Biol* 1986;**102**:1164-72.

542. REINHOLT FP, HULTENBY K, OLDBERG Å, HEINEGÅRD D. Osteopontin - a possible anchor of osteoclasts to bone. *Proc Natl Acad Sci USA* 1990;**87**:4473-75.

543. MIYAUCHI A, ALVAREZ J, GREENFIELD EM, et al. Recognition of osteopontin and related peptides by an alpha v beta 3 integrin stimulates immediate cell signals in osteoclasts. *J Biol Chem* 1991;**255**:20369-74.

544. OLDBERG Å, FRANZÉN A, HEINEGÅRD D. Cloning and sequence analysis of rat bone sialoprotein (osteopontin) cDNA reveals an Arg-Gly-Asp cell-binding sequence. *Proc Natl Acad Sci USA* 1986;**83**:8819-23.

545. GAY CV, MUELLER WJ. Carbonic anhydrase and osteoclasts: localization by labeled inhibitor autoradiography. *Science* 1974;**183**:432-34.

546. NEUMAN WF, MULRYAN BJ, MARTIN GR. A chemical view of osteoclasts based on studies with yttrium. *Clin Orthop* 1960;**17**:124-34.

547. VAES G. On the mechanisms of bone resorption. The action of parathyroid hormone on the excretion and synthesis of lysosomal enzymes and on the extracellular release of acids by bone cells. *J Cell Biol* 1968;**39**:676-97.

548. BARON R, NEFF L, LOUVARD D, COURTOY PJ. Cell-mediated extracellular acidification and bone resorption: evidence for a low pH in resorbing lacunae and localization of a 100-kD lysosomal membrane protein at the osteoclast ruffled border. *J Cell Biol* 1985;**101**:2210-22.

549. BARON R, NEFF L, LIPPINCOTT-SCHWARTZ M, et al. Distribution of lysosomal membrane proteins in osteoclasts and their relationship to acidic compartments. *J Cell Biol* 1985;**101**:53a.

550. BARON R, NEFF L, BROWN W, LOUVARD D, COURTOY PJ. Selective internalization of the apical plasma membrane and rapid redistribution of lysosomal enzymes and mannose 6-phosphate receptors during osteoclast inactivation by calcitonin. *J Cell Sci* 1990;**97**:439-47.

551. BLAIR HC, TEITELBAUM SL, GHISELLI R, GLUCK S. Osteoclastic bone resorption by a polarized vacuolar proton pump. *Science* 1989;**245**:855-57.

552. BEKKER PJ, GAY CV. Biochemical characterization of an electrogenic vacuolar proton pump in purified chicken osteoclast plasma membrane vesicles. *J Bone Min Res* 1990;**5**:569-79.

553. TETI A, BLAIR HC, TEITELBAUM SL, et al. Cytoplasmic pH regulation and chloride/bicarbonate exchange in avian osteoclasts. *J Clin Invest* 1989;**83**:227-33.

554. BLAIR HC, TEITELBAUM SL, TAN H-L, KOZIOL CM, SCHLESINGER PH. Passive chloride permeability charge coupled to H^+-ATPase of avian osteoclast ruffled membrane. *Am J Physiol* 1991;**260**:C1315-C1324.

555. HALL GE, KENNY AD. Role of carbonic anydrase in bone resorption induced by 1,25-dihydroxyvitamin D_3 *in vitro*. *Calcif Tissue Int* 1985;**37**:134-42.

556. GAY CV. Avian bone resorption at the cellular level. *CRC Crit Rev Poultry Biol* 1988;**1**:197-210.

557. GAY CV, FALESKI EJ, SCHRAER H, SCHRAER R. Localization of carbonic anhydrase in avian gastric mucosa, shell gland and bone by immunohistochemistry. *J Histochem Cytochem* 1974;**22**:819-25.

558. ANDERSON RE, SCHRAER H, GAY CV. Ultrastructural immunocytochemical localization of carbonic anhydrase in normal and calcitonin-treated chick osteoclasts. *Anat Rec* 1982;**204**:9-20.

559. KADOYA Y, NAGAHAMA S, KUWAHARA H, SHIMAZAKI M, SHIMAZU A, OGAWA Y, YAGI T. Isolation of avian carbonic anydrase and its immunohistochemical demonstration in medullary bone. *Osaka City Med J* 1987;**33**:111-119.

560. SUNDQUIST KT, LEPPILAMPI M, JÄRVELIN K, KUMPULAINEN T, VÄÄNÄNEN HK. Carbonic anhydrase isoenzymes in isolated rat peripheral monocytes, tissue macrophages, and osteoclasts. *Bone* 1987;**8**:33-38.

561. VÄÄNÄNEN HK, PARVINEN E-K. High active isoenzyme of carbonic anhydrase in rat calvaria osteoclasts. Immunohistochemical study. *Histochemistry* 1983;**78**:481-85.

562. VÄÄNÄNEN HK. Immunohistochemical localization of carbonic anhydrase isoenzymes I and II in human bone, cartilage and giant cell tumor. *Histochemistry* 1984;**81**:485-87.

563. JILKA RL, ROGERS JI, KHALIFAH RG, VAANANEN HK. Carbonic anhydrase isozymes of osteoclasts and erythrocytes of osteopetrotic micropthalmic mice. *Bone* 1985;**6**:445-49.

564. HUNTER SJ, ROSEN CJ, GAY CV. In vitro resorptive activity of isolated chick osteoclasts: effects of carbonic anhydrase inhibition. *J Bone Min Res* 1991;**6**:61-66.

565. HUNTER SJ, SCHRAER H, GAY CV. Characterization of isolated and cultured chick osteoclasts: the effects of acetazolamide, calcitonin and parathyroid hormone on acid production. *J Bone Min Res* 1988;**3**:297-303.

566. EMÅS S. Effect of acetazolamide on histamine-stimulated and gastrin-stimulated gastric secretion. *Gastroenterology* 1962;**43**:557-63.

567. BARON R, NEFF L, BROWN W, COURTOY PJ, LOUVARD D, FARQUHAR MG. Polarized secretion of lysosomal enzymes: co-distribution of cation-independent mannose-6-phosphate receptors and lysosomal enzymes along the osteoclast exocytic pathway. *J Cell Biol* 1988;**106**:1863-72.

568. BARON R, NEFF L, TRAN VAN P, NEFUSSI J-R, VIGNERY A. Kinetic and cytochemical identification of osteoclast precursors and their differentiation into multinucleated osteoclasts. *Am J Pathol* 1986;**122**:363-78.

569. EVERTS V, DELAISSÉ J-M, KORPER W, NIEHOF A, VAES G, BEERTSEN W. Degradation of collagen in the bone-resorbing compartment underlying the osteoclast involves both cysteine-proteinases and matrix metalloproteinases. *J Cellular Physiol* 1992;**150**:221-31.

570. FULLMER HM, LAZARUS G. Collagenase in human, goat and rat bone. *Israel J Med Sci* 1967;**3**:758-61.

571. FULLMER HM, LAZARUS GS. Collagenase in bone of man. *J Histochem Cytochem* 1969;**17**:793-98.

572. VAES G. The release of collagenase as an inactive proenzyme by bone explants in culture. *Biochem J* 1972;**126**:275-89.

573. SAKAMOTO S, SAKAMOTO M. Biochemical and immunohistochemical studies on collagenase in resorbing bone in tissue culture. *J Periodont Res* 1982;**17**:523-26.

574. EECKHOUT Y, DELAISSÉ J-M, VAES G. Direct extraction and assay of bone tissue collagenase and its relation to parathyroid-hormone-induced bone resorption. *Biochem J* 1986;**239**:793-96.

575. DELAISSE JM, EECKHOUT Y, VAES G. Bone-resorbing agents affect the production and distribution of procollagenase as well as the activity of collagenase in bone tissue. *Endocrinology* 1988;**123**:264-76.

576. DELAISSÉ J-M, EECKHOUT Y, SEAR C, GALLOWAY A, MCCULLAGH K, VAES G. A new synthetic inhibitor of mammalian tissue collagenase inhibits bone resorption in culture. *Biochem Biophys Res Commun* 1985;**133**:483-90.

577. SHIMIZU H, SAKAMOTO M, SAKAMOTO S. Bone resorption by isolated osteoclasts in living versus devitalized bone: differences in mode and extent and the effects of human recombinant tissue inhibitor of metalloproteinases. *J Bone Min Res* 1990;**5**:411-18.

578. HEATH JK, ATKINSON SJ, MEIKLE MC, REYNOLDS JJ. Mouse osteoblasts synthesize collagenase in response to bone resorbing agents. *Biochim Biophys Acta* 1984;**802**:151-54.

579. STRICKLIN GP, BAUER EA, JEFFREY JJ, EISEN AZ. Human skin collagenase: isolation of precursor and active forms from both fibroblast and organ cultures. *Biochemistry* 1977;**16**:1607-15.

580. BORNSTEIN P, SAGE H. Structurally distinct collagen types. *Annu Rev Biochem* 1980;**49**:957-1003.

581. DELAISSÉ JM, BOYDE A, MACONNACHIE E, et al. The effects of inhibitors of cysteine-proteinases and collagenase on the resorptive activity of isolated osteoclasts. *Bone* 1987;**8**:305-13.

582. RAISZ LG. Bone resorption in tissue culture. Factors influencing the response to parathyroid hormone. *J Clin Invest* 1965;**44**:103-16.

583. LUBEN RA, COHN DV. Effects of parathormone and calcitonin on citrate and hyaluronate metabolism in cultured bone. *Endocrinology* 1976;**98**:413-19.

584. DIETRICH JW, CANALIS EM, MAINA DM, RAISZ LG. Hormonal control of bone collagen synthesis *in vitro*: effects of parathyroid hormone and calcitonin. *Endocrinology* 1976;**98**:943-49.

585. RAISZ LG, KREAM BE. Hormonal control of skeletal growth. *Ann Rev Physiol* 1981;**43**:225-38.

586. HOCK JM, FONSECA J, GUNNESS-HEY M, KEMP BE, MARTIN TJ. Comparison of the anabolic effects of synthetic parathyroid hormone-related protein (PTHrP) 1-34 and PTH 1-34 on bone in rats. *Endocrinology* 1989;**125**:2022-27.

587. GUNNESS-HEY M, HOCK JM. Increased trabecular bone mass in rats treated with human synthetic parathyroid hormone. *Metab Bone Dis Relat Res* 1984;**5**:177-81.

588. HOCK JM, GERA I, FONSECA J, RAISZ LG. Human parathyroid hormone (1-34) increases bone mass in ovariectomized and orchidectomized rats. *Endocrinology* 1988;**122**:2899-904.

589. TAM CS, HEERSCHE JNM, MURRAY TM, PARSON JA. Parathyroid hormone stimulates the bone apposition rate independently of its resorptive action: differential effects of intermittent and continuous administration. *Endocrinology* 1982;**110**:506-12.

590. REEVE J, MEUNIER PJ, PARSONS SJA, et al. Anabolic effect of human parathyroid hormone fragment on trabecular bone in involutional osteoporosis: a multicentre trial. *Br Med J* 1980;**280**:1340-44.

RESPONSE OF ORAL TISSUE TO TRAUMA

591. SLOVIK DM, ROSENTHAL DI, DOPPELT SH, POTTS JT JR, DALY MA, CAMPBELL JA, NEER RM. Restoration of spinal bone in osteoporotic men by treatment with human parathyroid hormone (1-34) and 1,25-dihydroxyvitamin D. *J Bone Min Res* 1986;**1**:377-81.

592. FARLEY JR, TARBAUX NM, VERMEIDEN JPW, BAYLINK DJ. *In vitro* evidence that local and systemic skeletal effectors can regulate [^{3}H]-thymidine incorporation in chick calvarial cell cultures and modulate the stimulatory action(s) of embryonic chick bone extract. *Calcif Tissue Int* 1988;**42**:23-33.

593. VAN DER PLAS A, FEYEN JHM, NIJWEIDE PJ. Direct effect of parathyroid hormone on the proliferation of osteoblast-like cells: a possible involvement of cyclic AMP. *Biochem Biophys Res Commun* 1985;**129**:918-25.

594. MACDONALD BR, GALLAGHER JA, RUSSELL RGG. Parathyroid hormone stimulates the proliferation of cells derived from human bone. *Endocrinology* 1986;**118**:2445-49.

595. FINKELMAN RD, MOHAN S, LINKHART TA, ABRAHAM SM, BOUSSY JP, BAYLINK DJ. PTH stimulates the proliferation of TE-85 human osteosarcoma cells by a mechanism not involving either increased cAMP or increased secretion of IGF-I, IGF-II or TGF. *Bone Min* 1992;**16**:89-100.

596. SILVE CM, HRADEK GT, JONES AL, ARNAUD CD. Parathyroid hormone receptor in intact embryonic chicken bone: characterization and cellular localization. *J Cell Biol* 1982;**94**:379-86.

597. ROULEAU MF, WARSHAWSKY H, GOLTZMAN D. Parathyroid hormone binding *in vivo* to renal, hepatic, and skeletal tissues of the rat using a radioautographic approach. *Endocrinology* 1986;**118**:919-31.

598. CHAMBERS TJ. The pathobiology of the osteoclast. *J Clin Pathol* 1985;**38**:241-52.

599. TAKAHASHI N, YAMANA H, YOSHIKI S, et al. Osteoclast-like cell formation and its regulation by osteotropic hormones in mouse bone marrow cultures. *Endocrinology* 1988;**122**:1373-82.

600. KREAM BE, ROWE DW, GWOREK SC, RAISZ LG. Parathyroid hormone alters collagen synthesis and procollagen mRNA levels in fetal rat calvaria. *Proc Natl Acad Sci USA* 1980;**77**:5654-58.

601. RAISZ LG, KREAM BE, SMITH MA, SIMMONS HA. Comparison of the effects of vitamin D metabolites on collagen synthesis and resorption of fetal rat bone in organ culture. *Calcif Tissue Int* 1980;**32**:135-38.

602. ROWE DW, KREAM BE. Regulation of collagen synthesis in fetal rat calvaria by 1,25-dihydroxyvitamin D$_3$. *J Biol Chem* 1982;**257**:8009-15.

603. ABE E, MIYAURA C, TANAKA H, et al. 1α, 25-Dihydroxyvitamin D$_3$ promotes fusion of mouse alveolar macrophages both by a direct mechanism and by a spleen cell-mediated indirect mechanism. *Proc Natl Acad Sci USA* 1983;**80**:5583-87.

604. ABE E, MIYAURA C, SAKAGAMI H, et al. Differentiation of mouse myeloid leukemia cells induced by 1α, 25-dihydroxyvitamin D$_3$. *Proc Natl Acad Sci USA* 1981;**78**:4990-94.

605. TAKAHASHI N, AKATSU T, UDAGAWA N, et al. Osteoblastic cells are involved in osteoclast formation. *Endocrinology* 1988;**123**:2600-02.

606. NICHOLSON GC, MOSELEY JM, SEXTON PM, MENDELSOHN FAO, MARTIN TJ. Abundant calcitonin receptors in isolated rat osteoclasts. Biochemical and autoradiographic characterization. *J Clin Invest* 1986;**78**:355-60.

607. CHAMBERS TJ, MAGNUS CJ. Calcitonin alters behaviour of isolated osteoclasts. *J Pathol* 1982;**136**:27-39.

608. CHAMBERS TJ, FULLER K, MCSHEEHY PMJ. The effects of calcium regulating hormones on bone resorption by isolated human osteoclastoma cells. *J Pathol* 1985;**145**:297-305.

609. CHAMBERS TJ, CHAMBERS JC, SYMONDS J, DARBY JA. The effect of human calcitonin on the cytoplasmic spreading of rat osteoclasts. *J Clin Endocrinol Metab* 1986;**63**:1080-85.

610. ARNETT TR, DEMPSTER DW. A comparative study of disaggregated chick and rat osteoclast *in vitro*: effects of calcitonin and prostaglandins. *Endocrinology* 1987;**120**:602-08.

611. RAISZ LG. Calcium regulation. *Clin Biochem* 1981;**14**:209-12.

612. PENSLER JM, RADOSEVICH JA, HIGBEE R, LANGMAN CB. Osteoclasts isolated from membranous bone in children exhibit nuclear estrogen and progesterone receptors. *J Bone Min Res* 1990;**5**:797-802.

613. OURSLER MJ, OSDOBY P, PYFFEROEN J, RIGGS BL, SPELSBERG TC. Avian osteoclasts as estrogen target cells. *Proc Natl Acad Sci USA* 1991;**88**:6613-17.

614. PACIFICI R, RIFAS L, MCCRACKEN R, et al. Ovarian steroid treatment blocks a postmenopausal increase in blood monocyte interleukin 1 release. *Proc Natl Acad Sci USA* 1989;**86**:2398-02.

615. PACIFICI R, BROWN C, PUSCHECK E, et al. Effect of surgical menopause and estrogen replacement on cytokine release from human blood mononuclear cells. *Proc Natl Acad Sci USA* 1991;**88**:5134-38.

616. OURSLER MJ, CORTESE C, KEETING P, et al. Modulation of transforming growth factor-β production in normal human osteoblast-like cells by 17-β estradiol and parathyroid hormone. *Endocrinology* 1991;**129**:3313-20.

617. FINKELMAN RD, BELL NH, STRONG DD, DEMERS LM, BAYLINK DJ. Ovariectomy selectively reduces the concentration of transforming growth factor in rat bone: implications for estrogen deficiency-associated bone loss. *Proc Natl Acad Sci USA* 1992;**89**:12190-93.

618. ABE E, ISHIMI Y, TAKAHASHI N, et al. A differentiation-inducing factor produced by the osteoblastic cell line MC3T3-E1 stimulates bone resorption by promoting osteoclast formation. *J Bone Min Res* 1988;**3**:635-45.

619. LEMANN J JR, LITZOW JR, LENNON EJ. The effects of chronic acid loads in normal man: Further evidence for the participation of bone mineral in the defense against chronic metabolic acidosis. *J Clin Invest* 1966;**45**:1608-14.

620. RELMAN AS. The acidosis of renal disease. *Am J Med* 1968;**44**:706-13.

621. BARZEL US, JOWSEY J. The effects of chronic acid and alkali administration on bone turnover in adult rats. *Clin Sci* 1969;**36**:517-24.

622. CHAN Y-L, SAVDIE E, MASON RS, POSEN S. The effect of metabolic acidosis on vitamin D metabolites and bone histology in uremic rats. *Calcif Tissue Int* 1985;**37**:158-64.

623. DOMINGUEZ JH, RAISZ LG. Effects of changing hydrogen ion, carbonic acid, and bicarbonate concentrations on bone resorption in vitro. *Calcif Tissue Int* 1979;**29**:7-13.

624. BUSHINSKY DA, GOLDRING JM, COE FL. Cellular contribution to pH-mediated calcium flux in neonatal mouse calvariae. *Am J Physiol* 1985;**248**:F785-F789.

625. BUSHINSKY DA, KRIEGER NS, GEISSER DI, GROSSMAN EB, COE FL. Effects of pH on bone calcium and proton fluxes in vitro. *Am J Physiol* 1983;**245**:F204-F209.

626. ARNETT TR, DEMPSTER DW. Effect of pH on bone resorption by rat osteoclasts *in vitro*. *Endocrinology* 1986;**119**:119-24.

627. HORTON JE, RAISZ LG, SIMMONS HA, OPPENHEIM JJ, MERGENHAGEN SE. Bone resorbing activity in supernatant fluid from cultured human peripheral blood leukocytes. *Science* 1972;**177**:793-95.

628. MUNDY GR. Cytokines and local factors which affect osteoclast function. *Int J Cell Cloning* 1992;**10**:215-22.

629. IBBOTSON KJ, ROODMAN GD, MCMANUS LM, MUNDY GR. Identification and characterization of osteoclast-like cells and their progenitors in cultures of feline marrow mononuclear cells. *J Cell Biol* 1984;**99**:471-80.

630. ROODMAN GD, IBBOTSON KJ, MACDONALD BR, KUEHL TJ, MUNDY GR. 1,25-Dihydroxyvitamin D$_3$ causes formation of multinucleated cells with several osteoclast characteristics in cultures of primate marrow. *Proc Nat Acad Sci USA* 1985;**82**:8213-17.

631. MacDonald BR, Mundy GR, Clark S, et al. Effects of human recombinant CSF-GM and highly purified CSF-1 on the formation of multinucleated cells with osteoclast characteristics in long-term bone marrow cultures. *J Bone Min Res* 1986;1:227-33.

632. Yoneda T, Alsina MA, Chavez JB, Bonewald L, Nishimura R, Mundy GR. Evidence that tumor necrosis factor plays a pathogenetic role in the paraneoplastic syndromes of cachexia, hypercalcemia, and leukocytosis in a human tumor in nude mice. *J Clin Invest* 1991;87:977-85.

633. Takahashi N, Kukita T, MacDonald BR, et al. Osteoclast-like cells form in long-term human bone marrow but not in peripheral blood cultures. *J Clin Invest* 1989;83:543-50.

634. Yoneda T, Alsina MM, Garcia JL, Mundy GR. Differentiation of HL-60 cells into cells with the osteoclast phenotype. *Endocrinology* 1991;129:683-89.

635. Boyde A, Ali NN, Jones SJ. Resorption of dentine by isolated osteoclasts in vitro. *Brit Dent J* 1984;156:216-20.

636. Chambers TJ, Revell PA, Fuller K, Athanasou NA. Resorption of bone by isolated rabbit osteoclasts. *J Cell Sci* 1984;66:383-99.

637. Mc Sheehy PMJ, Chambers TJ. Osteoblastic cells mediate osteoclastic responsiveness to parathyroid hormone. *Endocrinology* 1986;118:824-828.

638. Boyde A, Jones SJ. Editorial: pitfalls in pit measurement. *Calcif Tissue Int* 1991;49:65-70.

639. Sabatini M, Boyce B, Aufdemorte T, Bonewald L, Mundy GR. Infusions of recombinant human interleukin 1α and 1β cause hypercalcemia in normal mice. *Proc Natl Acad Sci USA* 1988;85:5235-39.

640. Boyce BF, Aufdemorte TB, Garrett IR, Yates AJ, Mundy GR. Effects of interleukin-1 on bone turnover in normal mice. *Endocrinology* 1989;125:1142-50.

641. Boyce BF, Yates AJP, Mundy GR. Bolus injections of recombinant human interleukin-1 cause transient hypocalcemia in normal mice. *Endocrinology* 1989;125:2780-83.

642. Johnson RA, Boyce BF, Mundy GR, Roodman GD. Tumors producing human tumor necrosis factor induce hypercalcemia and osteoclastic bone resorption in nude mice. *Endocrinology* 1989;124:1424-27.

643. Black K, Garret IR, Mundy GR. Chinese hamster ovarian cells transfected with the murine interleukin-6 gene cause hypercalcemia as well as cachexia, leukocytosis and thrombocytosis in tumor-bearing nude mice. *Endocrinology* 1991;128:2657-59.

644. Mizel SB. Interleukin 1 and T cell activation. *Immunol Rev* 1982;63:51-72.

645. Gery I, Lupe-Zuniga JL. Interleukin 1: uniqueness of its production annd spectrum of activities. *Lymphokines* 1984;9:109-25.

646. March CJ, Mosley B, Larsen A, et al. Cloning, sequence and expression of two distinct human interleukin-1 complementary DNAs. *Nature* 1985;315:641-47.

647. Dewhirst FE, Stashenko PP, Mole JE, Tsurumachi T. Purfication and partial sequence of human osteoclast-activating factor: identity with interleukin 1β. *J Immunol* 1985;136:2562-68.

648. Bertolini DR, Nedwin GE, Bringman TS, Smith DD, Mundy GR. Stimulation of bone resorption and inhibition of bone formation *in vitro* by human tumor necrosis factors. *Nature* 1986;319:516-18.

649. Gowen M, Wood DD, Ihrie EJ, McGuire MKB, Russell RGG. An interleukin 1 like factor stimulates bone resorption *in vitro*. *Nature* 1983;306:378-80.

650. Stashenko P, Dewhirst FE, Rooney ML, Desjardins LA, Heeley JD. Interleukin-1β is a potent inhibitor of bone formation *in vitro*. *J Bone Min Res* 1987;2:559-65.

651. Pfeilschifter J, Chenu C, Bird A, Mundy GR, Roodman GD. Interleukin-1 and tumor necrosis factor stimulate the formation of human osteoclastlike cells in vitro. *J Bone Min Res* 1989;4:113-18.

652. Thomson BM, Saklatvala J, Chambers TJ. Osteoblasts mediate interleukin 1 stimulation of bone resorption by rat osteoclasts. *J Exp Med* 1986;164:104-12.

653. Keeting PE, Rifas L, Harris SA, et al. Evidence for interleukin-β production by cultured normal human osteoblast-like cells. *J Bone Min Res* 1991;6:827-33.

654. Fried RM, Voelkel EF, Rice RH, Levine L, Gaffney EV, Tashjian AH Jr. Two squamous cell carcinomas not associated with humoral hypercalcemia produce a potent bone resorption-stimulating factor which is interleukin-1α. *Endocrinology* 1989;125:742-51.

655. Sato K, Fujii Y, Kasono K, et al. Parathyroid hormone-related protein and interleukin-1α synergistically stimulate bone resorption *in vitro* and increase the serum calcium concentration in mice *in vivo*. *Endocrinology* 1989;124:2172-78.

656. Kawano M, Tanaka H, Ishikawa H, et al. Interleukin-1 accelerates autocrine growth of myeloma cells through interleukin-6 in human myeloma. *Blood* 1989;73:2145-48.

657. Cozzolino F, Torcia M, Aldinucci D, et al. Production of interleukin-1 by bone marrow myeloma cells. *Blood* 1989;74:380-87.

658. D'Souza R, Brown LR, Newland JR, Levy BM, Lachman LB. Detection and characterization of IL-1 in human dental pulps. *Arch Oral Biol* 1989;34:307-13.

659. Stashenko P, Jandinski JJ, Fujiyoshi P, Rynar J, Socransky SS. Tissue levels of bone resorptive cytokines in periodontal disease. *J Periodontol* 1991;62:504-09.

660. Stashenko P, Yu SM, Wang C-Y. Kinetics of immune cell and bone resorptive responses to endodontic infections. *J Endod* 1992;18:422-26.

661. Safavi KE, Rossomando EF. Tumor necrosis factor identified in periapical tissue exudates of teeth with apical periodontitis. *J Endod* 1991;17:12-14.

662. Barkhordar RA, Hussain MZ, Hayashi C. Detection of IL-1β in human periapical lesions. *Oral Surg Oral Med Oral Pathol* 1992;73:334-36.

663. Lim G, Torabinejad M, Kettering J, Linkhart T, Finkelman R. Concentration of interleukin 1β- in symptomatic and asymptomatic human periradicular lesions. *J Endodon* 1992;18:189 (Abs 10).

664. Schrader JW. The panspecific hemopoietin of activated T lymphocytes (interleukin-3). *Annu Rev Immunol* 1986;4:205-30.

665. Ihle JN, Weinstein Y. Immunological regulation of hematopoietic/lymphoid stem cell differentiation by interleukin 3. *Adv Immunol* 1986;39:1-50.

666. Barton BE, Mayer R. IL-3 induces differentiation of bone marrow precursor cells to osteoclast-like cells. *J Immunol* 1989;143:3211-16.

667. Hattersley G, Chambers TJ. Effects of interleukin 3 and of granulocyte-macrophage and macrophage colony stimulating factors on osteoclast differentiation from mouse hemopoietic tissue. *J Cellular Physiol* 1990;142:201-09.

668. Yoshie H, Taubman MA, Olson CL, Ebersole JL, Smith DJ. Periodontal bone loss and immune characteristics after adoptive transfer of *Actinobacillus*-sensitized T cells to rats. *J Periodont Res* 1987;22:499-505.

669. Kennedy AC, Lindsay R. Bone involvement in rheumatoid arthritis. *Clin Rheum Dis* 1977;3:403-20.

670. Kennedy AC, Lindsay R, Buchanan WW, Allan BF. Bone-resorbing activity in the sera of patients with rheumatoid arthritis. *Clin Sci Mol Med* 1976;51:205-07.

671. Billiau A, van Damme J, Ceuppens J, Baroja M. Interleukin 6, a ubiquitous cytokine with paracrine as well as endocrine functions. In: Fradelizi D, Bertoglio J, eds. *Lymphokine Receptor Interactions*, London: John Libby Eurotext, 1989:133-42.

672. FEYEN JHM, ELFORD P, DI PADOVA FE, TRECHSEL U. Interleukin-6 is produced by bone and modulated by parathyroid hormone. *J Bone Min Res* 1989;**4**:633-38.

673. KURIHARA N, BERTOLINI D, SUDA T, AKIYAMA Y, ROODMAN GD. IL-6 stimulates osteoclast-like multinucleated cell formation in long term human marrow cultures by inducing IL-1 release. *J Immunol* 1990;**144**:4226-30.

674. AL-HUMIDAN A, RALSTON SH, HUGHES DE, et al. Interleukin-6 does not stimulate bone resorption in neonatal mouse calvariae. *J Bone Min Res* 1991;**6**:3-8.

675. ISHIMI Y, MIYAURA C, JIN CH, et al. IL-6 is produced by osteoblasts and induces bone resorption. *J Immunol* 1990;**145**:3297-03.

676. ROODMAN GD, KURIHARA N, OHSAKI Y, et al. Interleukin 6. A potential autocrine/paracrine factor in Paget's disease of bone. *J Clin Invest* 1992;**89**:46-52.

677. KONO Y, BEAGLEY KW, FUJIHASHI K, et al. Cytokine regulation of localized inflammation. Induction of activated B cells and IL-6-mediated polyclonal IgG and IgA synthesis in inflamed human gingiva. *J Immunol* 1991;**146**:1812-21.

678. AL-BALAGHI S, STROM H, MÖLLER E. B cell differentiation factor in synovial fluid of patients with rheumatoid arthritis. *Immunol Rev* 1984;**78**:7-23.

679. THOMSON BM, MUNDY GR, CHAMBERS TJ. Tumor necrosis factors α and β induce osteoblastic cells to stimulate osteoclastic bone resorption. *J Immunol* 1987;**138**:775-779.

680. TASHJIAN AH JR, VOELKEL EF, LAZZARO M, GOAD D, BOSMA T, LEVINE L. Tumor necrosis factor–α (Cachectin) stimulates bone resorption in mouse calvaria via a prostaglandin-mediated mechanism. *Endocrinology* 1987;**120**:2029-36.

681. SABATINI M, YATES AJ, GARRETT IR, et al. Increased production of tumor necrosis factor by normal immune cells in a model of the humoral hypercalcemia of malignancy. *Lab Invest* 1990;**63**:676-682.

682. SABATINI M, CHAVEZ J, MUNDY GR, BONEWALD LF. Stimulation of tumor necrosis factor release from monocytic cells by the A375 human melanoma via granulocyte-macrophage colony stimulating factor. *Cancer Res* 1990;**50**:2673-78.

683. GARRETT IR, DURIE BGM, NEDWIN GE, et al. Production of lymphotoxin, a bone resorbing cytokine, by cultured human myeloma cells. *N Engl J Med* 1987;**317**:526-32.

684. STASHENKO P. The role of immune cytokines in the pathogenesis of periapical lesions. *Endod Dent Traumatol* 1990;**6**:89-96.

685. METCALF D. The molecular biology and functions of the granulocyte-macrophage colony-stimulating factors. *Blood* 1986;**67**:257-67.

686. BURGER EH, VAN DER MEER JWM, VAN DE GEVEL JS, et al. In vitro formation of osteoclasts from long-term cultures of bone marrow mononuclear phagocytes. *J Exp Med* 1982;**156**:1604-14.

687. HAGENAARS CE, VAN DER KRAAN AA, KAWILARANG-DE HAAS EW, VISSER JWM, NIJWEIDE PJ. Osteoclast formation from cloned pluripotent hemopoietic stem cells. *Bone Min* 1989;**6**:179-89.

688. ELFORD PR, FELIX R, CECCHINI M, TRECHSEL U, FLEISCH H. Murine osteoblastlike cells and the osteogenic cell MC3T3-E1 release a macrophage colony-stimulating activity in culture. *Calcif Tissue Int* 1987;**41**:151-56.

689. FELIX R, FLEISCH H, ELFORD PR. Bone-resorbing cytokines enhance release of macrophage colony-stimulating activity by the osteoblastic cell MC3T3-E1. *Calcif Tissue Int* 1989;**44**:356-60.

690. SHIINA-ISHIMI Y, ABE E, TANAKA H, SUDA T. Synthesis of colony-stimulating factor (CSF) and differentiation-inducing factor (D-factor) by osteoblastic cells, clone MC3T3-E1. *Biochem Biophys Res Commun* 1986;**134**:400-06.

691. SATO K, KASONO K, FUJII Y, KAWAKAMI M, TSUSHIMA T, SHIZUME K. Tumor necrosis factor type α (cachectin) stimulates mouse osteoblast-like cells (MC3T3-E1) to produce macrophage-colony stimulating activity and prostaglandin E₂. *Biochem Biophys Res Commun* 1987;**145**:323-29.

692. SATO K, FUJII Y, ASANO S, et al. Recombinant human interleukin 1 alpha and beta stimulate mouse osteoblast-like cells (MC3T3-E1) to produce macrophage-colony stimulating activity and prostaglandin E₂. *Biochem Biophys Res Commun* 1986;**141**:285-91.

693. FELIX R, CECCHINI MG, HOFSTETTER W, ELSFORD PR, STUTZER A, FLEISCH H. Impairment of macrophage colony-stimulating factor production and lack of resident bone marrow macrophages in the osteopetrotic op/op mouse. *J Bone Min Res* 1990;**5**:781-89.

694. YOSHIDA H, HAYASHI S-I, KUNISADA T, et al. The murine mutation osteopetrosis is in the coding region of the macrophage colony stimulating factor gene. *Nature* 1990;**345**:442-44.

695. FELIX R, CECCHINI MG, FLEISCH H. Macrophage colony stimulating factor restores in vivo bone resorption in the op/op osteopetrotic mouse. *Endocrinology* 1990;**127**:2592-94.

696. MARKS SC JR, WOJTOWICZ A, SZPERL M, et al. Administration of colony stimulating factor-1 corrects some macrophage, dental, and skeletal defects in an osteopetrotic mutation (toothless, *tl*) in the rat. *Bone* 1992;**13**:89-93.

697. EVANS DB, BUNNING RAD, RUSSELL RGG. The effects of recombinant human granulocyte-macrophage colony-stimulating factor (rhGM-CSF) on human osteoblast-like cells. *Biochem Biophys Res Commun* 1989;**160**:588-95.

698. FELIX R, ELFORD PR, STOERCKLÉ C, et al. Production of hemopoietic growth factors by bone tissue and bone cells in culture. *J Bone Min Res* 1988;**3**:27-36.

699. HOROWITZ MC, COLEMAN DL, RYABY JT, EINHORN TA. Osteotropic agents induce the differential secretion of granulocyte-macrophage colony-stimulating factor by the osteoblast cell line MC3T3-E1. *J Bone Min Res* 1989;**4**:911-21.

700. CARACCIOLO D, CLARK SC, ROVERA G. Human interleukin-6 supports granulocytic differentiation of hematopoietic progenitor cells and acts synergistically with GM-CSF. *Blood* 1989;**73**:666-70.

701. FELIX R, CECCHINI MG, HOFSTETTER W, GUENTHER HL, FLEISCH H. Production of granulocyte-macrophage (GM-CSF) and granulocyte colony-stimulating factor (G-CSF) by rat clonal osteoblastic cell population CRP 10/30 and the immortalized cell line IRC 10/30-myc1 stimulated by tumor necrosis factor α. *Endocrinology* 1991;**128**:661-67.

702. LINDEMANN A, RIEDEL D, OSTER W, LOEMS ZIEGLER-HEITBROCK HW, MERTELSMANN R, HERRMANN F. Granulocyte-macrophage colony-stimulating factor induces cytokine secretion by human polymorphonuclear leukocytes. *J Clin Invest* 1989;**83**:1308-12.

703. ZSEBO KM, YUSCHENKOFF VN, SCHIFFER S, et al. Vascular endothelial cells and granulopoiesis: interleukin-1 stimulates release of G-CSF and GM-CSF. *Blood* 1988;**71**:99-103.

704. SATO K, FUJII Y, KAKIUCHI T, et al. Paraneoplastic syndrome of hypercalcemia and leukocytosis caused by squamous carcinoma cells (T3M-1) producing parathyroid hormone-related protein, interleukin 1α, and granulocyte colony-stimulating factor. *Cancer Res* 1989;**49**:4740-46.

705. KLEIN DC, RAISZ LG. Prostaglandins: stimulation of bone resorption in tissue culture. *Endocrinology* 1970;**86**:1436-40.

706. DIETRICH JW, GOODSON JM, RAISZ LG. Stimulation of bone resorption by various prostaglandins in organ cultue. *Prostaglandins* 1975;**10**:231-40.

707. RAISZ LG, DIETRICH JW, SIMMONS HA, SEYBERTH HW, HUBBARD W, OATES JA. Effect of prostaglandin endoperoxides and metabolites on bone resorption *in vitro*. *Nature* 1977;**267**:532-34.

708. TASHJIAN AH JR, TICE JE, SIDES K. Biological activities of prostaglandin analogues and metabolites on bone in organ culture. *Nature* 1977;**266**:645-47.

CHAPTER 2

709. Dewhirst FE. 6-Keto-prostaglandin E_1-stimulated bone resorption in organ culture. *Calcif Tissue Int* 1984;**36**:380-83.

710. Chambers TJ, McShehy PMJ, Thompson BM, Fuller K. The effect of calcium-regulating hormones and prostaglandins on bone resorption by osteoclasts disaggregated from neonatal rabbit bones. *Endocrinology* 1985;**116**:234-39.

711. Chambers TJ, Ali NN. Inhibition of osteoclastic motility by prostaglandins I_2, E_1, E_2 and 6-oxo E_1. *J Pathol* 1983;**139**:383-97.

712. Okuda A, Taylor LM, Heersche JNM. Prostaglandin E_2 initially inhibits and then stimulates bone resorption in isolated rabbit osteoclast cultures. *Bone Min* 1989;**7**:255-66.

713. Collins DA, Chambers TJ. Effect of prostaglandins E_1, E_2, and $F_2\alpha$ on osteoclast formation in mouse bone marrow cultures. *J Bone Min Res* 1991;**6**:157-64.

714. Goodson JM, Dewhirst FE, Brunetti A. Prostaglandin E_2 levels and human periodontal disease. *Prostaglandins* 1974;**6**:81-85.

715. Offenbacher S, Odle BM, van Dyke TE. The use of crevicular fluid prostaglandin E_2 levels as a predictor of periodontal attachment loss. *J Periodont Res* 1986;**21**:101-12.

716. Cohen JS, Reader A, Fertel R, Beck M, Meyers WJ. A radioimmunoassay determination of the concentrations of prostaglandins E_2 and $F_2\alpha$ in painful and asymptomatic human dental pulps. *J Endod* 1985;**11**:330-35.

717. Lessard G, Torabinejad M, Swope D. Arachidonic acid metabolism in canine tooth pulps and the effects of non-steroidal anti-inflammatory drugs. *J Endod* 1986;**12**:146-49.

718. Jeffcoat MK, Williams RC, Wechter WJ, et al. Flurbiprofen treatment of periodontal disease in beagles. *J Periodont Res* 1986;**21**:624-33.

719. Robinson DR, Tashjian AH Jr, Levine L. Prostaglandin-stimulated bone resorption by rheumatoid synovia. *J Clin Invest* 1975;**56**:1181-88.

720. Voelkel EF, Tashjian AH Jr, Franklin R, Wasserman E, Levine L. Hypercalcemia and tumor prostaglandins: The VX_2 carcinoma model in the rabbit. *Metabolism* 1975;**24**:973-86.

721. Seyberth HW, Segre GV, Morgan JL, Sweetman BJ, Potts JT Jr, Oates JA. Prostaglandins as mediators of hypercalcemia associated with certain types of cancer. *N Engl J Med* 1975;**293**:1278-83.

722. Chyun YS, Raisz LG. Stimulation of bone formation by prostaglandin E_2. *Prostaglandins* 1984;**27**:97-103.

723. Rø S, Sudmann E, Marton PF. Effect of indomethacin on fracture healing in rats. *Acta Orthop Scand* 1976;**47**:558-599.

724. Tatakis DN, Schneeberger G, Dziak R. Recombinant interleukin-1 stimulates prostaglandin E2 production by osteoblastic cells: synergy with parathyroid hormone. *Calcif Tissue Int* 1988;**42**:358-62.

725. Mizel SB, Dayer J-M, Krane SM, Mergenhagen SE. Stimulation of rheumatoid synovial cell collagenase and prostaglandin production by partially purified lymphocyte-activating factor (interleukin 1). *Proc Natl Acad Sci USA* 1981;**78**:2474-77.

726. Knudsen PJ, Dinarello CA, Strom TB. Prostaglandins posttranscriptionally inhibit monocyte expression of interleukin 1 activity by increasing intracellular cyclic adenosine monophosphate. *J Immunol* 1986;**137**:3189-94.

727. Mitnick M, Isales C, Paliwal I, Insogna K. Parathyroid hormone-related protein stimulates prostaglandin E_2 release from human osteoblast-like cells: modulating effect of peptide length. *J Bone Min Res* 1992;**7**:887-96.

728. Metcalf D, Gearing DP. Fatal syndrome in mice engrafted with cells producing high levels of the leukemia inhibitory factor. *Proc Natl Acad Sci USA* 1989;**86**:5948-52.

729. Abe E, Tanaka H, Ishimi Y, et al. Differentiation-inducing factor purified from conditioned medium of mitogen-treated spleen cell cultures stimulates bone resorption. *Proc Natl Acad Sci USA* 1986;**83**:5958-62.

730. Abe E, Ishimi Y, Takahashi N, et al. A differentiation-inducing factor produced by the osteoblastic cell line MC3T3-E1 stimulates bone resorption by promoting osteoclast formation. *J Bone Min Res* 1988;**3**:635-45.

731. Mackie EJ, Trechsel U. Stimulation of bone formation in vivo by transforming growth factor-β: remodeling of woven bone and lack of inhibition by indomethacin. *Bone* 1990;**11**:295-300.

732. Noda M, Camilliere JJ. In vivo stimulation of bone formation by transforming growth factor-β. *Endocrinology* 1989;**124**:2991-94.

733. Joyce ME, Roberts AB, Sporn MB, Bolander ME. Transforming growth factor-β and the initiation of chondrogenesis and osteogenesis in the rat femur. *J Cell Biol* 1990;**110**:2195-207.

734. Beck LS, Deguzman L, Lee WP, Xu Y, McFatridge LA, Gillett NA, Amento EP. TGF-$β_1$ induces bone closure of skull defects. *J Bone Min Res* 1991;**6**:1257-65.

735. Chenu C, Pfeilschifter J, Mundy GR, Roodman GD. Transforming growth factor β inhibits formation of osteoclast-like cells in long-term human marrow cultures. *Proc Natl Acad Sci USA* 1988;**85**:5683-87.

736. Tashjian AH Jr, Voelkel EF, Lloyd W, Derynck R, Winkler ME, Levine L. Actions of growth factors on plasma calcium. Epidermal growth factor and human transforming growth factor-alpha cause elevation of plasma calcium in mice. *J Clin Invest* 1986;**78**:1405-09.

737. Gowen M, Nedwin GE, Mundy GR. Preferential inhibition of cytokine-stimulated bone resorption by recombinant interferon gamma. *J Bone Min Res* 1986;**1**:469-74.

738. Lerner UH, Ljunggren Ö, Ransjö M, Klaushofer K, Peterlik M. Inhibitory effects of γ-interferon on bradykinin-induced bone resorption and prostaglandin formation in cultured mouse calvarial bones. *Agents Actions* 1991;**32**:305-11.

739. Carter DB, Deibel MR, Dunn CJ, et al. Purification, cloning, expression and biological characterization of an interleukin-1 receptor antagonist protein. *Nature* 1990;**344**:633-38.

740. Hannum CH, Wilcox CJ, Arend WP, et al. Interleukin-1 receptor antagonist activity of a human interleukin-1 inhibitor. *Nature* 1990;**343**:336-40.

741. Eisenberg SP, Evans RJ, Arend WP, et al. Primary structure and functional expression from complementary DNA of a human interleukin-1 receptor antagonist. *Nature* 1990;**343**:341-46.

742. Arend WP, Joslin FG, Thompson RC, Hannum CH. An IL-1 inhibitor from human monocytes. Production and characterization of biologic properties. *J Immunol* 1989;**143**:1851-58.

743. Garrett IR, Black KS, Mundy GR. Interactions between interleukin-6 and interleukin-1 in osteoclastic bone resorption in neonatal mouse calvariae. *Calcif Tissue Int* 1990;**46**(suppl 2):140.

744. Seckinger P, Klein-Nulend J, Alander C, Thompson RC, Dayer J-M, Raisz LG. Natural and recombinant human IL-1 receptor antagonists block the effects of IL-1 on bone resorption and prostaglandin production. *J Immunol* 1990;**145**:4181-84.

CHAPTER 3

Classification, Etiology and Epidemiology

J. O. ANDREASEN & F. M. ANDREASEN

Classification

Dental injuries have been classified according to a variety of factors, such as etiology, anatomy, pathology, or therapeutic considerations (1-14, 62, 131, 132).

The present classification is based on a system adopted by the World Health Organization in its *Application of International Classification of Diseases to Dentistry and Stomatology*, (133). However, for the sake of completeness, it was felt necessary to define and classify certain trauma entities not included in the W. H. O. system. The following classification includes injuries to the teeth, supporting structures, gingiva, and oral mucosa and is based on anatomical, therapeutic and prognostic considerations. This classification can be applied to both the permanent and the primary dentitions.

The code number is according to the International Classification of Diseases (1992) (133).

Injuries to the Hard Dental Tissues and the Pulp (Fig. 3.1)

ENAMEL INFRACTION
(N 502.50) An incomplete fracture (crack) of the enamel without loss of tooth substance (Fig. 3.1, A).

ENAMEL FRACTURE (UNCOMPLICA-TED CROWN FRACTURE)
(502.50) A fracture with loss of tooth substance confined to the enamel (N 502.50) (Fig. 3.1 A).

ENAMEL-DENTIN FRACTURE (UN-COMPLICATED CROWN FRACTURE)
(N502.51) A fracture with loss of tooth substance confined to enamel and dentin, but not involving the pulp (Fig. 3.1 B).

COMPLICATED CROWN FRACTURE
(N502.52) A fracture involving enamel and dentin, and exposing the pulp (Fig. 3.1, C).

UNCOMPLICATED CROWN-ROOT FRACTURE
(N 502.54) A fracture involving enamel, dentin and cementum, but not exposing the pulp (Fig. 3.1, D).

COMPLICATED CROWN-ROOT FRAC-TURE
(N 502.54) A fracture involving enamel, dentin and cementum, and exposing the pulp (Fig. 3.1, E).

ROOT FRACTURE
(N 502.53) A fracture involving dentin, cementum, and the pulp (Fig. 3.1, F). Root fractures can be further classified according to displacement of the coronal fragment, see under luxation injuries.

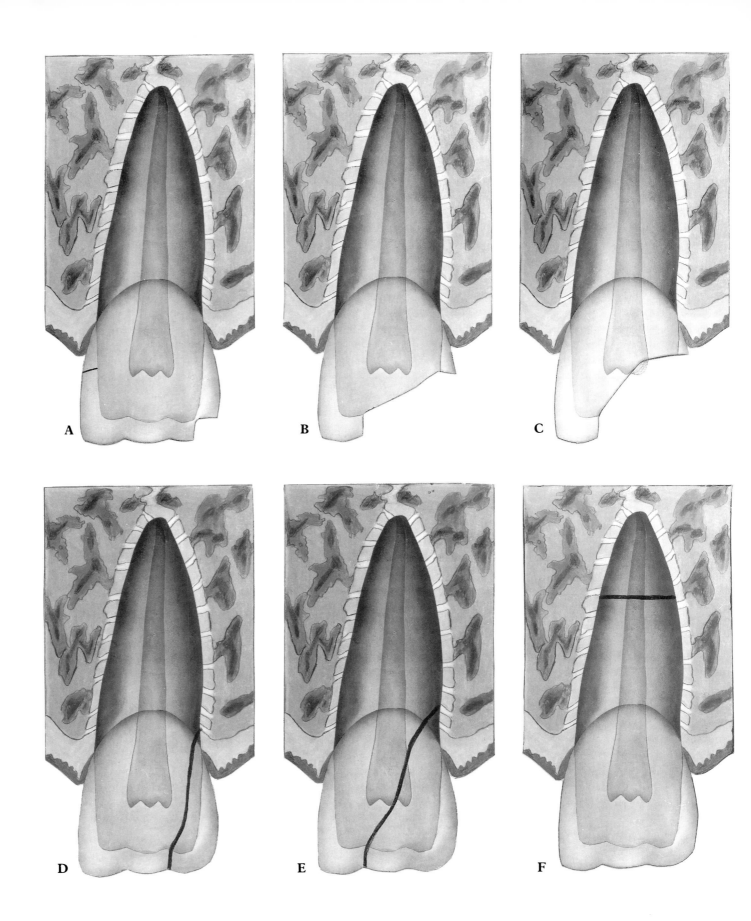

Fig. 3.1.
Injuries to the hard dental tissues and pulp. A. Crown infraction and uncomplicated fracture without involvement of dentin. B. Uncomplicated crown fracture with involvement of dentin. C. Complicated crown fracture. D. Uncomplicated crown-root fracture. E. Complicated crown-root fracture. F. Root fracture.

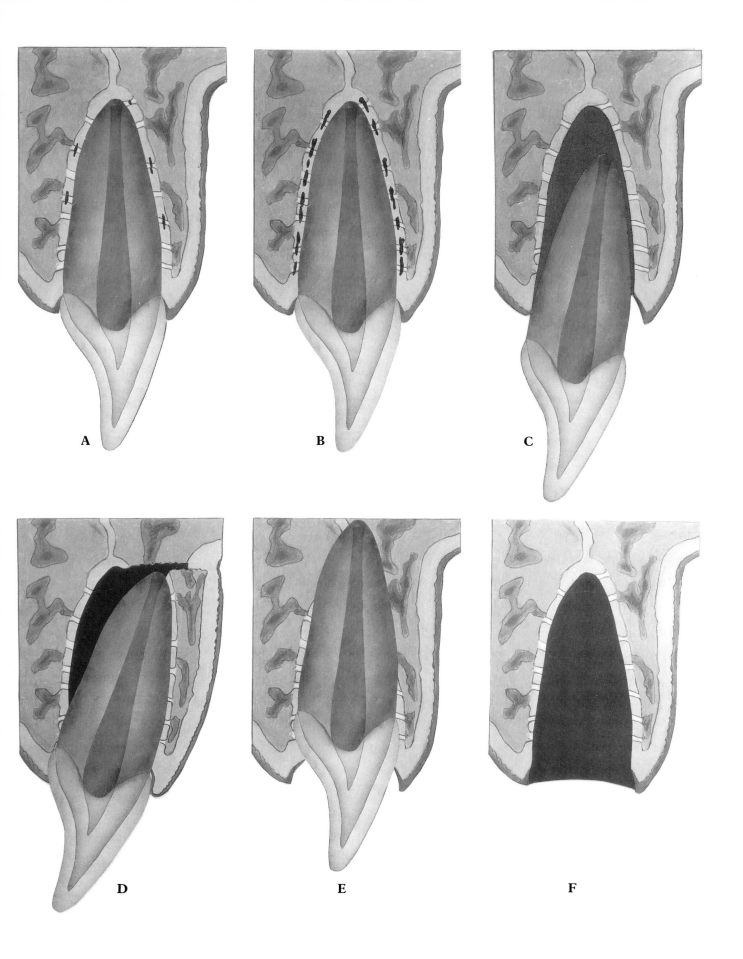

Fig 3.2.
Injuries to the periodontal tissues. A. Concussion. B. Subluxation. C. Extrusive luxation. D. Lateral luxation. E. Intrusive luxation. F. Exarticulation.

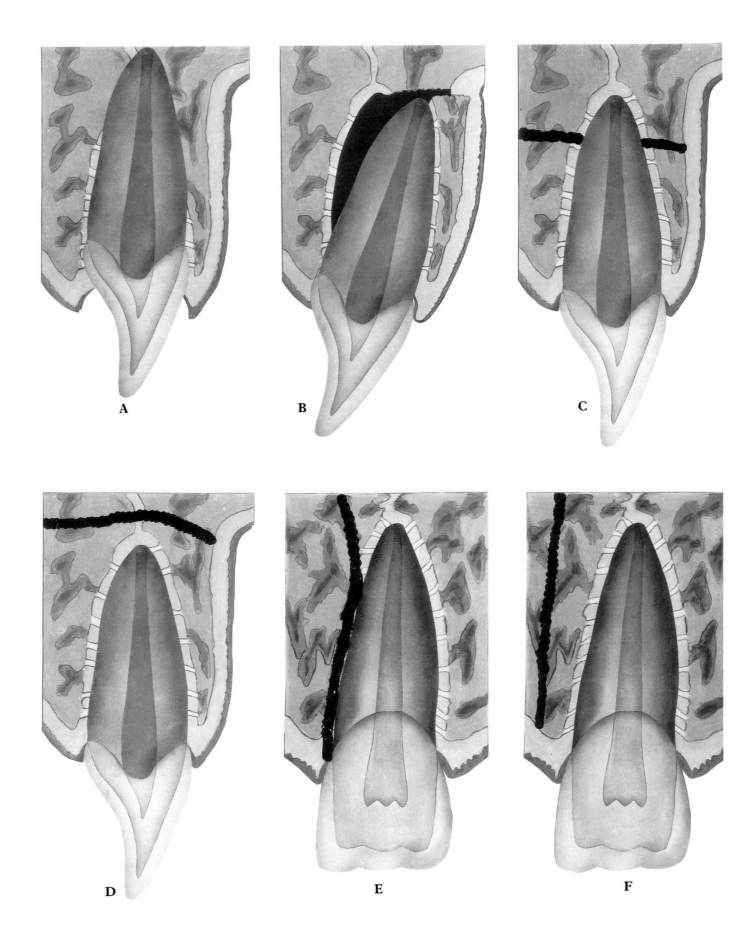

Fig.3.3.

Injuries to the supporting bone. A. Comminution of alveolar socket. B. Fractures of facial or lingual alveolar socket wall. C. and D. Fractures of alveolar process with and without involvement of the tooth socket. E. and F. Fractures of mandible or maxilla with and without involvement of the tooth socket.

Injuries to the Periodontal Tissues (Fig. 3.2).

CONCUSSION
(N 503.20) An injury to the tooth-supporting structures without abnormal loosening or displacement of the tooth, but with marked reaction to percussion (Fig. 3.2, A).

SUBLUXATION (LOOSENING)
(N 503.20) An injury to the tooth-supporting structures with abnormal loosening, but without displacement of the tooth (Fig. 3.2, B).

EXTRUSIVE LUXATION (PERIPHERAL DISLOCATION, PARTIAL AVULSION)
(N 503.20) Partial displacement of the tooth out of its socket (Fig. 3.2, C).

LATERAL LUXATION
(N 503.20) Displacement of the tooth in a direction other than axially. This is accompanied by comminution or fracture of the alveolar socket (Fig. 3.2, D).

INTRUSIVE LUXATION (CENTRAL DISLOCATION)
(N 503.21) Displacement of the tooth into the alveolar bone. This injury is accompanied by comminution or fracture of the alveolar socket (Fig. 3.2, E).

AVULSION (EXARTICULATION)
(N 503.22) Complete displacement of the tooth out of its socket (Fig. 3.2, F).

Injuries to the Supporting Bone (Fig. 3.3)

COMMINUTION OF THE MANDIBULAR (N 502.60) OR MAXILLARY (N 502.40) ALVEOLAR SOCKET
Crushing and compression of the alveolar socket. This condition is found concomitantly with intrusive and lateral luxations (Fig. 3.3, A).

FRACTURE OF THE MANDIBULAR (N502.60) OR MAXILLARY (N 502.40) ALVEOLAR SOCKET WALL
A fracture confined to the facial or oral socket wall (Fig. 3.3, B).

FRACTURE OF THE MANDIBULAR (N 502.60) OR MAXILLARY (N 502.40) ALVEOLAR PROCESS
A fracture of the alveolar process which may or may not involve the alveolar socket (Fig. 3.3, C and D).

FRACTURE OF MANDIBLE (N 502.61) OR MAXILLA (N 502.42)
A fracture involving the base of the mandible or maxilla and often the alveolar process (jaw fracture). The fracture may or may not involve the alveolar socket (Fig. 3.3, E and F).

Injuries to Gingiva or Oral Mucosa (Fig. 3.4)

LACERATION OF GINGIVA OR ORAL MUCOSA
(S 01.50) A shallow or deep wound in the mucosa resulting from a tear, and usually produced by a sharp object (Fig. 3.4, A).

CONTUSION OF GINGIVA OR ORAL MUCOSA
(S 00.50) A bruise usually produced by impact with a blunt object and not accompanied by a break in the mucosa, usually causing submucosal hemorrhage (Fig. 3.4, B).

ABRASION OF GINGIVA OR ORAL MUCOSA
(S 00.50) A superficial wound produced by rubbing or scraping of the mucosa leaving a raw, bleeding surface (Fig. 3.4, C).

Etiology

Iatrogenic Injuries in Newborns

Prolonged intubation in neonates is a procedure which is used in the care of prematurely born infants. The prolonged pressure of tubes against the maxillary alveolar process has been shown to lead to a high frequency of developmental enamel defects in the primary dentition [134-136] (see Chapter 12, p 461).

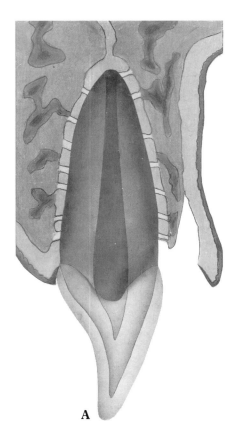 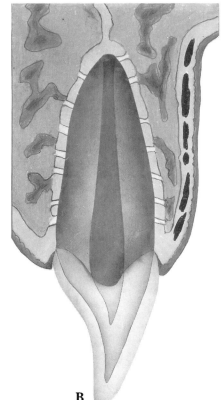 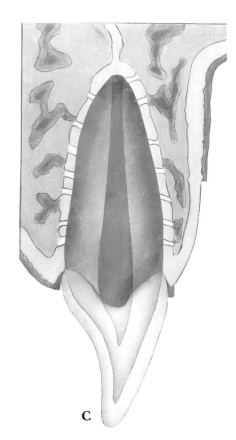

A   B   C

Fig. 3.4.
Injuries to gingiva or oral mucosa. A. Laceration of gingiva. B.Contusion of gingiva. C. Abrasion of gingiva

Fig. 3.5.
Battered child syndrome in a 2 1/2- year- old girl. The mother suffered from depression and shook the child violently against a fireplace. The child died and was found to have contusion of the brain with intracranial hemorrhage. The child also had partly healed fractures at the lower end of each radius, which had been treated by an orthopedic consultant one month previously; but battering was not suspected at that time. The oral injuries consisted of laceration of the mucosa of the lower lip and tearing of the frenum. From TATE (19) 1971

Falls in Infancy

Dental injuries are infrequent during the first year of life; but can occur, for example, due to a fall from a baby carriage. Injuries increase substantially with the child's first efforts to move about. The frequency increases as the child begins to walk and tries to run, due to lack of experience and coordination. The incidence of dental injuries reaches its peak just before school age and consists mainly of injuries due to falls and collisions (16, 18, 63-65).

Child Physical Abuse

A tragic cause of oral injuries in small children is manifested in the battered child syndrome (or non-accidental injuries (NAI)), a clinical condition in infants who have suffered serious physical abuse (19, 66-68, 74, 75, 137-147). The alarming frequency of child abuse can be seen in the following statistics:

It has been reported that child abuse occurs in approximately 0.6% of children (19, 142). In 1972, in New York City alone, 5,200 cases were reported. It has been estimated that in the entire U.S.A., 4,000 - 6,000 children yearly die as a result of maltreatment (69, 140). Approximately half of all children being exposed to physical abuse suffer facial or oral injuries. The outcome is often fatal due to intracranial hemorrhage (19, 72-74). (Fig. 3.5).

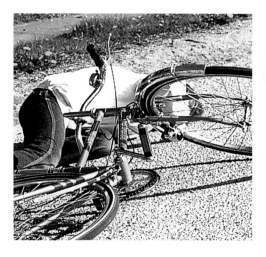

Fig. 3.6.
Bicycle accident usually results in multiple crown fractures and soft tissue injuries.

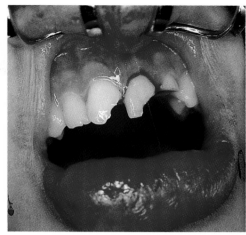

Facial trauma is often the principal reason for admission to a hospital (71, 74, 75). Up to 50% of child abuse injuries are to the face and involve the oral cavity. The etiologic and diagnostic aspects of child abuse are further described in Chapter 4.

Falls and Collisions

When the child reaches school age, accidents in the school playground are very common (20, 76, 77, 148). Most of the resultant injuries can be classified as fall injuries and are characterized by a high frequency of crown fractures (16, 78).

Bicycle Injuries

These injuries usually result in severe trauma to both the hard and soft tissues due to the high velocity at the time of impact (16, 151, 160).

Patients sustaining this type of trauma frequently experience multiple crown fractures in addition to injuries to the upper lip and chin (16) (Fig. 3.6).

Sports

Injuries during the teenage years are often due to sports (21, 22, 65, 78-84, 149-155). This especially applies to contact sports, such as ice-hockey, soccer, baseball, American football, basketball, rugby and wrestling (17, 23-27, 83, 85, 156-159) (Fig. 3.7). The severity of this problem has been elucidated in a number of studies which report that each year 1.5% to 3.5% of children participating in contact sports sustain dental injuries (26-29, 86). The injury profiles of various types of sports, as well as measures for their prevention, are described in Chapter 21.

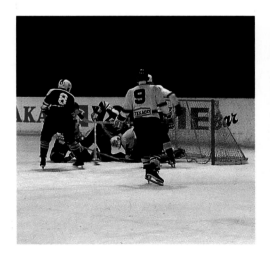

Fig. 3.7.
The unprotected ice hockey player runs a high risk of injuries due to collision with other players or being hit by a puck or a hockey stick.

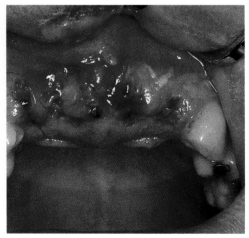

CLASSIFICATION, ETIOLOGY AND EPIDEMIOLOGY

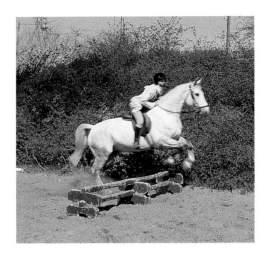
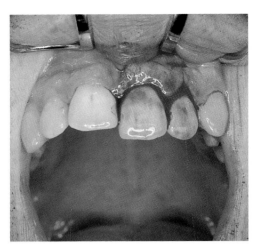

Horseback Riding

Horseback riding, a popular sport in many countries, is a significant source of injury. In a single season, 23% of all riders sustained injuries of various types, including dental and maxillofacial injuries (87, 88). Furthermore, this type of injury was the third most common source of sports-related injury recorded among 10 sporting activities registered (soccer and handball were the first and second most common sources of injuries) and represented the most severe types of trauma. Figs. 3.8 and 3.9 illustrate the typical trauma situations related to horseback riding. There is little doubt that special precautions, such as the use of sturdy helmets, can reduce the number and severity of these accidents (88).

Automobile Injuries

Facial and dental injuries resulting from automobile accidents are seen more frequently in the late teens (30-31) (Fig. 3.10). The front seat passenger is particularly prone to facial injuries. This trauma group is dominated by multiple dental injuries, injuries to the supporting bone, and soft tissue injuries to the lower lip and chin (16, 89, 161). This pattern of injury is seen when the front seat passenger or the driver hits the steering wheel or dashboard (32, 90). Children seated in - or standing on - the front seat are in a very dangerous position, since dental injuries often occur as a result of being thrown against the dashboard during sudden stops (33).

Fig. 3.9.
A kick by the horse normally results in serious injuries, e.g. exarticulation, intrusion and sometimes jaw fractures.

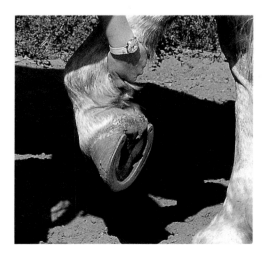
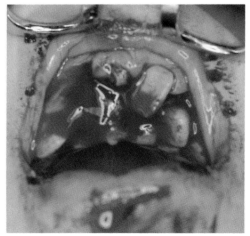

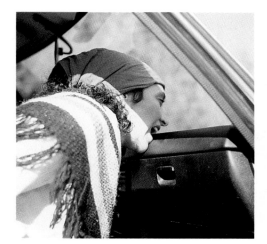

Fig. 3.10.
Automobile accidents in which the front seat passenger hits the dashboard result in soft tissue injuries and damage to the supporting bone.

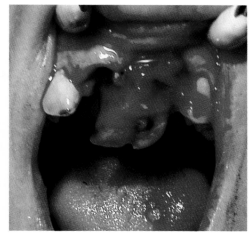

Assaults

Injuries from fights are prominent in older age groups and are closely related to alcohol abuse (89, 91, 92, 124, 162). This type of trauma usually results in a particular injury pattern characterized by luxation and exarticulation of teeth as well as fractures of roots and/or supporting bone (16).(Fig. 3.11) In this context, it should be mentioned that recent evidence has shown wife-beating to be a universal problem (124-130, 163, 164). These assaults often result in trauma to the facial region (Fig. 3.12). Establishing the victim as a battered wife is complicated by the fact that these women will seldom volunteer that information. There are no economic, educational or class predictors of wife abuse. Suspicion of abuse should be aroused if there is (1) a substantial delay between time of injury and presentation for treatment, (2) evidence of repeated injuries to the face and neck, or (3) a previous history of abuse. Social agencies for the care and counselling of these victims exist in many countries and should be used (128).

Although there are no economic, educational or class predictors of wife abuse, there are factors common to wife abusers that are significant. The man often has a history of crime, often involving violence. Alcohol abuse is a common factor.

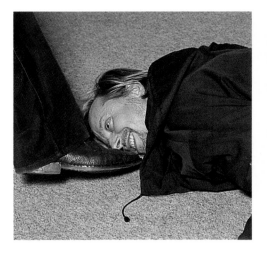

Fig. 3.11.
Kicks to the face during assaults result in severe damage to teeth and supporting structures.

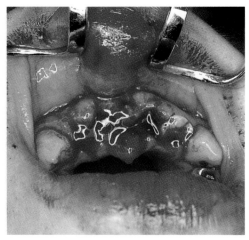

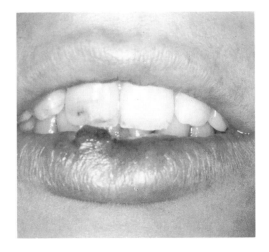
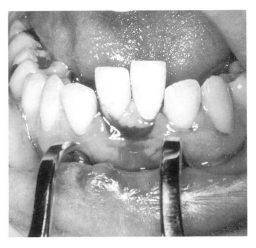

Fig. 3.12.
A 19-year-old woman battered by her husband. The patient was beaten around the face and suffered lacerations of the lower lip and an alveolar fracture confined to the mandibular incisor region.

Approximately half of all cases of repeated wife beating take place when the husband is under the influence of alcohol. Another tragic statistic shows that, in addition to wife beating, the children are also abused (124). When one considers that men who abuse their wives and children often have a childhood history of family violence, and that the battered wife also often has a history of abuse as a child (165), a vicious circle is apparent, which links being beaten as a child with violent behavior in adult life.

Torture

A disgraceful and apparently increasing type of injury is represented by trauma to the oral and facial regions of tortured prisoners. Recent investigations have shown that the majority of these victims, apart from other atrocities inflicted upon their persons, have suffered from torture involving the oral region (95-97) (Fig. 3.13). A recent study has described the findings from examinations of 34 former prisoners from 6 countries who had all been subjected to torture involving the facial region (95). The most common type of torture was beating, which resulted in loosening, avulsion or fracture of teeth and soft tissue laceration. Deliberate tooth fractures with forceps were also seen. Furthermore, electrical torture was described in which electrodes were attached to teeth, lips, tongue and the soft tissue over the temporomandibular joint (Fig. 3.13). In the latter instance, very forceful occlusion resulted due to muscle spasm. The result was loosening and fracture of teeth as well as severe pain in the muscles and the temporomandibular joint.

Under the auspices of Amnesty International, working groups of dentists and physicians have now been formed in sev-

Fig. 3.13.
A 35-year-old political refugee who was tortured by having live electrodes attached to the oral mucosa. Furthermore, lower incisors were avulsed during 'interrogation'. The patient still suffers profound pain in the masticatory muscles, 9 years after being tortured. B. A 35-year-old male political refugee who had been tortured during his imprisonment. The man was beaten by security police. During torture, he fell and fractured and luxated two central incisors. No treatment was given. The radiograph is indicative of his condition one year after torture. It was taken at an examination by the medical board of Amnesty International. Courtesy Drs. P. MARSTRAND, B. JERLANG & P. JERLANG, Amnesty International, Copenhagen.

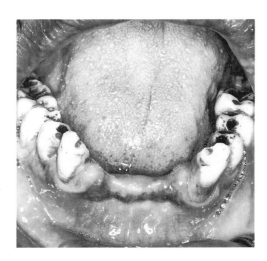
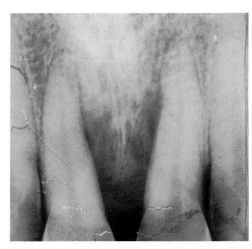

Fig. 3.14.
A 32-year-old male who has sustained 5 trauma episodes within 7 years due to epilepsy. These episodes involved multiple fractures of teeth and the mandible, as well as an alveolar fracture of the maxilla. A. Intruded maxillary incisors. B. Diagram with indication of fracture lines as well as missing teeth due to trauma. From BESSERMANN (93) 1978.

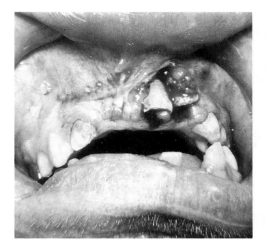
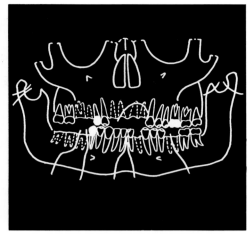

eral countries with the aim of gathering evidence to document the torture of prisoners.

Mental Retardation

A very high frequency of dental injuries has been found among mentally retarded patients (65, 123), a phenomenon probably related to various factors, such as lack of motor coordination, crowded conditions in institutions or concomitant epilepsy.

Epilepsy

Epileptic patients present special risks and problems with regard to dental injuries (34, 93). A study of 437 such patients in an institution showed that 52 % had suffered traumatic dental injuries, many of which were of a repetitive nature. In one-third of the cases, the injuries could be directly

related to falls during epileptic seizures (93) (Fig. 3.14).

Drug-Related Injuries

It has been reported that many drug addicts suffer from crown fractures of molars and premolars, apparently resulting from violent tooth clenching 3 to 4 hours after drug intake. Fractures are confined to the lingual or buccal cusps. Up to 5 or 6 fractured teeth have been found in the same individual (35, 94).

Dentinogenesis Imperfecta

An unusual type of injury is spontaneous root fracture affecting individuals with dentinogenesis imperfecta (36). The explanation for this phenomenon could be the decreased microhardness of dentin (37) and abnormal tapering of the roots (Fig. 3.15).

Fig. 3.15.
Spontaneous root fractures in a 15-year-old patient with osteogenesis and dentinogenesis imperfecta. A. Clinical view of incisors at the age of 14 years. The color of the teeth is bluish-brown. Note the marked attrition. The incisal edges of the incisors were later restored with cast inlays. B. Root fractures affecting three incisors and the left canine at the age of 15 years. There was no evidence of trauma in the history. The right central incisor was later extracted. From OVERVAD (38) 1969.

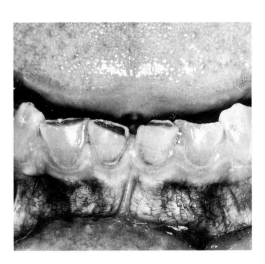
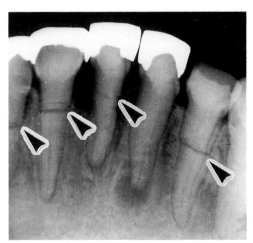

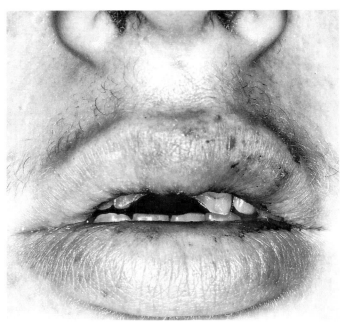

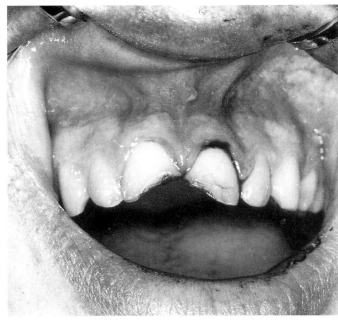

Fig. 3.16.
A. Direct tooth trauma without soft tissue injury. B. The impact was taken by the protruding central incisors. From ANDREASEN (16) *1970.*

Mechanisms of Dental Injuries

The *exact* mechanisms of dental injuries are, for the most part, unknown and without experimental evidence. Injuries can be the result of either direct or indirect trauma (2). *Direct trauma* occurs when the tooth itself is struck, e.g. against playground equipment, a table or chair (Fig. 3.16). *Indirect trauma* is seen when the lower dental arch is forcefully closed against the upper, as by a blow to the chin in a fight or a fall. While direct trauma usually implies injuries to the anterior region, indirect trauma favors crown or crown-root fractures in the premolar and molar regions (Fig. 3.17), as well as the possibility of jaw fractures in the condylar regions and symphysis. Another effect of a blow to the chin can be the forceful whiplash effect to the head and neck, occasionally leading to cerebral involvement. This condition can be revealed during the clinical examination (see later).

Fig. 3.17.
A. Trauma to the chin. B. The impact was transferred to the dental arches and inflicted crown-root fractures in both right premolars by the forceful occlusion. From ANDREASEN (16) *1970.*

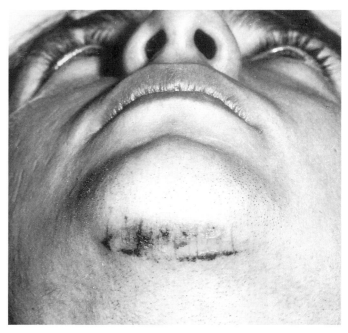

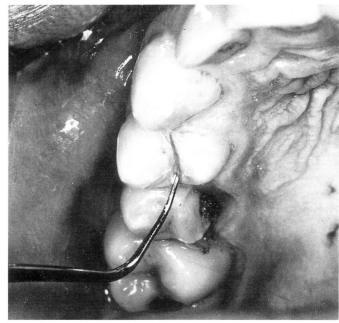

Fig. 3.18.
A. Direct trauma to the upper lip. B. The impact was transmitted through the lip, resulting in extrusive luxation of right incisors and laceration of gingiva. The upper surface of the lip shows minor lacerations in the area which was in contact with the tooth surfaces during transmission of the trauma (arrows), From ANDREASEN (16) 1970.

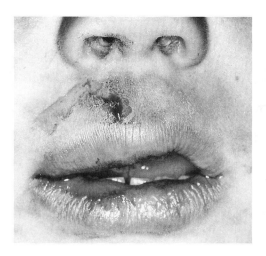

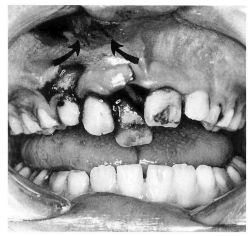

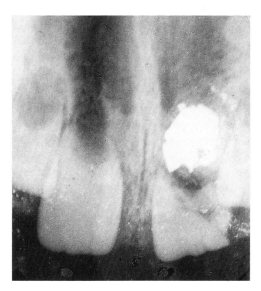

Fig. 3.19.
Multiple dental fractures caused by a gunshot.

The following factors characterize the impact and determine the extent of injury (42).

1. *Energy of impact.* This factor includes both mass and velocity. Examples of these combinations are a force of high velocity and low mass (gunshot) (Fig. 3.19) or of high mass and minimal velocity (striking the tooth against the ground). Experience has shown that low velocity blows cause the greatest damage to the supporting structures, whereas tooth fractures are less pronounced. In contrast, in high velocity impacts the resulting crown fractures are usually not associated with damage to the supporting structures. In these cases, the energy of the impact is apparently expended in creating the fracture and is seldom transmitted to any great extent to the root of the tooth (16).

Fig. 3.20.
A. Force of a frontal blow to the lower lip was transmitted through the lip to the lower incisor region, resulting in a fracture of the alveolar process. B. The oral mucosa is lacerated in areas where the incisal edges contacted the labial mucosa during impact (arrows). From ANDREASEN (16) 1970.

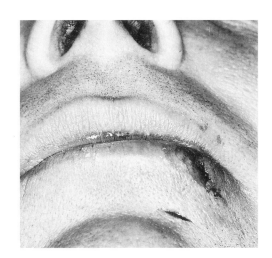

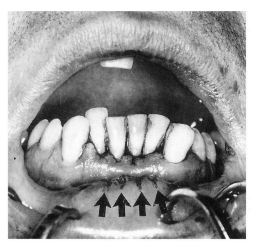

CLASSIFICATION, ETIOLOGY AND EPIDEMIOLOGY

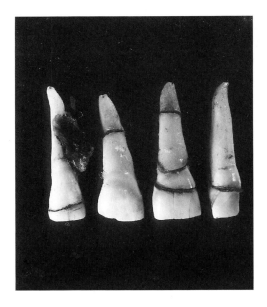
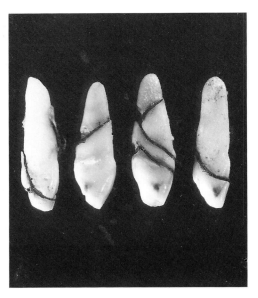

2. *Resilience of the impacting object.* If a tooth is struck with a resilient or cushioned object, such as an elbow during play, or if the lip absorbs and distributes the impact, the chance of crown fracture is reduced while the risk of luxation and alveolar fracture is increased (16) (Figs. 3.18 and 3.20).

3. *Shape of the impacting object.* Impact with a sharp object favors clean crown fractures with a minimum of displacement of the tooth, as the energy is spread rapidly over a limited area. On the other hand, with a blunt object impact increases the area of resistance to the force in the crown region and allows the impact to be transmitted to the apical region, causing luxation or root fracture.

4. *Direction of the impacting force.* The impact can meet the tooth at different angles, most often hitting the tooth facially, perpendicular to the long axis of the root. In this situation, typical cleavage lines will be encountered, as demonstrated in Fig. 3.21. With other angles of impact, other fracture lines will arise.

When considering the direction and position of fracture lines caused by frontal impacts, the fractures fall easily into four categories (Fig. 3.22).

1. Horizontal crown fractures.
2. Horizontal fractures at the neck of the tooth.
3. Oblique crown-root fractures.
4. Oblique root fractures.

Engineering principles can provide a de-

Fig. 3.22.
Facio-lingual orientation of 33 fracture lines.

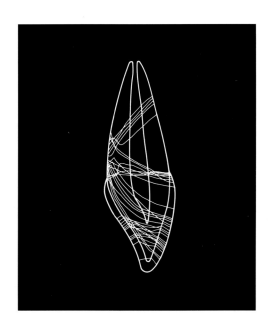

Fig. 3.23.

Fig. 3.23.
A. Frontal impact to the facial surface of an anterior tooth tends to displace the tooth lingually. B. If the energy is absorbed by the tooth-supporting structures, the tooth is displaced.

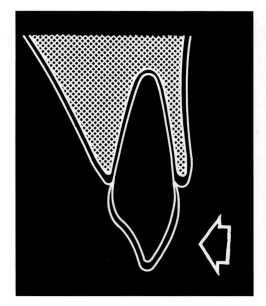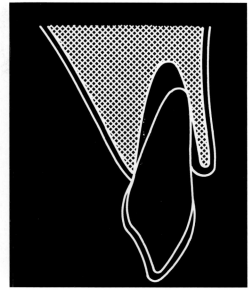

scription of the forces involved in injuries caused by frontal impacts.

Frontal impacts to anterior teeth generate forces which tend to displace the coronal portion orally. Under certain circumstances, such as blunt impacts and high resilience of tooth supporting structures in young individuals, a tooth is more likely to be displaced orally without fracturing, as the energy of the impact is absorbed by the supporting structures during displacement (Fig. 3.23).

A different situation arises if the bone and periodontal ligament resist displacement (Fig. 3.24, A). The root surface is forced against bone marginally and apically (a and b), creating high compressive forces. As the tensile and shearing strength of the brittle dental tissues are much lower than the compressive strength, shearing strains develop between the two zones of the opposing forces, and the root is fractured along the plane joining the two compression areas (a and b) (Fig. 3.24, B) [105].

Fig. 3.24.
A. Bone and periodontal ligament resist displacement from a frontal impact. Compressive forces are exerted upon the root surface at a and b and tensile strains develop across the line connecting a and b. B. A root fracture occurs in the shearing zone, at the area of tensile strain.

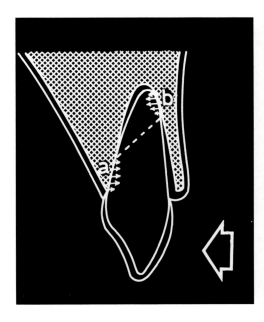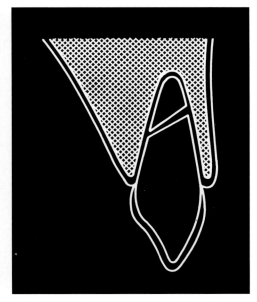

Fig. 3.25.
A. The tooth is firmly locked in its socket. B. A pure bending fracture occurs at the site of maximum bending stress.

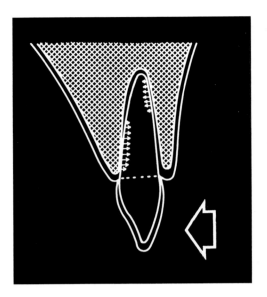 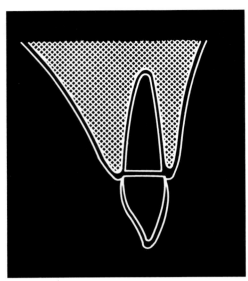

Fig. 3.25 illustrates a condition presumably leading to horizontal fractures at the level of the gingival margin. The tooth is firmly locked in its socket so that stresses in the shearing zone will not be as high as that shown in Fig. 3.24. The impact will, therefore, induce a pure bending fracture at the site of maximum bending stress, i.e. where the tooth emerges from its suppor-

ting structures (Fig. 3.25, B). Tensile strains on the facial surface of the crown usually result in horizontal infraction lines in the cervical enamel (Fig. 3.26). Horizontal fractures at the cervical area usually affect the maxillary lateral incisors, probably due to their firm, deep anchorage in alveolar bone.

Fig. 3.26.
A. Horizontal infraction lines in the cervical area of a fractured maxillary incisor. B. High magnification of the cervical area.

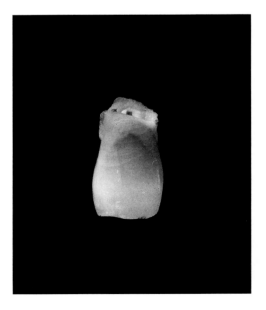 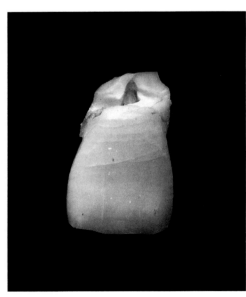

CHAPTER 3

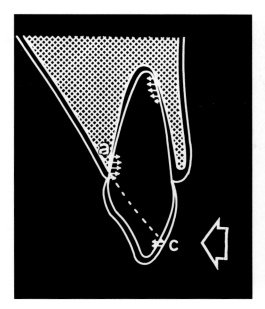
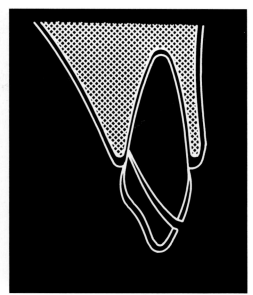

In Fig. 3.27, the stresses presumably causing oblique crown-root fractures are illustrated. The oblique fracture line follows a course along the inclined tensile stress lines developed between the compressive areas a and c. This line of fracture is supported by experiments using brittle materials such as concrete (Fig. 3.28).

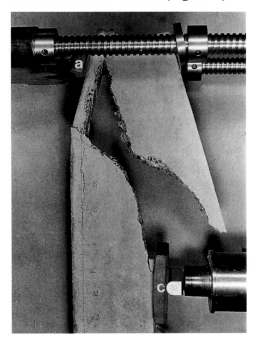

Fig. 3.28.
Experimental model in concrete showing an oblique fracture connecting the area of compression c and supporting area a. Courtesy of Dr. H.H. KRENCHEL, Structural Research Laboratory, Technical University, Copenhagen.

CLASSIFICATION, ETIOLOGY AND EPIDEMIOLOGY

167

Fig. 3.29.
A and B. Cleavage line takes the shortest route, resulting in a pure horizontal shear fracture of the crown.

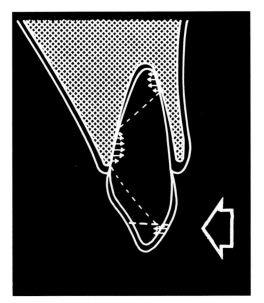 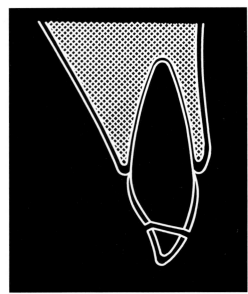

In Fig. 3.29, the same compressive forces and tensile strains as in Fig. 3.27 are presumably present, but are not great enough to cause an oblique fracture, so that the cleavage line follows the shortest possible route, resulting in a horizontal fracture of the crown. The area of contact between the impacting object and the enamel may show a shallow notch surrounded by radiating infraction lines (see Chapter 6, p. 223). The orientation of the enamel prisms determines the course of the fracture line in enamel, while the direction of the fracture in dentin is primarily perpendicular to the dentinal tubules (Fig. 3.30). The theoretical explanation for this has been sought in experimental procedures testing the fracture properties of enamel and dentin (106, 107). It has been found that enamel is weakest parallel to the enamel rods and that dentin is most easily fractured perpendicularly to the dentinal tubules (107)

Penetrating lip lesions occur when the impact direction is parallel to the axis of the mandibular or maxillary incisors (Figs. 3.31 and 3.32). In these cases, foreign bodies such as gravel and tooth fragments are frequently found in the lip lesion. The management of this type of wound is described in Chapter 13.

Fig. 3.30.
The orientation of the enamel prisms and, to a certain degree, the dentinal tubules determines the course of the fracture line. Ground section of a fractured maxillary central incisor.

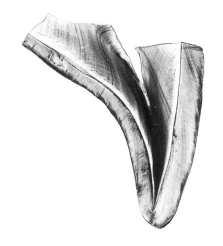 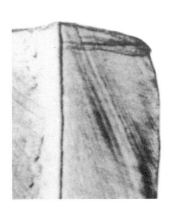

CHAPTER 3

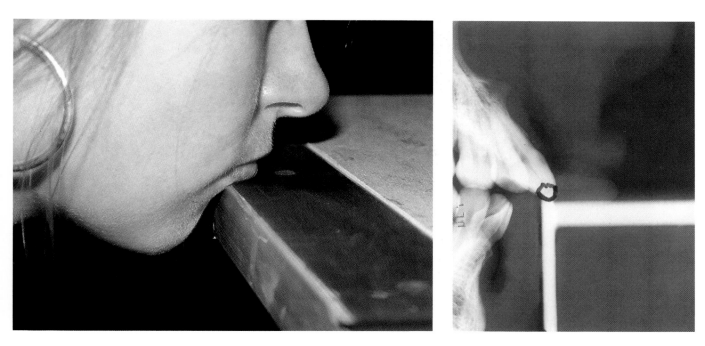

Fig. 3.31.
Etiology of a penetrating lip lesion. A. Impact direction parallel to the axis of the maxillary *incisors. B. The lower lip has been interposed between the incisal edges and the staircase.*

Fig. 3.32.
Etiology of a penetrating lip lesion. A. Impact direction is parallel to the axis of the mandibular *incisors. B. The lower lip has been interposed between incisal edges and the staircase.*

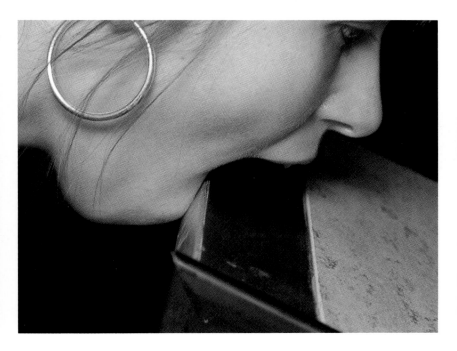 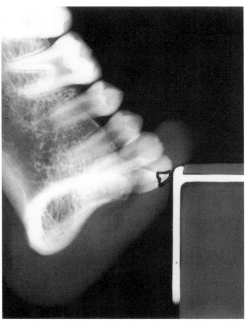

Table 3.1. Reported frequencies of traumatic dental injuries in various countries.

Examiner	Year	Country	Age groups	Sample Size	No. with dental injuries	
					No.	%
Kessler (47)	1922-37	Germany	?	40,203	1,857	4.6
Marcus (109)	1951	U.S.A.	8-17	150	25	16.0
Kessler (48)	1951-58	Germany	6-14	20,000		7-9.8
			10-18			13.8
Grundy (49)	1959	England	5-15	625	37	5.9
Ellis (6)	1960	Canada	?	4,251	178	4.2
McEwen et al. (46)	1967	England	13	2,905	239	8.2
Wallentin (45)	1967	Germany	?	11,966	893	7.5
Beck (50)	1968	New Zealand	15-21	2,145	201	9.4
Büttner (44)	1968	Switzerland	?	1,000	81	8.1
Akpata (51)	1969	Nigeria	6-25	2,819	410	14.5
Hargreaves & Craig (110)	1970	England	4-18	17,831		5.9
Lind et al. (111)	1970	Sweden	0-7	702	88	12.5
Schützmannsky (63)	1970	Germany	2-6	3,098	338	10.9
			7-18	22,708	1,202	5.2
Gutz (112)	1971	U.S.A.	6-13	1,166	236	20.2
O'Mullane (79)	1972	Ireland	6-19	2,792	357	12.8
Andreasen & Ravn (64)	1972	Denmark	3-7	487	147	30.2
			7-16	487	109	22.3
Bergink (113)	1972	Holland	11-16	943	142	15.1
Zadik et al. (122)	1972	Israel	6-14	10,903	948	8.7
Clarkson et al. (114)	1973	England	11-17	756	74	9.8
			15-59	1,604	148	9.2
Holm & Arvidsson (115)	1974	Sweden	3	208	50	24.0
Patkowska-Indyka & Plonka (101)	1974	Poland	10-15	1,946	191	9.8
Ravn (77)	1974	Denmark	14-15	75,000*	9,665	12.9
Wieslander & Lind (116)	1974	Sweden	6-16	2,065	180	8.7
Zadik (117)	1976	Israel	6-14	965		11.1
York et al. (118)	1978	New Zealand	11-13	430	72	16.7
Järvinen (108)	1979	Finland	6-16	1,614	?	19.8
Sanchez et al. (165)	1981	Dominican Republic	3-6	278	59	16.6
Baghady et al. (166)	1981	Iraq	6-12	6,090	467	7.6
Baghady et al. (166)	1981	Sudan	6-12	3,507	180	5.1
Garcia-Goday et al. (167)	1981	Domimican Republic	7-14	596	108	18.1
Garcia-Goday et al. (168)	1983	Dominican Republic	3-5	800	280	35.0
Garcia-Goday (169)	1984	Dominican Republic	5-14	1,633	81	10.0
Garcia-Goday et al. (170)	1985	Dominican Republic	6-17	1,200	146	12.2
Holland et al. (172)	1988	Ireland	15	1,106	403	16.4
Uji & Teramoto (173)	1988	Japan	6-18	15	822	21.8
Yagat et al. (174)	1988	Iraq	1-4	2,389	584	24.4
Kaba & Marechaux (175)	1989	Switzerland	6-18	262		10.8
Ravn (176)	1989	Denmark	6	391	86	22.0
Hunter et al. (177)	1990	U.K.	11-12	968		15.3
Forsberg & Tedestam (178)	1990	Sweden	7-15	1,635	483	30.0
Sanchez & Garcia-Goday. (179)	1990	Mexico	3-13	1,010	287	28.4
Bijella et al. (180)	1990	Brazil	1-6	576	174	30.2

*Personal communication, the number of participants is estimated.

Table 3.2. *Prevalence of traumatic dental injuries to primary teeth in 5-year-olds*

Author	Year	Country	♂ Sex	♀
Andreasen & Ravn (64)	1974	Denmark	31.3	24.6
Garcia-Goday et al. (168)	1983	Dominican Republic	33.6	28.9
Forsberg & Tedestam (178)	1990	Sweden	28.0	16.0
Sanchez & Garcia-Goday (179)	1990	Mexico	40.0	

Epidemiology

Prevalence and Incidence of Dental Injuries

As is shown in Table 3.1, the frequency of traumatic dental injuries varies considerably. This variation reflects a number of factors, such as differences in sampling criteria. However, the two most significant factors are differences in age and sex of the populations examined. Knowing the strong relationship between prevalence of trauma in both the primary and permanent dentitions, such variations as are demonstrated in Table 3.1 are to be expected, considering the age distribution involved.

One way to eliminate the influence of age is to study the prevalence of dental trauma at given stages of development, such as for the primary dentition at the age of 5 (i.e. prior to the mixed dentition period) and at the age of 12 (i.e. after the mixed dentition period and the period of high trauma incidence). See Table 3.2 and 3.3.

Most of these figures, however, are probably grossly underestimated because a number of children may have sustained minor injuries which were either not diagnosed or were routinely treated by a dentist. Apart from a few prospective studies (64, 77), most of the cited reports are cross sectional, which means that registration of previous injuries is to a certain extent dependent upon information from either the child or parent, which can entail a significant error. Thus, one clinical study demonstrated that parents in about half the cases of previously recorded injuries to primary teeth in a preschool dental clinic denied that such injuries had occurred in a questionnaire (64). In a prospective study where all dental injuries occurring from

Table 3.3 *Prevalence of traumatic dental injuries to permanent teeth in 12-year-olds*

Author	Year	Country	♂ Sex	♀
Andreasen & Ravn (64)	1972	Denmark	25.7	16.3
Clarkson et al. (114)	1973	U.K.	11.6	9.6
Todd (182)	1973	U.K.	22.0	12.0
Todd (183)	1983	U.K.	29.0	16.0
Järvinen (108)	1979	Finland	33.0	19.3
Baghdady et al. (166)	1981	Iraq	19.5	16.1
Baghdady et al. (170)	1981	Sudan	16.5	3.6
Garcia-Goday et al. (170)	1985	Dominican Republic	18.0	12.0
Garcia-Goday et al. (171)	1986	Dominican Republic	31.7	15.0
Holland (173)	1988	Ireland	21.2	12.1
Hunter et al. (177)	1990	U.K.	19.4	11.0
Forsberg & Tedestam (178)	1990	Sweden	27.0	12.0

Fig. 3.33.
Prevalence and incidence of traumatic dental injuries to primary teeth among children in Copenhagen. Prevalence indicates frequency (in percentage) of children who have sustained dental injuries at the various ages examined. Incidence indicates the number of new dental injuries (in percentage) arising per year at the various ages examined. From ANDREASEN & RAVN (64) 1972.

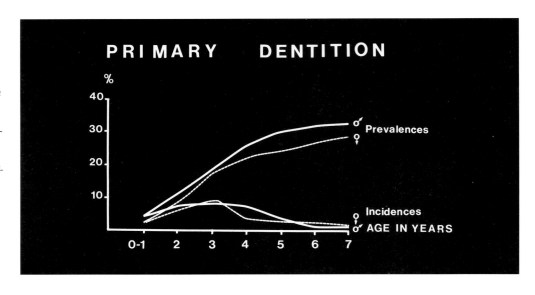

birth to the age of 14 years were carefully registered, it was found that 30% of the children had sustained injuries to the primary dentition and 22% to the permanent dentition. (Figs. 3.33 and 3.34.) Altogether, every second child by the age of 14 had sustained a dental injury (64). In a prospective incidence study from Australia, 2% per year of children aged 6 - 12 years suffered a traumatic dental injury (181).

Decade Variation

In a comparative study of the frequency of dental trauma in Germany from 1922 to 1937 and from 1951 to 1958, a 200 to 300% increase was found (47, 48). Likewise, in a similar study in England, a 5% increase in dental injuries among 15-year-olds could be demonstrated from 1973 to 1983 (182, 183). In the U.S.A., a doubling of

hospital admissions due to traumatic dental injuries was found in the period 1979 to 1987 (189). No increase in the frequency of dental trauma was found in Denmark between 1972 and 1991. However, in this country the frequency of traumas had already reached a very high level in the 1970's (64, 184) (see Fig. 3.33 and 3.34).

Sex and Age Distribution

In Tables 3.2 and 3.3, a comparison is made between prevalence of traumatic dental injuries in various countries for the primary and permanent dentitions for girls and boys. These age-corrected statistics indicate that in the *primary* dentition, the prevalence of injuries ranges from 31 to 40% in boys and from 16 to 30% in girls. In the *permanent* dentition, the prevalence of dental trauma in boys ranges from 12

Fig. 3.34.
Prevalence and incidence of traumatic dental injuries to permanent teeth among children in Copenhagen. Prevalence indicates frequency (in percentage) of children who have sustained dental injuries at the various ages examined. Incidence indicates the number of new dental injuries (in percentage) arising per year at the various ages examined. From ANDREASEN & RAVN (64) 1972.

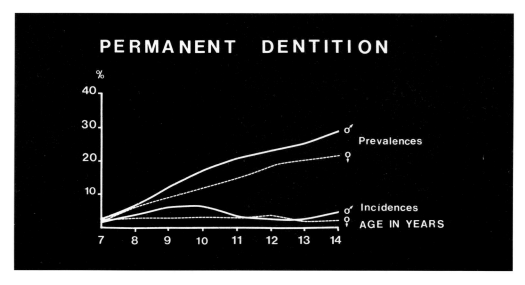

CHAPTER 3

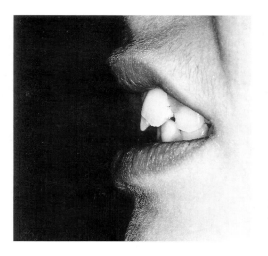

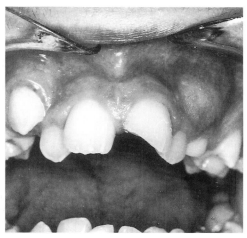

to 33% as opposed to 4 to 19% in girls. In various countries, the boy/girl of trauma frequency ratio differs significantly. The general finding that boys suffer dental traumas almost twice as often as girls in the *permanent* dentition is a fact which is no doubt related to their more active participation in contact games and sports (6, 16, 20-23, 40, 42-45, 49, 52-56, 64, 77, 78, 81, 82, 112, 116, 187).

The prevalence and incidence of traumatic injuries according to age and sex is shown in Figs. 3.33 and 3.34 for a group of children from Copenhagen that was followed continuously from the age of 2 years to the age of 14 years. It can be seen that the first peak appears at 2 to 4 years of age. By the age of 7 years, 28% of the girls and 32% of the boys have suffered a traumatic dental injury to the primary dentition. In the permanent dentition, a marked increase in the incidence of traumatic injuries is seen for boys aged 8 to 10 years, while the incidence is rather stable for girls (64, 77, 185). This peak incidence is probably related to the more vigorous play characteristic of this age group (17, 20-23, 40, 42, 43, 45, 52-54, 56, 77, 119, 120).

Location of Dental Injuries

The majority of dental injuries involve the anterior teeth, especially the maxillary central incisors; while the mandibular central incisors and maxillary lateral incisors are less frequently involved (6, 16-18, 20, 21, 42, 44, 45, 52-54, 56, 59, 60, 63, 77-79, 112, 120, 121). This preference for location also applies to the primary dentition (53, 58, 61).

Dental injuries usually affect only a single tooth (18, 20, 23, 49, 59, 63, 77); however, certain trauma types, such as automobile accidents and sports injuries, favor multiple tooth injuries (16, 78).

Predisposing Factors

Increased overjet with protrusion of upper incisors and insufficient lip closure are significant predisposing factors to traumatic dental injuries (18, 39, 40-46, 63, 65, 77, 79, 98-104, 172, 183, 186, 188, 191) (Fig. 3.35). Studies have shown that dental injuries are approximately twice as frequent among children with protruding incisors than in children with normal occlusion (41, 46), and that the greatest number of injured teeth in the individual patient is associated with protrusive occlusion (43). Concerning orthodontic evaluation of these patients, the reader is referred to the chapter on orthodontic treatment of traumatized teeth (Chapter 15, p. 587).

Various studies have shown that a number of patients treated for dental injuries appear to be accident-prone and sustain repeated trauma to the teeth; frequencies have been reported to range from 4 to 30% (16, 40, 54, 65, 77-79).

Type of Dental Injuries

Statistics concerning different types of dental injuries vary according to the place of treatment. Thus, Table 3.4 lists the frequencies of different types of dental injuries treated by a municipal school dental service and a hospital dental clinic in Copenhagen. It appears that the more severe injuries, such as luxations and bone fractures, dominate in the hospital material where there are fewer crown fractures (16, 20).

When injuries are registered, it is very

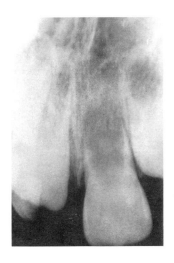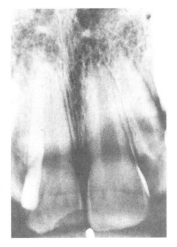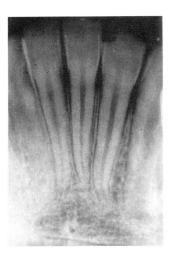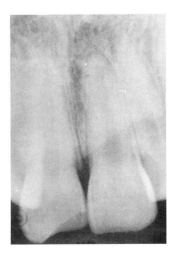

Fig. 3.36.
*Accident prone individual. A.
Avulsion of primary right maxillary central incisor at the age of
7. B. Crown fracture at the age of
9. C. Luxation of the right mandibular central incisor at the age
of 10. D. New trauma to the right
central incisor at the age of 12.*

important that both injury to hard dental tissues, to the periodontium and to associated soft tissues are registered (16, 190). In the hospital material, almost one-half of the cases were complicated by soft-tissue injuries (16, 189).

When injuries affecting primary and permanent teeth are compared, it appears that trauma to the primary dentition is usually confined to the supporting structures, i.e. luxation and exarticulation (16, 22, 58, 64, 191, 192), while the largest propor-

tion of injuries affecting the permanent dentition is represented by crown fractures (20, 22, 40, 49, 53, 54, 56, 59, 64, 77, 78, 112).

Place of Injury

The place of injury varies in different countries according to local customs. In studies examining dental trauma in Iraq, India, Australia and Norway, it was found that the majority of injuries occurred outside school grounds (185, 193, 194). Further-

Table 3.4. *Types of dental injuries to permanent dentition in two different treatment institutions in Copenhagen. From ANDREASEN (16) 1970 and RAVN & ROSSEN (20) 1969*

	Dental Clinic, University Hospital Copenhagen		Municipal School Dental Service, Copenhagen	
	No. of teeth	%	No. of teeth	%
Crown fracture without pulp exposure	433*	19	1,171	64
Crown fracture with pulp exposure	172*	8	89	5
Crown-root fracture	108*	5	0	0
Root fracture	156*	7	16	1
Concussion and subluxation	336*	15	324	18
Intrusive and extrusive luxation	691*	31	36	2
Exarticulation	350*	16	29	1
Contusion of alveolar socket and/or fracture of the facial or lingual alveolar socket wall	109*	5	0	0
Fracture of alveolar process	205*	9	0	0
Fracture of mandible or maxilla	36*	2	0	0
Other injuries or exact injury not specified	334*	15	169	9
Total number of injured teeth	**2,239**		**1,834**	

* The number of diagnoses exceeds the number of teeth due to multiple diagnosis for some teeth.

more, a greater number of severe injuries occurred after school hours (195).

Seasonal Variations

A relationship seems to exist between the time of year and prevalence of dental injuries. Thus, several studies have shown that the frequency of dental injuries increases during the winter months (43, 54, 77, 116). However, other reports indicate an increase in the summer months (148, 154, 196, 197). The reported variations seem to have been dependent upon the reporter. Thus, emergency room reports indicated a greater frequency of dental traumas in the summer months, whereas reports from Scandinavian school dental services indicated a drop in the same period (20, 153, 176). This disagreement could reflect differences in clinic activity in this period.

Treatment Demands

In various studies it has been shown that the treatment needs of traumatic dental injuries are not properly met. Thus, studies from Finland have shown that only 25% had received treatment (198), and in Britain only 10-15% (183, 199). The root of this problem would appear to be two-fold. First, information provided to the public as to appropriate first-aid and its relationship to improved long-term prognosis in many trauma situations might improve public awareness of the need for emergency care. Thus, in a public survey conducted in Australia, it was found that while most parents would seek emergency dental care if necessary, only 10% were informed of the correct emergency procedures in the case of acute trauma (199). Thus, 90% of the parents questioned had never received advice on what to do in the event of an accident where a permanent tooth was avulsed. The second problem involves lack of organization in the provision of emergency care. In centers where emergency care is lacking, public and professional awareness could be instrumental in creating such facilities.

Essentials

Terminology

INJURIES TO THE HARD DENTAL TISSUES AND THE PULP (FIG. 3.1)
   Enamel infraction
   Enamel fracture
   Enamel-dentin fracture
   Complicated crown fracture (i.e. with pulp exposure)
   Uncomplicated crown-root fracture
   Complicated crown-root fracture (i.e. with pulp exposure)
   Root fracture

INJURIES TO THE PERIODONTAL TISSUES (FIG. 3.2)
   Concussion
   Subluxation (loosening)
   Intrusive luxation (central dislocation)
   Extrusive luxation (peripheral dislocation, partial avulsion)
   Lateral luxation
   Avulsion (exarticulation)

INJURIES TO THE SUPPORTING BONE (FIG. 3.3)
   Comminution of alveolar socket
   Fracture of alveolar socket wall
   Fracture of alveolar process
   Fracture of mandible or maxilla (jaw fracture)

INJURIES TO THE GINGIVA OR ORAL MUCOSA (FIG. 3.4)
   Laceration of gingiva or oral mucosa
   Contusion of gingiva or oral mucosa
   Abrasion of gingiva or oral mucosa

Etiology

   Iatrogenic injuries in newborns
   Falls in infancy
   Child physical abuse
   Falls and collisions
   Sport
   Horseback riding
   Bicycle injuries
   Automobile injuries
   Assaults

Torture
Mental retardation
Epilepsy
Drug-related injuries
Dentinogenesis imperfecta

PREDISPOSING FACTORS
Protrusion of upper incisors
Insufficient lip closure

MECHANISM OF DENTAL INJURIES
Trauma type
a. Direct trauma
b. Indirect trauma

FACTORS CHARACTERIZING AN IMPACT TO THE TEETH
a. Energy of impact
b. Resilience of the impacting object
c. Shape of the impacting object
d. Angle of direction of the impacting force

Epidemiology

SEX AND AGE DISTRIBUTION
Boys affected almost twice as often as girls
Peak incidence of dental injuries at 2 to 4 and 8 to 10 years of age

PREVALENCE OF DENTAL INJURIES ACCORDING TO SEX (TABLES 3.2 AND 3.3)
Primary dentition (at 5 years of age):
Boys (31-40%).
Girls (16-30%)
Permanent dentition (at 12 years of age):
Boys (12-33%).
Girls (4-19%)

LOCATION OF INJURIES
Maxillary central incisors most commonly involved

TYPE OF DENTAL INJURIES (TABLE 3.2)
Permanent dentition: most often uncomplicated crown fractures
Primary dentition: most often luxations

SEASONAL VARIATIONS

Bibliography

1. ADAMS FR. Traumatized and fractured young teeth. *J Am Dent Assoc* 1944;**31**:241-8.

2. BENNETT DT. Traumatised anterior teeth. I - Assessing the injury and principles of treatment. *Br Dent J* 1963;**115**:309-11.

3. BRAUER JC. Treatment and restoration of fractured permanent anterior teeth. *J Am Dent Assoc* 1936;**23**:2323-36.

4. COWSON RA. Essentials of dental surgery and pathology. 2nd edn. London: J & A Churchill Ltd, 1968:90-9.

5. COOKE C, ROWBOTHAM TC. Treatment of injuries to anterior teeth. *Br Dent J* 1951;**91**:146-52.

6. ELLIS RG, DAVEY KW. *The classification and treatment of injuries to the teeth of children.* 5th edn. Chicago: Year Book Publishers Inc, 1970.

7. ESCHLER J, SCHILLI W, WITT E. *Die traumatischen Verletzungen der Frontzähne bei Jungendlichen.* 3rd edn. Heidelberg: Alfred Hüthig Verlag, 1972.

8. HOGEBOOM FE. *Practical pedodontia or juvenile operative dentistry and public health dentistry.* 5th edn. St. Louis: CV Mosby Company, 1946:288-314.

9. MCBRIDE WC. *Juvenile Dentistry.* 5th edn. London: Henry Kimpton, 1952:247-62.

10. INGLE JI, FRANK AL, NATKIN E, NUTTING EE. Diagnosis and treatment of traumatic injuries and their sequelae. In: INGLE JI, BEVERIDGE EE, eds. *Endodontics.* 2nd edn. Philadelphia: Lea & Febiger, 1976:685-741.

11. SOLEIL J. Essai de classification étiologie des lésions traumatiques des dents. *Rev Stomatol* 1960;**61**:633-6.

12. SWEET CA. A classification and treatment for traumatized anterior teeth *ASDC J Dent Child* 1955;**22**:144-9.

13. TOVERUD G. Traumatiske beskadigelser av incisiver i barnealderen og deres behandling. *Odontologisk Tidskrift* 1947;**55**:71-82.

14. THOMA KH, GOLDMAN HM. *Oral Pathology.* 5th edn. St. Louis: CV Mosby Company, 1960:231-41.

15. *Application of the International Classification of Diseases and Stomatology,* IDC-DA, 2nd edn. Geneva: WHO, 1978.

16. ANDREASEN JO. Etiology and pathogenesis of traumatic dental injuries. A clinical study of 1298 cases. *Scand J Dent Res* 1970;**78**:339-42.

17. NORD C-E. Tandskador hos skolbarn och ishockeyspelare. *Odontologisk Förenings Tidskrift* 1966;**30**:15-25.

18. SCHÜTZMANNSKY G. Unfallverletzungen an jugendlichen Zähnen. *Dtsch Stomatol* 1963;**13**:919-27.

19. TATE RJ. Facial injuries associated with the battered child syndrome. *Br J Oral Surg* 1971;**9**:41-5.

20. RAVN JJ, ROSSEN I. Hyppighed og fordeling af traumatiske beskadigelser af tænderne hos københavnske skolebørn 1967/68. *Tandlægebladet* 1969;**73**:1-9.

21. MAGNUSSON B, HOLM A-K. Traumatised permanent teeth in children - a follow-up. I. Pulpal complications and root resorp. In: NYGAARD J, ØSTBY B, OSVALD O, eds. *Nordisk Klinisk Odontologi.* Copenhagen: A/S Forlaget for Faglitteratur 1964: Chapter 11, III, 1-40.

23. EDWARD S, NORD C-E. Dental injuries of school-children. *Svensk Tandläkaras Tidskrift* 1968;**61**:511-6.

24. GRIMM G. Kiefer- und Zahnverletzungen beim Sport. *Zahnärztl* 1967;**76**:115-35.

25. HAWKE JE. Dental injuries in rugby football. *N Z Dent J* 1969;**65**:173-5.

26. KRAMER LR. Accidents occurring in high school athletics with special reference to dental injuries. *J Am Dent Assoc* 1941;**28**:1351-2.

27. ROBERTS JE. Wisconsin Interschlolastic Athletic Association 1970. *Benefit plan summary.* Supplement to the 47th Official Handbook of the Wisconsin Interscholastic Athletic Association 1970:1-77.

28. ROBERTS JE. *Dental guard questionaire summary.* Wisconsin Interscholastic Athletic Association report to the National Alliance Football Rules Committee 1962.

29. COHEN A, BORISH AL. Mouth protector project for football players in Philadelphia high schools. *J Am Dent Assoc* 1958;**56**:863-4.

30. KULOWSKI J. Facial injuries; a common denominator of automobile casualties. *J Am Dent Assoc* 1956;**53**:32-7.

31. KULOWSKI J. *Crash injuries.* Springfield, Illinois: CT Thomas, 1960:306-22.

32. SCHULTZ RC. Facial injuries from automobile accidents: a study of 400 consecutive cases. *Plast Reconstr Surg* 1967;**40**:415-25.

33. STRAITH CL. Guest passenger injuries. *J Am Dent Assoc* 1948;**137**:348-51.

34. RUSSELL BG. Personal communication, 1969.

35. WIKSTRÖM L. Narkotika och tänder. *Sveriges Tandläkaras - Förbunds Tidning* 1970;**62**:1152-5.

36. WILSON GW, STEINBRECHER M. Heriditary hypoplasia of the dentin. *J Am Dent Assoc* 1929;**16**:866-86.

37. HODGE HC. Correlated clinical and structural study of hereditary opalescent dentin. *J Dent Res* 1936;**15**:316-7.

38. OVERVAD H. Et tilfælde af osteogenesis imperfecta med dentinogenesis imperfecta. *Tandlægebladet* 1969;**73**:840-50.

39. GLUCKSMAN DD. Fractured permanent anterior teeth complicating orthodontic treatment. *J Am Dent Assoc* 1941;**28**:1941-3.

40. HARDWICK JL, NEWMANN PA. Some observations on the incidence and emergency treatment of fractured permanent anterior teeth of children. *J Dent Res* 1954;**33**:730.

41. LEWIS TE. Incidence of fractured anterior teeth as related to their protrusion. *Angle Orthod* 1959;**29**:128-31.

42. HALLET GEM. Problems of common interest to the paedodontist and orthodontist with special reference to traumatised incisor cases. *Eur Orthod Soc Trans* 1953;**29**:266-77.

43. EICHENBAUM IW. A correlation of traumatized anterior teeth to occlusion. *ASDC J Dent Child* 1963;**30**:229-36.

44. BÜTTNER M. Die Häufigkeit von Zahnunfällen im Schulalter. *Zahnärztl Prax* 1968;**19**:286.

45. WALLENTIN I. Zahnfrakturen bei Kindern und Jugendlichen. *Zahnärztl Mitt* 1967;**57**:875-7.

46. MCEWEN JD, MCHUGH WD, HITCHIN AD. Fractured maxillary central incisors and incisal relationships. *J Dent Res* 1967;**46**:1290.

47. KESSLER W. *Kinder-Zahnheilkunde und Jugendzahnpflege.* 3rd edn. München: Carl Hanser Verlag, 1953:144.

48. KESSLER W. Fratture dentarie nell'infanzia. *Riv Ital Stomatol* 1959;**14**:251-5.

49. GRUNDY JR. The incidence of fractured incisors. *Br Dent J* 1959;**106**:312-4.

50. BECK JJ. Dental health status of the New Zealand population in late adolescence and young adulthood. *Department of Health. Special report series 29.* Wellington: RE Owen Government Printer, 1968:65-9.

51. AKPATA ES. Traumatised anterior teeth in Lagos school children. *J Nigeria Med Assoc* 1969;**6**:1-6.

52. GAARE A, HAGEN AR, KANSTAD S. Tannfrakturer hos barn. Diagnostiske og prognostiske problemer og behandling. *Norske Tannlegeforenings Tidende* 1958;**68**:364-78.

53. PARKIN SF. A recent analysis of traumatic injuries to children's teeth. *ASDC J Dent Child* 1967;**34**:323-5.

54. GELBIER S. Injured anterior teeth in children. A preliminary discussion. *Br Dent J* 1967;**123**:331-5.

55. LIEBAN EA. Traumatic injuries to children's teeth. *N Y State Dent J* 1947;**13**:319-34.

56. ABRAHAM G. Über unfallbedingte Zahnschädigungen bei Jugendlichen. Thesis. Zürich, 1963.

57. SCHREIBER CK. The effect of trauma on the anterior deciduous teeth. *Br Dent J* 1959;**106**:340-3.

58. NORD C-E. Traumatiska skador i det primära bettet. *Odontolgisk Förenings Tidende* 1968;**32**:157-63.

59. DOWN CH. The treatment of permanent incisor teeth of children following traumatic injury. *Aust Dent J* 1957;**2**:9-24.

60. KRETER F. Klinik und Therapie extraalveolärer Frontzahnfrakturen. *Zahnärztl Prax* 1967;**18**:257-60.

61. TAATZ H. Verletzungen der Milchzähne und ihre Behandlung. In: REICHENBACK E, ed. *Kinderzahnheilkunde im Vorschulalter. Zahnärztliche Fortbildung.* No. 16. Leipzig: Johann Ambrosius Barth Verlag, 1967:363-86.

62. STICH E. Dentoalveoläre Verletzungen. *Zahnärztl Welt* 1970;**79**:554-6.

63. SCHÜTZMANNSKY G. Statistisches über Häufigkeit und Schweregrad von Unfalltraumen an der Corona Dentis im Frontzahnbereich des kindlichen und jugendlichen Gebisses. *Z Gesamte Hyg* 1970;**16**:133-5.

64. ANDREASEN JO, RAVN JJ. Epidemiology of traumatic dental injuries to primary and permanent teeth in a Danish population sample. *Int J Oral Surg* 1972;**1**:235-9.

65. JOHNSON JE. Causes of accidental injuries to the teeth and jaws. *J Public Health Dent* 1975;**35**:123-31.

66. LASKIN DM. The battered-child syndrome. *J Oral Surg* 1973;**31**:903.

67. SCHWARTZ S, WOOLRIDGE E, STEGE D. Oral manifestations and legal aspects of child abuse. *J Am Dent Assoc* 1977;**95**:586-91.

68. LASKIN DM. The recognition of child abuse. *J Oral Surg* 1978;**36**:349.

69. BENSEL RW, KING KJ. Neglect and abuse of children; historical aspects, identification, and management. *ASDC J Dent Child* 1975;**42**:348-58.

70. O'NEILL JA Jr, MEACHAM WF, GRIFFIN PP, SAWYERS JL. Patterns of injury in the battered child syndrome. *J Trauma* 1973;**13**:332-9.

71. HOLTER JC, FRIEDMAN SB. Child abuse; early case finding in the emergency department. *Pediatrics* 1968;**42**:128-38.

72. CAMERON JM, JOHNSON HRM, CAMPS FE. The battered child syndrome. *Med Sci Law* 1966;**6**:2-21.

73. SKINNER AE, CASTLE RL. *A retrospective study.* National Society for the Prevention of Cruelty to Children, London 1969.

74. BECKER DB, NEEDLEMAN HL, KOTELCHUCK M. Child abuse and dentistry; orofacial trauma and its recognition by dentist. *J Am Dent Assoc* 1978;**97**:24-8.

75. HAZLEWOOD AI. Child abuse. The dentist's role. *N Y Dent J* 1970;**36**:289-91.

76. CARTER AP, ZOLLER G, HARLIN VK, JOHNSON CJ. Dental injuries in Seattle's public school children - school year 1969-1970. *J Public Health Dent* 1972;**32**:251-4.

77. RAVN JJ. Dental injuries in Copenhagen schoolchildren, school years 1967-1972. *Community Dent Oral Epidemiol* 1974;**2**: 231-45.

78. HEDEGÅRD B, STÅLHANE I. A study of traumatized permanent teeth in children aged 7-15 years. Part I. *Swed Dent J* 1973;**66**:431-50.

79. O'MULLANE DM. Some factors predisposing to injuries of permanent incisors in school children. *Br Dent J* 1973;**134**:328-32.

80. KNYCHALSKA-KARWAN Z. Trauma to the anterior teeth in sportsmen in the light of statistics. *Czas Stomatol* 1975;**28**:479-84.

81. HAAVIKKO K, RANTANEN L. A follow-up study of injuries to permanent and primary teeth in children. *Proc Finn Dent Soc* 1976;**72**:152-62.

82. O'MULLANE DM. Injured permanent incisor teeth; An epidemiological study. *J Irish Dent Assoc* 1972;**18**:160-73.

83. LEES GH, GASKELL PH. Injuries to the mouth and teeth in an undergraduate population. *Br Dent J* 1976;**140**:107-8.

84. SZYMANSKA-JACHIMCZAK EI, SZPRINGER-NODZAK M. Statistical analysis of traumatic damage to permanent teeth in children and adolescents treated at the outpatient clinic of the department of pediatric stomatology institute of the medical academy in Warsaw in the years 1960-1975. *Czas Stomatol* 1977;**30**:689-93.

85. GRIMM G. Kiefer und Zahnverletzungen beim Sport. *Zahnärztl Rdsch* 1967;**76**:115-35.

86. DENNIS CG, PARKER DAS. Mouthguards in Australian sport. *Aust Dent J* 1972;**17**:228-35.

87. LIE HR, LUCHT U. Ridesportsulykker. I. Undersøgelse af en rytterpopulation med særligt henblik på ulykkesfrekvensen. *Ugeskr Læger* 1977;**139**:1687-9.

88. LUCHT U, LIE HR. Ridesportsulykker. II. Ulykkerne belyst gennem en prospektiv sygehusundersøgelse. *Ugeskr Læger* 1977;**139**:1689-92.

89. LINDAHL L, GRØNDAHL H-G. Traumatiserade tänder hos vuxna. *Tandläkartidningen* 1977;**69**:328-32.

90. HUELKE DF, SHERMAN HW. Automobile injuries - the forgotten area of public health dentistry. *J Am Dent Assoc* 1973;**86**:384-93.

91. LINDAHL L. Tand- och käkskador i Göteborg. Epidemiologisk och behandlingsmässig kartläggning. *Svensk Tandläkaras Tidning* 1974;**66**:1019-30.

92. LINDAHL L. Tand- och käkskador i Göteborg. Nogra sociala faktorers inverkan. *Svensk Tandläkaras Tidning* 1974;**66**:1011-4.

93. BESSERMANN K. Frequency of maxillo-facial injuries in a hospital population of patients with epilepsy. *Bull Nord Soc Dent Handicap* 1978;**5**:12-26.

94. VON GERLACH D, WOLTERS HD. Zahn- und Mundschleimhautbefunde bei Rauschmittelkonsumenten. *Dtsch Zahnärztl Z* 1977;**32**:400-4.

95. BØLLING P. Tandtortur. *Tandlægebladet* 1978;**82**;571-4.

96. DIEM CR, RICHLING M. Dental problems in Navy and Marine Corps repatriated prisoners of war before and after captivity. *Milit Med* 1978;**143**:532-7.

97. DIEM CR, RICHLING M. Improvisational dental first aid used by American prisoners of war in Southeast Asia. *J Am Dent Assoc* 1979;**98**:535-7.

98. BERZ H, BERZ A. Schneidezahnfrakturen und sagitale Schneidezahnstufe. *Dtsch Zahnärztl Z* 1971;**26**:941-4.

99. WOJCIAK L, ZIOLKIEWICS T, ANHOLCER H, FRANKOWSKA-LENARTOWSKA M, HABER-MILEWSKA T, ZYNDA B. Trauma to the anterior teeth in school-children in the city of Poznán with reference to masticatory anomalies. *Czas Stomatol* 1974;**27**:1355-61.

100. ANTOLIC I, BELIC D. Traumatic damages of teeth in the intercanine sector with respect to the occurrence with school children. *Zoboz Vestn* 1973;**28**:113-20.

101. PATKOWSKA-INDYKA E, PLONKA K. The effect of occlusal anomalies on fractures of anterior teeth. *Stomatol* 1974;**24**:375-9.

102. DE MUÑIZ BR, MUÑIZ MA. Crown fractures in children. Relationship with anterior occlusion. *Rev Asoc Odont Argent* 1975;**63**:153-7.

103. JÄRVINEN S. Incisal overjet and traumatic injuries to upper permanent incisors. A retrospective study. *Acta Odontol Scand* 1978;**36**:359-62.

104. FERGUSON FS, RIPA LW. Incidence and type of traumatic injuries to the anterior teeth of preschool children. *J Dent Res* 1975;**58**: *I.A.D.R.* Abstracts no. 401, 1979.

105. LEHMAN ML. Bending strength of human dentin. *J Dent Res* 1971;**50**:691.

106. RENSON CE, BOYDE A, JONES SJ. Scanning electron microscopy of human dentine specimens fractured in bend and torsion tests. *Arch Oral Biol* 1974;**19**:447-54.

107. RASMUSSEN ST, PATCHIN RE, SCOTT DB, HEUER AH. Fracture properties of human enamel and dentin. *J Dent Res* 1976;**55**:154-64.

108. JÄRVINEN S. Fractured and avulsed permanent incisors in Finnish children. A retrospective study. *Acta Odontol Scand* 1979;**37**:47-50.

109. MARCUS M. Delinquency and coronal fractures of anterior teeth. *J Dent Res* 1951;**30**:513.

110. HARGREAVES JA, CRAIG JW. *The management of traumatised anterior teeth in children.* London: E. & S. Livingstone Publishers, 1970.

111. LIND V, WALLIN H, EGERMARK-ERIKSSON I, BERNHOLD M. Indirekta traumaskador. Kliniska skador p- permanenta incisiver som följd av trauma mot temporära incisiver. *Sverig Tandläk Förb Tidning* 1970;**62**:738-56.

112. GUTZ DP. Fractured permanent incisors in a clinic population. *ASDC J Dent Child* 1971;**38**:94-121.

113. BERGINK AH. Tandbeschadigingen. *Maandschr Kindergeneesk* 1972;**40**:278-93.

114. CLARKSON BH, LONGHURST P, SHEIHAM A. The prevalence of injured anterior teeth in English school children and adults. *J Int Assoc Dent Child* 1973;**4**:21-4.

115. HOLM AK, ARVIDSSON S. Oral health in preschool Swedish children. 1. Three-year-old children. *Odontologisk Revy* 1974;**25**:81-98.

116. WIESLANDER I, LIND V. Traumaskador på permanenta tänder. Något om förekomst och behandlingsproblem. *Tandläkaratidningen* 1974;**66**:716-9.

117. ZADIK D. A survey of traumatized primary anterior teeth in Jerusalem preschool children. *Community Dent Oral Epidemiol* 1976;**4**:149-51.

118. YORK AH, HUNTER RM, MORTON JG, WELLS GM, NEWTON BJ. Dental injuries in 11- to 13-year-old children. *N Z Dent J* 1978;**74**:218-20.

119. IRMISCH B, HETZER G. Eine klinische Auswertung akuter Traumen im Milchgebiss und permanenten Gebiss. *Dtsch Stomatol* 1971;**21**:28-34.

120. HERFORTH A. Zur Frage der Pulpavitalität nach Frontzahntrauma bei Jugendlichen- eine Longitudinaluntersuchung. *Dtsch Zahnärztl Z* 1976;**31**:938-46.

121. WÖRLE M. Katamnestische Erhebung zur Prognose des Frontzahntraumas. *Dtsch Zahnärzl Z* 1976;**31**:635-7.

122. ZADIK D, CHOSACK A, EIDELMAN E. A survey of traumatized incisors in Jerusalem school children. *ASDC J Dent Child* 1972;**39**:185-8.

123. SNYDER JR, KNOOPS JJ, JORDAN WA. Dental problems of non-institutionalized mentally retarded children. *North-West Dent* 1960;**39**:123-33.

124. GAYFORD JJ. Wife battering: a preliminary survey of 100 cases. *Br Med J* Vol no I (5951) 1975;194-7.

125. PARKER B, SCHUMACHER DN. The battered wife syndrome and violence in the nuclear family of origin. A controlled pilot study. *Am J Public Health* 1977;**67**:760-1.

126. SCOTT PD. Battered wives. *Br J Psychiatry* 1974;**125**:433-41.

127. ROUNSAVILLE B, WEISSMANN MM. Battered women; A medical problem requiring detection. *Int J Psychiatry* 1977-78;**8**:191-202.

128. ROUNSAVILLE BJ. Battered wives. Barriers to identification and treatment. *Am J Orthopsychiatry* 1978;**48**:487-94.

129. PETRO JA, QUANN PL, GRAHAM WP. Wife abuse. The diagnosis and its implications. *J Am Dent Assoc* 1978;**240**:240-1.

130. PETERSSON B, JACOBSEN AT. Mishandlede kvinder (battered wives). *Ugeskr Læger* 1980;**142**:469-71.

131. JOHNSON R. Descriptive classification of traumatic injuries to the teeth and supporting structures. *J Am Dent Assoc* 1981;**102**:195-7.

132. GARCÍA-GODOY F. A classification for traumatic injuries to primary and permanent teeth. *J Pedodont* 1981;**5**:295-7.

133. *Application of the International Classification of Diseaseas and Stomatology,* IDC-DA, 3rd edn. Geneva: WHO, 1992.

134. MOYLAN FMB, SELDEN EB, SHANNON DC, TODRES JD. Defective primary dentition in survivors of neonatal mechanical ventilation. *J Paediatr* 1980;**96**:106-8.

135. BOICE JB, KROUS HF, FOLEY JM. Gingival and dental complication of orotracheal intubation. *J Am Med Assoc* 1976;**236**:957-8.

136. SEOW WK, BROWN JP, TUDEHOPE DI, O'CALLAGHAN M. Developmental defects in the primary dentition of low birthweight infants: adverse effects of laryngoscopy and prolonged endotracheal intubation. *Pediatr Dent* 1984;**6**:28-31.

137. BECKER DB, NEEDLEMAN HL, KOTELCHUCK M. Child abuse and dentistry: orofacial trauma and its recognition by dentists. *J Am Dent Assoc* 1978;**27**:24-8.

138. MALECZ RE. Child abuse, its relationship to pedodontics: a survey. *ASDC J Dent Child* 1979;**46**:193-4.

139. DAVIS GR, DOMOTO PK, LEVY RL. The dentists role in child abuse and neglect. *ASDC J Dent Child* 1979;**46**:185-92.

140. KITTLE PE, RICHARDSON DS, PARKER JW. Two child abuse/child neglect examinations for the dentist. *ASDC J Dent Child* 1981;**48**:175-80.

141. SCHMITT BD. Types of child abuse and neglect: an overview for dentists. *Pediatr Dent* 1986;**8**:67-71.

142. NEEDLEMAN HL. Orofacial trauma in child abuse: types, prevalence, management, and the dental professions involvement. *Pediatr Dent* 1986;**8**:71-80.

143. KITTLE PE, RICHADSON DS, PARKER JW. Examining for child abuse and child neglect. *Pediatr Dent* 1986;**8**:80-2.

144. SCHMITT BD. Physical abuse: specifics of clinical diagnosis. *Pediatr Dent* 1986;**8**:83-7.

145. DUBOWITZ H. Sequelae of reporting child abuse. *Pediatr Dent* 1986;**8**:88-92.

146. WAGNER GN. Bitemark identification in child abuse cases. *Pediatric Dent* 1986;**8**:96-100.

147. CASAMASSIMO PS. Child sexual abuse and the pediatric dentist. *Pediatr Dent* 1986;**8**:102-6.

148. ONEIL DW, CLARK MV, LOWE JW, HARRINGTON MS. Oral trauma in children: a hospital survey. *Oral Surg Oral Med Oral Pathol* 1989;**68**:691-6.

149. NYSETHER S. Dental injuries among Norwegian soccer players. *Community Dent Oral Epidemiol* 1987;**15**:141-3.

150. NYSETHER S. Tannskader i norsk idrett. *Norske Tannlegeforenings Tidende* 1987;**97**:512-4.

151. JÄRVINEN S. On the causes of traumatic dental injuries with special reference to sports accidents in a sample of Finnish children. A study of a clinical patient material. *Acto Odontol Scand* 1980;**38**:151-4.

152. HÄYRINEN-IMMONEN R, SANE J, PERKKI K, MALMSTRÖM M. A six-year follow-up study of sports-related dental injuries in children and adolescents. *Endod Dent Tramatol* 1990;**6**:208-12.

153. BHAT M, LI S-H. Consumer product-related tooth injuries treated in hospital emergency rooms: United States, 1979-87. *Community Dent Oral Epidemiol* 1990;**18**:133-8.

154. KENRAD B. Tandlægetjeneste på en spejderlejr. *Tandlægebladet* 1991;**95**:583-5.

155. SANDHAM A, DEWAR I, CRAIG J. Injuries to incisors during sporting activities at school. *Tandlægebladet* 1986;**90**:661-3.

156. HILL CM, CROCHER RF, MASON DA. Dental and facial injuries folowing sports accidents: a study of 130 patients. *Br J Oral Maxillofac Surg* 1985;**23**:268-74.

157. LINN EW, VRIJHOEF MMA, DE WIJN JR, COOPS RPHM,

CLITEUR BF, MEERLOO R. Facial injuries sustained during sports and games. *J Maxillofac Surg* 1986;**14**:83-8.

158. SEGUIN P, BEZIAT JL, BRETON P, FREIDEL M, NICOD C. Sports et traumatologie maxillo-faciale. Aspects étiologiqes et cliniqes à propos de 46 cas. Mesures de prévention. *Rev Stomatol Chir Maxillofac* 1986;**87**:372-5.

159. STOCKWELL AJ. Incidence of dental trauma in the Western Australian School Dental Service. *Community Dent Oral Epidemiol* 1988;**16**:294-8.

160. WIENS JP. Acquired maxillofacial defects from motor vehicle accidents: statistics and prosthodontic considerations. *J Prosthet Dent* 1990;**63**:172-81.

161. LAMBERG MA, TASANEN A, KOTILAINEN R. Maxillo-facial fractures caused be assault and battery. Victims and their injuries. *Proc Finn Dent Soc* 1975; **71**:162-75.

162. KORSGAARD GM, CARLSEN A. "Hustruvold". En prospektiv opgørelse af vold mod kvinder i parforhold. *Ugeskrift for Læger* 1983;**145**:443-6.

163. LASKIN DM. Looking out for the battered woman. *J Oral Surg* 1981;**39**:405.

164. YOUNG GH, GERSON S. New psychoanalytic perspectives on masochism and spouse abuse. *Psychotherapy* 1991;**28**:30-8.

165. SÁNCHEZ JR, SÁNCHEZ R, GARCÍA-GODOY F. Traumatismos de los dientes anteriores en ninos pre-escolares. *Acta Odontol Pediatr* 1981;**2**:17-23.

166. BAGHDADY VS, GHOSE LJ, ENKE H. Traumatized anterior teeth in Iraqi and Sudanese children - a comparative study. *J Dent Res* 1981;**60**:677-80.

167. GARCÍA-GODOY F, SÁNCHEZ R, SÁNCHEZ JR. Traumatic dental injuries in a sample of Dominican schoolchildren. *Community Dent Oral Epidemiol* 1981;**9**:193-7.

168. GARCÍA-GODOY F, MORBÁN-LAUCHER F, COROMINAS LR, FRANJUL RA, NOYOLA M. Traumatic dental injuries in pre-schoolchildren from Santo Domingo. *Community Dent Oral Epidemiol* 1983;**11**:127-30.

169. GARCÍA-GODOY FM. Prevalence and distribution of traumatic injuries to the permanent teeth of Dominican children from private schools. *Community Dent Oral Epidemiol* 1984;**12**:136-9.

170. GARCÍA-GODOY F, MORBÁN-LAUCER F, COROMINAS LR, FRANJUL RA, NOYOLA M. Traumatic dental injuries in schoolchildren from Santo Domingo. *Community Dent Oral Epidemiol* 1985;**13**:177-9.

171. GARCÍA-GODOY F, DIPRES FM, LORA IM, VIDAL ED. Traumatic dental injuries in children from private and public schools. *Community Dent Oral Epidemiol* 1986;**14**:287-90.

172. HOLLAND T, O'MULLANE DO, CLARKSON J, O'HICKEY SO, WHELTON H. Trauma to permanent teeth of children aged 8,12 and 15 years, in Ireland. *Paediatr Dent* 1988;**4**:13-6.

173. UJI T, TERAMOTO T. Occurrence of traumatic injuries in the oromaxillary region of children in a Japanese prefecture. *Endod Dent Traumatol* 1988;**4**:63-9.

174. YAGOT KH, NAZHAT NY, KUDER SA. Traumatic dental injuries in nursery schoolchildren from Baghdad, Iraq. *Community Dent Oral Epidemiol* 1988;**16**:292-3.

175. KABA AD, MARÉCHAUX SC. A fourteen-year follow-up study of traumatic injuries to the permanent dentition. *ASDC J Dent Child* 1989;**56**:417-25.

176. RAVN JJ. Dental traume epidemiologi i Danmark: en oversigt med enkelte nye oplysninger. *Tandlægebladet* 1989;**93**:393-6.

177. HUNTER ML, HUNTER B, KINGDON A, ADDY M, DUMMER PMH, SHAW WC. Traumatic injury to maxillary incisor teeth in a group of South Wales schoolchildren. *Endod Dent Traumatol* 1990;**6**:260-4.

178. FORSBERG C, TEDESTAM G. Traumatic injuries to teeth in Swedish children living in an urban area. *Swed Dent J* 1990;**14**:115-22.

179. SANCHEZ AV, GARCÍA-GODOY F. Traumatic dental injuries in 3- to 13-year-old boys in Monterrey, Mexico. *Endod Dent Traumatol* 1990;**6**:63-5.

180. BIJELLA MFTB, YARED FNFG, BIJELLA VT, LOPES ES. Occurrence of primary incisor traumatism in Brazilian children: a house-by house survey. *ASDC J Dent Child* 1990;**57**:424-7.

181. STOCKWELL AJ. Incidence of dental trauma in the Western Australian Shool Dental Service. *Community Dent Oral Epidemiol* 1988;**16**:294-8.

182. TODD JE. *Children's dental health in England and Wales.* London: social survey division and Her Majesty's Stationary Office, 1973.

183. TODD JE. *Children's dental health in England and Wales.* London: social survey division and Her Majesty's Stationary Office, 1983.

184. RAVN JJ. Stiger antallet af akutte trandtrumer? *Odontologia Practica* 1991;**3**:103-5.

185. HANSEN M, LOTHE T. Tanntraumer hos skolebarn og ungdom i alderen 7-18 år i Oslo. *Norske Tannlægeforenings Tidende* 1982;**92**:269-73.

186. GHOSE LJ, BAGHDADY VS, ENKE H. Relation of traumatized permanent anterior teeth to occlusion and lip condition. *Community Dent Oral Epidemiol* 1980;**8**:381-4.

187. OLUWOLE TO, LEVERETT DH. Clinical and epidemiological survey of adolescents with crown fractures of permanent anterior teeth. *Pediatr Dent* 1986;**8**:221-3.

188. HOLLAND T, O'MULLANE D, CLARKSON J, HICKEY SO, WHELTON H. Trauma to permanent teeth of children aged 8, 12 and 15 years, in Ireland. *J Paedia Dent* 1988;**4**:13-6.

189. GALEA H. An investigation of dental injuries treated in an acute care general hospital. *J Am Dent Assoc* 1984;**109**:434-8.

190. ANDREASEN FM, ANDREASEN JO. Diagnosis of luxation injuries: The importance of standardized clinical, radiographic and photographic techniques in clinical investigations. *Endod Dent Traumatol* 1985;**1**:160-9.

191. TETSCH P. Statistische Auswertung von 1588 traumatisierten Zähnen. *Dtsch Zahnärztl Z* 1983;**38**:474-5.

192. MORGANTINI J, MARÉCHAUX SC, JOHO JP. Traumatismes dentaires chez l'enfant en âge préscolaire et répercussions sur les dents permanentes. *Rev Mens Suisse Odontostomatol* 1986;**96**:432-40.

193. BAGHDADY VS, GHOSE LJ, ALWASH R. Traumatized anterior teeth as related to their cause and place. *Community Dent Oral Epidemiol* 1981;**9**:91-3.

194. DAVIS GT, KNOTT SC. Dental trauma in Australia. *Aust Dent J* 1984;**29**:217-21.

195. LIEW VP, DALY CG. Anterior dental trauma treated after-hours in Newcastle, Australia. *Community Dent Oral Epidemiol* 1986;**14**:362-6.

196. GARCÍA-GODOY F, GARCÍA-GODOY F, OLIVO M. Injuries to primary and permanent teeth treated in a private paedodontic practice. *J Canad Dent Assoc* 1979;**45**:281-4.

197. GARCÍA-GODOY F, GARCÍA-GODOY F, GARCÍA-GODOY FM. Primary teeth traumatic injuries at a private pediatric dental center. *Endod Dent Traumatol* 1987;**3**:126-9.

198. JÄRVINEN S. Extent to which treatment is sought for children with traumatized permanent anterior teeth. An epidemiological study. *Proc Finn Dent Soc* 1979;**75**:103-5.

199. RAPHAEL LSJ, GREGORY PJ. Parental awareness of the emergency management of avulsed teeth in children. *Australian Dent J* 1990;**35**:130-5.

CHAPTER 4

Child Physical Abuse

R. R. WELBURY

Child Physical Abuse - a Definition

A child is considered to be abused if he or she is treated in a way that is unacceptable in a given culture at a given time. The last two clauses are important, because not only are children treated differently in different countries, but also within a country and even within a city there are sub-cultures of behavior and variations of opinion as to what constitutes abuse.

Child Physical Abuse - Historical Aspects

Violence towards children has been noted between cultures and at different times within the same culture since early civilization. Infanticide has been documented in almost every culture so that it can almost be considered a universal phenomenon [1]. Ritualistic killing, maiming and severe punishing of children in an attempt to educate them, exploit them or rid them of evil spirits has been reported since early biblical times and ritualistic surgery or mutilation of children has been recorded as part of religious and ethnic traditions [2].

With the advent of urbanization and technological advancement in the 18th century, more economic value was placed upon the child by society and they were often used as a cheap source of labor. Harsh punishments for relatively minor misdemeanors were accepted and indeed expected in the courts, the school and the home [3].

In the 19th century, western societies became more protective towards children, and their lot gradually improved. However, the mortality rate remained high, and the isolated death of a child probably did not arouse suspicion. Lord SHAFTESBURY, who campaigned to create better conditions in Britain for children at work, recognized the problem of child abuse at home, but was powerless to intervene:

"The evils are enormous and indisputable, but they are so private, internal and domestic a character as to be beyond the reach of legislation and the subject would not, I think, be entertained in either House of Parliament"
Lord SHAFTESBURY 1880.

As more effective health care became available in the developed countries, more children survived poor living and working conditions. But in the middle of this century reports appeared in the USA of unexplained skeletal injury to children [4,5]. These reports described unexpected skeletal trauma, sometimes associated with subdural hematoma. The possibility that these injuries could have been inflicted by a parent was recognized by some authors but there appears to have been a general reluctance to accept that parents could wilfully abuse their offspring [6]. However, when KEMPE et al published their paper "The

Battered-Child Syndrome" in 1962 [7] the full impact of the physical maltreatment of children was brought to the attention of the medical community and subsequently the general public. The battered-child syndrome, which is now usually termed non-accidental injury (NAI) or child physical abuse, had such a profound effect upon the professions and the public that within a few years the majority of states in the USA had introduced laws which made it mandatory for physicians, dentists and other health related professionals to report suspected cases.

Prevalence

NAI is now recognized as an international issue and has been reported in many countries [8-18]. However, despite this global recognition, prevalence rates in most countries are still not available. It is estimated that in the USA 1.7 millon children per year will be subjected to maltreatment that is sufficiently serious to warrant attention by the child psychiatry services [19]. In Britain most departments of social services and child welfare are notified of more than 20 times as many cases of suspected child abuse as they were 10 years ago [20]. Although some of these reports will prove to be unfounded, the common experience is that proved cases of child abuse are four or five times as common as they were a decade ago [20].

In Britain, at least 1 child per 1000 under 4 years of age per year suffers severe physical abuse - for example fractures, brain hemorrhage, severe internal injuries or mutilation [21] and in the USA more than 95% of serious intracranial injuries during the 1st year of life are the result of abuse [22]. Studies analyzing the attendance of children in accident and emergency departments of hospitals have shown that in the USA 10% of children younger than 5 [23] and in Denmark 1.3 children per 1000 per year [24] will have injuries that were wilfully inflicted. Each year at least 4000 children in the U.S.A. [25] and 200 children in Britain [26] will die as a result of abuse or neglect. In Scandinavia, the estimated number of deaths from NAI is much lower, at about 10 annually giving an estimated frequency of 0.5 child deaths per million inhabitants per year [27]. A common finding in all countries is that the workers concerned with child abuse believe that many cases remain undetected and the real mortality figures are considerably higher.

Children of all ages are subject to physical abuse; but the majority of cases occur in younger children [21] (Fig. 4.1). This is partly because they are more vulnerable and partly because they cannot seek help elsewhere. Children under 2 years of age are most at risk from severe NAI. Death from abuse is rare after the age of 1 year. The number of boys subjected to violence slightly exceeds that of girls; and first-born children are more often affected. Within a family, it is common for just one of the children to be abused and the others to be free from such abuse.

Etiology

The etiology of NAI is based on the interaction between the personality traits of the parents or the abusing adult, the child's characteristics and the environmental conditions [28]. Due to the wide variation in behavioral characteristics, personality traits and psychiatric symptoms among abusive adults, a specific abusive personality does not exist. However, certain commonly recurring traits can be recognized [8,21,29-31].

NAI encompasses all social classes; but more cases have been identified in the poorer socio-economic groups. Many cases of NAI are by the child's parents or by persons known to the child [24]. Often the mother of the affected child may be divorced or single. It is also common for a cohabitant who is living in the home, but who is not related to the child, to be the perpetrator. Young parents, often of low intelligence, are more likely to be abusers. This is especially true if they have been exposed to such behavior during their own childhood [32]. Indeed, abuse is thought to be 20 times more likely if one of the parents was abused as a child [21]. A significant proportion of the perpetrators have a criminal record of some kind; and although they usually do not have an identified mental illness, they may exhibit personality traits predisposing to violent behavior. Contributing factors to abuse on behalf of the adults involved include alcohol and other drug abuse, poverty, unemployment and marital problems. Children

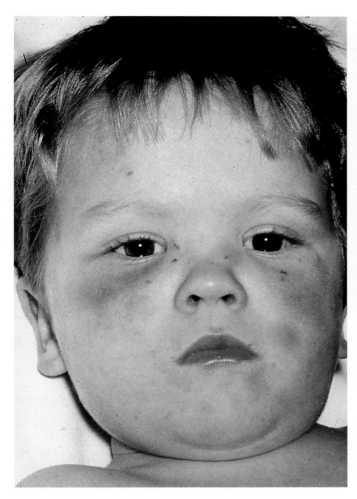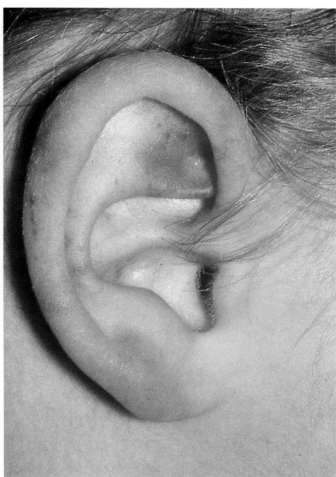

Fig. 4.1.

Three- year old boy suffering from physical abuse. Note bruising of different vintages involving the skin overlying the bony prominences of the cheekbones and the soft tissue areas of the cheek and circumoral region. This history was inconsistent with the amount, degree and vintage of the bruising. The 'pinch' type bruises on the superior surface of the right ear was a result of the ear being held between the fingers and thumb of the abuser and then pulled.

already at risk may add to the stress by continually crying, throwing tantrums, or soiling their clothes. In addition, the child may be handicapped, be the result of an unwanted pregnancy or may fail to attain the expectations of the parents. These factors can provoke frustration in the most stable parent. But in association with other stresses, they may lead to physical neglect or injury.

Diagnosis

The most important step in diagnosing NAI is to believe that it can happen in the first place. The diagnosis is a difficult intellectual and emotional exercise; and is one of the most consuming tasks for a pediatrician, requiring time, experience and emotional energy. Failure to spot the signs and make the diagnosis can vitally influence a child's future life. At worst, it is a matter of life or death for the child. Short of death, there may still be possible brain damage or handicap.

NAI is not a full diagnosis, it is merely a symptom of disordered parenting. The aim of intervention is to diagnose and cure (if possible) the disordered parenting. Simply to aim at preventing death is a lowly ambition. In the 1970's it was estimated that in the USA 5% of abused children who were returned to the home environment without some form of intervention died following further trauma [33] and 35-50% sustained serious re-injury [33,34]. However, by 1986 it was recognized that probably as many as 50% of severely abused children returned to the abuser would die of recurrent abuse if proper therapeutic measures were not introduced [35]. In some cases, the occurrence of

Fig. 4.2.
A slap mark bruise. Three parallel linear bruises at finger-width spacing can be seen to run through a more diffuse bruise.

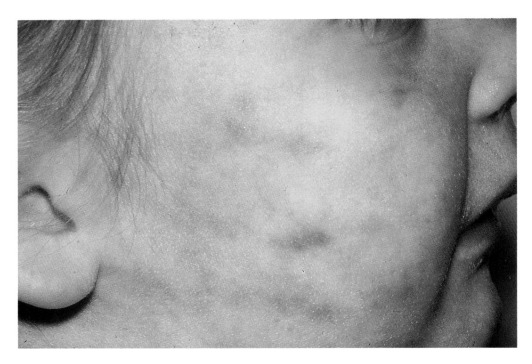

physical abuse may provide an opportunity for intervention. If this opportunity is missed, there may be no further opportunity for many years.

There are no hard-and-fast rules to make the diagnosis of NAI easier (36). The following list constitutes seven classic indicators to the diagnosis. None of them is pathognomonic on its own; neither does the absence of any of them preclude the diagnosis of NAI (37)

1. There is a delay in seeking medical help (or medical help is not sought at all).
2. The story of the "accident" is vague, is lacking in detail, and may vary with each telling and from person to person.
3. The account of the accident is not compatible with the injury observed.
4. The parents' mood is abnormal. Normal parents are full of creative anxiety for the child; while abusing parents tend to be more pre-occupied with their own problems - for example, how they can return home as soon as possible.
5. The parents' behavior gives cause for concern - for example they may become hostile and rebut accusations that have not been made.
6. The child's appearance and the interaction with their parents are abnormal. The child may look sad, withdrawn, or frightened.
7. The child may say something concerning the injury that is different to the parents' story.

Types of Orofacial Injuries in NAI

Approximately 50% of cases diagnosed as NAI have orofacial trauma , which may or may not be associated with injury elsewhere(8, 38-40). Although the face often seems to be the focus of impulsive violence, facial fractures are not frequent. The types and prevalence of orofacial injuries in child abuse have been reviewed by NEEDLEMAN (41). The largest and most detailed study was reported by BECKER ET AL. (1978) (40). The medical records of 260 cases of child abuse admitted to The Children's Hospital in Boston between 1970 and 1975 were reviewed. One-hundred-and-twenty-eight (49%) of the patients had facial and/or intra-oral trauma. An additional 16% of the children had injuries to the head, such as skull fractures, subdural hematomas, contusions and lacerations of the scalp. Of the 236 injuries sustained by the orofacial structures, 61% involved the face (66% contusions and ecchymoses, 28% abrasions and lacerations, 4% burns and bites, 2% fractures) and 6% the intraoral structures (43% contusions and ecchymoses, 28% abrasions and lacerations, 28% dental trauma). From these figures, it can be seen that soft tissue injuries, most frequently bruises, are the most common injury sustained to the orofacial structures in NAI.

184

CHAPTER 4

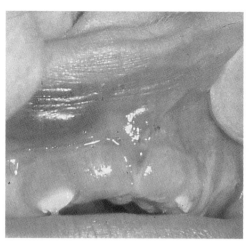

Fig. 4.3.
A torn labial frenum and bruising of the buccal sulcus, sustained during forceful feeding.

Bruising

Accidental falls rarely cause bruises to the soft tissues of the cheek; but instead involve the skin overlying bony prominences such as the forehead or cheekbone. Inflicted bruises occur at typical sites and/or fit recognizable patterns (Table 4.1) (25). The clinical dating of bruises usually conforms to the guidelines in Table 4.2 , but there is a wide variability(42). More accurate assessment may be possible by laboratory methods in forensic pathology (43,44). Bruises of different vintage indicate more than one episode of abuse and, together with extensive bruising and a history of minimal trauma, bruises of different vintages are almost pathognomonic of NAI (Fig. 4.1).

Bruises on the ear are commonly due to being pinched or pulled by the ear (Fig.4.1); and there will usually be a matching bruise on the posterior surface of the ear.

Bruises or cuts on the neck are almost always due to being choked or strangled by a human hand, cord or some sort of collar. Accidents to this site are extremely rare and should be looked upon with sus-

picion. "Resuscitation" attempts do not leave bruises on the face or neck.

Bruising and laceration of the upper labial frenum of a young child can be produced by forcible bottle feeding and is another injury of NAI, but one which may remain hidden unless the lip is carefully everted (Fig. 4.3). The same injury can also be caused by gagging or gripping and violent rubbing of the face; and may be accompanied by facial bruising/abrasions (Fig. 4.4). A frenum tear is not uncommon in the young child who accidently falls while learning to walk (generally between 8-18 months). However, a frenum tear in a very young non-ambulatory patient (less than 1 year) or an older more stable child (2 years) should arouse one's suspicion as to the possibility of this injury being non-accidental (41).

Human Hand Marks

The human hand can leave various types of pressure bruises: grab marks or fingertip bruises, linear marks or finger-edge bruises, hand prints, slap marks and pinch marks (25). The most common types are grab marks or squeeze marks which leave oval-shaped bruises that resemble fingerprints. Grab mark bruises can occur on the cheeks if an adult squeezes a child's face in an attempt to get food or medicine into his mouth. This action leaves a thumb mark bruise on one cheek and 2-4 fingermark bruises on the other cheek. Linear marks are caused by pressure from the entire finger. In slap marks to the cheek, parallel linear bruises at finger-width spacing will be seen to run through a more diffuse bruise (Fig. 4.2). These linear bruises are due to the capillaries rupturing at the edge of the injury (between the striking fingers), as a result of being stretched and receiving a sudden influx of blood.

Table 4.1. Typical sites for inflicted bruises

Buttocks and lower back (paddling)
Genitals and inner thigh
Cheek (slap marks)
Earlobe (pinch marks)
Upper lip and frenum (forced feeding)
Neck (choke marks)

Table 4.2. Dating bruises

Age	Color
0- 2 days	Swollen, tender
0- 5 days	Red, blue, purple
5- 7 days	Green
7-10 days	Yellow
10-14 days	Brown
2- 4 weeks	Cleared

Fig. 4.4 .
Tattoo bruising in the right fore-
head region of the child in Fig.
4.1. The exact object causing this
injury was not known.

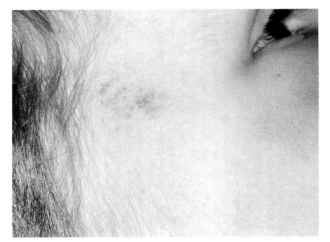
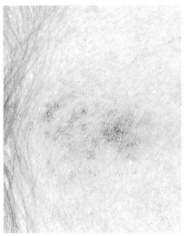

Bizarre Bruises

Bizarre-shaped bruises with sharp borders are nearly always deliberately inflicted. If there is a pattern on the inflicting imple- ment, this may be duplicated in the bruise – so-called tattoo bruising (Fig. 4.4).

Abrasions and Lacerations

Penetrating injuries to the palate, ves- tibule and floor of the mouth can occur during forceful feeding of young infants; these are usually caused by the feeding utensil.

Abrasions and lacerations on the face may be caused by a variety of objects, but are most commonly due to rings or finger- nails on the inflicting hand and injuries are rarely confined to the orofacial structures (Figs. 4.1 and 4.5).

Burns

Approximately 10% of physical abuse cases involve burns (45). Burns of the oral muccosa can be the result of forced inges- tion of hot or caustic fluids in young child- ren. Burns from hot solid objects applied to the face are usually without blister for- mation and the shape of the burn often resembles its agent. Cigarette burns give circular, punched out lesions of uniform size (Figs. 4.5 and 4.7). Lesions such as these are pathognomonic for child abuse.

Bite-marks

Human bite-marks are identified by their shape and size (Fig. 4.6). When necessary, serological techniques are available and may assist in identification. The nature and location of the bite is likely to change with increasing age of the child. In in- fants, bite-marks tend to be punitive and are often a response to soiling or crying. As a result, bite marks may appear any- where; but they tend to be concentrated on the cheek, arm, shoulders, buttocks or genitalia. In childhood, bite-marks tend to be less punitive and more a function of assault or defense. Sexually orientated bite-marks occur more frequently in ado- lescents and adults (46). However, a bite mark at any age should raise the suspicion of child sexual abuse.

The duration of a bite-mark is depend- ent on the force applied and the extent of tissue damage. Teeth-marks that do not break the skin are visible up to 24 hours. In those cases where the skin is broken, the borders or edges will be apparent for sev- eral days depending on the thickness of the tissue. Thinner tissues retain the marks longer (47).

CHAPTER 4

Fig. 4.5.
Multiple superficial lacerations, extensive facial bruising of different vintages, a cigarette burn of the forehead and a "pinch" injury of the left ear in a child subjected to repeated physical abuse.

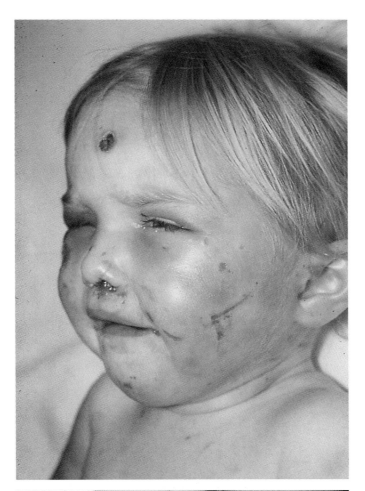

There are numerous pinch mark bruises over the chest and abdomen, extensive bruising over the suprapubic region and a number of small abrasions and lacerations.

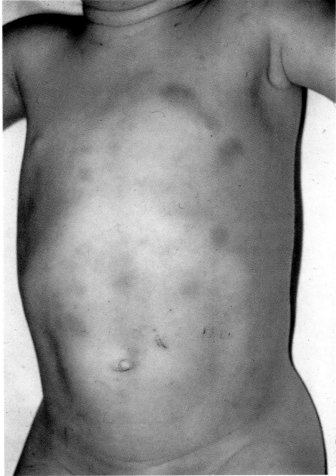

CHILD PHYSICAL ABUSE

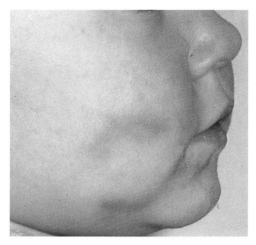

Fig. 4.6.
A human bite-mark injury on the right cheek.

Dental Trauma

Trauma either to the primary or permanent dentition in NAI can be due to blunt trauma (Fig. 4.7). A similar range of injuries to those found in accidental trauma is seen.

Eye Injuries

Most periorbital bruises caused by NAI involve both sides of the face. Ocular damage in NAI includes acute hyphema, dislocated lens, traumatic cataract and detached retina (48). More than half of these injuries result in permanent impairment of vision affecting one or both eyes.

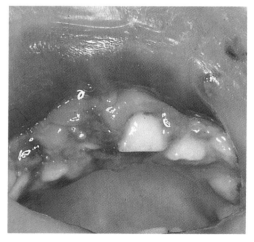

Fig. 4.7.
Luxation of four incisors and extensive bruising in the upper buccal sulcus sustained as a result of a blow to the mouth.

Bone Fractures

Fractures are among the most serious injuries sustained in NAI. They may occur in almost any bone and may be single or multiple, clinically obvious, or occult and detectable only by radiography. Most fractures in physically abused children occur under the age of 3 (49). In contrast, accidental fractures occur more commonly in children of school age.

Facial fractures are relatively uncommon in children. They can, however, occur during physical assault with nasal fractures occurring most frequently (45%), followed by mandibular fractures (32%), and zygomatic

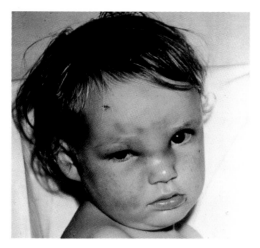

Fig. 4.8
A fracture of the nasoethmoidal complex caused by a heavy blow to the midface.

maxillary complex and orbit fractures (20%) (50).

The presence of a fracture of the facial skeleton in a case of NAI is an indication for a full skeletal radiographic survey (Fig. 4.8). Generally the force required to produce a facial fracture in a child is greater than that required to produce metaphyseal, epiphyseal, spiral, oblique and transverse fractures in long bones. A skeletal survey of a child who has suffered NAI may show evidence of multiple fractures at different stages of healing.

In some instances, a number of the varied features mentioned above may be present at any one time and the diagnosis of NAI will be clear. However, there are occasions when clinical evidence is inconclusive and the diagnosis merely suspected.

Differential Diagnosis

Although dental practitioners should be suspicious of all injuries to children, they should never consider the diagnosis of NAI on the basis of one sign, as various diseases can be mistaken for NAI. Impetiginous lesions may look similar to cigarette burns (Figs. 4.9 and 4.10); birthmarks can be mistaken for bruising; and conjunctivitis can be mistaken for trauma. All children who are said to bruise easily and extensively should have a full blood count, platelet estimation and blood coagulation studies to eliminate a blood dyscrasia (e.g. leukemia), a platelet deficiency (e.g. thrombocytopenia) or other hemorrhagic disorders (e.g. hemophilia, von Willebrand's disease).

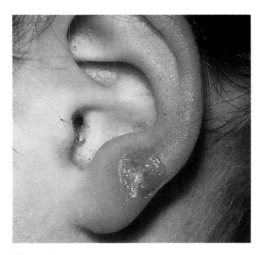

Fig. 4.9.
A discrete well demarcated lesion, typical of the appearance of a cigarette burn.

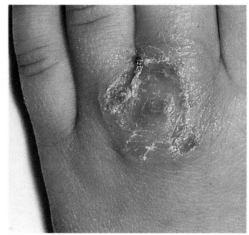

Fig. 4.10.
An impetiginous lesion which can resemble the appearance of a cigarette burn.

The Dentist's Role in the Management of Child Physical Abuse

The dental practitioner may be the first professional to suspect physical abuse as a result of injuries involving the orofacial structures (51-57). The primary aim of all professionals involved is to ensure the safety of the child. The secondary aim is to provide help and counseling for the parents or care givers so that the abuse stops. The method of liaison and referral between dental practitioners and the other health care professionals involved in child abuse cases will vary, not only from country to country, but also between cities and different regions within one country. Most regional child welfare departments now issue procedural guidelines for dental practitioners in suspected child abuse cases (58).

A child with a severe injury is usually referred immediately to a hospital-based consultant pediatrician. Where suspicions are aroused, the dentist should speak to the child's medical practitioner immediately and arrange for a medical examination within 24 hours. As far as possible, parents should accompany the child for the medical examination. If the parent is not available, the local child welfare department should be contacted.

Dental practitioners should ensure that their clinical records are completed immediately with illustrations of the size, position and type of injuries. Photographic documentation would be beneficial in this respect. These records may be referred to in any subsequent case conference or legal proceedings.

Dental practitioners should not feel any guilt about referring children with suspected NAI to a pediatrician or general medical practitioner. They are not accusing either parent; they are simply asking for a second opinion on an important and difficult diagnosis. It is neither in the interest of the child nor the parents for child abuse to be covered up. To do so leaves the parents at greater risk of inflicting more severe injuries next time, being imprisoned for causing more severe injuries, and long-term loss of custody of their children. Early intervention may help to prevent these events. Failure to follow up suspicions is a form of professional negligence. Dental practitioners should be aware that in the United States a doctor who fails to report suspected child abuse is guilty of a federal offence that is punishable by imprisonment.

This being said, it must be stressed that the diagnosis of non-accidental injury is a difficult one to make with certainty. Conflicting reports even in the same scientific journal confirm this statement (59, 60). Thus, there have been reports of various pathological or postmortem changes that have been mistakenly identified as NAI (59), while suspected child abuse and neglect might go undetected in connection with unexpected deaths in children (52) or facial or intraoral injuries (61).

Because of the high frequency of intraoral and facial injuries, dental professionals comprise a very important part of the team necessary for identifying and reporting child abuse and neglect (61, 62). However, the team approach is absolutely necessary, whereby members of multiple specialties collaborate to confirm the diagnosis of NAI.

In conclusion, the dental practitioner's contribution to the management of NAI. should be (31):

1. to recognize the possibility of physical abuse;
2. to provide essential emergency dental treatment and arrange further treatment if required;
3. to inform the appropriate authorities of his or her suspicions.

Essentials

Terminology

Non-Accidental Injury (NAI) or Child Physical Abuse

Frequency

Prevalences in children range from 0.1% to 10% in various countries

Clinical Findings

Delay in seeking treatment
Explanation for injury does not fit the clinical findings
Explanation for injury may differ with each telling and from person to person
Abnormal parental reaction and behavior
Type of relationship between parents and child
The child's reaction to other people
The child's story may differ from parents'
50% of NAI cases have oro-facial findings
Usually more than one sign present
Hematomas of different vintage suggest repeated trauma

Treatment

Recognize the possibility of physical abuse
Provide emergency dental treatmet
Refer the patient for a medical examination

Bibliography

1. BAKAN D. *Slaughter of the Innocents. A study of the Battered-Child Phenomenon.* Boston: Beacon Press, 1972.

2. RADBILL SX. A History of Child Abuse and Infanticide. In: *The Battered Child.* HERFER RE, KEMPE CH, eds. Chicago: The University of Chicago Press, 1968.

3. SOLOMON T. History and Demography of Child Abuse. *Paediatrics* 1973;**51**:773-6.

4. CAFFEY J. Multiple fractures in the long bones of infants suffering from chronic subdural haematoma. *Am J Roentgenology* 1946;**56**:162-73.

5. SILVERMAN FN. The roentgen manifestations of unrecognised skeletal trauma in infants. *Am J Roentgenology and Radium Therapy* 1953;**69**:413-27.

6. WOOLLEY PV, EVANS WA. Significance of skeletal lesions in infants resembling those of traumatic origin. *J Am Med Assoc* 1955;**158**:539-43.

7. KEMPE CH, SILVERMAN FN, STEELE BF, DROEGEMUELLER W, SILVER HK. The Battered-Child Syndrome. *J Am Med Assoc* 1962;**181**:105-12.

8. BAETZ K, SLEDZIEWSKI W, MARGETTS D. Recognition and management of the battered child syndrome. *J Dent Assoc S.Afr* 1977;**32**:13-18.

9. AGATHONOS H, STATHACOPOULOU N, ADAM H, NAKOU S. Child abuse and neglect in Greece: Sociomedical aspects. *Child Abuse and Neglect* 1982;**6**:307-11.

10. CREIGHTON S. An epidemiological study of abused children and their families in the United Kingdom between 1977 and 1982. *Child Abuse and Neglect* 1985;**9**:441-8.

11. FERRIER P, SCHALLER M, GIRARDET I. Abused children admitted to a paediatric in-patient service in Switzerland: a ten-year experience and follow up evaluation. *Child Abuse and Neglect* 1985;**9**:373-81.

12. MARZOUKI M, HADHFREDJ A, CHELLI M. L'enfant battu et les attitudes culturelles: L'exemple de la Tunisie. *Child Abuse and Neglect* 1987;**11**:137-41.

13. SYMONS AL, ROWE PV, ROMANIAK K. Dental aspects of child abuse: review and case reports. *Aust Dent J* 1987;**32**:42-7.

14. FINKELHOR D, KORBIN J. Child abuse as an international issue. *Child Abuse and Neglect* 1988;**12**:3-23.

15. MERRICK J, MICHELSEN N. Children at-risk: Child abuse in Denmark. *Int J Rehabil Res* 1985;**8**:181-8.

16. LARSSON G, EKENSTEIN G, RASCH E. Are the social workers prepared to assist a changing population of dysfunctional parents in Sweden? *Child Abuse and Neglect* 1984;**8**:9-14.

17. PELTONIEMI T. Child abuse and physical punishment of children in Finland. *Child Abuse and Neglect* 1983;**7**:33-36.

18. OLESEN T, EGEBLAD M, DIGE-PETERSEN H, AHLGREN P, NIELSEN AM, VESTERDAL J. Somatic manifestations in children suspected of having been maltreated. *Acta Paediatr Scand* 1988;**77**:154-60.

19. HART SN, BRASSARD MR. A major threat to children's mental health: Psychological maltreatment. *American Psychologist* 1987;**42**:160-5.

20. MEADOW R. Epidemiology. In: MEADOW R, ed. *The ABC of Child Abuse.* Br Med J London 1989.

21. CREIGHTON SJ. The incidence of child abuse and neglect. In: BROWNE K, DAVIES C, STRATTON P, eds. *Early prediction and prevention of child abuse.* Chichester, England: Wiley, 1988.

22. BILLMIRE ME, MYERS PA. Serious head injury in infants: accident or abuse? *Pediatrics* 1985;**75**:340-2.

23. HOLTER JC, FRIEDMAN SB. Child abuse, early case finding in the emergency department. *Pediatrics* 1968;**42**:128-38.

24. BREITING VB, HELWEG-LARSEN K, STAUGAARD H, et al. Injuries due to deliberate violence in areas of Denmark. *Forensic Sci Int* 1989;**41**:285-94.

25. SCHMITT BD. Physical abuse: specifics of clinical diagnosis. *Pediatric Dentistry* 1986;**8**:83-87.

26. CREIGHTON SJ, GALLAGHER B. *Child Abuse Deaths.* London: The National Society for the Prevention of Cruelty to Children. Information Briefing No.5 (revised) 1988.

27. GREGERSEN M, VESTERBY A. Child abuse and neglect in Denmark: medicolegal aspects. *Child Abuse and Neglect* 1984;**8**:83-91.

28. GREEN AH, GAINES RW, SANDRUND A. Child Abuse: pathological syndrome of family interaction. *Am J Psychiat* 1974;**131**:882-8.

29. LASKIN DM. The battered child syndrome. *J Oral Surg* 1973;**31**:903.

30. SOPHER IM. The dentist and the battered child syndrome. *Dent Clin North Am* 1977;**21**:113-22.

31. MACINTYRE DR, JONES GM, PINCKNEY RCN. The role of the dental practitioner in the management of non-accidental injury to children. *Br Dent J* 1986;**161**:108-10.

32. POLLOCK VE, BRIERE J, SCHNEIDER L, KNOP J, MEDNICK SA, GOODWIN DW. Childhood antecedents of antisocial behaviour: parental alcoholism and physical abusiveness. *Am J Psych* 1990;**147**:1290-3.

33. SCHMITT BD, KEMPE CH. Neglect and abuse of children. In: VAUGHAN VC, McKAY RJ, eds. *Nelson Textbook of Paediatrics* 10th edn, pp. 107-111. Philadelphia: WB Saunders 1975.

34. LASKIN DM. The recognition of child abuse. *J Oral Surg* 1978;**36**:349.

35. KITTLE PE, RICHARDSON DS, PARKER JW. Examining for child abuse and neglect. *Pediatric Dentistry* 1986;**8**:80-82.

36. SILVER LB, DUBLIN CC, LAURIE RS. Child abuse syndrome. The 'grey areas' in establishing a diagnosis. *Paediatrics* 1969;**44**:594-600.

37. SPEIGHT N. Non-Accidental Injury. In: MEADOW R, ed *The ABC of Child Abuse.* Br Med J London 1989.

38. CAMERON JM, JOHNSON HR, CAMPS FE. The battered child syndrome. *Med Sci Law* 1966;**6**:1-36.

39. SKINNER AE, CASTLE RL. *78 battered children: a retrospective study.* London - National Society for the Prevention of Cruelty to Children 1-21 1969.

40. BECKER DB, NEEDLEMAN HL, KOTELCHUCK M. Child abuse and dentistry; orofacial trauma and its recognition by dentists. *J Am Dent Assoc* 1978;**97**:24-28.

41. NEEDLEMAN HL. Orofacial trauma in child abuse: types, prevalence, management and the dental profession's involvement. *Pediatric Dentistry* 1986;**8**:71-79.

42. WILSON EF. Estimation of the age of cutaneous contusions in child abuse. *Pediatrics* 1977;**60**:750-2.

43. BERG VON S, EBEL R. Altersbestimmung subkutaner Blutungen. *Münchener Medizinische Wochenschrift* 1969;**21**:1185-90.

44. BERG VON SZ. Die Altersbestimmung von Hautverletzungen *Rechtsmedizin* 1972;**70**:121-35.

45. LENOSKI EF, HUNTER KA. Specific patterns of inflicted burn injuries. *J Trauma* 1977;**17**:842-46.

46. WAGNER GN. Bitemark identification in child abuse cases. *Paed Dentistry* 1986;**8**:96-100.

47. DINKEL EH. The use of bitemark evidence as an investigative aid. *J For Sci* 1974;**19**:535-47.

48. GAMMON JA. Ophthalmic manifestations of child abuse, In: ELLERSTEIN NS, ed. *Child Abuse and Neglect: A Medical Reference.* New York: John Wiley and Sons, 1981:121-39.

49. WARLOCK P, STOWER M, BARBOR P. Patterns of fractures in accidental and non-accidental injury in children: a comparative study. *Br Med J* 1986;**293**:100-2.

50. KABAN LB, MULLIKEN JB, MURRAY JE. Facial fractures in children. *Plast Reconstr Surg* 1977;**59**:15-20.

51. HAZELWOOD AI. Child abuse. The dentists role. *N.Y. State Dent J* 1970;**36**:289-91.

52. TATE RJ. Facial injuries associated with the battered child syndrome. *Br J Oral Surg* 1971;**9**:41-45.

53. BLUMBERG ML, KUNKEN FR. The dentists involvement with child abuse. *N.Y. State Dent J* 1981;**47**:65-69.

54. CROLL TP, MENNA VJ, EVANS CA. Primary identification of an abused child in the dental office: a case report. *Pediatric Dentistry* 1981;**3**:339-41.

55. KITTLE PE, RICHARDSON DS, PARKER JW. Two child abuse/child neglect examinations for the dentist. *ASDC J Dent Child* 1981;**48**:175-80.

56. WRIGHT JT, THORNTON JB. Osteogenesis imperfecta with dentinogenesis imperfecta: a mistaken case of child abuse. *Pediatric Dentistry* 1983;**5**:207-9.

57. SOBEL RS. Child abuse: a case report. *Pediatric Dentistry* 1986;**8**:93-95.

58. *North Tyneside Area Review Committee Information and Procedural Guidance for Child Abuse,* September 1987.

59. KIRSCHNER RH, STEIN RJ. The mistaken diagnosis of child abuse. *Am J Dis Child* 1985;**139**:873-5.

60. CHRISTOFFEL KK, ZIESERI EJ, CHIARAMONTE J. Should child abuse and neglect be considered when a child dies unexpectedly? *Am J Dis Child* 1985;**139**:876-80.

61. FONSECA MA, FEIGAL FJ, TEN BENSEL RW. Dental aspects of 1248 cases of child maltreatment on file at a major county hospital. *Pediatric Dentistry* 1992;**14**:152-7.

62. RASMUSSEN P. Tannlegens forhold til sykdom hos barn, barnemishandling og omsorgssvikt. *Odontologi '92.* Copenhagen: Munksgaard Publishers, 1992. pp. 81-92.

CHAPTER 5

Examination and Diagnosis of Dental Injuries

F. M. ANDREASEN & J. O. ANDREASEN

A dental injury should always be considered an emergency and be treated immediately to relieve pain, facilitate reduction of displaced teeth and improve prognosis.

Rational therapy depends upon a correct diagnosis, which can be achieved with the help of various examination techniques. While a dental injury can often present a complex picture, most injuries can be broken down into several smaller components. Information gained from the various examination procedures will assist the clinician in defining these trauma components and determining treatment priorities (1-18, 57-65, 97-107). It must be understood that an incomplete examination can lead to inaccurate diagnosis and less successful treatment (102). An excellent survey of examination procedures in children has been published by HALL (108) (1986).

An adequate history is essential to the examination and should include answers to the questions listed below. In order to save time, standardized charts are recommended (64) (See Appendices 1-4 p. 745-750 and Fig. 5.1). The recorded information is of value in insurance claims and for other medico-legal considerations.

Despite the importance of a systemic approach, which begins with an adequate medical and dental history, acute bleeding or respiratory problems and replantation of avulsed teeth will change this sequence.

The *pattern of injury* observed depends primarily upon factors such as (a) the en-

ergy of impact, (b) the direction and location of impact, and (c) the resilience of the periodontal structures.

Resilience of the periodontal structures appears to be the most significant factor in determining the *extent of injury*. Thus, impact in the very resilient skeleton supporting the primary dentition usually results in tooth displacement rather than fracture of hard tissues.

The opposite is true of injuries in the permanent dentition. Thus, with impact against the ground in an adult, either a *crown, crown-root* or *root fracture* may result, as the energy of impact will tend to produce a combination of zones of compression and tensile stress.

In the event that the lips intercept the initial blow, the energy delivered may be distributed over several teeth, resulting in *concussions, subluxations, lateral luxations* or *intrusions*.

If the course of impact is steeper and there is direct impact against the teeth, *crown fractures* can result. An indirect impact with the lips intervening may result in *extrusive luxation* with or without a *penetrating lip wound*.

In case of an axially directed impact against the chin, energy may be absorbed by the mandibular condyles or symphysis, and the premolars or molars of both dental arches. Such an impact can result in *fracture* or *luxation of the mandible* or *temporomandibular joint*, as well as *crown-* or *crown-root fractures* of the involved teeth. In the

UNIVERSITY HOSPITAL
(RIGSHOSPITALET)
Copenhagen

Diagram for dental and
maxillo-facial injuries

Name: Date:

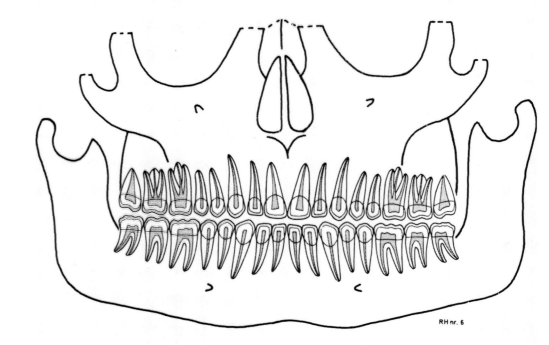

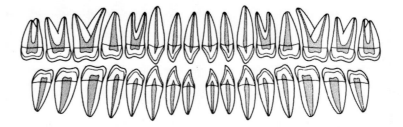

RH nr. 6

event of this type of impact, it should also be borne in mind that the axis of rotation of the head can be at the base of the skull. In these cases, *cerebral involvement* should also be considered. (See also under History).

The extent of the above-mentioned injuries will naturally be altered by the relative binding strength of the teeth to their supporting structures.

In conclusion, when examining a dental trauma, consider the following features with respect to determining the pattern of injury and the subsequent extent of injury:

1. The direction of impact (its relationship to the occlusal plane);

2. Possible lip involvement; and
3. Resilience of the periodontal structures.

In this regard, the patient's history will be valuable.

History

1. Patient's name, age, sex, address, and telephone number.
2. When did injury occur?
3. Where did injury occur?
4. How did injury occur?
5. Treatment elsewhere.
6. History of previous dental injuries.
7. General health.

Fig. 5.2.
Previous injury, primary dentition
This 4-year-old girl has suffered subluxation of her right central incisor. At the age of 1 year there was an injury affecting both central incisors resulting in pulp necrosis of the right central incisor and pulp canal obliteration of the left incisor.

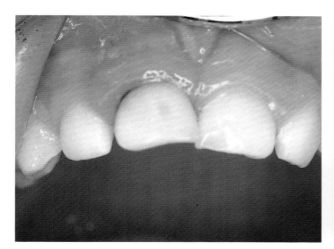
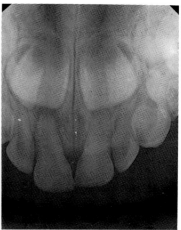

The implications of the answers to these questions are discussed separately:

Item 1. Apart from the obvious necessity of such information, the ability of the patient to provide the desired information might also provide clues to possible cerebral involvement or general mental status (e.g. inebriation) (see also Item 8).

Item 2. The time interval between the injury and treatment significantly influences the result of replantation of avulsed teeth (19). Furthermore, the result of treatment of luxated teeth (20), crown fractures with and without pulp exposures (21-23), as well as bone fractures, may be influenced by delay in treatment (24-25).

Item 3. The place of accident may indicate a need for of tetanus prophylaxis.

Item 4. As already indicated, the nature of the accident can yield valuable information on the type of injury to be expected, e.g. a blow to the chin will often cause fracture at the mandibular symphysis or condylar region as well as crown-root fractures in the premolar and molar regions. Accidents in which a child has fallen with an object in its mouth, e.g. a pacifier or toy, tend to cause dislocation of teeth in a labial direction.

In young children and women presenting multiple soft tissue injuries at different stages of healing, and where there is a marked discrepancy between the clinical findings and the past history, the battered child or battered wife syndromes should be considered (see Chapter 4, p. 181). In such cases the patient should be referred for a medical examination.

Item 5. Previous treatment, such as immobilization, reduction or replantation of teeth, should be considered before further treatment is instituted. It is also important to ascertain how the avulsed tooth was stored, e.g. tap water, sterilizing solutions, or dry.

Item 6. A number of patients may have sustained repeated injuries to their teeth. This can influence pulpal sensibility tests and the recuperative capacity of the pulp and/or periodontium (Fig. 5.2)

Item 7. A short medical history is essential for providing information about a number of disorders such as allergic reactions, epilepsy, or bleeding disorders, such as hemophilia (66-68). These conditions can

Fig. 5.3.

An 8-year-old boy with known hemophilia experiencing prolonged bleeding from the periodontal ligament around the left central incisor. The patient had suffered a subluxation injury 22 hours earlier. From BESSERMAN-NIELSEN (67) 1974.

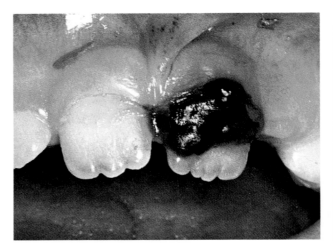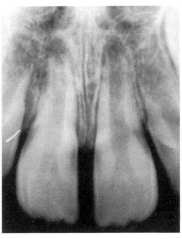

influence emergency as well as later treatment (Fig. 5.3).

The subjective complaints can provide the examiner with a clue to the injury. The following questions should be addressed.

8. Did the trauma cause amnesia, unconsciousness, drowsiness, vomiting, or headache?
9. Is there spontaneous pain from the teeth?
10. Do the teeth react to thermal changes, sweet or sour foods?
11. Are the teeth tender to touch, or during eating?
12. Is there any disturbance in the bite?

Item 8. Episodes of amnesia, unconsciousness, drowsiness, vomiting or headache indicate cerebral involvement. Amnesia can be disclosed by the patient's response to questions (e.g. Item 1), repetition of questions (e.g. "Where am I?", "What's happened?") and inability to recall events immediately before or after the accident. In such cases, the patient should immediately be referred for medical examination to establish priorities for further treatment (109). It should be noted, however, that most acute dental treatment (e.g. radiographic examination, repositioning of displaced teeth, application of fixation) can be performed at the patient's bedside. And, as previously mentioned, that early treatment will help to improve the long-term prognosis of dental injury.

Another type of trauma may occur in patients under general anesthesia who are slowly regaining consciousness. At a certain stage of recovery, strong masticatory muscle activity can take place with resultant clenching and biting which can lead to injury of the tongue, lips and teeth (108, 111, 112).

Item 9. Spontaneous pain can indicate damage to the tooth-supporting structures, e.g., hyperemia or extravasation of blood into the periodontal ligament. Damage to the pulp due to crown or crown-root fractures can also give rise to spontaneous pain.

Item 10. Reaction to thermal or other stimuli can indicate exposed dentin or pulp. This symptom is to some degree proportional to the area of exposure.

Items 11 and 12. If the tooth is painful during mastication or if the occlusion is disturbed, injuries such as extrusive or lateral luxation, alveolar or jaw fractures, or crown-root fractures should be suspected.

Clinical Examination

An adequate clinical examination depends upon a thorough examination of the entire injured area and the use of special examination techniques. The use of standardized examination charts can aid data registration (see Appendices 1-4 p. 745-750). These diagnostic procedures can be summarized as follows:

13. Recording of extraoral wounds and palpation of the facial skeleton.
14. Recording of injuries to oral mucosa or gingiva.

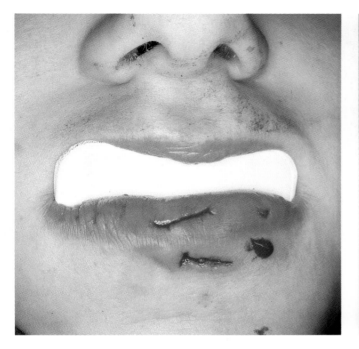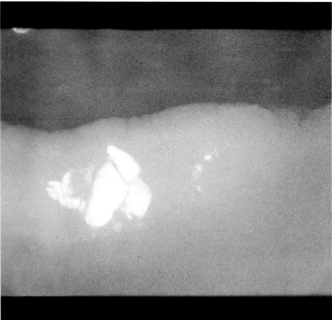

Fig. 5.4. Penetrating lip lesion
Two parallel lesions, either in the mucosa and skin or mucosa only, are an indication that teeth have penetrated tissue and that tooth fragments and other foreign bodies can be expected deep within the wound. A radiographic film is placed between the lips and the dental arch. The exposure time is 25% of the normal for a dental esposure.

15. Examination of crowns of teeth for the presence and extent of fractures, pulp exposures, or changes in color.
16. Recording of displacement of teeth (i.e. intrusion, extrusion, lateral displacement, or avulsion).
17. Disturbances in occlusion.
18. Abnormal mobility of teeth or alveolar fragments.
19. Palpation of the alveolar process.
20. Tenderness of teeth to percussion and change in percussion (ankylosis) tone.
21. Reaction of teeth to pulpal sensibility testing.

Item 13. Extraoral wounds are usually present in cases resulting from traffic accidents. The location of these wounds can indicate where and when dental injuries are to be suspected, e.g. a wound located under the chin suggests dental injuries in the premolar and molar regions and/or concomitant fracture of the mandibular condyle and/or symphysis. Palpation of the facial skeleton can disclose jaw fractures. Subcutaneous hematomas can also be an indication of fracture of the facial skeleton.

Item 14. Injuries of the oral mucosa or gingiva should be noted. Wounds penetrating the entire thickness of the lip can frequently be observed, often demarcated by two parallel wounds on the inner and/or outer labial surfaces (Fig. 5.4). If present, the possibility of tooth fragments buried between the lacerations should be considered (26, 27, 69-72). Such embedded fragments can cause acute or chronic infection and disfiguring fibrosis. The probable mechanism for these injuries is that the tooth, having penetrated the full thickness of the lip, is fractured as it emerges from the skin and strikes a hard object. The tooth fragment is retained within the soft tissue, which then envelops it at the moment of impact (26). These fragments can seldom be palpated, irrespective of size. Careful radiographic examination of the involved soft tissues is therefore necessary to disclose these fragments (Fig. 5.4). Along with tooth fragments, other foreign bodies can often be found within the soft tissue.

Gingival lacerations are often associated with displaced teeth. Bleeding from non-lacerated marginal gingiva indicates damage to the periodontal ligament .

Submucosal hematomas sublingually, in the vestibular region or in the palate can be indicative of a jaw fracture. Thorough radiographic examination, including examination of the border of the mandible and mobility of jaw segments en bloc, must accompany this finding, as a jaw

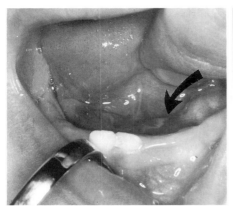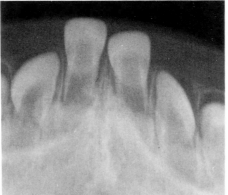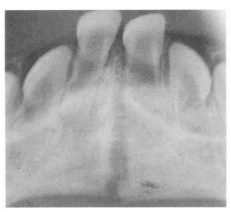

Fig. 5.5.
A 10-month old child referred for a luxated left primary central incisor. The clinical examination revealed slight loosening of the incisor and a sublingual hematoma (arrow). B. Radiographic examination of the involved incisors revealed no sign of jaw fracture. C. Because of the finding of a sublingual hematoma, a new radiograph including the border of the mandible was taken. This radiograph clearly demonstrated fracture of the symphysis.

fracture could otherwise be overlooked (Fig. 5.5).

Finally, it is essential that blood covering the alveolar process be removed, as this can sometimes reveal displacement of the mucoperiosteum into the buccal sulcus. Typically these patients demonstrate severe edema of the upper lip and sharp pain upon palpation of the exposed periosteal surface (108).

Item 15. Before examining traumatized teeth, the crowns should be cleaned of blood and debris.

Infraction lines in the enamel can be visualized by directing a light beam parallel to the long axis of the tooth or by shadowing the light beam with a finger or mouth mirror (see Chapter 6, p.220). When examining crown fractures, it is important to note whether the fracture is confined to enamel or includes dentin. The fracture surface should be carefully examined for pulp exposures; if present, the size and location should be recorded. In some cases, the dentin layer may be so thin that the outline of the pulp can be seen as a pinkish tinge beneath dentin. One should take care not to perforate the thin dentinal layer during the examination.

Crown-root fractures in the molar and premolar regions should be expected in the case of indirect trauma (see Chapter 7, p. 257). It is important to remember that crown-root fractures in one quadrant are very often accompanied by similar fractures on the same side of the opposing

jaw. It is therefore necessary to examine occlusal fissures of all molars and premolars to confirm the presence or absence of possible fractures.

Depending on the stage of eruption, fractures below the gingival margin can involve the crown alone or the cervical third of the root.

Color of the traumatized tooth should be noted, as changes can occur in the post-injury period. These color changes are most often prominent on the oral aspect of the crown at the cingulum. Moreover, examination with transillumination can reveal changes in translucency (see Chapter 9, p. 356).

Item 16. Displacement of teeth is usually evident by visual examination; however, minor abnormalities can often be difficult to detect. In such cases, it is helpful to examine the occlusion as well as radiographs taken at various angulations (see p.210).

The possibility of inhaling or swallowing teeth at the time of injury should always be considered when teeth or prosthetic appliances are missing and their presence elsewhere cannot be established (73-76).

Although inhalation of foreign bodies in connection with traumatic injuries is normally associated with a loss of protective reflexes in an unconscious patient, it may also occur in a conscious patient without producing symptoms (76). Consequently, if there is reason to suspect inhalation or swallowing of a tooth or dental appliance, it is important that radiographs of the

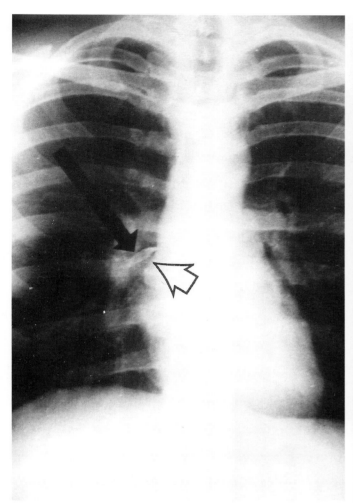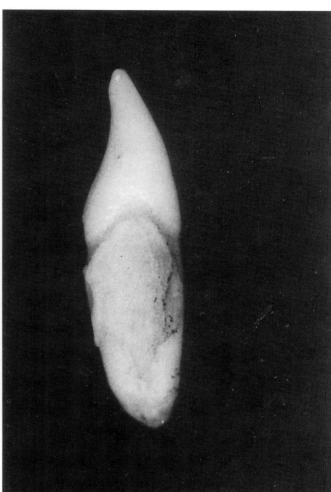

Fig. 5.6
A. Posteroanterior radiograph of chest showing foreign body in right middle lobe intermediate bronchus after maxillofacial injury. B. Tooth recovered from right lung via bronchoscopy.
From GILLILAND ET AL. (76) *1972.*

chest and the abdomen be taken as soon as possible (Fig. 5.6).

In case of tooth luxation, the direction of the dislocation as well as extent (in mm) should be recorded. In the primary dentition, it is of utmost importance to diagnose oral dislocation of the apex of a displaced primary tooth, as it can impinge upon the permanent successor.

It is important to remember that, apart from displacement and interference with occlusion, laterally luxated and intruded teeth present very few clinical symptoms. Moreover, these teeth are normally firmly locked in their displaced position and do not usually demonstrate tenderness to percussion. While radiographs can be of assistance, diagnosis is confirmed by the percussion tone (see Chapter 9, p. 321).

Item 17. Abnormalities in occlusion can indicate fractures of the jaw or alveolar process. In the former case, abnormal mobility of the jaw fragments can be demonstrated.

Item 18. All teeth should be tested for abnormal mobility, both horizontally and axially. Disruption of the vascular supply to the pulp should be expected in case of axial mobility.

It should be remembered that erupting teeth and primary teeth undergoing physiologic root resorption always exhibit some mobility.

The typical sign of alveolar fracture is movement of adjacent teeth when the mobility of a single tooth is tested.

In case of root fracture, location of the fracture determines the degree of tooth mobility. However, without radiographic examination, it is usually not possible to discriminate between luxation injuries and root fractures.

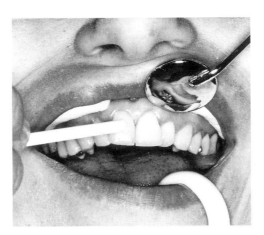

Fig. 5.7.
Pulp testing with heated gutta percha. The stick of guttapercha is applied to the middle third of the facial surface.

Item 19. Uneven contours of the alveolar process usually indicate a bony fracture. Moreover, the direction of the dislocation can sometimes be determined by palpation.

Item 20. Reaction to percussion is indicative of damage to the periodontal ligament (77). The test may be performed by tapping the tooth lightly with the handle of a mouth mirror, in a vertical as well as horizontal direction. Injuries to the periodontal ligament will result in pain. As with all examination techniques used at the time of injury, the percussion test should be begun on a non-injured tooth to assure a reliable patient response. In smaller children, the use of a fingertip can be a gentler

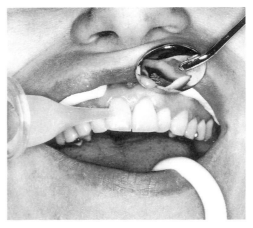

Fig. 5.8.
Pulp testing with ice. A cone of ice is applied to the middle third of the facial surface of the tooth: 5 to 8 seconds may be required to elicit a reaction.

diagnostic tool. In infants, this is neither possible nor reliable.

Recently, a calibrated percussion instrument has been introduced Periotest ® (112, 113). However, the force imparted by such an instrument might contribute to a new trauma, as in the case of root fractures.

The sound elicited by percussion is also of diagnostic value. Thus, a hard, metallic ring elicited by percussion in a horizontal direction indicates that the tooth is locked into bone; while a dull sound indicates subluxation or extrusive luxation. However, it should be noted that teeth with apical and marginal periodontal lesions can also give a dull percussion sound (77).

Item 21. Pulp testing following traumatic injuries is a controversial issue. These procedures require cooperation and a relaxed patient, in order to avoid false reactions. However, this is often not possible during initial treatment of injured patients, especially children.

Pulpal sensibility testing at the time of injury is important for establishing a point of reference for evaluating pulpal status at later follow-up examinations. A number of tests have been proposed. However, the value of these has recently been questioned (28-30, 114, 116). The principle of the tests involves transmitting stimuli to the sensory receptors of the dental pulp and registering the reaction.

Mechanical Stimulation

In crown fractures with exposed dentin pulpal sensibility can be tested by scraping with a dental probe. Some authors have proposed drilling a test cavity in the tooth in order to register the pain reaction when the bur advances into the dentin. However, in a study on sensibility reactions of replanted teeth, it was found that a pain reaction was not noted until the dentin-pulp border was reached (31).

In the case of crown fractures with exposed pulp tissue, the reaction of the pulp to mechanical stimuli can be tested by applying a pledget of cotton soaked in saline. Exploration with a dental probe must not be attempted as it may provoke severe pain and inflict additional injury to the pulp.

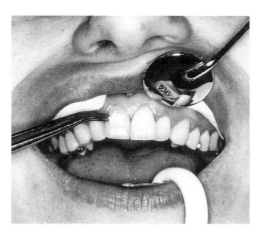

Fig. 5.9.
Pulp testing with ethyl chloride. A pledget of cotton is saturated with ethyl chloride and applied to the middle third of the facial surface.

Thermal Tests

Thermal stimulation of teeth has been used for many years and various methods have been advocated. Among these, the most frequently used are heated gutta percha, ethyl chloride, ice, carbon dioxide snow, and dichlor-difluormethane.

Thermal pulp testing results are not reproducible in terms of graded intensity, and normal pulp tissue may yield a negative response (29, 79). A positive reaction usually indicates a vital pulp, but it may also occur in a non-vital pulp, especially in cases of gangrene when heat produces thermal expansion of fluids in the pulp space, which in turn presumably exerts pressure on inflamed periodontal tissues (38).

HEATED GUTTA PERCHA
The following standardization has been advocated by MUMFORD (29). A stick of gutta percha is heated by holding about 5 millimeters of its length in a flame for 2 seconds, whereupon it is applied to the tooth on the middle third of the facial surface (Fig. 5.7). The value of this test has been questioned, as the intensity of sensation reported by the patient is not reproducible, and even non-injured teeth may fail to respond (29, 79).

ICE
This method involves the application of a cone of ice to the facial surface of the tooth (Fig. 5.8). Reaction depends on the duration of application; a period of 5 to 8 seconds increases the sensitivity of this test (33). The reliability of this procedure has also been questioned as non-injured teeth may not respond (32, 33, 78).

ETHYL CHLORIDE
Ethyl chloride can be applied by soaking a cotton pledget and then placing it on the facial surface of the tooth to be tested (Fig. 5.9) (CAUTION! flammable). The limitations described for heated gutta percha also apply to this method, although ethyl chloride gives more consistent results (29, 80, 81).

CARBON DIOXIDE SNOW
Because of its low temperature (-78°C, -108°F), carbon dioxide snow gives very consistent and reliable results, even in immature teeth (34-37, 78, 79, 82, 83) (Fig. 5.10). This method also allows pulp testing in cases where an injured tooth is completely covered with a temporary crown or splint (32, 82) (Fig. 5.10). However, a serious

Fig. 5.10.
Pulp testing with carbon dioxide snow. A. Disassembled model of a carbon dioxide snow pulp tester (Odontotest®, Fricar A. G., Zürich 1, Switzerland). B. Pulp testing with carbon dioxide snow of a fractured incisor covered with a stainless steel crown.

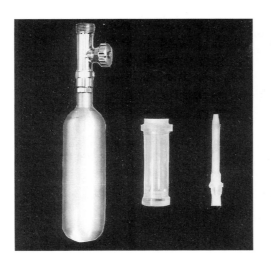

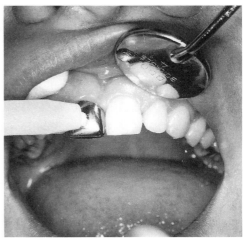

Fig. 5.11.
Scanning electron microscope view of the enamel surface before (A) and after (B) pulp testing with carbon dioxide snow. It is apparent that an infraction line has developed after testing (arrows). x 1200 From BACHMANN & LUTZ (85) 1976.

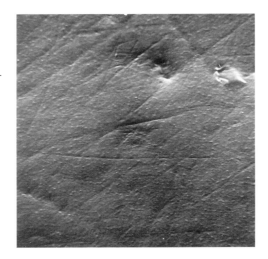 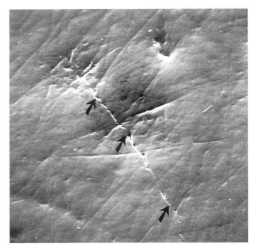

drawback to this procedure is that the very low temperature of the carbon dioxide snow can result in new infraction lines in the enamel (84, 85) (Fig. 5.11), although this finding has not been substantiated in later studies (116, 118). Furthermore, no changes could be found in the pulp in animal experiments (119). Only prolonged exposure to very low temperatures (i.e. -80°C for 1 to 3 minutes) has been shown to elicit transient pulpal changes (secondary dentin formation) (120).

DICHLOR-DIFLUORMETHANE

This is another cold test (e.g., Frigen[®] 109, Provotest[®]109) in which an aerosol is released at a temperature of -28°C, -18°F, onto the enamel surface (85, 86, 87, 109). Like carbon dioxide snow, it elicits a very reliable and consistent response from both mature and immature teeth (88). However, the same drawback has been recorded with this test as with carbon dioxide snow, although to a lesser degree; namely, infraction lines in the enamel caused by the thermal shock (85).

Electrometric Tests

ELECTRIC PULPTESTERS

Electric pulp testing should employ a current measurement instrument that allows control of the mode, duration, frequency, and direction of the stimulus (38, 121). Voltage measurement is not satisfactory because a given voltage produces varying currents as a result of differences in the electrical resistance of the tissues, espe-

cially enamel. Such variations can result from fissures, caries, and restorations (39). Experimental studies have shown that the current is presumably carried ionically through the electrolytes of the tooth (40, 41).

The stimulus should be clearly defined, as it significantly affects nerve excitation (42). Furthermore, the electrode area should be as large as the tooth shape will permit, allowing maximum stimulation (39, 43, 122). A stimulus duration of 10 milliseconds or more has been advocated (43). Recently, a digital pulp tester has been introduced which appears to produce very reliable readings (123).

Electrical sensibility testing is usually carried out in the following way (Fig. 5.12).

1. The patient is informed as to the purpose and nature of the test and is instructed to indicate when a sensation is first experienced.

2. The tooth surface is isolated with cotton rolls and air-dried. Saliva on the tooth surface can divert the current to the gingiva and periodontal tissue, giving false readings. However, the tooth should not be desiccated for long periods, as enamel can lose moisture with a resultant increase in electrical resistance (44, 45). Several media such as saline and toothpaste can be used as conductor between electrode and tooth surface (146).

3. The electrode is placed as far from the gingiva as possible, preferably on a fracture area or the incisal edge, where the strongest response can be obtained (78, 124, 125). The neutral electrode can

CHAPTER 5

Fig. 5.12.
Electrometric pulp testing. The tooth is air-dried and isolated with cotton rolls. A. and B. The electrode is placed on the incisal edge or on the incisal third of the facial surface of the crown.

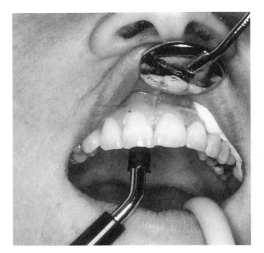 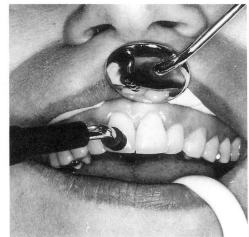

be held by the patient. A modification of this system involves the examiner completing the circuit by touching the patient's mouth with a finger or a mouth mirror. A metal dental instrument (e.g. dental explorer) can also serve as an electric conductor to the tooth (126).

The use of rubber gloves presents a clinical problem, as the correct use of the pulp tester requires that the dentist completes the electrical circuit by direct physical contact with the patient. One study has indicated that this problem can be overcome if the patient grasps the end of the pulp tester after it is positioned on the tooth (128); however, other studies suggest that such a procedure can produce unreliable results (129, 130). Recently, a clip to the lip has been developed which permits the dentist to conduct a test wearing rubber gloves (131).

4. The rheostat of the tester is advanced continuously until the patient reacts. If the current is then maintained at the existing level, adaptation occurs and the patient feels that the pain has disappeared, so that a further increase of current gives a higher threshold value. This phenomenon implies that the pain threshold cannot be regarded as constant (43). The threshold value should therefore be determined by a quick rather than a slow increase in current. However, the current should not be increased so quickly that it is painful. The value of the pain threshold of the tooth should be recorded for later comparison.

5. Splints and temporary crowns used in the treatment of traumatic dental injuries can alter the response to both thermal and electrometrical tests (79). Thus, contact between the gingiva and a stainless steel crown, a metal cap splint or arch bar significantly increases the pain threshold, as the current bypasses the tooth and is conducted to the gingiva or adjacent teeth (79). In order to obtain a reliable sensibility response to electrometric pulp testing, the electrode must be placed upon enamel and the tooth isolated from adjacent vital teeth (Fig. 5.13). A distance of at least 1 millimeter between the electrode and metal is recommended. If the temporary crown or splint cannot be altered in the above-mentioned manner, thermal pulp testing with carbon dioxide snow is a reliable alternative (79) (Fig. 5.13).

The value and reliability of electrometric pulp testing have been evaluated by comparison of the pain threshold with the histologic condition of the pulp (30, 46, 89-92). Apparently, there is not always a direct relationship; thus teeth which fail to respond to stimulation with maximum current can show a histologically normal pulp, while inflamed or even necrotic pulps can respond electrometrically within the normal range. A common belief has been that low readings indicate hyperemia or acute pulpitis while high readings indicate chronic pulpitis or degenerative changes. However, recent investigations do not support this view (30, 47).

The interpretation of pulpal sensibility

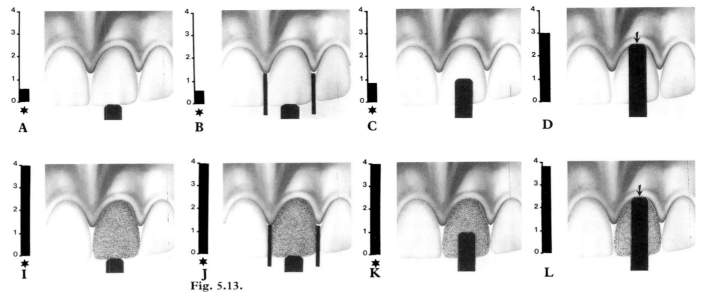

Fig. 5.13.

Influence of splints and temporary crowns upon electric pulp testing procedures. The schematic drawings illustrate the reactions recorded with a Siemens pulp tester (Sirotest II®) which has a scale from 0 to 4. The columns next to the drawing of the teeth indicate the average reaction to the specific testing circumstances. A to H illustrate testing of a vital tooth and I to P illustrate testing of a tooth with pulp necrosis. A. Electrode placed upon the incisal edge. B. Tooth isolated with an acetate strip. C. Electrode placed upon the middle third of the labial surface. D. Electrode contacting gingiva. E. Electrode contacting an open-faced steel crown. F. Electrode placed upon enamel on a tooth with an open-faced steel crown. G. Electrode placed upon the incisal edge of a tooth splinted with a metal arch bar. H. Electrode placed upon the metal arch bar. I. Electrode placed upon the incisal edge of a tooth with pulp necrosis. J. Tooth isolated with acetate strips. K. Electrode placed upon the middle third of the labial surface. L. Electrode contacting gingiva. M. Electrode contacting an open-faced steel crown, the current is passed on to the gingiva, giving a weak response. N. Electrode placed upon enamel on a tooth with an open-faced steel crown. The current is passed on to the adjacent teeth. O. Electrode placed upon the incisal edge of a tooth splinted with a metal arch bar. Current is passed on to neighboring vital teeth. P. Electrode placed upon the metal arch bar. The current is passed on to neighboring vital teeth. NOTE: all testing situations revealing a reliable response are indicated with an asterisk. From FULLING & ANDREASEN (79) 1976.

tests performed immediately after traumatic injuries is complicated by the fact that sensitivity responses can be temporarily or permanently decreased, especially after luxation injuries (132-135). However, repeated testing has shown that normal reactions can return after a few weeks or months (1, 32, 48-51, 81, 93, 133-135). Moreover, teeth which have been loosened can elicit pain responses merely from pressure of the pulp testing instrument. It is therefore important to reposition and immobilize, e.g., root-fractured or extruded incisors prior to pulp testing. If local anesthetics are to be administered for various treatment procedures, pulp testing should be performed prior to doing this.

Another factor to consider is the stage of eruption. Teeth react differently at various stages, sometimes showing no reaction at all when root formation is not complete (52-54, 78, 94, 95). However, the excitation threshold is gradually lowered to the normal range as maturation proceeds, although it increases again in adulthood when the pulp canal becomes partly obliterated (136, 137) (Fig. 5.14). One explanation could be incomplete communication between odontoblastic processes and nerve fibers in immature teeth (55). However, this has been questioned in a recent study where numerous myelinated nerve fibers were found in the coronal odontoblast layer irrespective of stage of development (138). Moreover, it is often difficult to isolate partially erupted teeth and the current may circumvent the tooth, passing directly to the gingiva (56).

Finally, teeth undergoing orthodontic movement display higher excitation thresholds (96).

Laser Doppler Flowmetry

Recently, a new method has been developed whereby a laser beam can be directed at the coronal aspect of the pulp. The reflected light scattered by moving blood cells undergoes a Doppler frequency shift. The fraction of light scat-

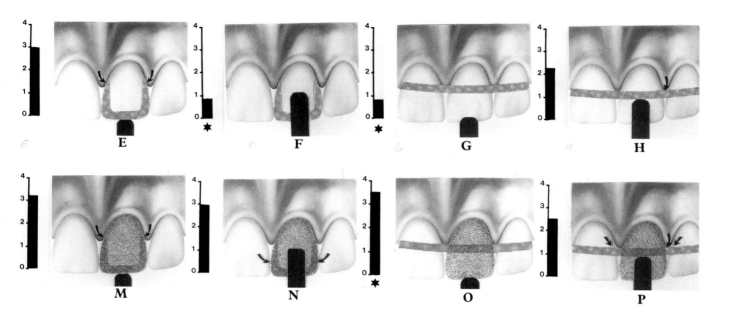

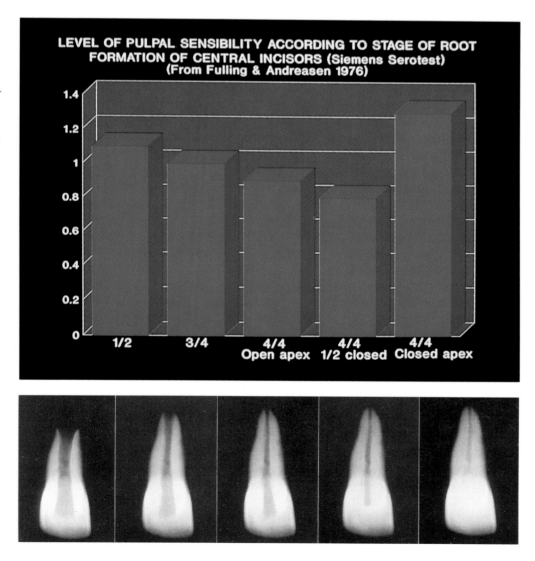

Fig. 5.14.
Variation in sensibility level according to stage of root development of permanent incisors. The diagram illustrates the reactions recorded with a Siemens pulp tester (Sirotest II® which has a scale from 0 to 4). It appears that early and late stages of root development are related to higher sensibility levels. From FULLING & ANDREASEN (78) 1976.

Fig. 5.15.
Pulp testing using a laser Doppler flowmeter. The probe is placed on the labial surface of the tooth.

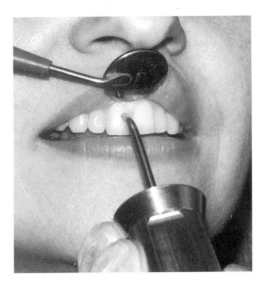
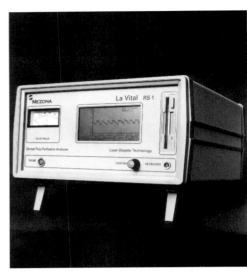

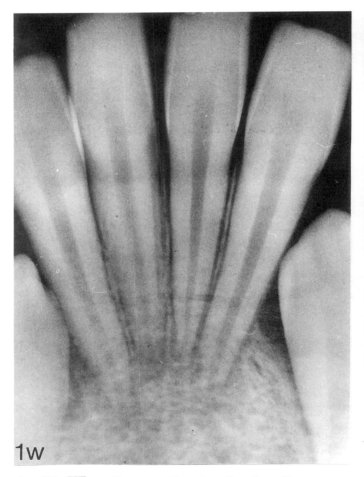
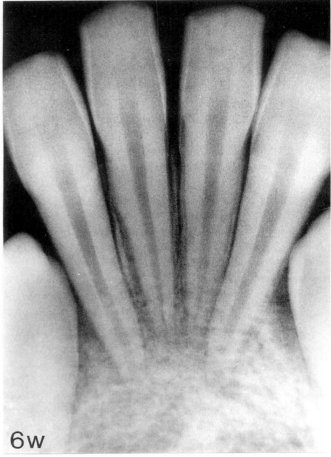

LDF 0.4 0.5 0.3 0.4   2.2 2.5 2.2 2.3

Sens —   —   —   —   —   —   —   —

Fig. 5.17.
Follow-up of 4 luxated incisors at 1 and 6 weeks, 9 and 12 months. LDF represents laser Doppler flow values and Sens *electrometric settings (Analytic Technology® pulp tester) at which sensory responses were obtained in each tooth. - indicates absence of sensory response at highest stimulus level. From GAZELIUS ET AL. (139) 1988.*

Fig. 5.16.
Laser Doppler flowmetry (LDF) recording from a non-vital tooth (A) and adjacent normal (control) tooth (B). Chart speed 600 mm/min. From GAZELIUS ET AL. (139) 1988.

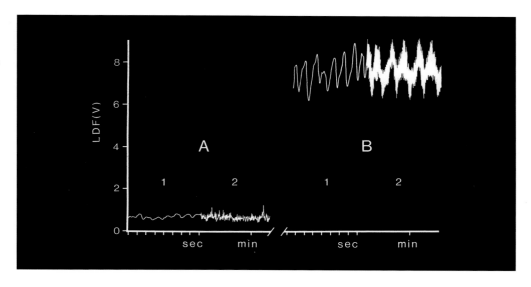

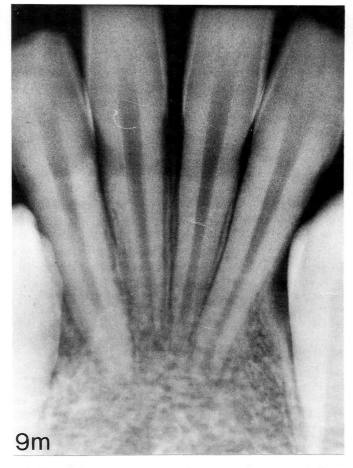

9m

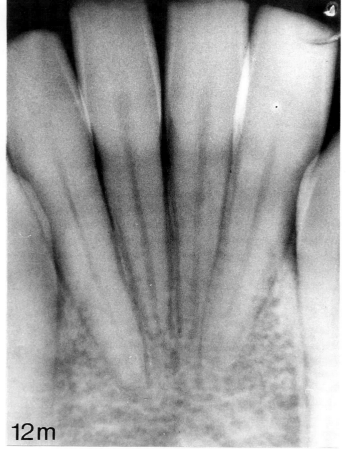

12m

LDF 5.5 5.0 5.3 6.5   3.0 3.1 4.0 2.5
Sens 65 69 77 42   48 61 55 38

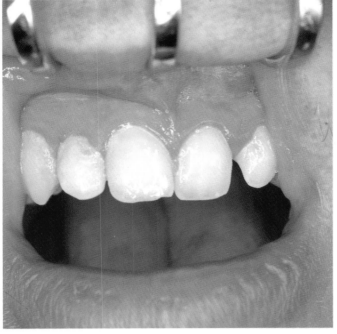
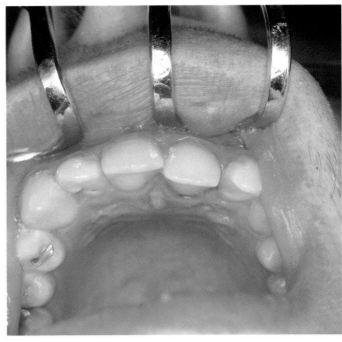

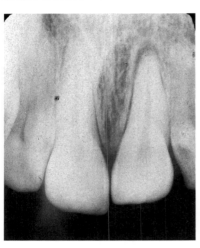
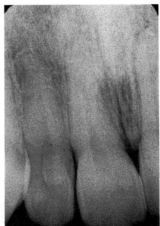
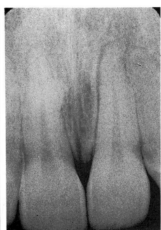
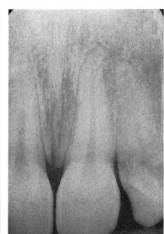

Fig. 5.18

A and B. Clinical examination reveals displacement of a left central incisor. C. to F. The radiographic examination of the anterior region consists of one occlusal film (C) and three periapical exposures, where the central beam is directed between the lateral and central incisors (D) and (F) and between the central incisors (E). Note that the displacement of the left central incisor is clearly shown on the occlusal exposure (C), whereas an apical exposure (E) shows hardly any displacement.

tered back from the pulp is detected and processed to yield a signal (Fig. 5.15). The value of this method has been demonstrated in two clinical studies where it was possible to diagnose the state of pulp revascularization before the traditional electrometric pulp sensitivity testing (139, 140).

In a recent clinical study it was found that in traumatized incisors which showed no electrometric sensibility reactions and where laser Doppler flowmetry (LDF) indicated no pulp vitality the reliability of LDF was 97%. Conversely in electrometric non-sensible teeth, where LDF showed the presence of blood perfusion, the accuracy of LDF in regard to pulp vitality was 100% (147).

Several problems must be solved before this method can be of general use. First it

has been found that blood pigment within a discolored tooth crown can interfere with laser light transmission (145). Second, the equipment necessary for this procedure needs further refinement before it can be of general clinical value. Thirdly the price of the equipment must be considerable lower than it is presently.

RADIOGRAPHIC EXAMINATION

All injured teeth should be examined radiographically. This examination serves two purposes: (1) it reveals the stage of root formation and (2) it discloses injuries affecting the root portion of the tooth and the periodontal structures. Most root fractures are disclosed by radiographic examination, as the fracture line usually runs

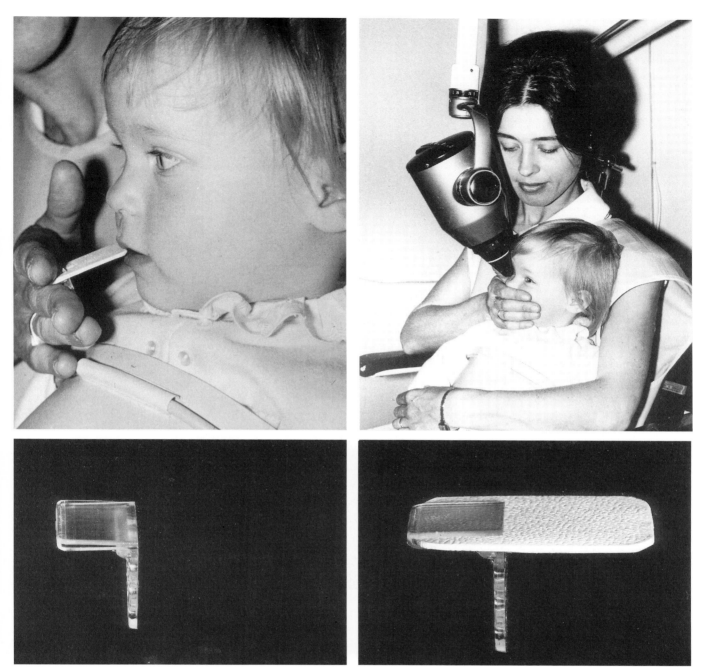

Fig. 5.19.
Radiographic examination of infants. A special film holder is used in combination with a standard dental film (3.8x5.1 cm) (Twix film holder®, A/B Svenska Dental Instrument, Stockholm, Sweden). The film holder is held between two fingers and the film placed between the dental arches. The mother holds the infant in position with her left arm while steadying the child's head with her right hand. The projection angle should be more vertical than normal in order not to have the index finger projected onto the film. Note that both mother and child are protected by lead aprons.

parallel to the central beam (102, 141) (see Chapter 8, p. 282).

The clinical diagnosis of tooth displacement is corroborated radiographically. There is a widening of the periodontal space in lateral and extrusive luxations, whereas intruded teeth often demonstrate a blurred periodontal space. However, determination of dislocation on the basis of radiographs is highly dependent on the angle of the central beam (20, 102). Radiographic demonstration of dislocation of permanent teeth normally requires the use of more than one exposure at differing angulations. The ideal method is the use of 3 different angulations for each traumatized tooth, using a standardized projection technique (102). Thus, a trau-

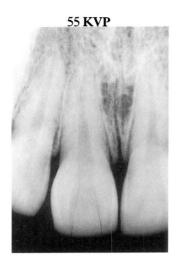 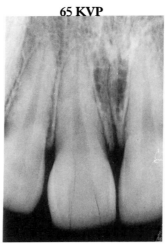 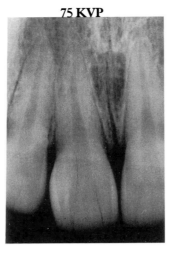 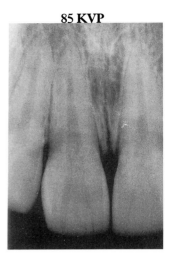

55 KVP **65 KVP** **75 KVP** **85 KVP**

Fig. 5.20.
An increase in KVP slightly reduces the contrast. The right central incisor in a skull was radiographed using ranges from 55-85 KVP. The infraction line in the crown which are clearly shown at 55 KVP are not so prominent at 85 KVP.

matized anterior region is covered by one occlusal film and 3 periapical exposures, where the central beam is directed between the lateral and central incisors and the two central incisors. This procedure ensures diagnosis of even minor dislocations or root fractures (Fig. 5.18). In this context, it is important to bear in mind that a steep occlusal exposure is of special value in the diagnosis of root fractures and lateral luxations with oral displacement of the crown (102, 141)(see Chapter 8, p. 282 and Chapter 9, p. 319).

Children under 2 years of age are often difficult to examine radiographically because of fear or lack of cooperation. With the parents' help and the use of special film holders, it is usually possible to obtain a radiograph of the traumatized area (Fig. 5.19). It should also be noted that exposure time can be reduced by 30% for each 10 KVP increase (Fig. 5.20). In this way, radiographs of diagnostic quality can be taken even with uncooperative patients.

Extraoral radiographs are of value in determining the direction of dislocation of intruded primary incisors (Fig. 5.21 and Chapter 9, p. 322). Bone fractures are usually discernible on intraoral radiographs unless the fracture is confined to the facial or lingual bone plate. If jaw fractures are suspected, extraoral radiographs should always be taken.

Dislocated tooth fragments within a lip laceration can be demonstrated radiographically by the use of an ordinary film placed between the dental arches and the lips (Fig. 5.4). A short exposure time (i.e. one-quarter to one-half normal exposure time) or the use of low kilovoltage is advocated for these exposures.

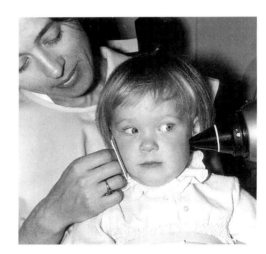

Fig. 5.21.
Extraoral lateral projection used to determine the position of displaced anterior teeth. The central beam is directed against the apical area and is parallel to the occlusal plane. A 6 x 7.5 cm film is held against the cheek perpendicular to the central beam.

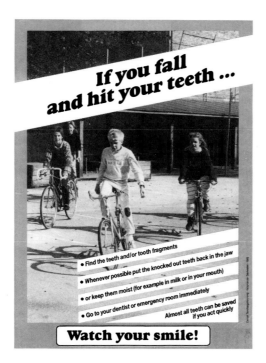

If you fall and hit your teeth ...

- Find the teeth and/or tooth fragments
- Whenever possible put the knocked out teeth back in the jaw
- or keep them moist (for example in milk or in your mouth)
- Go to your dentist or emergency room immediately

Almost all teeth can be saved if you act quickly

Watch your smile!

Fig. 5.22.
Example of a trauma campaign brochure.

All radiographs should be stored carefully as they provide a record for comparison at future controls.

Conducting a Trauma Propaganda Campaign

Investigations into the long-term prognosis of replanted permanent incisors have demonstrated that it is not the dentist, but those persons closest to the scene of the accident who play the most important role in improving the chances of successful healing following dental injury (142, 143).

Immediate replantation or extraoral storage in a physiological medium are essential for minimizing the risk of periodontal healing complications, as well as for improving the chances of pulpal revascularization in avulsed immature teeth. Information campaigns aimed at educating lay people on correct dental first-aid have been carried out in many countries, including Denmark, Australia, Brazil, Argentina and the USA (144) (Fig. 5.22)

The goals of such an information campaign should include:

- To raise public awareness concerning the active role non-professionals play in ensuring successful treatment of the acute dental injury

- To emphasize the need for cooperation between the public sector (e.g. emergency dental service) and private dental care

- To empasize the need for adequate emergency treatment if not already available (e.g. possibly a rotation among private practitioners during holiday periods to provide the necessary service)

The goals can be achieved via posters placed in strategic locations (e.g. sports' clubs, ambulance services, with the school physicians/nurses), via television spots and via radio. In Denmark, for example, when the reattachment of crown fragments with a dentin bonding agent was found to be a realistic treatment alternative, a spot on evening television news resulted in an enthusiastic public response, with patients retrieving tooth fragments for bonding (see Chapter 6, p. 230). Similar results can also be achieved with other injury groups if the population is well informed.

Essentials

History

Patient's name, age, sex, address, and telephone number
  When did the accident occur?
  Where did the accident occur?
  How did the accident occur?

Treatment elsewhere
History of previous dental injuries general health

Did the trauma cause amnesia, unconsciousness, drowsiness, vomiting, or headache?
Is there spontaneous pain from the teeth?

Do the teeth react to thermal changes, sweet or sour foods?

Are the teeth painful to touch or during eating?

Is there any disturbance in the bite?

Clinical Examination

Recording of extraoral wounds and palpation of the facial skeleton
Recording of injuries to oral mucosa or gingiva
Examination of the tooth crowns for the presence and extent of fractures, pulp exposures, or changes in color
Recording of displacement of teeth (i.e. intrusion, extrusion, lateral displacement, or avulsion)
Abnormalities in occlusion
Abnormal mobility of teeth or alveolar fragments
Palpation of the alveolar process
Reaction of teeth to percussion

Reaction of Teeth to Sensibility Tests

  a. Mechanical stimulation
  b. Heated gutta percha (Fig. 5.7)
  c. Ice (Fig. 5.8)
  d. Ethyl chloride (Fig. 5.9)
  e. Carbon dioxide snow (Fig. 5.10)
  f. Dichlor-difluormethane
  g. Electric vitalometers (Fig. 5.12 and 5.13)
  h. Laser Doppler flowmetry (Fig. 5.15)

Radiographic Examination

Intraoral radiographs (Figs. 5.18 and 5.19)
Extraoral radiographs (Fig. 5.21)

Bibliography

1. GAARE A, HAGEN AR, KANSTAD S. Tannfrakturer hos barn. Diagnostiske og prognostiske problemer og behandling. *Norske Tannlægeforenings Tidende* 1958;**68**:364-78.

2. MALONE AJ, MASSLER M. Fractured anterior teeth. Diagnosis, treatment, and prognosis. *Dent Dig* 1952;**58**:442-7.

3. ELLIS RG. Treatment of fractured incisors. *Int Dent J* 1953;**4**:196-208.

4. COOKE C, ROWBOTHAM TC. Treatment of injuries to anterior teeth. *Br Dent J* 1951;**91**:146-52.

5. CURRY VL. Fractured incisors. Dent Practit Dent Rec 1951;1:341-6.

6. DOUNIAU R. Traumatismes dentaires accidentels. *J Dent Belge* 1960;**5**:603-15.

7. RIPA LW, FINN SB. The care of injuries to the anterior teeth in children. In: FINN SB, ed. *Clinical Pedodontics.* Philadelphia London: W B Saunders Company, 1967:324-62.

8. SUNDVALL - HAGLAND I. Olycksfallsskador på tänder och parodontium under barnaåren. In: HOLST JJ, NYGAARD ØSTBY B, OSVALD O, eds. *Nordisk Klinisk Odontologi.* Copenhagen: A/S Forlaget for Faglitteratur, 1964:Chapter 11, III, 1-40.

9. RAVN JJ. *Ulykkesskadede fortænder på børn. Klassifikation og behandling.* Odontologisk Forening, Copenhagen 1966.

10. INGLE JI, FRANK AL, NATKIN E, NUTTING EE. Diagnosis and treatment of traumatic injuries and their sequelae. In: INGLE JI, BEVERIDGE EE, eds. *Endodontics.* 2nd edn. Philadelphia: Lea & Febiger, 1976:685-711.

11. ANDREWS RG. Emergency treatment of injured permanent anterior teeth. *Dent Clin North Am* 1965;**11**:703-10.

12. DOWN CH. The treatment of permanent incisor teeth of children following traumatic injury. *Aust Dent J* 1957;**2**:9-24.

13. KISLING E. Om behandlingen af skader som følge af akutte mekaniske traumer på unge permanente incisiver. *Tandlægebladet* 1953;**57**:61-9, 109-29.

14. KISLING E. Beskadigelser af tænder og deres ophængningsapparat ved akutte mekaniske traumata. In: TOVERUD G, ed. *Nordisk lærebog i Pedodonti.* Stockholm: Sveriges Tandläkarförbunds Förlagsförening, 1963:266-87.

15. WILBUR HM. Management of injured teeth. *J Am Dent Assoc* 1952;**44**:1-9.

16. BROWN WE. The management of injuries to young teeth. *J Dent Assoc South Afr* 1963;**18**:247-51.

17. OHLSSON Å. Behandling av olyckkesfallsskadade incisiver på barn. *Odontologisk Tidskrift* 1957;**65**:105-15.

18. ESCHLER J. Die traumatischen Verletzungen der Frontzähne bei Jugendlichen. Heidelberg: Alfred Hüthig Verlag, 1966.

19. ANDREASEN JO. Luxation of permanent teeth due to trauma. *Scand J Dent Res* 1970;**78**:273-86.

20. ANDREASEN JO. Luxation of permanent teeth due to trauma A clinical and radiographic follow-up study of 189 injured teeth. *Scand J Dent Res* 1970;**78**:273-86.

21. FIALOVÁ S, JURECEK B. Úrazy zubu u deti a naše zkušenosti s jejich lécením. *Prakt Zubni Lék* 1968;**16**:171-6.

22. ROZKOVCOVÁ E, KOMINEK J. Zhodnoceni vitálni amputace pri osetrováni úrazu stálych zubu udeti. Cs. *Stomatol* 1959;**59**:30-5.

23. HALLET GEM, PORTEOUS JR. Fractured incisors treated by vital pulpotomy. A report on 100 consecutive cases. *Br Dent J* 1963;**115**:279-87.

24. ANDREASEN JO. Fractures of the alveolar process of the jaw. A clinical and radiographic follow-up study. *Scand J Dent Res* 1970;**78**:263-72.

25. ROED - PETERSEN B, ANDREASEN JO. Prognosis of permanent teeth involved in jaw fractures. A clinical and radiographic follow-up study. *Scand J Dent Res* 1970;**78**:343-52.

26. ALLEN FJ. Incisor fragments in the lips. *Dent Practit Dent Rec* 1960-61;**11**:390-1.

27. JACOWSKI & COLAS Incarcération dentaire d'origine traumatique dans la langue et sous la muqueuse vestibulaire. *Rev Stomatol* 1952;**53**:909-12.

28. DEGERING CI. Physiologic evaluation of dental pulp testing methods. *J Dent Res* 1962;**41**:695-700.

29. MUMFORD JM. Evaluation of gutta-percha and ethyl chloride in pulp-testing. *Br Dent J* 1964;**116**:338-42.

30. MUMFORD JM. Pain perception threshold on stimulating human teeth and the histological condition of the pulp. *Br Dent J* 1967;**123**:427-33.

31. ÖHMAN A. Healing and sensitivity to pain in young replanted human teeth. An experimental, clinical, and histological study. *Odontologisk Tidskrift* 1965;**73**:165-228.

32. EHRMANN EH. Pulp testers and pulp testing with particular reference to the use of dry ice. *Aust Dent J* 1977;**22**:272-9.

33. DACHI SF, HALEY JV, SANDERS JE. Standardization of a test for dental sensitivity to cold. *Oral Surg Oral Med Oral Pathol* 1967;**24**:687-92.

34. OBWEGESER H, STEINHÄUSER E. Ein neues Gerät für Vitalitätsprüfung der Zähne mit Kohlensäureschnee. *Schweiz Monatschr Zahnheilk* 1963;**73**:1001-12.

35. FUHR K, SCHERER W. Prüfmethodik und Ergebnisse vergleichender Untersuchungen zur Vitalitätsprüfung von Zähnen. *Dtsch Zahnärztl Z* 1968;**23**:1344-9.

36. SCHILLER F. Ist die Vitalitätsprüfung mit Kohlensäureschnee unschädlich. *Öst Z Stomatol* 1937;**35**:1056-63.

37. SAUERMANN G. Die Vitalitätsprüfung der Pulpa bei überkronten Zähnen. *Zahnärztl Rdsch* 1952;**61**:14-9.

38. MUMFORD JM. Thermal and electrical stimulation of teeth in the diagnosis of pulpal and periapical disease. *Proc Roy Soc Med* 1967;**60**:197-200.

39. MUMFORD JM. Pain threshold of normal human anterior teeth. *Arch Oral Biol* 1963;**8**:493-501.

40. MUMFORD JM. Path of direct current in electric pulp-testing using two coronal electrodes. *Bri Dent J* 1959;**106**:243-5.

41. MUMFORD JM. Path of direct current in electric pulp-testing using one coronal electrode. *Br Dent J* 1959;**106**:23-6.

42. MUMFORD JM, BJÖRN H. Problems in electric pulp-testing and dental algesimetry. *Int Dent J* 1962;**12**:161-79.

43. MUMFORD JM. Pain perception threshold and adaptation of normal human teeth. *Arch Oral Biol* 1965;**10**:957-68.

44. NEWTON AV, MUMFORD JM. Transduction of square wave stimuli through human teeth. *Arch Oral Biol* 1968;**13**:831-2.

45. MUMFORD JM. Drying of enamel under rubber dam. *Br Dent J* 1966;**121**:178-9.

46. SELTZER S, BENDER IB, ZIONTZ M. The dynamics of pulp inflammation: Correlations between diagnostic data and actual histologic findings in the pulp. *Oral Surg Oral Med Oral Pathol* 1963;**16**:846-71, 969-77.

47. REYNOLDS RL. The determination of pulp vitality by means of thermal and electrical stimuli. *Oral Surg Oral Med Oral Pathol* 1966;**22**:231-40.

48. ANEHILL S, LINDAHL B, WALLIN H. Prognosis of traumatised permanent incisors in children. A clinical-roentgenological after-examination. Svensk Tandläkaras Tidning 1969;62:367-75.

49. SKIELLER V. Om prognosen for unge tænder med løsning efter akut mekanisk læsion. *Tandlægebladet* 1957;**1**:657-73.

50. MAGNUSSON B, HOLM A-K. Traumatised permanent teeth in children - a follow-up. I. Pulpal complications and root resorption. *Svensk Tandläkaras Tidning* 1969;**62**:61-70.

51. KRÖNCHE A. Über die Vitalerhaltung der gefährdeten Pulpa nach Fraktur von Frontzahn-kronen. *Dtsch Zahnärztebl* 1957;**11**:333-6.

52. ELOMAA M. Oireettomien ehjien ja pinnalta karioituneiden hampaiden reaktio sähköstimulaattoriin. *Suomi Hammaslääk*

Toim 1963;**59**:316-31.

53. ELOMAA M. Alaleuan pysyvien etuhampaiden reaktio sähkös-timulaattoriin 6-15 vuoden iässä. *Suomi Hammaslääk Toim* 1968;**64**:13-7.

54. STENBERG S. Vitalitetsprövning med elektrisk ström av incisiver i olika genombrottsstadier. *Svensk Tandläkaras Tidning.* 1950;**43**:83-6.

55. FEARNHEAD RW. The histological demonstration of nerve fibres in human dentine. In: ANDERSON DJ, ed. *Sensory mechanisms in dentine.* London: Pergamon Press, 1963:15-26.

56. MUMFORD JM. Personal communication, 1969.

57. ESCHLER J, SCHILLI W, WITT E. *Die Verletzungen der Frontzähne bei Jugendlichen.* Heidelberg: Alfred Hüthig Verlag, 1972.

58. HARGIS HW. Trauma to permanent anterior teeth and alveolar processes. *Dent Clin North Am* 1973;**17**:505-21.

59. HERFORTH A. Notfall: Frontzahntrauma. Hinweise zur Therapie der esten Stunde. *Zahnärztl Mitt* 1973;**63**:317-320.

60. HARGREAVES JA. Emergency treatment for injuries to anterior teeth. *Int Dent J* 1974;**24**:18-29.

61. INGLE JJ, FRANK AL, NATKIN E, NUTTING EE. Diagnosis and treatment of traumatic injuries and their sequelae. In: INGLE JJ, BEVERIDGE EE, eds. *Endodontics.* Philadelphia: Lea & Febiger, 1976.

62. SNAWDER KD. Traumatic injuries to teeth of children. *J Prev Dent* 1976;**3**:13-20.

63. BRAHAM RL, ROBERTS MW, MORRIS ME. Management of dental trauma in children and adolescents. *J Trauma* 1977;**17**:857-65.

64. GRANATH L-E. Traumatologi. In: HOLST JJ, NYGAARD ØSTBY B, OSVALD O, eds. *Nordisk Klinisk Odontologi.* Copenhagen: A/S Forlaget for Faglitteratur, 1978: Chapter 11:79-100.

65. RAVN JJ. *Ulykkesskadede fortænder på børn. Klassifikation og behandling.* Copenhagen: Odontologisk Boghandels Forlag, 1970.

66. SHUSTERMAN S. Treatment of Class III fractures in the hemophiliac patient. A case report. *J Acad Gen Dent* 1973;**21**:25-8.

67. BESSERMANN-NIELSEN M. Orale blødninger hos hæmofilipatienter. *Tandlægebladet* 1974;**78**:756-61.

68. POWELL D. Management of a lacerated frenum and lip in a child with severe hemophilia and an inhibitor: report of case. *J Dent Child* 1976;**43**:272-5.

69. SNAWDER KD, BASTAWI AE, O'TOOLE TJ. Tooth fragments lodged in unexpected areas. *J Am Med Assoc* 1976;**236**:1378-9.

70. SNAWDER KD, O'TOOLE TJ, BASTAWI AE. Broken-tooth fragments embedded in soft tissue. *ASDC J Dent Child* 1979;**46**:145-8.

71. MADER C. Restoration of a fractured anterior tooth. *J Am Dent Assoc* 1978;**96**:113-5.

72. GILBERT JM. Wrinkle corner: traumatic displacement of teeth into the lip. *Injury* 1977;**9**:64-5.

73. BOOTH NA. Complications associated with treatment of traumatic injuries of the oral cavity - aspiration of teeth - report of case. *J Oral Surg* 1953;**11**:242-4.

74. BUSCHINGER K. Dens in pulmone. *Dtsch Zahnärztl Z* 1955;**10**:1302-4.

75. BOWERMAN JE. The inhalation of teeth following maxillo-facial injuries. *Br Dent J* 1969;**127**:132-4.

76. GILLILAND RF, TAYLOR CG, WADE WM JR. Inhalation of a tooth during maxillofacial injury: report of a case. *J Oral Surg* 1972;**30**:839-40.

77. REICHBORN-KJENNERUD I. Development, etiology and diagnosis of increased tooth mobility and traumatic occlusion. *J Periodontol* 1973;**44**:326-38.

78. FULLING H-J, ANDREASEN JO. Influence of maturation status and tooth type of permanent teeth upon electrometric and thermal pulp testing. *Scand J Dent Res* 1976;**84**:286-90.

79. FULLING HJ, ANDREASEN JO. Influence of splints and temporary crowns upon electric and thermal pulp-testing procedures. *Scand J Dent Res* 1976;**84**:291-6.

80. TEITLER D, TZADIK D, EIDELMAN E, CHOSACK A. A clinical evaluation of vitality tests in anterior teeth following fracture of enamel and dentin. *Oral Surg Oral Med Oral Pathol* 1972;**34**:649-52.

81. ZADIK D, CHOSACK A, EIDELMAN E. The prognosis of traumatized permanent anterior teeth with fracture of the enamel and dentin. *Oral Surg Oral Med Oral Pathol* 1979;**47**:173-5.

82. MAYER R, HEPPE H. Vergleichende klinische Untersuchungen unterschiedlicher Mittel und Methoden zur Prüfung der Vitalität der Zähne. *Zahnärztl Welt* 1974;**83**:777-81.

83. HERFORTH A. Zur Frage der Pulpavitalität nach Frontzahntrauma bei Jugendlichen - eine Longitudinaluntersuchung. *Dtsch Zahnärztl Z* 1976;**31**:938-46.

84. LUTZ R, MÖRMANN W, LUTZ T. Schmelzsprünge durch die Vitalitätsprüfung mit Kohlensäureschnee. *Schweiz Monatsschr Zahnheilk* 1974;**84**:709-25.

85. BACHMANN A, LUTZ F. Schmelzsprünge durch die Sensibilitätsprüfung mit CO2- Schnee und Dichlor - difluormethan - eine vergleichende In-vivo-Untersuchung. *Schweiz Monatsschr Zahnheilk* 1976;**86**:1042-59.

86. MAYER R. Neues über die Vitalitätsprüfung mit Kältemitteln. *Dtsch Zahnärztl Z* 1971;**26**:423-8.

87. FERGER P, MATTHIESSEN J. Untersuchungen über die Sensibilitätsprüfung mit Provotest. *Zahnärztl Welt* 1974;**83**:422-3.

88. EIFINGER FF. Sensibilitätstest am menschlichen Zahn mit Kälteaerosolen. *Dtsch Zahnärztebl* 1970;**70**:26-32.

89. JOHNSON RH, DACHI SF, HALEY JV. Pulpal hyperemia - a correlation of clinical and histological data of 706 teeth. *J Am Dent Assoc* 1970;**81**:108-17.

90. BHASKAR SN, RAPPAPORT HM. Dental vitality tests and pulp status. *J Am Dent Assoc* 1973;**86**:409-11.

91. MATTHEWS B, SEARLE BN, ADAMS D, LINDEN R. Thresholds of vital and non-vital teeth to stimulation with electric pulp testers. *Br Dent J* 1974;**137**:352-5.

92. CONSTANTIN I, SEVERINEAU V, TUDOSE N. Die Prüfung des elektrischen Widerstandes als objektiver Diagnosetest bei Pulpaerkrankungen. *Zahn Mund Kieferheilkd* 1976;**64**:550-60.

93. BARKIN PR. Time as a factor in predicting the vitality of traumatized teeth. *ASDC J Dent Child* 1973;**40**:188-92.

94. BADZIAN-KOBOS K, WOCHNA-SOBANSKA M, SZOSLAND E, CICHOCKA D. Application of certain tests for assessment of reactions of dental pulp in permanent anterior teeth of children aged from 7 to 11. *Czas Stomatol* 1975;**28**:1155-62.

95. KLEIN H. Pulp responses to an electric pulp stimulator in the developing permanent anterior dentition. *ASDC J Dent Child* 1978;**45**:199-202.

96. BURNSIDE RR, SORENSON FM, BUCK DL. Electric vitality testing in orthodontic patients. *Angle Orthod* 1974;**44**:213-7.

97. HAUN F. Unfallfolgen mit Spätkomplikationen bei Kindern und Jugendlichen. *ZWR* 1974;**83**:927-31.

98. VEIGEL W, GARCIA C. Möglichkeiten und Grenzen der Erhaltung traumatisch geschädigter Milchzähne. *Dtsch Zahnärztl Z* 1976;**31**:271-73.

99. KRETER F, KLÄHN K-H. Das akute extraalveoläre Zahntrauma des Milch- und Wechselgebisses. *Zahnärztl Prax* 1975;**26**:228-32.

100. JOHO J-P, MARECHAUX SC. Trauma in the primary dentition: a clinical presentation. *ASDC J Dent Child* 1980;**47**:167-74.

101. JACOBSEN I. Clinical problems in the mixed dentition: traumatized teeth - evaluation, treatment and prognosis. *Int Dent J* 1981;**31**:99-104.

102. ANDREASEN FM, ANDREASEN JO. Diagnosis of luxation injuries: The importance of standardized clinical, radiographic and photographic techniques in clinical investigations. *Endod*

Dent Traumatol 1985;**1:**160-9.

103. CAPRIOGLIO D, FALCONI A. I traumi dei denti anteriori in stomatologia infantile. *Dental Cadmos* 1985;**52:**21-47 and 1986;**53:**21-44.

104. MOSS SJ, MACCARO H. Examination, evaluation and behavior management following injury to primary incisors. *N Y State Dent J* 1985;**51:**87-92.

105. MACKIE IC, WARREN VN. Dental trauma: 1. General aspects of management, and trauma to the primary dentition. *Dent Update* 1988;**15:**155-9.

106. HOTZ PR. Accidents dentaires. Accidents aux dents permanentes en denture jeune. *Rev Mens Odontostomatol* 1990;**100:**859-63.

107. FRENKEL G, ADERHOLD L. Das Trauma im Frontzahnbereich des jugendlichen Gebisses aus chirurgischer Sicht. *Fortschr Kieferorthop* 1990;**51:**138-44.

108. HALL RK. Dental management of the traumatized child patient. *Ann Roy Aust Coll Dent Surg* 1986;**9:**80-99.

109. KOPEL HM, JOHNSON R. Examination and neurologic assessment of children with oro-facial trauma. *Endod Dent Traumatol* 1985;**1:**155-9.

110. TURLEY PK, HENSON JL. Self-injurious lip-biting etiology and management. *J Pedodont* 1983;**7:**209-20.

111. NGAN PWH, NELSON LP. Neuropathologic chewing in comatose children. *Pediatr Dent* 1985;**7:**302-6.

112. GUDAT H, MARKL M, LUKAS D, SCHULTE W. Analyse von Perkussionssignalen an Zähnen. *Dtsch Zahnärztl Z* 1977;**32:**169-72.

113. WEISMAN MI. The use of a calibrated percussion instrument in pulpal and periapical diagnosis. *Oral Surg Oral Med Oral Pathol* 1984;**57:**320-2.

114. CHAMBERS IG. The role and methods of pulp testing in oral diagnosis: a review. *Int Endod J* 1982;**15:**1-5.

115. LADO EA, RICHMOND AF, MARKS RG. Reliability and validity of a digital pulp tester as a test standard for measuring sensory perception. *J Endod* 1988; **14:**352-6.

116. ROWE AHR, PITT FORD TR. The assessment of pulpal vitality. *Int Endod J* 1990;**23:**77-83.

117. PETERS DD, LORTON L, MADER CL, AUGSBURGER RA, INGRAM TA. Evaluation of the effects of carbon dioxide used as a pulpal test. 1. In vitro effect on human enamel. *J Endod* 1983;**9:**219-27.

118. PETERS DD. MADER Cl, DONNELLY JC. Evaluation of the effects of carbon dioxide used as a pulpal test. 3. In vivo effect on human enamel. *J Endod* 1986;**12:**13-20.

119. INGRAM TA, PETERS DD. Evaluation of the effects of carbon dioxide used as a pulpal test. Part 2. In vivo effect of canine enamel and pulpal tissues. *J Endod* 1983;**9:**296-303.

120. DOWDEN WE, EMMINGS F, LANGELAND K. The pulpal effect of freezing temperatures applied to monkey teeth. *Oral Surg Oral Med Oral Pathol* 1983;**55:**408-18.

121. MCGRATH PA, GRACELY RH, DUBNER R, HEFT MW. Nonpain and pain sensations evoked by tooth pulp stimulation. *Pain* 1983;**15:**377-88.

122. COOLEY RL, ROBISON SF. Variables associated with electric pulp testing. *Oral Surg Oral Med Oral Pathol* 1980;**50:**66-73.

123. COOLEY RL, STILLEY J, LUBOW RM. Evaluation of a digital pulp tester. *Oral Surg Oral Med Oral Pathol* 1984;**58:**437-42.

124. JACOBSON JJ. Probe placement during electric pulp-testing procedures. *Oral Surg Oral Med Oral Pathol* 1984;**58:**242-7.

125. BENDER IB, LANDAU MA, FONSECCA S, TROWBRIDGE HO. The optimum placement-site of the electrode in electric pulp testing of the 12 anterior teeth. *J Am Dent Assoc* 1989;**118:**305-10.

126. PANTERA EA, ANDERSON RW, PANTERA CT. Use of dental instruments for bridging during electric pulp testing. *J Endod* 1992;**18:**37-41.

127. KOLBINSON DA, TEPLITSKY PE. Electric pulp testing with examination gloves. *Oral Surg Oral Med Oral Pathol* 1988;**65:**122-6.

128. ANDERSON RW, PANTERA EA. Influence of a barrier technique on electric pulp testing. *J Endod* 1988;**14:**179-80.

129. BOOTH DQ, KIDD EAM. Unipolar electric pulp testers and rubber gloves. *Br Dent J* 1988;**165:**254-5.

130. TREASURE P. Capacitance effect of rubber gloves on electric pulp testers. *Int Endod J* 1989;**22:**236-40.

131. STEIMAN HR. Endodontic diagnostic techniques. *Current Science* 1991;**1:**723-28.

132. BHASKAR SN, RAPPAPORT HM. Dental vitality tests and pulp status. *J Am Dent Assoc* 1973;**86:**409-11.

133. ANDREASEN FM, VESTERGAARD PEDERSEN B. Prognosis of luxated permanent teeth - the development of pulp necrosis. *Endod Dent Traumatol* 1985;**1:**207-20.

134. ANDREASEN FM. Transient apical breakdown and its relation to color and sensibility changes after luxation injuries to teeth. *Endod Dent Traumatol* 1986;**2:**9-19.

135. ANDREASEN FM. Pulpal healing after luxation injuries and root fracture in the permanent dentition. *Endod Dent Traumatol* 1989;**5:**111-31.

136. BRANDT K, KORTEGAARD U, POULSEN S. Longitudinal study of electrometric sensitivity of young permanent incisors. *Scand J Dent Res* 1988;**96:**334-8.

137. ANDREASEN JO, PAULSEN HU, YU Z, AHLQUIST R, BAYER T, SCHWARTZ O. A long-term study of 370 autotransplanted premolars. Part 1. Surgical procedures and standardized techniques for monitoring healing. *Eur J Orthod* 1990;**12:**3-13.

138. PECKHAM K, TORABINEJAD M, PECKHAM N. The presence of nerve fibres in the coronal odontoblast layer of teeth at various stages of root development. *Int Endod J* 1991;**24:**303-7.

139. GAZELIUS B, OLGART L, EDWALL B, EDWALL L. Non-invasive recordings of blood blow in human dental pulp. *Endod Dent Traumatol* 1986;**2:**219-21.

140. WILDER-SMITH PEEB. A new method for the non-invasive measurement of pulpal blood flow. *Int Endod J* 1988;**21:**307-12.

141. ANDREASEN FM, ANDREASEN JO. Resorption and mineralization processes following root fracture of permanent incisors. *Endod Dent Traumatol* 1988;**4:**202-14.

142. ANDREASEN JO, BORUM M, JACOBSEN HL, ANDREASEN FM. Replantation of 400 avulsed permanent incisors. II. Factors related to pulp healing. *Endod Dent Traumatol* 1993. To be submitted.

143. ANDREASEN JO, BORUM M, JACOBSEN HL, ANDREASEN FM. Replantation of 400 avulsed permanent incisors. IV. Factors related to periodontal ligament healing. *Endod Dent Traumatol* 1993. To be submitted.

144. BOOTH JM. "It's a knock-out" - an avulsed tooth campaign. *J Endod* 1980;**6:**425-7.

145. HERTHERSAY GS, HIRSCH RS. Tooth discoloration and resolution following a luxation injury: Significance of blood pigment in dentin to laser doppler flowmetry readings. *Quintessence Int* 1993 (in press).

146. MARTIN H, FERRIS C, MAZZELLA W. An evaluation of media used in electric pulp testing. *Oral Surg Oral Med Oral Pathol* 1969;**27:**374-8.

147. GAZELIUS B. Personal communication

CHAPTER 6

Crown Fractures

F. M. ANDREASEN & J. O. ANDREASEN

Terminology, Frequency and Etiology

The following classification of crown fractures is based upon anatomic, therapeutic and prognostic considerations (Fig. 6.1).

1. *Enamel infraction,* an incomplete fracture (crack) of the enamel without loss of tooth substance.
2. *Enamel fracture,* a fracture with loss of tooth substance confined to enamel (uncomplicated crown fracture).
3. *Enamel-dentin fracture,* a fracture with loss of tooth substance confined to en-amel and dentin, but not involving the pulp (uncomplicated crown fracture).
4. *Complicated crown fracture,* an enamel-dentin fracture involving the pulp (complicated crown fracture).

In the *permanent dentition,* crown fractures comprise 26 to 76% of dental injuries (1-4, 111-113). The frequency ranges from 4 to 38% in the *primary dentition* (1, 2, 111).

The most common etiologic factors of crown and crown-root fractures in the permanent dentition are injuries caused by falls, contact sports, automobile accidents or foreign bodies striking the teeth (1, 112).

Fig. 6.1.
Schematic drawings illustrating different types of crown fractures. A. Crown infraction and uncomplicated crown fracture without involvement of dentin. B. Uncomplicated crown fracture with involvement of dentin. C. Complicated crown fracture.

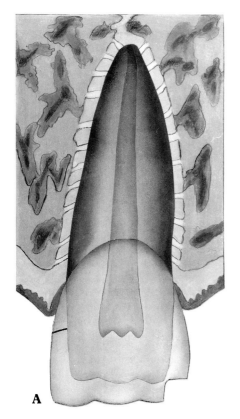
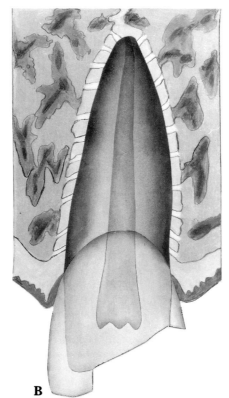
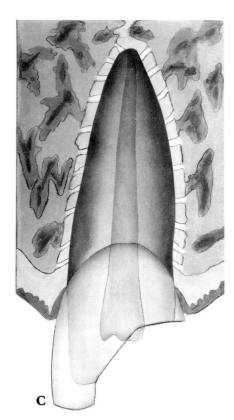

A   **B**   **C**

Fig. 6.2.
Infraction lines involving the right central and lateral incisors. The use of indirect illumination reveals the infraction lines (A) although they are barely visible by direct illumination (B).

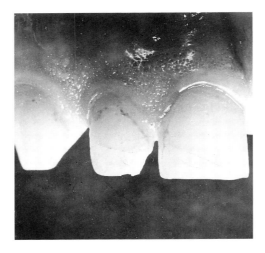 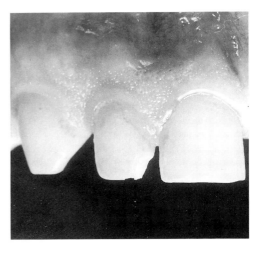

Enamel fractures comprise a very common occupational hazard among glassblowers, presumably due to impact by the blowpipe (192).

Clinical Findings

Enamel infractions are very common but often overlooked. These fractures appear as crazing within the enamel substance which do not cross the dentino-enamel junction and may appear with or without loss of tooth substance (i.e. uncomplicated or complicated crown fractures) (5, 6, 114, 194). Infractions are caused by direct impact to the enamel (e.g. traffic accidents and falls, which explains their frequent occurrence on the labial surface of upper incisors (194). Various patterns of infraction lines can be seen depending on the direction and location of the trauma, i.e. horizontal, vertical or diverging. Infractions are often overlooked if direct il-

lumination is used, but are easily visualized when the light beam is directed perpendicular to the long axis of the tooth from the incisal edge (Fig. 6.2). Fiber optic light sources are also very useful in detecting infractions. By modifying the intensity of the light beam, many infractions become readily visible (193). Infractions are often the only evidence of trauma, but can be associated with other types of injury. Thus the presence of infraction lines should draw attention to the possible presence of associated injuries, especially to the supporting structures.

Fractures without pulpal involvement occur more often than complicated crown fractures in both the permanent and primary dentitions (3, 7-9, 111, 115, 116). They are often confined to a single tooth, usually the maxillary central incisors (7, 10, 115), especially the mesial or distal corners (7) (Fig. 6.3). Fractures can be horizontal, extending mesiodistally. Occasionally only the central lobe of the incisal edge is in-

Fig. 6.3.
Central incisors with typical uncomplicated crown fractures involving the mesial corners. A. Primary dentition. B. Permanent dentition.

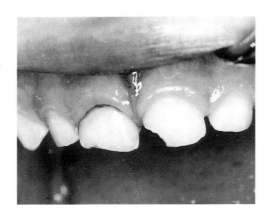 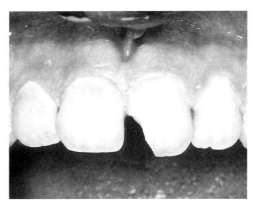

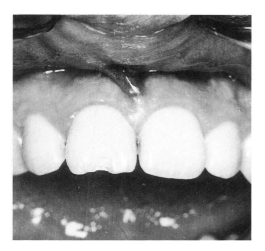

Fig. 6.4.
Uncomplicated crown fracture involving the central lobe of the incisal edge.

volved (Fig. 6.4). In rare cases, the fracture can involve the entire facial or oral enamel surface (Fig. 6.5).

Although not frequently found in combination with luxation injuries (195, 196), crown fractures can be seen concomitant to subluxations, extrusions and intrusions (1, 197, 198). This combination of luxation injury and crown fracture is of prognostic importance (see later).

A very unusual finding is crown fractures of non-erupted permanent teeth due to trauma transmitted from impact to the primary dentition (118, 119) (see Chapter 12, p. 475).

Examination of fractured teeth should be preceded by thorough cleansing of the injured teeth with a water spray. This is followed by an assessment of the extent of exposed dentin as well as a careful search for minute pulp exposures.

Dentin exposed after crown fracture usually gives rise to symptoms such as sensitivity to thermal changes and mastication, which are to some degree proportional to the area of dentin exposed and the maturity of the tooth (199).

The layer of dentin covering the pulp may be so thin that the outline of the pulp is seen as a pinkish tinge. In such cases, it is important not to perforate the dentin with a dental probe during the search for pulp exposures. Clinical examination should also include sensibility testing as a point of reference for later evaluation of pulpal status (120) (see Chapter 5, p.202).

Complicated crown fractures usually present slight hemorrhage from the exposed part of the pulp (Fig. 6.6). Proliferation of pulp tissue (i.e. pulp polyp) can occur when treatment in young teeth is delayed for days or weeks (Fig. 6.6).

Pulp exposure is usually followed by symptoms, such as sensitivity to thermal changes.

Radiographic Findings

The radiographic examination adds important information to the clinical evaluation which can influence future treatment, such as the size of the pulp and the stage of root development (200-202). Moreover, the radiograph serves as a record for comparison at later visits. This is especially true in the verification of a hard tissue barrier over an exposed pulp when clinical verification is not possible. How-

Fig. 6.5.
Frontal view of a crown fracture involving the entire lingual enamel.

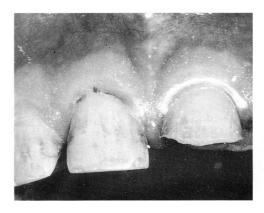

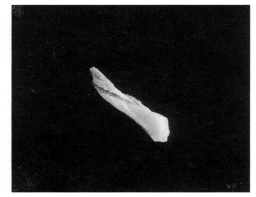

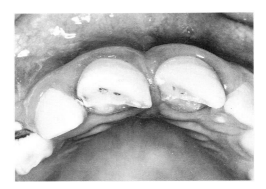
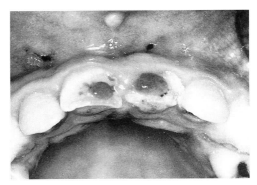

ever, it should be borne in mind that a radiograph can only provide an estimate of pulpal dimensions; and that the pulp cavity is usually larger and the distance of pulp horns from the incisal edge is usually smaller than that shown radiographically (200).

Pathology

Enamel infractions can be seen in ground sections, where they appear as dark lines running parallel to the enamel rods and terminate at the dentino-enamel junction (11) (Fig. 6.7).

Enamel-dentin crown fractures expose a large number of dentinal tubules. It has been estimated that the exposure of one square millimeter of dentin exposes 20,000 to 45,000 dentinal tubules (12, 121). These tubules constitute a pathway for bacteria and thermal and chemical irritants which can provoke pulpal inflammation, for which reason dentin-covering procedures described later in this chapter and in Chapter 14 are necessary. The speed of bacterial penetration into prepared dentin left exposed to saliva and plaque formation *in vivo* was found by LUNDY & STANLEY (203) to be 0.03-0.36 mm 6-11 days after preparation and 0.52 mm after approximately 84 days. Moreover, bacterial penetration into dentinal tubules is more rapid in teeth where dentin is exposed due to fracture rather than grinding , presumably due to the absence of the barrier formed by a smear layer (204, 205).

Finally, this bacterial penetration is more rapid where impeding hydrostatic pressure from an outward pulpal fluid flow is minimal or nonexistent, as after concomitant luxation injuries where there is a compromised pulpal blood supply (205-210). Experimental studies *in vivo* in the cat

have thus demonstrated an increased fluid flow from exposed dentinal tubules with an intact pulpal blood supply, presumably due to a chain of events involved in neurogenic inflammation arising from dentinal irritation following exposure and subsequent stimulation of, e.g., the inferior alveolar nerve (206-210). This fluid flow might mechanically inhibit bacterial ingress through patent dentinal tubules, and also distribute antibodies (205).

This increase in fluid flow after dentin exposure might also have clinical implications with respect to moisture control in the use of dentin bonding agents. Thus, it might seem advisable to administer a local anesthetic prior to such procedures to reverse dentinal fluid flow due to neurogenic stimulation (211). However, further investigation is necessary to test this theory before it can be advocated universally.

Little information exists about pulpal changes after *enamel-dentin crown fractures*. Experimental studies have demonstrated inflammatory changes when artificially exposed dentin was left uncovered for one week (13, 14). However, recent research suggests that the inflammatory changes are of a transient nature, if the pulpal vascular supply remains intact and bacterial invasion is prevented (212) (see later).

Histologically, exposed pulp tissue in *complicated crown fractures* is quickly covered by a layer of fibrin. Eventually the superficial part of the pulp shows capillary budding, numerous leukocytes and proliferation of histiocytes (Fig. 6.8, A to C). This inflammation spreads apically with increasing observation periods (Fig. 6.8, D to F). However, experimental studies in permanent teeth of monkeys have shown that the inflammatory process does not usually penetrate more than approximately 2 mm in an apical direction (122, 213), a finding which is of clinical signific-

Fig. 6.7.
Histologic features of a permanent central incisor showing crown infractions. A. Gross specimen. Note the point of impact (arrow) with irradiating infraction lines. B. Low-power view of ground section through the impact area. x 8. C. Lingual aspect of the crown exhibiting an infraction line. x 30. D. Higher magnification of (C) reveals that the line follows the direction of the enamel prisms. x 195. E. Infraction line in area of impact. The line terminates at the dentino-enamel junction. x 30. F. Higher magnification of (E). Foreign material is lodged in the enamel substance at the point of impact. x 195.

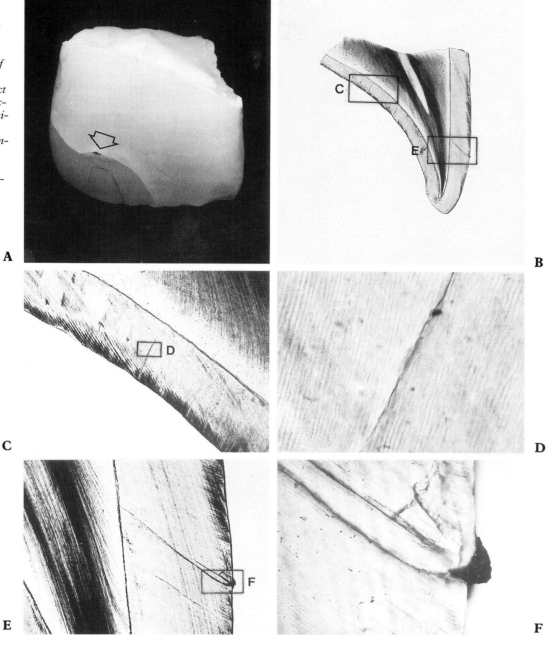

A   B

C   D

E   F

ance in treatment planning (see Chapter 14).

Complicated crown fractures which are left untreated for longer periods of time normally show extensive proliferation of granulation tissue at the exposure site (Fig. 6.6). However, instances of spontaneous closure of the perforation with hard tissue have been reported (15, 123).

Treatment

Many authors have discussed treatment principles for crown fractures in the *permanent dentition* (16-59). Therapeutic considerations comprise *pulpal* response to injury and treatment as well as the *prosthetic* considerations arising at the time of injury and final, definitive treatment. The reader is referred to Chapter 14 regarding pulpal considerations following crown fracture; while emphasis in the present chapter will be placed upon emergency treatment procedures. Final restorative treatment using composite resin will be described in Chapter 16.

Fig. 6.8.
*Pulp reactions following compli-
cated crown fractures in maxillary
primary incisors. A. Low-power
view of incisor removed 19 hours
after injury. Moderate inflammatory changes are present in the coronal part of the pulp while the
apical part shows only minor
changes, such as hyperemia and
perivascular bleeding. x 9. B. Hyperemia and perivascular bleeding. x 75. C. Moderate inflammatory changes. x 75.*

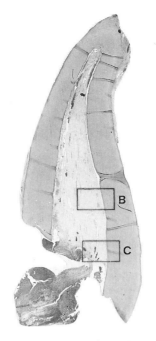

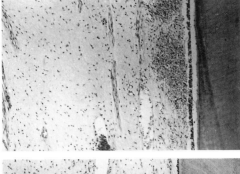

A

*D. Low-power view of incisor
removed 41 hours after injury.
Marked inflammatory changes
are present in the coronal part of
the pulp and spread of the inflammation apically is evident. x 9.
E. Moderate inflammation. x
75. F. Marked inflammatory
changes. x 75.*

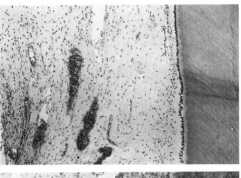

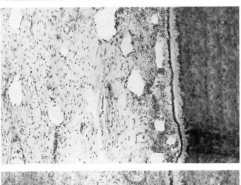

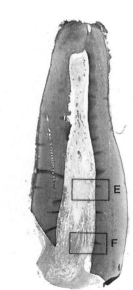

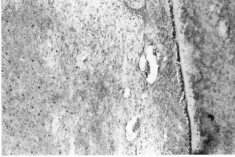

D

Permanent Teeth

ENAMEL INFRACTIONS

While infractions in both enamel, dentin and cementum in the *posterior* region are often implicated in "the cracked tooth syndrome," enamel infractions in *anterior* teeth following acute trauma do not appear to imply the same risk to tissue integrity due to the fact that these infractions are usually limited to enamel, stopping at the dentino-enamel junction. However, due to frequently associated injuries to periodontal structures, sensibility tests should be carried out in order to disclose possible damage to the pulp.

As a rule, enamel infractions do not require treatment. However, in case of multiple infraction lines, the indication might be to seal the enamel surface with

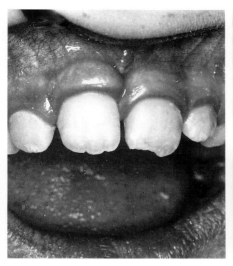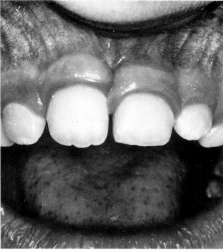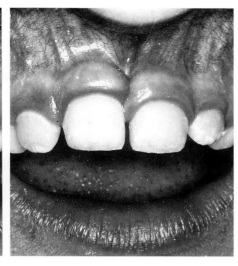

Fig. 6.9.
Grinding procedure used in the treatment of an uncomplicated crown fracture confined to enamel. A. Before treatment. B. After grinding of injured tooth. C. Grinding of the non-injured incisor in order to restore symmetry.

an unfilled resin and acid etch technique, as these lines might otherwise take up stain from tobacco, food, drinks, or other liquids (e.g. tea, red wine, cola drinks, chlorhexidine mouthwashes).

ENAMEL AND ENAMEL-DENTIN CROWN FRACTURES

Immediate treatment of crown fractures *confined to enamel* can be limited to smoothing of sharp enamel edges to prevent laceration of the tongue or lips. Selective reduction can be undertaken at the same time or at a later visit with good esthetic results, especially in imitating an accentuated rounding of a distal corner (47,

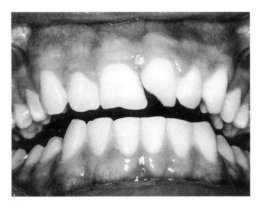

Fig. 6.10.
Untreated crown fracture. Note drifting and tilting of adjacent teeth into the fracture area. Courtesy of Dr. J. J. RAVN, Department of Pedodontics, Royal Dental College, Copenhagen, Denmark.

60) (Fig. 6.9). However, because of esthetic demands for midline symmetry, a fractured mesial corner can usually not be corrected in the same way. Selective reduction can in some cases be combined with orthodontic extrusion of the fractured tooth in order to restore incisal height. However, cervical symmetry must also be considered (61, 214) (see Chapter 7, p. 269)

When the shape or extent of the fracture precludes recontouring, a restoration is necessary.

Whatever treatment is decided, it is essential that the crown's anatomy and occlusion be restored immediately in order to prevent labial protrusion of the fractured tooth, drifting or tilting of adjacent teeth into the fracture site (6, 34, 63, 124) or overeruption of opposing incisors (60, 64) (Fig. 6.10).

Immediate reattachment of the original fragment (see p. 230) or restoration with a composite resin (see Chapter 16, p. 636) is normally to be preferred over a temporary crown for several reasons. These procedures are usually esthetically superior and are probably less traumatic to the injured tooth than adaptation of temporary crowns. The most significant disadvantage of temporary crowns is the potential risk of leakage which permits access of bacteria to the exposed dentin and thereby represents a significant threat to the recovery of the pulp.

An isolated fracture of enamel does not appear to represent any hazard to the pulp (See p. 245). However, in crown fractures with *exposed dentin*, therapeutic measures should be directed towards dentin coverage in order to avoid bacterial ingress and thereby permit the pulp to recover and elicit repair.

It was in the 1970's that the impact on pulpal healing of bacterial invasion and colonization in the gap between the tooth and the restorative material after exposure of dentin was appreciated (204, 215-240).

Thus, when bacteria are excluded from the tooth/restoration interface experimentally by placement of a superficial layer of zinc oxide-eugenol cement over the restorations or liners, healing with formation of a hard tissue bridge can be achieved even after direct pulp capping with silicate cement, zinc-phosphate cement, amalgam and light-cured composite resin (236, 237,241-244) (Fig. 6.11). It would therefore seem that the initial cytotoxic effect of these materials placed on or near the human pulp is not greater than that which is seen after capping with calcium hydroxide (199).

Experimentally it has been found that in teeth with vital pulp tissue, dentin can provide considerable resistance to bacterial invasion and that dentin which has been exposed to the oral environment for longer periods of time appears to be less permeable than fresh dentinal wounds (240). Furthermore, bacterial irritation via an area of exposed dentin causes limited pulpal inflammation and with little permanent damage (245).

As support for these findings, long-term clinical studies have shown very little pulpal response (e.g. pulp necrosis, or pulp canal obliteration) to either crown fracture with or without pulp exposure or subsequent restorative procedures as long as there was not a concomitant periodontal injury (233, 246-253) (Table 6.1).

Fig. 6.11.
Biocompatibility of dental materials in the absence of infection. A. Dentin bridge seen 7 days after pulp exposure and direct pulp capping with a composite resin and surface seal of zinc oxide-eugenol cement. B. Dentin bridge seen 21 days after pulp exposure and direct pulp capping with silicate cement and surface seal of zinc oxide-eugenol cement. Courtesy of Dr. C. F. COX, School of Dentistry, Birmingham, Alabama, USA.

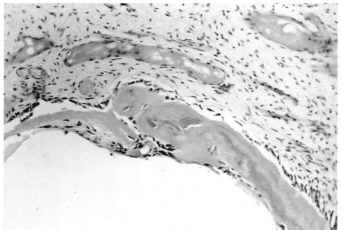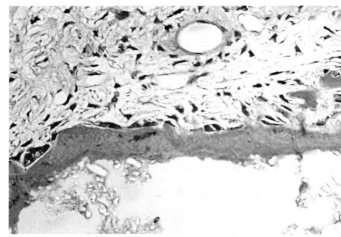

CHAPTER 6

Fig. 6.12.
Adaptation of a stainless steel crown
Selection of correct size is based upon measurements of the width of the fractured tooth itself or its contralateral with a millimeter gauge. The heights of the facial and proximal aspects of the crown are marked. The crown is trimmed with a curved crown scissors. (e.g. Rocky Mountain® No. i-25 curved crown scissors).

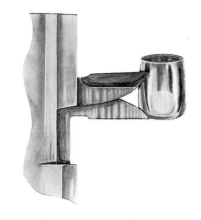 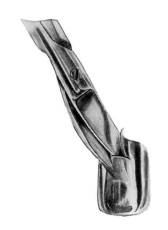

Contouring the cingulum
The cingulum can be contoured with contouring pliers (e.g. Rocky Mountain® No. i-114 Johnson contouring pliers). The area above the cingulum is depressed with the same pliers but with the ball placed outside. Facial and proximal aspects of the crown can be contoured, if necessary, with special contouring pliers (e.g. Rocky Mountain® No. i-137 Gordon contouring pliers).

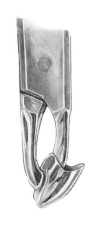 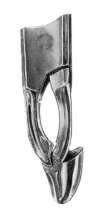

Finishing the gingival margin
The gingival margin of the crown can be contoured to fit slight undercuts by using bending pliers (e.g. Rocky Mountain® No. 1-139 Angle wire bending pliers) or contouring pliers (e.g. Rocky Mountain® No. i-114 Johnson contouring pliers). The gingival edge of the crown can be thinned by using a rotating diamond wheel towards the inside of the crown.

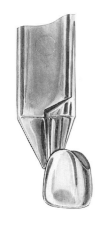 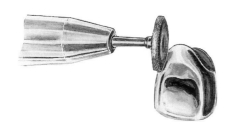

CROWN FRACTURES

Treatment Strategy

In light of current knowledge concerning the role of bacterial influences associated with marginal leakage, one must conclude that the primary objective of restorative procedures following crown fractures which expose dentin is to prevent injury to the pulp that is initiated by bacteria and bacterial components in the event that the restoration will not provide a proper marginal seal (250).

THE USE OF DENTIN BONDING AGENTS: SHOULD EXPOSED DENTIN BE LINED?

Until recently, strategy for the treatment of enamel-dentin fractures without pulp exposure has been dentin coverage with a hard-setting calcium hydroxide containing liner. Clinical experience, however, indicates that hard setting calcium hydroxide cements disintegrate beneath dental restorations with time. This finding has been confirmed both experimentally *in vitro* (255, 256) and *in vivo* (230, 257). Moreover, cultivable and stainable bacteria have been found within the calcium hydroxide liners used in both exposed and pulp capped and non-exposed control teeth and these are thus unable to provide a permanent barrier against microleakage (230, 257). Finally, it has been found *in vitro* that calcium hydroxide liners can have the same softening effect on composite resins as zinc oxide-eugenol liners (258). The long-term benefit of their use is therefore questionable (259). While a light-cured calcium hydroxide liner might prove more stable clinically, no long-term data exists at present.

What appears to be critical to pulpal healing is how effectively the dentin is sealed from bacterial irritants. If deeply exposed dentin is adequately sealed, the nonexposed pulp will form reparative dentin even without calcium hydroxide.

Microleakage around composite resin restorations is one of the major causes of restoration failure (260). Microleakage can be counteracted in part by a strong micromechanical bond arising between a composite resin and acid-etched *enamel* (261-263). If *dentin* bonding is also employed, it has been shown experimentally that the bonding strength of reattached crown fragments is approximately 3 times greater than if only acid-etched enamel is the source of retention (264).

The goal of a dentin bonding agent is, therefore, to supplement enamel acid etching by mediating a bond between an adhesive resin and the dentin surface. This would imply a hermetic seal against the oral flora and optimize pulpal healing after fracture.

As the bond strength of any dentin bonding system is proportional to the surface area of available unlined dentin for bonding, it is important that a calcium hydroxide liner not cover more dentin than is absolutely necessary.

Research into the impact of bacteria on pulpal healing (versus the impact of restorative material toxicity) has led to the concept of a single-step total etch technique (i.e. simultaneous enamel and dentin conditioning) (265-268).

Such an approach greatly simplifies the bonding procedures. Moreover, experimental results indicate little adverse pulpal response (266). However, long-term *clinical* pulpal response to such procedures has not yet been documented. An important key to the success of either the total-etch or dual step approach appears to be the chemical and physico-chemical aspects of the (dentin) bonding system employed.

Thus, it has been demonstrated that the chemical reactions needed for dentin bonding require compatibility between dentin or conditioned dentin and the adhesive resin with respect to polarity and solubility parameters (269). For example, to achieve minimum gap formation (270) and maximum bond strength with the original Gluma ® dentin bonding system (Bayer Corp., Leverkusen BRD), a neutral dentin surface is necessary (271, 272). Simultaneous acid etching the dentin and enamel thus lowers the pH of the dentin surface and weakens bond strength (273, 274).

The above findings might imply that a calcium hydroxide liner could be eliminated and a dentin bonding agent used to maximize bonding area and minimize gap formation between the tooth surface and the composite resin restoration to ensure pulpal healing. However, at present, the clinical durability of the bond achieved is unknown. Clinical failure might arise due to polymerization contraction, thermally induced dimensional changes or mechanical stress or fatigue of the material used. This may imply renewed contamination of the dentin surface and subsequent risk to pulpal integrity. Until further data exists, treatment strategy of deep dentin fractures would, therefore, imply application of a hard-setting calcium hydroxide liner or a glass ionomer cement to the deepest aspect of the fracture and then use of a dentin bonding agent to complete the hermetic seal against the oral environment.

While the use of dentin bonding agents would immediately appear to be easier, modern restorative dentistry involves the use of unforgivingly demanding dental materials. And such an approach implies great sensitivity of technique and places responsibility upon the clinician for meticulous tissue and moisture control and attention to detail that is required for treatment succeed.

ENAMEL-DENTIN CROWN FRACTURES WITH PULP EXPOSURE

The principles for the restoration of crown fractures with pulpal involvement differ from those of uncomplicated crown fractures only with respect to treatment of the exposed dental pulp. This implies pulp capping, partial pulpotomy or pulpal extirpation which are described in Chapter 14.

PROVISIONAL TREATMENT OF CROWN FRACTURES

Stainless Steel Crowns

These crowns were of particular value prior to the advent of enamel and dentin bonding systems (65, 67, 68, 86, 87). Since then, their application in the treatment of acute trauma has become very limited, primarily due to their esthetic shortcomings and the need of repeated trials in order to achieve adequate adaptation, which possibly elicits further damage to an already traumatized periodontium and pulp (275). However, in the case of extensive crown fractures with pulpal involvement, their use might still be warranted. The crown is finished short of the gingival margin in order to permit optimal gingival health and prevent cement from being forced into the injured periodontal ligament (Figs. 6.12 and 6.13). The fracture surface is cleaned with saline once the crown has been adapted and the occlusion checked. The application of potent irritants for the purpose of sterilizing or drying exposed dentin, or extended air

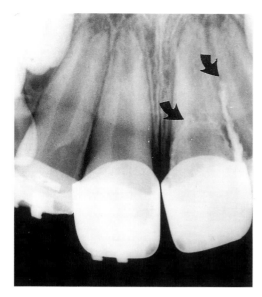

Fig. 6.13.
Cement displaced into the periodontal ligament after cementation of a steel crown on a luxated central incisor.

drying of the dentin, are harmful to the odontoblasts, impairing or destroying their ability to deposit a protective layer of secondary dentin. A hard-setting calcium hydroxide-containing liner is placed over the entire fracture surface and the adapted crown is cemented with a carboxylate cement, a material which has been shown to exert only a mild temporary irritation to the pulp (182-185). The crowns can later be removed by cutting a vertical groove in the lingual or facial surface, starting at the gingival margin.

Composite Resin

When esthetic demands are foremost, a temporary acrylic crown should be considered. Various types of prefabricated temporary crowns are available. Resin or celluloid crown forms have too little strength for this purpose and should only be used as a mold for the crown. After placement of a calcium hydroxide liner over the fracture surface, a suitable crown form is selected and contoured to fit the fractured tooth. A hole is made with a sharp explorer through the mesial or distal incisal corner to permit escape of excess crown material during placement. The fitted form is then filled with a composite resin, seated, and excess resin removed. When polymerized, the crown is removed, finished and cemented (60, 186).

Splints

In case of concomitant injuries to the periodontium, pulp protection must be incorporated into the splint. In these instances, it is a good idea for ease of splint removal and later restoration to cover the exposed enamel and dentin with a calcium hydroxide liner before application of an acid-etch/resin splint (Fig. 6.14). Enamel coverage with a liner is especially important in the case of later reattachment of the fractured crown fragment to ensure an intact enamel margin to which the fragment can be bonded (see later). In the case of profound crown fracture and simultaneous need for splinting, a fiber-reinforced splint can be the solution for satisfactory retention until splint removal and final restoration (276, 277).

DEFINITIVE TREATMENT OF CROWN FRACTURES

Because of the recent improvements in dental materials available, the boundary between provisional and definitive treatment has become less and less distinct.

Various cast semipermanent restorations (e.g. basket crowns, gold-acrylic open-faced crowns and pinledge inlays) have been designed in the past to meet the esthetic demands of a young traumatized permanent dentition until such time as definitive treatment was considered appropriate (60, 64, 70, 74-87, 99-110, 188). However, with the advent of composite resin materials and the acid etch technique (129-169, 180, 181, 261-263, 278, 279), the indications for these restorations has been eliminated. Moreover, in many situations, considering the life expectancy of these new materials, other definitive treatments of the past might not be necessary or might actually be overtreatment.

Definitive restoration of crown fractures presently consists of composite restorations (see Chapter 16, p. 636), reattachment of the original crown fragment (see later), full crown coverage (70, 76. 80. 94, 99-110), or laminate veneers (280, 281) (see later).

REATTACHMENT OF THE ORIGINAL CROWN FRAGMENT

Reattachment of the fragment provides several advantages over other forms of dental restoration following crown fracture. It results in exact restoration of crown and surface morphology in a material that abrades at the same rate as adjacent teeth. Chair time for the completion of the restoration is minimal, normally requiring less time than that needed for completion of a temporary restoration (Fig. 6.15).

Prior to the advent of dentin bonding agents, the only available method of fragment reattachment was by the use of enamel acid etching. Preparation of the tooth and avulsed fragment included either an internal bevel of enamel on both fracture surfaces (282) or simply hollowing out of the dentin of the fragment fracture surface to accommodate a thickness of hard-setting calcium hydroxide liner on the fracture surface of the tooth. This was then followed by enamel etching and adhesion of fragments using a creamy mixture of unfilled and filled composite resin on both fracture surfaces (282-295). Reports of these procedures have been anecdotal and with mixed long-term success. The concept of fragment reattachment was, therefore, reevaluated with the development of the new dentin bonding agents in the mid-1980's (296-303).

Reattachment of fractured enamel-dentin crown fragments using the original Gluma® dentin bonding system was begun as a routine treatment of complicated and uncomplicated crown fractures by the authors and co-workers in 1984 (304,305). As already mentioned, *in vitro* studies demonstrated a three-fold increase in fracture strength if a dentin bonding agent supplemented retention from acid-etched enamel (264). However, the bonding strengths achieved were only 50-60% that of intact teeth (264).

In animal studies, the bonding system has been proved safe for pulpal tissues as long as a 0.2 mm thickness of dentin remained between the pulp and the bonding surface. However, the adverse pulpal response seen after 8 days when the remaining dentin thickness was less than 0.2 mm was not evident at 90 days (306).

At the time the Gluma® dentin bonding system was introduced and crown fracture bonding initiated, it was one of the most

Fig 6.14. Combined splint and temporary crown for treatment of concomitant crown fractures and tooth luxation
This patient has suffered uncomplicated crown fractures and subluxation of 3 maxillary incisors. There is uncertain pulpal response to sensibility testing of the central incisors.

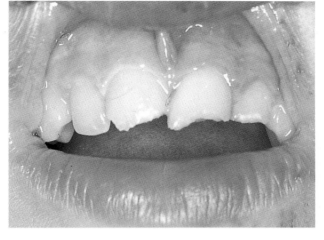 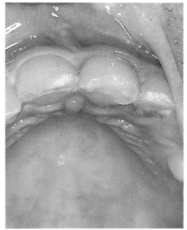

Dentin coverage
The entire fracture surface is covered with a hard-setting calcium hydroxide liner (Dycal®).

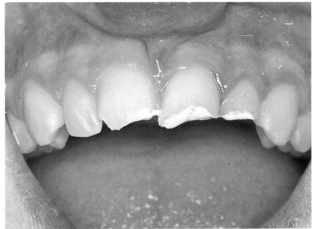 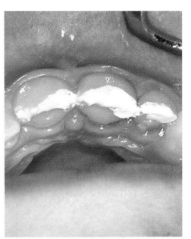

Enamel etching
The labial and lingual enamel is etched with phosphoric acid gel.

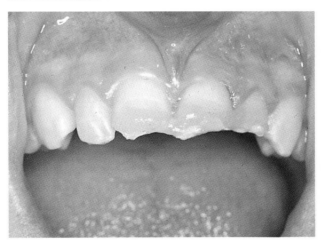 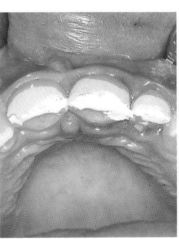

Coverage of the fracture surfaces with a temporary crown and bridge material
The fracture surfaces and labial enamel of the involved incisors are covered with a temporary crown and bridge material (Protemp®. Espe Corp.).

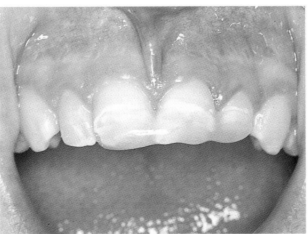 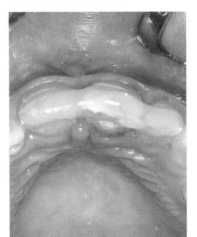

CROWN FRACTURES

Fig. 6.15. Reattaching a crown fragment with a dentin bonding agent and reinforcement of the bonding site with composite resin.
This 10-year-old boy has fractured his central incisor after a fall from his skateboard. The fracture is very close to the mesial pulp horn.

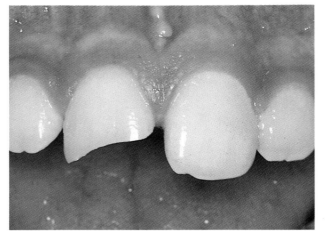 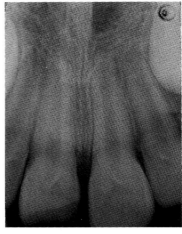

Testing pulpal sensibility
Pulpal response to sensibility testing is normal. The radiographic examination shows no displacement or root fracture.

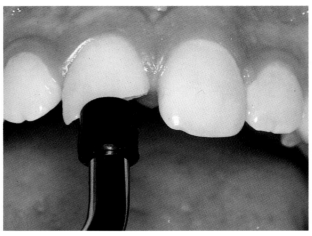 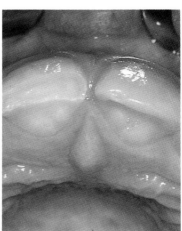

Testing the fit of the fragment
The fragment fits exactly. The enamel surface is intact, with no apparent defect at the enamel margins.

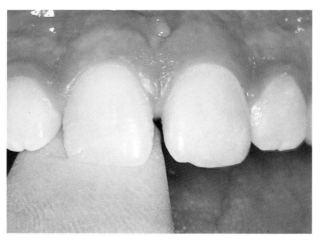 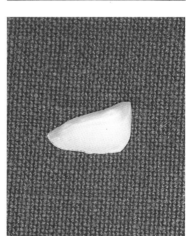

Temporary dentin coverage with calcium hydroxide
Due to the close proximity of the fracture surface to the pulp, a temporary calcium hydroxide fracture surface, including enamel, is prepared prior to placement of the temporary restoration.

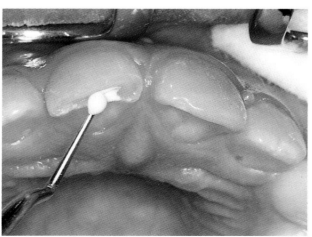 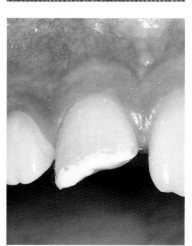

CHAPTER 6

Etching the enamel
A 2-mm wide zone of enamel around the fracture surface is etched.

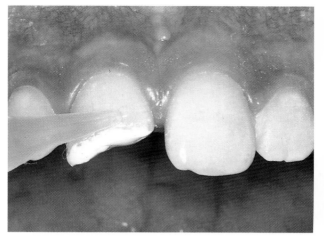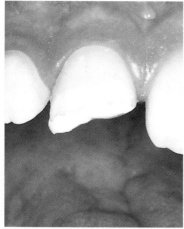

Covering the fracture surface
The tooth is temporarily restored with a temporary crown and bridge material. To provide greater stability, the restoration may be extended to adjacent teeth.

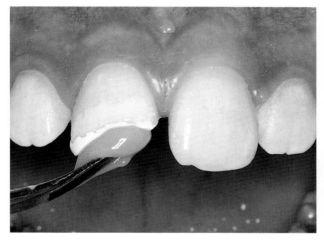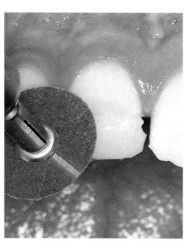

Storage of the crown fragment
The tooth is stored in physiologic saline for 1 month. The patient is given the fragment and is instructed to change the solution once a week to reduce contamination.

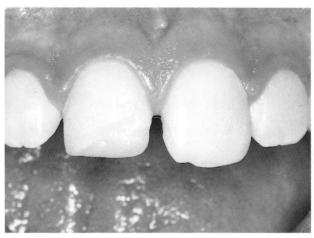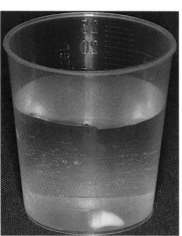

Bonding of the fragment after 1 month
The temporary cover is removed and the fragment is fastened to a piece of sticky wax for ease of handling.

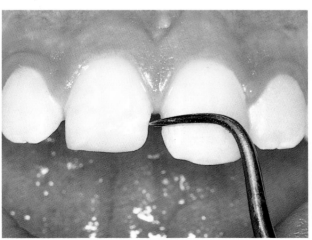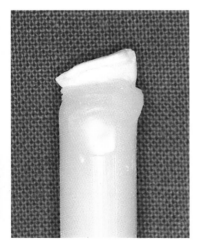

CROWN FRACTURES

Preparing for bonding

Pulpal sensibility is monitored and the fracture surfaces (of the tooth and crown fragment) are cleansed with a pumice-water slurry and a rubber cup.

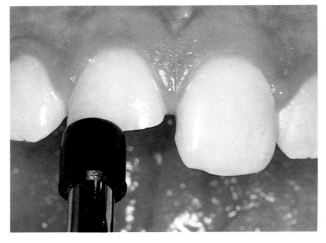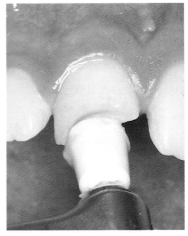

Etching enamel

Enamel on both fracture surfaces as well as a 2-mm wide collar of enamel cervical and incisal to the fracture are etched for 30 seconds with 35% phosphoric acid being sure that the etchant does not come in contact with dentin.

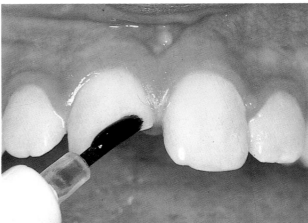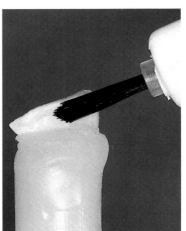

Removal of the etchant

The fracture surfaces are rinsed thoroughly with a copious flow of water for 20 seconds.

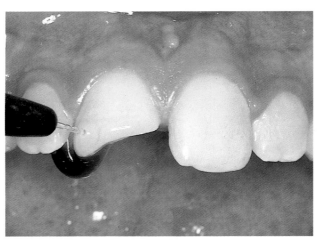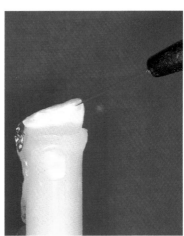

Drying the fracture surfaces

The fracture surfaces are air-dried for 10 seconds. NOTE: To avoid entrapment of air in the dentinal tubules and a subsequent chalky mat discoloration of the fragment, the air stream must be directed parallel with the fracture surface and not perpendicular to it.

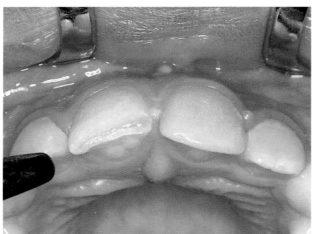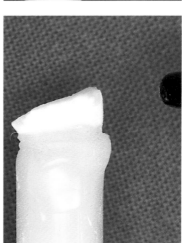

CHAPTER 6

Conditioning the dentin with EDTA and GLUMA

The fracture surfaces are conditioned with EDTA for 20 seconds, followed by 10 seconds water rinse and 10 seconds air drying. Thereafter 20 seconds GLUMA® and 10 seconds air drying.

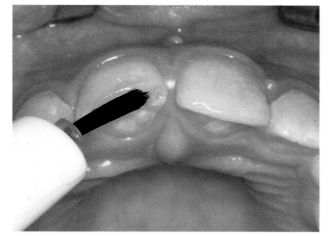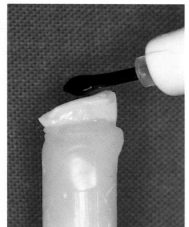

Bonding the fragment

The fracture surfaces are covered with a creamy mixture of a filled composite and its unfilled resin. After repositioning of the fragment, the composite is light-polymerized.

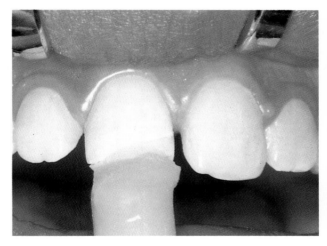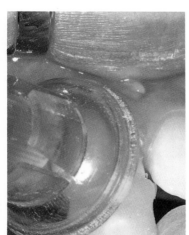

Light polymerization

The composite is light polymerized 60 seconds facially and 60 seconds orally.

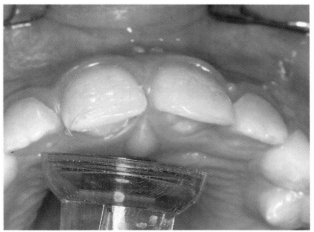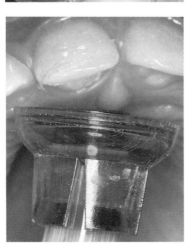

Removal of surplus composite

With a straight scalpel blade or composite finishing knives surplus composite is removed from the fracture site. The interproximal contacts are finished with finishing strips.

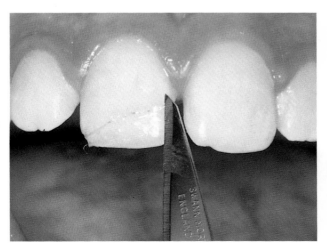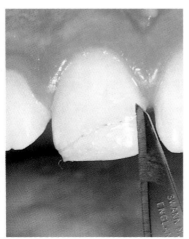

Reinforcing the fracture site
A round diamond bur is used to create a "double chamfer" margin 1 mm coronally and apically to the fracture line. To achieve optimal estitics, the chamfer follows an undulating path along the fracture line.

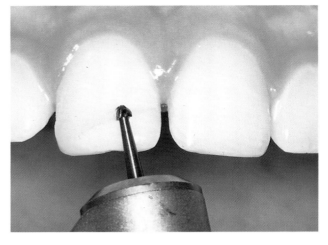 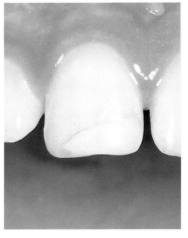

Finishing the labial surface
After restoring the labial aspect with composite, the restoration is contoured using abrasive discs.

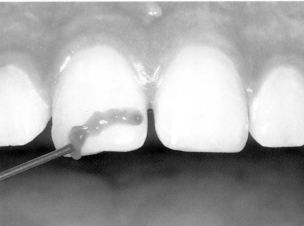 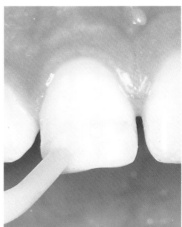

Reinforcing the palatal aspect of the fracture
The palatal aspect of the fracture is reinforced using the same procedure. Due to its position, esthetic consideration is less. The preparation can, therefore, follow the fracture line exactly.

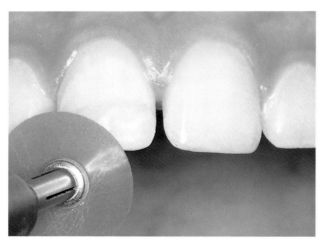 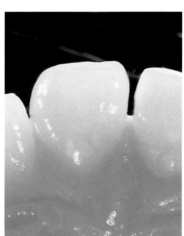

The final restoration
The condition 1 month after reattachment of the crown fragment.

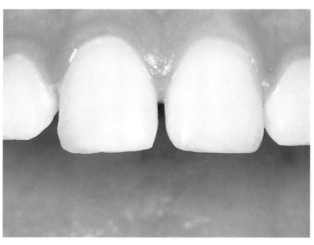 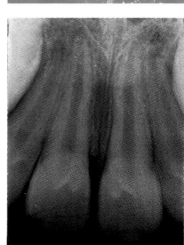

promising of the dentin bonding agents available. Since then, significant advances have been made in the area of dentin bonding agents and bond strength to dentin (307-311). However, at least in the case of reattachment of crown fragments, recent experiments have shown that successful fragment bonding can be achieved irrespective of the dentin bonding agent used as long as the manufacturer's directions are followed closely (264, 312).

INDICATIONS

It goes without saying that successful fragment reattachment is dependent upon fragment retrieval at the time of injury. As in the correct treatment of tooth avulsions, fragment retrieval requires an informed public. In Scandinavia, public information campaigns in the form of television spots and posters have proved successful in informing patients of their role in treatment success.

An intact enamel-dentin fragment is the sole indication for reattachment. That is, the majority of the enamel margin should be present so that the fragment can rest firmly against the fracture surface when it is tried against the fractured tooth. Small defects, however, can be restored with composite resin at the time of or following the bonding procedure. Moreover, if the fragment is in 2 pieces, these fragments can be bonded together prior to bonding the final fragment (Fig. 6.16).

TREATMENT STRATEGY

Treatment strategy for fragment reattachment without pulpal involvement is dependent upon the distance between the fracture surface and pulp. If the distance is small (i.e. the pulp can be seen through the thin dentinal floor), the entire fracture surface (enamel and dentin) is covered with a hard-setting calcium hydroxide liner and a provisional restoration placed for approximately one month to permit hard tissue deposition in the pulp horn and the pulpal inflammation to subside. Placement of liner on enamel and dentin facilitates later removal of the provisional restoration and ensures a fresh enamel surface for bonding. In the interim period, the crown fragment is kept moist, e.g. in tap water or physiologic saline which is changed weekly. If the distance between the fracture surface and the pulp is great (i.e. no pink dentin), fragment reattachment can proceed at the time of injury, as long as no other injuries (e.g. luxations) contraindicate such an approach, due to difficulty in moisture control. In the latter situation, placement of provisional restorations can be incorporated in the necessary splints and bonding performed at the time of splint removal. The bonding procedure is illustrated in Fig. 6.15.

Treatment strategy for crown fractures with pulpal involvement includes pulpotomy (see Chapter 14 p. 525), provisional restoration and a 3-month observation period to permit formation of a hard tissue barrier at the exposure site; or direct bonding can be performed after pulpotomy

It should be considered that the use of eugenol-containing liners or cements is not recommended on teeth where *dentin/resin* bonding is anticipated, as bonding strength can be reduced (301) presumably due to the complexing action of eugenol with calcium in sound dentin (313). However, the deleterious effect of eugenol-containing provisional cements on *enamel bonding* is presumably eliminated if the bonding surface is cleaned with pumice and etched with phosphoric acid prior to restoration due to the mechanical nature of the bond (314). Thus, a non-eugenol cement is recommended in situations where provisional therapy is indicated (e.g. crown fractures with concomitant luxation injuries and cases of multiple dental injuries).

Fig. 6.16. Reinforcement of fragment bonding

Condition at time of injury
This 20-year-old woman suffered complicated crown fractures of both maxillary central incisors as well as a penetrating lip lesion.

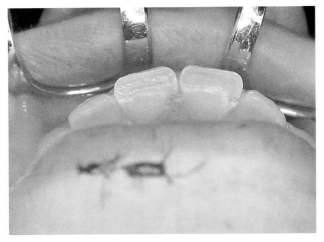 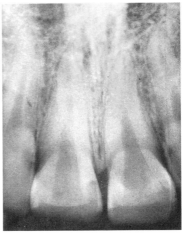

Radiographic examination of penetrating lip lesion

Radiographic examination reveals tooth fragments embedded in the lower lip. The crown fragments were retrieved and bonded. Two smaller fragments were bonded prior to fragment reattachment. Pulpal vitality was maintained.

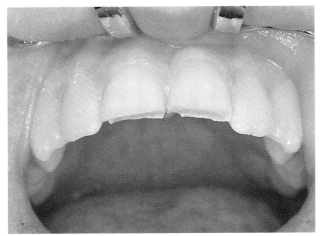 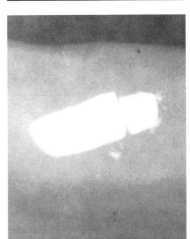

Four-year follow-up control

Clinical and radiographic conditions are normal. There is color harmony between the bonded fragments and the teeth; the fracture lines are just visible. Because of the relatively short half-life (50% re-fracture after fragment reattachment within 5 years), it was decided to reinforce the bonded fragments with veneers.

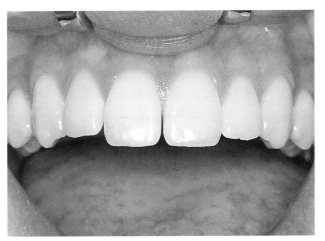 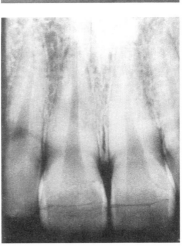

Final restoration

Dicor veneers in place after cementation and at 2-year follow-up. (Technique: Flügge's Dental Laboratory, Copenhagen)

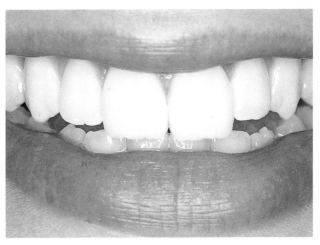 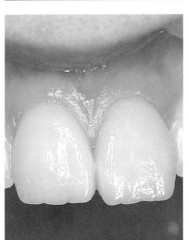

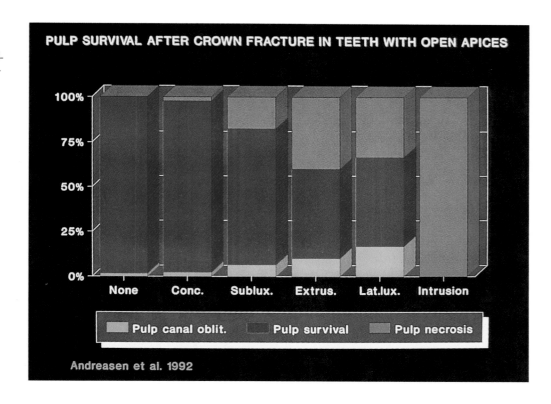

Fig. 6.17.
Pulp survival following crown fracture in the permanent dentition with immature root formation (open apices). From AN-DREASEN ET AL (246). 1992.

Clinical Results of Fragment Reattachment

With respect to the long-term success of fragment reattachment, factors such as pulpal response, esthetics and retention of the fragment should be considered.

PULPAL RESPONSE TO FRAGMENT REATTACHMENT
The reattachment of enamel-dentin crown fragments has not been found to lead to pulpal complications in three larger long-term studies (251-253). The few cases of pulp necrosis and pulp canal obliteration were all found in relation to concomitant luxation injuries. This low complication rate is more likely a response to the injury itself than to the treatment procedure (Figs. 6.17 and 6,18).

Fig. 6.18.
Pulp survival following crown fracture in the permanent dentition with mature root formation (closed apices). From AN-DREASEN ET AL (246) 1992.

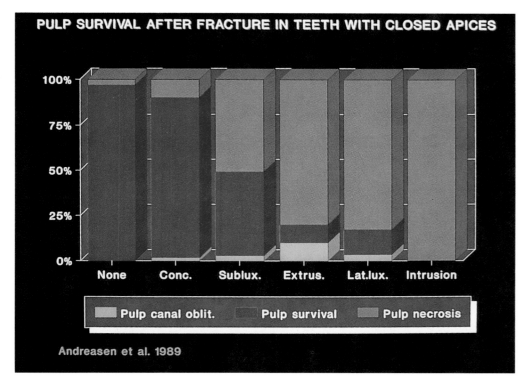

Fig. 6.19.
Esthetic problems following crown fragment reattachment: Discoloration of the composite bonding material at the fracture line.
Left: appearance at the time of fragment bonding of the maxillary left central incisor. Right: appearance one year later. There is discoloration of the bonding material.

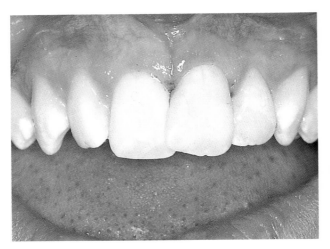
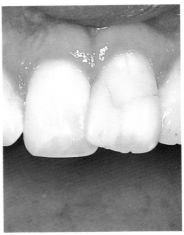

ESTHETICS FOLLOWING FRAGMENT REATTACHMENT

Approximately half of the teeth bonded demonstrate acceptable esthetics at long-term follow-up (251). Esthetic problems at the follow-up controls include discoloration or degradation of the composite bonding material at the fracture line (Figs. 6.19 and 6.21) or discoloration of the incisal fragment with time. The problem of discoloration of the fracture line is most pronounced in earlier cases of bonding, due to discoloration of the catalyst system of the chemically-cured resins used. This problem has been solved in part by the use of light-cured composite materials. Esthetics have also been enhanced by the use of a double chamfer preparation along the fracture line after fragment bonding and restoration with a composite resin (Fig. 6.15).

The problem of fragment discoloration, usually to a mat white color, is presumably due to dehydration of the underlying dentin (280). This is more difficult to manage clinically, as direct composite facings tend not to mask the color disharmony between the tooth and bonded fragment.

FRAGMENT RETENTION

Preliminary results from three Scandinavian studies indicate that 50% of the bonded fragments are lost by the end of the observation period of at least 5 years due primarily to a new trauma or non-physiological use of the restored teeth (251-253). Fragment debonding occurred irrespective of the use of enamel acid etch alone or supplemented with Gluma dentin bonding agent; also irrespective of the use of composite resin along the fracture line for esthetic revision and reinforcement of the restoration. While fragment debonding represents a practical inconvenience, it has no impact on pulpal vitality since debonding occurs as a cohesive failure within the bonding resin and not in dentin. Thus, the fracture surfaces of teeth with debonded fragments are glossy from retained resin plugs within the treated dentin. For this reason, the dentin must be freed of bonded resin, e.g. with a slurry of pure pumice and water, prior to rebonding of fragments.

It would seem that at present reattachment of the original incisal fragment can only be considered as an acceptable semi-permanent anterior restoration whereby gross and surface anatomy are restored perfectly with a material that abrades at a rate identical to adjacent teeth and which does not threaten pulpal vitality (305, 315, 316). Development of new dentin bonding systems and/or resins might provide improved fragment retention.

Fragment reattachment or restoration with a composite build-up are realistic treatment alternatives in the young (pre-teen and teenage) patient groups. These treatments serve to postpone the time of definitive treatment until an age when the gingival marginal contours are relatively stable (i.e. 20 years of age). (Figs. 6.16, 6.20 and 6.21).

Finally, it should be mentioned that laminate veneers under laboratory conditions can restore or even increase the strength of a fractured incisor treated by reattachment of the original fragment to attain the strength of an intact tooth (see later) (280, 281).(Figs 6.16 and 6.20).

Fig. 6.20. Improved esthetics achieved by ceramic veneering after fragment reattachment

Clinical and radiographic condition one year after fragment following an uncomplicated enamel-dentin fracture in a 25-year-old man. Note color harmony between tooth and fragment. Because of porcelain's very low affinity for stain and plaque accumulation, it is necessary to determine shade prior to stain removal, otherwise there is a serious risk that the veneer will always be too light in relation to adjacent teeth.

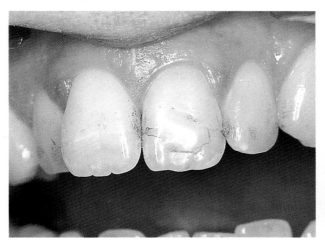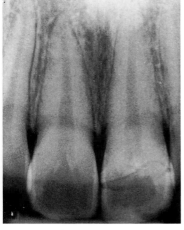

Veneer preparation

There is uniform enamel reduction mesiodistally following the curve of the facial surface and the proximal contacts.

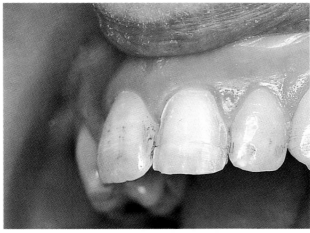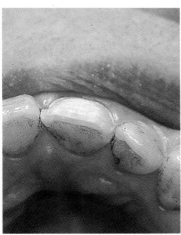

Finished restoration

The veneer in place after cementation. Note the facial "discoloration" incorporated into the surface to mimic tobacco stain, as well as the hypoplastic striae, similar to those seen on the surface of the right central incisor. Note gingival health and harmony of the restoration within the dental arch at the one-year follow-up. (Technique:Flügge's Dental Laboratory, Copenhagen)

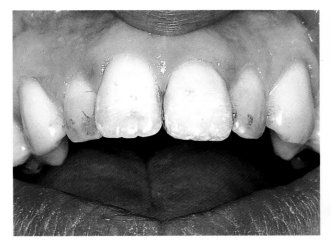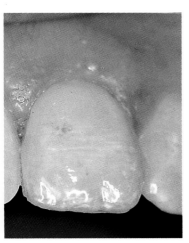

Laminate Veneers in the Treatment of Crown Fractures

INDICATIONS

Clinical experience seems to indicate expanded areas of application for ceramic veneering. Ceramic veneers can be used with advantage in the treatment of traumatic dental injuries in cases of acquired discoloration (pulp necrosis and pulp canal obliteration), crown fractures and crown defects due to developmental disturbances (317), as well as restoration of autotransplanted premolars to the anterior region due to anterior tooth loss (see Chapter 19, p. 682). Furthermore, veneers can be used as an important supplement in the treatment of crown fractures following reattachment of the enamel-dentin fragment. Thus, recent experimental studies demonstrated that fracture strength of fractured incisors with bonded fragments can be increased from half, to equal to or sometimes exceeding the fracture strength of intact teeth if restored with porcelain or cast ceramic veneers respectively, as long as the preparation was limited to enamel (281) (see later). Moreover, the fracture strength of a fractured incisor restored *in vitro* with a cast ceramic veneer alone (i.e. no preliminary composite build-up or fragment reattachment) is on average more than 1.5 times greater than intact control teeth (281). These experimental studies indicate that a conservative treatment approach (i.e. versus full crown coverage) might be justified in restoring esthetics and function to the traumatized anterior dentition and at the same time preserve tooth substance, maintain occlusal relationships and maintain pulpal vitality.

Because of optical properties which are similar to enamel, ceramic veneers have the advantage over direct composite veneering of consistently good esthetic results. Moreover, there is good marginal adaptation, minimal plaque retention, long-term stability with respect to color and anatomy, inherent strength of veneering material and reasonably limited chair time to complete treatment in comparison to direct composite veneering (318-320). Fabrication of ceramic veneers, however, is a technically demanding procedure. There must be a high level of cooperation and communication between patient, dentist and laboratory technician if the patient's subjective and objective functional and esthetic needs are to be fulfilled (321).

CONTRAINDICATIONS

In cases of malposed teeth, where a direct access line of insertion cannot be secured, veneering is not recommended (322, 323). Moreover, ceramic veneers are contraindicated in patients who are bruxers or with parafunctional activity or habits (e.g. nail biters, pipe smokers) (317, 324, 325). Ceramic veneers are fragile and the shearing stresses elicited by such habits may be too great for the veneer to withstand. Moreover, they are contraindicated in teeth that are composed predominantly of dentin and cementum (317, 322). This is due to compromised bonding to dentin with the presently available dentin bonding agents. Finally, teeth showing grey discoloration are very difficult to mask, and the success of ceramic veneers in these cases can be limited (325).

While some reports seem to indicate

acceptable success as long as the bulk of the preparation and margins remain in enamel under experimental conditions (317, 322, 326), preparation into dentin has shown reduced strength (281). Furthermore greater microleakage was recorded at the cervical dentin/composite resin interface than at the cervical enamel/composite interface of bonded ceramic veneers (327).

There has been some debate concerning whether or not enamel should be reduced prior to the taking of impressions (328-332). It would seem that at least gingival health is improved if enamel is reduced in order to diminish the risk of overcontouring of the restoration as well as to provide a well-defined finishing line for the fabrication of the restoration. The resultant accuracy of fit, especially with castable ceramics (333), reduces the need for marginal finishing at the time of cementation and thereby produces a smooth surface which is less plaque-retentive.

PATIENT SELECTION: TREATMENT PROBLEMS TO BE SOLVED

As many crown fractures occur in the younger age groups, the question arises as to when to provide ceramic veneering as a treatment option. The porcelain veneer has been considered a useful cosmetic procedure or for correction of minor functional problems in the young dentition (e.g. rotated or lingually inclined incisors, spacing and defects in mineralization) (321).

If it is decided to build the incisor up in a composite resin prior to veneering (e.g. to achieve uniform ceramic thickness in the final restoration), at least 2 weeks should elapse prior to taking impressions for the veneer to allow for dimensional stability of the composite (334).

In the patients illustrated in Figs. 6.16, 6.20 and 6.21, the fractured crown fragments were bonded and the teeth thereafter veneered. However, experimental results might justify a more direct treatment approach in adult patients (281).

Some situations require earlier definitive treatment. This can be in the situation of congenital enamel malformations where due to their superior esthetic properties and very low plaque retention ceramic veneers can be a realistic treatment option.

In the case of severe trauma leading to

Fig. 6.21. Use of veneer to improve esthetics after fragment reattachment
Clinical appearance after fragment reattachment following a complicated crown fracture in a 9-year-old girl. Six years after treatment, there is discoloration of the composite bonding resin.

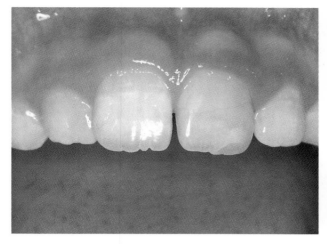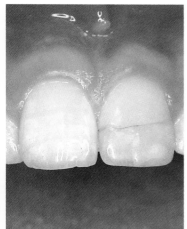

Preparation of tooth
Gingival retraction cord is used to permit a slightly subgingival placement of margins to ensure optimal esthetics. Mounted diamonds used for enamel reduction.

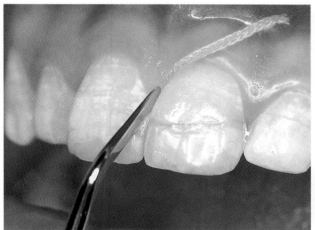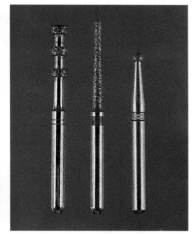

Initial enamel reduction
The incisor is isolated with a dead soft metal matrix strip and the triple cutting diamond is used for initial depth cuts of 0.5 mm facially.

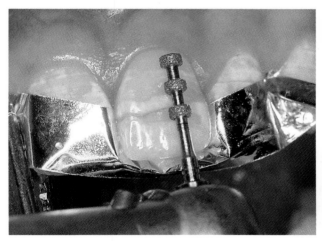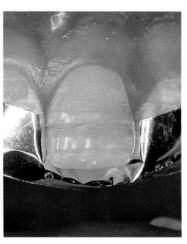

Final enamel reduction
To ensure uniform enamel reduction, the tapered diamond is used to reduce only one-half of the facial surface at a time. Approximately 1 mm is removed incisally to permit optimal porcelain translucency in this region. Finishing lines are enhanced using a round diamond, which also permits additional veneer bulk at the margins.

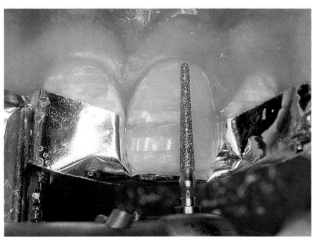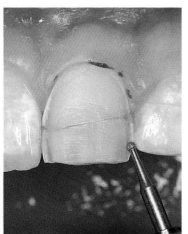

CROWN FRACTURES

Completed preparation
Note uniform tissue reduction following the curve of the tooth. A second cord is placed to ensure adequate tissue retraction, which is removed immediately prior to impression taking, while the first cord is removed once a satisfactory impression has been obtained.

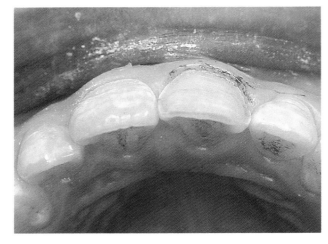
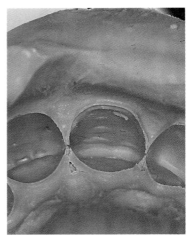

Final restoration
Dicor veneer cemented using a light-activated dual cement (Dicor LAC®) (Technique: Flügge's Dental Laboratory, Copenhagen). Radiographic condition 6 years after injury. Pulp vitality has been maintained.

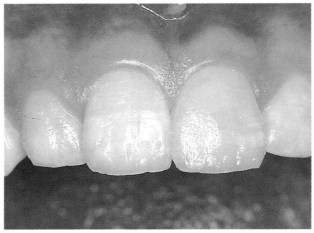
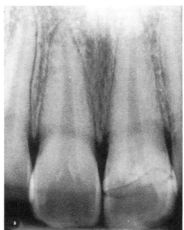

anterior tooth loss, autotransplantation can be a treatment solution. Such teeth can also be restored with veneers (see Chapter 19, p. 682).

Clinical evaluation of porcelain veneers has shown very promising results with respect to longevity of restorations, fractures, and secondary caries (322, 325, 331, 332, 335) (Table 6.1).

Table. 6.1. Long-term survival of ceramic veneer restorations.

Examiner	Observation period months	No. of veneers	Veneer debonding	Veneer fracture	Caries
Calamia et al. (328) 1987	6-36	116	0	3	1
Clyde & Gilmore (322) 1988	30	200	0	2	not reported
Reid & Murray (330) 1988	48	217	29	16	not reported
Jordan et al. (334) 1989	48	72	2	?	0
Strassler & Nathanson (331) 1989	18-42	291	0	5	0
Andreasen et al. (335) 1992	6-36	89	2	0	0
			0	1	0

Table 6.2. Prevalence of pulp necrosis after crown infraction

Examiner	No. of teeth	No. with pulp necrosis
Stålhane & Hedegård (116)1975	656	23 (3.5%)
Ravn (194) 1981	174	0 (0%)

Table 6.3. Prevalence of pulp necrosis after enamel fracture

Examiner	No. of teeth	No. with pulp necrosis
Fiolová & Jurecek (62) 1968	31	0 (0%)
Stålhane & Hedegård (116) 1975	876	2 (0.2%)
Ravn (195) 1981	2862	29 (1%)

Table 6.4. Prevalence of pulp necrosis after crown fracture with exposed dentin

Examiner	No. of teeth	No. with pulp necrosis
Stålhane & Hedegård (116) 1975	413	3 (1%)
Zadik et al. (120) 1979	123	7 (6%)
Ravn (196) 1981	3144	250 (25%)

Prognosis

Permanent Teeth

Follow-up after Trauma

Pulpal sensibility reactions in crown fractured teeth are often lowered immediately after injury (7, 72, 187, 195). Usually 1 to 8 weeks can elapse before a normal pulpal response can be elicited. However, greater observation periods can be required. Pulp testing can usually be carried out during this observation period without removing the temporary restoration (see Chapter 5, p. 206).

Enamel Infractions

The prognosis of isolated infractions with respect to risk of pulp necrosis appears to be very good (Table 6.2). Thus, two studies have shown risks between 0 and 3.5%, which is about the same as for "non-injured control teeth" (193, 195-197); which implies that pulp necrosis in these cases possibly reflects overlooked concussion or subluxation injuries.

Enamel Fractures

In two studies, the risk of pulp necrosis was found to range from 0.2 to 1.0% (Table 6.3). Using the above-mentioned rationale, these figures would imply virtually no risk to the pulp.

Enamel-Dentin Fractures without Pulpal Involvement

The overall risk of pulp necrosis irrespective of the extent of fracture and type of treatment ranges from 1 to 6% (Table 6.4). In this regard, it should be noted that factors, such as associated luxation injuries, stage of root development, type of treatment and extent of fracture exert significant influence upon the risk of pulp necrosis. A detailed study on the combined effects of these factors has been reported by RAVN (196).

With respect to the effect of *stage of root development* on the risk of pulp necrosis after uncomplicated crown fracture with or without concomitant luxation injury, it has been found that teeth with constricted

Table 6.5. Relation between associated luxation injuries to enamel-dentin fractures upon frequency pulp necrosis. After RAVN (196) 1981

	No. of teeth	No. with pulp necrosis
Enamel dentin fracture	3144	100 (3%)
Enamel dentin fracture + concussion	327	19 (6%)
Enamel dentin fracture + subluxation	423	106 (25%)

Table 6.6. Relation between extension of fracture in enamel-dentin fracture upon pulp necrosis. After RAVN (196) 1981

	No. of teeth	No. with pulp necrosis
Small mesial fracture	1034	26 (0.2%)
Comprehensive mesial fracture	435	30 (7%)
Fracture involving the entire incisal edge	1019	38 (0.4%)

Table 6.7. Relation between treatment upon frequency of pulp necrosis in teeth with extensive mesial or distal fractures. After RAVN (196) 1981

	No. of teeth	No. with pulp necrosis
No treatment	24	13 (54%)
Dentin coverage	620	30 (8%)

Table 6.8. Prevalence of pulp canal obliteration and root resorption after crown fracture. After STÅLHANE & HEDEGÅRD (116) 1975

	No. of teeth	No. with pulp canal obliteration	No. with external root resorption
Enamel infraction	174	0 (0%)	0 (0%)
Enamel fracture	876	4 (0.5%)	2 (0.2%)
Enamel and dentin fracture	413	2 (0.5%)	1 (0.2%)

apices have a greater risk of pulp necrosis than do teeth with open apices (316). Furthermore that the extent of periodontal ligament injury as revealed by the *luxation diagnosis* is significantly related to pulp survival after injury (Table 6.5).

Another factor to be considered is the *extent* and *location* of the fracture. Thus, horizontal and proximal superficial (corner) fractures demonstrate a very low frequency of pulp necrosis; whereas deep proximal fractures show increased risk (Table 6.6).

Only a single study has examined the *effect of treatment* (i.e. untreated versus treated crown fractures). A treatment effect was only in operation for deep proximal fractures (Table 6.7). In this connection, *no treatment* was found to be associated with 54% pulp necrosis; whereas *dentinal coverage* resulted in a decrease to 8% (196).

The effect of *time interval* between injury and dentin coverage and subsequent risk of pulp necrosis has yet to be examined.

REATTACHMENT OF THE CROWN FRAGMENT

With respect to pulp survival, fragment retention and esthetics, preliminary findings from a long-term clinical study indicate the following (251):

PULP SURVIVAL

Pulp survival without radiographic change was the predominant finding, whereby only 1 out of 198 bonded incisors (0.5%) developed pulp necrosis and 4 developed pulp canal obliteration (2%). All 5 teeth had suffered concomitant luxation injuries (251).

PULP CANAL OBLITERATION

In one study, pulp canal obliteration (PCO) was analyzed subsequent to crown fractures without associated luxation injury (116) (Table 6.8). The paucity of PCO cases possibly implies non-diagnosed luxation injuries. It seems safe to assume that a crown fracture *per se* does not elicit PCO.

ROOT RESORPTION

In one study, where only crown fractures without associated luxation injuries were examined, root resorption was a rare finding (116) (Table 6.8). Thus, like pulp canal obliteration, root resorption is probably not related to crown fractures *per se*.

Primary Teeth

Treatment of fractured primary teeth presents special problems due to their diminutive size and relatively large pulps. (58, 59).

Treatment of *enamel* and *enamel-dentin fractures* can usually be confined to grinding of sharp enamel edges. In case of extensive loss of tooth substance, the use of stainless steel crowns or retention pin restorations has previously been advocated (58, 59). However, the use of a dentin bonding agent precludes such an approach.

Treatment of *enamel-dentin fractures with pulpal involvement* consists of pulp-capping, pulpotomy or pulpectomy; however, in some cases, the treatment of choice is extraction, due to lack of co-operation of children

Essentials

Terminology (Fig. 6.1)

Enamel infraction
Enamel fracture
Enamel-dentin fracture
Enamel-dentin fracture with pulp exposure

Frequency

Permanent dentition:
  26 to 76% of dental injuries
Primary dentition:
  4 to 38% of dental injuries

Etiology

Usually falls with direct impact on the crown

History

Symptoms

Clinical Examination

Extent of fracture
Pulp exposure
Dislocation of tooth
Reaction to sensibility tests

Radiographic Examination

Size of pulp cavity
Stage of root development
Concomitant root fracture or luxation

Pathology

If the pulp is exposed, pulp inflammation normally confined close to the exposure site

Treatment of Permanent Teeth

Enamel Infraction

TREATMENT
a. Pulpal sensibility control after 6 to 8 weeks

Prognosis:

Pulp necrosis (0 to 3.5%)

Pulp canal obliteration (0%)
Root resorption (0%)

Enamel Fracture (no Dentin exposed)

Treatment

a. Removal of sharp enamel edges
b. Radiographic and sensibility controls
c. Corrective grinding (Fig. 6.11) or restoration with a composite resin

Prognosis:

Pulp necrosis (0.2 to 1.0%)
Pulp canal obliteration (0.5%)
Root resorption (0.2%)

Enamel-Dentin Fracture, no Pulp Exposure

IMMEDIATE (PROVISIONAL) TREATMENT (FIG. 6.14)
a. Place a calcium hydroxide liner (e.g. Dycal®, or Life®) over the exposed dentin and enamel to permit optimal bonding of the restorative material at the time of definitive therapy.
b. Adapt a temporary crown (e.g. acrylic crown). Crown cemented with a non-eugenol containing luting agent. Alternatively, an intermediate composite or epimine restoration can be placed using an acid-etch technique but without preparing the fracture margins (Fig. 6.16).
c . Check the occlusion
d. Control the tooth radiographically and with sensibility tests after 6 to 8 weeks

Prognosis:

Pulp necrosis (1-6%)
Pulp canal obliteration (0%)
Root resorption (0%)

PERMANENT TREATMENT
  Reattachment of the crown fragment (Fig. 6.15)
  Restoration with laminate veneer (Fig. 6.21)
  Restoration with composite resin (see Chapter 16, p. 636)
  Restoration with full crown coverage

Enamel-Dentin Fracture with Pulp Exposure

IMMEDIATE TREATMENT
Exposed pulp tissue is treated by pulp capping, pulpotomy or pulpectomy (see Chapter 14 p. 525)

Treatment of primary teeth

Enamel Infraction

Radiographic control after 6 weeks

Enamel and Enamel-Dentin Fractures

No treatment, selective grinding or composite restoration

Enamel-Dentin Fracture with Pulp Exposure

Usually extraction; however, if the patient is cooperative and physiologic root resorption not too advanced, pulp capping and pulpotomy may be carried out (see Chapter 14 p. 525)

Bibliography

1. ANDREASEN JO. Etiology and pathogenesis of traumatic dental injuries. A clinical study of 1,298 cases. *Scand J Dent Res* 1970;**78:**329-42.

2. SUNDVALL-HAGLAND I. Olycksfallsskador på tänder och parodontium under barna-åren. In: HOLST JJ, NYGAARD ØSTBY B, OSVALDO, eds. *Nordisk Klinisk Odontologi.* Copenhagen: A/S Forlaget for Faglitteratur, 1964: Chapter 11, III:1-40.

3. RAVN JJ, ROSSEN I. Hyppighed og fordeling af traumatiske beskadigelser af tænderne hos københavnske skolebørn 1967/68. *Tandlægebladet* 1969;**78:**1-9.

4. MAGNUSSON B, HOLM A-K. Traumatised permanent teeth in children - a follow-up. I. Pulpal complications and root resorption. *Svensk Tandläkaras Tidning* 1969;**62:**61-70.

5. SUTTON PRN. Transverse crack lines in permanent incisors of Polynesians. *Aust Dent J* 1961;**6:**144-50.

6. SUTTON PRN. Fissured fractures; 2,501 transverse crack lines in permanent incisors. *Aust Dent J* 1969;**14:**18-21.

7. KRÖNCKE A. Über die Vitalerhaltung der gefährdeten Pulpa nach Fraktur von Frontzahn-kronen. *Dtsch Zahnärztebl* 1957;**11:**333-6.

8. HARDWICK JL, NEWMAN PA. Some observations on the incidence and emergency treatment of fractured permanent anterior teeth of children. *J Dent Res* 1954;**33:**730.

9. GELBIER S. Injured anterior teeth in children. A preliminary discussion. *Br Dent J* 1967;**123:**331-5.

10. SOBKOWIAK E-M. Unser Standpunkt zur Versorgung frakturierter jugendlicher Zähne. *Zahnärztl Welt* 1965;**66:**502-9.

11. BODECKER CF. Enamel lamellae. A consultant article. *Oral Surg Oral Med Oral Pathol* 1951;**4:**787-98.

12. ORBAN B. *Oral histology and embryology.* 3rd edn. St. Louis: C V Mosby Company, 1953:124.

13. BRÄNNSTRÖM M. Observations on exposed dentine and the corresponding pulp tissue. A preliminary study with replica and routine histology. *Odontologisk Revy* 1962;**13:**235-45.

14. BRÄNNSTRÖM M, ÅSTRÖM A. A study on the mechanism of pain elicited from the dentin. *J Dent Res* 1964;**43:**619-25.

15. WILLIGER. Zähne und Trauma: *Deutsche Zahnheilkunde in Vorträgen,* No. 16, Verlag von Georg Thieme, Leipzig 1911.

16. DOW PR, Thompson ML. Pulp management for the immature fractured anterior tooth. *J Canad Dent Assoc* 1960;**26:**5-9.

17. KOMINEK J. Úrazy frontálních zubu u detí. *Cs. Stomatol* 1954;239-60.

18. MALONE AJ, MASSLER M. Fractured anterior teeth. Diagnosis, treatment, and prognosis. *Dent Dig* 1952;**58:**442-7.

19. HARRIS SD. Fractured incisors. Primary and permanent. *ASDC J Dent Child* 1954;**21:**205-7.

20. BERK H. Maintaining vitality of injured permanent anterior teeth. *J Am Dent Assoc* 1954;**49:**391-401.

21. FRENTZEN H. Die prothetische Behandlung von Frontzahnfrakturen bei Kindern und Jugendlichen. *Dtsch Stomatol* 1964;**14:**904-11.

22. DUNN NA, EICHENBAUM IW. Diagnosis and treatment of fractured anterior teeth. *J Am Dent Assoc* 1952;**44:**166-72.

23. KISLING E. Om behandlingen af skader som følge af akutte mekaniske traumer på unge permanente incisiver. *Tandlægebladet* 1953;**57:**61-9,109-29.

24. ROTTKE R. Zeitgerechte Behandlung der Schneidezahnfraktur im Wechselgebiss. *Zahnärztl Prax* 1954;**5:**1-4.

25. ANDREWS RG. Emergency treatment of injured permanent anterior teeth. *Dent Clin North Am* 1965;703-10.

26. NOLDEN R. Die konservierende Behandlung der Traumafolgen im Wachstumsalter. *Zahnärztl Welt* 1967;**68:**19-24.

27. RABINOWITCH BZ. The fractured incisor. *Pediatr Clin North Am* 1956;**3:**979-94.

28. NOTERMAN F. Restauration des traumatismes dentaires chez les jeunes. *Rev Belge Stomatol* 1951;**48:**367-81.

29. NOTERMAN F. Les fractures d'incisives en pratique courante. *Rev Belg Sci Dent* 1961;**16:**499-513.

30. CURRY VL. Fractured incisors. *Dent Practit Dent Rec* 1951;**1:**341-6.

31. BROGLIA ML, RE G. Le lesioni traumatiche dei denti permanenti nell'età infantile. *Minerva Stomatatol* 1959;**8:**161-80.

32. SWEET CA. A classification and treatment for traumatized anterior teeth. *ASDC J Dent Child* 1955;**22:**144-9.

33. BRAUER JC. The treatment of children's fractured permanent anterior teeth. *J Am Dent Assoc* 1950;**41:**399-407.

34. BENNETT DT. Traumatised anterior teeth. *Br Dent J* 1963;**115:**346-8,392-4,432-5,487-9.

35. BENNETT DT. Traumatised anterior teeth. *Br Dent J* 1964;**116:**96-8.

36. LENCHNER NH. A diagnosis and treatment plan for traumatized anterior teeth. *ASDC J Dent Child* 1957;**24:**197-205.

37. PALMER JD. Simple emergency treatment of fractured incisors. *Dent Practit Dent Rec* 1969;**20:**102-4.

38. PARRET J, VINCENT R. Fracture de l'incisive centrale permanente entre 7 et 12 ans. *Odont Stomatol Maxillofacial* 1950;**6:**74-7.

39. BROWN WE. The management of injuries to young teeth. *Aust Dent J* 1967;**12:**99-104.

40. TOVERUD G. Traumatiske beskadigelser av incisiver i barnealderen og deres behandling. *Odontologisk Tidskrift* 1947;**55:**71-82

41. ELLIS RG. Treatment of fractured incisors. *Int Dent J* 1953;**4:**196-208.

42. OHLSSON Å. Behandling av olycksfallsskadade incisiver på barn. *Odontologisk Tidskrift* 1957;**65:**105-15.

43. McBRIDE WC. *Juvenile Dentistry.* 5th edn. London: Henry Kimpton, 1952:247-62.

44. ADAMS FR. Traumatized and fractured young teeth. *J Am Dent Assoc* 1944;**31:**241-8.

45. COOKE C, ROWBOTHAM TC. Treatment of injuries to anterior teeth. *Br Dent J* 1951;**91:**146-52.

46. BRUCE RH. Inlays for fractured teeth. *Dent J Aust* 1947;**19:**309-14.

47. PANTKE H. Kronenfrakturen permanenter Frontzähne bei Jugendlichen. *Zahnärztl Prax* 1963;**14:**253-6.

48. RIPA LW, FINN SB. The care of injuries to the anterior teeth in children. In: FINN SB, ed. *Clinical Pedodontics.* 3rd edn. Philadelphia and London: W B Saunders Company, 1967:324-62.

49. HARTSOOK JT. Management of young anterior teeth which have been involved in accidents. *J Am Dent Assoc* 1948;**37:**554-64.

50. RAVN JJ. *Ulykkesskadede fortænder på børn. Klassifikation og behandling.* Copenhagen: Odontologisk Forening, 1966.

51. HORSNELL AM. Everyday procedure. Trauma to the incisor teeth. *Br Dent J* 1952;**93:**105-10.

52. RITZE H. Die Traumen im Frontzahngebiet. *Zahnärztl Prax* 1964;**15:**1-4.

53. STRASSBURG M. Zahnerhaltung nach Trauma im kindlichen Gebiss. *Dtsch Zahnärztl Z* 1968;**23:**1235-43.

54. NEGRO GC. Contributo alla conoscenza dell'eziologia e del trattamento conservativo delle fratture traumatiche dentarie nella età infantile. *Minerva Stomatol* 1967;**16:**165-9.

55. MUGNIER A. Traumatologie dentaire en stomatologie infantile. *Actual Odontostamtol* 1967;**77:**87-119.

56. OVERDIEK HF. Die Versorgung tiefer Kronenfrakturen an bleibenden Frontzähnen bei jugendlichen Patienten. *Zahnärztl Welt* 1956;**11:**56-7.

57. Giusti C. Contributo alla conoscenza delle affezioni traumatiche dei denti. *Minerva Stomatol* 1957;**6**:10-25.

58. Rapp R. Restoration of fractured primary incisor teeth. *Bull Acad Gen Dent* 1968;**2**:6-31.

59. Hawes RR. Traumatized primary teeth. *Dent Clin North Am* 1966;391-404.

60. Ellis RG, Davey RG. *The classification and treatment of injuries to the teeth of children.* 5th edn. Chicago: Year Book Publishers Inc., 1970.

61. Kisling E. Beskadigelser af tænder og deres ophængningsapparat ved akutte mekaniske traumata. In: Toverud G, ed. *Nordisk lærebog i Pedodonti.* Stockholm: Sveriges Tandläkarförbunds Förlagsförening, 1963:266-87.

62. Fialová S, Jurecek B. Úrazy zubu udeti a nase zkusenosti s jejich lécenim. *Prakt Zubni Lék* 1968;**16**:171-6.

63. Berger H. Do fractured incisors migrate? *ASDC J Dent Child* 1964;**27**:178-9.

64. Prophet AS, Rowbotham TC, James PMC. Symposium: Traumatic injuries of the teeth. *Br Dent J* 1964;**116**:377-85.

65. Winter GB. Temporary restoration of fractured incisor teeth. *Br Dent J* 1966;**120**:249-50.

66. Starkey P. The use of self-curing resin in the restoration of young fractured permanent anterior teeth. *ASDC J Dent Child* 1967;**34**:25-9.

67. Stewart DJ. Protective caps for fractured incisors. *Br Dent J* 1957;**102**:404-6.

68. Dana F, Pejrone CA. Uso delle corone fenestrate per la ricostruzione degli incisivi fratturati nei giovani pazienti. *Minerva Stomatol* 1967;**16**:775-80.

69. Glucksman DD. Fractured permanent anterior teeth complicating orthodontic treatment. *J Am Dent Assoc* 1941;**28**:1941-3.

70. Down CH. The treatment of permanent incisor teeth of children following traumatic injury. *Aust Dent J* 1957;**2**:9-24.

71. Dannenberg JL. Emergency covering for a fractured anterior tooth in children. *J Am Dent Assoc* 1965;**71**:853-5.

72. Gaare A, Hagen A, Kanstad S. Tannfrakturer hos barn. Diagnostiske og prognostiske problemer og behandling. *Norske Tannlegeforenings Tidende* 1958;**68**:364-78.

73. Lieban EA. Traumatic injuries to children's teeth. *N Y State Dent J* 1947;**13**:319-34.

74. Lawrence KE. Restoration of fractured anterior teeth for the young patient. *North West Dent* 1965;**44**:269-73.

75. Kelsten LB. Modern methods of managing injuries of children's anterior teeth. *Dent Dig* 1952;**58**:310-5.

76. Kelsten LB. A simple and rapid technic for restoring the fractured young incisor. *J Am Dent Assoc* 1950;**40**:455-6.

77. Magnusson B, Holm A-K, Berg H. Traumatised permanent teeth in children - a follow-up. II. The crown fractures. *Svensk Tandläkaras Tidning* 1969;**62**:71-7.

78. Gausch K, Waldhart E. Zur vitalerhaltenden Therapie der Kronenfrakturen bei Frontzähnen Jugendlicher. *Zahnärztl Welt* 1969;**78**:718-21.

79. Goldstein-Jourdan VB. Contribution a la dentisterie opératioire infantile - Traitement des fractures dentaires chez l'enfant. *Rev Fr Odontostomatol* 1954;**1**:62-70.

80. Noonan MA. A shoulder preparation and veneered gold jacket for fractured young vital permanent incisors. *ASDC J Dent Child* 1955;**22**:167-9.

81. Warnick ME. The use of porcelain-fused-to-gold in the restoration of fractured young permanent anterior teeth. *ASDC J Dent Child* 1962;**29**:3-8.

82. Mumford JM, Goose DH. Anterior crowns for young people. *Dent Practit Dent Rec* 1967;**18**:45-8.

83. Holloway PJ. The basket crown. *Dent Practit Dent Rec* 1953;**4**:308-11.

84. Slotosch H, Eschrich D, Stanka E. Die Versorgung frakturierter Frontzahnkronen mit vitaler Pulpa bei jugendlichen Patienten. *Zahnärztl Welt* 1968;**69**:473-7.

85. Anehill S, Lindahl B, Wallin H. Prognosis of traumatised permanent incisors in children. A clinical-roentgenological after-examination. *Svensk Tandläkaras Tidning* 1969;**62**:367-75.

86. Gelbier S. Stainless-steel preformed crowns in children's dentistry. *Dent Practit Dent Rec* 1965;**15**:448-50.

87. Humphrey WP, Fleege F. Restoration of fractured anterior teeth with steel crowns. *ASDC J Dent Child* 1953;**20**:178-9.

88. Dogon L. A technic for long term temporary repair of fractured anterior teeth. *ASDC J Dent Child* 1968;**35**:322-7.

89. Goldstein PM. Retention pins are friction locked without use of cement. *J Am Dent Assoc* 1966;**73**:1103-6.

90. McCormich EM. Use of stainless steel pins in the esthetic repair of fractured anterior teeth. *Dent Dig* 1968;**74**:218-20.

91. Sutter W. Frakturierte Frontzahn-Ecke bei Kindern. *Schweiz Monatsschr Zahnheilk* 1957;**67**:823.

92. Dietz WH. Means of saving mutilated teeth. *J Prosthet Dent* 1961;**11**:967-72.

93. Johnson DF. Anterior tooth fracture repair using Addent 12. *Dent Dig* 1968;**74**:340-2.

94. Kanter JC, Kanter EL. A restoration for fractured anterior teeth. *Dent Dig* 1964;**70**:159-63.

95. Liatukas EL. Branched pin restoration of anterior teeth with one penetration into tooth structure. *J Am Dent Assoc* 1969;**78**:1010-2.

96. Watson RJ. Pin retention in pedodontics. *ASDC J Dent Child* 1968;**35**:476-82.

97. Starkey P. Personal communication, 1971.

98. Laswell HR, Welk DA, Regenos JW. Attachment of resin restorations to acid pretreated enamel. *J Am Dent Assoc* 1971;**82**:558-63.

99. Kreter F. Klinik und Therapie extraalveolärer Frontzahnfrakturen. *Zahnärztl Prax* 1967;**18**:257-60.

100. Hogeboom FE. *Practical pedodontia or juvenile operative dentistry and public health dentistry.* 5th edn. St. Louis: CV Mosby Company, 1946:288-314.

101. Engelhardt JP. Die prothetische Versorgung des traumatisch geschädigten Jugendgebisses aus klinischer Sicht. *Zahnärztl Welt* 1968;**69**:264-70.

102. Marxkors R. Die prothetische Versorgung traumatisch geschädigter Frontzähne Jugendlicher. *Dtsch Zahnärztebl* 1965;**19**:74-6.

103. Brown WE. The management of injuries to young teeth. *J Dent Assoc South Afr* 1963;**18**:247-51.

104. Crabb HSM. Direct acrylic restorations in fractured incisors. Their use and limitations. *Int Dent J* 1952;**3**:10-2.

105. Wilbur HM. Management of injured teeth. *J Am Dent Assoc* 1952;**44**:1-9.

106. Vest G. Über die Behandlung von Unfallschäden des Gebisses mit Kronen- und Brüchenprothesen bei Jugendlichen. *Schweiz Monatsschr Zahnheilk* 1941;**51**:369-79.

107. Hampson EL. Fractured anterior teeth. *Dent Practit Dent Rec* 1950;**1**:34-41.

108. Voss R. Die Möglichkeiten der prothetischen Versorgung von Traumafolgen im Wachstumsalter. *Zahnärztl Welt* 1967;**68**:11-5.

109. Olsen NH. The family dentist and injured teeth in children. *Practical Dental Monographs.* Chicago: Year Book Medical Publishers, Inc, 1964:1-29.

110. Law DB. Prevention and treatment of traumatized permanent anterior teeth. *Dent Clin N Am* 1973;**66**:431-50.

111. Andreasen JO, Ravn JJ. Epodemiology of tramatic dental injuries to primary and permanent teeth in a Danish population sample. *Int J Oral Surg* 1972;**1**:235-39.

112. Hedegård B, Stålhane I. A study of traumatized permanent teeth in children aged 7-15 years. Part I. *Swed Dent J*

1973;**66**:431-50.

113. RAVN JJ. Dental injuries in Copenhagen school children, school years 1967-1972. *Community Dent Oral Epidemiol* 1974;**2**:231-45.

114. DOMINKOVICĖ T. Total reflection in tooth substance and diagnosis of cracks in teeth: A clinical study. *Swed Dent J* 1977;**1**:163-72.

115. GUTZ DP. Fractured permanent incisors in a clinic population. *ASDC J Dent Child* 1971;**38**:94-121.

116. STÅLHANÉI, HEDEGÅRD B. Traumatized permanent teeth in children aged 7-15 years. Part II. *Swed Dent J* 1975;**68**:157-69.

117. MACKO DJ, GRASSO JE, POWELL EA, DOHERTY NJ. A study of fractured anterior teeth in a school population. *ASDC J Dent Child* 1979;**46**:130-3.

118. ANDREASEN JO, SUNDSTRÖM B, RAVN JJ. The effect of traumatic injuries to primary teeth on their permanent successors. I. A clinical and histologic study of 117 injured permanent teeth. *Scand J Dent Res* 1971;**79**:219-83.

119. CLAUSEN BR, CRONE AS. To tilfælde af kronefraktur på permanente tænder som følge af traume på tilsvarende primære tænder. *Tandlægebladet* 1973;**77**:611-5.

120. ZADIK D, CHOSACK A, EIDELMAN E. The prognosis of traumatized permanent anterior teeth with fracture of the enamel and dentin. *Oral Surg Oral Med Oral Pathol* 1979;**47**:173-5.

121. GARBEROGLIO R, BRÄNNSTRÖM M. Scanning electron microscopic investigation of human dentinal tubules. *Arch Oral Biol* 1976;**21**:355-62.

122. CVEK M, CLEATON-JONES PE, AUSTIN JC, ANDREASEN JO. Pulp reactions to exposure after experimental crown fractures in adult monkeys. *J Endod* 1982;**8**:391-7.

123. MICHON FJ, CARR RF. Repair of a coronal fracture that involved the pulp of a deciduous incisor report of case. *J Am Dent Assoc* 1978;**87**:1416-7.

124. BARRETT BE, O'MULLANE D. Movement of permanent incisors following fracture. *J Irish Dent Assoc* 1973;**19**:145-8.

125. MJÖR IA. Histologic demonstration of bacteria subjacent to dental restorations. *Scand J Dent Res* 1977;**85**:169-74.

126. MJÖR IA. Bacteria in experimentally infected cavity preparations. *Scand J Dent Res* 1977;**85**:599-605.

127. QVIST J, QVIST V, LAMBJERG-HANSEN H. Bacteria in cavities beneath intermediary base materials. *Scand J Dent Res* 1977;**85**:313-9.

128. ERIKSEN HM, LEIDAHL TI. Monkey pulpal response to composite resin restorations in cavities treated with various cleansing agents. *Scand J Dent Res* 1979;**87**:309-17.

129. BUONOCORE MG. *The use of adhesives in dentistry.* Illinois: CC Thomas, 1975.

130. LASWELL HR, WELK DA, REGENOS JW. Attachment of resin restorations to acid pretreated enamel. *J Am Dent Assoc* 1972;**82**:558-63.

131. GOURION GRE. Une nouvelle méthode de restauration des fractures d'angles incisifs. Etude comparative des forces d'adhesion developpees entre une resine auto-polymerisante et l'email dentaire traite a l'acide orthophosphorique. *Rev Odontostomatol* 1972;**19**:19-25.

132. ROBERTS MW, MOFFA JP. Restoration of fractured incisal angles with an ultraviolet-light-activated sealant and a composite resin - a case report. *ASDC J Dent Child* 1972;**39**:364-5.

133. STAFFANOU RS. Restoration of fractured incisal angles. *J Am Dent Assoc* 1972;**84**:146-50.

134. WARD GT, BUONOCORE MG, WOOLRIDGE ED. Preliminary report of a technique using Nuva-seal in the treatment and repair of anterior fractures without pins. *N Y State Dent J* 1972;**38**:264-74.

135. BUONOCORE MG, DAVILA J. Restoration of fractured anterior teeth with ultraviolet-light-polymerized bonding materials: a new technique. *J Am Dent Assoc* 1973;**86**:1349-54.

136. DOYLE WA. Acid etching in pedodontics. *Dent Clin North Am* 1973;**17**:93-104.

137. HELLE A, SIRKKANEN R, EVÄLAHTI M. Repair of fractured incisal edges with UV-light polymerized and self-polymerized fissure sealants and composite resins. Two-year report of 93 cases. *Proc Finn Dent Soc* 1975;**71**:87-90.

138. HINDING JH. The acid-etch restoration: a treatment for fractured anterior teeth. *ASDC J Dent Child* 1973;**40**:21-4.

139. LEE HL Jr, ORLOWSKI JA, KOBASHIGAWA A. In vitro and in vivo studies on a composite resin for the repair of incisal fractures. *J Calif Dent Assoc* 1973;**1**:42-7.

140. ULVESTAD H, KEREKES K, DANMO C. Kompositkronen. En ny type semipermanent krone. *Norske Tannlægeforenings Tidende* 1973;**83**:281-4.

141. GÖLAND U, KOCH G, PAULANDER J, RASMUSSEN C-G. Principer for "självretinerende" plastmaterial jämte nogra användingsområden. *Tandläkartidningen* 1974;**66**:109-14.

142. MEURMAN JH, HELMINEN KJ. Repair of fractured incisal edges with ultraviolet-light activated fissure sealant and composite resin. *Proc Finn Dent Soc* 1974;**70**:186-90.

143. OPPENHEIM MN, WARD GT. The restoration of fractured incisors using a pit and fissure sealant resin and composite material. *J Am Dent Assoc* 1974;**89**:365-8.

144. RAVN JJ, NIELSEN LA, JENSEN IL. Plastmaterialer til restaurering af traumebeskadigede incisiver. En foreløbig redegørelse. *Tandlægebladet* 1974;**78**:233-40.

145. RAVN JJ, NIELSEN LA, JENSEN IL. Plastmateriale til restaurering af traumebeskadigede incisiver. Fortsatte observationer. *Tandlægebladet* 1976;**80**:185-6.

146. THYLSTRUP A. Ætsteknik og plastmaterialer anvendt som semipermanent erstatning på traumatiserede fortænder. *Tandlægebladet* 1974;**78**:225-32.

147. McLUNDIE AC, MESSER JG. Acid-etch incisal restorative materials. A comparison. *Br Dent J* 1975;**138**:137-40.

148. MANNERBERG F. Etsningsteknik ved klas IV restaurationer. Några synpunkter. *Tandläkartidningen* 1975;**67**:735-40.

149. RULE DC, ELLIOTT B. Semi-permanent restoration of fractured incisors in young patients. A clinical evaluation of one 'acid-etch' technique. *Br Dent J* 1975;**139**:272-5.

150. SCHEER B. The restoration of injured anterior teeth in children by etch-retained resin. A longitudinal study. *Br Dent J* 1975;**139**:465-8.

151. BROWN JP, KEYS JC. The clinical assessment of two adhesive composite resins. *J Dent* 1976;**4**:179-282.

152. KOCH G, PAULANDER J. Klinisk uppföljning av compositrestaureringar utförda med emaljetsningsmetodik. *Swed Dent J* 1976;**69**:191-6.

153. SHEYKHOLESLAM Z, OPPENHEIM M, HOUPT MI. Clinical comparison of sealant and bonding systems in the restoration of fractured anterior teeth. *J Am Dent Assoc* 1977;**95**:1140-4.

154. HILL FJ, SOETOPO. A simplified acid-etch technique for the restoration of fractured incisors. *J Dent* 1977;**5**:207-12.

155. JORDAN RE, SUZUKI M, GWINNETT AJ, HUNTER JK. Restoration of fractured and hypoplastic incisors by the acid etch resin technique: a three-year report. *J Am Dent Assoc* 1977;**95**:795-803.

156. LUTZ F, OCHSENBEIN H, LÜSCHER B. Nachkontrolle von 1¼ jährigen Adhäsivfüllungen. *Schweiz Monatsschr Zahnheilk* 1977;**87**:125-36.

157. RAU G. Klinische Erfahrungen mit der adhäsiven Restauration nach dem Nuva-System. *Zahnärztl Welt* 1977;**86**:296-304.

158. SMALES RJ. Incisal angle adhesive resins: a two-year clinical survey of three materials. *Aust Dent J* 1977;**22**:267-71.

159. STOKES AN, BROWN RH. Clinical evaluation of the restoration of fractured incisor teeth by an acid-etch retained composite resin. *N Z Dent J* 1977;**73**:31-3.

160. WATKINS JJ, ANDLAW RJ. Restoration of fractured incisors with an ultra-violet light-polymerised composite resin: a clini-

cal study. *Br Dent J* 1977;**142**:249-52.

161. FUKS AB, SHAPIRA J. Acid-etch/composite resin restoration of fractured anterior teeth. *J Prosthet Dent* 1977;**37**:639-42.

162. FUKS AB, SHAPIRA J. Acid-etch/composite resin restoration of fractured anterior teeth: Part II. *J Prosthet Dent* 1978;**39**:637-9.

163. WEGELIN H. Die Behandlung traumatisch geschädigter Frontzähne. *Schweiz Monatsschr Zahnheilk* 1978;**88**:623-9.

164. GWINNET AJ. Structural changes in enamel and dentin of fractured anterior teeth after acid conditioning in vivo. *J Am Dent Assoc* 1973;**86**:117-22.

165. JÖRGENSEN KD, SHIMOKOBE H. Adaptation of resinous restorative materials to acid etched enamel surfaces. *Scand J Dent Res* 1975;**83**:31-6.

166. JÖRGENSEN KD. Contralateral symmetry of acid etched enamel surfaces. *Scand J Dent Res* 1975;**83**:26-30.

167. ASMUSSEN E. Penetration of restorative resins into acid etched enamel. I. Viscosity, surface tension and contact angle of restorative resin monomers. *Acta Odontol Scand* 1977;**35**:175-82.

168. ROBERTS MW, MOFFA JP. Repair of fractured incisal angles with an ultraviolet-light-activated fissure sealant and a composite resin: two-year report of 60 cases. *J Am Dent Asssoc* 1973;**87**:888-91.

169. CRIM GA. Management of the fractured incisor. *J Am Dent Assoc* 1978;**96**:99-100.

170. BROSE J, COOLEY R, MOSER JB, MARSHAL GW, GREENER EH. In vitro strength of repaired fractured incisors. *Dent J* 1976;**45**:273-7.

171. BRÄNNSTRÖM M, NYBORG H. Pulpal reaction to composite resin restorations. *J Prosthet Dent* 1972;**27**:181-9.

172. ERIKSEN HM. Protective effect of different lining materials placed under composite resin restorations in monkeys. *Scand J Dent Res* 1974;**82**:373-80.

173. STANLEY HR, GOING RE, CHAUNCEY HH. Human pulp response to acid pretreatment of dentin and to composite restoration. *J Am Dent Assoc* 1975;**91**:817-25.

174. VOJINOVIC O, NYBORG H, BRÄNNSTRÖM M. Acid treatment of cavities under resin fillings: bacterial growth in dentinal tubules and pulpal reactions. *J Dent Res* 1973;**52**:1189-93.

175. RETIEF DH, AUSTIN JC, FATTI LP. Pulpal response to phosphoric acid. *J Oral Pathol* 1974;**3**:114-22.

176. KARJALAINEN S, FORSTEN L. Sealing properties of intermediary bases and effect on rat molar pulp. *Scand J Dent Res* 1975;**83**:293-301.

177. HEYS DR, HEYS RJ, COX CF, AVERY JK. Pulpal response to acid etching agents. *J Michigan Dent Assoc* 1976;**58**:221-32.

178. MACKO DJ, RUTBERG M, LANGELAND K. Pulpal response to the application of phosphoric acid to dentin. *Oral Surg Oral Med Oral Pathol* 1978;**45**:930-46.

179. SUZUKI M, GOTO B, JORDAN RE. Pulpal response to pin placement. *J Am Dent Assoc* 1973;**87**:636-40.

180. ULVESTAD H. A 5-year evaluation of semipermanent composite resin crowns. *Scand J Dent Res* 1978;**86**:163-8.

181. BROWN JP, KEYS JC. The clinical assessment of two adhesive composite resins. *J Dent* 1976;**4**:279-82.

182. STANLEY HR, SWERDLOW H, BUONOCORE MG. Pulp reactions to anterior restorative materials. *J Am Dent Assoc* 1967;**75**:132-41.

183. PLANT CG. The effect of polycarboxylate cement on the dental pulp. *Br Dent J* 1970;**129**:424-6.

184. TRUELOVE EL, MITCHELL DF, PHILLIPS RW. Biologic evaluation of a carboxylate cement. *J Dent Res* 1971;**50**:166.

185. JENDRESEN MP, TROWBRIDGE HO. Biologic and physical properties of a zinc polycarboxylate cement. *J Prosthet Dent* 1972;**28**:264-71.

186. KOPEL HM, BATTERMAN SC. The retentive ability of various cementing agents for polycarbonate crown. *ASDC J Dent Child* 1976;**43**:333-9.

187. BARKIN PR. Time as a factor in predicting the vitality of traumatized teeth. *ASDC J Dent Child* 1973;**40**:188-92.

188. PALMER JD. The care of fractured incisors and their restoration in children. *Dent Pract* 1971;**21**:395-400.

189. ASMUSSEN E. Factors affecting the color stability of restorative resins. *J Dent Res* (Special Issue A) 1981;**60**:(Abstract)1088.

190. WILLIAMS HA, GARMAN TA, FAIRHURST CW, ZWEMER JD, RINGLE RD. Surface characteristics of resin-coated composite restorations. *J Am Dent Assoc* 1978;**97**:463-7.

191. SIMONSEN RJ. *Clinical applications of the acid etch technique.* Chicago: Quintessence Publishing Co. Inc., 1978.

192. SCHIÖDT M, LARSEN V, BESSERMANN M. Oral findings in glassblowers. *Community Dent Oral Epidemiol* 1980;**8**:195-200.

193. BEDI R. The use of porcelain veneers as coronal splints for traumatised anterior teeth in children. *Restorative Dentistry* 1989;*August*:55-8.

194. RAVN JJ. Follow-up study of permanent incisors with enamel craks as a result of an acute trauma. *Scand J Dent Res* 1981;**89**:117-23.

195. RAVN JJ. Follow-up study of permanent incisors with enamel fractures as a result of acute trauma. *Scand J Dent Res* 1981;**89**:213-7.

196. RAVN JJ. Follow-up study of permanent incisors with enamel-dentin fractures after acute trauma. *Scand J Dent Res* 1981;**89**:355-65.

197. ANDREASEN FM, VESTERGAARD PEDERSEN B. Prognosis of luxated permanent teeth - the development of pulp necrosis. *Endod Dent Traumatol* 1985;**1**:207-20.

198. ANDREASEN FM, BROHOLM FAHRNER A, BORUM M, ANDREASEN JO. Long-term prognosis of crown fractures treated by reattachment of the original fragment using the Gluma dentin bonding system. 1992. Manuscript in preparation.

199. BRÄNNSTRÖM M. Dentin and pulp in restorative dentistry. Nacka, Sweden: Dental Therapeutics AB, 1981. 127 pp.

200. JUNG OJ. The value of radiographs in the preparation of teeth for crowns. *Proceedings of 3rd International Congress of Maxillofacial Radiology*, Kyoto, Japan, 1974.

201. ANDREASEN FM, ANDREASEN JO. Diagnosis of luxation injuries. The importance of standardized clinical, radiographic and photographic techniques in clinical investigations. *Endod Dent Traumatol* 1985;**1**:160-9.

202. ANDREASEN FM, YU Z, THOMSEN BL. The relationship between pulpal dimensions and the development of pulp necrosis after luxation injuries in the permanent dentition. *Endod Dent Traumatol* 1986;**2**:90-8.

203. LUNDY T, STANLEY HR. Correlation of pulpal histopathology and clinical symptoms in human teeth subjected to experimental irritation. *Oral Surg, Oral Med, Oral Pathol* 1969;**27**:187-201.

204. VOJINOVIC Q, NYBORG H, BRÄNNSTRÖM M. Acid treatment of cavities under resin fillings: bacterial growth in dentinal tubules and pulp reactions. *J Dent Res* 1973;**52**:1189-93.

205. OLGART L, BRÄNNSTRÖM M, JOHNSON G. Invasion of bacteria into dentinal tubules. Experiments in vivo and in vitro. *Acta Odontol Scand* 1974;**32**:61-70.

206. VONGSAVAN N, MATTHEWS B. The permeability of cat dentine *in vivo* and *in vitro*. *Archs oral Biol* 1991;**36**:641-6.

207. VONGSAVAN N, MATTHEWS B. Fluid flow through cat dentine *in vivo*. *Archs Oral Biol* 1992;**37**:175-85.

208. VONGSAVAN N, MATTHEWS B. Changes in pulpal blood flow and in fluid flow through dentine produced by autonomic and sensory nerve stimulation in the cat. *Proc Finn Dent Soc* 1992;**8**:(Suppl I):491-7.

209. VONGSAVAN N, MATTHEWS B. Changes in the rate of fluid flow through exposed dentine produced by sympathetic and inferior alveolar nerve stimulation in anesthetized cats. *J Physiol (London)* 1993: In press.

210. MATTHEWS B. Sensory physiology: a reaction. *Proc Finn Dent Soc* 1992;**8**:*(Suppl I)*:529-32.

211. MATTHEWS B. Personal communication 1992.

212. COX CF. Effects of adhesive materials on the pulp. Presented at the International Symposium on Adhesives in Dentistry, Creighton University, Omaha, Nebraska, 11-13 July 1992. *Operative Dentistry* 1992; *Supplement* 5:156-76.

213. HEIDE S, MJÖR IA. Pulp reactions to experimental exposures in young permanent monkey teeth. *Int Endod J* 1983;**16**:11-9.

214. INGBER JS. Forced eruption: Part II. A method of treating nonrestorable teeth - periodontal and restorative considerations. *J Periodont* 1976;**47**:203-16.

215. WAERHAUG J, ZANDER HA. Reaction of gingival tissues to self-curing acrylic restorations. *J Am Dent Assoc* 1957; **54**:760-8.

216. ZANDER HA. Pulp response to restorative materials. *J Am Dent Assoc* 1959;**59**:911-5.

217. BRÄNNSTRÖM M, NYBORG H. The presence of bacteria in cavities filled with silicate cement and composite resin materials. *Swed Dent J* 1971;**64**:149-55.

218. BRÄNNSTRÖM M, NYBORG H. Cavity treatment with a microbicidal fluoride solution: growth of bacteria and effect on the pulp. *J Prosthet Dent* 1973;**30**:303-10.

219. BRÄNNSTRÖM M, NYBORG H. Pulp reaction to a temporary zinc oxide/eugenol cement. *J Prosthet Dent* 1976;**35**:185-91.

220. FRANK RM. Reactions of dentin and pulp to drugs and restorative materials. *J Dent Res* 1975;**54**:*(Spec Issue B)*:176-87.

221. HEYS RJ, HEYS DR, COX CF, AVERY JK. The histological effects of composite resin materials on the pulps of monkey teeth. *J Oral Pathol* 1977;**6**:63-81.

222. HEYS RJ, HEYS DR, COX CF, AVERY JK. Histopathologic evaluation of three ultraviolet-activated composite resins on monkey pulps. *J Oral Pathol* 1977;**6**:317-30.

223. QVIST J, QVIST V, LAMBJERG-Hansen H. Bacteria in cavities beneath intermediary base materials. *Scand J Dent Res* 1977;**85**: 313-9.

224. MEJÀRE B, MEJÀRE I, EDWARDSSON S. Bacteria beneath composite restorations - a culturing and histobacteriological study. *Acta Odontol Scand* 1979;**37**:267-75.

225. BERGENHOLTZ G, COX CF, LOESCHE WJ, SYED SA. Bacterial leakage around dental restorations: its effect on the dental pulp. *J Oral Pathol* 1982;**11**:439-50.

226. COX CF, BERGENHOLTZ G, FITZGERALD M, et al. Capping of the dental pulp mechanically exposed to the oral microflora - a 5 week observation of wound healing in the monkey. *J Oral Pathol* 1982;**11**:327-39.

227. HEYS RJ, HEYS DR, COX CF, AVERY JK. Experimental observations on the biocompatibility of composite resins. In: SMITH DC, WILLIAMS DF, eds. *Biocompatibility of dental materials* Vol. III Boca Raton: CRC Press Inc., 1982: 131-50.

228. TORSTENSON B, NORDENVALL KJ, BRÄNNSTRÖM M. Pulpal reaction and microorganisms under Clearfil Composite Resin in deep cavities with acid etched dentin. *Swed Dent J* 1982;**6**:167-76.

229. BROWNE RM, TOBIAS RS, CROMBIE IK, PLANT CG. Bacterial microleakage and pulpal inflammation in experimental cavities. *Int Endod J* 1983;**16**:147-55.

230. COX CF, BERGENHOLTZ G, HEYS DR, SYED SA, FITZGERALD M, HEYS RJ. Pulp capping of dental pulp mechanically exposed to oral microflora: a 1-2 year observation of wound healing in the monkey. *J Oral Pathol* 1985;**14**:156-68.

231. LEIDAHL TI, ERIKSEN HM. Human pulpal response to composite resin restorations. *Endod Dent Traumatol* 1985;**1**:66-8.

232. BROWNE RM, TOBIAS RS. Microbial microleakage and pulpal inflammation: a review. *Endod Dent Traumatol* 1986;**2**:177-83.

233. GERKE DC. Pulpal integrity of anterior teeth treated with composite resins. A long-term clinical evaluation. *Australian Dent Assoc* 1988;**33**;133-5.

234. HÖRSTED PB, SIMONSEN A-M, LARSEN MJ. Monkey pulp reactions to restorative materials. *Scand J Dent Res* 1986;**94**:154-63.

235. COX CF. Biocompatibility of dental materials in the absence of bacterial infection. *Oper Dent* 1987;**12**:146-52.

236. COX CF, KEALL CL, KEALL HJ, OSTRO E, BERGENHOLTZ G. Biocompatability of surface-sealed dental materials against exposed pulps. *J Prosthet Dent* 1987;**57**:1-8.

237. CVEK M, GRANATH L, CLEATON-JONES P, AUSTIN J. Hard tissue barrier formation in pulpotomized monkey teeth capped with cyanoacrylate or calcium hydroxide for 10 and 60 minutes. *J Dent Res* 1987;**66**:1166-74.

238. FUSAYAMA T. Factors and prevention of pulp irritation by adhesive composite resin restorations. *Quintessence Int* 1987;**18**:633-41.

239. COX CF, WHITE KC, RAMUS DL, FARMER JB, SNUGGS HM. Reparative dentin: factors affecting its deposition. *Quintessence Int* 1992;**23**:257-70.

240. BERGENHOLTZ G. Bacterial leakage around dental restorations - impact on the pulp. In: ANUSAVICE KJ, ed. *Quality evaluation of dental restoration.Criteria for Placement and Replacement of Dental Restorations* Chicago: Quintessence Publishing Co, 1989: pp. 243-54.

241. BRÄNNSTRÖM M, NYBORG H. Pulpal reaction to polycarboxylate and zinc phosphate cements used with inlays in deep cavity preparations. *J Am Dent Assoc* 1977;**94**:308-10.

242. BRÄNNSTRÖM M, VOJINOVIC O, NORDENVALL K-J. Bacteria and pulpal reactions under silicate cement restorations. *J Prosthet Dent* 1979;**41**:290-4.

243. WATTS A. Bacterial contamination and the toxicity of silicate and zinc phosphate cements. *Br Dent J* 1979;**146**:7-13.

244. COX CF, WHITE KC. Biocompatability of amalgam on exposed pulps employing a biological seal. *J Dent Res* 1992;**71**: *(AADR Abstracts)*: Abstract no. 656.

245. WARFVINGE J, BERGENHOLTZ G. Healing capacity of human and monkey dental pulps following experimentally-induced pulpitis. *Endod Dent Traumatol* 1986;**2**:256-62.

246. KISLING E. Om behandlingen af skader som følge af akute mekaniske traumer på unge permanente incisiver. *Tandlægebladet* 1953;**57**:61-9, 109-29.

247. GAARE A, HAGEN A, KANSTAD S. Tannfrakturer hos barn, Diagnostiske og prognostiske problemer og behandling. *Norske Tannl Tid* 1958;**68**:364-78.

248. STÅLHANE I, HEDEGÅRD B. Traumatized permanent teeth in children aged 7-15. Part II. *Svenske Tandläk-T* 1975;**68**:157-69.

249. ZADIK D, CHOSAK A, EIDELMAN E. The prognosis of traumatized permanent incisor teeth with fracture of the enamel and dentin. *Oral Surgery Oral Medicine Oral Pathology* 1979; **47**:173-5.

250. ANDREASEN FM, BROHOLM FAHRNER A, BORUM M, ANDREASEN JO. Long-term prognosis of crown fractures: pulp survival after injury. 1992: Manuscript in preparation.

251. ANDREASEN FM, BROHOLM FAHRNER A, BORUM M, ANDREASEN JO. Long-term prognosis of crown fractures treated by reattachment of the original fragment using a dentin bonding agent. 1993: Manuscript in preparation.

252. ENGELHARDTSEN S, STØRMER K. Long-term prognosis of crown fractures treated by reattachment of the original fragment using enamel acid-etch retention. Report from Scandinavian Trauma Study Group. 1993: Manuscript in preparation.

253. LINDH-STRÖMBERG U, CVEK M, MEJARE I. Long-term prognosis of crown fractures treated by reattachment of the original fragment using enamel acid-etch retention. Report from Scandinavian Trauma Study Group. 1992: Manuscript in preparation.

254. BERGENHOLTZ G. Iatrogenic injury to the pulp in dental procedures: Aspects of pathogenesis, management and preventive measures. *Int Dent J* 1991;**41**:99-110.

255. MCCOMB D. Comparison of physical properties of commer-

cial calcium hydroxide lining cements. *J Am Dent Assoc* 1983;**107**:610-13.

256. HWAS M, SANDRICK JL. Acid and water solubility and strength of calcium hydroxide bases. *J Am Dent Assoc* 1984;**108**:46-8.

257. COX CF, WHITE KC, RAMUS DL, FARMER JB, SNUGGS HM, DELGADO AA. Tunnel defects in dentine bridges: their formation following direct pulp capping. Manuscrpit in preparation.

258. REINHARDT JW, CHALKEY Y. Softening effects of bases on composite resins. *Clinical Preventive Dentistry* 1983;**5**:9-12.

259. HÖRSTED PB, SIMONSEN A-M, LARSEN MJ. Monkey pulp reactions to restorative materials. *Scand J Dent Res* 1986;**94**:154-63.

260. RETIEF DH. Dentin bonding agents: a deterrent to microleakage? In: ANUSAVICE KJ, ed. *Quality evaluation of dental restorations. Criteria for placement and replacement.* Chicago: Quintessence Publishing Co., Inc. 1989: pp.185-98.

261. BUONOCORE MG. A simple method of increasing the adhesion of acrylic filling materials to enamel surfaces. *J Dent Res* 1955;**34**:849.

262. BUONOCORE MG. Adhesives in the prevention of caries. *J Am Dent Assoc* 1973;**87**:1000-5.

263. BUONOCORE MG, SHEYKHOLESLAM Z, GLENA R. Evaluation of an enamel adhesive to prevent marginal leakage: an in vitro study. *J Dent Child* 1973;**40**:119-24.

264. MUNKSGAARD EC, HØJTVED L, JØRGENSEN EHW, ANDREASEN FM, ANDREASEN JO. Enamel-dentin crown fractures bonded with various bonding agents. *Endod Dent Traumatol* 1991;**7**:73-7.

265. FUSAYAMA T. *New concepts in operative dentistry* Chicago: Quintessence Publishing Co., 1980.

266. INOKOSHI S, IWAKU M, FUSAYAMA T. Pulpal response to a new adhesive restorative resin. *J Dent Res* 1982;**61**:1014-9.

267. KANKA J. A method for bonding to tooth structure using phosphoric acid as a dentin-enamel conditioner. *Quintessence Int* 1991;**22**:285-90.

268. WHITE KC, COX CF, KANCA III J, FARMER JB, RAMUS DL, SNUGGS HM. Histologic pulpal response of acid etching vital dentin. *J Dent Res* 1992;**71**:(AADR Abstracts):188, Abstr. no. 658.

269. ASMUSSEN E, UNO S. Adhesion of restorative resins to dentin: chemical and physico-chemical aspects. Proceedings of the International Symposium on Adhesives in Dentistry, Creighton University, Omaha, Nebraska, 11-13 July 1991. *Operative Dentistry* 1992; *Supplement* 5:68-74.

270. HANSEN EK. Effect of Gluma in acid-etched dentin cavities. *Scand J Dent Res* 1987;**95**:181-4.

271. ASMUSSEN E, BOWEN RL. Effect of acid pretreatment on adhesion to dentin mediated by Gluma. *J Dent Res* 1987;**66**:1386-8.

272. ASMUSSEN E, BOWEN RL. Adhesion to dentin mediated by Gluma: Effect of pretreatment with various amino acids. *Scand J Dent Res* 1987;**95**:521-5.

273. NATHANSON D, AMIN F, ASHAYERI N. Dentin etching vs. priming: effect on bond strength *in vitro*. *J Dent Res* 1992;**71**: *(AADR abstracts)*: Abstract no. 1192.

274. NATHANSON D, L'HERAULT R, FRANKL S. Dentin etching vs priming: surface element analysis. *J Dent Res* 1992;**71**: *(AADR abstracts)*: Abstract no. 1193.

275. ANDREASEN FM, YU Z, THOMSEN BL, ANDERSEN PK. The occurrence of pulp canal obliteration after luxation injuries in the permanent dentition. *Endod Dent Traumatol* 1987;**3**:103-15.

276. HENRY PJ, BISHOP BM, PURT RM. Fiber-reinforced plastics for interim restorations. *Quintessence of Dental Technology (QDT)* 1990/1991:110-23.

277. OIKARINEN K, ANDREASEN JO, ANDREASEN FM. Rigidity of various fixation methods used as dental splints after tooth dislocation. *Endod Dent Traumatol* 1992;**8**:113-9.

278. BEECH DR. Adhesion to teeth: Principles and mechanism. In: SMITH DC, WILLIAMS DF, eds. *Biocompatibility of dental materials*, Vol. II p. 87. Boca Raton: CRC Press 1982.

279. SILVERSTONE CM. The structure and characteristics of human dental enamel. In: SMITH DC, WILLIAMS DF, eds. *Biocompatibility of dental materials*, Vol. I, p. 39. Boca Raton: CRC Press 1982.

280. ANDREASEN FM, DAUGAARD-JENSEN J, MUNKSGAARD EC. Reinforcement of bonded crown fractures with porcelain laminate veneers. *Endod Dent Traumatol* 1991;**7**:78-83.

281. ANDREASEN FM, FLÜGGE E, DAUGAARD-JENSEN J, MUNKSGAARD EC. Treatment of crown fractured incisors with laminate veneer restorations. *Endod Dent Traumatol* 1992;**8**:30-35.

282. SIMONSEN RJ. Restoration of a fractured central incisor using original tooth fragment. *J Am Dent Assoc* 1982;**105**:646-8.

283. MADER C. Restoration of a fractured anterior tooth. *J Am Dent Assoc* 1978;**96**:113-5.

284. TENNERY TN. The fractured tooth reunified using the acid-etch bonding technique. *Texas Dent J* 1978;**96**:16-7.

285. SIMONSEN RJ. Traumatic fracture restoration: an alternative use of the acid-etch techique. *Quintess Int* 1979;**10**:15-22.

286. STARKEY PE. Reattachment of a fractured fragment to a tooth. *J Indiana Dent Assoc* 1979;**58**:37-8.

287. MCDONALD RE, AVERY DR. *Dentistry for the child and adolescent* 4th edn. St. Louis: CV Mosby Co., 1983, pp. 436-8.

288. AMIR E, BAR-GIL B, SARNAT H. Restoration of fractured immature maxillary central incisors using the crown fragments. *Pediatr Dent* 1986;**8**:285-8.

289. DEAN JA, AVERY DR, SWARTZ ML. Attachment of anterior tooth fragments. *Pediatr Dent* 1986;**8**:139-43.

290. RICCITIELLO F, CARLOMAGNO F, INGENITO A, DE FAZIO P. Nuova metodica di reincollamento di un frammento di corona su dente trattato endodonticamente. *Min Stom* 1986;**35**:1057-63.

291. DIANGELIS AJ, JUNGBLUTH MA. Restoration of an amputated crown by the acid-etch technique. *Quintessence International* 1987;**18**:829-33.

292. LIEW VP. Re-attachment of original tooth fragment to a fractured crown. Case report. *Aust Dent J* 1988;**33**:47-50

293. EHRMANN EH. Restoration of a fractured incisor with exposed pulp using original tooth fragment: report of case. *J Am Dent Assoc* 1989;**118**:183-5.

294. KOTSANOS N. Restoring fractured incisors with the original fragments. Abstract, *12th Congress of the International Association of Dentistry for Children*, Athens, Greece, June 1989. p. 83.

295. BARATIERI LN, MONTEIRO S, JR. CALDEIRA DE ANDRADA MA. The "sandwich" technique as a base for reattachment of dental fragments. *Quintessence International* 1991;**22**:81-5.

296. ASMUSSEN E, MUNKSGAARD EC. Formaldehyde as bonding agent between dentin and restorative resins. *Scand J Dent Res* 1984;**92**:480-3.

297. MUNKSGAARD EC, ASMUSSEN E. Bond strength between dentin and restorative resins mediated by mixtures of HEMA and glutaraldehyde. *J Dent Res* 1984;**63**:1087-90.

298. MUNKSGAARD EC, HANSEN EK, ASMUSSEN E. Effect of five adhesives on adaptation of resin in dentin cavities. *Scand J Dent Res* 1984;**92**:187-91.

299. MUNKSGAARD EC, IRIE M, ASUMSSEN E. Dentin-polymer bond promoted by Gluma and various resins. *J Dent Res* 1985; **64**:1409-11.

300. FINGER WJ, OHSAWA M. Effect of bonding agents on gap formation in dentin cavities. *Operative Dentistry* 1987;**12**:100-4.

301. HANSEN EK, ASMUSSEN E. Comparative study of dentin adhesives. *Scand J Dent Res* 1985;**93**:280-7.

302. MUNKSGAARD EC, IRIE M. Dentin-polymer bond established by Gluma and tested by thermal stress. *Scand J Dent Res* 1987;**95**:185-90.

303. ALBERS HF (ed). Dentin-resin bonding. *ADEPT Report* 1990;**1**:33-41.

304. RINDUM JL, MUNKSGAARD EC, ASMUSSEN E, HØRSTED P, ANDREASEN JO. Pålimning af tandfragmenter efter fraktur: en foreløbig redegørelse. *Tandlægebladet*1986;**90**:397-403.

305. ANDREASEN FM, RINDUM JL, MUNKSGAARD EC, ANDREASEN JO. Bonding of enamel-dentin crown fractures with GLUMA^R and resin. Short communication. *Endod Dent Traumatol* 1986;**2**:277-80.

306. HÖRSTED-BINDSLEV P. Monkey pulp reactions to cavities treated with Gluma Dentin Bond and restored with a microfilled composite. *Scand J Dent Res* 1987;**95**:347-55.

307. SETCOS JC. Dentin bonding in perspective. *Am J Dent* 1988;1 (Spec.Issue):173-5.

308. ROULET J-F, BLUNCK U. Effectiveness of dentin bonding agents. *Scanning Microscopy* 1989;**3**:1013-22.

309. EICK JD. Materials interaction with smear layer. *Proc Finn Dent Soc* 1992;**8**(Suppl I).

310. EICK JD, COBB CM, CHAPPELL RP, SPENCER P, ROBINSON SJ. The dentin surface - its influence on dentin adhesion. Part I. *Quintessence Int* 1991; **22**:967-77.

311. GWINNETT AJ, KANCA III J. The micromorphology of the bonded dentin interface and its relationship to bond strength. *Am J Dent* 1992;**5**:73-7.

312. ANDREASEN FM, STEINHARDT U, BILLE M, MUNKSGAARD EC. Reattachment of dentin-enamel tooth fragments. Comparison of bond strengths using various dentin bonding agents. An experimental study. 1993. Submitted for publication.

313. ROTBERG SJ, DE SHAZER DO. The complexing action of eugenol on sound dentin. *J Dent Res* 1966;**45**:307-10.

314. SCHWARTZ R, DAVIS R, MAYHEW R. The effect of a ZOE temporary cement on the bond strength of a resin luting cement. *Am J Dent* 1990;**3**:28-30.

315. ANDREASEN FM, ANDREASEN JO, RINDUM JL, MUNKSGAARD EC. Preliminary clinical and histological results of bonding dentin-enamel crown fragments with GLUMA technique. Presented at the *Nordic Association of Pedodontology*, Annual Congress, Bergen, Norway, June 1988.

316. ANDREASEN JO, ANDREASEN FM. *Essentials of Traumatic Injuries to the Teeth*, Copenhagen: Munksgaard, 1990. 168 pp.

317. GARBER DA, GOLDSTEIN RE, FEINMAN RA. *Porcelain laminate veneers* Chicago: Quintessence Publishing Co., Inc. 1988. 136 pp.

318. SMITH DC, PULVER F. Aesthetic dental veneering materials. *Int Dent J* 1982;**32**:223-39.

319. WALLS AWG, MURRAY JJ, McCABE JF. Composite laminate veneers: a clinical study. *J Oral Rehab* 1988;**15**:439-54.

320. MEUNINGHOFF LA, O'NEAL SJ, RAMUS DL. Six months evaluation of clinical esthetic veneers. *J Dent Res* 1990;**69**:Abstr.no.1542.

321. McLEAN JW. Ceramics in clinical dentistry. *Br Dent J* 1988;**164**:187-94.

322. CLYDE JS, GILMOUR A. Porcelain veneers: a preliminary review. *Br Dent J* 1988;**164**:9-14.

323. NASEDKIN JN. Current perspectives on esthetic restorative dentistry. Part I. Porcelain laminates. *J Canad Dent Assoc* 1988;**54**:248-55.

324. QUINN F, McCONNELL RJ, BYRNE D. Porcelain laminates: a review. *Br Dent J* 1986;**161**:61-5.

325. ANDREASEN FM, FLÜGGE E, DAUGAARD-JENSEN J, MUNKSGAARD EC. Reinforcement of crown fractured incisors with laminate veneer restorations. Presented at the *Nordic Pedodontic Association*, Turku, Finland, August 15, 1992.

326. DOERING JV, JENSEN ME, SHETH J, TOLLIVER D, CHAN DCN. Fracture resistance of resin-bonded etched porcelain full veneer crowns. *J Dent Res* 1987;**66**:207 (Abstr. no. 803).

327. TJAN AHL, DUNN JR, SANDERSON IR. Microleakage patterns of porcelain and castable ceramic laminate veneers. *J Prosthet Dent* 1989;**61**:276-82.

328. PLANT CG, THOMAS GD. Do we need to prep porcelain veneers? *Br Dent J* 1987;**163**:231-4.

329. CALAMIA JR, CALAMIA S, LEMLER J, HAMBURG M, SCHERER W. Clinical evaluation of etched porcelain laminate veneers: Results at (6 months - 3 years). *J Dent Res* 1987;**66** (Spec Iss):245 (Abstr.no. 1110).

330. NORDBØ H. Individuelle porselenslaminater - et alternativ til kompositfasader og kroner? *Norske Tannlaegeforenings Tid* 1987;**97**:194-200.

331. REID JS, MURRAY MC, POWER SM. Porcelain veneers - a four-year follow-up. *Restorative Dentistry* 1988;*August*:60-6.

332. STRASSLER HE, NATHANSON D. Clinical evaluation of etched porcelain veneers over a period of 18 to 42 months. *Esthetic Dent* 1989;**1**:21-8.

333. TAY WM, LYNCH E, AUGER D. Effects of some finishing techniques on cervical margins of porcelain laminates. *Quint Int* 1987;**18**:599-602.

334. OLIVA RA, LOWE JA. Dimensional stability of composite used as a core material. *J Prosthet Dent* 1986;**56**:554-61.

335. JORDAN RE, SUZUKI M, SENDA A. Four year recall evaluation of labial porcelain veneer restorations. *J Dent Res* 1989;**68** (Spec Iss):240 (Abstr. no. 544).

CHAPTER 7

Crown-Root Fractures

J. O. ANDREASEN & F. M. ANDREASEN

Terminology, Frequency and Etiology

A crown-root fracture is defined as a fracture involving enamel, dentin, and cementum. The fractures may be grouped according to pulpal involvement into *uncomplicated* and *complicated*.

In most classification systems, this type of injury is not recognized as a special entity and is, therefore, classified as either a crown or a root fracture. In the authors' material, however, crown-root fractures comprised 5% of injuries affecting the permanent dentition and 2% in the primary dentition (1).

The most common etiologic factors are injuries caused by falls, bicycle and auto- mobile accidents and foreign bodies striking the teeth (1).

Crown-root fractures in the anterior region are usually caused by *direct trauma* (see Chapter 3, p. 162). The direction of the impacting force determines the type of fracture. A frontal blow results in the typical fracture line shown in Fig. 7.1. In the posterior regions, fractures of the buccal or lingual cusps of premolars and molars may occur (2, 21). These fractures extend below the gingival crevice, often without pulp exposure (uncomplicated). (Fig. 7.2). The causes of such injuries are often *indirect trauma* (see Chapter 3, p. 162).

For the sake of completeness, it should be mentioned that crown-root fractures can also have an iatrogenic etiology, such

Fig. 7.1.
Complicated crown-root fracture of a right central incisor due to direct trauma. A. Clinical condition. B. Lateral view of crown portion after removal. Note extension below gingival crevice lingually.

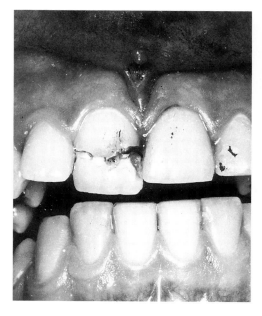
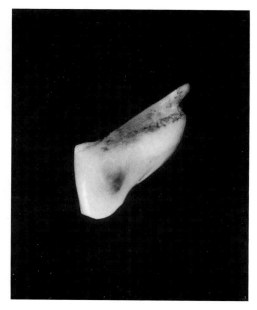

Fig. 7.2

A and B. Uncomplicated crown-root fractures involving lingual cusps in the maxilla and buccal cusps in the mandible (arrows) due to forceful occlusion from a blow to the chin. Note that the fractures of the lingual cusps in the maxilla correspond to the fractures of the buccal cusps in the mandible.

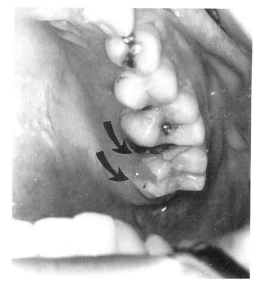
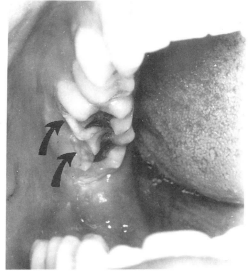

Fig. 7.3.

Complicated crown-root fractures of right second and first premolars (arrow) following indirect trauma (blow to the chin). A. Minimal displacement of fragments in the first premolar. B. Lateral view of extracted first premolar.

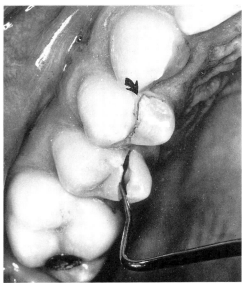
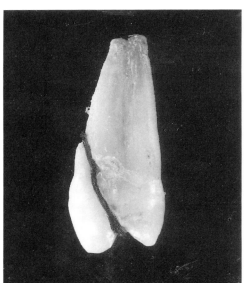

as longitudinal crown-root fractures, especially in the premolar and molar regions, caused by lateral pressure during root filling procedures, cementation of posts, corrosion of posts or improperly designed restorations (22-33). The clinical and radiographic signs of these fractures have recently been described (54).

Clinical Findings

Most commonly, the fracture line begins a few millimeters incisal to the marginal gingiva on the facial aspect of the crown, following an oblique course below the gingival crevice orally. The fragments are usually only slightly displaced, the coronal fragment being kept in position by fibers of the periodontal ligament on the oral aspect (Fig. 7.3).

Displacement of the coronal fragment is often minimal, which explains why these fractures are frequently overlooked, particularly in the posterior regions (Fig. 7.3).

In rare cases, a crown-root fracture may occur prior to eruption of the permanent tooth due to a trauma transmitted by displacement of a primary incisor (55).

The fracture line is usually *single*, but *multiple* fractures can occasionally be seen (Fig. 7.4, A). A rare type of injury is a vertical fracture running along the axis of the tooth (34) (Fig. 7.4, B), or deviating in a mesial or distal direction.

Crown-root fractures of anterior teeth often expose the pulp in fully erupted teeth, while fractures of teeth in earlier stages of eruption can be uncomplicated.

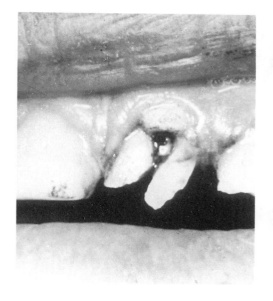 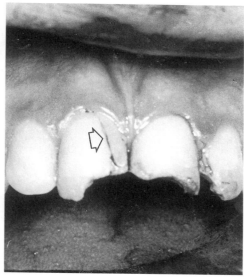

Fig. 7.5.
Schematic drawings of radiographic orientation in a complicated crown-root fracture A. The normal projection angle is almost perpendicular to the fracture surface. B. Radiographic determination of the lingual part of the fracture is obscured due to the perpendicular relationship between fracture line and central x-ray beam.

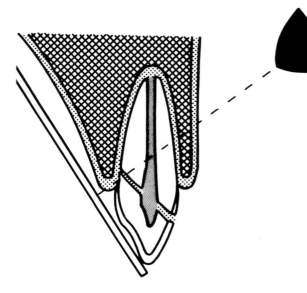 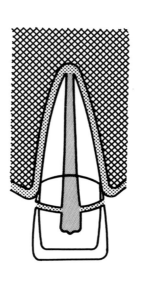

Symptoms are normally few, even with pulp exposure, and are usually limited to slight pain due to mobility of the crown fragment during mastication.

Radiographic Findings

Radiographic examination of crown-root fractures following the usual course seldom contributes to the clinical diagnosis, as the oblique fracture line is almost perpendicular to the central beam (Fig. 7.5). Radiographic determination of the oral limit of the fracture is frequently unsuccessful due to close proximity of the fragments at this level. On the other hand, the facial limit is always visible (Fig. 7.6).

Vertical fractures are easily demonstrated if oriented in a facio-oral direction.

This also applies to superficial vertical fractures deviating in a mesial or distal direction (chisel fractures) (Fig. 7.7). However, vertical root fractures running in a mesio-distal direction are seldom disclosed radiographically (Fig. 7.10).

Pathology

Communication from the oral cavity to the pulp and periodontal ligament in these fractures permits bacterial invasion and subsequent inflammation (3-5).

Early histological changes consist of acute pulpal inflammation located close to the fracture area, caused by invasion of bacteria into the fracture line (56) (Fig. 7.8). Later, proliferation of marginal gingival epithelium into the pulpal chamber

CROWN-ROOT FRACTURES

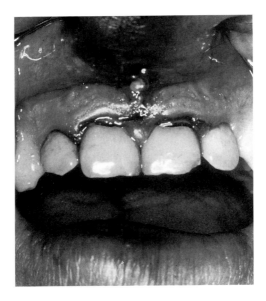
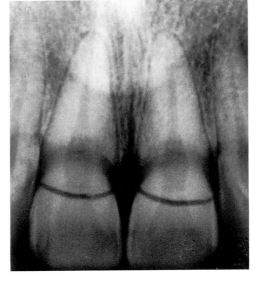

can be seen (Figs. 7.9 and 7.10). Repair of the fracture by deposition of osteo-dentin along the fracture line is exceptionally rare (5-7) (Fig. 7.11).

Treatment

Emergency treatment can include stabilization of the coronal fragment with an acid-etch/resin splint to adjacent teeth (Fig. 7.12). Despite contamination from saliva via the fracture line to the pulp, the tooth will generally remain symptom-free. However, it is essential that definitive treatment is begun within a few days after injury. In case of multiple uncomplicated crown-root fractures in the premolar and molar region, immediate provisional treatment can include removal of loose fragments and coverage of exposed supragingival dentin with glass ionomer cement.

Vertical crown-root fractures must generally be extracted. However, it should be mentioned that cases have been reported where bonding of the coronal fragment has led to consolidation of the intraalveolar part of the fracture (58,59). The type of healing in these cases has not yet been established.

Finally, it should be mentioned that in the case of vertical fractures of *immature permanent incisors*, the fractures are usually incomplete, stopping at or slightly apical to the level of the alveolar crest. These fractures are amenable to orthodontic extrusion, whereby the level of the fracture is brought to a level where pulp capping and restoration are possible.

Definitive conservative therapy in the *permanent dentition* comprises one of four different treatment modalities. The choice is determined primarily by exact information on the site and type of fracture, but cost and complexity of treatment can be deciding factors (Table 7.1). In the following, conservative treatment of various

Fig. 7.7.
Radiographic demonstration of longitudinal crown-root fractures. A. Complicated crown-root fracture running along the axis of a left primary incisor. B. Vertical complicated longitudinal crown-root fracture affecting a right central incisor. C. Uncomplicated crown-root fracture located in the mesial part of a right central incisor (chisel fracture).

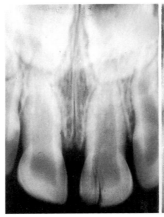
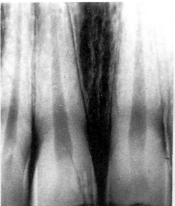
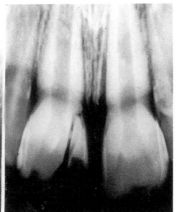

Fig. 7.8.
Early histologic reactions following complicated crown-root fracture of a left central incisor. A. Clinical condition. The tooth was extracted 4 days after injury. B. Low-power view of sectioned incisor. Interruption of the pulp tissue at the fracture site is an artifact. x 3. C. A marked acute inflammation is present close to the fracture site, while only slight inflammation is found more apically. x 75. D. Incomplete fracture extending halfway through the dentin. x 20.

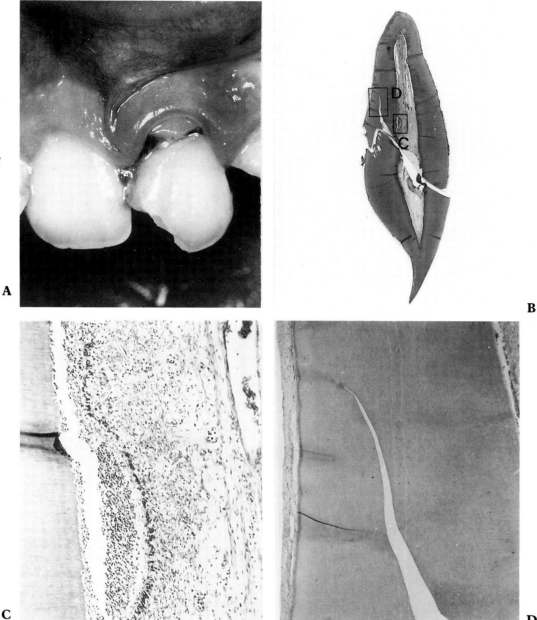

A

B

C

D

types of crown-root fractures will be described.

Removal of Coronal Fragment and Supragingival Restoration

Treatment principle. To allow gingival healing (presumably with formation of a long junctional epithelium), whereafter the coronal portion can be restored (Fig. 7.13).

In regard to restoration the following procedures can be used: bonding the original tooth fragment, where the subgingival portion of the fragment has been removed, composite build-up using dentin and en-

amel bonding agents; or full crown coverage.

Pulpal considerations are identical to those that apply to treatment of crown fractures (see Chapter 6).

Indication. This procedure should be limited to superficial fractures that do not involve the pulp (i.e. chisel fractures).

Treatment procedure. The loose fragment is removed as soon as possible after injury. Rough edges along the fracture surface below the gingiva may be smoothed with a chisel. The remaining crown is temporarily restored supragingivally (Fig. 7.14). Optimal oral hygiene should be maintained during the healing period (e.g. daily chlorhexidine rinsing). Once gingival

Fig. 7.9.
Late histologic reactions following uncomplicated crown-root fracture of a right central incisor. The tooth was left untreated and extracted 3 weeks after injury. A. Low-power view of sectioned incisor. x 3. B. Proliferation of connective tissue into the fracture line. x 75. C. Marked inflammation in the coronal part of the pulp. x 30.

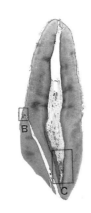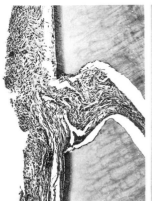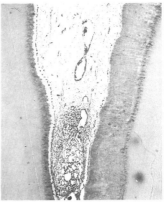

Table: 7.1. Comparison between various treatment modalities of crown-root fractures

Procedure	Indications	Advantages	Disadvantages
Fragment removal only	Superficial fractures (chisel fractures)	Easy to perform. Definitive restoration can be completed soon after injury.	Long-term prognosis has not been established.
Fragment removal and gingivectomy (sometimes ostectomy)	Fractures where denudation of the fracture site does not compromise esthetics (i.e. fractures with palatal extension)	Relatively easy procedure. Restoration can be completed soon after injury.	The restored tooth may migrate labially. Health of palatal gingiva not optimal.
Orthodontic extrusion of apical fragment	All types of fractures, assuming that reasonable root length can be achieved	Stable position of the restored tooth. Optimal gingival health★.	Technically time consuming procedure, with later completion of treatment.
Surgical extrusion of apical fragment	All types of fractures supposing that a reasonable long root length can be secured	Rapid procedure. Stable position of the tooth. The method allows inspection of the root for extra fractures.	Small risk of the root resorption and marginal breakdown of periodontium.

★Note: Cervical gingival fibers must be incised once tooth is at desired position to prevent return of tooth to original position.

CHAPTER 7

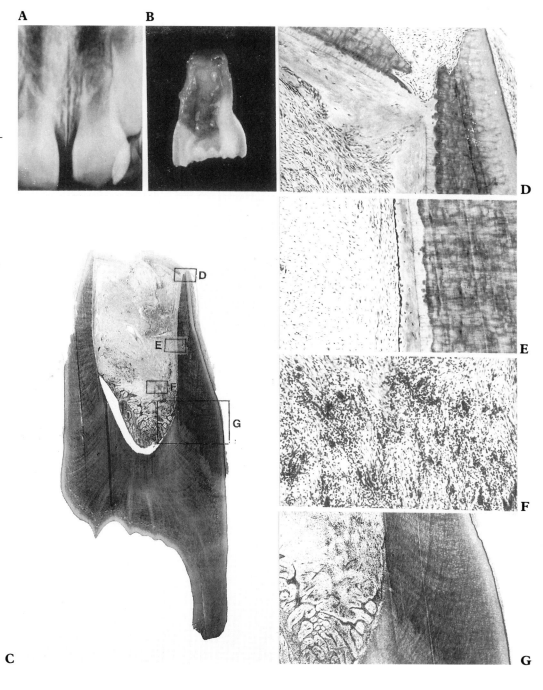

Fig. 7.10.
Late histologic reactions follow-ing complicated crown-root frac-ture of a left central incisor. The tooth was traumatized 2 months earlier. A. Radiograph taken at the time of extraction. The frac-ture line is not seen on the radio-graph due its mesio-distal orienta-tion. B. Lingual fragment. C. Low-power view of sectioned tooth. x 8. D. Apex of the root is fractured and forced into the pulp. Note pulpal repair with new dentin. x 75. E. Deposition of cellular dentin x 75. F. In-flammatory changes in the coro-nal part of the pulp. x 75. G. Proliferation from the cuff epithe-lium. x 30. From NEIMANN-SØRENSEN & PINDBORG (4) 1955.

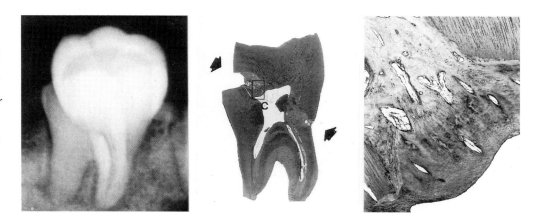

Fig. 7.11.
Healing of a crown-root fracture with calcified tissue. Radiograph of a right second molar taken 10 months after crown-root fracture. The tooth was immobilized after the injury. Fourteen months after injury, the tooth was extracted for prosthetic reasons. Note that the fracture communicating with the oral cavity is united by new dentin with vascular inclusions. x 30. From LOSEE (7) 1948.

Fig. 7.12.
Emergency treatment of a crown-root fracture of a right central incisor. The coronal fragment was stabilized using an acid-etch/resin splint.

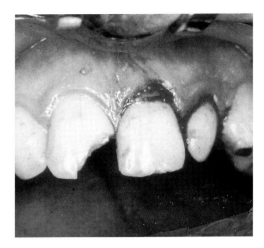
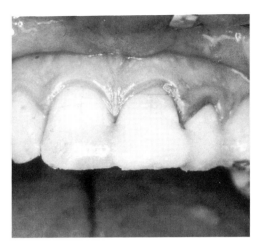

Fig. 7.13.
Removal of the coronal fragment and supragingival restoration.

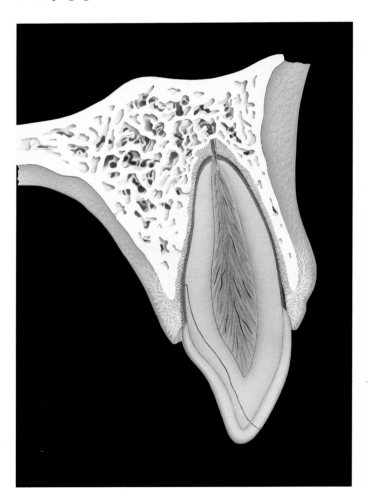
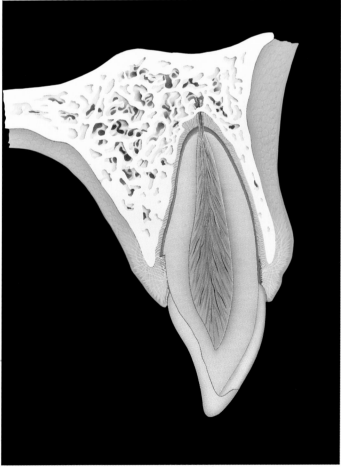

Fig. 7.14. Removal of the coronal fragment and supragingival restoration
This 16-year-old girl has suffered a crown-root fracture which has exposed the palatal root surface. The clinical condition is shown after fragment removal.

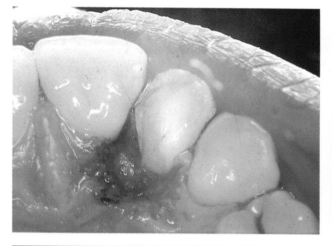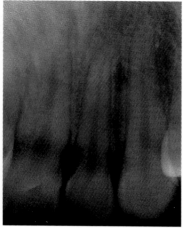

Condition 1 week later
The palatal fragment has been removed and the exposed root dentin smoothed with a chisel; the exposed dentin covered with calcium hydroxide and a temporary crown. Two weeks later creeping reattachment is seen and the palatal of the crown restored with a dentin-bonded composite resin restoration.

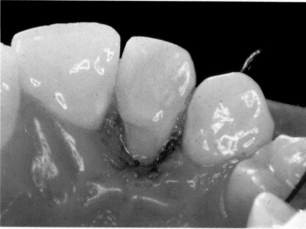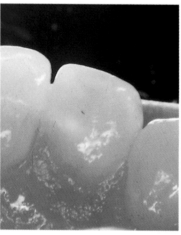

Follow-up
Clinical and radiographic condition 4 years after treatment. (Courtesy of Dr. B. MALMGREN, Eastman Institute, Stockholm, Sweden).

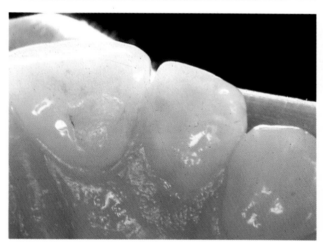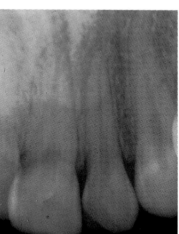

healing is seen (after 2-3 weeks), the crown can be restored with a dentin and enamel-bonded composite.

Reattachment of an incisal fragment of a crown-root fractured tooth basically follows the same principles as reattachment of the incisal fragment of a crown-fractured incisor (see Chapter 6). However, due to the subgingival placement of the fracture margin palatally, certain preliminary steps must be followed (Fig. 7.15). The subgingival aspect of the incisal fragment should be reduced to a sharp,

smooth margin ending at the free gingival margin and then bonded to the remaining tooth (Fig. 7.15).

Cost-benefit. While the pulp has been shown to respond well to this form of conservative treatment, the immediate shortcoming is frequent refracture of the reattached fragment or loss of the composite resin build-up due to the steep, non-retentive inclination of the fracture surface. Thus, these treatments can possibly best be described as provisional until definitive treatment can be provided.

CROWN-ROOT FRACTURES

Fig. 7.15. Condition before fragment bonding
The subgingival part of the fragment is reduced with diamonds and aluminum oxide discs. As the facio oral dimension of the fracture surface exceeded 5 mm and thereby exceeding the maximum depth of light penetration by a curing lamp (2.5 mm from each direction), a self-curing composite resin is chosen.

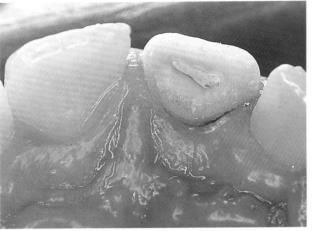
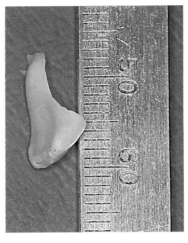

Condition after fragment bonding
Treatment resulted in complete restoration of coronal dental anatomy. However, with maxillary growth the cervicopalatal contour can be restored with a composite restoration.

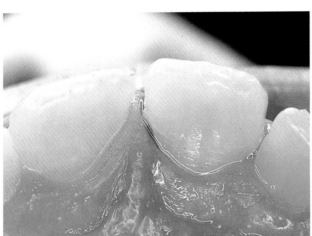
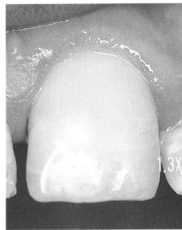

Surgical Exposure of Fracture Surface

Treatment principle. To convert the subgingival fracture to a supragingival fracture with the help of gingivectomy and osteotomy (8-11, 37-42, 57) (Fig. 7.16).

Indication. Should only be used where the surgical technique does not compromise the esthetic result, i.e. only the palatal aspect of the fracture must be exposed by this procedure.

Treatment procedure. After administration of a local anesthetic, the coronal fragment is removed and the fracture surface carefully examined. It is important to remember that most crown-root fractures contain a lingual step (Fig. 7.16). In some cases, this step is a part of an incomplete or complete fracture extending apically (Fig. 7.8). It is therefore essential to determine whether the lingual step in the root is part of a secondary fracture. This can be done during the gingivectomy by placing a sharp explorer or similar instrument at the base of the step and, with a gentle palatal movement, check whether abnormal mobility can be detected. Axial fracture lines running from the pulp chamber to the root surface should also be carefully explored. If these fractures are overlooked, an inflammatory reaction in the periodontium will develop after completion of the restoration (43, 45). The use of a conventional cast core and separate crown instead of a single unit restoration has the advantage that future changes in the position of the gingiva and subsequent loss of esthetics can easily be corrected.

Cost-benefit. Treatment time is short. The long-term prognosis of these restorations has been evaluated and the following results obtained (45). After gingivectomy, regrowth of the gingiva often takes place, leading to development of a pathologic lingual pocket and inflammation of the surrounding gingiva despite good marginal adaptation. After some years, this will result in facial migration of the restored teeth. Migration has been found to be approximately 0.5 mm in a 5-year period (45) (Fig. 7.17).

Fig. 7.16. Removal of the coronal fragment and surgical exposure of the fracture
Clinical and radiograpic appearance of a complicated crown-root fracture.

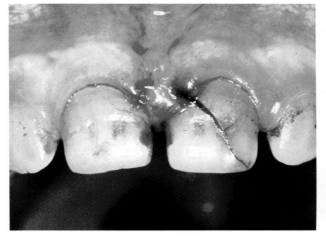 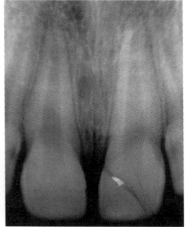

Exposing the fracture site
The coronal fragment is removed. A combined gingivectomy and osteotomy expose the fracture surface.

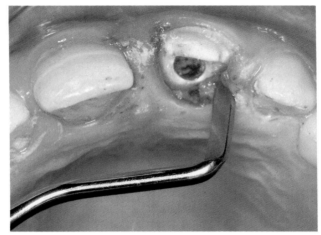 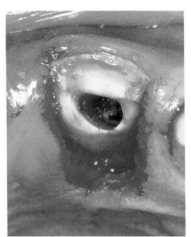

Constructing a post-retained crown
After taking an impression, a post-retained full crown is fabricated.

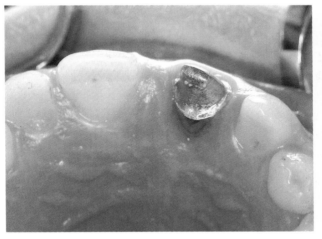 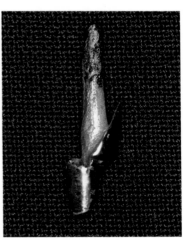

The finished restoration
The clinical and radiographic condition 2 months after insertion of the crown.

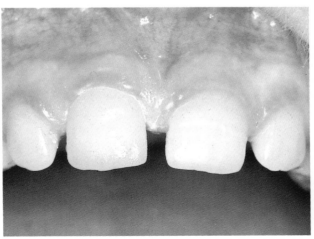 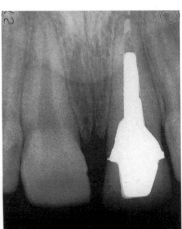

CROWN-ROOT FRACTURES

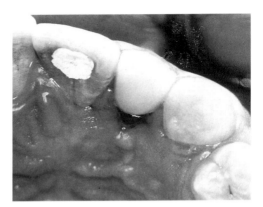
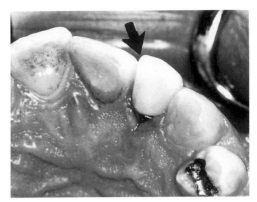

Fig. 7.17.
Labial movement of a crown-root fractured tooth, restored after surgical exposure of the fracture surface. A. Condition immediately after restoration of the right lateral incisor. B. Condition after 6 years. From BESSERMANN (45) 1980

Orthodontic Extrusion of Apical Fragment

Treatment principle. To move the fracture to a supragingival position orthodontically (Fig. 7.18).

This treatment procedure was introduced in 1973 by HEITHERSAY (44) and since then several clinical studies have supported its value (42, 46-50, 60-67).

Indication. The same as for surgical extrusion, but is more time-consuming.

Treatment procedure. In teeth with *completed root formation* and a crown-root fracture, the loose fragment(s) is removed, the pulp in the root extirpated and the root canal enlarged with reamers and files. Subsequently, the apical portion of the root canal is filled with guttapercha and a sealer. Alternatively, the endodontic therapy can be performed prior to the removal of the coronal fragment (i.e. while the coronal fragment is splinted to the adjacent teeth). This might facilitate the en-

Fig. 7.18.
Removal of the coronal fragment and orthodontic extrusion of the root.

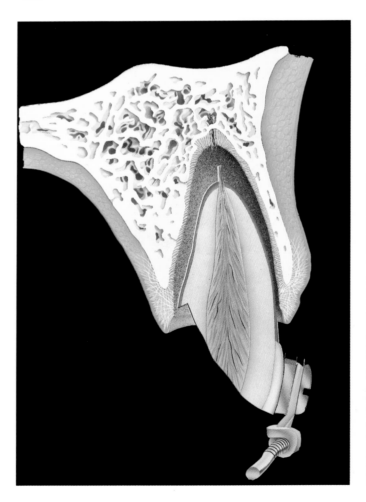
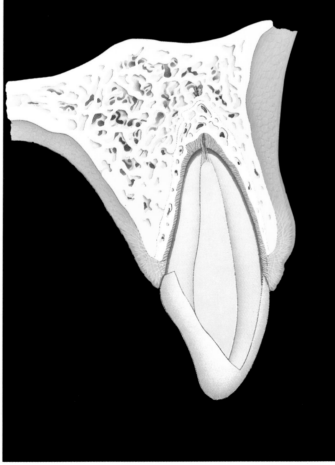

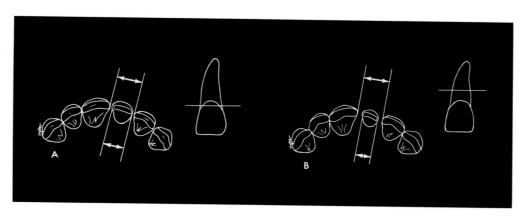

Fig. 7.19.
A. Tooth preparation at the level of the cemento-enamel junction is directly related to the fixed amount of space between the teeth. B. Tooth preparation after eruption of the apical root fragment, the diameter of the preparation is small relative to the fixed amount of space between the teeth. Restoration will thus require greater attention. From INGBER (47) *1976.*

dodontic procedure. Thereafter orthodontic extrusion is performed. This procedure is described in Chapter 15, p 603.

In teeth with *incomplete root formation*, pulp capping or pulpotomy may be performed. Thereafter, orthodontic traction is carried out; this technique is further described in Chapter 15, p. 603.

In cases of *incomplete vertical fracture* of *immature incisors* (see later), it can be difficult to gain access to the pulp and to control moisture and hemorrhage in order to perform a pulpotomy. It could then be an advantage to seal the fracture lines facially and orally with an acid-etch technique and an unfilled resin while the tooth is being extruded. Once the fracture is at a level where access is possible, the fragment can be removed, and pulp capping or pulpotomy performed (see Chapter 14, p. 525) and the crown restored.

An important question is: how much can a tooth be extruded and still maintain reasonable periodontal support? This can best be answered by considering the crown-root ratio. If the goal of extrusion is a crown-root ratio of approximately 1:1, a central incisor can be extruded 2-4 mm, while a lateral incisor can be extruded 4-6 mm. However, it should be noted that, as yet, no study has confirmed that a crown-root ratio of 1:1 cannot be exceeded while maintaining stable periodontal support. Clinical experience with long-term observations of root fractures showing healing with interposition of connective tissue indicates that a relatively large deviation from a crown-root ratio of 1:1 can be effected without resulting in excessive mobility or breakdown of the periodontium.

After extrusion and stabilization, restorative procedures can be carried out as described under the surgical approach.

However, special restorative problems arise when dealing with a root which has been moved coronally. Thus, it should be realized that the extruded root will normally present a smaller cervical diameter for restoration than a root in its normal position (47, 65) (Fig. 7.19). If conventional restorative techniques are employed, the final restoration will have greater divergence from the gingival margin incisally. However, experience gained by the restoration of single tooth implants has shown that conventional porcelain techniques can be used to restore anterior symmetry.

Concerning the prognosis of teeth treated by forced eruption, nothing definitive can be said at the present time. However, experience to date has shown that this procedure leads to stable periodontal conditions (45).

Cost-benefit. The procedure is slow and cumbersome. However, it can provide excellent esthetic results and the gingival health appears to be optimal. Moreover, pulpal vitality can in some cases be maintained where indicated.

Surgical Extrusion of Apical Fragment

Treatment principle. To surgically move the fracture to a supragingival position (Fig. 7.20).

This treatment procedure was introduced by TEGSJÖ ET AL. (53) (1978), (69) (1987), and the method further developed by BÜHLER (70) (1984), (71) (1987), and KAHNBERG (72-75) (1982, 1985, 1988, 1990).

Indication. Should only be used where there is completed root development and the apical fragment is long enough to accommodate a post-retained crown.

CROWN-ROOT FRACTURES

Table 7.2. Long-term results of surgical extrusion of crown-root fractured anterior teeth

	Observation period yr. (mean)	Age of patient yr. (mean)	No. of teeth	Tooth survival %	Healing		
					PDL %	Periapical %	Gingiva %
Tegsjö et al.(69) 1987	4 (4.0)	9-33 (15.0)	56	91	88	98	
Kahnberg et al.(74) 1988	5.5	13-75 (31.0)	17[1]	100	65[3]	94	100
	(2.4)	13-75 (31.0)	41[2]	100	74[3]	95	100

[1]Transplant performed via apical exposure
[2]Transplant performed via coronal approach
[3]Including cases with surface resorption that resulted in only slight shortening of the roots

Treatment. Clinical experience has shown that the time factor for removal of the coronal fragment is not critical for success of treatment. Thus, fragment removal can be instituted days or weeks after injury. The pulp can be extirpated and the tooth rootfilled at this time. However, clinical studies have shown that postponement of endodontic therapy for 3-4 weeks gives better results (76). If the latter approach is chosen, the pulp canal is sealed with zinc oxide-eugenol cement. Moreover, experience has shown that postponement of the surgical procedure for 2-3 weeks facilitates treatment due to inflammatory processes arising in the periodontal ligament.

The apical fragment is luxated with a

Fig. 7.20.
Removal of the coronal fragment and surgical extrusion of the root.

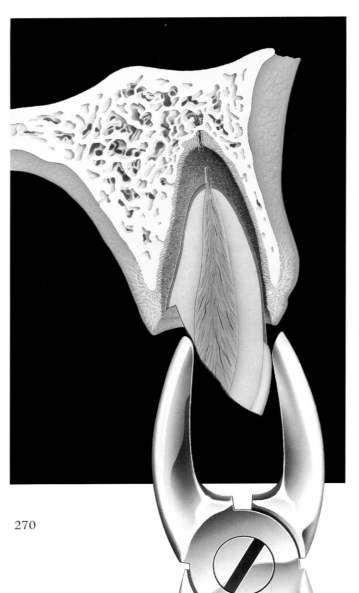
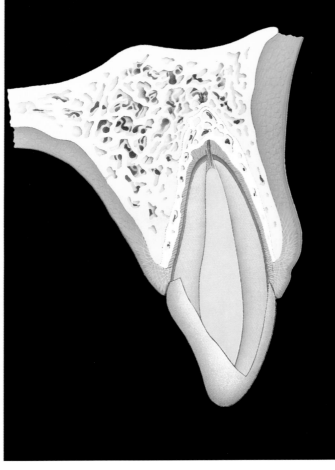

Fig. 7.21. Removal of the coronal fragment and surgical extrusion of the root

A complicated crown-root fracture in a 13-year-old boy. The loose fragment is stabilized immediately after injury with a temporary crown and bridge material using the acid-etch technique.

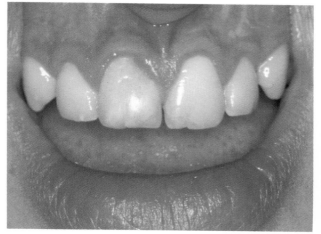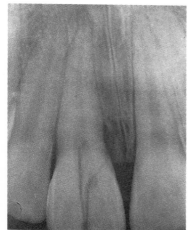

Incision of the PDL

After a local anesthesia the PDL is incised using a specially contoured surgical blade, the PDL is incised as far apically as possible.

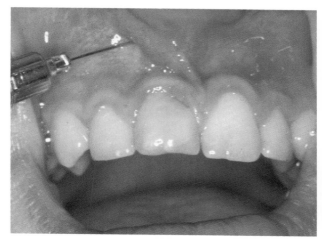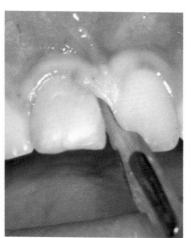

Luxation of the root

The root is then luxated with a narrow elevator which is placed at the mesiopalatal and distopalatal corners respectively.

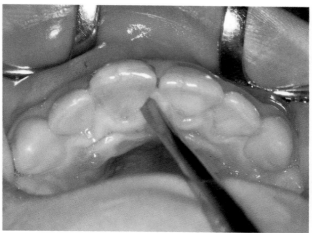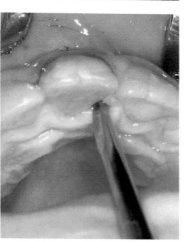

Extracting the root

The root is extracted and inspected for additional fractures.

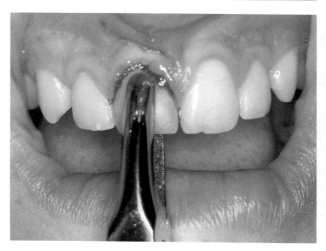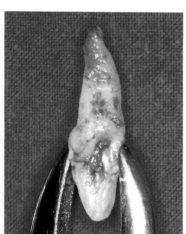

CROWN-ROOT FRACTURES

Replanting the apical fragment

The root is tried in different positions in order to establish where the fracture is optimally exposed, yet with minimal extrusion. In this instance, optimal repositoning was achieved by rotating the root 45°.

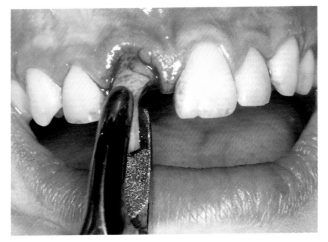 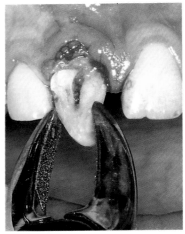

Stabilization of the apical fragment during healing

The root is splinted to adjacent teeth. The pulp is extirpated and the access cavity to the root canal closed.

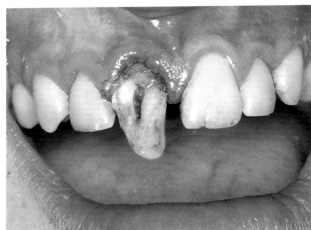 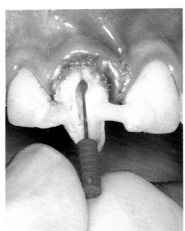

Root filling

Two weeks after initial treatment, endodontic therapy can be continued, in the form of an interim dressing with calcium hydroxide. The root canal is obturated with gutta percha and sealer as far apically as possible 1 month after surgical extrusion.

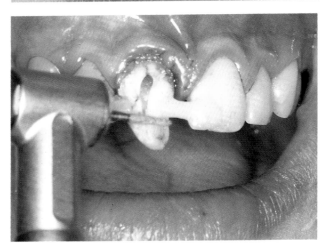 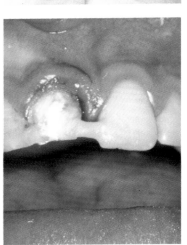

Completion of the restoration

Two months after surgical extrusion, healing has occurred and it is possible to complete the restoration.

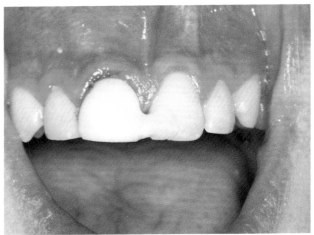 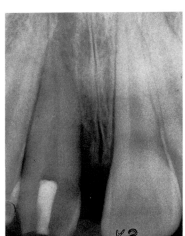

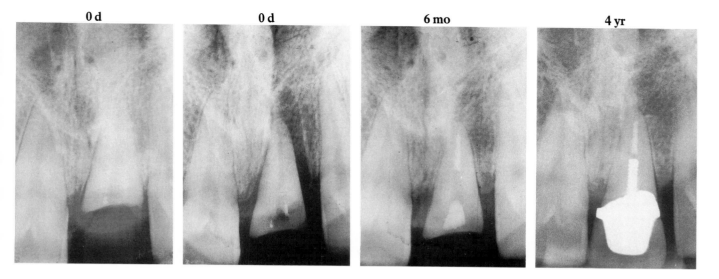

Fig. 7.22.

Intra-alveolar transplantation of a crown-root fractured central incisor. No sign of root resorption is seen 4 years after transplantation. From KAHNBERG (73) *1985.*

Fig. 7.23.

Tooth survival of 68 intraalveolar transplanted anterior teeth with completed root formation at time of surgery. From KAHNBERG (75) *1990.*

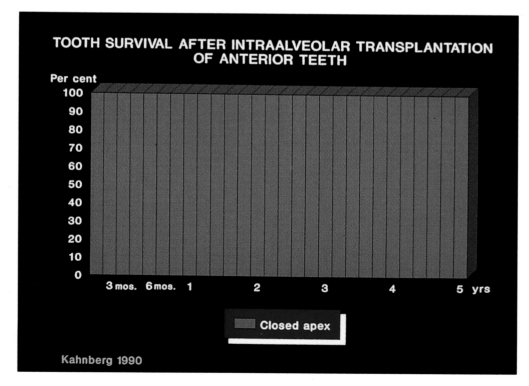

CROWN-ROOT FRACTURES

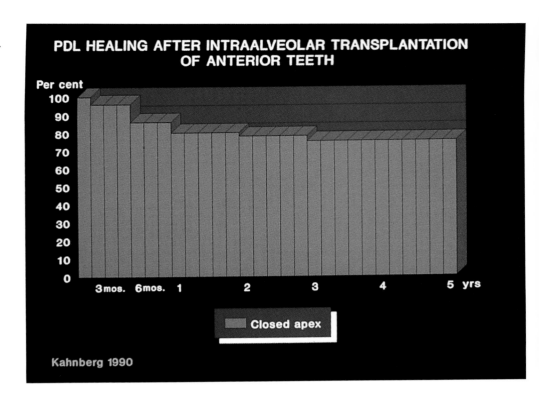

PDL HEALING AFTER INTRAALVEOLAR TRANSPLANTATION OF ANTERIOR TEETH

Kahnberg 1990

thin periosteal elevator (Fig. 7.21). The extracted root is then inspected for incomplete fractures which will contraindicate repositioning of the root. The root is then moved into a more coronal position and secured in that position with interproximal sutures and/or a splint. In case of palatally inclined fractures, 180° rotation can often imply that only slight extrusion is necessary to accommodate crown preparation due to the difference in position of the enamel cementum junction labially and palatally. The exposed pulp is covered with a zinc oxide-eugenol cement. After 3-4 weeks, the tooth can be treated endodontically. After another 1-2 months, the tooth can be restored with a post-retained crown.

Prognosis. In the reported series of patients treated, with up to 5-year observation periods, either no or slight root resorption (surface resorption) was seen (Table 7.2 and Figs.7.22-7.24) (69,74).

Cost-benefit. Several clinical studies have indicated that this is a safe and rapid method for the treatment of crown-root fractures. However, pulp vitality must be sacrificed

PRIMARY DENTITION
In the *primary dentition*, the treatment of choice in case of complicated crown-root fractures is extraction.

Essentials
Treatment of Permanent Teeth

EMERGENCY PROCEDURES
Fragments of crown-root fractured teeth can be temporarily splinted to alleviate pain from mastication (Fig. 7.12). Definitive treatment should be provided within a few days.

DEFINITIVE TREATMENT
The level of the fracture determines the type of therapy (i.e. extraction of the root, surgical exposure of the fracture surface or orthodontic or surgical extrusion of the root).

Extraction of the Tooth

Indicated in teeth where the coronal fragment comprises more than 1/3 of the clinical root and in case of fractures following the long axis of the tooth.

Removal of Coronal Fragment and Supragingival Restoration

Indicated in superfacial fractures that do not involve the pulp (Fig. 7.13).
a) Administer local anesthesia.
b) Remove loose fragments.
c) Smooth rough subgingival fracture surface with a chisel.
d) Cover supragingival exposed dentin.
e) When gingival healing has occurred a supragingival restoration is made using bonded composite or the original fragment where the subgingival portion has been restored.

Surgical Exposure of Fracture Surface

Indicated in teeth where the coronal fragment comprises 1/3 or less of the clinical root (Fig. 7.16).
a) Administer local anesthesia.
b) Remove loose fragments.
c) Perform a pulpectomy and obturate the root canal with gutta-percha and a sealer.
d) Expose the fracture surface with a gingivectomy and ostectomy.
e) Restore the tooth with a post-retained porcelain jacket crown.

Orthodontic Extrusion of Apical Fragment

Indicated in teeth where the coronal fragment comprises 1/3 or less of the clinical root (Fig. 7.18).
a) Administer local anesthesia.
b) Remove loose fragments.
c) In teeth with *mature root formation*, perform pulpectomy and obturate the root canal with gutta percha and a sealer. In teeth with *immature root formation*, perform a cervical pulpotomy (see Chapter 14, p. 524).
d) Expose the fracture surface via orthodontic extrusion of the root (see also Chapter 15, p. 603).
e) When the root is extruded, perform a gingivectomy and ostectomy, if needed, to restore symmetry of gingival contour.
f) Restore the tooth temporarily and splint to neighboring teeth for a retention period of 6 months.
g) After the retention period, restore definitively.

Surgical Extrusion of Apical Fragment

Indicated in teeth where the coronal fragment comprises less than 1/2 root length (Fig. 7.20).
a) Administer antibiotics and local anesthesia.
b) The pulp can be extirpated and the root canal filled with gutta-percha and a sealer prior to intra-alveolar transplantation; or endodontics can be postponed and the root canal entrance sealed with a zinc oxide-eugenol cement.
c) The PDL is incised, the tooth luxated with an elevator and the tooth extracted with forceps.
d) The root surface is inspected for incomplete root fractures, which would contraindicate transplantation.
e) The root is repositioned at a level 1 mm coronal to the alveolar crest. If desirable, the root can be rotated to achieve a maximum periodontal surface area within the socket.
f) The tooth is stabilized using interproximal sutures.
g) Take a postoperative radiograph.
h) After 2 to 3 weeks, the transplant is usually firm. If the root canal has not been filled, calcium hydroxide can be used as an interim dressing which will ensure apical hard tissue closure. A temporary restoration can now be fabricated.
i) After 6 months, a permanent root filling as well as a definitive crown restoration can be completed.
j) If a gutta-percha root filling has been made prior to transplantation, the tooth can be restored after 2 months.

Treatment of Primary Teeth

Extraction is usually the treatment of choice.

Bibliography

1. ANDREASEN JO. Etiology and pathogenesis of traumatic dental injuries. A clinical study of 1,298 cases. *Scand J Dent Res* 1970;**78**:329-42.

2. SUTHER T, FIXOTT HC. Multiple accidental fractures of posterior primary teeth. A case report. *ASDC J Dent Child* 1952;**19**: 115-7.

3. BEVELANDER G. Tissue reactions in experimental tooth fracture. *J Dent Res* 1942;**21**:481-7.

4. NEIMANN-SØRENSEN E, PINDBORG JJ. Traumatisk betingede forandringer i ikke færdigdannede tænder. *Tandlægebladet* 1955;**59**:230-43

5. LINDEMANN H. Histologische Untersuchung einer geheilten Zahnfraktur. *Dtsch Zahn Mund Kieferheilk* 1938;**5**:915-25.

6. RITCHIE GM. Repair of coronal fractures in upper incisor teeth. *Br Dent J* 1962;**112**:459-60.

7. LOSEE FL. Untreated tooth fractures. Report of three cases. *Oral Surg Oral Med Oral Pathol* 1948;**1**:464-73.

8. CLYDE JS. Transverse-oblique fractures of the crown with extension below the epithelial attachment. *Br Dent J* 1965;**119**:402-6.

9. LANGDON JD. Treatment of oblique fractures of incisors involving the epithelial attachment. A case report. *Br Dent J* 1968;**125**:72-4.

10. FELDMAN G, SOLOMON C, NOTARO PJ. Endodontic management of traumatized teeth. *Oral Surg Oral Med Oral Pathol* 1966;**21**:100-12.

11. NATKIN E. Diagnosis and treatment of traumatic injuries and their sequelae. In: INGLE JI, ed. *Endodontics*. Philadelphia: Lea & Febiger, 1965:566-611.

12. ELLIS RG. Fractured anterior teeth. Natural crown restoration. *J Canad Dent Assoc* 1940;**6**:339-44.

13. GRAZIDE, COULOMB, BOISSET & DASQUE. L'embrochage et le collage dans le traitement des fractures dentaires. *Rev Stomatol* (Paris) 1956;**57**:428-44.

14. KISLING E. Om behandlingen af skader som følge af akutte mekaniske traumer på unge permanente incisiver. *Tandlægebladet* 1953;**57**:61-9,109-29.

15. LEE EC. Total fracture of the crown. *Br Dent J* 1966;**120**:139-40.

16. CURRY VL. Fractured incisors. *Dent Practit Dent Rec* 1951;**1**:341-6.

17. PROPHET AS, ROWBOTHAM TC, JAMES PMC. Traumatic injuries of the teeth. *Br Dent J* 1964;**116**:377-85.

18. RAVN JJ. *Ulykkesskadede fortænder på børn. Klassifikation og behandling.* Copenhagen: Odontologisk Forening, 1966.

19. CHOSACH A, EIDELMAN E. Rehabilitation of a fractured incisor using the patient's natural crown. Case report. *ASDC J Dent Child* 1964;**31**: 3119-21.

20. TAKIUCHI H, NOBUHARA A, NOHMI A. Repair of the total fracture of anterior tooth crown and its fluorination. Three case reports. *Jpn J Conserv Dent* 1967;**10**:37-41.

21. NEEDLEMAN HL, WOLFMAN MS. Traumatic posterior dental fractures Report of a case. *ASDC J Dent Child* 1976;**43**:262-4.

22. RUD J, OMNELL K-Å. Root fractures due to corrosion. Diagnostic aspect. *Scand J Dent Res* 1970;**78**:397-403.

23. PIETROKOVSKI J, LANTZMAN E. Complicated crown fractures in adults. *J Prosthet Dent* 1973;**30**:801-7.

24. SNYDER DE. The cracked tooth syndrome and fractured posterior cusp. *Oral Surg Oral Med Oral Pathol* 1976;**41**:698-704.

25. CAMERON CE. The cracked tooth syndrome additional findings. *J Am Dent Assoc* 1976;**93**:971-5.

26. SILVESTRI AR Jr. The undiagnosed split-root syndrome. *J Am Dent Assoc* 1976;**92**:930-5.

27. BOUCHON F, HERVÉ M, MARMASSE A. Propos empiriques fractures dentaires spontanées' *Actual Odontostomatatol* 1977;**118**:221-39.

28. HIATT WH. Incomplete crown-root fracture in pulpal-periodontal disease. *J Periodontol* 1973;**44**:369-79.

29. MAXWELL EH, BRALY BV. Incomplete tooth fracture. Prediction and prevention. *J Calif Dent Assoc* 1977;**5**:51-5.

30. POLSON AM. Periodontal destruction associated with vertical root fracture. Report of four cases. *J Periodontol* 1977;**48**:27-32.

31. LOMMEL TJ, MEISTER F Jr, GERSTEIN H, DAVIES EE, TILK MA. Alveolar bone loss associated with vertical root fractures. Report of six cases. *Oral Surg Oral Med Oral Pathol* 1978;**45**:909-19.

32. WECHSLER SM, VOGEL RI, FISHELBERG G, SHOWLING FE. Iatrogenic root fractures: a case report. *J Endod* 1978;4:251-3.

33. WEISMAN MI. The twenty-five cent crack detector. *J Endod* 1978;4:222.

34. MICHANOWICZ AE, PERCHERSKY JL, McKIBBEN DH. A vertical fracture of the crown and root. *ASDC J Dent Child* 1978;**45**:54-6.

35. TODD HW. Avulsed natural crown as a temporary crown: report of case. *J Am Dent Assoc* 1971;**82**:1398-1400.

36. STERN N. Provisional restoration of a broken anterior tooth, with its own natural crown. *J Dent* 1975;2:217-8.

37. FELDMAN G, SOLOMON C, NOTARO P, MOSKOWITZ E. Endodontic management of the subgingival fracture. *Dent Radio Photogr* 1972;**45**:3-9.

38. GOLDSTEIN RE, LEVITAS TC. Preservation of fractured maxillary central incisors in an adolescent: report of case. *J Am Dent Assoc* 1972;**84**:371-4.

39. TALIM ST, GOHIL KS. Management of coronal fractures of permanent posterior teeth. *J Prosthet Dent* 1974;**31**:172-8.

40. GOERIG AC. Restoration of teeth with subgingival and subosseous fractures. *J Prosthet Dent* 1975;**34**:634-9.

41. FEDERICK DR. Klinische Wiederherstellung der Kronenlänge durch parodontal-prothetische Verfahren. *Quintessenz* 1976;3:47-53.

42. BESSERMANN M. Ny behandlingsmetode af krone-rodfrakturer. *Tandlægebladet* 1978;**82**:441-4.

43. LINABURG RG, MARSHALL FJ. The diagnosis and treatment of vertical root fractures report of case. *J Am Dent Assoc* 1973;**86**:679-83.

44. HEITHERSAY GS. Combined endodontic-orthodontic treatment of transverse root fractures in the region of the alveolar crest. *Oral Surg Oral Med Oral Pathol* 1973;**36**:404-15.

45. BESSERMANN-NIELSEN M. Personal communication, 1980.

46. WOLFSON EM, SEIDEN L. Combined endodontic-orthodontic treatment of subgingivally fractured teeth. *J Canad Dent Assoc* 1975;**11**:621-4.

47. INGBER JS. Forced eruption Part II. A method of treating nonrestorable teeth - periodontal and restorative considerations. *J Periodontol* 1976;**47**:203-16.

48. PERSSON M, SERNEKE D. Ortodontisk framdragning av tand med cervikal rotfraktur för att möjliggöra kronersättning. *Tandläkartidningen* 1977;**69**:1263-69.

49. DELIVANIS P, DELIVANIS H, KUFTINEC MM. Endodontic-orthodontic management of fractured anterior teeth. *J Am Dent Assoc* 1978;**97**:483-5.

50. SIMON JHS, KELLY WH, GORDON DG, ERICKSEN GW. Extrusion of endodontically treated teeth. *J Am Dent Assoc* 1978;**97**:17-23.

51. STENVIK A. The effect of extrusive orthodontic forces on human pulp and dentin. *Scand J Dent Res* 1971;**79**:430-5.

52. REITAN K. Initial tissue behavior during apical root resorption. *Angle Orthod* 1974;**44**:68-82.

53. TEGSJÖ U, VALERIUS-OLSSON H, OLGART K. Intra-alveolar

transplantation of teeth with cervical root fractures. *Swed Dent J* 1978;2:73-82.

54. PITTS DL, NATKIN E. Diagnosis and treatment of vertical root fractures. *J Endod* 1983;**9**:338-46.

55. BODNER L, LUSTMANN J. Intra-alveolar fracture of a developing permanent incisor. *Pediatr Dent* 1988;**10**:1379.

56. WALTON RE, MICHELICH RJ, SMITH GM. The histopatogenesis of vertical root fractures. *J Endod* 1984;**10**:48-56.

57. McDONALD FL, DAVIS SS, WHITBECK P. Periodontal surgery as an aid to restoring fractured teeth. *J Prosthet Dent* 1982;**47**:366-72.

58. MICHANOWICZ AE, PERCHERSKY JL, McKIBBEN DH. A vertical fracture of the crown and root. *J Dent Child* 1978;**45**:310-2.

59. SPETALEN E. Behandling av komplisert vertikal krone-rot fraktur. Kasusrapport. *Norske Tannlegeforenings Tidende* 1985;**95**:301-3.

60. BIELAK S, BIMSTEIN E, EIDELMAN E. Forced eruption: the treatment of choice for subgingivally fractured permanent incisors. *J Dent Child* 1982;**49**:186-90.

61. LEMON RR. Simplified esthetic root extrusion techniques. *Oral Surg Oral Med Oral Pathol* 1982;**54**:93-9.

62. COOKE MS, SCHEER B. Extrusion of fractured teeth. The evolution of practical clinical techniques. *Brit Dent J* 1980;**149**:50-3.

63. MANDEL RC, BINZER WC, WITHERS JA. Forced eruption in restoring severely fractured teeth using removable orthodontic appliances. *J Prosthet Dent* 1982;**47**:269-74.

64. GARRETT GB. Forced eruption in the treatment of transverse root fractures. *J Am Dent Assoc* 1985;**111**:270-2.

65. FEIGLIN B. Problems with the endodontic-orthodontic management of fractured teeth. *Int Endod J* 1986;**19**:57-63.

66. WILLIAMS S, DIETZ B. Kieferorthopädische Zahnverlängerung im Rahmen der Restaurierung eines frakturierten Frontzahns. *Z Stomatol* 1986;**83**:555-9.

67. INGBER JS. Forced eruption: alteration of soft tissue cosmetic deformities. *Int J Periodont Rest Dent* 1989;**9**:417-25.

68. MALMGREN O, MALMGREN B, FRYKHOLM A. Rapid orthodontic extrusion of crown root and cervical root fractured teeth. *Endod Dent Traumatol* 1991;**7**:49-54.

69. TEGSJÖ U, VALERIUS-OLSSON H, FRYKHOLM H, OLGART K. Clinical evaluation of intra-alveolar transplantation of teeth with cervical root fractures. *Swed Dent J* 1987;**11**:235-50.

70. BÜHLER H. Nachuntersuchung wurzelseparierter Zähne. (Eine röntgenologische Langzeitstudie). *Quintessenz Int* 1984;**35**:1825-37.

71. BÜHLER H. Intraalveoläre Transplantation von Einzelwurzeln. *Quintessenz Int* 1987;**38**:1963-70.

72. KAHNBERG K-E, WARFVINGE J, BIRGERSSON B. Intraalveolar transplantation (I). The use of autologous bone transplants in the periapical region. *Int J Oral Surg* 1982;**11**:372-9.

73. KAHNBERG K-E. Intraalveolar transplantation of teeth with crown-root fractures. *J Oral Surg* 1985;**43**:38-42.

74. KAHNBERG K-E. Surgical extrusion of root-fractures teeth - a follow-up study of two surgical methods. *Endod Dent Traumatol* 1988;**4**:85-9.

75. KAHNBERG 1990. Personal communication.

76. WARFVINGE J, KAHNBERG K-E. Intraalveolar transplantation of teeth. IV. Endodontic considerations. *Swed Dent J* 1989;**13**:229-33.

CROWN-ROOT FRACTURES

CHAPTER 8

Root Fractures

F. M. ANDREASEN & J. O. ANDREASEN

Terminology, Frequency and Etiology

Root fractures, defined as fractures involving dentin, cementum and pulp, are relatively uncommon among dental traumas, comprising 0.5 to 7% of the injuries affecting the permanent dentition (1-8, 88, 89, 132) and 2 to 4% in the primary dentition (1, 4). Frequent causes of root fractures in the permanent dentition are fights and foreign bodies striking the teeth (1).

The mechanism of root fractures is usually a frontal impact which creates compression zones labially and lingually. The resulting shearing stress zone then dictates the plane of fracture. The result on a histologic level is a periodontal ligament injury (rupture and/or compression) usually confined to the coronal fragment and usually stretching or laceration of the

pulp at the fracture level (Figs. 8.1 and 8.2).

Clinical Findings

Root fractures involving the *permanent dentition* predominantly affect the maxillary central incisor region in the age group of 11 to 20 years (1, 9-12). In younger individuals, with the permanent incisors in various stages of eruption and with incomplete root development, root fractures are unusual (13), a finding possibly related to the elasticity of the alveolar socket which renders such teeth more susceptible to luxation injuries than to fractures (90). However, careful scrutiny of radiographs following luxation injuries in this age group can sometimes reveal incomplete root fractures (see later). In the *primary dentition*, root fractures are also uncommon before completion of root develop-

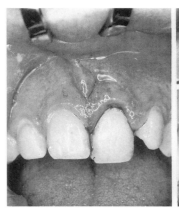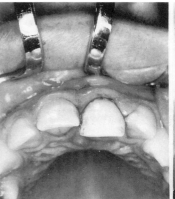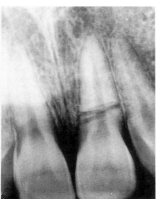

Fig. 8.1.
Lingual and incisal displacement of left central incisor due to root fracture.

ment and are most frequent at the age of 3-4 years where physiologic root resorption has begun, thereby weakening the root (91).

Root fractures are often associated with other types of dental injury; among these, concomitant fracture of the alveolar process, especially in the mandibular incisor region, is a common finding (1).

Clinical examination of teeth with root fractures usually reveals a slightly extruded tooth, frequently displaced in a lingual direction (Fig. 8.1). While the site of the fracture determines the degree of tooth mobility, it is usually not possible to distinguish clinically between displacement due to root fracture and luxation injury. Diagnosis is entirely depend-

Fig. 8.2.
Pathogenesis of root fracture. A frontal impact displaces the tooth orally and results in a root fracture and displacement of the coronal fragment. This results in both pulpal and PDL damage coronally. The pulp in the apical part of the root usually remains vital.

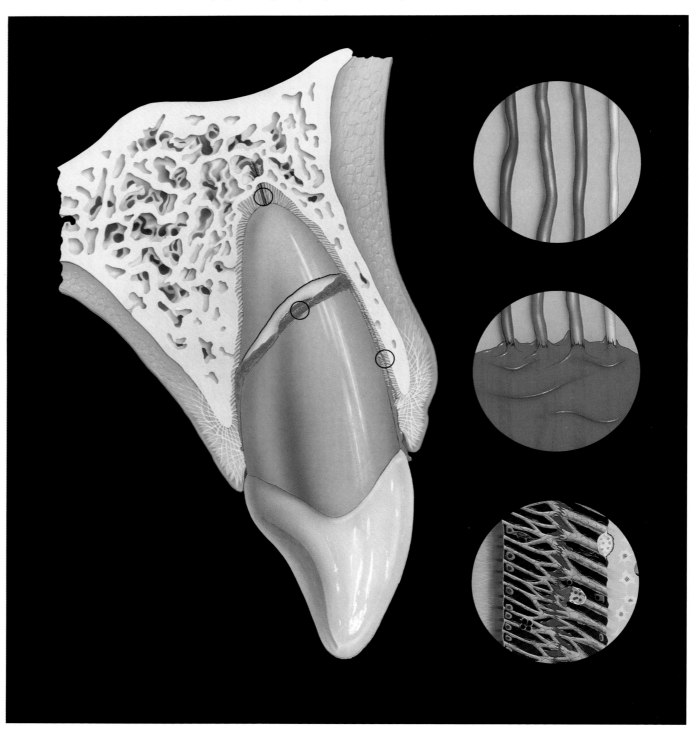

ent upon radiographic examination (see later).

Radiographic Findings

Radiographic demonstration of root fractures is facilitated by the fact that the fracture line is most often oblique and at an optimal angle for radiographic disclosure (13) (Figs. 8.3 and 8.4). In this context, it should be remembered that a root fracture will normally be visible only if the central beam is directed within a maximum range of 15-20° of the fracture plane (133, 134). Thus, if an elipsoid radiolucent line is seen on a radiograph, two additional periapical radiographs should be taken -

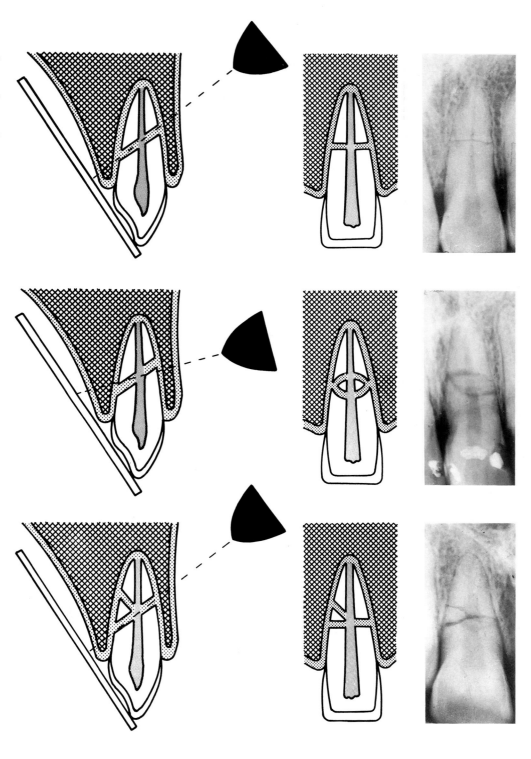

Fig. 8.3. Radiographic demonstration of root fractures
The normal projection angle is parallel to the fracture surface, resulting in a single transverse line on the radiograph. Decrease or increase of the projection angle results in an ellipsoid fracture line on the radiograph. The fracture line in multiple root fractures shows an irregular shape on the radiograph.

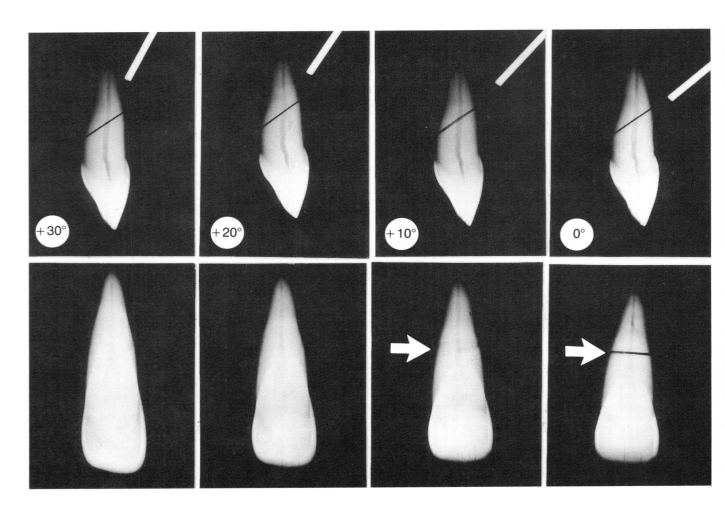

Fig. 8.4.
Radiographs taken of a human tooth with an artificial root fracture. The top row of radiographs indicates the direction of the central beam. The 0° beam corresponds to the direction of the central beam used in ordinary occlusal exposures. It appears from the bottom row that the fracture line was only disclosed with an angulation of the central beam from +10° to -20° in relation to the occlusal angulation of 0°. It also appears that deviations of the central beam from the fracture plane tend to depict the fracture as an ellipsoid structure mimicking an intermediary fragment.

one with an increased angulation of 15° to the original and the second at a negative angulation of 15° to the original (92) (Fig. 8.4).

Root fractures occasionally escape detection immediately after injury, while later radiographs clearly reveal the fracture (4, 16-18, 93, 94) (Fig. 8.5). This can be due to the development of either hemorrhage or granulation tissue between the fragments, which displaces the coronal fragment incisally or due to resorption at the fracture line which is a part of the healing process (see later) (134).

In previous clinical studies, root fractures were seen to occur most often in the apical or middle third of the root, and only rarely in the coronal one-third (11-13, 93, 94). However, in a recent clinical study, frac-tures of the middle third of the root were the most frequent, while fractures of the apical and cervical thirds occurred with equal frequency (135, 136). A single transverse fracture is the usual finding; however, oblique or multiple fractures can occur (Fig. 8.6). The direction of the fracture can vary considerably. Thus, the typical apical or mid-root fracture follows a steep course facio-orally in an incisal direction, while fractures of the cervical third tend to be more horizontal. This change in direction dictates a radiographic technique which involves multiple exposures, including a steep occlusal exposure, which is optimal for detecting fractures of the apical third of the root (134). (See Chapter 5, p.210).

Root fractures of teeth with incomplete

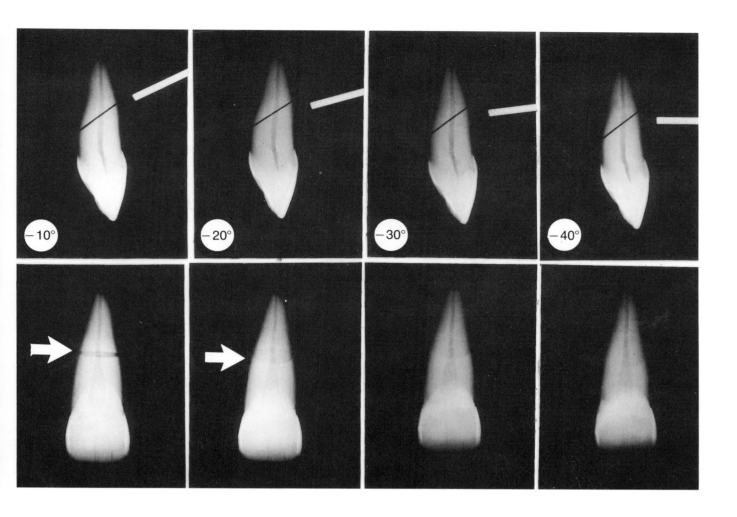

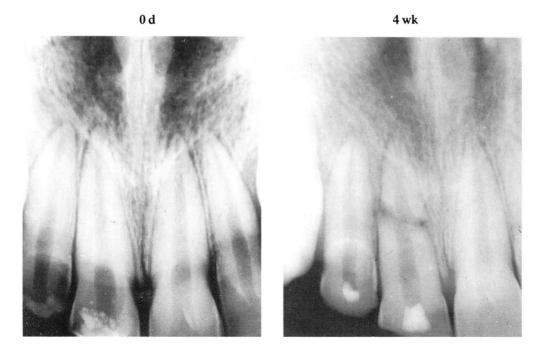

0 d　　　　　　**4 wk**

Fig. 8.5.
Radiograph taken immediately after injury. The root fracture of the right central incisor is barely discernible. Four weeks later a fracture line is clearly visible.

ROOT FRACTURES

Fig. 8.6.
Oblique root fracture of a left canine and multiple root fractures of left central incisor.

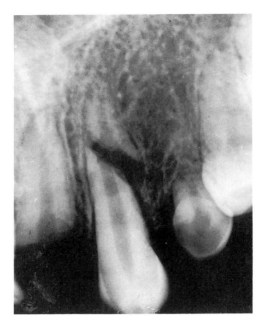
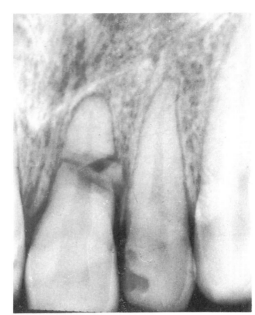

root formation can demonstrate a partial root fracture, a possible analogue to "green stick" fractures of long bones (4, 19). These fractures are usually seen as a unilateral break in the continuity of the thin root canal wall/root surface of the immature root (Fig. 8.7). In a recent clinical study, these fractures were seen to heal with subsequent hard tissue formation (136).

The primary dentition presents special radiographic problems due to superimposition of permanent teeth, which often makes detection of fractures near the apex difficult, if not impossible (Fig. 8.8).

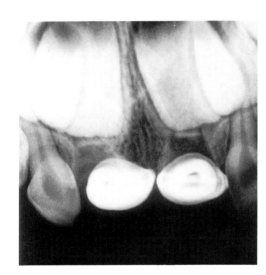

Fig. 8.8.
Apical fragments of fractured primary central incisors superimposed over the crowns of the permanent successors.

Fig. 8.7.
Incomplete root fracture of a left central incisor. 12 years later the fracture line is hardly visible.

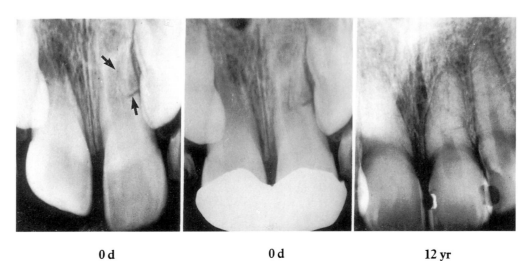

| 0 d | 0 d | 12 yr |

Pathology

Root Fracture Healing

Healing events following root fracture are initiated at the site of pulpal and periodontal ligament involvement and this creates two types of wound healing response (22-24, 96, 134-139) (Fig. 8.9). These processes apparently occur independently of each other and are sometimes even competitive in their endeavor to close the injury site with either pulpal or periodontally derived tissue.

On the pulpal side of the fracture, two healing events might occur, depending upon the integrity of the pulp at the level of fracture. Thus, if the pulp is intact at the fracture site, it will react in a manner analogous to a coronal pulp exposure under optimal conditions (i.e. with an intact vascular supply and absence of infection) (Fig. 8.10). Odontoblast progenitor cells will be recruited and create a hard tissue bridge which will unite the apical

and coronal fragments after 2 to 3 months (23). This bridge forms the initial callus which will stabilize the fracture. Callus formation is followed by deposition of cementum derived by ingrowth of tissue from the periodontal ligament (23) at the fracture line, first centrally and gradually obliterating the fracture site. Hard tissue union of the fractured root fragments cannot be diagnosed clinically earlier than 3 months after injury and may take several years to be completed (134-136).

In the event that the pulp is severed or severely stretched at the level of the fracture, a revascularization process in the coronal aspect of the pulp is initiated. In the absence of bacteria, this process will result in obliteration of the coronal pulp canal. While this revascularization process is under way, periodontally derived cells can dominate root fracture healing, resulting in "union" of the coronal and apical root fragments by interposition of connective tissue (Fig. 8.11).

Fig. 8.9.
Healing sequence after experimental root fractures in dogs. A. Eight days postoperatively, proliferation of odontoblasts and pulpal cells. B. and C. After 2 weeks a dentinal callus is formed, uniting the fragments. D. Nine months after experimental fracture, connective tissue separates the fragments in the peripheral part of the fracture. From HAMMER (23) 1939.

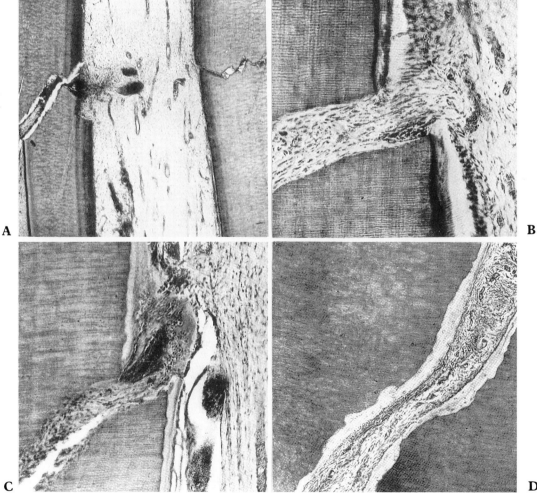

A

B

C

D

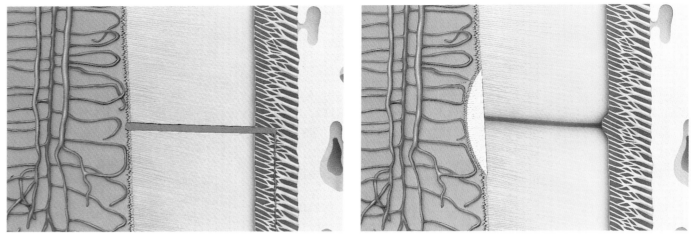

Fig. 8.10. Hard tissue healing after root fracture
Due to minimal displacement of the coronal fragment, the pulp is probably only slightly stretched at the level of the fracture. Fracture healing with ingrowth of cells originating from the apical half of the pulp ensures hard tissue union of the fracture.

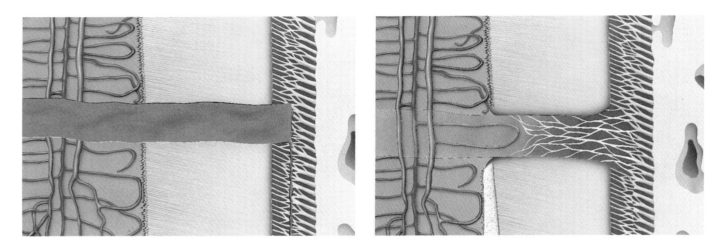

Fig. 8.11. Connective tissue healing after root fracture
The pulp is ruptured or severely stretched at the level of the fracture following displacement of the coronal fragment. Healing is dominated by ingrowth of cells originating from the periodontal ligament and results in interposition of connective tissue between the two fragments.

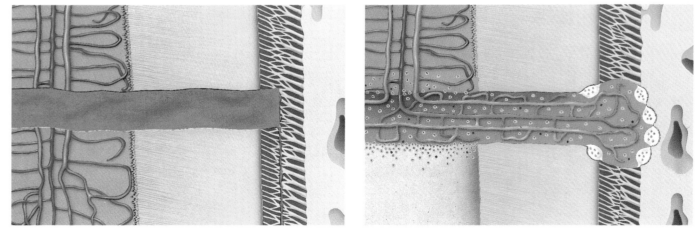

Fig. 8.12. Non-healing due to infection in the line of fracture
Infection occurs in the avascular coronal aspect of the pulp. Granulation tissue is soon formed which originates from the apical pulp and peridontal ligament. Accumulation of cells between the two fragments causes separation of the fragments and loosening of the coronal fragment.

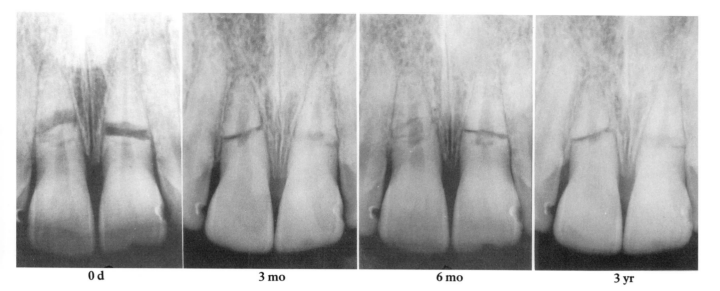

| 0 d | 3 mo | 6 mo | 3 yr |

Fig. 8.13.
Root fracture of the right and left maxillary central incisors of a 22-year-old woman, with extrusion of the fragments. Two months after injury, there is evidence of internal surface resorption (ISR) at the junction of the pulp canal and fracture line of both teeth and external surface resorption (ESR) of the right central incisor. After 3 years, there is resolution of ISR and pulp canal obliteration of the coronal canal can be seen. Healing is by interposition of connective tissue. From ANDREASEN & ANDREASEN (135) 1988.

Finally, if bacteria gain access - usually to the coronal pulp - an infected pulp necrosis results, with accumulation of inflamed, granulation tissue between the two root fragments (Fig. 8.12).

During the initial stages of wound healing, traumatized pulpal and hard dental tissues can stimulate an inflammatory response and thereby trigger the release of a series of osteoclast-activating factors (138) (see Chapter 2, p. 114).

Thus, root resorption processes beginning either at the periphery of the fracture line adjacent to the periodontal ligament or centrally at the border of the root canal were observed in 60% of a clinical material of root-fractured permanent incisors (134).

These processes could usually be detected within the 1st year after injury and preceded fracture healing and obliteration of the apical and/or coronal portions of the root canals. The changes observed represented three resorption entities:

1) *external surface resorption* (i.e. rounding of proximal fracture edges at the periodontal side of the fracture) (Fig. 8.13);

2) *internal surface resorption* (i.e. rounding of fracture edges centrally, at the pulpal side of the fracture) (Fig. 8.14)

3) *internal tunneling resorption* (i.e. resorption which burrows behind the predentin layer and along the root canal walls of the coronal fragment) (Figs. 8.14 and 8.15).

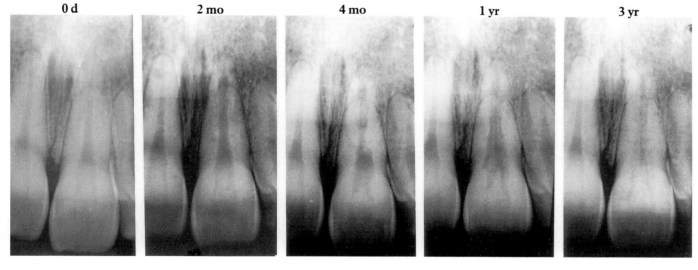

| 0 d | 2 mo | 4 mo | 1 yr | 3 yr |

Fig. 8.14.
Root fracture of the left maxillary central incisor in a 19-year-old man with extrusion of the coronal fragment. Two months after injury, there is evidence of resorption of the pulp canal walls (internal surface resorption (ISR)). Six months after injury, simultaneous resorption and deposition of hard tissue can be seen. Internal tunneling resorption (ITR) can be clearly seen after 1 year. After 2 years, arrest of the resorption process and obliteration of the apical and coronal pulp canals can be seen. Healing is by interposition of connective tissue. From ANDREASEN & ANDREASEN (135) 1988.

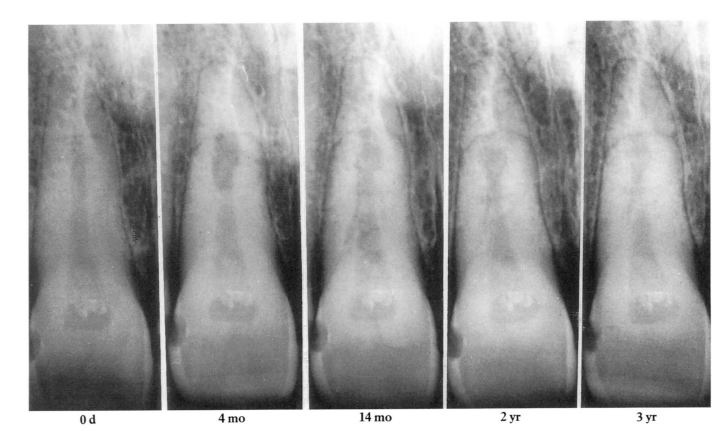

| 0 d | 4 mo | 14 mo | 2 yr | 3 yr |

Fig. 8.15.
Root fracture of the right maxillary central incisor in a 32-year-old man with extrusion of the coronal fragment. Four months after injury, there is evidence of ISR. One year after injury, ITR can be seen. After 2 years, arrest of the resorption process and obliteration of the apical and coronal pulp canals can be seen. Healing is by interposition of connective tissue. From ANDREASEN & ANDREASEN (135) 1988.

It has been speculated that the various root resorption entities represent osteoclastic activity connected with ingrowth of new highly vascularized connective tissue into the fracture site or coronal aspect of the root canal, as revasculularization processes are known to elicit transient osteoclast activity (134).(see Chapter 2, p. 114)

The resorption processes were all self-limiting, usually resolving within the first 1-2 years after injury, and therefore requiring no interceptive treatment. The pattern of resorption and pulp canal obliteration appeared to be decisive for fracture healing. Thus, all resorption entities collectively were significantly related to healing by interposition of connective tissue between fragments. However, when seen alone, internal surface resorption was significantly related to hard tissue union. Pulp canal obliteration in both aspects of the root canal indicated interposition of connective tissue; when seen only in the apical aspect, healing was by hard tissue union (134).

It should be emphasized that the pathogenesis of root fracture healing, while suggested by retrospective clinical studies (13, 93, 134), is only weakly supported by experimental research and revision of this hypothesis should be expected when future studies examine the specific roles of the pulp and periodontium in root fracture healing.

So far, radiographic and histological observations in *human subjects* have revealed that the final outcome after root fracture can be divided into the events listed below (13, 26) (Fig. 8.16).

Healing with Calcified Tissue

A uniting callus of hard tissue has been demonstrated histologically in a number of cases (9, 13, 19, 27-36, 97-100) (Figs. 8.17 and 8.18). Varying opinions exist on the na-

Fig. 8.16.
Radiographs and diagrams illustrating various modalities of healing after root fracture. A. Healing with calcified tissue. B. Interposition of connective tissue. C. Interposition of bone and connective tissue. D. Interposition of granulation tissue. From AN-DREASEN & HJØRTING-HANSEN (13) 1967.

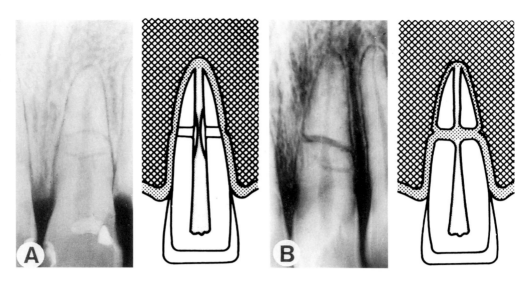

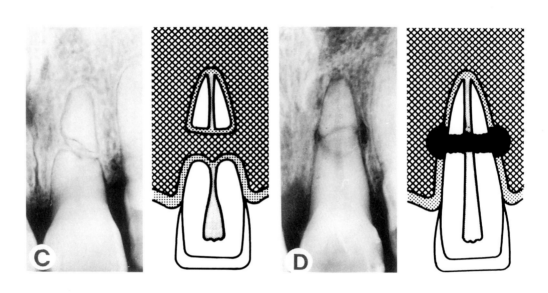

Fig. 8.17.
Complete healing with calcified tissue after root fracture. A. Radiographic condition 8 years after root fracture of both central incisors. Fracture lines are still visible. B. Histologic examination of left central incisor reveals a complete hard tissue callus. From SCHULZE (36) 1957.

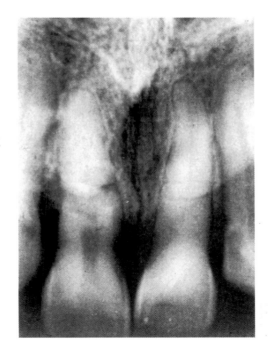

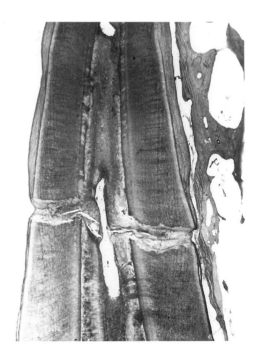

ROOT FRACTURES

Fig. 8.18.
Incomplete healing with calcified tissue after root fracture of a left central incisor. A. and B. Radiographs taken 3 and 10 months after injury. C. Low-power view of sectioned incisor removed 1 year after trauma. The lingual part of the fracture line shows repair with calcified tissue. x 6. D. Interposition of connective tissue. x 30. E. Uniting callus of hard tissue. x 30. F. Higher magnification of E. There is a distinct demarcation between dentin and cementum (arrows). A few tubules are found in the dentin. The cementum is probably formed after resorption of root fragments. x 75. G. Barely visible hard tissue formation at the peripheral part of fracture. x 30. From AN-DREASEN & HJØRTING-HANSEN (13) 1967.

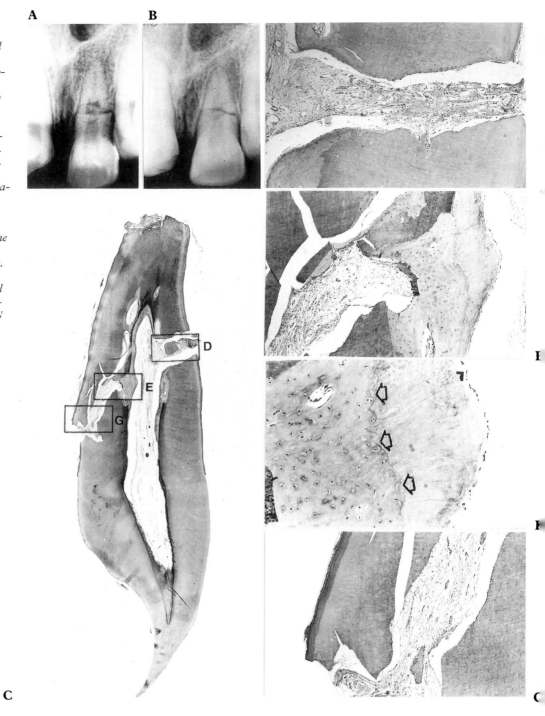

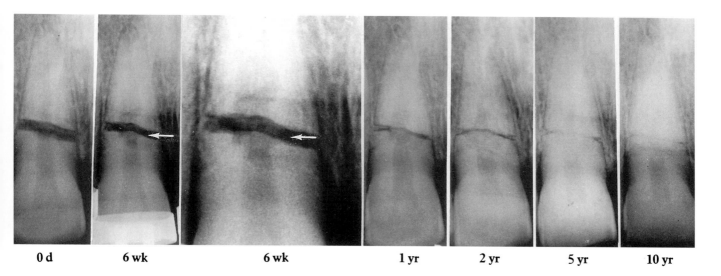

| 0 d | 6 wk | 6 wk | 1 yr | 2 yr | 5 yr | 10 yr |

Fig. 8.19.
Healing with calcified tissue of a fracture located at the gingival third of the root of a left lateral incisor. At the 1-month control visit, evidence of widening of the root canal close to the fracture site (arrow). At controls 1 and 5 years later, the resorption cavity in the pulp canal as well as the fracture site show repair with calcified tissue.

ture of the hard tissue found uniting the fragments. Dentin (36), osteodentin (27), or cementum (28, 29, 33, 34) have all been found in the repair site. In most cases, the innermost layer of repair seems to be dentin (Fig. 8.18 F), while the more peripheral part of the fracture is incompletely repaired with cementum (9, 13, 30-32, 36) (Fig. 8.18 E, F). The first layer of dentin is often cellular and atubular, later followed by normal tubular dentin (31, 36). Cementum deposition in the fracture line is often preceded by resorptive processes both centrally and peripherally (Fig. 8.18 E). Most often, cementum will not completely bridge the gap between the fracture surfaces, but is interspersed with connective tissue originating from the periodontal ligament (Fig. 8.18 G). This, combined with the greater radiodensity of cementum as compared with dentin, could explain why a fracture line is often discernible radiographically although the fragments are in close apposition and the fracture is completely consolidated (Fig. 8.19).

Occasionally, a slight widening of the root canal close to the fracture site is seen (i.e. *internal surface resorption* (134)), followed by hard tissue formation (101, 102) (Fig. 8.19). Moreover, it is characteristic that there is limited peripheral rounding of the fracture edges *(external surface resorption* (134))*.

Partial pulp canal obliteration, confined to the apical fragment, is a frequent finding.

Clinical examination of teeth within this healing group reveals normal mobility, as compared with non-injured adjacent teeth; moreover, there is normal reaction to percussion and normal or slightly decreased response to pulpal sensibility testing (13, 103).

This type of healing is dependent upon an intact pulp and is seen primarily in cases with little or no dislocation (i.e. concussion or subluxation) of the coronal fragment and most often in teeth with immature root formation (13, 90, 103, 134) (Fig. 8.20).

Fig. 8.20.

Upper. *Probability of the various healing modalities after root fracture of the maxillary right central incisor (arrows) in an 8-year-old boy based on the following information from the time of injury: the coronal fragment was subluxated, with first-degree loosening; the diameter of the apical foramen was 2.8 mm; antibiotics were administered due to avulsion and replantation of the maxillary left central incisor. Fixation was with an acid-etch splint. The times on the horizontal axis of the probability curves are the intervals defined in the statistical analysis. The times given on the radiographs are the exact observation periods, which correspond to the defined intervals.*

Lower. *The radiographic appearance at the various observation periods. At 39 days, the diagnosis of hard tissue union (HT) was made (asterisk). From AN-DREASEN ET AL. (136) 1989*

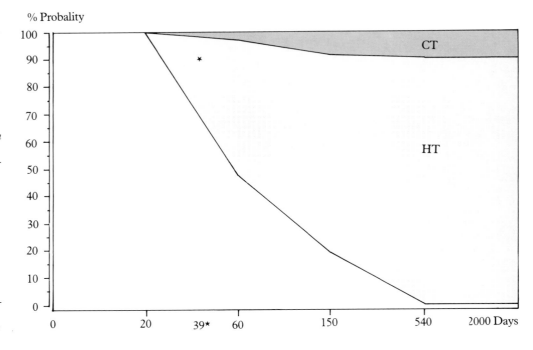

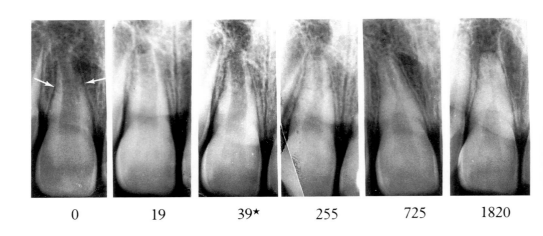

| 0 | 19 | 39★ | 255 | 725 | 1820 |

Interposition of Connective Tissue

This type of healing is apparently related to a moderately injured pulp (i.e. extrusion or lateral luxation of the coronal fragment), whereby pulpal revascularization and/or reinnervation must be completed prior to pulpal participation in fracture healing. In the interim, periodontal ligament cells are able to dominate the healing process (136). Histologically, this is characterized by the presence of connective tissue between the fragments (13, 37, 48) (Fig. 8.21). The fracture surfaces are covered by cementum, often deposited after initial resorption (38, 39, 43, 99), with connective tissue fibers running parallel to the fracture surface or from one fragment to the other. By means of secondary dentin formation, a new "apical foramen" is created at the fracture level (32, 45, 134, 135). A common finding is peripheral rounding of the fracture edges (*external surface resorption* (134)), sometimes with slight ingrowth of bone into the fracture area (13, 27) (Fig. 8.16). The width of the periodontal space around the fragments reflects the functional activity of the two fragments. The periodontal space surrounding the apical fragment is narrow, with fibers oriented parallel to the root surface, while the space around the coronal fragment is wide, with normal fiber arrangement (37, 41).

The radiographic features in this type of healing consist of peripheral rounding of the fracture edges and a radiolucent line separating the fragments (Fig. 8.16 B).

Fig. 8.21.
Interposition of connective tissue after root fracture of left central and lateral incisors. A. One week after injury. B. Radiograph at time of removal 6 weeks after injury. C. Low-power view of sectioned central incisor shows interposition of connective tissue. x 30. D. Vital pulp tissue in crown portion. x 75. E. Connective tissue in fracture line. x 30. F. Higher magnification of E. Note active resorption on surface of fragments (arrows) x 75. G. Comminuted fracture in apical region. Note formation of cementum on fragments. x 30. From ANDREASEN & HJØRTING-HANSEN *(13) 1967.*

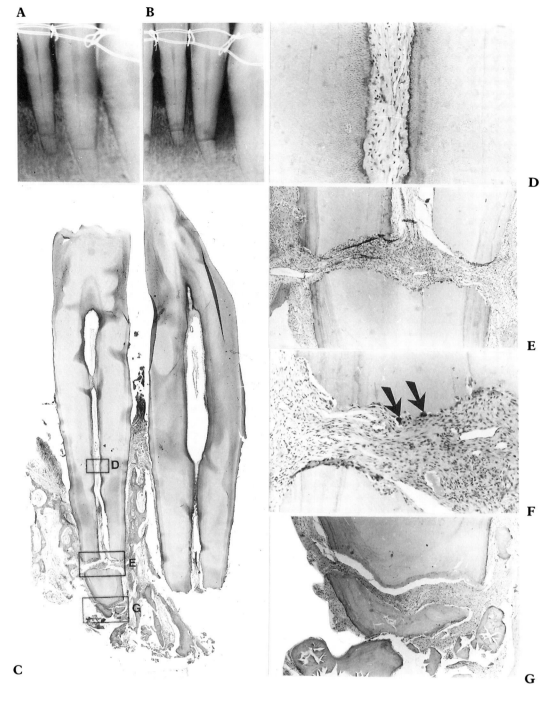

Initially, *external* and *internal surface resorption* are often seen (134), as well as *pulp canal obliteration* of both apical and coronal aspects of the root canal (136).

Clinically, the teeth are normally firm or slightly mobile and with a weak pain response to percussion. The response to sensibility testing is usually within the normal range (13, 93, 134-135). Although no interceptive therapy is required at the ap-

pearance of the above-mentioned resorption processes, it should be mentioned that a few cases have been observed whereby the post-resorptive mineralization process resulted in *ankylosis*. Thus, longer observation periods as well as more frequent follow-up examinations during the 1st year after injury might be advisable when these resorption processes are diagnosed. (see Appendix 4, p. 750).

ROOT FRACTURES

Interposition of Bone and Connective Tissue

Histologically teeth in this healing group demonstrate interposition of a bony bridge and connective tissue between the apical and coronal fragments, with a normal periodontal ligament surrounding both fragments (27, 49-53). In some instances, bone can be seen extending into the root canals (49-51) (Fig. 8.22).

This mode of healing is apparently a result of trauma prior to completed growth of the alveolar process; thus the coronal fragment continues to erupt, while the apical fragment remains stationary in the jaw (13) (Fig. 8.23).

Radiographically, a bony bridge is seen separating the fragments, with a periodontal space around both fragments. Total *pulp canal obliteration* of the root canals in both fragments is a common finding (Fig. 8.16 C).

Clinically, the teeth are firm and react normally to pulp tests.

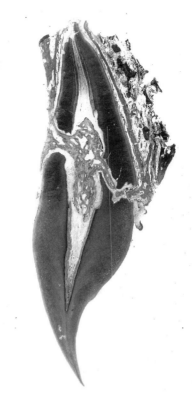

Fig. 8.22.
Interposition of bone and connective tissue between fragments of a permanent incisor removed 6 months after root fracture. Note extension of bone into the pulp canal. x 7. From BLACKWOOD *(49) 1959.*

Fig. 8.23.
The growth of the alveolar process leaves the apical fragment behind in its original position.

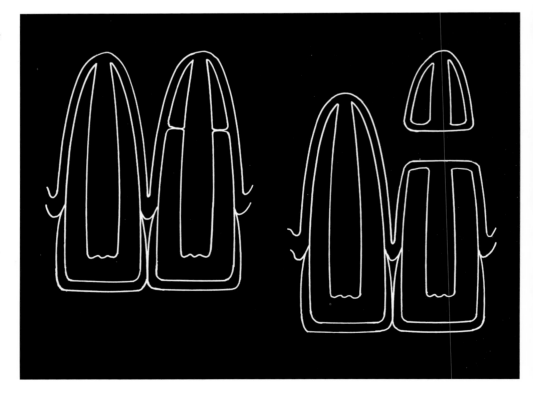

Fig. 8.24.
Interposition of granulation tissue between fragments of a left central incisor. A. Immediately after injury. B. Radiographs at the time of removal 6 months after injury. C. Low-power view of sectioned incisor. x 6. D. Vital pulp tissue in apical fragment. x 75. E. Granulation tissue with epithelial proliferation and chronic inflammation. x 30. F. Higher magnification of E. Area with newly formed cementum. x 195. G. Necrotic pulp tissue in coronal fragment. x 30. From ANDREASEN & HJØRTING-HANSEN (13) *1967.*

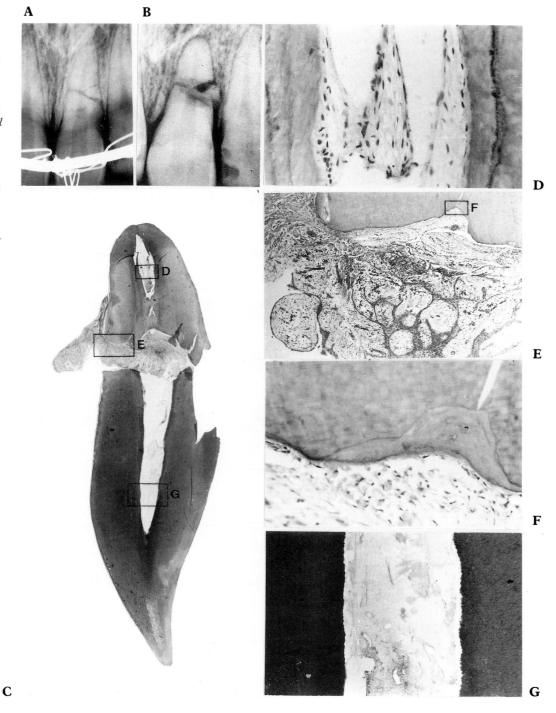

A B D E F G C

Interposition of Granulation Tissue

Histologic examination of teeth in this group reveals inflamed granulation tissue between the fragments (13, 37, 53-57, 140) (Figs. 8.24 and 8.25). The coronal portion of the pulp is necrotic, while the apical fragment usually contains vital pulp tissue (16) (Fig. 8.24 D and G). The necrotic and infected pulp tissue is responsible for the inflammatory changes along the fracture line. In some cases, however, communication between the fracture line and the gingival crevice is the source of inflammation (13, 47, 57) (Fig. 8.25).

Radiographically, widening of the fracture line and rarefaction of the alveolar bone corresponding to the fracture line are typical findings (141) (Fig. 8.16 D). If the tooth is not splinted, the coronal fragment is loose, slightly extruded and sensitive to

Fig. 8.25.
Interposition of granulation tissue between fragments of a left central incisor. A. and B. Radiographs taken 2 months after trauma. Note the periradicular radiolucency adjacent to the fracture line (arrow). C. Low-power view of sectioned incisor. The tooth was removed 2 months after injury. x 6. D. Downward proliferation of epithelium from gingival crevice. x 75. E and F. Palatal fracture with epithelial proliferation. x 30 and x 75. G. Necrotic pulp tissue in coronal fragment. x 30. From ANDREASEN *&* HJØRTING-HANSEN (13) *1967.*

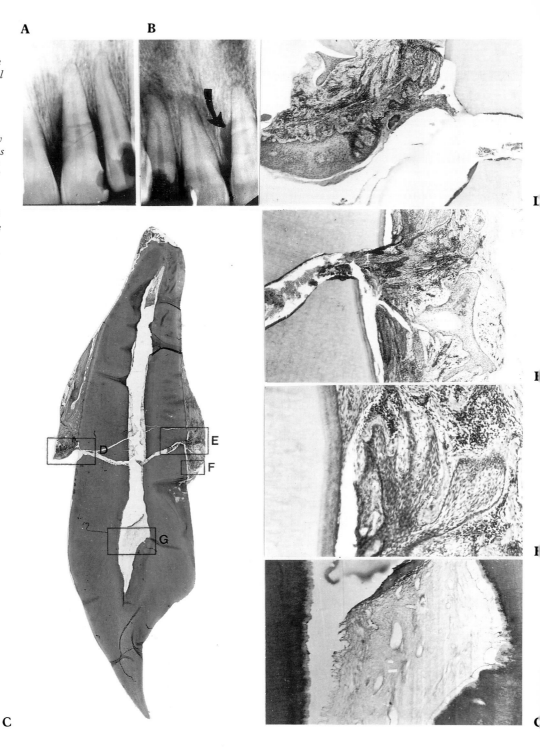

percussion. If splinted, the apical fragment becomes displaced in apical direction. Fistulae at a level on the labial mucosa corresponding to the fracture line are an occasional finding (13).

It has been found that negative pulpal sensibility at the time of injury was significantly related to later pulp necrosis, presumably a reflection of severe pulpal injury. However, a positive pulpal response was not able to predict healing by hard tissue union or interposition of connective tissue

(136). Moreover, fixation by the forceful application of orthodontic bands (a splinting technique employed prior to the advent of the passively applied acid-etch splints) played an important role in the development of coronal pulp necrosis following root fracture (136). This adverse effect was presumably due to an additional trauma, including possible dislocation of the coronal fragment, during splint application.

Treatment

The principles of treating *permanent teeth* are reduction of displaced coronal fragments and firm immobilization (Fig. 8.26). If treatment is instituted immediately after injury, repositioning of the fragment by digital manipulation is easily achieved (Fig. 8.27). If resistance is felt upon repositioning, it is most likely due to fracture of the labial socket wall. In this case, repositioning of the fractured bone is necessary before further attempts are made to reduce the root fracture (Fig. 8.28). After reduction, the position should be checked radiographically.

Immobilization of teeth with root fractures is achieved with rigid fixation, e.g. an acid etch/resin splint (see Chapter 9, p. 347). As previously mentioned, forceful application of, e.g. orthodontic bands for the purpose of immobilizing the coronal fragment is contraindicated, due to its traumatic influence on the already traumatized pulp that could result in pulp necrosis. A passively applied splint (e.g. using the acid-etch technique) is advised. The fixation period should be 2-3 months to ensure sufficient hard tissue consolidation. However, no studies to date have established the influence of the length of the splinting period upon fracture healing.

It should be noted that immature teeth with incomplete root fractures require no fixation and will heal by hard tissue union. However, these teeth may be included in a splint if multiple tooth injuries so require. During this period, it is important that the tooth be observed radiographically and with sensibility tests in order to detect pulp necrosis. See Appendix 4, p. 750 for a suggested schedule for recall examinations.

Fig. 8.26. Principles for treatment of root fractures
Treatment of root fractures consists of complete repositioning and firm, immobile splinting, preferably with a passively applied splint until a hard tissue callus is formed, usually after 3 months.

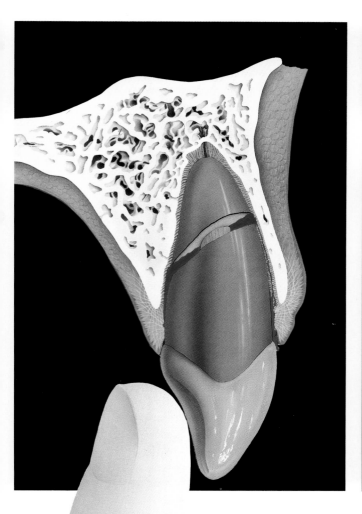
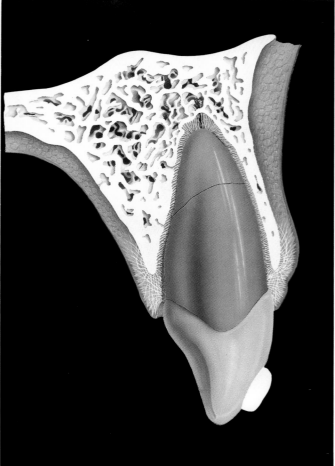

Fig. 8.27. Treatment of a laterally luxated root fracture

This 13-year-old boy received a horizontal blow to the left maxillary central incisor.

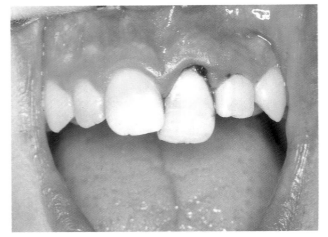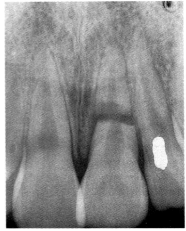

Examining the tooth

The tooth reacts to SENSITIBILITY TESTING, indicating an intact vascular supply. There is a high metallic sound elicited by the PERCUSSION TEST, indicating lateral luxation of the coronal fragment. The tooth is locked firmly in its displaced position, confirming the luxation diagnosis.

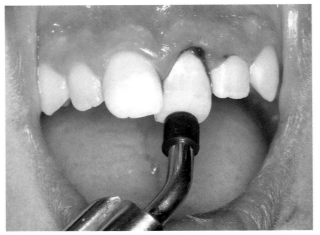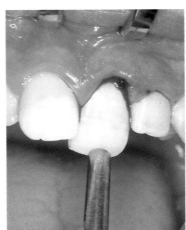

Repositioning

Because of the force necessary to reposition a laterally luxated tooth, local anesthesia is administered prior to repositioning. Firm pressure is applied to the facial bone plate at the fracture level in order to displace the coronal fragment out of its alveolar "lock." This is followed by horizontal (forward) pressure at the palatal aspect of the incisal edge, which repositions the coronal fragment into its original position.

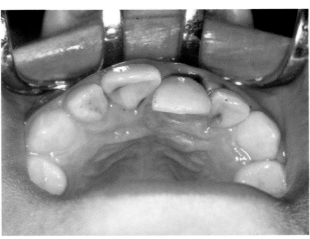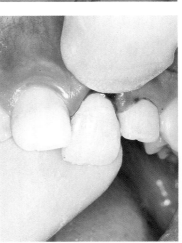

Verifying repositioning

The correct position of the coronal fragment is confirmed radiographicaly.

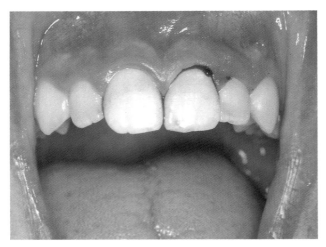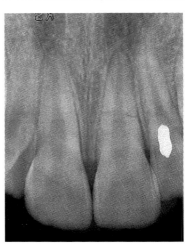

Fixation procedure

The acid-etch technique and a temporary crown and bridge material are used. Phosphoric acid gel is applied for 30 seconds to the facial surfaces of the injured and adjacent non-injured teeth. The tooth surfaces are then rinsed thoroughly with a stream of water for 20-30 seconds and blown dry. A mat enamel surface indicates adequate etching.

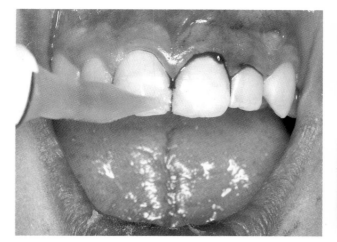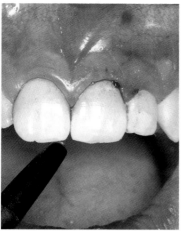

Applying the splinting material

Temporary crown and bridge material is applied to the etched enamel surfaces. The bulk of the material should be placed on the mesial and distal corners of the traumatized and adjacent, non-injured incisors. After setting, any irregularity in the surface is removed with abrasive discs or a scalpel blade.

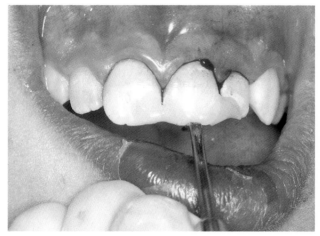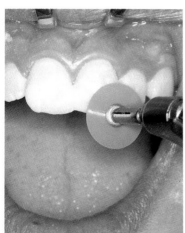

Removing the splint

The healing events are monitored radiographically 1, 2 and 3 months after injury. If, after these periods, the tooth reacts to sensibility testing and there is no sign of infection in the bone at the level of the fracture, the splint may be removed.

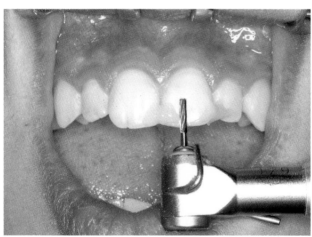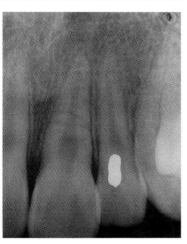

One year after injury

The tooth reacts normally to sensibility testing and the radiograph shows increasing radiopacity of the fracture line.

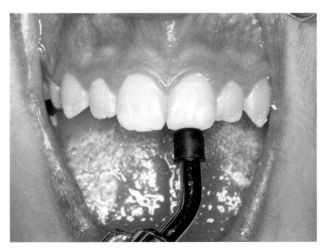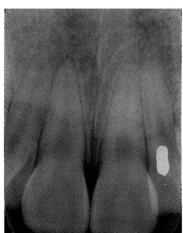

ROOT FRACTURES

Fig. 8.28. Treatment of a severely extruded root fracture

This 20-year-old woman has suffered a frontal blow to the left central incisor, resulting in extreme displacement of the coronal fragment.

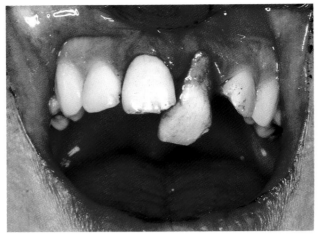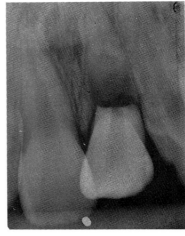

Examining the displaced coronal fragment

After cleansing the exposed root surface with saline, it can be seen that the coronal fragment has been forced past the cervical margin of the labial bone plate. The stretched pulp is seen within the socket area.

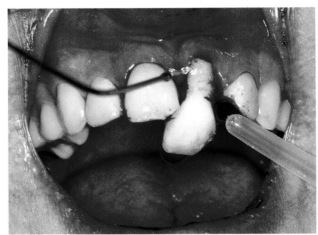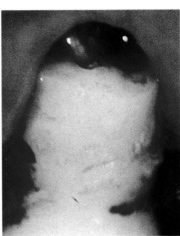

Repositioning

After local anesthetic infiltration, the coronal fragment is repositioned. To guide the root fragment into place, an amalgam carver is inserted beneath the cervical bone margin and used like a shoe horn.

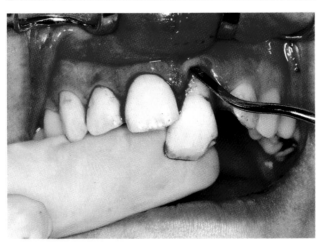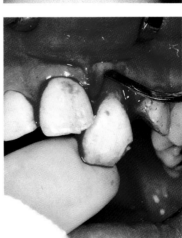

Splinting

The acid-etch technique is employed once optimal repositioning has been verified radiographically. The labial surfaces are etched and a splinting material (e.g. composite resin or a temporary crown and bridge material) is applied. The patient is given penicillin (2 million IU daily for 4 days) to safeguard healing.

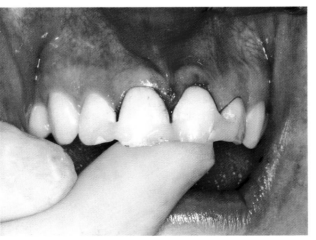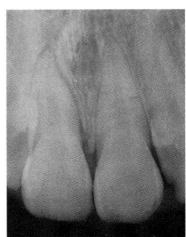

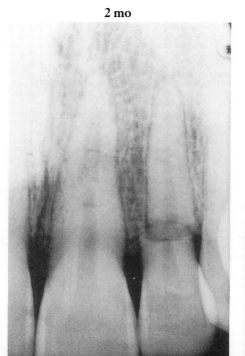
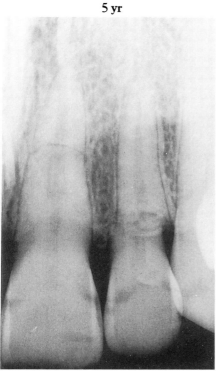

Fig. 8.29.
Hard tissue healing of a root fracture located at the marginal third of the root of a left incisor.

Close proximity of the root fracture to the gingival crevice may dictate treatment, as the chance of healing with calcified tissue is poorest when a cervical fracture line is very close to the gingival crevice. A treatment option which could then be considered is the removal of the coronal fragment and subsequent orthodontic (106) or surgical extrusion of the remaining apical fragment. These techniques are described in more detail in relation to treatment of complicated crown-root fractures (see Chapters 7 and 15, p. 269 and p. 603).

If the fracture is located at the cervical third of the root and below the alveolar crest, various studies have shown that healing is possible and a conservative approach justified (13, 26, 58) (Figs. 8.28 and 8.29). In cases where oral hygiene is optimal, treatment can be permanent fixation of the coronal fragment to adjacent non-injured teeth at the contact areas proximally with a filled composite resin (Fig. 8.30).

In cases where it is not possible to treat the fractured tooth conservatively and the

Fig. 8.30.
Permanent fixation of the coronal fragment of a root fractured lateral incisor healed with interposition of connective tissue. At the contact areas proximally, filled composite resin is placed. Radiograph shows 10 year follow-up.

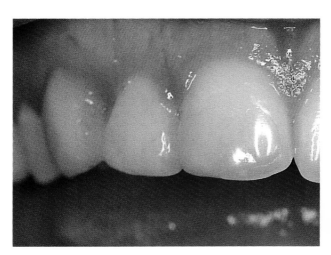
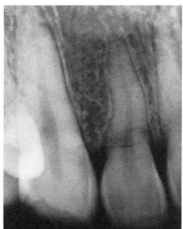

Fig. 8.31.
Atrophy of the alveolar process after surgical removal of a root fractured tooth. A. Condition after trauma. The right central incisor shows a root fracture close to the gingival crevice. The tooth was surgically removed. During this procedure the labial bone plate was also removed. B. and C. Marked atrophy of the alveolar process is evident 1 year later.

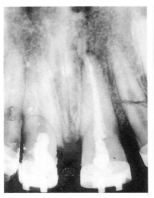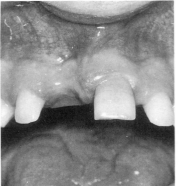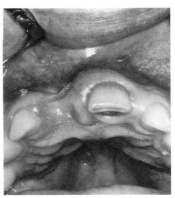

tooth must be extracted, it should be remembered that careless extraction procedures will result in extensive damage to the alveolar process and subsequent severe atrophy, especially in the labio-lingual direction, ultimately resulting in a compromised esthetic restorative treatment. This problem can be prevented to a certain degree by careful removal of the apical fragment with no or minimal sacrifice of labial bone. Thus, if removal of the apical fragment is not possible via the socket, surgical removal should be undertaken by raising a flap and making an osteotomy over the apical area, thereby pushing the apex out of its socket. Under no circumstance should the marginal socket wall be removed, as this can lead to labio-lingual collapse of the alveolar process (Fig. 8.31).

A preferred alternative to the above situation is the preservation of the apical fragment, which normally contains vital pulp tissue. Experimental evidence seems to indicate that intentionally submerged root fragments with vital pulps prevent or retard resorption of the alveolar process. These roots are usually covered along the fractured surface with a new layer of cementum as well as a thin layer of new bone. Moreover, the pulp retains its vitality (107-109). Preliminary clinical experience seems to indicate that the intentionally buried apical fragment resulting from root fracture acts similarly (Fig. 8.32). This is presumably analogous to the sub-

Fig. 8.32.
Apical fragment left in situ. The 2 central incisors were avulsed. A. Condition at the time of injury. B. At a follow-up 5 years after injury, the pulp canal in the apical fragment shows complete obliteration and bone covers the fractured surface of the root.

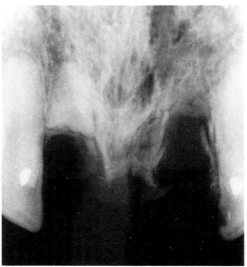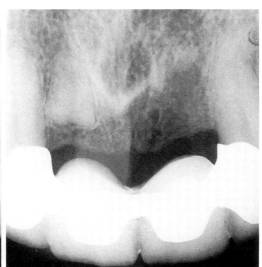

0 days   5 yr

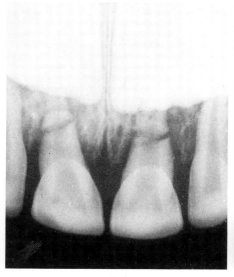

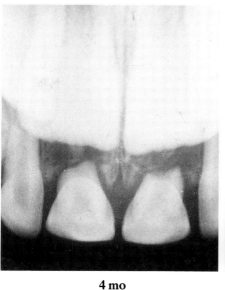

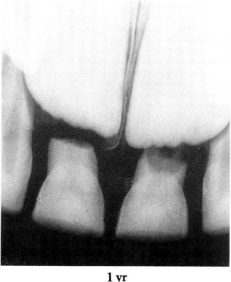

| 0 d | 4 mo | 1 yr |

Fig. 8.33.
Normal physiologic resorption after root fracture of both primary central incisors in a 4-year-old child. Note apparently normal physiologic resorption of the traumatized incisors. From AN-DREASEN & HJØRTING-HANSEN (13) 1967.

Fig. 8.34.
Lateral luxation of a right central incisor and root fracture of left central incisor in a 5-year-old child. The right incisor was extracted, as was the coronal portion of the left central incisor. Condition after 1 year. After 2 years, both permanent central incisors are erupting and the apex of the left primary incisor has been resorbed.

mergence of the apical fragment which is seen after healing by interposition of bone and connective tissue. Whether this treatment procedure is reliable must await the results of long-term clinical studies.

Primary teeth with root fractures without dislocation may be preserved and normal shedding of injured teeth anticipated (Fig. 8.33). It is usually not possible to splint these teeth; nor has the value of this procedure been demonstrated. The coronal fragments of primary teeth with severe dislocation should generally be removed, as pulp necrosis is likely to develop. In order to avoid trauma to the permanent tooth germ, no effort should be made to remove the apical fragment, as normal physiologic resorption can be expected (Fig. 8.34) (13, 91).

Prognosis

Several clinical reports have demonstrated successful treatment of root fractures (13, 26, 37, 59-71, 90-92, 100, 103, 110, 111, 133, 136, 142-144). However, follow-up examinations can disclose deviations in pulpal and periodontal healing. In this context, radiographic findings, such as *pulp canal obliteration, external and internal surface resorption* have been found to be related to specific healing modalities (134).

Pulpal Healing

Clinical experience has shown that the pulp is more likely to survive after root fracture than after luxation with no frac-

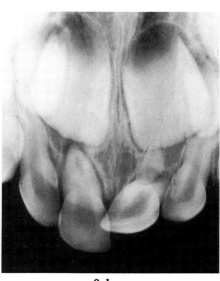

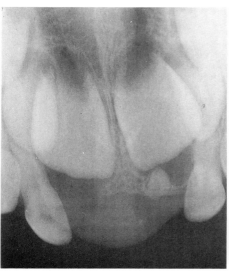

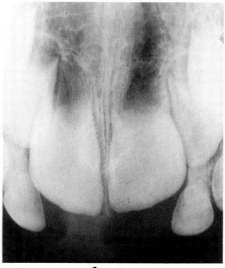

| 0 d | 1 yr | 2 yr |

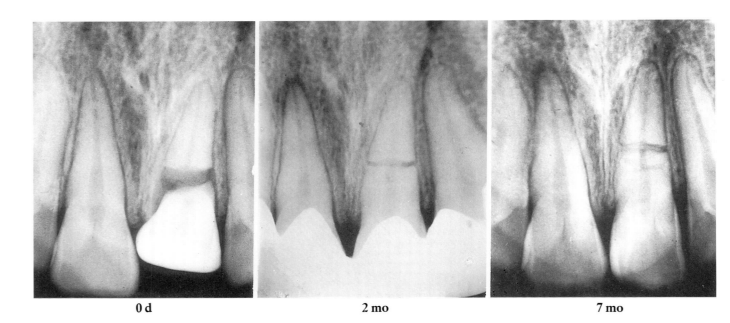

| 0 d | 2 mo | 7 mo |

Fig. 8.35.
Pulp necrosis and periapical involvement after subluxation and pulp survival after root fracture. Left central incisor showed root fracture and dislocation while the right central incisor was subluxated. The subluxated tooth has developed pulp necrosis but the tooth with the root fracture has remained vital.

ture of the root (41, 61, 65, 72-74, 135) (Fig. 8.35). An explanation could be that the fate of the injured pulp depends in part upon revascularization from the periodontal ligament. Such revascularization in luxation injuries is limited to the periapical tissues, whereas a fractured root offers broader communication from the pulp canal to the periodontal tissues, facilitating re-establishment of the blood supply. Moreover, if one assumes that only the coronal aspect of the pulp has been dam-

aged, the extent of tissue requiring revascularization is considerably reduced following root fracture than after luxation injuries. Another important factor could be the development of pulpal edema, which can escape through the fracture, minimizing pressure upon the delicate pulpal vessels. Furthermore, the root fracture itself could prevent transmission of the impact to the apical area, thus reducing damage to the vulnerable area at the constricted apical foramen (65).

Fig. 8.37.
Dislocation of a root fracture leading to pulp necrosis. Note that the left maxillary incisor is dislocated more than the right incisor. Three months later, the right central incisor was found to be vital whereas pulp necrosis and periapical rarefaction was diagnosed in the left central incisor (arrow).

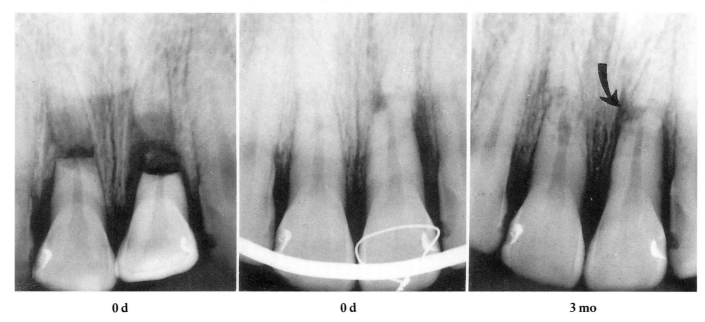

| 0 d | 0 d | 3 mo |

Examiner	No. of teeth	No. with pulp necrosis
Austin (12) 1930	40	8 (20%)
Douniau & Werelds (10) 1955	24	5 (21%)
Lindahl (11) 1958	25	6 (24%)
Andreasen & Hörting-Hansen (13) 1967	48	21 (44%)
Stålhane & Hedegård (111) 1975	18	4 (18%)
Zachrisson & Jacobsen (93) 1975	64	13 (20%)
Ravn (94) 1976	50	11 (22%)
Andreasen et al.(136) 1989	95	25 (26%)

Close clinical and radiographic follow-ups are necessary to disclose pulp necrosis (141). Extrusion of the coronal fragment, tenderness to percussion and, most significantly, radiographic signs of pulp necrosis, such as development of radiolucencies within bone adjacent to the fracture line (Figs. 8.36 and 8.37), can usually be detected within the first 2 months after injury.

A negative sensibility response immediately after injury does not necessarily indicate pulp necrosis, as a slow return to normal vitality is often observed (103). However, it has been found that teeth which did not respond to pulp testing immediately following root fracture demonstrated a significantly greater risk of later pulp necrosis than those which responded positively at the time of injury (136). The diagnosis of pulp necrosis should therefore always be based upon clinical and radiographic evaluation.

Table 8.1 lists various reports on the prevalence of pulp necrosis after root fracture. Factors contributing to necrosis are *displacement of the coronal fragment* (13, 93, 136) (Fig. 8.36), the *forceful application of splints* (136), *non-splinting,* and teeth with *completed root formation* at the time of injury (90, 93,136).

It has previously been supposed that

Fig. 8.36.
Radiographic demonstration of pulp necrosis after root fracture. The enlargement of the periodontal space adjacent to the fracture line indicates pulp necrosis (arrows).

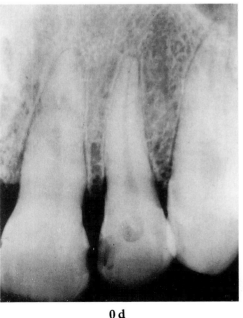

0 d

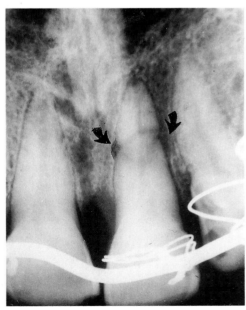

2 mo

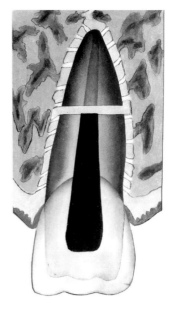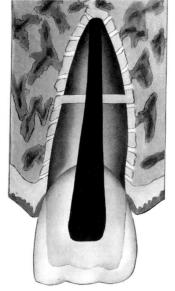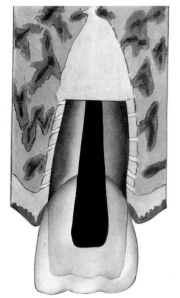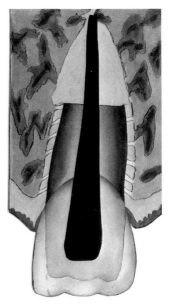

Fig. 8.38.
Schematic drawings illustrating various types of treatments of pulp necrosis after root fracture. A. Root canal filling of coronal fragment. B. Intraradicular splinting with a metal pin used as root canal filling. C. Surgical removal of apical fragment together with root canal filling of coronal fragment. D. Metal implant replacing the apical fragment and acting as root canal filling. From AN-DREASEN (87) *1968.*

root fractures located at the marginal one-third of the root had a very poor prognosis, thus indicating extraction therapy. However, this assumption has not been supported by recent studies where no relationship could be demonstrated between the frequency of pulp necrosis and the position of the fracture line (13, 90, 93, 94, 103, 136).

Other factors which have been found to be predictive of the type of fracture healing have included the presence of *restorations* at the time of injury as well as the presence of *marginal periodontitis* (136). Thus, if either of these factors were present, there was a significantly greater risk of healing by interposition of connective tissue than healing by hard tissue union. It was impossible to determine whether this finding reflected an age phenomenon or reduced pulpal defence due to disease or operative procedures.

Many types of treatment have been proposed for the management of pulp necrosis in root-fractured teeth (26) (Fig. 8.38). The most important feature to consider is that the apical fragment normally contains vital pulp tissue (13). This is the basis for treatment where only the coronal fragment is root-filled, a treatment form which has been shown to result in a high rate of healing (26, 83, 112, 141). This form of therapy is described in detail in Chapter 14, p. 532.

If the fracture line is situated in the cervical third of the root and the pulp is necrotic, the coronal fragment will

become quite mobile. Intraradicular splinting, with a metal pin uniting the fragments and serving as a root canal filling has been tried (113, 115-118, 145-147). So far, only limited clinical data have been reported concerning long-term prognosis of these forms of therapy. However, the failure rate appears to be as high as half of all treated cases (146, 147).

Another suggested method of stabilizing the coronal fragment involves using metal endodontic implants which replace the apical fragment (74, 85-87, 104, 119-126, 148-156). Prefabricated implants are normally used in association with standardized endodontic intracanal instruments (85) (Fig. 8.39). The purpose of the implant is to shift the fulcrum of transverse movements to a more apical position. Clinically, this shift is evident in the stability of the fractured tooth immediately after implantation. However, successful long-term prognosis for these implants is dubious. Thus, in the authors' experience, 12 implants which originally were considered to have a good prognosis failed at later follow-ups (87) (Fig. 8.40). Moreover, increasing numbers of experimental studies have demonstrated evidence of corrosion of the pins as well as severe inflammation in the soft tissues adjacent to these implants (127-130, 157). Only a single experimental study found implants in teeth with no initial periapical inflammation to be accepted with no evidence of inflammation after 6 months (157).

Another treatment procedure has been

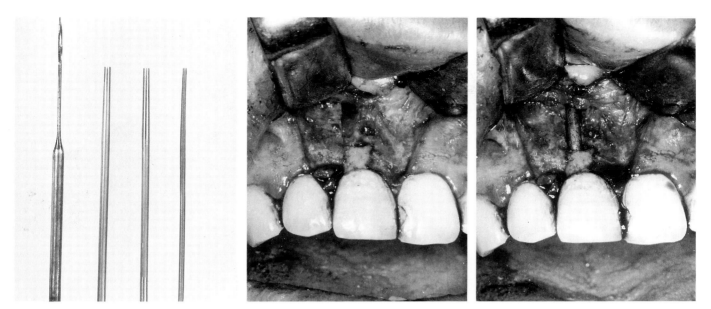

Fig. 8.39.
Surgical removal of apical fragment and insertion of a metal implant in a central incisor. A. Prefabricated cobalt-chromium implants and standardized endodontic instruments (Endodontic implant Starter Kit-B3, Star Dental Mfg. Co. Inc., Philadelphia, Pa., 19139, U.S.A).
B. A mucoperiosteal flap has been raised and the apical fragment removed. The entire root canal of the coronal fragment is enlarged to the level of the fracture. C. A cobalt-chromium implant of proper size is inserted into the root canal and the course taken by the implant noted. Subsequently, a cavity is created in the alveolar bone, ensuring that the length of the implant exceeds the original length of the root by 2 to 4 millimeters. The length of the implant is adjusted to the bone cavity and, in addition, to the level of the lingual surface of the crown. Finally, the implant is cemented into the root canal with a root canal sealer and special care is taken to remove excess cement.

Fig. 8.40.
Treatment of root fracture by removal of apical fragment and insertion of a metal implant. At a follow-up 12 years later, inflammation around the implant is evident and a fistula is present.

advocated whereby the coronal fragment is extracted and the apical fragment removed. The root canal in the coronal fragment is enlarged and a combined root filling/root elongation is performed using an aluminum oxide implant which extends outside the apical foramen (see Chapter 10, p. 405). However, to date (158, 159) the long-term results of this procedure do not suggest that this procedure will be better than endontic treatment of the coronal fragment only (112). In this connection it should be borne in mind that root fractured incisors which heal after endodontic treatment of the coronal fragment tend to show decreasing mobility because of the physiologic decrease in tooth mobility with age (131, 160).

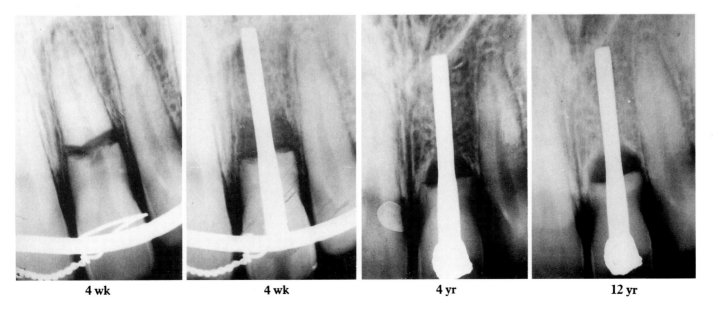

| 4 wk | 4 wk | 4 yr | 12 yr |

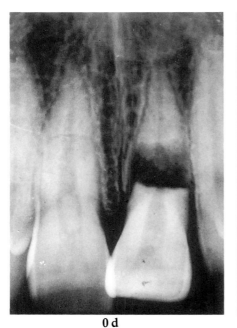 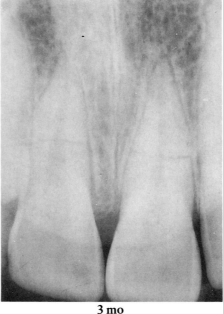 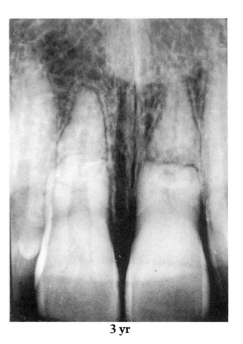

| **0 d** | **3 mo** | **3 yr** |

Fig. 8.41.

Effect of displacement of the coronal fragment on root fracture healing. Pulp canal obliteration after root fracture of both central incisors. The teeth were repositioned and splinted for 3 months. At the control appointment 3 years later, the right central incisor showed healing, with calcified tissue and partial pulp canal obliteration confined to the apical fragment and at the fracture site whereas the left central incisor demonstrated healing with interposition of connective tissue and complete pulp canal obliteration.

Fig. 8.42.

External inflammatory resorption following root fracture of a right central incisor. External resorption is evident at re-examination 2 years after injury. Mesial and distal radiographic projections revealed the external nature of this resorption process. Pulp necrosis was diagnosed at the clinical examination.

Pulp Canal Obliteration

Partial or complete obliteration of the pulp canal is a common finding after root fracture (Fig. 8.41) (132, 134-136). Thus, in recent studies of root-fractured permanent incisors, pulp canal obliteration was found in 69-73% of the teeth (93, 103, 136). *Partial* pulp canal obliteration is seen most often in the fracture region and the apical fragment. In addition, partial obliteration extends 1-2 mm into the coronal fragment. *Complete* pulp canal obliteration is seen as an even decrease in the size of the entire pulp

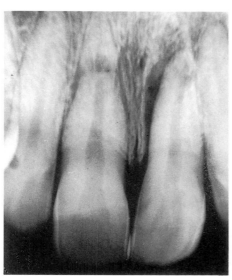 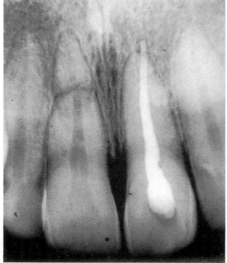 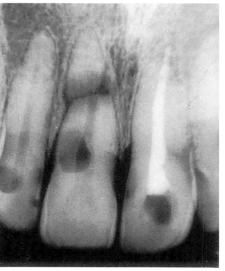

| **0 d** | **9 mo** | **24 mo** |

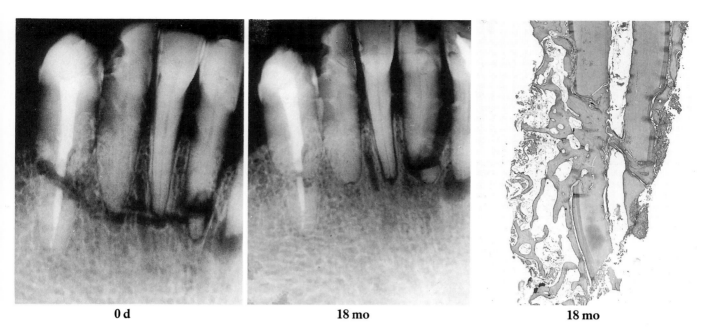

0 d **18 mo** **18 mo**

Fig. 8.43.
External replacement resorption following root fracture of right canine as well as fracture of the alveolar process. At re-examination 18 months later, external replacement resorption is evident. Histologic examination of extracted canine demonstrates marked replacement resorption. x 6.

cavity, leading to total obliteration. Both obliteration types progress at the same rate and are normally well advanced after 9-12 months and approach full density 1-2 years later (103). Obliteration of the apical root canal alone is commonly seen in cases of healing with calcified tissue, while obliteration of the apical and coronal aspects of the root canal is often seen in cases with interposition of connective tissue, as well as in teeth with interposition of connective tissue and bone (103, 136). In this context, however, one should be aware that in cases of pulp necrosis, while the coronal root canal is usually the only part of the root canal affected, the apical root canal can be completely obliterated. Thus, one must use other criteria (i.e. resorption of bone at the level of the fracture, loss of sensibility, loosening of the coronal fragment) for the determination of pulpal status. Clinically, a slight yellowish discoloration of the crown is sometimes seen in the case of coronal pulp canal obliteration. Pulpal sensibility testing is in most cases normal, but a negative response can be registered. In contrast to pulp canal obliteration after luxation injuries, secondary pulp necrosis is a rare finding (103).

Root Resorption

Root resorption has been found to occur in approximately 60% of root-fractured permanent incisors and can usually be detected within 1 year after injury. These processes often precede fracture healing and obliteration of the coronal and/or apical aspects of the root canal and should be distinguished from resorption of bone at the level of root fracture which is indicative of coronal pulp necrosis. Root resorption appears in the following types:

1) *External surface resorption,* characterized by the rounding of the fracture edges mesially and/or distally (Fig. 8.13)
2) *External inflammatory resorption* (Fig. 8.42)
3) *External replacement resorption* (Fig. 8.43)
4) *Internal surface resorption,* manifested as rounding of the fracture edges centrally, in the apical and coronal root canals, at the intersection between the root canal and fracture line (Fig. 8.13)
5) *Internal tunneling resorption,* going behind the pre-dentin layer and burrowing along the root canal walls of the coronal fragment (Fig. 8.14).

Orthodontic Treatment of Root Fractured Teeth

This problem is discussed in detail in Chapter 15 (see p. 606).

Essentials

Treatment of Permanent Teeth

a. If the fracture is located very close to the gingiva, extraction of the coronal fragment may be indicated, followed by orthodontic or surgical extrusion of the apical fragment. (see Chapter 7 p. 218). However, in the case of optimal oral hygiene, a conservative approach comprising permanent proximal fixation may be attempted.

b. Otherwise, reposition the coronal fragment, if displaced (Figs. 8.27 and 8.28).

c. Check position of the coronal fragment radiographically.

d. Immobilize the tooth with a rigid splint (e.g. acid-etch/resin splint). Forceful application of splints should be avoided.

e. Control the tooth radiographically and with sensibility tests.

f. Maintain the splint for 2-3 months.

g. Follow-up period minimum 1 year.

Prognosis

Pulp necrosis: 20-44%
Risk groups: Mature, dislocated and non-splinted teeth
> Treatment of pulp necrosis
a. Root canal treatment of coronal fragment (see Chapter 14, p. 532)

Pulp canal obliteration: 69%

Root resorption: 60%
Considered to be a link in fracture healing and requires no treatment

Treatment of Primary Teeth

Treatment principles are generally the same as for permanent teeth. Important features are:

a. Apical fragments should not be removed if extraction is decided upon

b. Splinting can be omitted

Bibliography

1. ANDREASEN J O. Etiology and pathogenesis of traumatic dental injuries. A clinical study of 1,298 cases. *Scand J Dent Res* 1979;**78**:329-42.

2. HARDWICK JL, NEWMAN PA. Some observations on the incidence and emergency treatment of fractured permanent anterior teeth of children. *J Dent Res* 1954;**33**:730.

3. DOWN CH. The treatment of permanent incisor teeth of children following traumatic injury. *Aust Dent J* 1957;**2**:9-24.

4. SUNDVALL-HAGLAND I. Olycksfallsskador på tänder och parodontium under barnaåren. In: Holst JJ, Nygaard Østby B, Osvald O. *Nordisk Klinisk Odontologi.* Copenhagen: A/S Forlaget for Faglitteratur, 1964, Chapter 11, III:1-40.

5. GELBIER S. Injured anterior teeth in children. A preliminary discussion. *Br Dent J* 1967;**123**:331-5.

6. RAVN JJ, ROSSEN I. Hyppighed og fordeling af traumatiske beskadigelser af tænderne hos københavnske skolebørn 1967/68. *Tandlægebladet* 1969;**73**:1-9.

7. FIALOVÁ S, JURECEK B. Urazy zubu udeti a nase zkusenosti s jejich lécenim. *Prakt zubni Lék* 1968;**16**:171-6.

8. MAGNUSSON B, HOLM A-K. Traumatised permanent teeth in children - a follow-up. I. Pulpal complications and root resorption. *Svensk Tandläkars Tidning* 1969;**62**:61-70.

9. ENGELHARDT H-G, HAMMER H. Pathologie und Therapie der Zahnwurzelfrakturen. *Dtsch Zahnärztl Z* 1959;**14**:1278-89.

10. DOUNIAU R, WERELDS RJ. La consolidation des fractures radiculaires. Observations cliniques, radiographiques et histologiques. *Rev Belge Stomatol* 1955;**52**:621-43.

11. LINDAHL B. Transverse intra-alveolar root fractures: Roentgen diagnosis and prognosis. *Odontologisk Revy* 1958;**9**:10-24.

12. AUSTIN LT. A review of forty cases of retained fractured roots of anterior teeth. *J Am Dent Assoc* 1930;**17**:1930-2.

13. ANDREASEN JO, HJØRTING-HANSEN E. Intraalveolar root fractures: radiographic and histologic study of 50 cases. *J Oral Surg* 1967;**25**:414-26.

14. FREZIERES H, PONS J, LARTIGAU G. Traumatismes accidentels des incisives superieures chez l'adulte jeune. *Rev Fr Odonto- Stomatol* 1965;**12**:1017-27.

15. DUCLOS J, BRUGIRARD J. Diagnostic radiologique des fractures radiculaires (Loi des épasseurs du Professeur Duclos). *Ann Odontostomatol* 1955;**12**:59-71.

16. MARSHALL FJ. Root fracture. Report of a case. *Oral Surg Oral Med Oral Pathol* 1960;**13**:1485-7.

17. BOUCHER A. Fractures dentaires et radiographie. *Rev Fr Odontostomatatol* 1956;**3**:1015-7.

18. GOOSE DH. Invisible root fracture. *Dent Practit Dent Rec* 1964;**14**:271-2.

19. BLACKWOOD HJJ. Metaplasia or repair of the dental pulp as a response to injury. *Br Dent J* 1957;**102**:87-92.

20. SARNAT BG, SCHOUR I. Effect of experimental fracture on bone, dentin, and enamel. Study of the mandible and the incisor in the rat. *Arch Surg* 1944;**49**:23-38.

21. DREYER CJ, BLUM L. Effect of root fracture on the epithelial attachment. *J Dent Assoc South Afr* 1967;**22**:103-5.

22. BEVELANDER G. Tissue reactions in experimental tooth fracture. *J Dent Res* 1942;**21**:481-7.

23. HAMMER H. Die Heilungsvorgänge bei Wurzelbrücken. *Dtsch Zahn Mund Kieferheilk* 1939;**6**:297-317.

24. ROTTKE B, HATIFOTIADIS D. Spätergebnisse experimentell gesetzter Zahnfrakturen im Tierversuch. *Fortschr Kiefer Gesichtschir* 1967;**12**:271-4.

25. BROSCH F. Über die Anwendbarkeit der Gesetze der traumatischen Entzündung auf die Vorgänge nach dem Zahnwurzelbruch. *Dtsch Zahn Mund Kieferheilk* 1961;**36**:169-86.

26. ANDREASEN JO. Treatment of fractured and avulsed teeth. *ASDC J Dent Child* 1971;**38**:29-48.

27. ARWILL T. Histopathologic studies of traumatized teeth. *Odontologisk Tidsskrift* 1962;**70**:91-117.

28. BOUYSSOU M, CHANCHUS P, BADER J, VIVES J. Observations histologiques sur deux fractures radiculo-dentaires spontanément consolidées. *Rev Stomatol(Paris)*;**57**:417-27.

29. BRAUER JC. Treatment and restoration of fractured permanent anterior teeth. *J Am Dent Assoc* 1936;**23**:2323-36.

30. OMNELL KÅ. Study of a root fracture. *Br Dent J* 1953;**95**:181-5.

31. OTTOLENGUI R. Further consideration of the possible results of the fracture of the root of a tooth which contains a living pulp. *Dent Items Interest* 1927;**49**:79-90.

32. PRITCHARD GB. The reparative action of the dental tissues following severe injury. *Br Dent J* 1933;**54**:517-25.

33. REITAN K. Om vevsreaksjonen ved tilheling av rotfrakturer. *Norske Tannlægeforenings Tidende* 1947;**57**:367-73.

34. ZILKENS K. Beiträge zur traumatischen Zahnschädigung. In: WANNENMACHER E, ed. *Ein Querschnitt der deutschen wissenschaftlichen Zahnheilkunde.* No. 33. Leipzig: Hermann Meusser Verlag, 1938:43-70.

35. SCHULZE C. Klinisch-röntgenologischer Beitrag zur Frage der Heilungsvorgänge bei Wurzelbrüchen vitaler Zähne. *Dtsch Zahnärztl Z* 1951;**6**:595-601.

36. SCHULZE C. Über die Heilungsvorgänge nach intraalveolären Frakturen vitaler Zähne. *Dtsch Zahnärztl Z* 1957;**12**:666-73.

37. PINDBORG JJ. Clinical, radiographic and histological aspects of intraalveolar fractures of upper central incisors. *Acta Odontol Scand* 1955;**13**:41-71.

38. BENNETT DT. Repair following root fracture. *Br Dent J* 1959;**107**:217-20.

39. BOULGER EP. Histologic studies of a specimen of fractured roots. *J Am Dent Assoc* 1928;**15**:1778-89.

40. EVERETT CC, ORBAN B. Fractured vital teeth. *Oral Surg Oral Med Oral Pathol* 1953;**6**:605-13.

41. KRONFELD R. A case of tooth fracture, with special emphasis on tissue repair and adaptation following traumatic injury. *J Dent Res* 1936;**15**:429-46.

42. KÖNIG A. Über Heilungsvorgänge bei Zahnfrakturen. *Dtsch Zahn Mund Kieferheilk* 1939;**6**:273-87.

43. LEHNERT S. Ein Beitrag zur Pathologie der Zahnwurzelfrakturen. *Dtsch Zahnärztebl* 1964;**18**:451-8.

44. MALLESON HC. Fractured upper lateral incisor extracted after being splinted for three months. *Dent Cosmos* 1923;**65**:492-4.

45. MANLEY EB, MARSLAND EA. Tissue response following tooth fracture. *Br Dent J* 1952;**93**:199-203.

46. GOLDMAN HM, BLOOM J. A collective review and atlas of dental anomalies and diseases. *Oral Surg Oral Med Oral Pathol* 1949;**2**:874-905.

47. DAWKINS J. Two transverse root fractures. *Aust Dent J* 1959;**4**:27-30.

48. BOUYSSOU M, WERELDS RJ. Histomorphologic assessment of the three possible patterns of hard callus in the healing of dental root fractures. *J Dent Res* 1969;**48**:1143-4.

49. BLACKWOOD HJJ. Tissue repair in intra-alveolar root fractures. *Oral Surg Oral Med Oral Pathol* 1959;**12**:360-70.

50. AISENBERG MS. Repair of a fractured tooth. *Dent Cosmos* 1932;**74**:382-5.

51. GOTTLIEB B. Histologische Untersuchung einer geheilten Zahnfraktur. Ein weiterer Beitrag zur Biologie der Zähne. *Z Stomatol* 1922;**20**:286-300.

52. LEFKOWITZ W. The formation of cementum. *Am J Orthod* 1944;**30**:224-40.

53. TULLIN B. Three cases of root fractures. *Odontologisk Revy* 1968;**19**:31-43.

54. KOVÁCS G, REHÁK R. Das Verhalten wurzelfrakturierter Zähne. *Österr Z Stomatol* 1955;**52**:570-6.

55. OVERDIEK HF. Zur Auswirkung von Traumen auf Wurzeln bleibender Zähne unter besonderer Berücksichtigung der histologischen Befunde. *Dtsch Zahnärztl Z* 1957;**12**:1057-61.

56. STEINHARDT G. Pathologisch-anatomische Befunde nach Wurzelspitzenresektionen und Wurzelfrakturen beim Menschen. *Dtsch Zahnärztl Wochenschr* 1933;**36**:541-5.

57. MILES AEW. Resolution of the pulp following severe injury. *Br Dent J* 1947;**82**:187-9.

58. VERGARA-EDWARDS I. Fractures radiculaires au tiers cervical. *Rev Stomatol(Paris)* 1960;**61**:794-8.

59. ROY M. Les fractures radiculaires intra-alvéolaires. *Odontologie* 1938;**6**:601-13.

60. SCHUG-KÖSTERS M. Frakturen und Subluxationen der Zähne mit lebender Pulpa und ihre Behandlung. *Dtsch Zahn Mund Kieferheilk* 1954;**21**:187-96.

61. SIBLEY LC. Management of root fracture. *Oral Surg Oral Med Oral Pathol* 1960;**13**:1475-84.

62. FLIEGE H, MÖLLENHOFF P. Ueber die Ausheilung interalveolärer Zahnfrakturen bei lebender Pulpa. *Dtsch Zahnärztl Wochenschr* 1933;**36**:479-81.

63. SCHINDLER J. Kasuistischer Beitrag zum Problem der Heilung von Zahnwurzelfrakturen mit Erhaltung der Vitalität der Pulpa. *Schweiz Monatschr Zahnheilkd* 1941;**51**:474-86.

64. HERVÉ M. Les fractures dentaires classification et traitement. *Actual Odontostomatol* 1951;**4**:157-91.

65. ANDERSON BG. Injuries to the teeth: Contusions and fractures resulting from concussion. *J Am Dent Assoc* 1944;**31**:195-200.

66. BRUSZT P. Intraalveoläre Frakturen der bleibenden Zähne und deren Behandlung. *Schweiz Monatschr Zahnheilkd* 1955;**65**:1103-10.

67. DRIAK F. Kasuistischer Beitrag zur Heilung von Zahnwurzelfrakturen. *Österr Z Stomatol* 1958;**55**:2-7.

68. JUNG F. Therapie bei Luxationen und Wurzelfrakturen. *Zahnärztl Prax* 1953;**4**:1-4.

69. OVERDIEK HF. Ein Beitrag zur Frage der Wurzelfrakturen insbesondere an Frontzähnen jugendlicher Patienten. *Dtsch Zahnärztl Z* 1957;**12**:1172-8.

70. FISCHER R. Zur Behandlung von Zahnwurzelfrakturen bei Jugendlichen. *Österr Z Stomatol* 1968;**65**:104-10.

71. CWIORA F, RZESZUTKO R. Przyczynek do leczenia zlaman korzeni zebow przednich. *Czas Stomatol* 1968;**21**:199-203.

72. ELLIS RG, DAVEY KW. *The classification and treatment of injuries to the teeth of children.* 5th edn. Chicago: Year Book Publishers, Inc. 1970.

74. BRUGIRARD MJ. Réflexions sur 100 cas de traumatismes des régions incisives et canine. *Ann Odontostomatatol* 1960;17:55-72.

75. GRAZIDE, COULOMB, BOISSET & DASQUE. L'embrochage et le collage dans le traitement des fractures dentaires. *Rev Stomatol (Paris)*;**57**:428-44.

76. STACY GC. Intra-alveolar root re-fracture treated by internal splinting. *Br Dent J* 1965;**118**:210-2.

77. NAUJOKS R. Zahnfrakturen und ihre Therapie. *Dtsch Zahnärztebl* 1957;**11**:408-11.

78. NOLDEN R. Die konservierende Behandlung der Traumafolgen im Wachstumsalter. *Zahnärztl Welt* 1967;**68**:19-24.

79. ESCHLER J, SCHILLI W, WITT E. *Die traumatischen Verletzungen der Frontzähne bei Jugendlichen.* 3 edn. Heidelberg: Alfred Hüthig Verlag, 1972.

80. INGLE JI, FRANK AL, NATKIN E, NUTTING EE. Diagnosis and treatment of traumatic injuries and their sequelae. In: INGLE JI, BEVERIDGE EE. eds. *Endodontics.* 2nd edn. Philadelphia: Lea & Febiger, 1976:685-741.

81. WEISKOPF J, GEHRE G, GRAICHEN K-H. Ein Beitrag zur Behandlung von Luxationen und Wurzelfrakturen im Front-

zahngebiet. *Stoma (Heidelberg)* 1961;**14**:100-13.

82. COHEN S. A permanent internal splint for a fractured incisor root. *Dent Dig* 1968;**74**:162-5.

83. MICHANOWICZ AE. Root fractures. A report of radiographic healing after endodontic treatment. *Oral Surg Oral Med Oral Pathol* 1963;**16**:1242-8.

84. FELDMAN G, SOLOMON C, NOTARO PJ. Endodontic management of traumatized teeth. *Oral Surg Oral Med Oral Pathol* 1966;**21**:100-12.

85. FRANK AL. Improvement of the crown-root ratio by endodontic endosseous implants. *J Am Dent Assoc* 19667;**74**:451-62.

86. FRANK AL, ABRAMS AM. Histologic evaluation of endodontic implants. *J Am Dent Assoc* 1969;**78**:520-24.

87. ANDREASEN JO. Treatment of intra-alveolar root fractures by cobalt-chromium implants. *Br J Oral Surg* 1968;**6**:141-6.

88. HEDEGÅRD B, STÅLHANE I. A study of traumatized permanent teeth in children aged 7-15 years. Part I. *Swed Dent J* 1973;**66**:431-50.

89. RAVN JJ. Dental injuries in Copenhagen schoolchildren, school years 1967-1972. *Community Dent Oral Epidemiol* 1974;**2**:231-45.

90. JACOBSEN I. Root fractures in permanent anterior teeth with incomplete root formation. *Scand J Dent Res* 1976;**84**:210-7.

91. DYNESEN H, RAVN JJ. Rodfrakturer i det primære tandsæt. *Tandlægebladet* 1973;**77**:865-8.

92. DEGERING CI. Radiography of dental fractures. An experimental evaluation. *Oral Surg Oral Med Oral Pathol* 1970;**30**:213-9.

93. ZACHRISSON BU, JACOBSEN I. Long-term prognosis of 66 permanent anterior teeth with root fracture. *Scand J Dent Res* 1975;**83**:345-54.

94. RAVN JJ. En klinisk og radiologisk undersøgelse af 55 rodfrakturer i unge permanente incisiver. *Tandlægebladet* 1976;**80**:391-6.

95. HARGREAVES JA, CRAIG JW. *The management of traumatised anterior teeth in children.* London: E. & S. Livingstone, 1970.

96. WALDHART E. Röntgenologische und histologische tierexperimentelle Untersuchungen nach Zahnwurzelverletzungen. *ZWR* 1973;**82**:624-8.

97. BOUYSSOU M. Les calc de fractures dentaires compares aux calc de fracture osseuses. *Rev Fr Odontostomatol* 1970;**17**:1293-316.

98. BOUYSSOU M, WERELDS RJ, LEPP FH, SOLEILHAVOUP JP, PEYRE J. Histologie comparative de la formation d'un cal dans les fractures dentaires et dans les fractures osseuses. *Bull Group Int Rech Soc Stomatol* 1970;**13**:317-68.

99. FISCHER C-H. Beobachtungen bei intra- und extraalveolärer Verletzung der Pulpa nach einem Frontzahntrauma. *Dtsch Zahnärztl Z* 1970;**25**:1135-40.

100. MICHANOWICZ AE, MICHANOWICZ JP, ABOU-RASS M. Cementogenic repair of root fractures. *J Am Dent Assoc* 1971;**82**:569-79.

101. HANSEN P. Et tilfælde af rodfraktur med usædvanligt helingsforløb. *Tandlægebladet* 1971;**75**:28-31.

102. HARTNESS JD. Fractured root with internal resorption, repair and formation of callus. *J Endod* 1975;**1**:73-5.

103. JACOBSEN I, ZACHRISSON BU. Repair characteristics of root fractures in permanent anterior teeth. *Scand J Dent Res* 1975;**83**:355-64.

104. TETSCH P, ESSER E. Die transdentale Fixation traumatisch geschädigter Frontzähne. *Österr Z Stomatol* 1974;**71**:59-65.

105. FISCHER R, KELLNER G. Klinische und histologische Befunde bei Zahnwurzelfrakturen. *Zahnärztl Welt* 1971;**80**:501-11.

106. HEITHERSAY GS. Combined endodontic-orthodontic treatment of transverse root fractures in the region of the alveolar crest. *Oral Surg Oral Med Oral Pathol* 1973;**36**:404-15.

107. JOHNSON DL, KELLY JF, FLINTON RJ, CORNELL MT. Histologic evaluation of vital root retention. *J Oral Surg* 1974;**32**:829-33.

108. WHITAKER DD, SHANKLE RJ. A study of the histologic reaction of submerged root segments. *Oral Surg Oral Med Oral Pathol* 1974;**37**:919-35.

109. COOK RT, HUTCHENS LH, BURKES EJ JR. Periodontal osseous defects associated with vitally submerged roots. *J Periodontol* 1977;**48**:249-60.

110. LUSTMANN J, AZAZ B. Roentgenographic study of mid root fractures. *Israel J Dent Med* 1976;**24**:23-8.

111. STÅLHANE I, HEDEGÅRD B. Traumatized permanent teeth in children aged 7-15 years. Part II. *Swed Dent J* 1975;**68**:157-69.

112. CVEK M. Treatment of non-vital permanent incisors with calcium hydroxide. IV. Periodontal healing and closure of the root canal in the coronal fragment of teeth with intra-alveolar fracture and vital apical fragment. A follow-up. *Odontologisk Revy* 1974;**25**:239-46.

113. KRÖNCKE A. Zur Problematik der endodontalen Schienung frakturierter Zahnwurzeln. *Dtsch Zahnärztl Z* 1969;**24**:49-53.

114. KOZLOWSKA I, GRATKOWSKA H. Transverse fractures of roots of permanent teeth. *Czas Stomatol* 1975;**28**:681-6.

115. LUTTERBERG B, GÖTZE G. Die Behandlung intraalveolärer Frakturen sowie parodontalgeschädigter Frontzähne mit der Stiftverbolzung. *Zahn Mund Kieferheilkd* 1978;**66**:669-73.

116. LUHR H-G. Endodontale Kompressionsverschraubung bei Zahnwurzelfrakturen. *Dtsch Zahnärztl Z* 1972;**27**:927-8.

117. GALITZIEN M-A. Die perkanaläre Kompressionschraube zur Versorgung von Zahnwurzelfrakturen im mittleren Drittel. *Dtsch Zahnärztl Z* 1978;**33**:665-7.

118. LUHR H-G, BULL H-G, MOHAUPT K. Histologische Untersuchungen nach endodontaler Kompressionsverschraubung bei Zahnwurzelfrakturen. *Dtsch Zahnärztl Z* 1973;**28**:365-9.

119. FRANK AL. Resorption, perforations and fractures. *Dent Clin North Am* 1974;**18**:465-87.

120. DIETZ G. Apex und periapikales Parodont endodontisch enossal stiftfixierter Zähne. *Dtsch Zahnärztl Z* 1975;**30**:481-2.

121. DIETZ G. Endodontischer enossaler Fixations - und Stumpfaufbaustift. *Dtsch Zahnärztl Z* 1975;**30**:483-5.

122. CRANIN AN, RABKIN M. Endosteal oral implants. A retrospective radiographic study. *Dent Radio Photography* 1976;**49**:3-12.

123. CRANIN AN, RABKIN MF, GARFINKEL L. A statistical evaluation of 952 endosteal implants in humans. *J Am Dent Assoc* 1977;**94**:315-20.

124. DIETZ G. Perkanaläre Schienung im Knochen von Frontzähnen mit horizontaler Wurzelfraktur im mittleren Drittel. *Dtsch Zahnärztl Z* 1977;**32**:450-2.

125. GÖDDE HJ. Ein kasuistischer Beitrag zur transdentalen Fixation. *ZWR* 1978;**87**:841-3.

126. SILVERBAND H, RABKIN M, CRANIN AN. The uses of endodontic implant stabilizers in posttraumatic and periodontal disease. *Oral Surg Oral Med Oral Pathol* 1978;**45**:920-9.

127. SELTZER S, GREEN DB, DE LA GUARDIA R, MAGGIO J, BARNETT A. Vitallium endodontic implants: a scanning electron microscope, electron microscope, histologic study. *Oral Surg Oral Med Oral Pathol* 1973;**35**:828-60.

128. LANGELAND K, SPÅNGBERG L. Methodology and criteria in evaluation of dental endosseous implants. *J Dent Res* 1975;**54**(Special Issue B):158-65.

129. NEUMAN G, SPÅNGBERG L, LANGELAND K. Methodology and criteria in the evaluation of dental implants. *J Endod* 1975;**1**:193-202.

130. SELTZER S, MAGGIO J, WOLLARD R, GREEN D. Titanium endodontic implants: a scanning electron microscope, electron microprobe and histologic investigation. *J Endod* 1976;**2**:267-76.

131. SCOPP IW, DICTROW RL, LICHTENSTEIN B, BLECHMAN H. Cellular response to endodontic endosseous implants. *J Periodontol* 1971;**42**:717-20.

132. BIRCH R, ROCK WP. The incidence of complications following root fracture in permanent anterior teeth. *Br Dent J* 1986;**160**:119-22.

133. BENDER IB, FREEDLAND JB. Clinical considerations in the diagnosis and treatment of intra-alveolar root fractures. *J Am Dent Assoc* 1983;**107**:595-600.

134. ANDREASEN FM, ANDREASEN JO. Resorption and mineralization processes following root fracture of permanent incisors. *Endod Dent Traumatol* 1988;**4**:202-14.

135. ANDREASEN FM. Pulpal healing after luxation injuries and root fracture in the permanent dentition. *Endod Dent Traumatol* 1989;**5**:111-31.

136. ANDREASEN FM, ANDREASEN JO, BAYER T. Prognosis of root-fractured permanent incisors - prediction of healing modalities. *Endod Dent Traumatol* 1989;**5**:11-22.

137. MICHANOWICZ AE. Histologic evaluation of experimentally produced intra-alveolar root fractures. In: GUTMANN JL, HARRISON JW, eds. *Proceedings of the International Conference on Oral Trauma.* American Association of Endodontists Endowment & Memorial Foundation, Chicago, Illinois 1986:101-28.

138. ANDREASEN JO. Review of root resorption systems and models. Etiology of root resorption and the homeostatic mechanisms of the periodontal ligament. In: DAVIDOVITCH Z ed. *The Biological Mechanisms of Tooth Eruption and Root Resorption.* 1988:9-21.

139. HERWEIJER JA, TORABINEJAD M, BAKLAND LK. Healing of horizontal root fractures. *J Endod* 1992;**18**:118-22.

140. SCHMITZ R, DONATH K. Morphologische Veränderungen an traumatisierten Zähnen. Eine klinische und patho-histologische Studie. *Dtsch Zahnärztl Z* 1983;**38**:462-5.

141. JACOBSEN I, KEREKES K. Diagnosis and treatment of pulp necrosis in permanent anterior teeth with root fracture. *Scand J Dent Res* 1980;**80**:370-6.

142. ENGELHARDTSEN S. Rotfraktur i midtre tredjedel på rotåpen tann med luksasjon av koronale fragment. *Norske Tannlegeforenings Tidende* 1990;**100**:102-3.

143. HAGEN SO. Rotfraktur i cervikale tredjedel på rotåpen tann - med tilheling. *Norske Tannlegeforenings Tidende* 1990;**100**:104-5.

144. SUNDNES SK. Rotfraktur i midtre tredjdel med luksasjon og utvikling av pulpanekrose. *Norske Tannlegeforenings Tidende* 1990;**100**:106-7.

145. BULL H, NEUGEBAUER W. Transdentale Kompressionsverschraubung zur Stabiliserung wurzelfrakturierter Zähne. *Zahnärztl Prax* 1983;**34**:258-60.

146. REUTER E, WEBER W. Sekundäre Schienung von Zahnwurzelfrakturen durch endodontale Zugschraube. Langzeitergebnisse. *Dtsch Zahnärztl Z* 1987;**42**:308-10.

147. BECHTOLD H, BULL H-G, SCHUBERT F. Ergebnisse der transdentalen Stabilisierung gelockerter und wurzelfrakturierter Zähne. *Dtsch Zahnärztl Z* 1987;**42**:295-8.

148. BERGER F. Transdental Fixation bei noch weitem Apikalforamen. *Zahnärztl Prax* 1980;**31**:456-7.

149. ZINNER R, GLIEN W. Die transdentale Fixation mit Aluminiumoxidkeramik. *Stomatol DDR* 1986;**36**:385-8.

150. HERFORTH A. Zur Stabilisierung gelockerter Zähne durch transdentale Fixation. *Dtsch Zahnärztl Z* 1983;**38**:129-30.

151. SCHRAMM-SCHERER B, TETSCH P, TRIPPLER S, BRÜDERLE U. Stabilisierung einwurzeliger Zähne durch Transfixationsstifte. *Dtsch Zahnärztl Z* 1987;**42**:302-4.

152. HÄUSSLER F, MAIER KH. Indikationen und Erfahrungen der chirurgischen Zahnerhaltung durch transdentale Fixation. *Dtsch Zahnärtzl Z* 1987;**42**:290-1.

153. VOSS A. Kronen- und Wurzelfrakturen im bleibenden Gebiss. *Zahnärztl Mitt* 1989;**79**:2600-5.

154. FRENKEL G, ADERHOLD L. Das Trauma im Frontzahnbereich des jugendlichen Gebisses aus chirurgischer Sicht. *Fortschr Kieferorthop* 1990;**51**:138-44.

155. HERFORTH A. Wurzelfrakturen und Luxationen von Zähnen - I. Teil. *ZWR* 1990;**99:**440-4.

156. HERFORTH A. Wurzelfrakturen und Luxationen von Zähnen - II. Teil. *ZWR* 1990;**99:**604-8.

157. STRUNZ V, KIRSCH A. Transfization von Zähnen mit Titan-plasma-beschichteten Stiften im Tierexperiment. *Dtsch Zahnärztl Z* 1987;**42:**292-4.

158. BRINKMANN E. Indikation und Anwendung der chirurgischen Zahnerhaltung. *Zahnärztl Mitt* 1982;**72:**1-12.

159. HERFORTH A. Zur Stabilisierung gelockerter Zähne durch transdental Fixation. *Dtsch Zahnärztl Z* 1983;**38:**129-30.

160. ANDREASEN JO, ANDREASEN FM. Long term tooth mobility testings of non-healed rootfractures. A study of 100 cases. In preparation 1993.

161. DIETZ G. Experimentell horizontal wurzelfrakturierte Affen-frontzähne und deren perkanaläre enossale Stiftfixation. *Dtsch Zahnärztl Z* 1976;**31:**89-91.

CHAPTER 9

Luxation Injuries

F. M. ANDREASEN & J. O. ANDREASEN

Terminology, Frequency and Etiology

From a therapeutic, anatomic and prognostic point of view, five different types of luxation injuries can be recognized (Fig. 6.1).

1. *Concussion*: An injury to the tooth-supporting structures without abnormal loosening or displacement but with marked reaction to percussion (Fig. 9.1, A).

2. *Subluxation (loosening)*: An injury to the tooth-supporting structures with abnormal loosening but without clinically or radiographically demonstrable displacement of the tooth (Fig. 9.1, B).

3. *Extrusive luxation (peripheral displacement, partial avulsion)*: Partial displacement of the tooth out of its socket (Fig. 9.1, C). Radiographic examination always reveals increased width of the periodontal ligament space (Fig. 9.4).

4. *Lateral luxation*: Eccentric displacement of the tooth. This is accompanied by comminution or fracture of the alveolar socket (Fig. 9.1, D and E). Depending on the angulation of the central beam, radiographic examination may or may not demonstrate increased width of the periodontal ligament space (Fig. 9.5) (148).

5. *Intrusive luxation (central dislocation)*: Displacement of the tooth deeper into the alveolar bone. This injury is ac-companied by comminution or fracture of the alveolar socket (Fig. 9.1, F). The direction of dislocation follows the axis of the tooth. Radiographic examination reveals dislocation of the tooth and sometimes a missing or diminished periodontal space. In the adult dentition, an apical shift of the cemento-enamel junction of the involved tooth can be seen.

The most important clinical difference between intrusive and extrusive luxation is that in the latter the apex is displaced out of its socket and not through the alveolar bone as in intrusive luxation. Moreover, extrusive luxation can imply complete rupture or stretching/tearing of the neurovascular supply to the pulp at the apical foramen and the periodontal ligament fibers are to a great extent severed; whereas the supporting bone is not affected.

The factors which determine the type of luxation injury appear to be the force and direction of impact (Fig. 9.2).

Luxation injuries comprise 15 to 61% of dental traumas to permanent teeth, (1, 2, 92-94, 149); while frequencies of 62 to 73% have been reported for the primary dentition (1, 92, 149). Predominant etiologic factors of luxation injuries in the permanent dentition are bicycle injuries, falls, fights and sports injuries (1, 150); whereas falls dominate in the primary dentition (1, 95, 96, 149, 151, 152).

**Fig. 9.1.Injuries to the peri-
odontal tissues**
*A. Concussion. B. Subluxation.
C. Extrusive luxation. D and E.
Lateral luxation. F. Intrusive lux-
ation.*

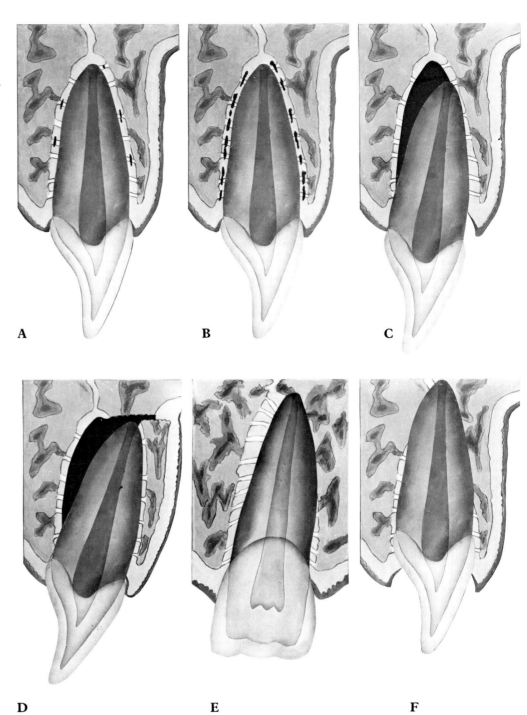

A   B   C

D   E   F

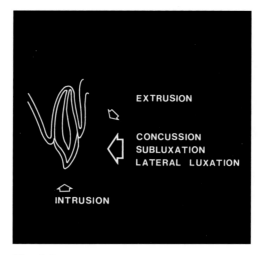

Fig. 9.2.
The energy and direction of the impact determine the type of luxation injury.

Clinical Findings

In both the primary and permanent dentitions, tooth luxations primarily involve the maxillary central incisor region and are seldom seen in the mandible (2-4, 93, 163).

With increasing age, the frequency and pattern of injury change. In the primary dentition, intrusions and extrusions comprise the majority of all injuries, a finding which is possibly related to the resilience of the alveolar bone at this age. In contrast, in the permanent dentition the number of intrusive luxation injuries is considerably reduced and usually seen in younger individuals (1, 5, 92).

Most frequently, two or more teeth are luxated simultaneously (1, 3, 7); a number of luxations show concomitant crown or root fractures (1, 93, 97) (Fig. 9.3).

While the diagnosis of luxation injuries is based upon the combination of radiographic and clinical findings including sensibility testings (Table 9.1), diagnostic accuracy increases with multiple radiographic exposures, where angulation of the central beam is altered (148).

Concussion

In concussions, only minor injuries have been sustained by the periodontal structures so that no loosening is present. The patient complains that the tooth is tender to touch. Clinical examination reveals a marked reaction to percussion in horizontal and/or vertical direction (Fig. 9.3).

Subluxation

Subluxated teeth retain their normal position in the dental arch; however, the tooth is mobile in a horizontal direction and sensitive to percussion and occlusal forces. Hemorrhage from the gingival crevice is usually present, indicating damage to the periodontal tissues (Fig. 9.3).

Fig. 9.3. Clinical and radiographic features of concussion and subluxation
The right and left maxillary central incisors have received a blow and are tender to percussion. The right central incisor is firm in its socket (concussion, with a concomitant crown fracture). While the left central incisor is loose with bleeding from the gingival sulcus (subluxation).

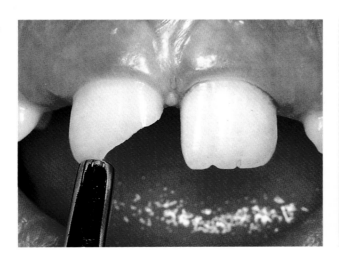

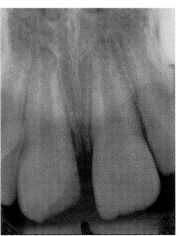

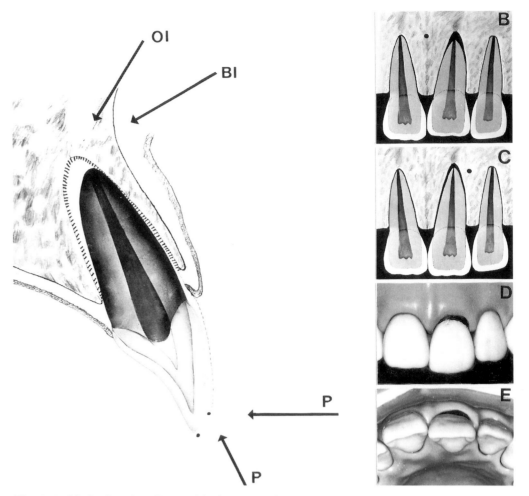

Fig. 9.4. Clinical and radiographic features of extrusive luxation
The standard bisecting angle periapical radiographic technique is more useful than an occlusal exposure in revealing axial displacement. From ANDREASEN & ANDREASEN (148) 1985

Extrusion

Extruded teeth appear elongated and most often with lingual deviation of the crown, being suspended only by the palatal gingiva (Fig. 9.4). There is always bleeding from the periodontal ligament. The percussion sound is dull.

Lateral Luxation

Laterally luxated teeth usually have their crowns displaced lingually and are often associated with fractures of the vestibular part of the socket wall (Fig. 9.5). Displacement of teeth after lateral luxation is normally evident by visual inspection. However, in case of marked inclination of maxillary teeth, it can be difficult to decide

whether the trauma has caused minor abnormalities in tooth position. In such cases, occlusion should be checked. The findings revealed by percussion and mobility tests are identical with those found in intruded teeth because of the frequent locked position of the tooth in the alveolus (Table 9.1 p. 321).

Intrusion

Intruded teeth often show marked displacement, especially in the primary dentition. Most intruded teeth, because of their locked position in the socket, are not sensitive to percussion and are completely firm (Fig. 9.6). The percussion test often elicits a high-pitched metallic sound, similar to an ankylosed tooth. The latter test is

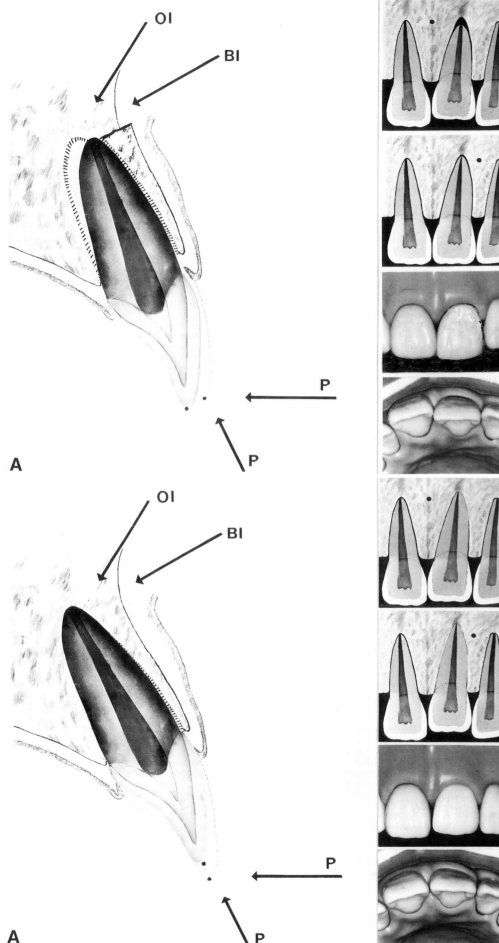

Fig. 9.5. Clinical and radiographic features of lateral luxation
The occlusal radiographic exposure or an eccentric periapical bisecting angle exposure are more useful than an orthoradial bisecting technique in revealing lateral displacement. From ANDREASEN & ANDREASEN (148) 1985.

Fig. 9.6. Clinical and radiographic features of intrusive luxation
The occlusal and periapical bisecting angle exposures reliably reproduce the extent of displacement, with slight preference in favor of the eccentric bisecting angle technique. From ANDREASEN & ANDREASEN (148) 1985.

LUXATION INJURIES

Fig. 9.7.Displacement of an intruded central incisor into the nasal cavity
Clinical and radiographic condition. The tooth is completely intruded.

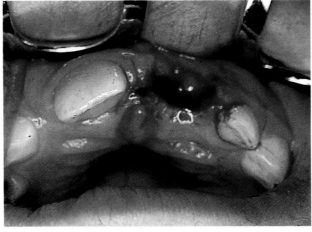
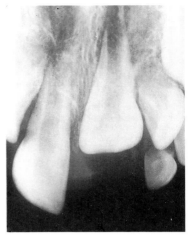

Nasal inspection
Inspection of the right nostril with a nasal speculum shows protrusion of the apex through the floor of the nose (arrow).

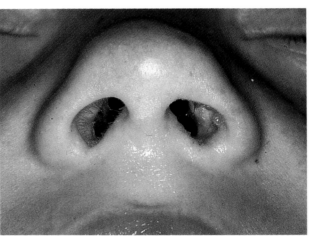
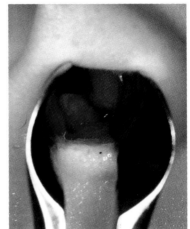

of great importance in determining whether or not erupting teeth are intruded (Table 9.1). The tooth may be completely buried in the alveolar process and be erroneously considered avulsed until a radiograph shows the intruded position. Palpation of the alveolar process often reveals the position of the displaced tooth.

If a permanent central incisor is completely intruded, it should be considered that the apex is most likely forced into the nasal cavity, resulting in bleeding from the nose. Examination of the floor of the nostril will reveal the protruding apex (Fig. 9.7).

In the primary dentition, the apices of intruded primary teeth will usually be driven through the thin vestibular bone, the direction probably being determined by the direction of the impact and the labial curve of the root (Fig. 9.9).

For later comparison, the degree of dislocation should be recorded in millimeters (i.e. the distance between the incisal edge of the intruded incisor and the non-intruded adjacent tooth), with the direction of dislocation indicated as well. Especially in the primary dentition, it is of great importance to determine whether the apex is dislocated facially or orally because in the latter case, the permanent successors can be directly involved (see p. 323).

Radiographic Findings

Radiographic examination is an important adjunct to the clinical examination, as it can disclose minor dislocations. It has been shown experimentally that error in the radiographic recording of the distance of dislocation is minimal if the bisecting angle technique is used. Moreover, in order to obtain reproducible radiographs, filmholders should be employed to standardize exposure technique. Thus, an average of 6.9% error in measurement of tooth length was encountered if filmholders were not used compared to a 2.0% average error if they were (148). And the probability

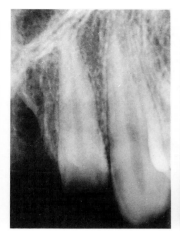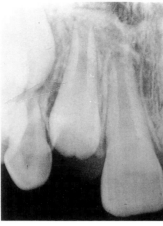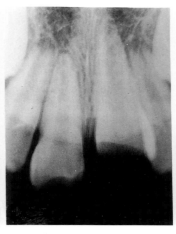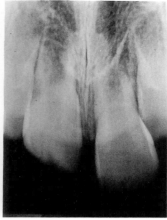

Fig. 9.8.
A. Intrusive luxation of lateral incisor. Note disappearance of the periodontal space around the displaced tooth. B. Intruded lateral incisor. Note that a periodontal space is present along most of the root surface. C and D. Intrusion of teeth with incomplete and complete root formation. Note the difference in position of the cemento-enamel junction compared with the adjacent tooth.

of diagnosing displacement (irrespective of direction) is increased if multiple radiographic exposures with varying vertical and horizontal angulations of the central beam are taken of the injured region (148).

The width of the periodontal ligament space is increased on radiographs of *extrusive luxations* (Fig. 9.4).

A *laterally luxated* tooth likewise shows an increased periodontal space apically when the apex is displaced labially. However, this will usually be seen only in an occlusal exposure; an orthoradial exposure will give little or no evidence of dis-

placement. The radiographic picture, which imitates extrusive luxation, is explained by the relation between the dislocation and direction of the central beam (Fig. 9.5).

In *intrusive luxations*, the periodontal ligament space will partially or totally disappear (Fig. 9.8). However, it should be noted that in some cases of obvious displacement, a periodontal space of normal width can still be seen radiographically (Fig. 9.8 B).

In the primary dentition, radiographs can reveal the position of displaced teeth

Table 9.1. Typical clinical and radiographic findings with different types of luxation injuries

	Type of luxation injury				
	Concussion	**Subluxation**	**Extrusion**	**Intrusion**	**Lateral luxation**
Abnormal mobility	-	+	+	-(+)[1]	-(+)
Tenderness to percussion	+	+(-)	+(-)	-(+)	-(+)
Percussion sound	normal[2]	dull	dull	metallic	metallic
Positive response to sensibility testing	+/-	+/-	-	-	-
Radiographic dislocation	-	-(+)	+	+	+

[1] A sign in parentheses indicates a finding of rare occurrence.
[2] Teeth with incomplete root formation and teeth with marginal or periapical inflammatory lesions will also elicit a dull percussion sound (98).

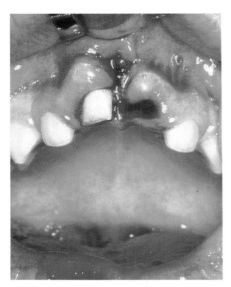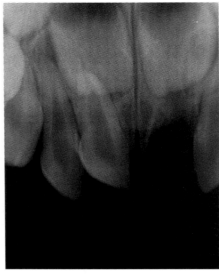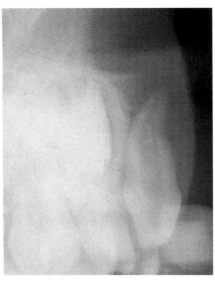

Fig. 9.9.

Radiographic demonstration of the direction of displacement in a case of intrusive luxation of a primary central incisor. A. Clinical condition. B. Right central incisor appears shorter than right lateral incisor due to displacement in apico-labial direction of the former. C. Lateral radiograph reveals the relationship between the apex of the displaced tooth and the permanent tooth germ as well as the direction of dislocation. Note that the apex of the primary tooth has been forced through the facial bone plate (arrow). At later examination, re-eruption of the intruded incisor is seen. There is no sign of pulp necrosis.

Fig. 9.10.

Schematic illustration of the geometric relationship between an intruded primary incisor and the developing tooth germ and the resultant radiographic image.

If the primary tooth is intruded AWAY from the developing tooth germ, the radiographic image will be FORESHORTENED. If the primary tooth is intruded INTO the developing tooth germ, the radiographic image will be ELONGATED.

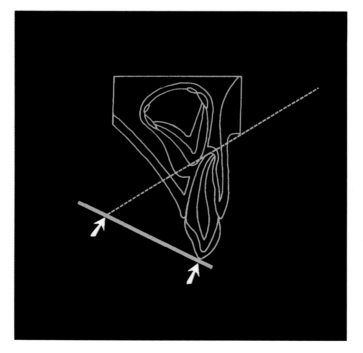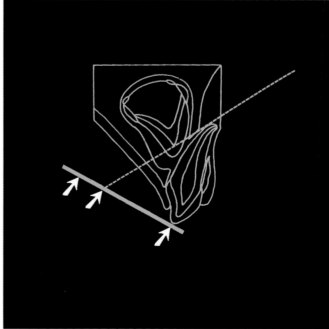

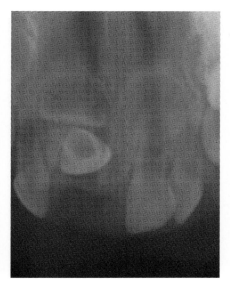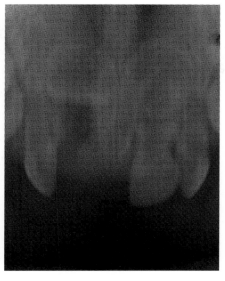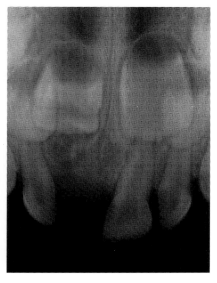

Fig. 9.11. Radiographic demonstration of displacement of the developing permanent tooth germ following intrusion of the primary incisor.
The distance between the incisal edge and mineralization front of the involved developing tooth germ is shorter than the same distance in the non-involved tooth germ, implying luxation of the involved tooth germ. Although the displaced primary tooth was removed, a slight dilaceration of the permanent crown developed.

in relation to the permanent successors and the direction of dislocation (Fig. 9.9). In intrusion with dislocation apico-facially, the injured tooth appears shorter than its contralateral, whereas elongation of the involved tooth is noted when the apex is displaced towards the permanent tooth germ (Fig. 9.10). However, these guidelines can only be applied when the central beam is oriented exactly at the midline between the two incisors to be compared. Apart from this, lateral projections can be of assistance in determining the direction of dislocation (Fig. 9.9) (see Chapter 5, p. 210).

In the evaluation of radiographs of displaced primary teeth, it is also important to determine whether the permanent tooth germ has been displaced in its crypt (Fig. 9.11). Intruded primary incisors are sometimes forced into the follicle of the permanent tooth germ. If clinical examination arouses suspicion of such displacement, radiographic examination including lateral and occlusal projections is necessary (Fig. 9.9).

Pathology

Most luxations represent a combined injury to the pulp and periodontium. However, the pathology of luxation injuries has received little attention. At present, only a few specific changes can be ascribed to the periodontal ligament after luxation injury (153-158); whereas pulpal changes have been studied to a certain extent (6, 91, 99-102, 157-160).

Periodontal Ligament (PDL)

The histologic response in the periodontal ligament has only been sparsely studied experimentally. *Concussion* and *subluxation* have been induced in rat molars (153, 157, 158) and in monkey incisors (155). Furthermore, *extrusive luxations* have been studied in monkeys (156, 161), whereas *intrusions* have been analyzed in monkeys (162) and in dogs (154). These studies have revealed the following PDL changes after trauma (see also Chapter 2, p. 95).

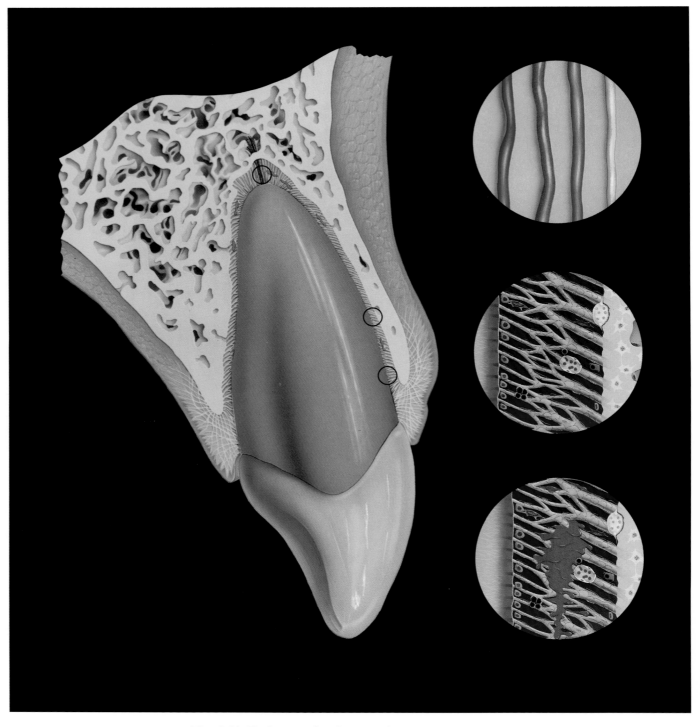

Fig. 9.12. Pathogenesis of concussion
A frontal impact leads to hemorrhage and edema in the periodontal ligament.

CONCUSSION/SUBLUXATION

The general feature is edema, bleeding and sometimes laceration of PDL fibers. The neurovascular supply to the pulp may or may not be intact (Figs. 9.12 and 9.13). The PDL changes 1 hour after trauma were characterized by hemorrhage, stretched, torn or compressed PDL fibers, cell destruction and edema (158). After 1 day, cell-free zones could be seen in the PDL, bordered by a zone of inflammation. In the bony socket 1 day after trauma, osteoclastic activity had begun. After 1 week, this had reached the root surface. After 10 days, the resorption activity was arrested, leaving healed surface resorption cavities along the root surface (158).

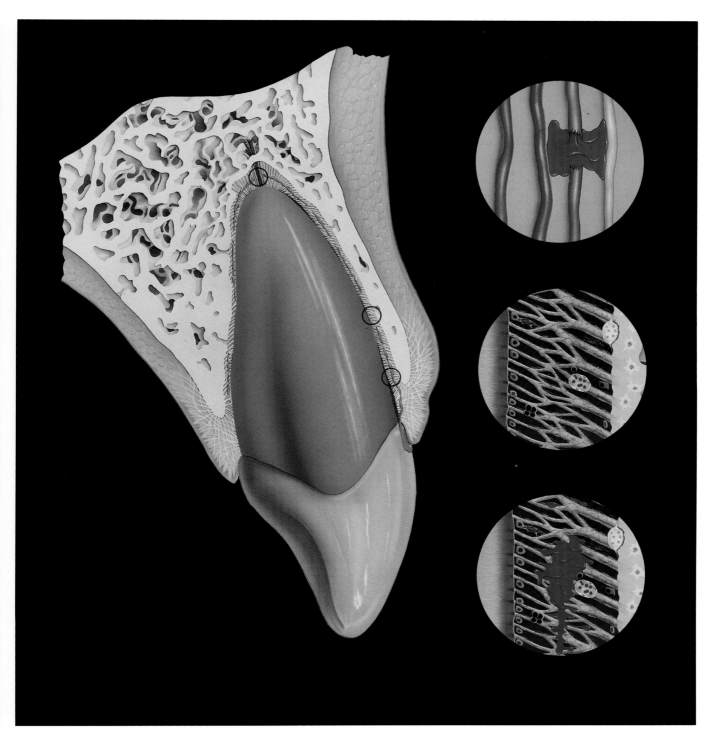

Fig. 9.13. Pathogenesis of subluxation.
If the impact has greater force, periodontal ligament fibers may be torn, resulting in loosening of the injured tooth.

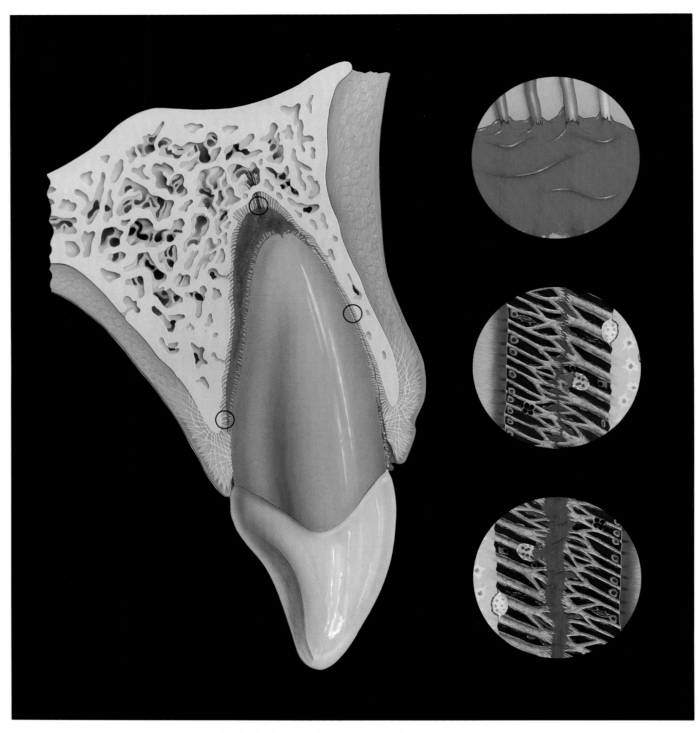

Fig. 9.14. Pathogenesis of extrusive luxation
Oblique forces displace the tooth out of its socket. Only the palatal gingival fibers prevent the tooth from being avulsed. Both the PDL and the neurovascular supply to the pulp are ruptured.

EXTRUSIVE LUXATION
Immediate changes are characterized by a complete rupture of the PDL fibers and the neurovascular supply to the pulp (Fig. 9.14). After 3 days, in monkeys, the split in the PDL, which is usually seen midway between bone and root surface, is filled in with a tissue dominated by endothelial cells and young fibroblasts. In some areas, cell-free zones indicate infarcted tissue (161). After 2 weeks, newly formed collagen fibers are seen. After 3 weeks, the PDL appears normal (156).

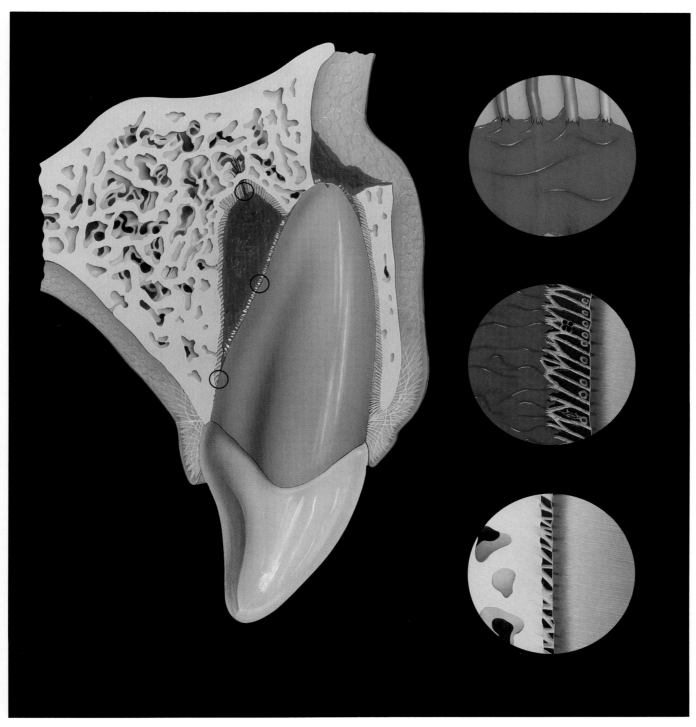

Fig. 9.15. Pathogenesis of lateral luxation
Horizontal forces displace the crown palatally and the root apex labially. Apart from rupture of the PDL and the neurovascular supply to the pulp, compression of the PDL is found on the palatal aspect of the root.

LATERAL LUXATION
This comprises a complex injury involving rupture or compression of PDL fibers, severance of the neurovascular supply to the pulp and fracture of the alveolar socket wall (Fig. 9.15).

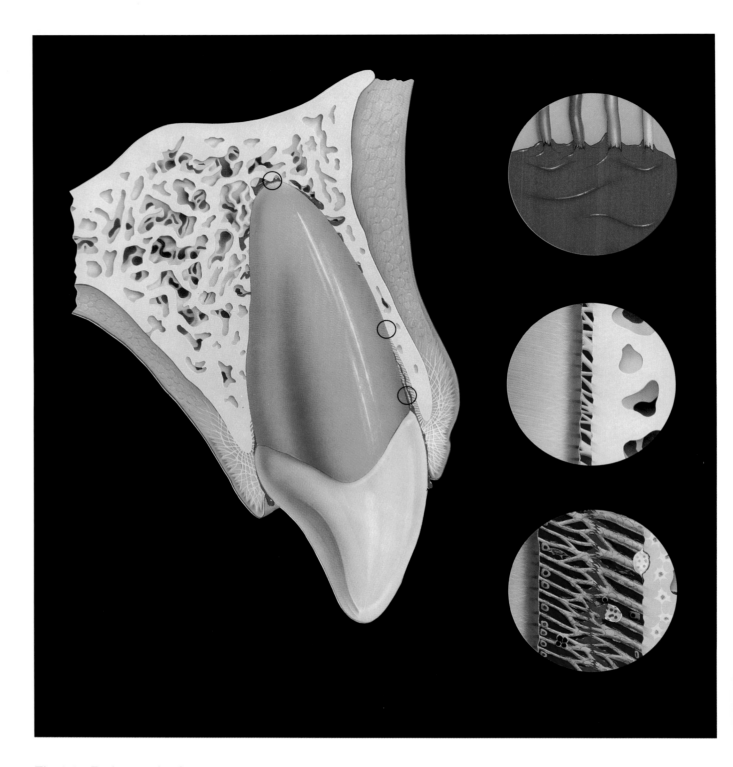

Fig. 9.16. Pathogenesis of intrusion

Axial impact leads to extensive injury to the pulp and periodontium.

INTRUSIVE LUXATION

The immediate response to intrusion in monkeys appears to be an extensive crushing injury to the PDL and alveolar socket and rupture of the neurovascular supply to the pulp (Fig. 9.16) (162). After an observation period of 3 months, some intruded teeth in dogs showed extensive ankylosis; whereas others showed areas with surface resorption and otherwise normal PDL (154).

Pulp

Changes seen in the pulp soon after injury are edema and disorganization of the odontoblast layer as well as nuclear pyknosis of pulp cells (6) (Fig. 9.17). Perivascular hemorrhage can be demonstrated within a few hours in human subjects (Fig. 9.18). Such bleeding could be the result of a partially severed vascular supply. However, in most cases a complete arrest of pulpal circulation occurs, which leads to ischemia, breakdown of vessel walls,

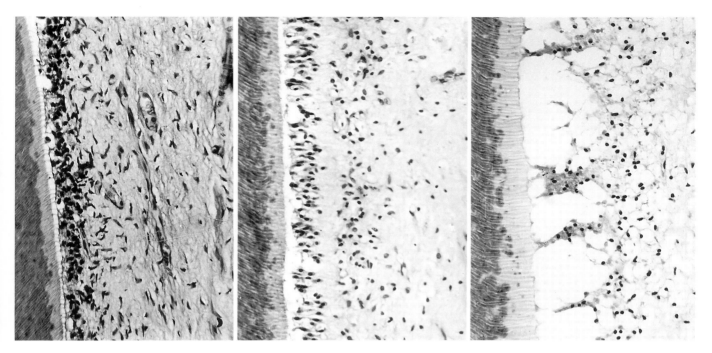

Fig. 9.17.
Pulp changes at various time intervals following intrusive luxation of primary incisors. A. Two hours after injury, pulpal structures-including the odontoblasts-are without significant change, apart from edema. x 195. B. After 13 hours nuclear pyknosis and disintegration of odontoblast layer is evident. x 195. C. Six days after injury only pyknotic nuclei are seen within a stroma of autolyzed pulp tissue. x 195.

Fig. 9.18.
Early histologic changes following subluxation. A. Radiograph of left central incisor following subluxation. The tooth was extracted 6 hours after injury. B. Perivascular bleeding is evident in the apical part of the pulp. x 30. C. Higher magnification of B. x 75.

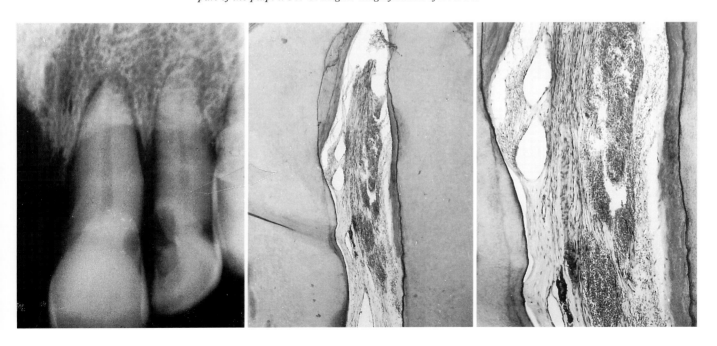

LUXATION INJURIES

escape of erythrocytes and the eventual conversion of hemoglobin to red granular debris which permeates the pulp tissue and gives it a scarlet red color (102). Ultrastructurally as well, blood vessels with disrupted or absent endothelium and erythrocyte remnants can be seen (159).

Histologic evidence of pulp necrosis, including nuclear pyknosis, disappearance of odontoblasts and stromal elements can be seen 6 days after injury (Fig. 9.17). This reponse is related to either partial or total rupture of the pulpal neurovascular supply. The later events of pulpal healing after luxation injury are presently unknown. However, based on experimental findings after extraction and replantation of teeth, it might be expected that a gradual revascularization and reinnervation of the pulp occurs if the size of the apical foramen is adequate to permit vascular ingrowth and that intervening infection of the ischemic pulp does not occur. This process is further described in Chapter 2, p. 104.

If the pulp survives or becomes revascularized, a number of regressive pulp changes can occur, such as hyalinization and deposition of amorphous, diffuse calcifications (6, 9, 10). Furthermore, the injury usually interferes with normal dentin formation. This interference is apparently related to a number of clinical factors, among which the stage of root formation and the type of luxation injury seem to be decisive (3, 104, 105, 163, 164).

In teeth with incomplete root development, a distinct incremental line usually indicates arrest of normal tubular dentin formation at the time of injury. Most of the dentinal tubules stop at this line, while the original predentin layer is often preserved.

After a certain period, apposition of new hard tissue is resumed, but without the normal tubular structure (Fig. 9.19). This tissue often contains cell inclusions which maintain their tubular connections with dentin formed before the injury (11, 15), as well as vascular inclusions. The junction between old and new dentin is rather weak, explaining the separation which may occur in this area during extraction (12-14). This hard tissue formation often continues to the point of total obliteration of the root canal (15, 17-25, 106) (Fig. 9.20).

Although the calcified cellular tissue which is formed in response to the injury may resemble bone and cementum, it lacks the cellular organization characteristic of these tissues. Due to its tendency to convert to tubular dentin, the repair tissue has been termed *cellular dentin* (16). This tendency to return to tubular dentin could be related to differentiation of new odontoblasts from the primitive mesenchymal cells of the pulp. This response is especially marked in the apical portion of the root canal, possibly due to the rapid re-establishment of blood supply in this area after injury (16).

The rate of hard tissue formation is accelerated after injury, resulting in large amounts of newly formed hard tissue, especially in the coronal portion.

In the case of luxation of young permanent teeth, bone can be deposited within the pulp after trauma and is usually connected to the root canal walls by a collagenous fiber arrangement imitating a periodontal ligament. (see Chapter 2, p. 91). This form of healing has been found to be related to damage or destruction of Hertwig's epithelial root sheath (HERS). Such damage can arise from either incomplete repositioning, whereby HERS suffers injury due to ischemia, or by forceful repositioning, whereby all or parts of HERS is crushed (165).

In mature teeth, the disturbance of the odontoblast layer can be more severe, with resorption sometimes preceding deposition of new hard tissue (17, 18). Presumably, the time required for re-establishing vascularization after injury is longer in a tooth with complete root formation, thus increasing the damage to the pulp. The cellular hard tissue formed after the injury rarely assumes a tubular appearance; this applies especially to the coronal portion.

In a clinical luxation material, temporary resorption of bone surrounding the root apex and of dentin within the apical foramen of extruded and laterally luxated mature incisors has been described. Mineralization of these resorption processes could be associated with normalization of coronal discoloration and/or restoration of pulpal sensibility and was significantly related to later pulp canal obliteration (166). (see Chapter 2, p. 104)

Teeth with incomplete root formation at the time of injury sometimes show pulp necrosis confined to the coronal part of the pulp, while the apical portion apparently survives for some time, ensuring occlusion

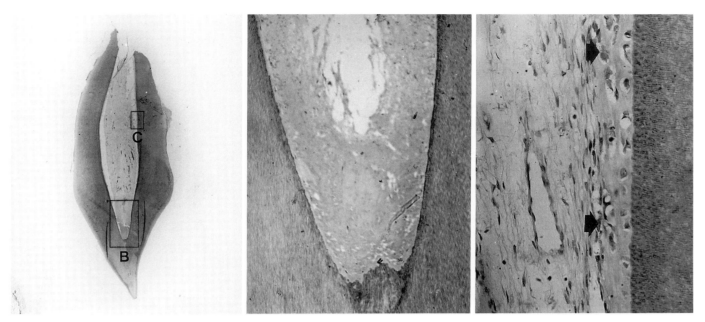

Fig. 9.19.
Early histologic changes following extrusive luxation of a primary right central incisor. A. Low-power view of sectioned incisor. The tooth was extracted 4 weeks after injury. x 6. B. Complete necrosis of the coronal part of the pulp. x 30. C. More apically, formation of new hard tissue with numerous cell inclusions (arrows). x 195.

Fig. 9.20.
Pulp canal obliteration in a primary central incisor following luxation injury. A. Radiographic condition at time of extraction. No pulp cavity is discernible. B. Low-power view of sectioned specimen. Obliteration of the pulp canal is evident. x 10. C. Note atubular dentin deposited immediately after trauma followed by a return to tubular dentin (arrows). x 75.

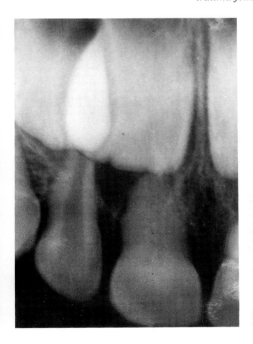
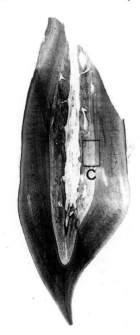
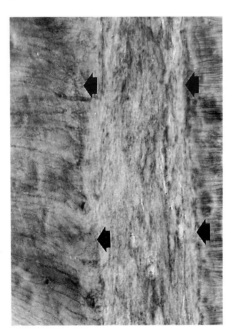

of the wide apex with calcified tissue (8,103) (see Chapter 2, p. 104).

Treatment

Therapeutic measures vary greatly from the primary to the permanent dentitions and according to the type of injury to the tooth-supporting structures. In this context, it should be borne in mind that repositioning and sometimes even splinting procedures can elicit further trauma. Before repositioning of a displaced tooth, it is therefore worth considering whether the repositioning procedure achieves any of the following goals:

1. Facilitates pulpal healing?
2. Facilitates periodontal ligament healing?
3. Eliminates occlusal interferences?
4. Improves esthetics?

At least one or more of these objectives should be achieved by the repositioning procedure, especially if this procedure, as in the case of lateral luxation, results in further damage to the site of injury.

Fig. 9.21. Treatment principles for concussion/subluxation
Relief of occlusal interferences by selective grinding of opposing teeth may be necessary. Teeth may be splinted in the case of severe loosening and/or multiple tooth injuries. Otherwise, a soft diet for 14 days is recommended.

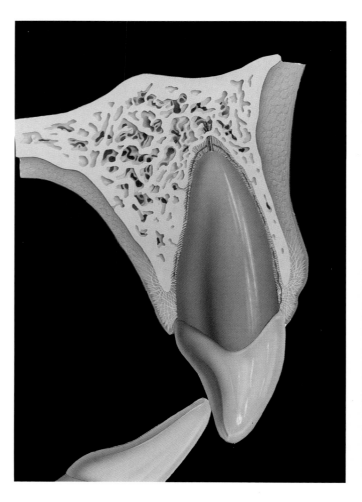
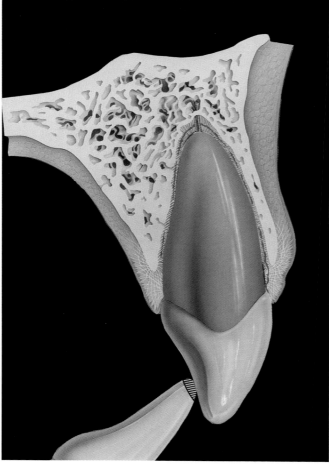

Permanent Dentition

CONCUSSION/SUBLUXATION

In the permanent dentition, if there is no displacement, i.e. *concussion* and *subluxation*, the treatment may be confined to occlusal grinding of the opposing teeth, supplemented by repeated pulp tests during the follow-up period (see Appendix 4 p. 750) for follow-up schedule for the various types of luxation injuries) (Fig. 9.21). While fixation is not needed following these minor injuries, in the case of multiple tooth injuries these teeth may be included in the splint with no risk of damage to the periodontal ligament by the splinting procedure or splinting period.

The treatment of *extruded* permanent teeth seen soon after injury consists of careful repositioning, whereby the coagulum formed between the displaced root and the socket wall can be slowly extruded along the gingival crevice (Figs 9.22 and 9.23). Administration of local anesthetic is not necessary. As the repositioned tooth often has a tendency to migrate incisally, a flexible splint should be applied for 2-3 weeks (see later).

Fig. 9.22.
Treatment principles for extrusive luxation: repositioning and splinting

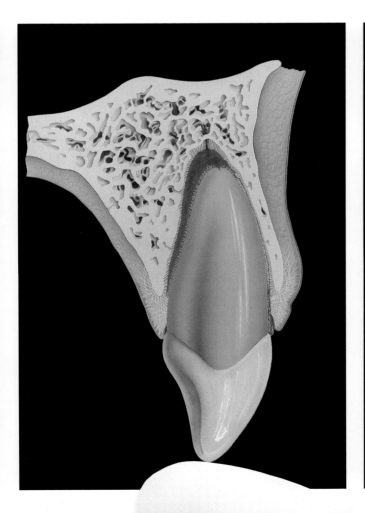
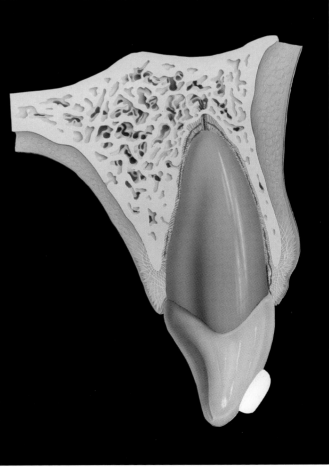

Fig. 9.23.Diagnosis and treatment of extrusive luxation

This 17-year-old man has extruded the left central incisor and avulsed the lateral incisor, which could not be retrieved.

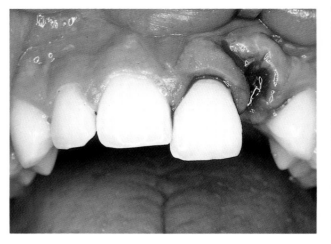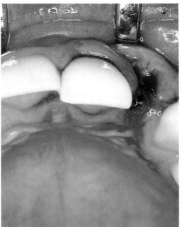

Mobility and percussion testing

The tooth is very mobile and can be moved in horizontal and axial direction. The percussion test reveals slight tenderness and there is a dull percussion tone.

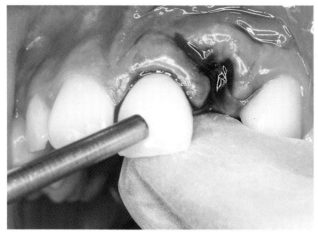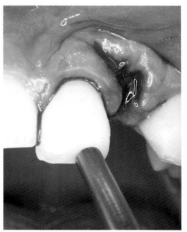

Sensibility testing and radiographic examination

The tooth does not respond to sensibility testing. The radiographic examination shows coronal displacement of the tooth.

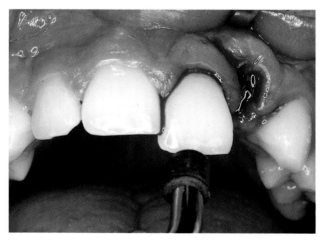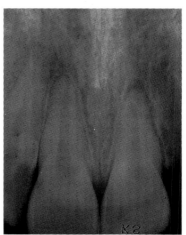

Repositioning

The tooth is gently pushed back into its socket. Thereafter the labial surfaces of both central incisors are etched in preparation for splinting.

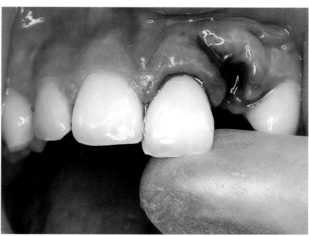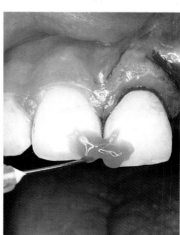

Applying splinting material
After rinsing the labial surfaces with water and drying with compressed air, the splinting material (Protemp®) is applied.

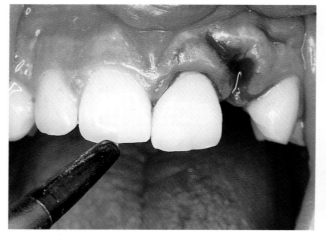
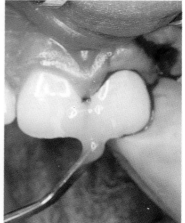

Polishing the splint
The surface of the splint is smoothed with abrasive discs and contact with the gingiva eliminated with a straight scalpel blade.

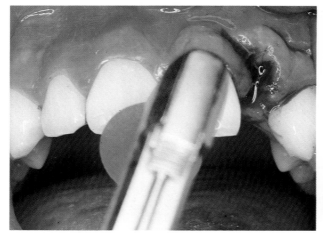
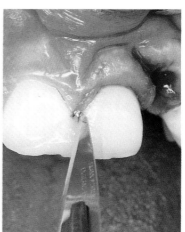

The finished splint
Note that the splint allows optimal oral hygiene in the gingival region which is the most likely port of entry for bacteria which may complicate periodontal and pulpal healing.

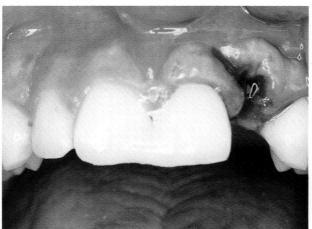
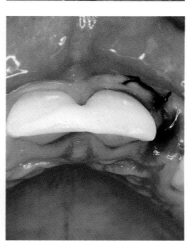

Suturing the gingival wound
The gingival wound is closed with interrupted silk sutures. The final radiograph shows optimal repositioning of the tooth.

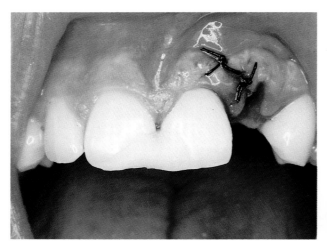
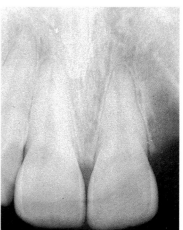

In case of *lateral luxation*, repositioning is usually a very forceful and, therefore, a traumatogenic procedure (Figs. 9.24 and 9.25). Prior to this procedure, it is necessary to anesthetize the area. An infraorbital regional block anesthesia on the appropriate side of the maxilla is the most effective. As indicated, this type of luxation is characterized by the forceful displacement of the root tip through the facial alveolar wall, which complicates the repositioning procedure. In order to dislodge the root tip from its bony lock, firm digital pressure in an incisal direction must first be applied immediately over the displaced root. This structure can be localized by palpating the corresponding bulge in the sulcular fold. Once the tooth is dislodged, it can be maneuvered apically into its correct position.

If manual repositioning is not possible, a forceps can be applied, whereby the tooth is first slightly extruded past the bony alveolar lock and then directed back into its correct position.

Once the tooth is repositioned, the labial and palatal bone plates should also be compressed, to ensure complete repositioning in order to facilitate periodontal healing. Lacerated gingiva should then be re-adapted to the neck of the tooth and sutured. The tooth should be splinted in its normal position and a radiograph taken to verify this and to register the level of the alveolar bone for later comparison. This is recommended in order to monitor eventual loss of marginal bone support in the follow-up period (see later).

If treatment of a laterally luxated or extruded permanent tooth is delayed (i.e.

Fig. 9.24.
Treatment principles for lateral luxation: repositioning and splinting

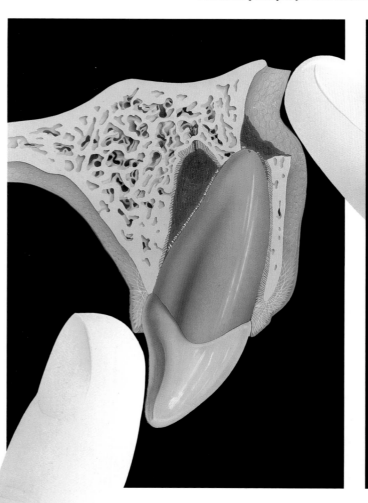 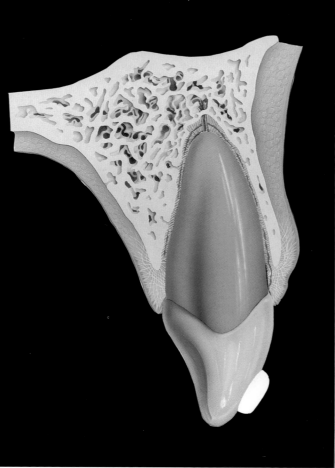

Fig. 9.25. Diagnosis and treatment of lateral luxation
This 23-year-old man suffered a lateral luxation of the left central incisor.

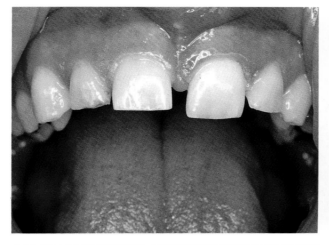 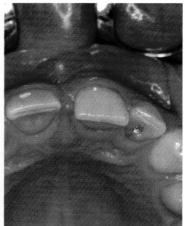

Percussion test
Percussion of the injured tooth will reveal a high-pitched metallic sound.

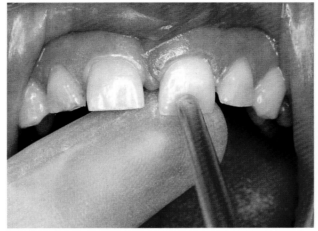 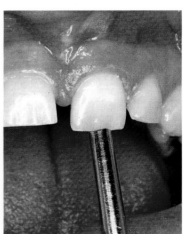

Mobility and sensibility testing
Mobility testing, using either digital pressure or alternating pressure of two instrument handles facially and orally, reveals no mobility of the injured tooth. There is no response to pulpal sensibility testing.

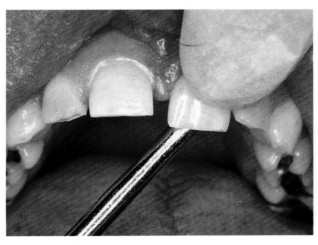 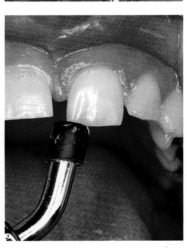

Radiographic examination
A steep occlusal radiographic exposure reveals, as expected, more displacement than the bisecting angle technique. A lateral radiograph reveals the associated fracture of the labial bone plate.

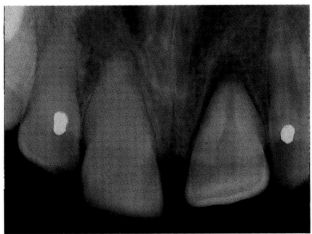 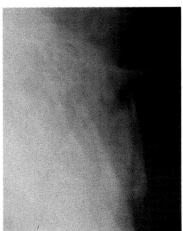

LUXATION INJURIES

Anesthesia

An infraorbital regional block is placed and supplemented with anesthesia of the nasopalatinal nerve.

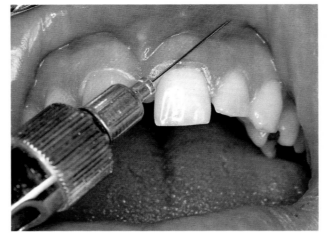
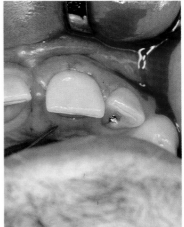

Repositioning

The tooth is repositioned initially by forcing the displaced apex past the labial bone lock and thereby disengaging the root. Thereafter, axial pressure apically will bring the tooth back to its original position. It should be remembered that the palatal aspect of the marginal bone has also been displaced at the time of impact. This must be repositioned with digital pressure to ensure optimal periodontal healing.

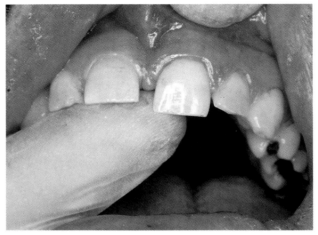
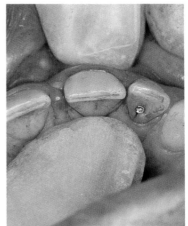

Verifying repositioning and splinting with the acid-etch technique

Occlusion is checked and a radiograph taken to verify adequate repositioning. The incisal one-third of the labial aspect of the injured and ajacent teeth are acid-etched (30 seconds) with phosphoric acid gel.

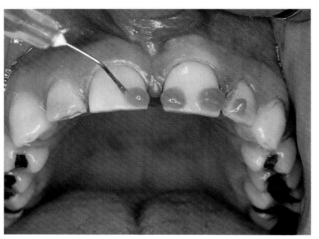
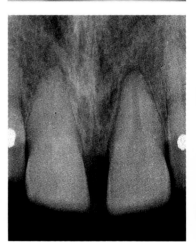

Preparing the splinting material

The etchant is removed with a 20-seconds water spray. The labial enamel is dried with compressed air, revealing the mat, etched surface.

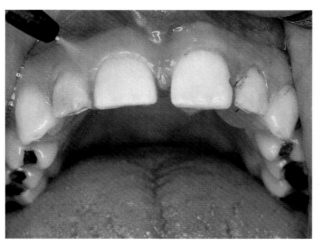
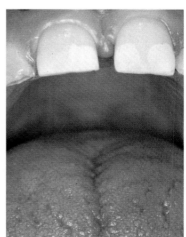

Applying the splinting material

A temporary crown and bridge material (e.g. Protemp®) is then applied. Surplus material can be removed after polymerization using a straight scalpel blade, abrasive discs or a fissure bur.

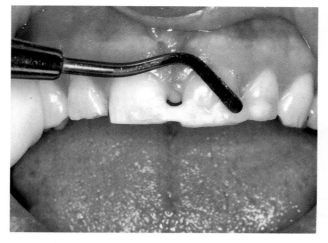
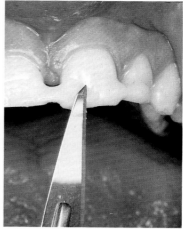

Three weeks after injury

At this examination, a radiograph is taken to evaluate periodontal and pulpal healing. That is, neither periapical radiolucency nor breakdown of supporting marginal bone, as compared to the radiograph taken after repositioning.

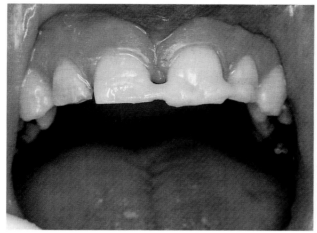
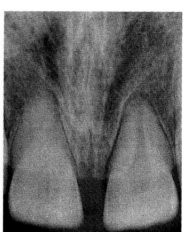

Splint removal

The splint is removed using fissure burs, by reducing the splinting material interproximally and thereafter thinning the splint uniformly across its total span. Once thinned out, the splint can be removed using a sharp explorer.

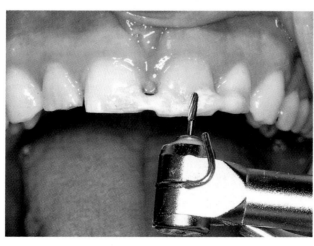
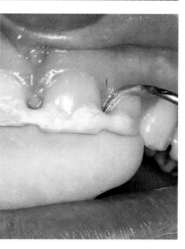

Six months after injury

After 6 months, there is a weak sensibility reaction and normal radiographic conditions.

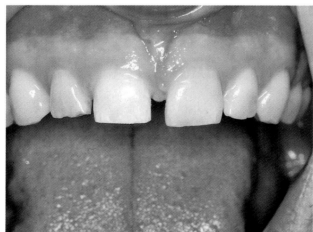
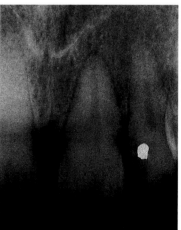

more than 48 hours after injury), it is usually found that the tooth is extremely difficult to reposition. Recent studies seem to indicate that reduction procedures should be deferred and the tooth allowed to realign itself or that this should be accomplished orthodontically (3, 5, 26-28) (see Chapter 15, p. 617).

The optimal treatment for *intruded* permanent teeth has not yet been determined (28-31, 107, 170-174). Intruded immature teeth will normally re-erupt spontaneously, as has also been observed in teeth with completed root formation (170, 173, 174).

Prevention of complications such as external root resorption and loss of marginal bone support determine the choice of treatment. In this context, it should be noted that immediate repositioning (surgical repositioning) has been found to increase the frequency of these complications. The treatment of choice for both immature and mature teeth, therefore, appears in most cases to be orthodontic repositioning over a period of 3-4 weeks

(Figs. 9.26 and 9.27). Ideally, orthodontic extrusion should be accomplished at a pace that keeps up with the repair of marginal bone. Furthermore, it is important that the tooth be sufficiently repositioned within 2-3 weeks to assure access to the pulp chamber should endodontic treatment be necessary. This is important as external root resorption will be initiated by this time and the only way to arrest this process is endodontic therapy (see Chapter 14, p. 557). This is also the reason for not awaiting spontaneous eruption. This process can take 2-3 months. In the meantime, root resorption can become quite advanced and, due to the semi-buried position of the tooth, there is no possibility of endodontic intervention.

Orthodontic movement of intruded permanent teeth can begin at the initial examination at the time of injury, or some days later when swelling has subsided. If the tooth has been completely intruded, it is essential that it is partially repositioned so that half of the crown is exposed. This will

Fig. 9.26.
Treatment principles for intrusive luxation: spontaneous eruption or orthodontic extrusion.

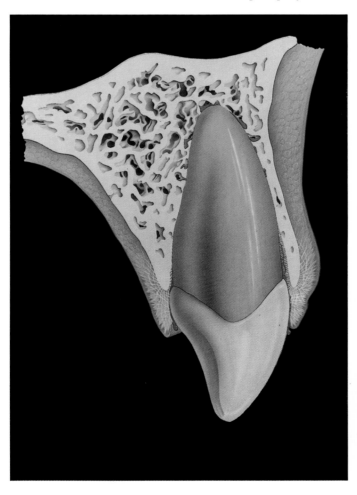 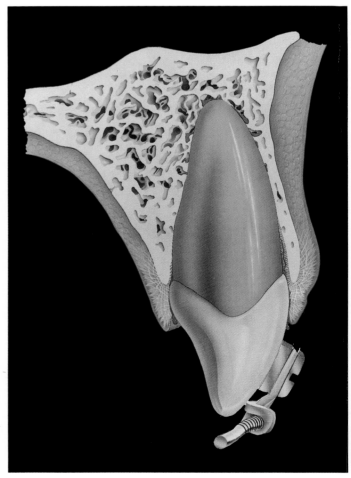

CHAPTER 9

Fig. 9.27. Orthodontic extrusion of an intruded incisor
Clinical and radiographic condition in a 22-year-old woman after an axial impact.

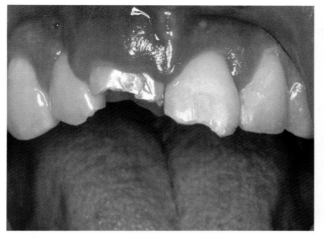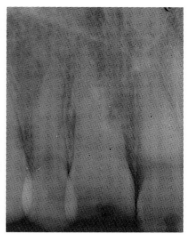

Covering exposed dentin
The exposed dentin of both central incisors is covered with a hard-setting calcium hydroxide cement (e.g. Dycal®).

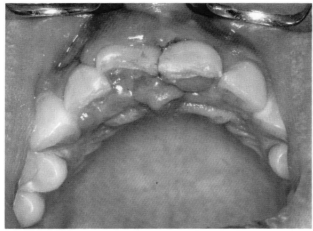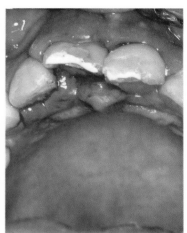

Applying orthodontic traction
A 0.5-mm thick semi-rigid orthodontic wire is bent to follow the curvature of the dental arch, including two adjacent teeth on either side of the intruded incisor. The orthodontic wire is fastened to the adjacent teeth using an acid-etch technique. In the area where elastic traction is exerted, a coil spring (e.g. 0.228 x 0.901, Elgiloy®) is placed in order to prevent slippage of the elastic.

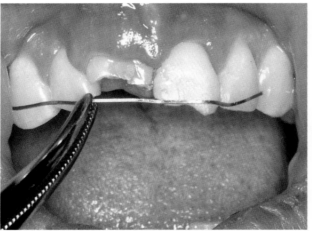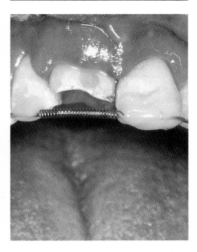

Placing the bracket
A bracket is placed on the labial surface and the fractured incisal edge is covered with a temporary crown and bridge material.

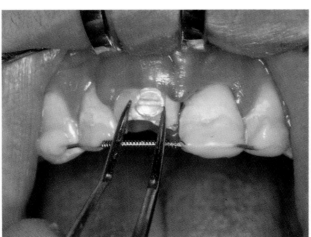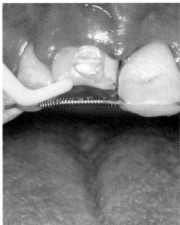

LUXATION INJURIES

Orthodontic traction

Elastic traction of 70-100 grams is activated. The direction of traction should extrude the tooth out of its socket in a purely axial direction.

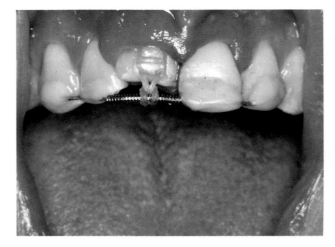 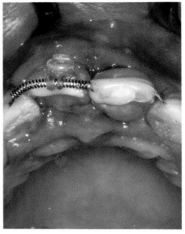

Extrusion initiated

After approximately 10 days, osteoclastic activity around the intruded tooth has usually resulted in loosening; and extrusion can then occur. If extrusion has not yet begun after 10 days, a local anesthetic is administered and the tooth is luxated slightly with a forceps. After 2-3 weeks, a rubber dam is applied and the pulp extirpated. The root canal is filled with calcium hydroxide paste.

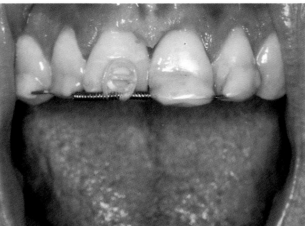 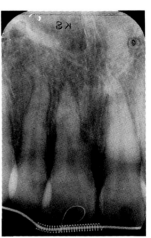

Extrusion complete

After 4 weeks, the intruded tooth is extruded to its original position and the tooth retained in its new position for 2-4 weeks. Thereafter, the orthodontic appliance can be removed.

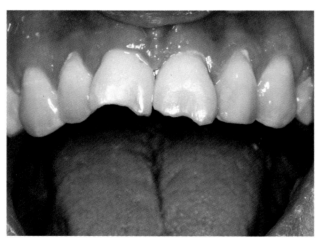 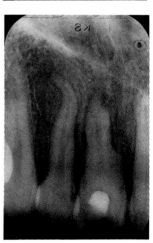

Crown restoration

The fractured crowns are restored with composite resin.

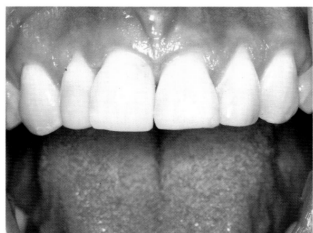 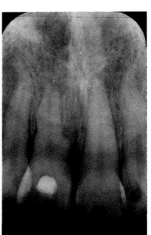

hasten the final re-eruption and facilitate application of an orthodontic bracket to the labial surface. The orthodontic appliances used for extrusion are similar to those used for extrusion of crown-root fractured teeth (cf. Chapter 15, p. 600).

Before orthodontic extrusion is initiated, it may be an advantage to luxate the tooth slightly with forceps after administration of local anesthesia. If this alternative is chosen, orthodontic extrusion should be postponed for a few days to avoid avulsion of the tooth upon activation of the appliance.

Primary Dentition

Concussion and *subluxation* injuries in the primary dentition require no treatment apart form a clinical and radiographic follow-up. *Extruded* primary teeth can either be repositioned or extracted. In some cases of extrusion and lateral luxation, there might be occlusal interference. In these cases, either repositioning or extraction is necessary (Figs. 9.28 and 9.30).

The treatment of *intruded* and *laterally luxated* primary teeth is still debated. The essential problem is the prevention of injuries to the developing permanent teeth. In experimental studies in monkeys, where primary incisors were intruded, it appeared that extraction of the intruded primary incisor led to minor damage to the reduced enamel epithelium of the permanent successor compared to when the intruded primary incisor was preserved (108). However, in a similar macroscopic study, it was found that the frequency and extent of the macroscopic enamel hypoplasias were almost identical in the two groups (109). Clinical studies in humans have also demonstrated only small and insignificant differences in the extent and frequency of developmental disturbances in the permanent dentition when preservation and extraction of the intruded primary incisor were compared (32, 107, 110). Consequently,

until further studies have appeared, it seems appropriate that conservative therapy be favored.

Intruded or *laterally luxated* primary teeth will usually reerupt or reposition themselves spontaneously within a period of 1 to 6 months (Fig. 9.28) (4, 33-35) and impactions are very rare (175, 176). However, before a decision is made to await spontaneous repositioning, the direction of displacement should be considered. Only teeth whose apices are displaced facially (i.e. away from the permanent tooth germ) should be allowed to re-erupt. Where clinical and radiographic evidence indicates that the apex is displaced towards the permanent successor, the primary tooth should be extracted immediately and atraumatically (Fig. 9.29).

During the re-eruption phase of intruded primary teeth, there is a risk of acute inflammation around the displaced tooth. This is manifested clinically as swelling and hyperemia of the gingiva, sometimes with abscess formation and oozing of pus from the gingival crevice (Fig. 9.31). There is a rise in temperature and complaint of pain from the traumatized region. In these cases, immediate extraction and antibiotic therapy are essential in order to prevent the spread of inflammation to the permanent tooth germ.

In this context, it is important to consider that a proper extraction technique be employed so as to avoid further injury, especially to the developing dentition. Elevators should never be used due to the risk of their entering the follicular space. Moreover, it is necessary that the intruded incisor be grasped proximally with the forceps and removed without further luxation of the root. These precautions are necessary in order to avoid collision with the developing tooth germ. Finally, once the tooth has been removed, the palatal and facial bone plates should be repositioned with slight digital pressure. A su-

Fig. 9.28. Spontaneous re-eruption of an intruded primary incisor

This 2-year-old boy suffered an intrusion of the right central incisor. The foreshortened appearance of the intruded tooth implies labial displacement. Spontaneous re-eruption is therefore anticipated.

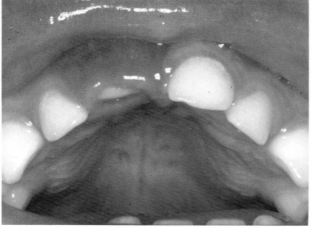 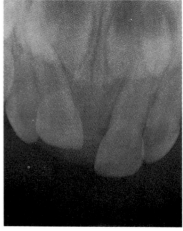

Follow-up, 2 months after injury

The tooth has erupted approximately 2 mm coronally.

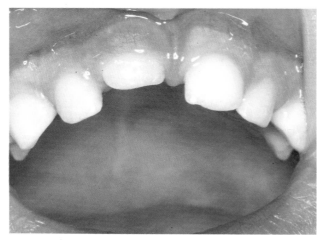 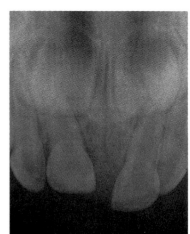

Follow-up, 3 months after injury

The tooth lacks 1 mm for complete eruption.

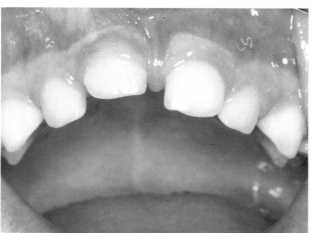 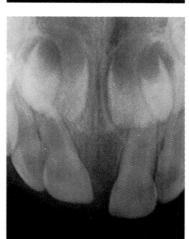

Follow-up, 1 year after injury

The tooth is in normal position. Crown color is normal and the radiographs show no sign of pathology.

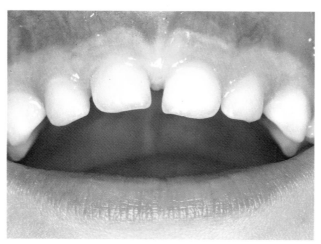 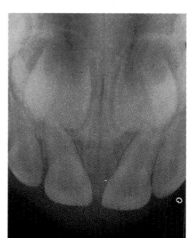

CHAPTER 9

Fig. 9.29. Intrusion, severe follicle invasion

This 1-year-old boy sustained an axial impact, resulting in complete intrusion of the central incisor. Note the displacement of the permanent tooth germ in the follicle. Removal of the primary incisor is mandatory.

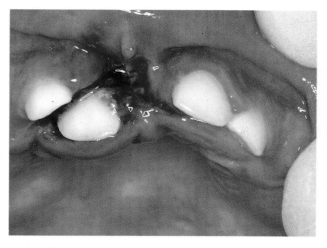 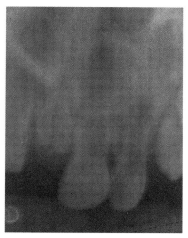

Removing the displaced tooth

Using sedation and topical anesthesia, the tooth is grasped proximally with forceps and removed in a labial direction. The fractured and displaced palatal bone is repositioned with digital pressure and a suture placed to close the entrance to the socket.

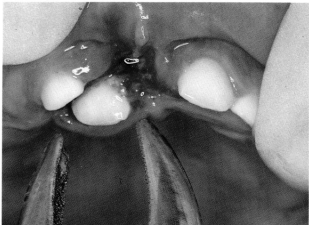 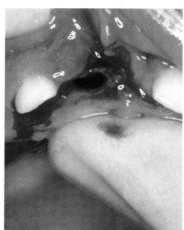

Follow-up

At examination 1 week later, a slight change in the position of the tooth germ is seen.

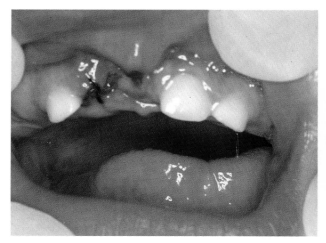 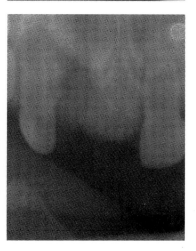

Disturbance in eruption

At the age of 6 years, it is evident that a crown dilaceration has developed.

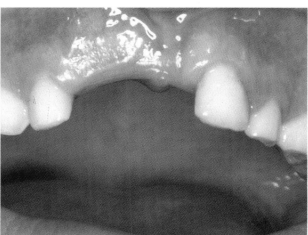 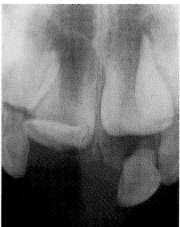

LUXATION INJURIES

Fig. 9.30. Repositioning of a laterally luxated primary central incisor
This 4-year-old boy suffered a lateral luxated of the left maxillary primary central incisor. Repositioning is indicated due to occlusal interference.

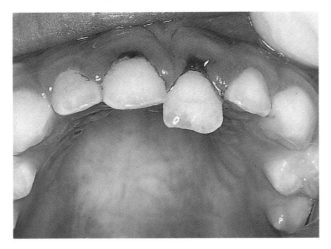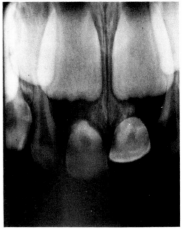

Treatment evaluation
Due to interference with occlusion and the distance between the apex of the primary tooth to the permanent tooth germ, repositioning is indicated.

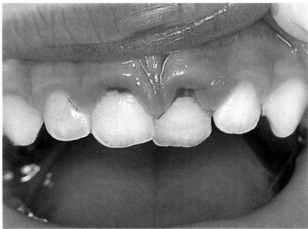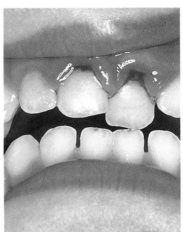

Repositioning
After application of a topical anesthetic, the tooth is repositioned with combined labial and palatal pressure.

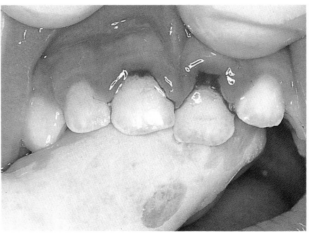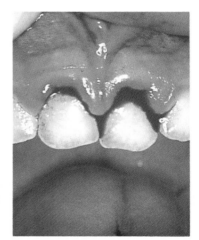

Post-operative condition
The tooth has been adequately repositioned, as revealed both clinically and radiographically.

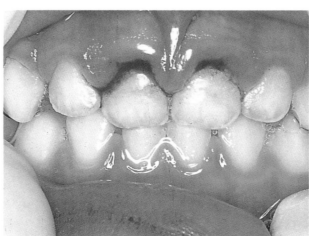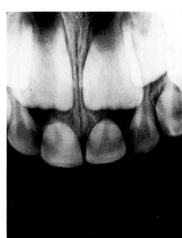

Fig. 9.31. Acute infection following intrusion
This 3-year-old boy suffered intrusion of 2 central incisors. As the root tips were displaced away from the developing tooth germs, spontaneous eruption was anticipated.

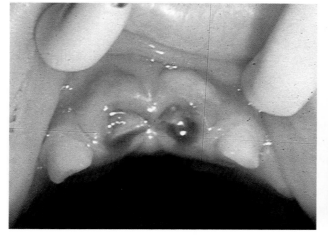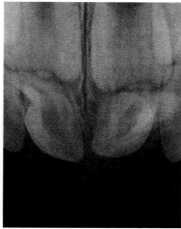

Follow-up, 2 weeks after injury
Acute infection with swelling and pus formation around the displaced incisors has developed.

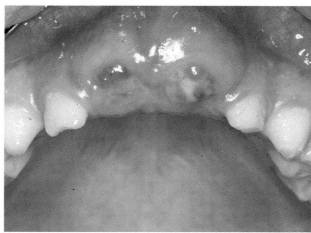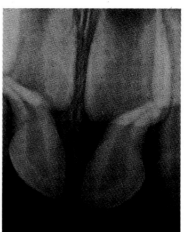

ture to close the wound might be appropriate.

Splinting

When a tooth is loose or repositioned after displacement, the question arises as to whether a splint will aid periodontal or pulpal healing. To date, this issue has not been adequately researched. However, both experimental and clinical data indicate that the efficacy of splinting is dubious. Thus, in experimental studies, rigid splinting had a negative influence on pulpal revascularization after autotransplantation (177) and had no effect on periodontal ligament healing after extrusive luxation (156). In clinical studies, the effect of splinting upon luxated teeth appeared to lead to an increase in pulp necrosis (178) and pulp canal obliteration (163, 178). Only a few guidelines with a weak scientific foundation can be given. In Appendix 4, p. 750 a suggested splinting regimen is listed for the various luxation entities in the permanent dentition.

A number of different splinting methods have been developed, especially in recent years (179-181). There are certain requirements that a splint should fulfill for it to be acceptable in a trauma situation (36):

1. It should be able to be applied directly in the mouth without delay due to laboratory procedures.
2. It should not traumatize the tooth during application or removal.
3. It should stabilize the injured tooth in a normal position.
4. It should provide adequate fixation throughout the entire period of immobilization (37).
5. It should neither damage the gingiva nor predispose to caries.
6. It should not interfere with occlusion or articulation.
7. It should not interfere with any required endodontic therapy.
8. It should preferably fulfill esthetic demands.
9. In case of fixation after luxation injuries

and replantation of avulsed teeth, the splint should allow a certain (not yet defined) mobility to aid periodontal ligament healing (179, 181), whereas after root fracture the splint should be rigid to permit optimal formation of a dentin callus to unite the root fragments.

10. It should be easily removed.

Only one type of splint comes close to fulfilling these demands today. That is the acid-etch/resin splint or variants of this technique. After the introduction of etching techniques to conservative dentistry, this technique was soon used for the purpose of splinting loose teeth (111-115, 182-192). This type of splinting has become very popular in recent years and is, in the majority of cases, to be preferred over other methods such as wiring, arch bars and cap splints. In the following, descriptions will be given for the various recommended techniques.

Techniques such as arch bars, interdental wiring, orthodontic bands/resin and cap splints have outlived their usefulness and have therefore been excluded from this edition.

ACID-ETCH/RESIN SPLINT

This splint is applied directly after etching the incisal half of the labial surfaces of the traumatized and adjacent teeth (Figs. 9.23 and 9.25). It is essential that the labial surfaces are as clean as possible when the etching solution is applied. With a water spray and cotton rolls, the labial surfaces should be cleansed of blood and debris. Thereafter, the etchant gel should be applied to the incisal third of the labial surface for 30 seconds, avoiding the interproximal contact areas. The etchant is then removed with a 20-second water spray and the teeth are air-dried.

The etched surface should appear mat white. Several types of splinting materials can be used. However, it should be noted that they have slightly different properties. Temporary crown and bridge materials have been found to be very useful for this purpose, being slightly flexible, easy to remove and having a minimal effect upon the pulp if inadvertently applied to exposed dentin (116, 191). A slight disadvantage is that fracture of the material sometimes occurs, as it is rather brittle when exposed to occlusal stress. The cold cure resins (e.g. Sevriton® and Paladur®),

offer great stability for prolonged splinting periods (i.e. after root fracture). Composite resins also offer great stability and esthetics, but their complete removal is cumbersome, especially as it can be difficult to distinguish enamel from the composite material.

Before application of the splinting material, it is important to consider that concomitant crown fractures with exposed dentin should be covered with a calcium hydroxide liner (e.g. Dycal® or Life®) before etching to prevent damage to the pulp (Fig. 9.32). To facilitate later restoration of the fracture, it is a good idea to cover not only dentin but also enamel on the fracture surface with liner prior to etching. This will prevent bonding of the splinting material to enamel in this location. In the case of fragment reattachment (see Chapter 6, p. 230), this precaution will ensure an intact enamel surface at the time of later treatment.

After drying the etched area, it is important that the enamel is not contaminated with blood or saliva during application of the splint. Profuse bleeding from the gingiva can be controlled by suction or compression of the gingival margin with cotton rolls. In cases of missing teeth or in a mixed dentition where teeth are not fully erupted, it is necessary to span the edentulous area. In these cases, reinforcement is necessary. This can be accomplished with metal bars (117, 118, 182-186), orthodontic wires (180, 187), nylon lines (188, 189), fiber glass (190), polycarbonate (192), or any one of the synthetic fibers or tapes presently on the market (e.g. Kevlar®, DuPont Corp., Fiber-splint®, Polydent Corp., Mezzovico, Switzerland) which can fuse with a composite resin. If these are not available, even paper clips can be straightened out for the purpose. The splinting material is then applied to the incisal half of the labial surfaces.

In the lower jaw with normal occlusion, the splint is applied to the lingual surfaces in order not to interfere with occlusion. Slight digital pressure incisally or the patient's occlusion will prevent movement of the repositioned teeth under the splint during polymerization. In the case of multiple luxations, where it can be difficult to reposition and splint all involved teeth at once, a stepwise fixation technique is suggested whereby a single luxated tooth can be repositioned and

Fig. 9.32. Treatment of a concomitant crown fracture and lateral luxation

This 11-year-old boy has suffered lateral luxation and crown fracture of the right central incisor due to a fall.

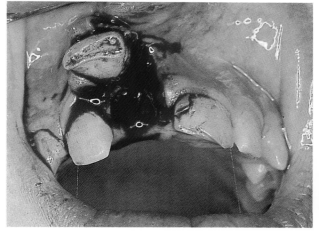
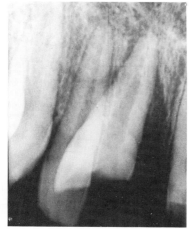

Repositioning the displaced incisor

After administration of regional anesthetic, the incisor is repositioned and a radiograph is taken to verify repositioning.

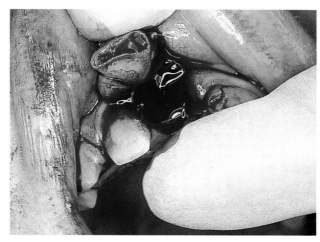
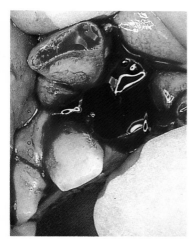

Suturing gingival wounds and dentin coverage

The gingival wound is sutured and exposed dentin covered with a hard-setting calcium hydroxide liner.

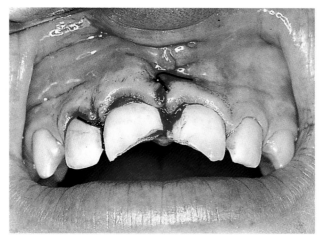
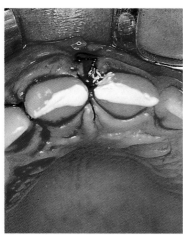

Completed treatment

A combination injury (luxation and crown fracture) has been splinted and covered with a temporary crown and bridge material.

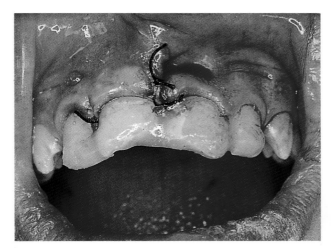
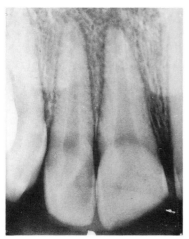

splinted to the adjacent non-injured tooth and the procedure repeated until all teeth are stabilized.

In cases of multiple tooth injuries with conflicting requirements of short fixation periods (e.g. after replantation) and longer fixation periods for the various luxation types, as well as for root fractures, splints using bonded orthodontic brackets (not bands) and a totally passive wire or the use of a wire applied to the facial surfaces of the injured and adjacent teeth with composite resin can solve this problem (187).

After polymerization of the splinting material, it is necessary to ensure that the splint does not interfere with occlusion. The splint is also checked for any interferences with the gingiva, so that optimal oral hygiene can be maintained during the healing period.

Finally, the patient should be instructed to avoid using the anterior teeth as much as possible while the splint is in place.

At the end of the fixation period, the splint is removed using a tapered fissure bur at low speed by thinning the resin universally and cutting through it interproximally. Remnants can then be removed with a scaler while the teeth are supported by digital pressure. After splint removal, the facial surfaces should be polished with pumice in order to remove residual resin. Following injuries where teeth have been displaced, repositioned and splinted, one should remember that the teeth might still be slightly loose and tender to touch following splint removal. Therefore, the polishing procedure might well be postponed to a later visit.

SPLINTING PERIOD

The optimal splinting period for luxated teeth is, to date, empirically-based. Thus, the following guidelines are subject to future revision. A splinting period of 2-3 weeks is normally sufficient in case of isolated injury to the periodontal ligament (i.e. *extrusion*). If injury to the periodontal ligament is combined with a fracture of bone, 3-4 weeks is recommended. Finally, in case of comminution of bone, as seen in connection with *lateral luxation* and *intrusion*, a splinting period of 6-8 weeks may be necessary due to initial resorption of injured bone which retards periodontal healing.

During the splinting period, it is essential that good oral hygiene be maintained. Careful toothbrushing and rinsing with chlorhexidine are recommended.

The application of splints in the primary dentition is usually not feasible. In these cases, a soft diet is recommended in the post-trauma period to avoid further damage to the injured tissues.

Prognosis

The follow-up period can disclose a number of complications, such as pulp canal

Table 9.2. *Prevalence of pulp necrosis after luxation of permanent teeth*

Examiner	No. of teeth	No. with pulp necrosis
Skieller (7) 1960	107	44 (41%)
Weiskopf et al. (74) 1961	121	72 (59%)
Anehill et al. (75) 1969	76	18 (24%)
Andreasen (3) 1970	189	98 (52%)
Stålhane & Hedegård (104) 1975	1116	172 (15%)
Rock et al. (97) 1974	200	75 (38%)
Rock & Grundy (178) 1981	517	192 (37%)
Wepner & Bukel (195) 1981	142	30 (21%)
Andreasen & Vestergaard Pedersen (163) 1985	637	156 (24%)
Oikarinen et al. (196) 1987	147	74 (50%)
Herforth (197) 1990	319	81 (25%)

Table 9.3. Prevalence of pulp necrosis according to type of luxation of permanent teeth. From ANDREASEN & VESTERGAARD PEDERSEN (163) 1985

Type of luxation	No. of teeth	No. with pulp necrosis
Concussion	178	5 (3%)
Subluxation	223	14 (6%)
Extrusive luxation	53	14 (26%)
Lateral luxation	122	71 (58%)
Intrusive luxation	61	52 (85%)

obliteration, pulp necrosis, root resorption and loss of marginal bone support. A follow-up schedule whereby healing complications can be diagnosed and interceptively treated is presented in Appendix 4, p. 750. However, in order to utilize the suggested recall schedule to full advantage, certain information must be gathered at the time of injury in order to identify those cases in which healing complications can be anticipated. The information needed for such clinical decisions will be discussed in the following.

"Tooth luxation" as a clinical diagnosis covers a broad spectrum of injury from a therapeutic, anatomic and prognostic point of view. A multivariate analysis of clinical and radiographic data registered at the time of injury confirmed the relevance of the current classification system, in that each type of injury could be described by a unique survival curve with respect to the development of pulp necrosis following injury (163) (see later). The same classification system was found useful in describing the luxation injury to the coronal fragment

of a root fracture (193, 194) (see Chapter 8, p. 305).

Pulp Necrosis

PERMANENT DENTITION
The frequency of pulp necrosis after luxation injuries in the permanent dentition has been found to range from 15 to 59% (Table 9.2).

Two factors have been found to be significantly related to the development of pulp necrosis: the *type of luxation injury* and *stage of root development* (3, 163, 196, 197) (Tables 9.3 and 9.4). In these investigations, it was not possible to demonstrate any effect of treatment in the development of PN (e.g. repositioning, fixation, antibiotic therapy).

TYPE OF LUXATION INJURY
The greatest frequency of pulp necrosis is encountered among intrusions followed by lateral luxation and extrusion (Fig. 9.33) while the least frequent occurrence of pulp necrosis was after concussion and subluxation (3, 7, 104, 136, 163) (Table 9.3).

Table 9.4. Prevalence of pulp necrosis after luxation of permanent teeth according to stage of root development. From ANDREASEN & VESTERGAARD PEDERSEN (163) 1985

Stage of root development	No. of teeth	No. with pulp necrosis
Incomplete	279	21 (8%)
Complete	358	135 (38%)

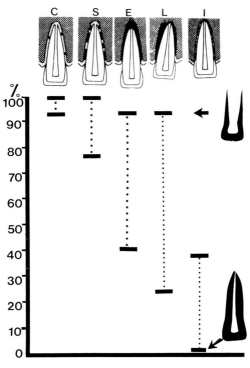

Fig. 9.33.
Relationship between luxation diagnosis, stage of root development and pulpal healing after trauma. From ANDREASEN (193) *1989.*

STAGE OF ROOT DEVELOPMENT
Pulp necrosis occurs more frequently in teeth with fully developed roots (3, 7, 104, 136, 163). (Table 9.4 and Fig 9.33). In teeth with immature root development, slight movements of the apex can presumably occur without disruption of the blood vessels passing through the apical foramen. Moreover, the process of revascularization is more easily achieved in teeth with a wide apical foramen, thus favoring the chance of pulp survival.

Fig. 9.33 shows survival curves following luxation injury according to type of injury and stage of root development (defined by quarters' of anticipated root growth and patency of the apical foramen). It can be seen that teeth with a constricted apical foramen which have been displaced run a greater risk of pulp necrosis than do teeth with patent root apices, where there is a greater possibility of pulpal revascularization. If the stage of root development is expressed as the mesiodistal diameter of the apical foramen at the time of injury it is also possible to demonstrate an improved revascula-

rization potential following extrusion and lateral luxation with an increase in apical diameter, presumably reflecting the area of the pulpo-periodontal interface from which new vessels could proliferate (198).

Regarding the diagnosis of pulp necrosis following luxations, different chronological patterns are followed for the various luxation types. Thus, pulp necrosis can be diagnosed within the first 6 months after concussion and subluxation; and up to 2 years after injury following extrusion, lateral luxation and intrusion (163) (Chapter 22), presumably due to difficulties in radiographic diagnosis related to the extent of damage to the periodontal structures.

DIAGNOSIS OF PULP NECROSIS
In the permanent dentition, the development of pulp necrosis can be associated with symptoms such as spontaneous pain or tenderness to percussion or occlusion. In a clinical material, where it was possible to compare pulpal histology with clinical and radiographic parameters, it was found that *tenderness to percussion* was the only sign which was significantly related to infected pulp necrosis following tooth luxation (193). However, pulp necrosis following luxation injuries and root fractures is normally asymptomatic and the diagnosis must therefore be based on clinical and radiographic parameters alone. Transillumination might reveal decreased translucency (Fig. 9.37, C). Grey color change in the crown can be seen, which is especially prominent on the lingual surface (Fig. 9.37, B). This may be accompanied by a periapical radiolucency which can be observed as early as 2-3 weeks after injury; but many cases show no sign of periodontal involvement radiographically. In these cases, a sterile necrosis might be suspected. Teeth with periapical rarefaction almost always represent pulpal infection, which is dominated by anaerobic microorganisms (133-135). The diagnosis of pulp necrosis should be further confirmed by pulpal sensibility tests. However, these findings can be difficult to interpret or can even be misleading. But if a pulpal response changes from positive to negative, pulp necrosis should be strongly suspected.

From previous studies, there appears to be general agreement that lack of pulpal sensibility alone (7, 199-202) or coronal dis-

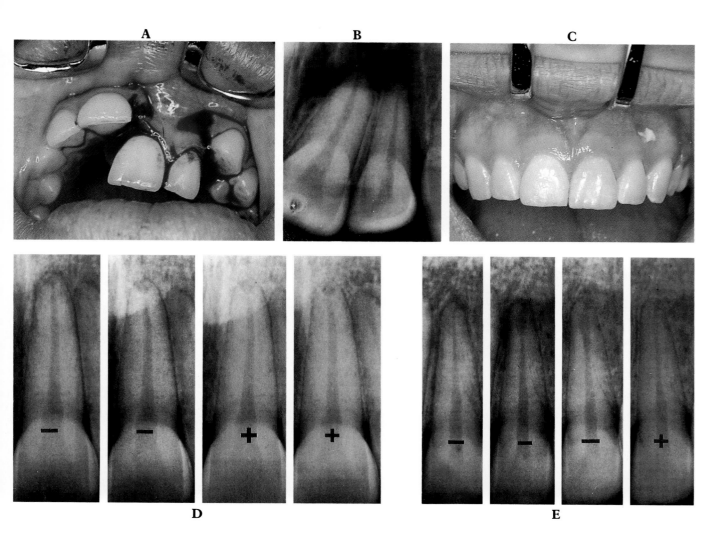

Fig. 9.34.
Internal surface resorption of the apical foramen after fracture of the alveolar process and extrusion of the left maxillary central and lateral incisors in a 21-year-old woman. A and B. Clinical and radiographic appearance at the time of injury. C. Clinical appearance 2 months after injury. The crown of the left central incisor has become grey. D and E. Orthoradial exposures of the central and lateral incisors respectively at 2 months, 9 months, 1 year and 2 years after injury. Plus and minus signs on the radiographs indicate positive or negative responses to pulp testing. At the 2-year control, the color of the left central incisor is almost normal. From ANDREASEN (193) 1989.

coloration alone (199, 201) are not enough to justify a diagnosis of pulp necrosis. The development of periapical radiolucency (199, 201, 202) has so far been considered the only "safe" sign of pulp necrosis. However, more recent investigations have cast doubt on the validity of the presently accepted diagnostic criteria (193). Even the concomitant presence of all three classical signs of pulp necrosis (coronal discoloration, loss of pulpal sensibility and periapical radiolucency) could still be followed by pulpal repair (193) (Figs. 9.34 and 9.35).

ELECTRICAL PULP TESTING
Pulpal sensibility tests have many limita-

tions in diagnosing pulp necrosis after traumatic dental injuries. Immediately following trauma approximately half of the teeth with luxation injuries do not respond to sensibility tests (7, 130, 164) (Fig. 9.36). In a recent clinical study, it was found that a negative response to pulp testing at the time of injury was closely related to the type of pulpal healing achieved. Thus, there were significantly more teeth that did not react to electrical stimulation at the time of injury whose root canals ultimately became obliterated than teeth that survived injury with no radiographic change (164, 193).

An explanation for the temporary loss of

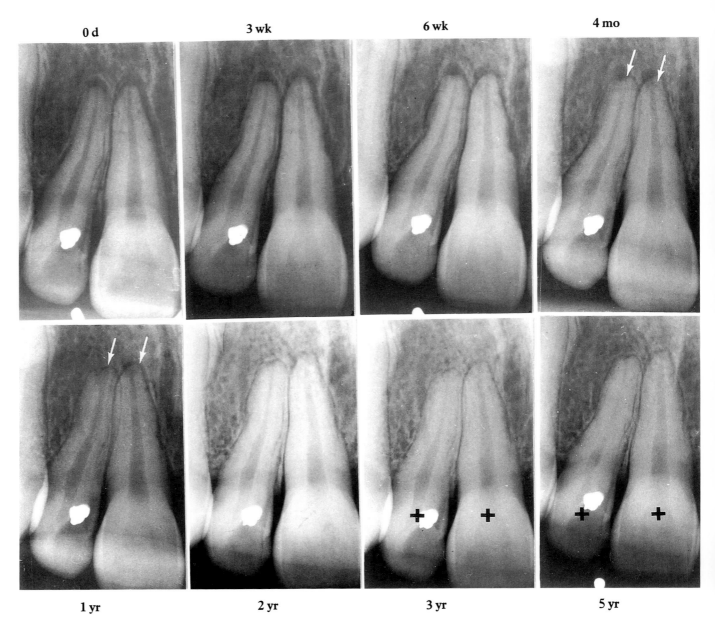

Fig. 9.35.

Transient apical breakdown after extrusive luxation of the maxillary right central and lateral incisors in a 19-year-old man. There is coronal discoloration of both teeth at the 1- and 2-year controls. Note internal surface resorption of both teeth at the apical foramina (arrows) 4 months and 1 year after injury, which is later followed by apical blunting (external surface resorption) and pulp canal obliteration of the lateral incisor. Plus signs on radiographs indicate when the incisors regained normal pulpal sensibility. From ANDREASEN (166) 1986.

normal excitability could be pressure or tension on the nerve fibers in the apical area. If complete rupture of nerve fibers has occurred, a period of at least 36 days is required before a positive response can be expected in immature permanent teeth (67, 130). In mature incisors, the observation period can be much greater (i.e. 1 year or more) prior to a return of a positive sensibility response (7, 66, 97, 131, 166, 193) (Fig. 9.36).

At later follow-up examinations, a previously negative reaction can return to positive, usually within the first 2 months after injury (130); but a period of at least 1 year can elapse before pulp excitability returns (7, 66, 166, 193). While this change in reaction is much more common in teeth with incomplete root formation than those with completely formed roots, longer observation periods can demonstrate restoration of pulpal sensibility in many mature permanent incisors (7, 97, 131, 193) (Fig. 9.36).

46 subluxated teeth with incomplete root formation

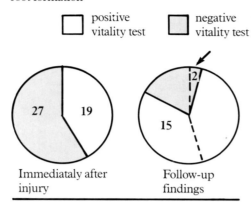

☐ positive vitality test   ▨ negative vitality test

Immediataly after injury   Follow-up findings

37 subluxated teeth with completed root formation

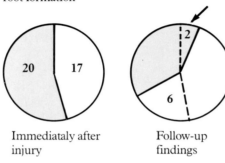

Immediataly after injury   Follow-up findings

Fig. 9.36.
Diagrams illustrating electrometric vitality reactions following subluxation of permanent teeth. After SKIELLER (7) 1960.

In rare cases, a previously positive response can become negative, a phenomenon usually evident within 2 months. However, cases have been reported in which a year or more elapsed before an avital response was recorded (7, 130).

PULP TESTING USING LASER DOPPLER FLOWMETRY

Lately, a new method has been developed whereby a laser beam can be directed against the coronal aspect of the pulp. The reflected light scattered by moving erythrocytes undergoes a Doppler frequency shift. The fraction of light scattered back from the pulp is detected and processed to yield a signal. The value of this method in determining pulp vitality has been demonstrated clinically (203-207).(see Chapter 5, p. 206). However, the equipment necessary for this procedure is quite costly and needs further refinement before it can be of general clinical value. Moreover, recent work has demonstrated false negative responses in the case of dis-

colored vital teeth (HEITHERSAY 1992, (see Chapter 5 p. 206).

Clearly, the diagnosis of pulp necrosis cannot be based upon sensibility tests alone, but should include additional findings, such as progressive grey discoloration of the crown, reaction to percussion, periapical radiolucency or cessation of root development.

COLOR CHANGES IN THE CROWN

Post-traumatic color change is a well-known phenomenon (9, 68-70). These changes can range from a lack of translucency to pink, bluish or grey discoloration (Fig. 9.37). FISH (71) offered an explanation for the pathogenesis of some of these changes, suggesting that an injury that was not strong enough to rupture the arteries passing through the apical foramen could occlude or sever the thin-walled veins. Hence, blood continues to be pumped into the canal, causing hemorrhage in the pulp and later diffusion into the hard dental tissues. Another explanation has been that occlusion or rupture of the apical vessels due to trauma leads to ischemia with breakdown of capillaries and subsequent escape of erythrocytes into the pulpal tissue (102).

When the injury displaces the tooth (e.g. intrusive or extrusive luxation), apical vessels are instantly severed with no extravasation of blood into the pulpal tissue and, thus, no immediate discoloration (73). In the case of moderate injury, where disruption of the vascular supply is less than total, ischemia can lead to increased vascular permeability. However, the same phenomenon could occur in the case of healing, as the immature vessels invading the avascular, traumatized pulp lack a basement membrane and are thereby incompetent until vessels mature (208-214). In this case, the ingrowing vessels can still carry blood to pulpal tissues, but blood and blood products could spill out into the stroma (193). In a recent clinical study, temporary grey coronal discoloration following luxation of mature permanent incisors was described (166, 193). These changes and their normalization could be associated with concomitant loss and restoration of pulpal sensibility, appearance and disappearance of apical radiolucencies and ultimately with pulp canal obliteration. It was suggested that, in the absence of infection, these transient changes could be links in a chain of events leading to pulpal healing. However, if bacteria gained access to the injured avascular pulp, permanent coronal discoloration might then be attributed to autolysis of the necrotic pulp and extravasation of these products into dentin.

Experimental findings indicate that hemoglobin breakdown products enter dentinal tubules (72). This penetration initially alters the crown color to a pinkish hue (Fig. 9.37 E). As the hemocomponents disintegrate, the color turns bluish which, when seen through the grey enamel, gives a greyish-blue tinge (Fig. 9.37 A and B). This shift from pink to greyish-blue takes approximately 2 weeks in the permanent dentition (9). A certain fading of the grey-blue tint can occur, or an opaque grey hue can persist (9). If the pulp survives, the stain can disappear (70) (Fig. 9.37 D and E).

Late color changes can occur if the pulp canal becomes obliterated (see p. 362). In these cases, the color of the crown shifts to a yellow hue (3) (Fig. 9.37 D to F).

Fig. 9.37. A. Color changes following luxation injuries in the permanent dentition
Grey discoloration 3 months after lateral luxation of a right central incisor.

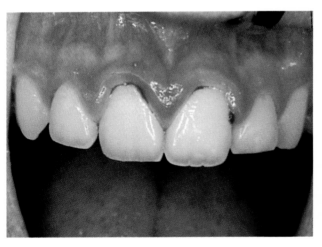 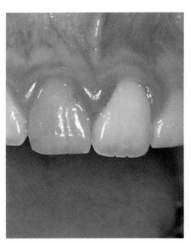

B. Influence of the direction of the light beam on the appearance of coronal discoloration
The color of the tooth is almost normal when the beam of light is perpendicular to the long axis of the tooth. Only the palatal surface is discolored, whereas the labial surface of the tooth appears normal.

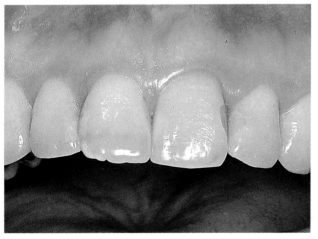 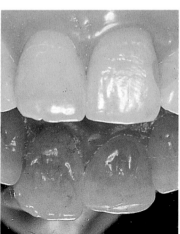

C. Changing the axis of the light beam

A shift in color to grey appears when the light beam is parallel to the long axis of the tooth. Furthermore, a change in translucency is evident.

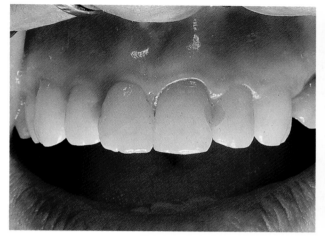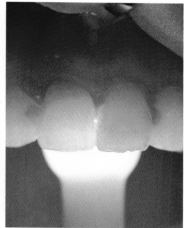

D. Reversibility of grey discoloration

This laterally luxated left central incisor shows marked grey discoloration which becomes normal at a later follow-up examination.

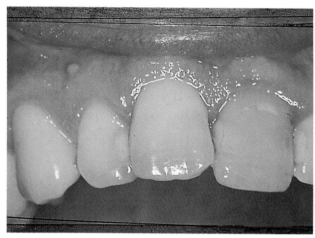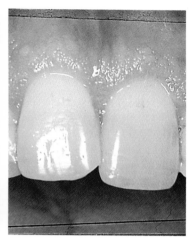

E. Reversibility of red discoloration

The clinical condition is shown 11 days after injury and at the 5-year follow-up.

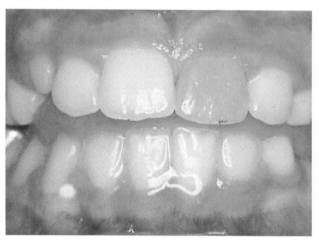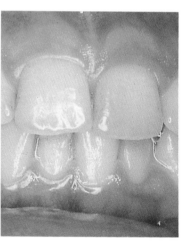

F. Yellow discoloration due to pulp canal obliteration

Yellow coronal discoloration seen 10 years after luxation.

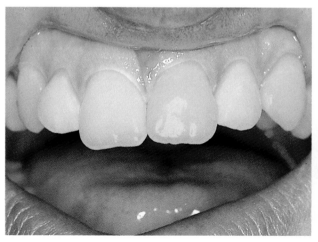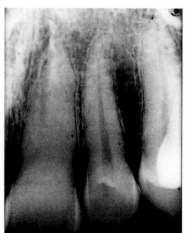

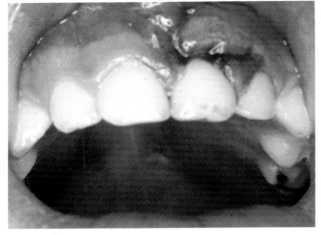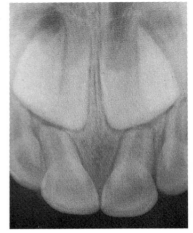

Follow-up, 3 weeks after injury
Intense reddish brown discoloration is seen.

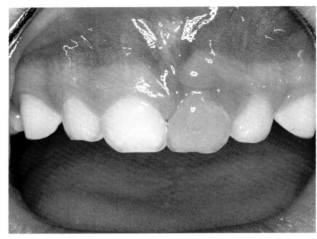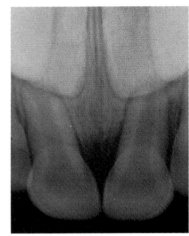

Follow-up, 1 year after injury
The color has changed to yellow and the radiographs demonstrate pulp canal obliteration.

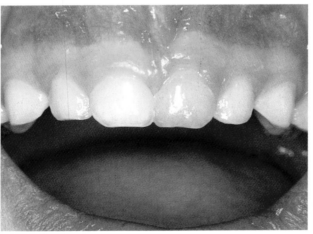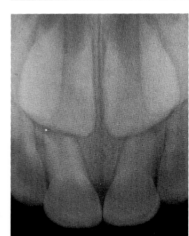

In the primary dentition, color changes are very frequent (132) (Fig. 9.38). In a clinical material, where the pulps in discolored primary teeth were extirpated within the first 8 months after injury, two-thirds of the pulps showed evidence of pulp necrosis (215). In another clinical material, approximately two-thirds returned to normal color within the first 6 months after trauma (151). However, the long-term outcome, i.e. infected pulp necrosis or pulpal revascularization has not yet been determined (216). Discoloration of a primary tooth after luxation should therefore not be used as the only criterion for interceptive pulpal therapy.

RADIOGRAPHIC CHANGES

The typical change reflecting a necrotic and infected pulp is a widened periodontal ligament space or an apical radiolucency. These changes may develop 2 to 3 weeks after injury and are caused by infection-induced release of a number of osteoclast activating factors [217] (see Chapter 2, p. 112).

In recent years, however, temporary apical radiographic changes in the region of the apical foramen following acute dental trauma and in connection with healing have been described [166, 193, 217]. It would seem that as a result of displacement of the root after luxation (or of the coronal fragtment of a root fracture), the vascular supply at the apical foramen (or "fracture foramen") could be partially or totally severed, leading to ischemic changes in the pulp. This would in turn lead to wound healing response and release of osteoclast-activating factors (see Chapter 2, p. 112). Subsequent resorption of hard tissue (dentin, cementum and alveolar bone), presumably at the interface between the vital and necrotic tissue, could then result either in an increase in the periodontal ligament space immediately adjacent to the injured apical foramen or an increase in the diameter of the apical foramen in the case of *extrusion* or *lateral luxation* of teeth with completed root formation. This event might be seen as a way to gain space to accommodate vascular ingrowth into the root canal.

Presumably once repair has reached the remodelling phase, the resorption processes resolve. This can be seen as a normalization of the radiographic condition within the root canal (i.e. hard tissue deposition in the previous resorption process and occasionally pulp canal obliteration) and restoration of a normal apical periodontal ligament space [217] (Figs. 9.34 and 9.35).

It might be speculated whether delay in treatment after the appearance of an apical radiolucent zone would worsen the prognosis of future endodontic therapy. However, it has been found that the success rate of endodontic therapy of teeth demonstrating periapical radiolucencies can be equal to the success rate of teeth treated before the development of manifest radiographic change, at least when the former are initially treated with calcium hydroxide prior to final guttapercha root filling (versus immediate guttapercha root filling) [218]. Thus, it appears that there would be imited risk of healing complications in the event of late endodontic therapy (i.e. up to 1 year after injury), delayed in anticipation of pulpal repair in selected patient categories (i.e. extrusive and lateral luxation of mature incisors).

TREATMENT GUIDELINES

Traditionally, diagnosis of pulp necrosis following luxation injuries has been based on clinical and radiographic findings. In fact, most teeth demonstrating such findings can be shown to contain a necrotic pulp.

However, as indicated, none of these signs can be considered pathognomonic of pulp necrosis. In selected cases, a conservative approach might be indicated, whereby active treatment can be avoided. [193].

As long as the following conditions are met, a tooth with one or more signs of pulp necrosis could be observed for pulpal repair over a longer period of time (up to approximately 1 year):

1. The patient is at low risk of inflammatory resorption (i.e. over 10 years of age, has completed root formation and has not suffered intrusive luxation) [193, 219].
2. The injury type and stage of root development (extrusion and lateral luxation of teeth with completed root development) imply that transient apical changes might be anticipated [166].
3. Neither prosthetic treatment nor orthodontic therapy is planned to immediately involve the injured tooth. As the clinical and radiographic signs previously described are assumed to reflect healing processes within the pulp, presumably because of a temporary disruption of the neurovascular supply, the additional trauma of crown preparation or orthodontic tooth movement might be anticipated to shift the balance of pulpal survival unfavorably.
4. As it is not presently possible to adequately evaluate pulpal status following dental luxations, the possibility of *asymptomatic* sterile pulp necrosis must not be ignored. It is therefore of utmost importance that the patient be thoroughly informed regarding the diagnostic problems involved and the

Fig. 9.39.
Relationship between pulp canal obliteration, pulp survival with no radiographic change and pulp necrosis in teeth with incomplete and completed root formation. From ANDREASEN ET AL. (164) 1987.

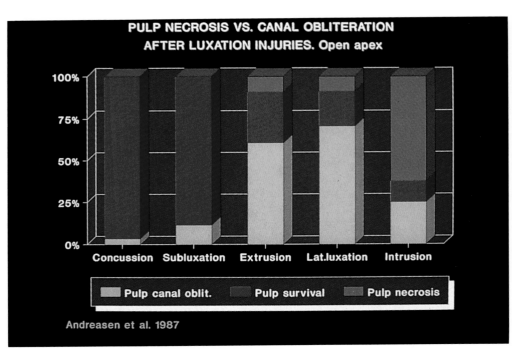

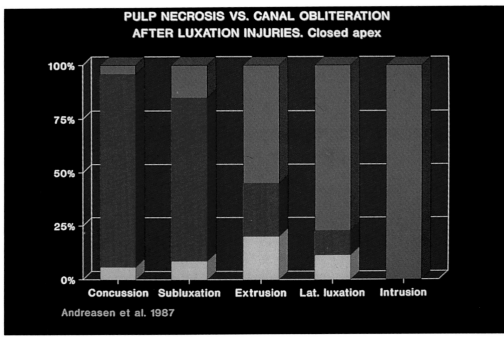

consequent need for extra follow-up examinations - and is willing and able to cooperate. If there is any doubt as to the possibility of recalling the patient, endodontic therapy rather than "observation therapy" should be the treatment of choice (193).

Primary Dentition

In the *primary dentition*, the frequency of pulp necrosis seems to parallel that in the permanent dentition (32, 132, 137, 138). As for the influence of age, a lower frequency of pulp necrosis is found among patients under 3 years of age (4). The influence of other clinical factors, such as type of injury and root development, has not yet been clarified.

It should be noted that intruded and later re-erupted primary and permanent incisors can develop pulp necrosis, a complication found in approximately one-third of re-erupted primary teeth (34).

As in the permanent dentition, there is no correlation between clinical/radio-

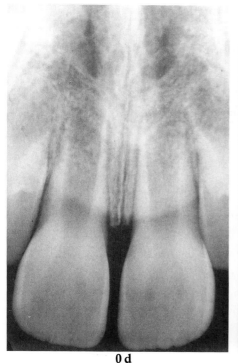 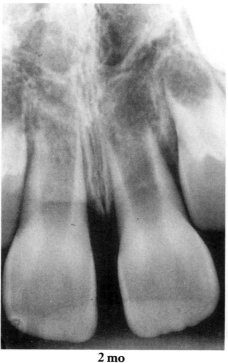 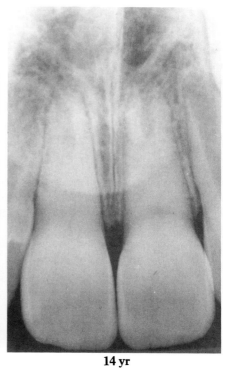

| 0 d | 2 mo | 14 yr |

Fig. 9.40.
Partial pulp canal obliteration after extrusion of 2 central incisors. Partial canal obliteration is evident after one year.

graphic observations and the histopathological changes in the pulp and periapical tissues (216). However, the diagnosis of pulp necrosis of primary teeth is based primarily on radiographic evidence of periapical rarefaction. This diagnosis can usually be made 6-8 weeks after injury. A therapeutic problem could be whether, during the observation period, pulp necrosis could inflict damage to the permanent tooth germ. Admittedly, there is a long-term effect of pulp necrosis and chronic periapical inflammation upon permanent successors (see Chapter 2, p. 83); however, an experimental study in monkeys has shown that pulp necrosis and periapical inflammation of primary incisors of only 6 weeks' duration do not lead to developmental disturbances of the permanent successors (139). Thus, a short observation period appears to be justified, thereby facilitating a diagnosis of pulp necrosis.

Another question concerns how to deal with primary teeth which become discolored after trauma. Histological studies have demonstrated pathological change in approximately one-half of such teeth. These changes include pulp necrosis and acute or chronic inflammatory changes. Grey discoloration was related to slightly more frequent pathological changes (215,

216). It is therefore recommended that an adequate follow-up schedule is maintained for discolored teeth; that is, control appointments 1 and 2 months after injury. If the grey discoloration persists in the presence of normal periodontal structures, further controls 6 and 12 months later are indicated (132). The treatment of these teeth is still open to debate, as no study to date has examined whether extraction therapy, mere observation therapy or endodontic treatment of the primary incisor is the optimal procedure with respect to the safety of the developing permanent successors.

In clinical studies, however, it has been shown that the majority of discolored primary teeth do not develop radiographic or clinical signs of infection and are exfoliated at the expected time (132, 143, 220). In one clinical study, it was shown that pulpotomies (using formocresol) and pulpectomy (using zinc oxide-eugenol) had success rates of 86% and 78% respectively (221). In another clinical study, the success rate of pulpotomy was 76% (222). Concerning pulpectomy, a disturbing finding was that the majority of cases showed incomplete resorption of the zinc oxide-eugenol dressing (221).

An important issue is whether endodontic treatment *per se* may induce developmental disturbances in the permanent dentition (221, 223, 224). In one clinical study it was found that root-filling of primary teeth with zinc-oxide eugenol resulted in 60% disturbance in enamel formation compared with only 21% in a non-treated group. However, the enamel disturbances were usually minute in both groups (224). In conclusion, endodontic treatment appears to be a realistic treatment procedure. However, the problem of resorbable root filling materials for use after pulp extirpation remains to be solved.

Pulp Canal Obliteration

Pulp canal obliteration can be regarded as a response to a severe injury to the neurovascular supply to the pulp which, after healing, leads to an accelerated dentin deposition and is frequently encountered after luxation injuries of permanent teeth (3, 20, 34, 35, 76, 77, 104-106, 141-143, 164, 178, 196, 225-227) (Table 9.5). Pulp canal obliteration is strongly related to the severity of the luxation injury, being especially common in severely mobile or dislocated teeth (104, 164, 178). It would appear to be a phenomenon which is closely related to the loss and reestablishment of pulpal neural supply (193), as it is rarely seen when there is no tooth displacement and thus little damage to the pulpal neurovascular supply (i.e. concussion and subluxation). Moreover, this complication mainly involves teeth injured before completion of root formation (3, 164) (Fig. 9.39).

A clinical manifestation of pulp canal obliteration is a yellow discoloration of the crown (Fig. 9.37 F). Response to thermal sensibility tests has been reported to be lowered or absent (78, 130); and response to electrical stimulation is also reported decreased and often absent (78, 105, 141). However, a recent clinical investigation could find no difference in sensibility threshold between paired incisors with and without pulp canal obliteration up to 5 years after injury (164). Nevertheless, with longer observation periods there is a tendency to higher thresholds or absence of reaction in pulp canal obliterated teeth.

The first radiographic sign of obliteration is reduction in the size of the coronal pulp chamber, followed by gradual narrowing of the entire root canal, occasionally leading to partial or complete obliteration (Figs. 9.40 and 9.41). However, histologic examination of these teeth always shows a persisting narrow root canal. Normalization of temporary apical radiolucencies, as described earlier, has been found to be significantly related to pulp canal obliteration in mature permanent incisors. This apparently reflects the wound healing processes involved in revascularization and reinnervation of the injured pulp (166) (Fig. 9.42).

Pulp canal obliteration usually appears between 3 to 12 months after injury (Fig. 9.41). It has been shown that two types of pulp canal obliteration exist. In *partial canal obliteration*, the coronal part of the pulp chamber is not discernible, while the

Table 9.5. Prevalence of pulp canal obliteration after luxation of permanent teeth

Examiner	No.of teeth	No. with pulp canal obliteration
Andreasen (3) 1970	189	42 (22%)
Gröndahl et al. (140) 1974	320	77 (24%)
Herforth (130) 1976	161	57 (35%)
Stålhane & Hedegård (104) 1975	1116	67　(6%)
Rock & Grundy (178) 1981	517	83 (16%)
Wepner & Bukel (194) 1981	142	12　(8%)
Lawnik & Tetsch (225) 1983	246	20　(8%)
Posukidis & Lehmann (226) 1983	162	25 (15%)
Andreasen et al. (164) 1987	637	96 (15%)
Oikarinen et al. (195) 1987	147	40 (27%)
Herforth (196) 1990	319	106 (33%)

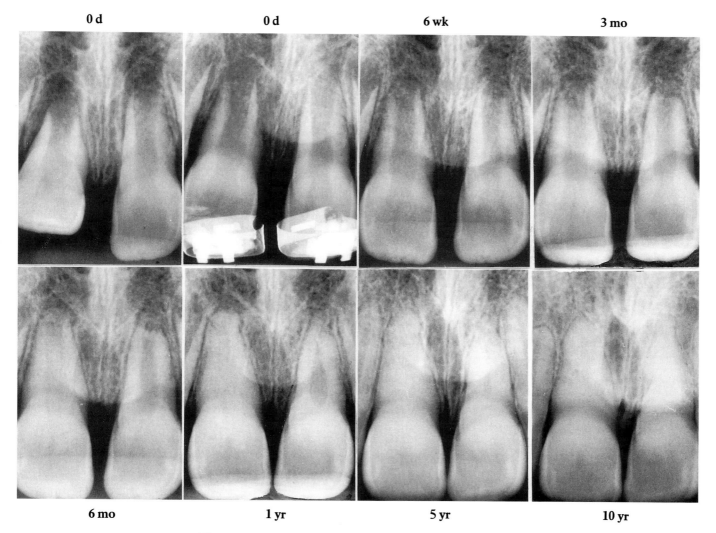

Fig. 9.41.
Radiographic definition of the various stages in pulp canal obliteration (PCO). Extrusive luxation of the maxillary right central incisor and avulsion of the maxillary left central incisor in a 6-year-old boy. Onset of PCO is seen 6 months after injury. Total PCO of right incisor, partial PCO of left incisor is found 1 year after injury. From ANDREASEN ET AL. (164) 1987.

Fig. 9.42.
Transient apical breakdown (TAB) in the form of a persistent expansion of the apical PDL of an immature root beyond the time of apical closure after extrusive luxation of the maxillary right lateral incisor and lateral luxation of the maxillary right central incisor in an 8-year-old boy. In both teeth, TAB is followed by obliteration of the pulp canal. From ANDREASEN (166) 1986.

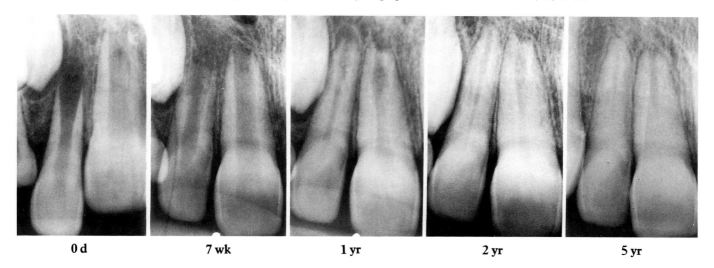

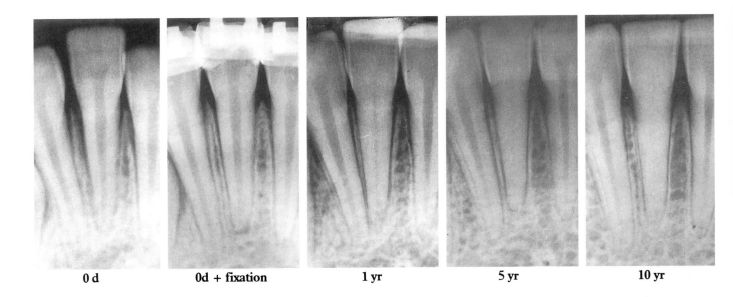

| 0 d | 0d + fixation | 1 yr | 5 yr | 10 yr |

Fig. 9.43.
Radiographic definition of the various stages in pulp canal obliteration (PCO). Lateral luxation of a mandibular right central incisor in a 10-year-old boy. Partial PCO is seen 1 year after injury and total PCO after 5 years. From ANDREASEN ET AL. (164) 1986.

apical part is markedly narrowed but still discernible (Fig. 9.40). In *total canal obliteration, the* pulp chamber and root canal are hardly (or not at all) discernible (105) (Fig. 9.41).

As with pulp necrosis, pulp canal obliteration is determined by the type of luxation injury and stage of root development at the time of injury (164). In contrast to pulp necrosis, however, where no treatment effect could be established, pulp canal obliteration was found to be signifi-

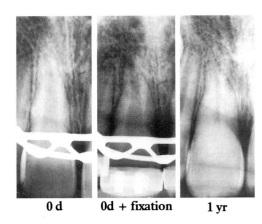

| 0 d | 0d + fixation | 1 yr |

Fig. 9.44.
The probable effect of orthodontic splinting. Subluxated maxillary right central incisor in a 9-year-old girl. After orthodontic band fixation, it can be seen that the root apex is displaced. There is pulp canal obliteration 1 year after injury. From ANDREASEN ET AL. (164) 1986.

cantly related to the type of fixation used (164). Prior to the use of acid-etched splinting techniques, orthodontic bands were cemented onto the traumatized and adjacent teeth and united with cold-curing acrylic (Figs. 9.43 and 9.44). There was a significant relationship between the use of this type of splint and this healing complication, presumably reflecting additional injury to the already traumatized periodontium due to forceful placement of the bands. In some cases, displacement of initially non-displaced traumatized incisors could be demonstrated after orthodontic band/acrylic fixation (Fig. 9.44). This effect has also been documented following forceful orthodontic extrusion of ectopic canines (228).

A late complication following pulp canal obliteration is the development of pulp necrosis and the occurrence of periapical changes (3, 78, 79, 164) (Figs. 9.45 and 9.46, Table 9.6). The pathogenesis of this complication is still obscure; but minor injuries are probably able to sever the vulnerable vascular supply at the constricted apical foramen, or the pulp vessels are progressively occluded due to hard tissue formation. Caries and restorative treatment apparently also contribute to the frequency of secondary pulp necrosis (Table 9.6). Several clinical investigations have recorded secondary pulp necrosis following pulp canal obliteration in 7-16% of cases. However, no distinction was

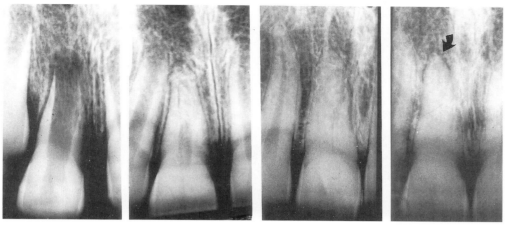

Fig. 9.45.
Pulp canal obliteration (PCO) followed by secondary pulp necrosis. The extruded central incisor develop is seen to develop PCO. At the 20-year follow-up examination, pulp necrosis and a periapical rarefaction have developed.

Fig. 9.46.
Extrusive luxation of permanent incisors leading to pulp obliteration and complicating pulp necrosis. A. Condition immediately after reduction and fixation. B. At follow-up 12 years later pulp canal obliteration and periapical inflammation are evident. C. Histologic specimen including apex of left central incisor. x 10. D. Periapical inflammation. x 30. E. Extensive hard tissue formation following injury. The pulp tissue is necrotic. x 75. F. Higher magnification of E. A few dentinal tubules in the post-traumatic hard tissue can be recognized (arrows). x 195.

A   **B**   **D**

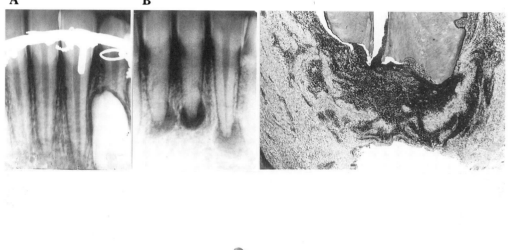

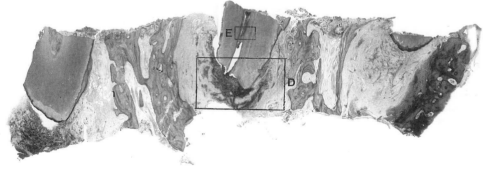

C

E   **F**

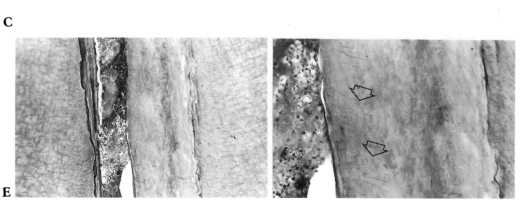

Table 9.6. *Frequency of necrosis secondary to pulp canal obliteration in permanent teeth*

Examiner	Observation period yr. (mean)	No. of teeth	No. of teeth developing pulp necrosis
Holcomb & Gregory (78) 1967	4	41	3 (7%)
Andreasen (3) 1970	1-12 (3.4)	42	3 (7%)
Stålhane (141) 1971	13-21	76	12 (16%)
Jacobsen & Kerekes (105) 1977	10-23 (16.0)	122	16 (13%)
Andreasen et al. (164) 1987	1-10 (3.6)	96	1 (1%)

made between between new trauma, secondary caries and/or crown preparation. A recent clinical investigation reported a frequency of secondary pulp necrosis of 1% with an observation period of up to 10 years. A greater frequency might be expected with longer observation periods (164).

It has also been reported that secondary pulp necrosis was only found in teeth with *total canal obliteration* and especially in those teeth which showed rapid obliteration after injury (i.e. total canal obliteration within 2 years after injury). Moreover, complicating pulp necrosis was common in teeth with completed root formation and with severe periodontal injury at the time of trauma (105).

While early prophylactic pulp extirpation and endodontic intervention can prevent periapical lesions, the rather low frequency of this complication does not support such measures (164, 229-232). The endodontic considerations of pulp canal obliteration are further discussed in Chapter 14, p. 567.

In the *primary dentition*, pulp canal obliteration is a frequent sequel to luxation injuries (132, 143, 227). Most of these teeth initially show a greyish discoloration, which later fades and then becomes yellow, concomitant with radiographic evidence of canal obliteration. Secondary pulp necrosis can occur, with reported frequencies of 10 to 13% (132, 143). This complication is seen as a periapical rarefaction. It is important to consider that pulp canal obliteration does not interfere with physiological root resorption; the permanent successors erupt without complication (143).

TREATMENT OF PULP NECROSIS
This subject is discussed in detail in Chapter 14, p. 567.

Root Resorption

A late complication following luxation injuries in both the primary and permanent dentitions is root resorption (29, 70, 80, 163, 217, 233), (Table 9.7). Root resorption can be classified into various types such as root surface resorption and root canal resorption (Figs. 9.47 and 9.52).

Root Surface Resorption (External Root Resorption)

The damage inflicted to the periodontal structures and the pulp by luxation injuries can result in various types of root surface resorption. The etiology and pathogenesis of these complications seem to be identical to root resorption following replantation of avulsed teeth (see Chapter 10, p. 388). Three types of esternal root resorption can be recognized.

SURFACE RESORPTION
The root surface shows superficial resorption lacunae repaired with new cementum. These lacunae have been termed surface resorption. It has been suggested that they occur as a response to a localized injury to the periodontal ligament or cementum (3, 81). In contrast to other types of resorption, surface resorption is self-limiting and shows spontaneous repair. Surface resorptions are not usually seen on radiographs due to their small size; however, it is sometimes possible to recognize small excavations of the root surface delineated by a normal lamina dura (3) (Fig. 9.48). When visible, these resorption cavities are usually confined to the lateral surfaces of the root, but may also be found apically, resulting in a slight shortening of the root.

Fig. 9.47. External root surface resorption.

Three types of root surface (external) resorption may develop subsequent to trauma: surface resorption, inflammatory resorption and ankylosis. After AN-DREASEN & ANDREASEN (217) 1992.

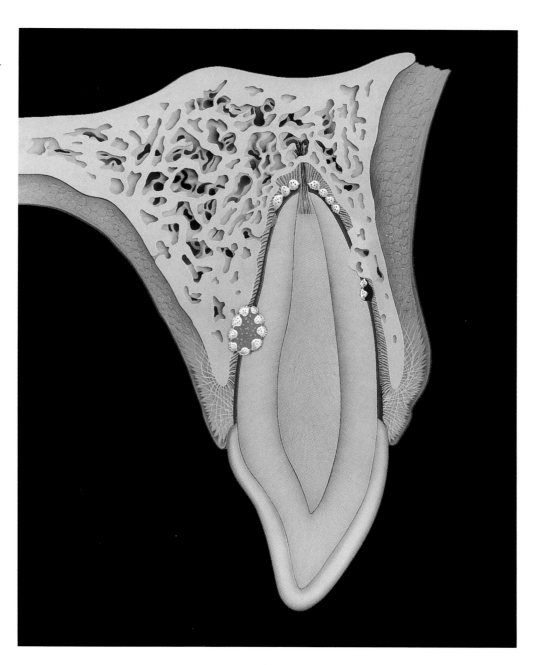

Fig. 9.48.

Surface resorption following intrusive luxation of right central incisor. A. Condition at time of injury. B. Six weeks after injury. Multiple small resorption cavities are evident along the root surface (arrows). C. One year later. Repair is evident with re-establishment of the periodontal space adjacent to the resorption areas. From ANDREASEN (3) 1970.

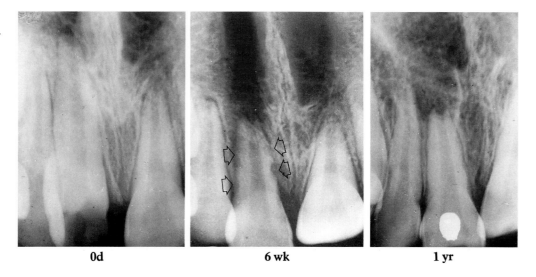

0d   6 wk   1 yr

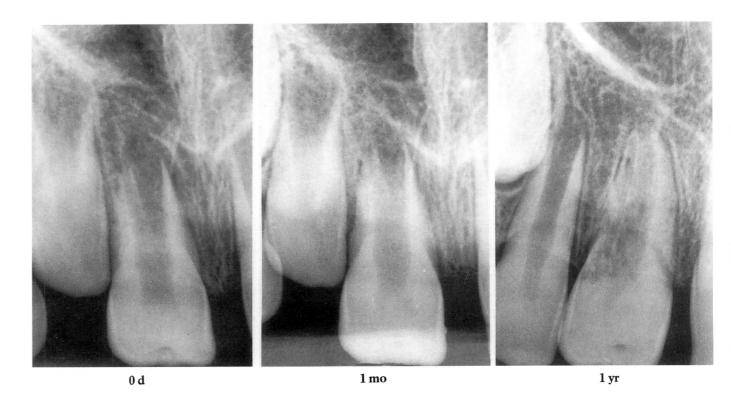

| 0 d | 1 mo | 1 yr |

Fig. 9.49.
External replacement resorption as a sequel to lateral luxation. At the time of removal of the splint one month later there is no evidence of root resorption. At the one-year follow-up, ankylosis is evident distally.

REPLACEMENT RESORPTION

A direct union between bone and root substance is seen, with the root substance gradually being replaced by bone (Figs. 9.47 and 9.49). Disappearance of the periodontal space and progressive root resorption are typical radiographic findings (3) (Fig. 9.50).

INFLAMMATORY RESORPTION

Histologically, bowl-shaped areas of resorption of both cementum and dentin are seen together with inflammation of adjacent periodontal tissue. The inflammation and resorption activity are appar-

ently related to the presence of infected, necrotic pulp tissue in the root canal (Figs. 9.47 and 9.51). Radiographically, root resorption with an adjacent radiolucency in bone is the typical finding (3) (Fig. 9.51).

External root resorption is most commonly seen after intrusive luxation. However, this can also be found following severe lateral luxations (163). Subluxation yields the lowest frequency of resorption, primarily in the form of surface resorption and intrusion the highest frequency and with frequent occurrence of inflammatory and replacement resorption (3, 7, 93, 104, 163,

Table 9.7. Frequency of progressive root resorption after luxation of permanent teeth

Examiner	No. of teeth	No. with progressive root resorption (ankylosis and inflammatory resorption)
Skieller (7) 1960	107	6 (6%)
Andreasen (3) 1970	189	21 (11%)
Stålhane & Hedegård (104) 1975	1116	16 (1%)
Rock & Grundy (178) 1981	517	37 (8%)
Andreasen & Vestergaard Pedersen (163) 1975	637	47 (7%)
Oikarinen et al. (196) 1987	147	27 (18%)

CHAPTER 9

Fig. 9.50.
Replacement resorption following intrusive luxation of the left permanent incisors. Progression of replacement resorption is seen over 21/2 year period. At this time both incisors were extracted. E. Low-power view of sectioned lateral incisor. x 8. F. Vital pulp tissue. x 75. G. Marked posttraumatic dentin formation containing few dentinal tubules (arrows). x 75. H. Ankylosis area with apposition of bone. x 30.

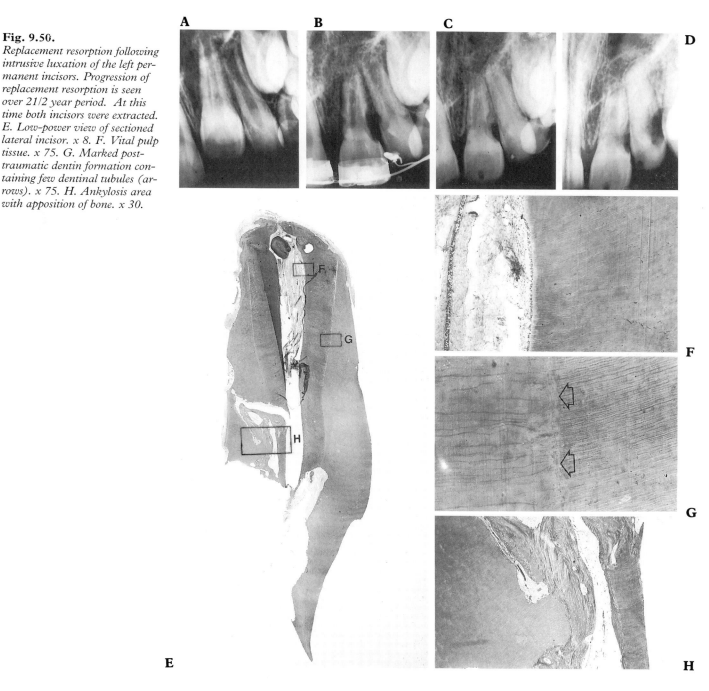

Tabel 9.8. Prevalence of external root resorption related to luxation diagnosis. From ANDREASEN & VESTERGAARD PEDERSEN (163) 1985

	No. of teeth	No. with surface resorption	No. with inflammatory resorption	No. with ankylosis
Concussion	178	8 (4%)	0 (0%)	0 (0%)
Subluxation	223	4 (2%)	1 (0,5%)	0 (0%)
Extrusive Luxation	53	3 (6%)	3 (6%)	0 (0%)
Lateral luxation	122	32 (26%)	4 (3%)	1 (1%)
Intrusive luxation	61	15 (24%)	23 (38%)	15 (24%)

Fig. 9.51.

Inflammatory resorption following extrusive luxation of a left lateral incisor. A. Condition immediately after reduction and splinting. B. Six months later. Note periradicular radiolucency as well as root resorption. C. Low-power view of sectioned incisor removed 6 months after injury. x 7. D. Resorption area with inflammation in the connective tissue and epithelial proliferation. x 75. E. Abscess bordering coronal necrotic pulp tissue. x 195. F and G. Surface resorption repaired with new cementum. x 195. H. Complete autolysis of pulp tissue. x 75.

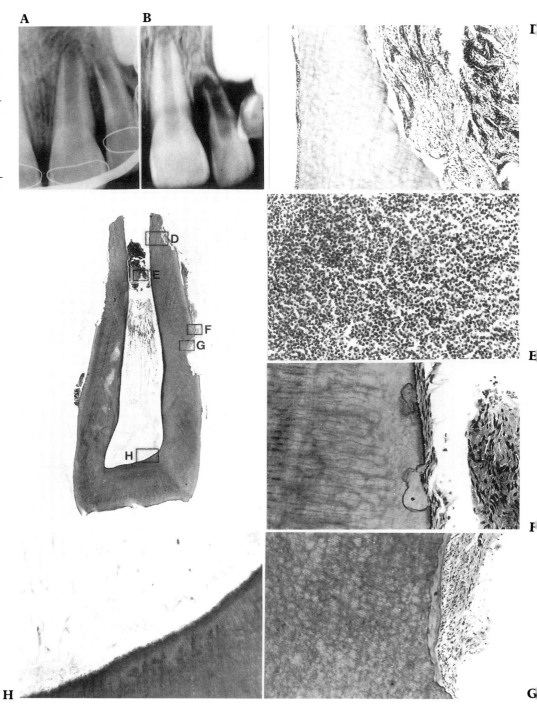

170) (Table 9.8). This reflects a correlation between the degree of injury to the periodontal structures and root resorption (see Chapter 2, p. 95).

The time interval from injury to repositioning of displaced teeth appears to be related to root surface resorption. Thus, teeth treated within 90 minutes after injury show a very low frequency of root resorption compared to teeth treated at a later time (3).

For treatment of external root resorption, see Chapter 14, p. 557.

Root Canal Resorption (Internal Root Resorption)

Root canal resorption is a rather unusual finding (35, 82, 83, 217) and has been recorded in only 2% of re-examined luxated permanent teeth (3). This resorption type is also seen in the primary dentition (144). In the radiographic diagnosis of internal root resorption, one must consider that root surface resorption located labially or lingually on the root can mimic internal

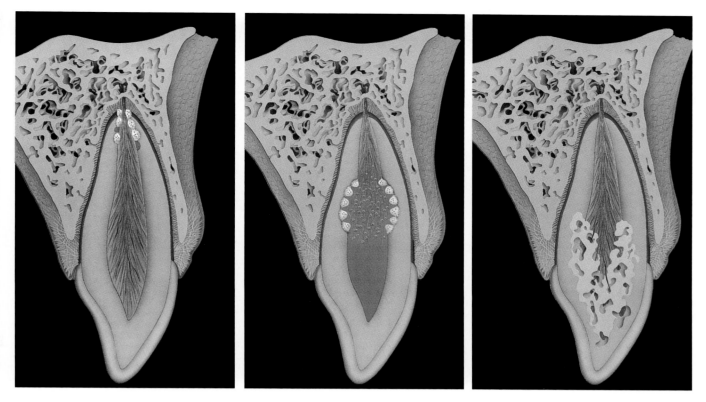

Fig. 9.52. Root canal resorption
Three types of root canal (internal) resorption may develop subsequent to trauma: internal surface resorption, internal inflammatory resorption, and internal ankylosis. After ANDREASEN & ANDREASEN (217) 1992.

resorption as it is superimposed over the root canal (145-147). It is therefore necessary to take supplementary mesial and distal eccentric radiographs of the root. If the resorption cavity does not change position, it is root canal resorption.

Root canal resorption can be classified as follows (Fig. 9.52).

ROOT CANAL REPLACEMENT RESORPTION
This resorption type is characterized

Fig. 9.53.
Internal replacement resorption as a sequel to extrusive luxation. At re-examination 10 years later internal replacement resorption is evident (arrow). From ANDREASEN (3) 1970.

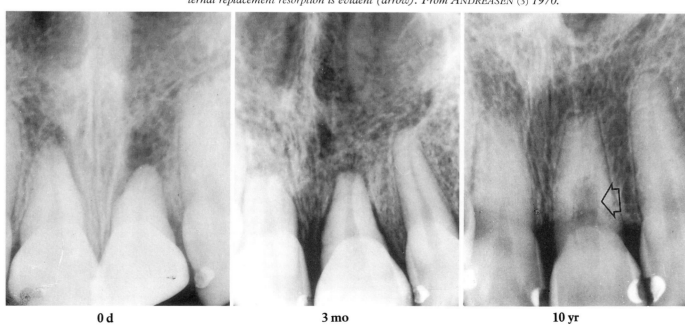

| 0 d | 3 mo | 10 yr |

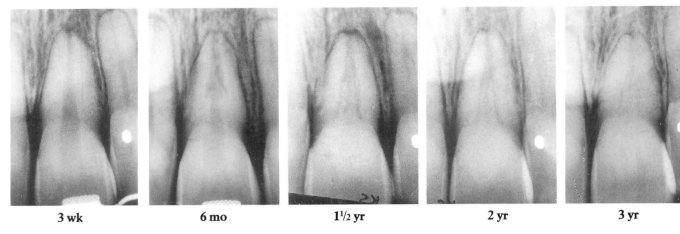

| 3 wk | 6 mo | 1½ yr | 2 yr | 3 yr |

Fig. 9.54.
Internal replacement resorption (tunneling resorption variant) developed in an extruded and repositioned left central incisor. Tunneling resorption is evident after 6 months, but gradually disappears. Courtesy of Dr. B. MALMGREN, Eastman Institute, Stockholm.

radiographically by an irregular enlargement of the pulp chamber (84, 85) (Fig. 9.53). A variant has been termed *internal tunneling resorption*. This resorption is usually found in the coronal fragment of root fractures (234), but may also occur after luxation (Fig. 9.54). The typical feature of this resorption is a tunnelling resorption process next to the root canal. After some time the resorption process becomes arrested and complete pulp canal obliteration takes place.

Histologically, the teeth show metaplasia of the normal pulp tissue into cancellous bone. The continuous rebuilding of bone at the expense of dentin is responsible for the gradual enlargement of the pulp chamber (15, 86).

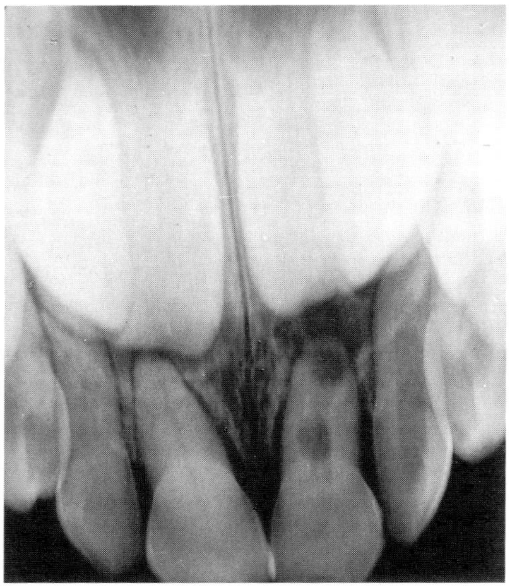

ROOT CANAL INFLAMMATORY RESORPTION

This resorption type is radiographically characterized by an oval-shaped enlargement within the pulp chamber (87-89, 91, 113, 129) (Fig. 9.55). This type of resorption is usually found in the cervical aspect of the pulp. If initial resorption is located in the apical aspect, it is often a sign of active revascularization (internal surface resorption) (166, 193, 234)(see p. 353).

Histologically, a transformation is seen of normal pulp tissue into granulation tissue with giant cells resorbing the dentinal walls of the root canal, advancing from the dentinal surface towards the periphery (Fig. 9.56). A zone of necrotic pulp tissue is usually found coronal to the resorbing tissue. This necrotic zone, or dentinal tubules containing bacteria, are apparently responsible for maintaining the resorptive process.

It should be emphasized that progression of root canal resorption depends upon the interaction between necrotic and vital pulp tissue at their interface. Consequently, root canal treatment should be instituted as soon as possible after root canal resorption has been diagnosed unless the resorption cavity is located in the vicinity of the apical foramen and suspected of being related to pulpal revascularization (see Chapter 14. p. 563).

Fig. 9.55.
Internal inflammatory resorption of primary left central incisor following injury 3 years previously.

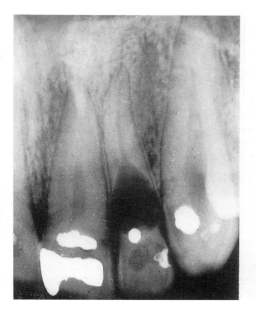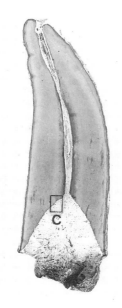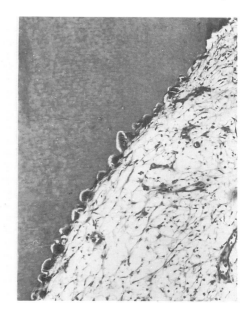

Fig. 9.56.
Internal inflammatory root resorption in a lateral incisor possibly caused by a luxation injury sustained 18 years previously. A. Radiograph showing marked internal inflammatory resorption. B. Histologic section of removed incisor. x 6. C. Active resorption of dentin by multinucleated cells. x 195.

LOSS OF MARGINAL BONE SUPPORT
The post-traumatic course following intrusive or lateral luxation is often complicated by temporary or permanent changes in the marginal periodontium. A frequency of 5-24% was found among luxated permanent teeth (3, 163) (Table 9.9). If broken down according to specific luxation categories, 5% of laterally luxated and 31% of intruded permanent incisors demonstrated this complication (163). It has been found that the repositioning procedure following intrusive luxation plays an important role in periodontal healing. Thus, immediate surgical repositioning (i.e. complete repositioning at the time of injury) of the intruded mature incisors results in significantly greater loss of marginal bone and a higher frequency of ankylosis than orthodontic extrusion.

Loss of marginal support is a common healing complication following lateral luxation. It becomes clinically evident with the appearance of granulation tissue in the gingival crevice and sometimes secretion of pus from the pocket. Probing the pocket reveals a loss of attachment. Radiographically, rarefaction and loss of supporting bone is seen. This clinical situation represents the first part of the healing sequence in a traumatized periodontium, namely the resorption of traumatized bone. After 6-8 weeks, repair of the periodontium takes place with reattachment of new periodontal fibers (Fig. 9.57). If signs of marginal bone loss are evident, the fixation period following lateral luxation may be extended until the situation has resolved.

If there has been injury to the marginal bone, it is essential that optimal oral hygiene be maintained throughout the healing period. If there is secretion of pus, the

Table 9.9. Frequency of loss of marginal bone support after luxation of permanent teeth

Examiner	No. of teeth	No. with loss of marginal bone support
Andreasen & Vestergaard Pedersen (163) 1985	637	34 (5%)
Oikarinen et al. (196) 1987	147	35 (24%)

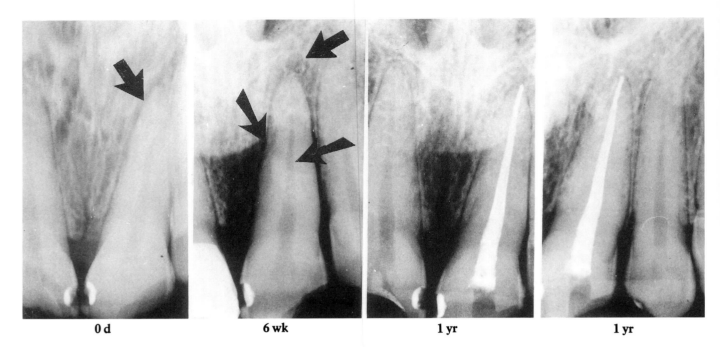

| 0 d | 6 wk | 1 yr | 1 yr |

Fig. 9.57.
Transient destruction of marginal bone around a left central incisor after lateral luxation. Note displacement of the tooth in its socket (arrow). Six weeks later, extensive marginal and apical bone destruction is evident (arrows). Clinically, a pathologic deepening of the gingival crevice of 10 mm is found lingually. At follow-up one year later, marginal bone formation can be seen accompanied by normal pocket depth.

pocket should be rinsed with saline. Moreover, oral rinsing with chlorhexidine should be instituted.

Where sequestration of bone occurs during the healing period, permanent loss of marginal bone can be expected (Fig. 9.58).

Delayed reduction of luxated teeth seems to increase the risk of damage to the supporting structures (3) (Fig. 9.59). Further, it has been found that loss of marginal bone support increases with increasing age of the patient (140, 196) and the duration of the splinting period (196).

Fig. 9.58.
Loss of marginal supporting bone as a result of intrusive luxation. A. Radiograph at the time of injury reveals intrusive luxation of both right incisors. The teeth were repositioned and splinted. B. Three months later a marked loss of supporting marginal bone has occurred. From ANDREASEN (3) 1970.

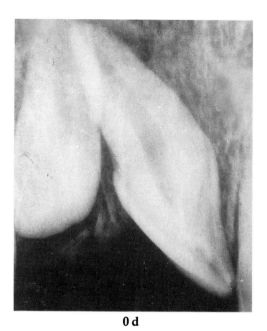 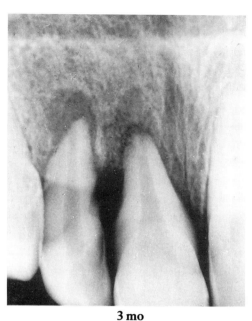

0 d   **3 mo**

Fig. 9.59.
Loss of supporting bone as a result of delayed reduction of an extruded central incisor. A. Condition at time of admission. The tooth had been luxated 7 days previously. B. Two months later a periodontal pocket extends to the apex. A gutta-percha point is inserted in the periodontal pocket lingually.

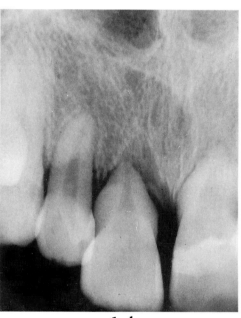 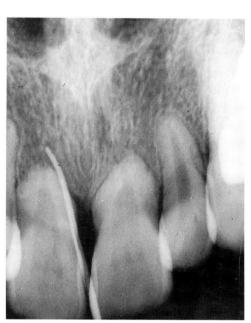

1 wk   **2 mo**

LUXATION INJURIES

Essentials

Terminology (Fig. 9.1)

Concussion
Subluxation (loosening)
Intrusive luxation (central dislocation)
Extrusive luxation (peripheral dislocation, partial avulsion)
Lateral luxation

Frequency

Permanent dentition: 15 to 40% of dental injuries
Primary dentition: 62-69% of dental injuries

Etiology

Fall injuries
Fight injuries

History

Symptoms

Pain with occlusion

Clinical Examination (Table 9.1)

Direction of dislocation
Mobility testing
Response to percussion
Response to vitality tests

Radiographic Examination (Figs. 9.4-9.6)

Several projections necessary

Pathology

PDL changes not known
Pulp changes, depending upon interference with the neurovascular supply (i.e. partial or total ischemia), leading to:
Pulpal healing
Pulpal revascularization
Partial pulp necrosis
Total pulp necrosis

ROOT SURFACE (EXTERNAL) RESORPTION (Fig. 9.47)

Surface resorption
Replacement resorption (ankylosis)
Inflammatory resorption

ROOT CANAL (INTERNAL) RESORPTION (Fig. 9.52)

Internal replacement resorption
Internal inflammatory resorption

Treatment of Permanent Teeth

Concussion and Subluxation

a. Relief of the occlusion upon injured teeth and/or immobilization may be indicated, especially in the case of marked loosening. Otherwise, a soft diet for 14 days
b. Control the tooth radiographically and with sensibility testing
c. Follow-up period: minimum 1 year

Extrusive and Lateral Luxation

a. Administer local anesthesia if forceful repositioning is anticipated
b. Reposition the tooth into normal position (Figs. 9.23-25). In case of delayed treatment, the teeth should be allowed to realign spontaneously into normal position or be moved orthodontically
c. Splint the tooth with an acid-etch/resin splint
d. Control the tooth radiographically
e. Splinting period:
   Extrusion: 2-3 weeks
   Lateral luxation: 3 weeks; in case of marginal bone breakdown, 6-8 weeks
f. Follow-up period: minimum 1 year

Intrusion

a. Repositioning should either be anticipated (i.e. teeth with incomplete root formation) or be carried out orthodontically over a period of 3-4 weeks (Figs. 9.26 and 9.27)
b. Suture gingival lacerations
c. Radiographic controls during the re-eruption phase
d. Follow-up period of 5 years (risk of late healing complications, i.e. root surface resorption)

Prognosis

Pulp Necrosis: 15-59%
   Risk groups: dislocated mature teeth
   Treatment of pulp necrosis: see Chapter 14, p. 543.
Pulp Canal Obliteration: 6-35%
   Risk groups: extremely mobile or dislocated teeth with immature root formation

Root surface resorption: 1-18%
  Risk groups: intrusions
  Treatment of external root resorption:
  see Chapter 14, p. 557.

Root canal resorption: 2%
  Treatment of internal root resorption:
  see Chapter 14, p. 563.

Loss of supporting bone: 10%
  Risk groups: intrusions and lateral
  luxations

Treatment of Primary Teeth

Concussion and Subluxation

  a. Control the tooth clinically and radiographically after 1 and 2 months
  b. Follow-up period: 1 year

Extrusion

  Extraction is usually the treatment of
  choice

Intrusive and Lateral Luxation

a. Intruded and laterally luxated teeth
   should generally be allowed to readjust
   spontaneously. However, if radiographic examination reveals that the
   intruded or laterally luxated tooth has
   been forced into the follicle of the permanent tooth germ, extraction of the
   primary tooth is indicated.
b. Control of the luxated tooth clinically
   and radiographically after 1 and 2
   months.
c. Follow-up period: minimum 1 year

Prognosis

  Pulp necrosis, pulp canal obliteration
  and root resorption occur with frequencies rather similar to luxated permanent teeth.

Bibliography

1. ANDREASEN JO. Etiology and pathogenesis of traumatic dental injuries. A clinical study of 1,298 cases. *Scand J Dent Res* 1970;**78**:329-42.

2. RAVN JJ, ROSSEN I. Hyppighed og fordeling af traumatiske beskadigelser af tænderne hos københavnske skolebørn 1967/68. *Tandlægebladet* 1969;**73**:1-9.

3. ANDREASEN JO. Luxation of permanent teeth due to trauma. A clinical and radiographic follow-up study of 189 injured teeth. *Scand J Dent Res* 1970;**78**:273-86.

4. DOBRZANSKA A, SZPRINGER M. Obserwacje zebow mlecznyck, dotknietych urazem mechanicznym. *Czas Stomatol* 1966;**19**:167-172.

5. SUNDVALL-HAGLAND I. Olycksfallsskador på tänder och parodontium under barnaåren. In: Holst JJ, Nygaard Østby B, Osvald O. *Nordisk Klinisk Odontologi*. Copenhagen: A/S Forlaget for Faglitteratur, 1964:Chapter 11, 1-40.

6. LINK K. Über Veränderungen der Pulpa bei luxierten Zähnen. *Frankfurt Z Pathol* 1957;**68**:596-612.

7. SKIELLER V. The prognosis for young teeth loosened after mechanical injuries. *Acta Odontol Scand* 1960;**18**:171-81.

8. STEWART DJ. Traumatised incisors. An unusual type of response. *Br Dent J* 1960;**108**:396-9.

9. ARWILL T, HENSCHEN B, SUNDVALL-HAGLAND I. The pulpal reaction in traumatized permanent incisors in children aged 9-18. *Odontologisk Tidsskrift* 1967;**75**:130-47.

10. CHIRNSIDE IM. A bacteriological and histological study of traumatised teeth. *N Z Dent J* 1967;**53**:176-91.

11. BLACKWOOD HJJ. Metaplasia or repair of the dental pulp as a response to injury. *Br Dent J* 1957;**102**:87-92.

12. MAIN DMG. Segmentation of teeth. *Br Dent J* 1968;**124**:275-277.

13. PAYNE JL. An unusual case of fracture of a tooth. *Proc Roy Soc Med* 1912;**5**:141-2.

14. TAMMOSCHEIT UG. The two-pieced tooth. *Quintessence Int* 1969;**1**:117-8.

15. ARWILL T. Histopathologic studies of traumatized teeth. *Odontologisk Tidsskrift* 1962;**70**:91-117.

16. BLACKWOOD HJJ. Tissue repair in intra-alveolar root fractures. *Oral Surg Oral Med Oral Pathol* 1959;**12**:360-70.

17. RUSHTON MA. Some late results of injury to teeth. *Br Dent J* 1956;**100**:299-305.

18. MORRIS ME. Pulpal changes in traumatized primary central incisors. *IADR abstracts* 1966;**135**:135.

19. HERBERT WE. Calcification of pulp following trauma. *Br Dent J* 1953;**94**:127-8.

20. PATTERSON SS, MITCHELL DF. Calcific metamorphosis of the dental pulp. *Oral Surg Oral Med Oral Pathol* 1965;**20**:94-101.

21. FISCHER C-H. Die Wurzelkanalbehandlung bei nichtinfiziertem Wurzelkanal. *Dtsch Zahnärztl Z* 1957;**12**:1729-42.

22. HARNDT E. Die körpereigene Hartgewebsausfüllung des Wurzelkanals. *Dtsch Zahnärztl Z* 1960;**15**:392-9.

23. HARNDT E. Milchzahnstudien. II. Zur Pathologie der Milchzahnpulpa. *Dtsch Zahn Mund Kieferheilk* 1948;**11**:97-121.

24. LUND G. Et tilfælde af tanddannelsesforstyrrelse på traumatisk basis. *Tandlægebladet* 1951;**55**:102-14.

25. BUBENIK J. Der Heilungsprocess der verletzten Zahnpulpa nach einem Trauma der Milchzähne. *Dtsch Stomatol* 1966;**16**:159-66.

26. ESCHLER J, SCHILLI W, WITT E. *Die traumatischen Verletzungen der Frontzähne bei Jugendlichen*. 3 ed. Heidelberg: Alfred Hüthig Verlag, 1972.

27. KLOEPPEL J. Diagnosis and treatment of traumatic injuries of the teeth among children. *Int Dent J* 1963;**13**:684-7.

28. TRÄNKMANN J. Zur Prognose zentral luxierter Frontzähne im Wechselgebiss. *Dtsch Zahnärztl Z* 1966;**21**:999-1005.

29. MÜLLER GH, OVERDIEK HF. Das parodontale Trauma beim Jugendlichen. *Dtsch Zahnärztl Z* 1965;**20**:94-105.

30. BRUSZT P. Secondary eruption of teeth intruded into the maxilla by a blow. *Oral Surg Oral Med Oral Pathol* 1958;**11**:146-9.

31. BRUSZT P. L'avenir des dents atteintes de luxation interne au niveau du maxillaire supérieur. Bilan dix ans après le traumatisme. *Actual Odontostomatol* 1967;**78**:139-46.

32. ANDREASEN JO, Ravn JJ. The effect of traumatic injuries to primary teeth on their permanent successors. II. A clinical and radiographic follow-up study of 213 injured teeth. *Scand J Dent Res* 1971;**79**:284-94.

33. SCHREIBER CK. The effect of trauma on the anterior deciduous teeth. *Br Dent J* 1959;**106**:340-3.

34. RAVN JJ. Sequelae of acute mechanical traumata in the primary dentition. *ASDC J Dent Child* 1968;**35**:281-9.

35. GAARE A, HAGEN A, KANSTAD S. Tannfrakturer hos barn. Diagnostiske og prognostiske problemer og behandling. *Norske Tannlegeforenings Tidende* 1958;**68**:364-78.

36. ANDREASEN JO. Fiksation med ortodontisk bånd-akryl skinne. En ny fiksationsmetode til traumatisk løsnede permanente tænder. (Orthodontic band-acrylic splint: a new fixation method for luxated permanent teeth) *Tandlægebladet* 1971;**75**:404-7.

37. SHARGUS G. Experimentelle Untersuchungen über den Halt verschiedener Schienungssysteme. *Dtsch Zahn Mund Kieferheilk* 1969;**53**:378-88.

38. HUMPHREY WP. A simple technique for splinting displaced anterior teeth in children. *ASDC J Dent Child* 1967;**33**:359-62.

39. BURLEY MA, CRABB HSM. Replantation of teeth. *Br Dent J* 1960;**108**:190-3.

40. SMITH DC. A new dental cement. *Br Dent J* 1968;**125**:381-4.

41. HIRSCHFELD L. The use of wire and silk ligatures. *J Am Dent Assoc* 1950;**41**:647-56.

42. RUD J. Provisoriske fiksationer med akryl. *Tandlægebladet* 1965;**69**:385-90.

43. HAMILTON A. A method of arch wiring for displaced anterior teeth. In: Husted E,& Hjørting-Hansen E, eds. *Oral Surgery Transactions, 2nd Congress of the International Association of Oral Surgeons*. Copenhagen: Munksgaard Ltd., 1967:333-5.

44. BEHRMAN SJ. A new method of splinting loose, fractured and evulsed teeth. *N Y State Dent J* 1960;**26**:287-96.

45. LEHNERT S. Zur chirurgischen Therapie traumatisch geschädigter Frontzähne. *Dtsch Zahnärztebl* 1964;**18**:352-8.

46. VAN DE VYVER LM. Traumata van de fronttanden. *Acta Stomatol Belge* 1964;**61**:499-513.

47. TILLMAN HH. A method of stabilizing loosened and displaced anterior teeth. *J Am Dent Assoc* 1962;**65**:378-80.

48. DUCLOS J, FAROUZ R. Fixation des dents réimplantées apres luxations accidentelles. *Rev Stomatol (Paris)* 1947;**48**:434-6.

49. WILBUR HM. Management of injured teeth. *J Am Dent Assoc* 1959;**44**:1-9.

50. SCHUCHARDT K. Ein Vorschlag zur Verbesserung der Drahtschienenverbände. *Dtsch Zahn Mund Kieferheilk* 1956;**24**:39-44.

51. SCHUCHARDT K, KAPOVITS M, SPIESSL B. Technik und Anwendung des Drahtbogenkunststoffverbandes. *Dtsch Zahnärztl Z* 1961;**16**:1241-9.

52. ROTZLER J. Die Fixation von frakturierten oder luxierten Zähnen mit der Drahtkunstharzschiene. *Schweiz Monatschr Zahnheilk* 1962;**72**:162-5.

53. ROTTKE B, SHIMIZU M. Der Draht-Kunststoffschienenverband nach Schuchardt und seine Wirkung auf Gingiva und Periodontium. *Zahnärztl Rdsch* 1966;**75**:451-4.

54. HUGET EF, BRAUER GM, KUMPULA JW, CIVJAN S. A filled cold-curing acrylic resin as a splinting material. *J Am Dent Assoc* 1969;**79**:645-8.

55. EPSTEIN LI. Traumatic injuries to anterior teeth in children. *Oral Surg Oral Med Oral Pathol* 1969;**15**:334-44.

56. PFEIFER G. Freihändige Kunststoffschienung bei Alveolarfortsatzfrakturen und Luxationen im Milchgebiss. *Fortschr Kiefer Gesichtschir* 1959;**5**:328-32.

57. HERING H-J, VON DOMARUS H. Die Biegungsbelastbarkeit von Kieferbruchschienen aus Kunststoffen. *Stoma (Heidelberg)* 1968;**21**:231-6.

58. HOLLMANN K, FISCHER R. Zur Schienung traumatisch gelockerter Zähne. *Österr Z Stomatol* 1965;**62**:452-5.

59. RAVN JJ. Fiksationsskinne i kunststof. En direkte fremstillingsmetode. *Tandlægebladet* 1968;**72**:264-6.

60. FREEDMAN GL, HOOLEY JR. Immobilization of anterior alveolar injuries with cold curing acrylic resins. *J Am Dent Assoc* 1968;**76**:785-6.

61. SEELA W. Eine freihändig anzufertigende, einfache Kappenschiene unter Verwendung selbsthärtender Kunststoffe. *Zahnärztl Rdsch* 1966;**75**:411-3.

62. STEWART DJ. Stabilising appliances for traumatised incisors. *Br Dent J* 1964;**115**:416-8.

63. KATTERBACH R. Eine einfache Methode zur Schienung traumatisch oder infektiös gelockerter Zähne stwie von Alveolarfortsatzfrakturen. *Dtsch Zahnärztebl* 1968;**22**:338-44.

64. MILLER J. IX.-First aid for fractured permanent incisors. *Br Dent J* 1962;**112**:435-7.

65. NORDENRAM Å. Omnivac, en tandteknisk apparat med mångsidig användning. *Sveriges Tandläkaras Förbunds Tidning* 1966;**58**:961-3.

66. TAMMOSCHEIT U-G. Klassifikation und Behandlung unfallverletzter Milchfrontzähne. *Zahnärztl Rdsch* 1967;**76**:190-3.

67. ÖHMAN A. Healing and sensitivity to pain in young replanted human teeth. An experimental, clinical and histological study. *Odontologisk Tidskrift* 1965;**73**:165-228.

68. AUSLANDER WP. Discoloration. A traumatic sequela. *N Y State Dent J* 1967;**33**:534-8.

69. GLUCKSMAN DD. Fractured permanent anterior teeth complicationg orthodontic treatment. *J Am Dent Assoc* 1941;**28**:1941-3.

70. HOTZ R. Die Bedeutung, Beurteilung und Behandlung beim Trauma im Frontzahngebiet vom Standpunkt des Kieferorthopäden. *Dtsch Zahnärztl Z* 1958;**13**:42-51, 401-16.

71. FISH EW. *Surgical pathology of the mouth.* London: Sir Isaac Pitman & Sons Ltd., 1948:123.

72. FORSHUFVUD S. A study of the paracapillary nutrition canals and their possible sympathetic innervation. *Acta Odontol Scand* 1946-7;**7**:1-57.

73. COOKE C, ROWBOTHAM TC. Treatment of injuries to anterior teeth. *Br Dent J* 1951;**91**:146-52.

74. WEISKOPF J, GEHRE G, GRAICHEN K-H. Ein Beitrag zur Behandlung von Luxationen und Wurzelfrakturen im Frontzahngebiet. *Stoma (Heidelberg)* 1961;**14**:100-13.

75. ANEHILL S, LINDAHL B, WALLIN H. Prognosis of traumatised permanent incisors in children. A clinical-roentgenological after-examination. *Svensk Tandläkara Tidskrift* 1969;**62**:367-75.

76. WENZEL H. Ein Beitrag zur Patho-Biologie der Zahnpulpa nach Trauma. *Dtsch Zahn Mund Kieferheilk* 1934;**1**:278-83.

77. SMYTH KC. Obliteration of the pulp of a permanent incisor at the age of 13-9/12 years. *Dent Rec* 1950;**70**:218-9.

78. HOLCOMB JB, GREGORY WB. Calcific metamorphosis of the pulp: Its incidence and treatment. *Oral Surg Oral Med Oral Pathol* 1967;**24**:825-30.

79. LUKS S. Observed effects of traumatic injuries upon anterior teeth. *N Y State Dent J* 1962;**28**:65-70.

80. LANGELAND K. The histopathologic basis in endodontic treatment. *Dent Clin North Am* 1967;491-520.Index 1965-l967. (nov 1967)

81. ANDREASEN JO, HJØRTING-HANSEN E. Replantation of teeth. II. Histological study of 22 replanted anterior teeth in humans. *Acta Odontol Scand* 1966;**24**:287-306.

82. COHEN S. Internal tooth resorption. *ASDC J Dent Child* 1965;**32**:49-52.

83. MENZEL G. Seltene Folgen eines Traumas an 2 Zähnen. *Dtsch Zahnärztl Wochenschr* 1942;**45**:249.

84. ZILKINS K. Beiträge zur traumatischen Zahnschädigung. In: Wannenmacher E. *Ein Querschnitt der deutschen Wissenschaftlichen Zahnheilkunde.* No. 33. Leipzig: Verlag von Hermann Meusser, 1938:43-70.

85. OEHLERS FAC. A case of internal resorption following injury. *Br Dent J* 1951;**90**:13-6.

86. GOLDMAN HM. Spontaneous intermittent resorption of teeth. *J Am Dent Assoc* 1954;**49**:522-32.

87. BRAUER JC, LINDAHL RL. Fractured and displaced anterior teeth. In: Brauer JC, Higley LB, Lindahl RL, Massler M, Schour I. *Dentistry for Children.* 5 ed. New York, Toronto London: McGraw-Hill Book Company, 1964:530-53.

88. HAWES RR. Traumatized primary teeth. *Dent Clin North Am* 1966; 391-404.

89. BERCHER J, PARRET J, FAROUZ R. Les effets des traumatismes sur les pulpes des dents en cours de croissance. *Rev Stomatol (Paris)* 1952;**53**:99-106.

90. PENICK EC. The endodontic management of root resorption. *Oral Surg Oral Med Oral Pathol* 1963;**16**:344-52.

91. LORBER CG. Zur Behandlung bei Kiefergesichtsverletzungen traumatisch geschädigter Zähne unter besonderer Berücksichtigung ihres histologischen Befundes. *Stoma (Heidelberg)* 1968;**21**:25-34.

92. ANDREASEN JO, RAVN JJ. Epidemiology of traumatic dental injuries to primary and permanent teeth in a Danish population sample. *Int J Oral Surg* 1972;**1**:235-9.

93. HEDEGÅRD B, STÅLHANE I. A study of traumatized permanent teeth in children aged 7-15 years. Part I. *Swed Dent J* 1973;**66**:431-50.

94. RAVN JJ. Dental injuries in Copenhagen schoolchildren, school years 1967-1972. *Community Dent Oral Epidemiol* 1974;**2**:231-45.

95. HAAVIKO K, RANTANEN L. A follow-up study of injuries to permanent and primary teeth in children. *Proc Finn Dent Soc* 1976;**72**:152-62.

96. GUZNER N, LUSTMANN J, SHTEYER A. Trauma to primary teeth. *IADR* Abstracts 1978;**58**: abstract no. 469.

97. ROCK WP, GORDON PH, FRIEND LA, GRUNDY MC. The relationship between trauma and pulp death in incisor teeth. *Br Dent J* 1974;**136**:236-9.

98. REICHBORN-KJENNERUD I. Development, etiology and diagnosis of increased tooth mobility and traumatic occlusion. *J Periodontol* 1973;**6**:326-38.

99. LORBER CG. Einige Untersuchungen zur Pathologie unfallgeschädigter Zähne. *Schweiz Monatschr Zahnheilk* 1973;**83**:990-1014.

100. ACETOZE PA, SABBAG Y, RAMALHO AC. Luxaçao dental. Estudo das Alteraçoes Teciduais em Dentes de Crescimento Continuo. *Rev Fac Farm Odont Araraquara* 1970;**4**:125-45.

101. LORBER CG. Röntgenologische und histologische Befunde an traumatisierten Zähnen. *Zahnärztl Welt* 1972;**81**:215-20.

102. STANLEY HR, WEISMAN MI, MICHANOWICZ AE, BELLIZZI R. Ischemic infarction of the pulp: sequential degenerative changes of the pulp after traumatic injury. *J Endod* 1978;**4**:325-35.

103. BARKER BCW, MAYNE JR. Some unusual cases of apexification subsequent to trauma. *Oral Surg Oral Med Oral Pathol* 1975;**39**:144-50.

104. STÅLHANE I, HEDEGÅRD B. Traumatized permanent teeth in children aged 7-15 years. Part II. *Swed Dent J* 1975;**68**:157-169.

105. JACOBSEN I, KEREKES K. Long-term prognosis of traumatized permanent anterior teeth showing calcifying processes in the pulp cavity. *Scand J Dent Res* 1977;**85**:588-98.

106. KÜNZEL W. Die hartgewebige Metaplasie des Zahnmarkes nach akutem Trauma. *Dtsch Stomatol* 1970;**20**:617-24.

107. RAVN JJ. Intrusion af permanente incisiver. *Tandlægebladet* 1975;**79**:643-6.

108. ANDREASEN JO. The influence of traumatic intrusion of primary teeth on their permanent successors. A radiographic and histologic study in monkeys. *Int J Oral Surg* 1976;**5**:207-19.

109. THYLSTRUP A, ANDREASEN JO. The influence of traumatic intrusion of primary teeth on their permanent succesors in monkeys. A macroscopic, polarized light and scanning electron miscroscopic study. *J Oral Pathol* 1977;**6**:296-306.

110. SELLISETH N-E. The significance of traumatised primary incisors on the development and eruption of permanent teeth. *Trans Eur Orthod Soc* 1970;**46**:443-59.

111. IRANPOUR B. Application of enamel adhesives in oral surgery. *Int J Oral Surg* 1974;**3**:223-6.

112. McEVOY SA, MINK JR. Acid-etched resin splint for temporarily stabilizing anterior teeth. *ASDC J Dent Child* 1974;**41**:439-41.

113. KELLY JR, WEBB EE, NEWTON JA. Use of acid-etch resins to splint traumatized anterior teeth. *Dent Surv* 1977;**53**:24-31.

114. KIN PJ. A simple technic for treatment of dental trauma. *Dent Surv* 1977;**53**:40-1.

115. SIMONSEN RJ. Splinting of traumatic injuries using the acid etch system. *Dent Surv* 1977;**53**:26-33.

116. SAYEGH FS, KIM HW, KAZANOGLU A. Pulp reactions to Scutan in monkeys' and dogs' teeth. *AADR* Abstracts B 1977:142.

117. RÖTHLER G, KRENKEL C, RICHTER M. Die Schienung luxierter Zähne mit Hilfe der Schmelzklebetechnik. *Zahnärztl Prax* 1977;**28**:507-8.

118. WIKKELING OE. Luxated teeth: a new way of splinting. *Int J Oral Surg* 1978;**7**:221-3.

119. BERMAN RG, BUCH TM. Utilization of a splint combining bracket-type orthodontic bands and cold-curing resin for stabilization of replaced avulsed teeth: report of case. *ASDC J Dent Child* 1973;**40**:475-8.

120. HOVLAND EJ, GUTMANN JL. Atraumatic stabilization for traumatized teeth. *J Endod* 1976;**2**:390-2.

121. MACKO DJ, KAZMIERSKI MR. Stabilization of traumatized anterior teeth. *ASDC J Dent Child* 1977;**44**:46-8.

122. FISCHER R. Nachuntersuchungen geschienter, traumatisch gelockerter Zähne. *Österr Z Stomatol* 1976;**67**:439-42.

123. TASANEN A. Eräs kappakiskomenatelmä hammasluksaatioiden ja dento-alveolaaristen murtumien hoidossa. *Suomi Hammaslääk Toim* 1971;**67**:199-201.

124. MEGQUIER RJ. Splint technique for dental-alveolar trauma. *J Am Dent Assoc* 1972;**85**:634-6.

125. BIVEN GM, RITCHIE GM, GERSTEIN H. Acrylic splint for intentional replantation. *Oral Surg Oral Med Oral Pathol* 1970;**30**:537-9.

126. SIMPSON TH, HARRINGTON GW, NATKIN E. A splinting method for replantation of teeth in a noncontiguous arch. *Oral Surg Oral Med Oral Pathol* 1974;**38**:104-8.

127. KERNOHAN DC, BEIRNE LR. Conservative treatment of severely displaced permanent incisors: a case report. *Br Dent J* 1971;**131**:111-2.

128. SAUNDERS IDF. Removable appliances in the stabilisation of traumatised anterior teeth - a preliminary report. *Proc Br Paedod Soc* 1972;**2**:19-22.

129. HERFORTH A, MÜNZEL H-J. Zur Frage der Ätiologie intradentärer Resorptionen. *Dtsch Zahnärztl Z* 1974;**29**:971-80.

130. HERFORTH VA. Zur Frage der Pulpavitalität nach Frontzahntrauma bei Jugendlichen - eine Longitudinaluntersuchung. *Dtsch Zahnärztl Z* 1976;**31**:938-46.

131. BARKIN PR. Time as a factor in predicting the vitality of traumatized teeth. *ASDC J Dent Child* 1973;**40**:188-92.

132. SCHRÖDER U, WENNBERG E, GRANATH L-E, MÖLLER H. Traumatized primary incisors-follow-up program based on frequency of periapical osteitis related to tooth color. *Swed Dent J* 1977;**70**:95-8.

133. BERGENHOLZ G. Micro-organisms from necrotic pulp of traumatized teeth. *Odontologisk Revy* 1974;**25**:347-58.

134. CVEK M, NORD C-E, HOLLENDER L. Antimicrobial effect of root canal debridément in teeth with immature root. A clinical and microbiologic study. *Odontologisk Revy* 1976;**27**:1-10.

135. CVEK M, HOLLENDER L, NORD C-E. Treatment of non-vital permanent incisors with calcium hydroxide. VI. A clinical microbiological and radiological evaluation of treatment in one sitting of teeth with mature or immature root. *Odontologisk Revy* 1976;**27**:93-108.

136. EKLUND G, STÅLHANE I, HEDEGÅRD B. A study of traumatized permanent teeth in children aged 7-15 years. Part III. A multivariate analysis of post-traumatic complications of subluxated and luxated teeth. *Swed Dent J* 1976;**69**:179-189.

137. HETZER G, IRMISCH B. Einige Beobachtungen nach Milchzahnintrusionen. *Dtsch Stomatol* 1971;**21**:35-9.

138. VEIGEL W, GARCIA C. Möglichkeiten und Grenzen der Erhaltung traumatisch geschädigter Milchzähne. *Dtsch Zahnärztl Z* 1976;**31**:271-3.

139. ANDREASEN JO, RIIS I. Influence of pulp necrosis and periapical inflammation of primary teeth on their permanent successors. Combined macroscopic and histologic study in monkeys. *Int J Oral Surg* 1978;**7**:178-87.

140. GRÖNDAHL H-G, KAHNBERG K-E, OLSSON G. Traumatiserade tänder. En klinisk och röntgenologisk efterundersökning. *Göteborg Tandläkare Sällskaps Årsbok* 1974;38-50.

141. STÅLHANE I. Permanente tænder med reducerat pulpalumen som följd av olycksfallsskada. *Svensk Tandläkare Tidskrift* 1971;**64**:311-6.

142. FISCHER CH. Hard tissue formation of the pulp in relation to treatment of traumatic injuries. *Int Dent J* 1974;**24**:387-96.

143. JACOBSEN I, SANGNES G. Traumatized primary anterior teeth. Prognosis related to calcific reactions in the pulp cavity. *Acta Odontol Scand* 1978;**36**:199-204.

144. SHARPE MS. Internal resorption in a deciduous incisor: an unusual case. *J Am Dent Assoc* 1970;**81**:947-8.

145. LEPP FH. Progressive internal resorption. *Oral Surg Oral Med Oral Pathol* 1969;**27**:184-5.

146. VINCENTELLI R, LEPP FH, BOUYSSOU M. Les "tàches rosées de la couronne" ("pink spots") - leurs localisations intra- et extra-camérales. *Schweiz Monatschr Zahnheilk* 1973;**83**:1132-50.

147. GARTNER AH, MACK T, SOMMERLOTT RG, WALSH LC. Differential diagnosis of internal and external root resorption. *J Endod* 1976;**2**:329-34.

148. ANDREASEN FM, ANDREASEN JO. Diagnosis of luxation injuries: The importance of standardized clinical, radiographic and photographic techniques in clinical investigations. *Endod Dent Traumatol* 1985;**1**:160-9.

149. HAAVIKKO K, RANTANEN L. A follow-up study of injuries to permanent and primary teeth in children. *Proc Finn Dent Soc* 1976;**72**:152-62.

150. CRONA-LARSSON G, NORÉN JG. Luxation injuries to permanent teeth - a retrospective study of etiological factors. *Endod Dent Traumatol* 1989;**5**:176-9.

151. KENWOOD M, SEOW WK. Sequelae of trauma to the primary dentition. *J Pedodont* 1989;**13**:230-8.

152. VON ARX T. Traumatologie im Milchgebiss (I). Kliniche und therapeutische Aspekte. *Schweiz Monatsschr Zahnmed* 1990;**100**:1195-1204.

153. BIRKEDAL-HANSEN H. External root resorption caused by luxation of rat molars. *Scand J Dent Res* 1973;**81**:47-61.

154. TURLEY PK, JOINER MW, HELLSTROM S. The effect of orthodontic extrusion on traumatically intruded teeth. *Am J Orthod* 1984;**85**:47-56.

155. TZIAFAS D. Pulpal reaction following experimental acute trauma of concussion type on immature dog teeth. *Endod Dent Traumatol* 1988;**4**:27-31.

156. MANDEL U, VIIDIK A. Effect of splinting on the mechanical and histological properties of the healing periodontal ligament in the vervet monkey (cercopithecus aethiops). *Arch Oral Biol* 1989;**34**:209-17.

157. MIYASHIN M, KATO J, TAKAGI Y. Experimental luxation injuries in immature rat teeth. *Endod Dent Traumatol* 1990;**6**:121-8.

158. MIYASHIN M, KATO J, TAKAGI Y. Tissue reations after experimental luxation injuries in immature rat teeth. *Endod Dent Traumatol* 1991;**7**:26-35.

159. CIPRIANO TJ, WALTON RE. The ischemic infarct pulp of traumatized teeth: A light and electron microscopic study. *Endod Dent Traumatol* 1986;**2**:196-204.

160. ANDREASEN FM. Histological and bacteriological study of pulps extirpated after luxation injuries. *Endod Dent Traumatol* 1988;**4**:170-81.

161. OIKARINEN K, ANDREASEN JO. The influence of conventional forceps extraction and extraction with an extrusion instrument on cementoblast damage and root resorption of replanted monkey incisors. 1993. In preparation.

162. ANDREASEN JO, ANDREASEN FM. Immediate histologic periodontal ligament response to traumatic intrusion of incisiors in monkeys. 1993. In preparation.

163. ANDREASEN FM, VESTERGAARD PEDERSEN B. Prognosis of luxated permanent teeth - the development of pulp necrosis. *Endod Dent Traumatol* 1985;**1**:207-20.

164. ANDREASEN FM, YU Z, THOMSEN BL, ANDERSON PK. Occurrence of pulp canal obliteration after luxation injuries in the permanent dention. *Endod Dent Traumatol* 1987;**3**:103-15.

165. ANDREASEN JO, KRISTERSON L, ANDREASEN FM. Damage to the Hertwigs epithelial root sheath: effect upon growth after autotransplantation of teeth in monkeys. *Endod Dent Traumatol* 1988;**4**:145-151.

166. ANDREASEN FM. Transient apical breakdown and its relation to color and sensibility changes after luxation injuries to teeth. *Endod Dent Traumatol* 1986;**2**:9-19.

167. MORLEY KR, BELLIZZI R. Management of subluxative and intrusive injuries to the permanent dentition: a case report. *Ontario Dentist* 1981;**58**:28-31.

168. PEREZ B, BECKER A, CHOSACK A. The repositioning of a traumatically intruded mature, rooted permanent incisor with a removable orthodontic appliance. *J Pedodontics* 1982;**6**:343-54.

169. HELING I. Intrusive luxation of an immature incisor. *J Endod* 1984;**10**:387-90.

170. JACOBSEN I. Long term evalution, prognosis and subsequent management of traumatic tooth injuries. In: Gutmann JL, Harrison JW, eds. *Proceedings of the International Conference on Oral Trauma*. Illinois: American Association of Endodontists Endowment & Memorial Foundation, 1986: 129-38.

171. VINCKIER F, LAMBRECHTS W, DECLERCK D. Intrusion de l'incisive définitive. *Rev Belge Med Dent* 1989;**44**:99-106.

172. KINIRONS MJ, SUTCLIFFE J. Traumatically intruded permanent incisors: a study of treatment and outcome. *Br Dent J* 1991;**170**:144-6.

173. SHAPIRA J, REGEV L, LIEBFELD H. Re-eruption of completely intruded immature permanent incisors. *Endod Dent Traumatol* 1986;**2**:113-6.

174. TRONSTAD L, TROPE M, BANK M, BARNETT F. Surgical access for endodontic treatment of intruded teeth. *Endod Dent Traumatol* 1986;**2**:75-8.

175. BELOSTOKY L, SCHWARTZ Z, SOSKOLNE WA. Undiagnosed intrusion of a maxillary primary incisor tooth: 15-year follow-up. *Pediatric Dent* 1986;**8**:294-6.

176. NIELSEN LA, RAVN JJ. Intrusion af primære tænder: et kasuistisk bidrag. *Tandlægebladet* 1989;**93**:441-4.

177. KRISTERSON L, ANDREASEN JO. The effect of splinting upon periodontal and pulpal healing after autotransplantation of mature and immature permanent incisors i monkeys. *Int J Oral Surg* 1983;**12**:239-49.

178. ROCK WP, GRUNDY MC. The effect of luxation and subluxation upon the prognosis of traumatized incisor teeth. *J Dent* 1981;**9**:224-30.

179. OIKARINEN K. Comparison of the flexibility of various splinting methods for tooth fixation. *J Oral Maxillofac Surg* 1988;**17**:125-7.

180. OIKARINEN K. Tooth splinting: a review of the literature and consideration of the versatility of a wire-composite splint. *Endod Dent Traumatol* 1990;**6**:237-50.

181. OIKARINEN K, ANDREASEN JO, ANDREASEN FM. Rigidity of various fixation methods used as dental splints. *Endod Dent Traumatol* 1992; **8**:113-9.

182. KRENKEL C, RICHTER M, RÖTHLER G. Die Silcadraht-Klebeschiene - eine neue Methode zur Behandlung luxierter Zähne. *Dtsch Zahnärzztl Z* 1979;**34**:280-2.

183. BELL O, STØRMER K, ZACHRISSON BU. Ny metode for fiksering av traumatiserte tenner. *Norske Tannlegeforenings Tidende* 1984;**94**:49-55.

184. LOWNIE JF, REA MA. Splinting a traumatically avulsed tooth. *J Dent* 1980;**8**:260-2.

185. WEISMAN MI. Tooth out! Tooth in! Simplified Splinting. *CDS Review* 1984:30-7.

186. HAGEN M, FRITZEMEIER CU. Unterschiedliche Schienungstechniken und deren Indikation zur chirurgischen Zahnerhaltung. *Dtsch Zahnärztl Z* 1987;**42**:194-7.

187. OIKARINEN K. Functional fixation for traumatically luxated teeth. *Endod Dent Traumatol* 1987;**3**:224-8.

188. ANTRIM DD, OSTROWSKI JS. A functional splint for traumatized teeth. *J Endod* 1982;**8**:328-32.

189. NORDENVALL K-J. Fixering av traumaskada. *Tandläkartidningen* 1991;**83**:770-1.

190. ANDERSSON L, FRISKOP J, BLOMLÖF L. Fiber-glass splinting of traumatized teeth. *ASDC J Dent Child* 1983;**50**:21-4.

191. FLEISCH L, CLEATON-Jones P, FORBES M, van Wyk J, FAT C. Pulpal response to a bis-acryl-plastic (Protemp) temporary crown and bridge material. *J Oral Pathol* 1984;**13**:622-31.

192. POLSON AM, BILLEN JR. Temporary splinting of teeth using ultraviolet light-polymerized bonding materials. *J Am Dent Assoc* 1974;**89**:1137-9.

193. ANDREASEN FM. Pulpal healing after luxation injuries and root fracture in the permanent dentition. *Endod Dent Traumatol* 1989;**5**:111-31.

194. ANDREASEN FM, ANDREASEN JO, BAYER T. Prognosis of root-fractured permanent incisors - prediction of healing modalities. *Endod Dent Traumatol* 1989;**5**:11-22.

195. BUCHHORN I. *Følger efter behandling af palatinalt retinerede hjørnetænder. En efterundersøgelse.* Thesis: Royal Dental College, Copenhagen 1985.

196. OIKARINEN K, GUNDLACH KKH, PFEIFER G. Late complications of luxation injuries to teeth. *Endod Dent Traumatol* 1987;**3**:296-303.

197. HERFORTH A. Wurzelfrakturen und Luxationen von Zähnen - III. Teil. *ZWR* 1990;**99**:784-91.

198. ANDREASEN FM, YU Z, THOMSEN BL. Relationship between pulp dimensions and development of pulp necrosis after luxation injuries in the permanent dentition. *Endod Dent Traumatol* 1986;**2**:90-8.

199. MAGNUSSON B, HOLM A-K. Traumatised permanent teeth in children - a follow-up. I. Pulpal considerations and root resorption. *Svensk Tandläk Tid* 1969;**62**:61-70.

200. BHASKAR SN, RAPPAPORT HM. Dental vitality tests and pulp status. *J Am Dent Assoc* 1973;**86**:409-11.

201. JACOBSEN I. Criteria for diagnosis of pulp necrosis in traumatized permanent incisors. *Scand J Dent Res* 1980;**88**:306-12.

202. ZADIK D, CHOSAK A, EIDELMAN E. The prognosis of traumatized permanent anterior teeth with fracture of the enamel and dentin. *Oral Surg Oral Med Oral Pathol* 1979;**47**:173-5.

203. GAZELIUS B, OLGART L, EDWALL B, EDWALL L. Non-invasive recording of blood flow in human dental pulp. *Endod Dent Traumatol* 1986;**2**:219-22.

204. GAZELIUS B, OLGART L, EDWALL B. Restored vitality in luxated teeth assessed by laser Doppler flowmeter. *Endod Dent Traumatol* 1988;**4**:265-8.

205. EDWALL B, GAZELIUS B, BERG JO, EDWALL L, HELLANDER K, OLGART L. Blood flow changes in the dental pulp of the cat and rat measured simultaneously by laser Doppler flowmetry and local I clearance. *Acta Physiol Scand* 1987;**131**:81-92.

206. OLGART L, GAZELIUS B, LINDH-STRÖMBERG U. Laser Doppler flowmetry in assessing vitality in luxated permanent teeth. *Int Endod J* 1988;**21**:300-6.

207. WILDER-SMITH PEEB. A new method for the non-invasive measurement of pulpal blood flow. *Int Endod J* 1988;**21**:307-12.

208. CONVERSE JM, RAPAPORT FT. The vascularization of skin autografts and homografts; experimental study in man. *Ann Surg* 1956;**143**:306-15.

209. CLEMMESEN T. The early circulation in split skin grafts. *Acta Chir Scand* 1962;**124**:11-8.

210. MARCKMANN A. Autologous skin grafts in the rat. Vital microscopic studies of microcirculation. *Angiology* 1966;**17**:475-82.

211. HALLER JA, BILLINGHAM RE. Studies of the origin of the vasculature in free skin grafts. *Ann Surg* 1967;**166**:896-901.

212. CLEMMESEN T. Experimental studies on the healing of free skin autografts. *Ugeskr Læger* 1967;14(Suppl II):1-74.

213. HINSHAW JR, MILLER ER. Histology of healing split-thickness, full-thickness autogenous skin grafts and donor sites. *Arch Surg* 1965;**91**:658-70.

214. ZAREM HA, ZWEIFACH BW, MCGEHEE JM. Development of microcirculation in full thickness autogenous skin grafts in mice. *Am J Physiol* 1967;**212**:1081-5.

215. SOXMAN JA, NAZIF MM, BOUGUOT J. Pulpal pathology in relation to discoloration of primary anterior teeth. *ASDC J Dent Child* 1984;**51**:282-4.

216. CROLL TP, PASCON EA, LANGELAND K. Traumatically injured primary incisors: a clinical and histological study. *ASDC J Dent Child* 1987;**54**:401-22.

217. ANDREASEN JO, ANDREASEN FM. Root resorption following traumatic dental injuries. *Proc Finn Dent Soc* 1991;**88**:95-114.

218. KEREKES K, JACOBSEN I. Follow-up examination of endodontic treatment in traumatized juvenil incisors. *J Endod* 1980;**6**:744-8.

219. ANDREASEN JO. External root resorption: its implication in dental traumatology, paedodontics, periodontics, orthodontics and endodontics. *Int Endod J* 1985;**18**:109-18.

220. SONIS AL. Longitudinal study af discolored primary teeth and effect on succedaneous teeth. *J Pedodont* 1987;**11**:247-52.

221. COLL JA, JOSELL S, NASSOF S, SHELTON P, RICHARDS MA. An evaluation of pulpal therapy in primary incisors. *Pediatr Dent* 1988;**10**:178-84.

222. FLAITZ CM, BARR ES, HICKS MJ. Radiograhic evaluation of pulpal treatment for anterior primary teeth in a pediatric dentistry practice. *Pediatr Dent* 1987;**9**:171-2.

223. PRUHS RJ, OLEN GA, SHARMA PS. Relationship between formocresol pulpotomies on primary teeth and enamel defects on their permanent successors. *J Am Dent Assoc* 1977;**94**:698-700.

224. HOLAN G, TOPF J, FUKS AB. Effect of root canal infection and treatment of traumatized primary incisors on their permanent successors. *Endod Dent Traumatol* 1992;**8**:12-5.

225. LAWNIK D, TETSCH P. Spätfolgen nach Frontzahnverletzungen - Ergebnisse einer Nachuntersuchung. *Dtsch Zhnärztl Z* 1983;**38**:476-7.

226. POSUKIDIS T, LEHMANN W. Die Prognose des traumatisierten Zahnes. *Dtsch Zahnärztl Z* 1983;**38**:478-9.

227. RAVN JJ. Dental traume epidemiologi i Danmark: en oversigt med enkelte nye oplysninger. *Tandlægebladet* 1989;**93**:393-6.

228. WEPNER F, BUKEL J. Problematik und Therapie der traumatischen Zahnluxation im Kindesalter. *Quintessenz* 1981;**32**:1541-7.

229. SMITH JW. Calcific metamorphosis: a treatment dilemma. *Oral Surg Oral Med Oral Pathol* 1982;**54**:441-4.

230. RAVN JJ. Obliteration af tænder. En litteraturoversigt. *Tandlægebladet* 1982;**86**:183-7.

231. STRONER WF. Pulpal dystrophic calcification. *J Endod* 1984;**10**:202-4.

232. SCHINDLER WG, GULLICKSON DC. Rationale for the management of calcific metamorphosis secondary to traumatic injuries. *J Endod* 1988;**14**:408-12.

233. MOULE AJ, THOMAS RP. Cervical external root resorption following trauma - a case report. *Int Endod J* 1985;**18**:277-81.

234. ANDREASEN FM, ANDREASEN JO. Resorption and mineralization processes following root fracture of permanent incisors. *Endod Dent Traumatol* 1988;**4**:202-14.

235. WALL WH. Universal polycarbonate fracture splint and its direct bonding potential. *Int J Oral Maxillofac Surg* 1986;**15**:418-21.

Avulsions

J. O. ANDREASEN & F. M. ANDREASEN

Terminology, Frequency and Etiology

Tooth avulsion (exarticulation) implies total displacement of the tooth out of its socket.

Various statistics have shown that exarticulation of teeth following traumatic injuries is relatively infrequent, ranging from 0.5 to 16% of traumatic injuries in the permanent dentition (1-5, 125, 126) and from 7 to 13% in the primary dentition (1, 3).

The main etiologic factors in the *permanent* dentition are fights and sports injuries (1, 127), while falls against hard objects are a frequent cause in the *primary* dentition (1).

Clinical Findings

In both the primary and permanent dentitions, the maxillary central incisors are the most frequently avulsed teeth, while the lower jaw is seldom affected (6-8, 128, 129, 199-203).

Avulsion of teeth occurs most often in children from 7 to 9 years of age, when the permanent incisors are erupting (6-8, 199-203). At this age, the loosely structured periodontal ligament surrounding erupting teeth provides only minimal resistance to an extrusive force.

Most frequently, avulsion involves a single tooth; but multiple avulsions are occasionally encountered (6-8, 199-202). Other types of injuries are often associated with avulsions; among these, fractures of the alveolar socket wall and injuries to the lips are the most common (1).

Radiographic Findings

Radiographs should be taken if the clinical examination arouses suspicion of bone fracture (Fig. 10.1). In the primary dentition, radiographs will often reveal that a

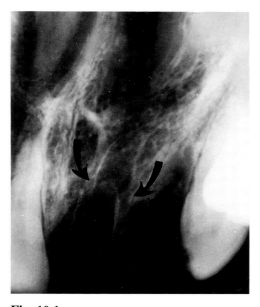

Fig. 10.1.
Radiograph illustrating an alveolar fracture (arrows) following avulsion of both central incisors.

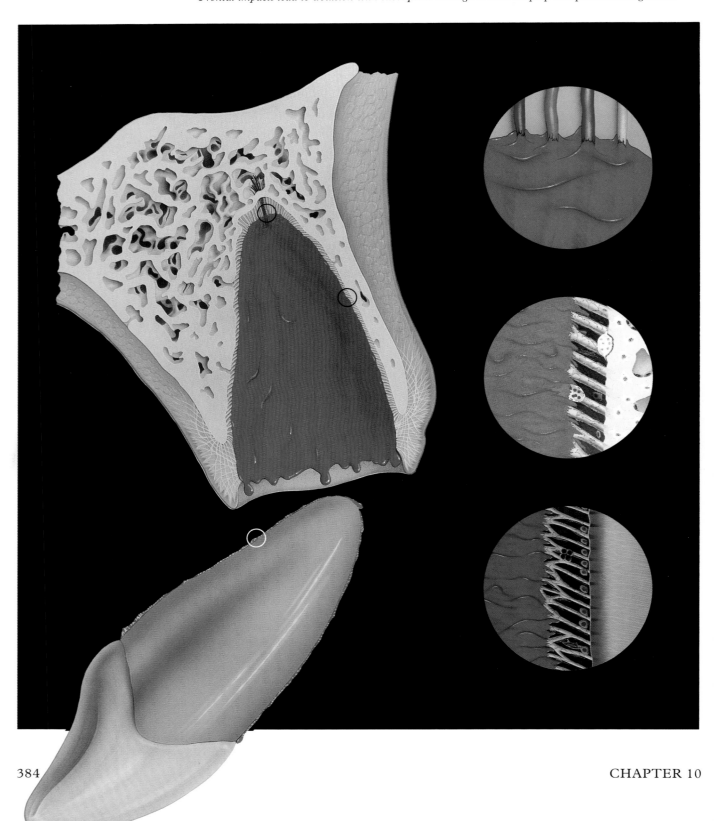

suspected avulsion is actually an intrusion, where the primary tooth is buried in the jaw.

Pathology

The pathology of *tooth replantation* can be divided into pulpal and periodontal reactions. Both the pulp and the periodontal ligament suffer extensive damage during an extra-alveolar period with healing reactions almost entirely dependent upon the extra-alveolar period and extra-alveolar handling (Fig. 10.2).

The healing reactions after replantation of teeth have been the subject of numerous experiments using mice (35), hamsters (36-42), rats (167-169), guinea pigs (170), rabbits (27), cats (204-208), dogs (9-29, 130-137, 209-212) and monkeys (17, 24, 31-34, 138-166, 213-226).

Pulpal Reactions

Studies on *pulp reactions* have mainly been performed in *animals* such as cats (204, 205), dogs (136, 137, 209-212) and monkeys (225, 226). Experimental studies have disclosed various distinct pulpo-dentinal responses which can occur after immediate replan-

tation and have been classified as follows (29) (Fig. 10.3):

I. Regular tubular reparative dentin.
II. Irregular reparative dentin with diminished tubular structures.
III. Irregular reparative dentin with encapsulated cells (osteodentin).
IV. Irregular immature bone.
V. Regular lamellated bone or cementum.
VI Internal resorption.
VII Pulp necrosis.

It is uncertain whether all of these reactions are encountered in humans; however, pulpal reactions observed in human patients after luxation injuries seem to support at least part of this classification (see Chapter 9, p. 323).

Several comprehensive studies of pulp reactions of extracted and immediately replanted permanent premolars in *human* patients have been published (43, 227-229). Extensive pulpal changes could be observed as early as 3 days after replantation. The most severe damage was usually observed in the coronal part of the pulp. Signs of healing were seen within 2 weeks after replantation. Damaged coronal pulp

Fig. 10.3.
Schematic drawing illustrating the various pulp reactions following experimental replantation of incisors in dogs. From ANDERSON, SHARAV & MASSLER (29) 1968.

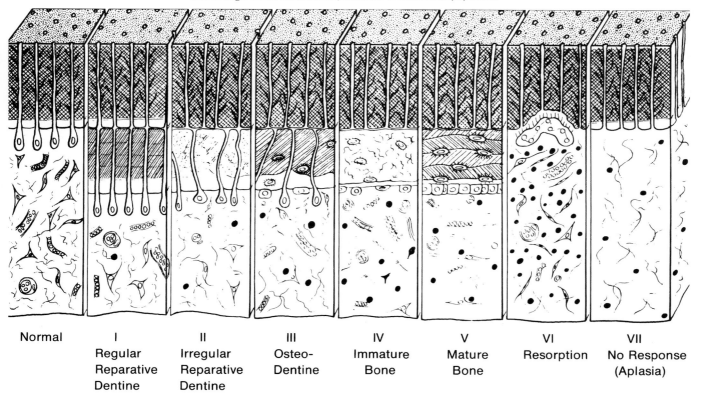

Normal	I	II	III	IV	V	VI	VII
	Regular Reparative Dentine	Irregular Reparative Dentine	Osteo-Dentine	Immature Bone	Mature Bone	Resorption	No Response (Aplasia)

Fig. 10.4.
A. Diagram illustrating initial pulp changes after replantation. N = necrotic pulp tissue, M = mesenchymal cells, H = healing zone, P = preserved vital pulp tissue. B. Proliferating mesenchymal cells along the root canal wall at the level of necrotic and vital pulp tissue 10 days after replantation. x 410. C. Karyorrhexis and pyknosis in the coronal part of the pulp 3 days after replantation. x 200. From ÖHMAN (43) 1965.

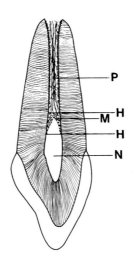

A

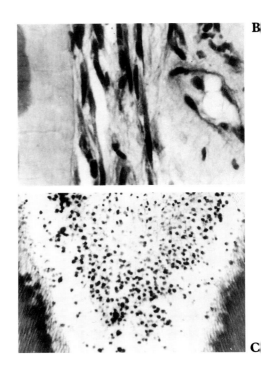

B

C

tissue was gradually replaced by proliferating mesenchymal cells and capillaries (Figs. 10.4 and 10.5). In the border zone between vital and necrotic tissue, neutrophils and round cells were present in some cases.

In the majority of cases with long observation periods, more advanced healing was found. This healing process led to the formation of a new cell layer along the dentinal wall in regions where the odonto-

blasts had been destroyed. The mesenchymal cells along the dentinal wall usually did not have processes extending into the dentinal tubules (Fig. 10.5, B). New hard tissue formation along the dentinal walls was noted after 17 days; but in most cases matrix formation started somewhat later. In the early stages of healing, a tissue was formed without dentinal tubules but with occasional cell inclusions (Fig. 10.6). Gradually, the cells along the pulp walls

Fig. 10.5. A.
Diagram illustrating late pulp changes after replantation. New mesenchymal cells proliferate into the injured zones during the first months of the healing period. R = regenerated pulp tissue, P = preserved vital pulp tissue. B. The cells adjacent to the predentin in the apical part of the pulp appear to send no processes into the dentinal tubules (observation period = 17 days). x 430. C. Regenerated pulp cells are aligned nearly parallel with the long axis of the tooth. x 520. From ÖHMAN (43) 1965.

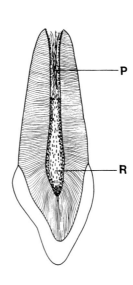

A

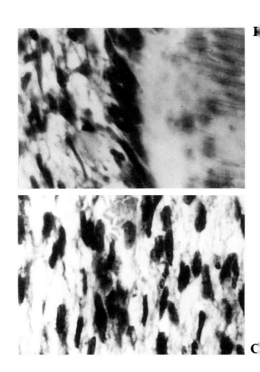

B

C

Fig. 10.6.
A. Diagram illustrating late pulp changes after replantation. Extensive obliteration of the pulp chamber with hard tissue and strands of vital pulp tissue extending into the hard tissue. V = vital regenerated pulp tissue, T = newly formed hard tissue, P = preserved vital pulp tissue. B. Two phases of repair. First, irregular atubular matrix (arrows), second atubular dentin (observation period = 101 days). x 180. C. Irregular new hard tissue formation in an area with severe pulp damage (observation period = 158 days). x 125. D. Nerve fibers coursing through newly-formed hard tissue in the pulp chamber (observation period = 360 days). Palmgren's silver stain. x 275. E. Nerve fibers with mitosis of Schwann cells (arrow) (observation period = 14 days). x 450. From ÖHMANN (43) 1965.

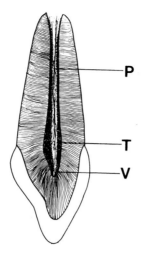

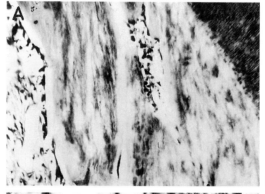

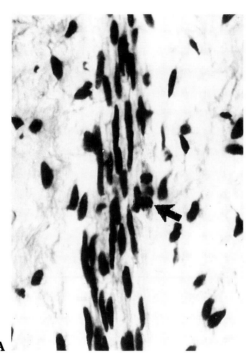

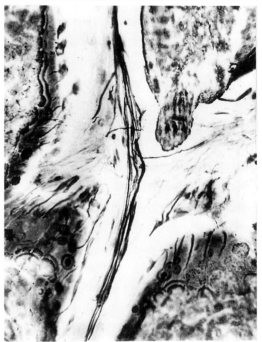

began to show similarities to odontoblasts with cytoplasmic processes within the newly formed matrix. This apparently corresponded to the degree of differentiation; however, in areas where new hard tissue formation indicated total primary destruction of the original odontoblasts, completely normal conditions were never found.

Severe primary pulpal damage was more often found in teeth with completed root formation than in those with an open apex, where the pulpal repair seemed also to be more rapid. Mitoses were seen in bands of Schwann cells 14 days after replantation (Fig. 10.6, E). Regenerating nerve fibers were observed after 1 month. In teeth with irregular hard tissue formation in the pulp

Fig. 10.7.

Healing sequence in the periodontal structures following experimental tooth replantations in dogs. A. Condition immediately after replantation. The line of separation is situated in the middle of the periodontal ligament. x 75. B. Three days later proliferating connective tissue cells invade the coagulum of the severed periodontal ligament. x 75. C. Two weeks later new collagenous fibers have bridged the periodontal space. x 75. D. Normal periodontal conditions 8 months after replantation. x 75.

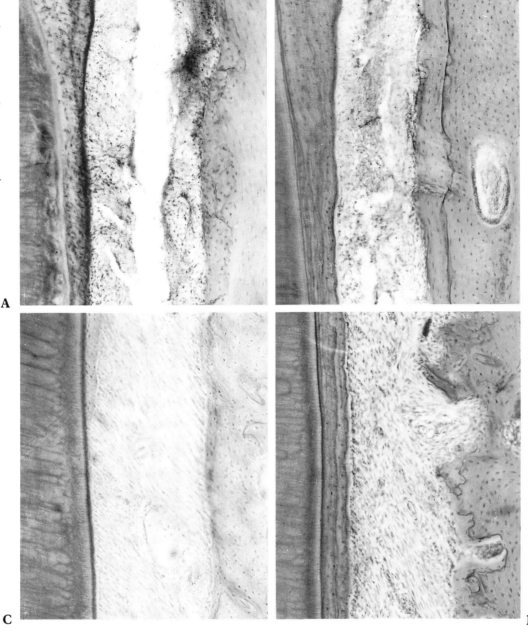

chamber, bundles of nerve fibers passed between the trabeculae of hard tissue; separate fibers could be followed to the newly formed layer of irregular odontoblasts. However, neither the number nor the caliber of the nerve fibers reached normal levels. In microangiographic studies of the revascularization process after replantation of teeth in dogs, it was demonstrated that ingrowth of new vessels could be seen 4 days after replantation. After 10 days, vessels were seen in the apical half of the pulp and, after 30 days, in the entire pulp (136, 137).

Periodontal Healing Reactions

The following healing sequence in the periodontal structures has been demonstrated after experimental immediate replantation in dogs (24), monkeys (138, 162), and humans (230).

Immediately after replantation, a coagulum is found between the two parts of the severed periodontal ligament (Fig. 10.7, A). The line of separation is most often situated in the middle of the periodontal ligament, although separation can occur at the insertion of Sharpey's fibers into cementum or alveolar bone. Proliferation of connective tissue cells soon occurs and, after 3 to 4 days, the gap in the periodontal ligament is obliterated by young connective tissue (Fig. 10.7, B). After 1 week, the epithelium is reattached at the cemento-enamel junction (138). This is of clinical

Fig. 10.8.
Healing with a normal periodontal ligament following replantation of a left lateral incisor. A. Apex removed 31/2 months after replantation. B. Normal periodontal ligament and cementum. x 12 and x 195. From AN-DREASEN & HJØRTING-HANSEN (44) 1966.

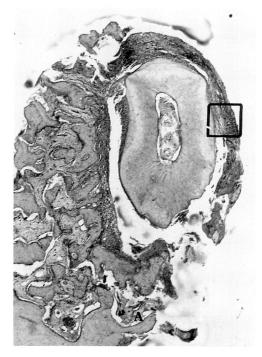

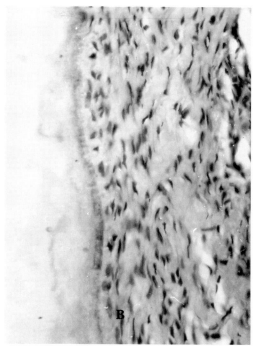

importance because it may imply a reduced risk of gingival infection and/or reduced risk of bacterial invasion of either the root canal or periodontal ligament via the gingival pocket. Gingival collagen fibers are usually spliced, while the infrabony fibers are united in only a few areas at this time (138). The first superficial osteoclast attack can now be seen along the root surface (140).

After 2 weeks, the split line in the periodontal ligament is healed and collagen fibers are seen extending from the cemental surface to the alveolar bone (Fig. 10.7, C). Resorption activity can now be recognized along the root surface (140).

Histologic examination of replanted human and animal teeth has revealed four different healing modalities in the periodontal ligament (44, 45, 147, 221, 222, 231, 232).

1. HEALING WITH A NORMAL PERIODONTAL LIGAMENT
Histologically, this is characterized by complete regeneration of the periodontal ligament (10, 24, 36, 44, 47, 48), which usually takes about 2 - 4 weeks to complete (233) (Fig. 10.8). This type of healing will only occur if the innermost cell layers along the root surface are vital (142, 215).

Radiographically, there is a normal periodontal ligament space without signs of root resorption (Fig. 10.9).

Clinically, the tooth is in a normal position and a normal percussion tone can be elicited.

Fig. 10.9.
Periodontal ligament healing after replantation of right central incisor. From ANDREASEN ET AL. (203) 1993.

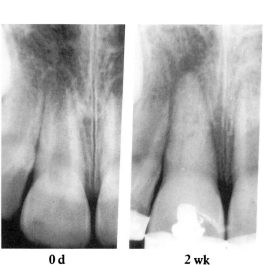

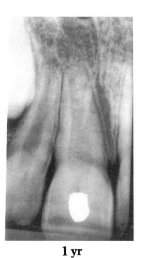

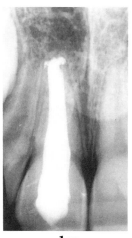

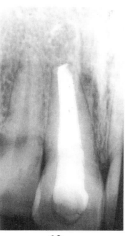

| 0 d | 2 wk | 1 yr | 1 yr | 10 yr |

Fig. 10.10.
Healing with a normal periodontal ligament and marked surface resorption after replantation of a left central incisor. Extra-alveolar period 95 minutes. A. Immediately after replantation. B. Five months later. Surface resorption of the root is evident (arrows). C. and D. Condition 2 and 4 years later. No progression of surface resorption has occurred whereas the pulp canal has become obliterated. For orthodontic reasons the tooth was later extracted. E. Low-power view of sectioned incisor. x 4. F. Large surface resorption defect repaired with new cementum (arrows). The periodontal ligament is normally structured. x 75. G. Area without surface resorption. x 75. H. Minor surface resorption areas repaired with cementum. x 75. I. Bone formation in the central part of the pulp. An internal periodontal ligament connects this structure with the hard tissue deposited on the canal walls. x 75.

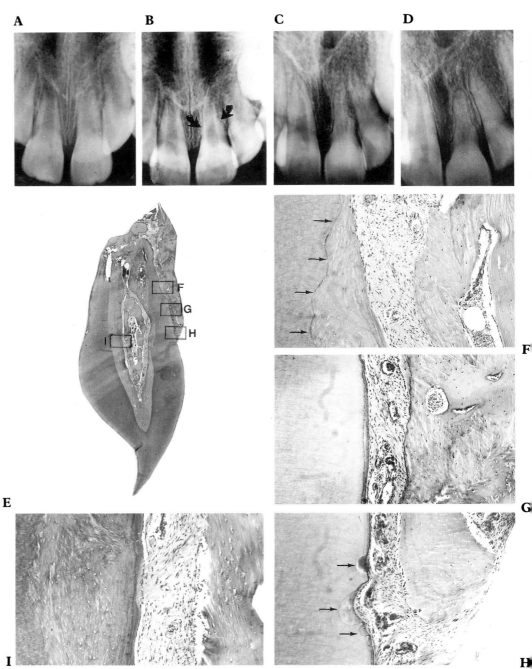

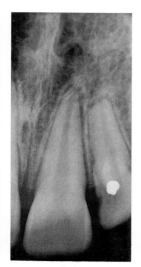
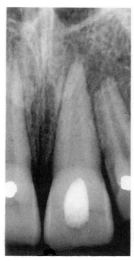
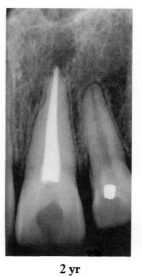
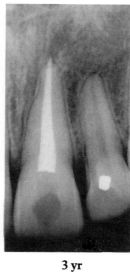
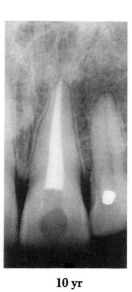

0 d   1 wk   2 yr   3 yr   10 yr

Fig. 10.11.
Surface resorption (arrow) of a replanted right central incisor. Note the superficial appearance on the root and sparse involvement on the lamina dura. The resorption cavity is stationary during the entire observation period. From ANDREASEN ET AL. (202) 1993.

This type of healing will probably never take place under clinical conditions (i.e. after tooth avulsion), as trauma will result in at least minimal injury to the innermost layer of the periodontal ligament, leading to surface resorption. (see Chapter 2, p. 100)

2. HEALING WITH SURFACE RESORPTION

Histologically, this type of healing is characterized by localized areas along the root surface which show superficial resorption lacunae repaired by new cementum. This condition has been termed *surface resorption*, presumably representing localized areas of damage to the periodontal ligament or cementum which have been healed by periodontal ligament-derived cells (44, 140, 142, 146, 222, 231). In contrast to other types of resorption, surface resorption is self-limiting and shows repair with new cementum (Fig. 10.10). Most resorption lacunae are superficial and confined to the cementum. In cases of deeper resorption cavities, however, healing occurs, but without restoration of the original outline of the root. It should be noted that resorption lacunae with similar morphology and location have been reported on

non-traumatized root surfaces with a frequency as high as 90% of all teeth examined (49).

Due to their small size, surface resorptions are usually not disclosed *radiographically*. However, with ideal angulation of the central beam it is sometimes possible to recognize small excavations of the root surface with an adjacent periodontal ligament space of normal width (Fig. 10.11) .

Clinically, the tooth is in a normal position and a normal percussion tone can be elicited.

3. HEALING WITH ANKYLOSIS (REPLACEMENT RESORPTION)

Histologically, ankylosis represents a fusion of the alveolar bone and the root surface and can be demonstrated 2 weeks after replantation (138). The etiology of replacement resorption appears to be related to the absence of a vital periodontal ligament cover on the root surface (141-143, 216, 221, 231, 234). Replacement resorption develops in two different directions, depending upon the extent of damage to the periodontal ligament cover of the root: either *progressive replacement resorption*, which gradually resorbs the entire root, or *transient replacement resorption*, in which a

Fig. 10.12.
Permanent replacement resorption. Mobility values indicated that an ankylosis was established 4 weeks after replantation. Replacement resorption was first radiographically demonstrable 6 weeks after replantation (arrow). From ANDREASEN (171) 1975.

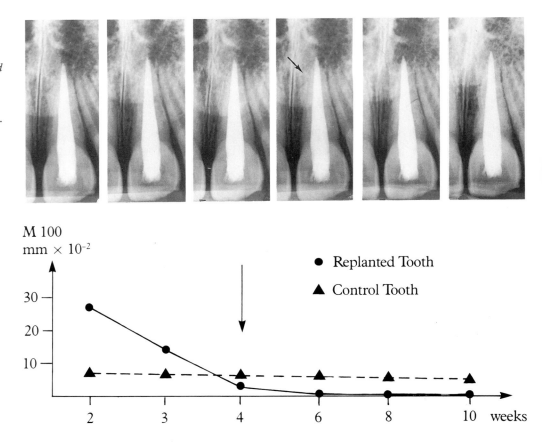

Fig. 10.13.
Transient replacement resorption. Mobility testing indicated an ankylosis 16 weeks after replantation. Ankylosis also demonstrable radiographically (arrow). A normal periodontal space was restored at later controls. From AN-DREASEN (171) 1975.

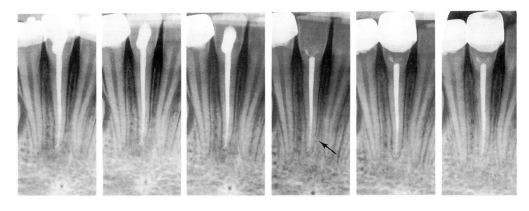

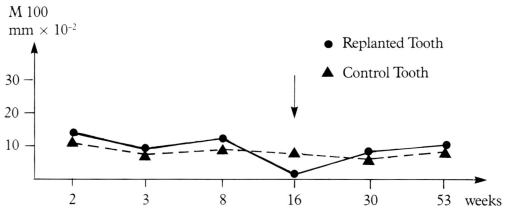

Fig. 10.14.
Ankylosis (replacement resorp-tion) after replantation of a right central incisor. A. Radiograph taken immediately after replanta-tion. B. Condition at the time of extraction 2 years after injury. C. Low-power view of sectioned incisor. x 5. D. Bony union be-tween root surface and surround-ing alveolar bone. Note resorp-tion lacunae with osteoclasts. x 75. E. and F. Replacement re-sorption with apposition of bone and active resorption (arrows). x 75. G. Surface resorption re-paired with cellular cementum. x 195. H. Area with normal perio-dontal ligament. x 195. From ANDREASEN & HJØRTING-HAN-SEN (44) *1966.*

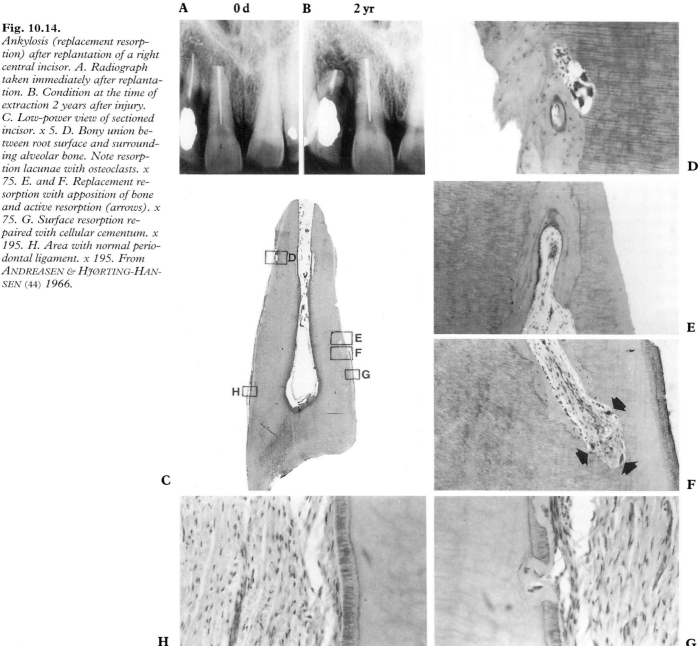

once-established ankylosis later disap-pears (144,171) (Figs. 10.12 and 10.13).

Progressive ankylosis is always elicited when the entire periodontal ligament is removed before replantation (143) or after extensive drying of the tooth before re-plantation (143, 146). It is assumed that the damaged periodontal ligament is repopu-lated from adjacent bone marrow cells, which have osteogenic potential and will consequently form an ankylosis (172). *Transient replacement resorption* is possibly related to areas of minor damage to the

root surface. In these cases, the ankylosis is formed initially and later resorbed by adjacent areas of vital periodontal liga-ment. This theory is supported ex-perimentally by research in which the ef-fect of limited drying or limited removal of the periodontal ligament upon periodon-tal healing after replantation was studied (144).

Figure 10.14 demonstrates an initial phase of replacement resorption. The an-kylosed root becomes part of the normal bone remodelling system and is gradually

Fig. 10.15.
Advanced ankylosis (replacement resorption) after replantation of upper left central and lateral incisors. A. Radiograph immediately after replantation. B. Condition at time of removal of the central incisor 3 years after replantation. C. Low-power view of sectioned incisor. x 12. D. Apical part of root canal filling surrounded by bone and connective tissue. x 30. E. Haversian canal under remodelling. The walls consist of both dentin and bone. Note tunneling resorption along the root canal filling (arrows). x 30. F. Fragment of dentin incorporated in bone (arrows). x 30. G. Higher magnification of F. x 195. H. Area with normal cementum and periodontal tissue including epithelial rests of Mallassez. x 195. From AN-DREASEN & HJØRTING-HANSEN (44) 1966.

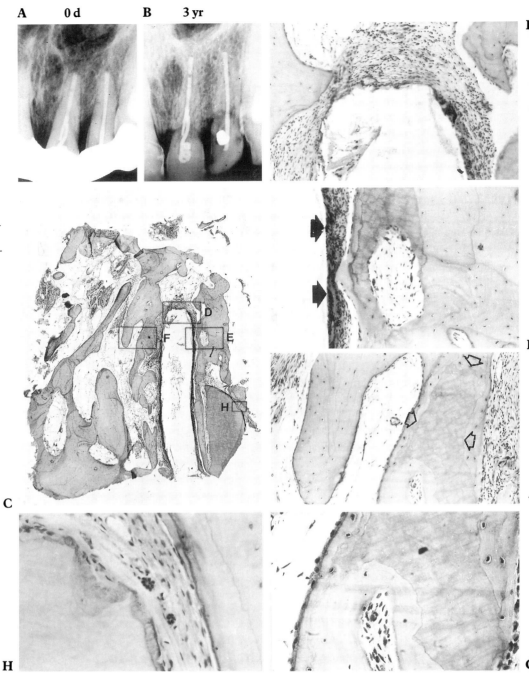

replaced by bone. After some time, little of the tooth substance remains (Fig. 10.15). At this stage, the resorptive processes are usually intensified along the surface of the root canal filling, a phenomenon known as *tunneling resorption* (Fig. 10.15, E).

Radiographically, ankylosis is characterized by disappearance of the normal periodontal space and continuous replacement of root substance with bone (Fig. 10.16, A to D).

Replacement resorption can usually first be recognized radiographically 2 months after replantation; however, in most cases 6 months or 1 year elapses (202) (Fig. 10.17).

Fig. 10.16.
Schematic and radiographic appearance of replacement and inflammatory resorption. A to D. Progression of replacement resorption. E to H. Progression of inflammatory resorption. From ANDREASEN & HJØRTING-HANSEN (6) 1966.

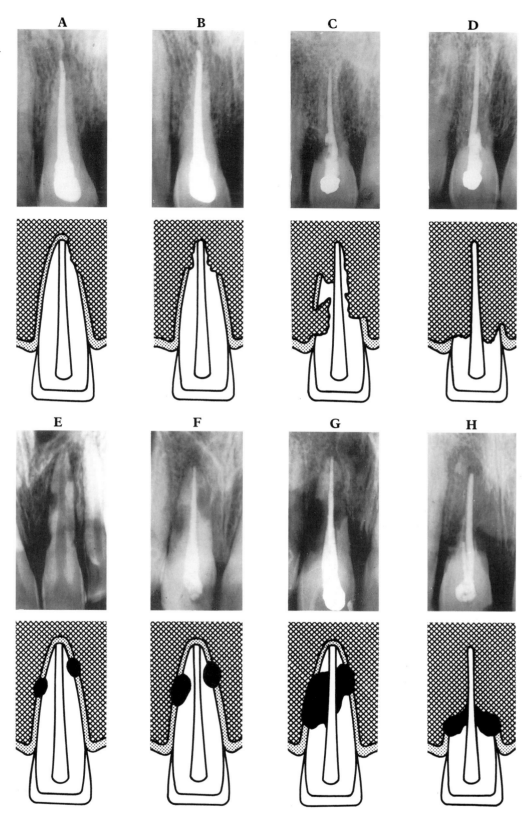

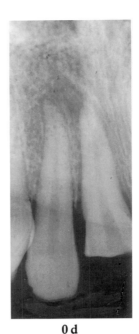 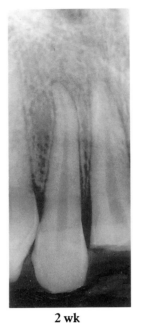 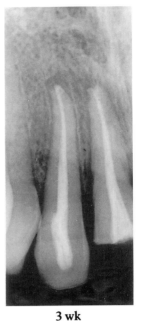 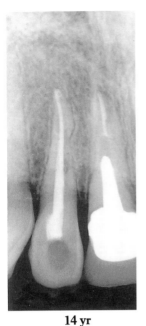 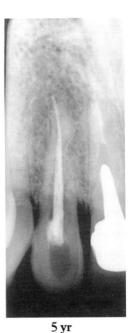

| 0 d | 2 wk | 3 wk | 14 yr | 5 yr |

Fig. 10.17.
Progression of replacement resorption is followed by tunneling inflammatory resorption along the root filling. From ANDREASEN ET AL. (203) 1991.

Fig. 10.18.
Late appearance of ankylosis. Resorption activity is suspected after 3 and 5 years and becomes manifest after 10 years. From ANDREASEN ET AL. (203) 1991.

Most cases can be diagnosed within 2 years but it has been found that up to 10 years may elapse before a radiographic diagnosis can be made (202) (Fig. 10.18). This problem of diagnosing ankylosis has also been verified in experimental studies where histologic findings were compared with radiography (235, 236).

Clinically, the ankylosed tooth is immobile and in children frequently in infraposition. The percussion tone is high, differing clearly from adjacent non-injured teeth. The percussion test can often reveal replacement resorption in its initial phases before it can be diagnosed radiographically (171, 202, 235).

Cases of transient replacement resorp-

tion can sometimes be demonstrated radiographically as small areas where the periodontal ligament space has disappeared (Fig. 10.13). Most often this type of ankylosis is demonstrated by its high percussion tone. Disappearance of the ankylosis, which always happens within the first year, is followed by the return of a normal percussion tone (171).

4. HEALING WITH INFLAMMATORY RESORPTION
Histologically, inflammatory resorption is characterized by bowl-shaped resorption cavities in cementum and dentin associated with inflammatory changes in the adjacent periodontal tissue (44, 53-57, 139, 147, 237) (Fig.

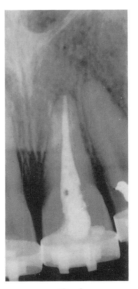 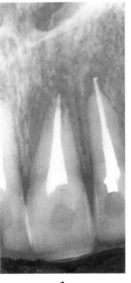 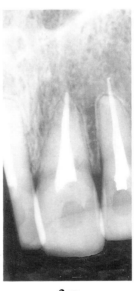 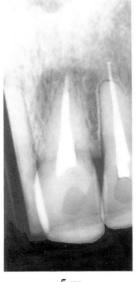 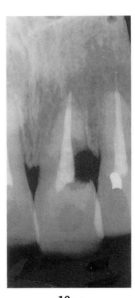

| 2 wk | 1 yr | 3 yr | 5 yr | 10 yr |

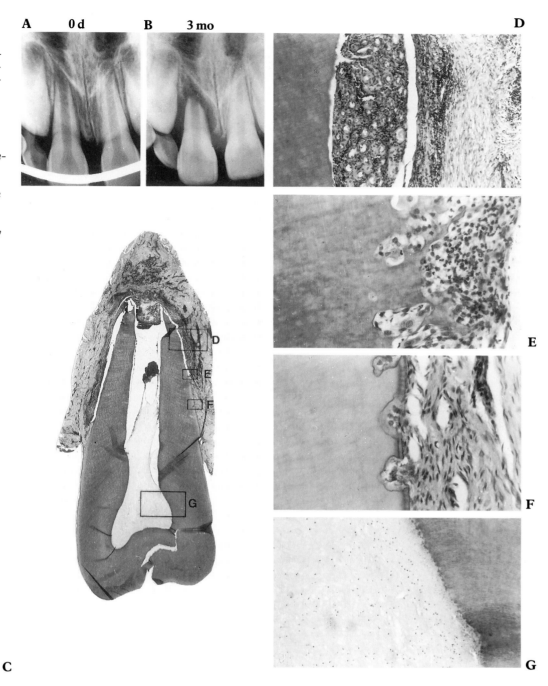

Fig. 10.19.
Inflammatory resorption after replantation of a right central incisor. A. Radiograph taken immediately after replantation. B. Condition at time of removal 3 months later. C. Low-power view of sectioned incisor. The pulp shows complete necrosis with autolysis. An intense inflammatory reaction is seen around the apical half of the root. x 7. D. Granulation tissue in relation to resorbed root surface. x 30. E. Area with active resorption. x 195. F. Surface resorption partly repaired with new cementum. x 195. G. Necrotic pulp tissue. x 30. From ANDREASEN & HJØRTING-HANSEN (44) 1966.

A 0 d

B 3 mo

D

E

F

G

C

10.18). The inflammatory reaction in the periodontium consists of granulation tissue with numerous lymphocytes, plasma cells, and polymorphonuclear leukocytes. Adjacent to these areas, the root surface undergoes intense resorption with numerous Howship's lacunae and osteoclasts.

The pathogenesis of inflammatory resorption can be described as follows (139): Minor injuries to the periodontal ligament and/or cementum due to trauma or contamination with bacteria induce small resorption cavities on the root surface, presumably in the same manner as in surface resorption. If these resorption cavities expose dentinal tubules and the root canal contains infected necrotic tissue, toxins from these areas will penetrate along the dentinal tubules to the lateral periodontal tissues and provoke an inflammatory response. This in turn will intensify the resorption process which advances towards the root canal (44, 139). The resorption process can progress very rapidly, i.e. within a few months the entire root can be resorbed.

Inflammatory resorption is especially frequent and aggressive after replantation in patients from 6 to 10 years of age. The explanation for this is probably a combination of wide dentinal tubules and/or a

Fig. 10.20.

Replacement and inflammatory resorption after replantation of a left central incisor. A. Radiograph taken immediately after replantation. B. Condition at time of removal 2 years later. C. Low-power view of sectioned incisor. Note partial pulp necrosis and root resorption. x 5. D. Arrested external root resorption. x 195. E. Acellular hard tissue (presumably cementum) deposited on the canal walls. x 195. F. Area with replacement resorption. x 75. G. Area with active inflammatory resorption. x 30. H. Border zone between vital and necrotic pulp tissue. x 30.

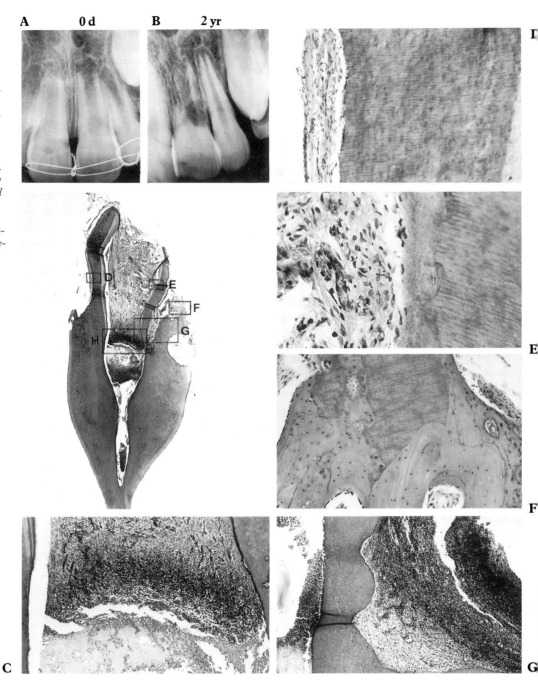

thin protective cementum cover (6, 139). In older age groups, the resorption process follows a more protracted course.

It should be noted that replanted teeth can show simultaneous inflammatory and replacement resorption (Fig. 10.20). Moreover, if the resorption process is allowed to progress and involve large areas of the root surface, *replacement resorption* can take over once inflammatory resorption has been arrested by endodontic therapy.

Radiographically, inflammatory resorption is characterized by radiolucent bowl-shaped cavitations along the root surface with corresponding excavations in the adjacent bone (Fig. 10.16, E to H). The first radiographic sign of inflammatory resorption can be demonstrated as early as 2 weeks after replantation and is usually first recognized at the cervical third of the root (6) (Fig. 10.21). As in the case of ankylosis, this resorption type is usually evident within the first 2 years after replantation.

Clinically, the replanted tooth is loose and extruded. Moreover, the tooth is sensitive to percussion and the percussion tone is dull (vs. ankylosis).

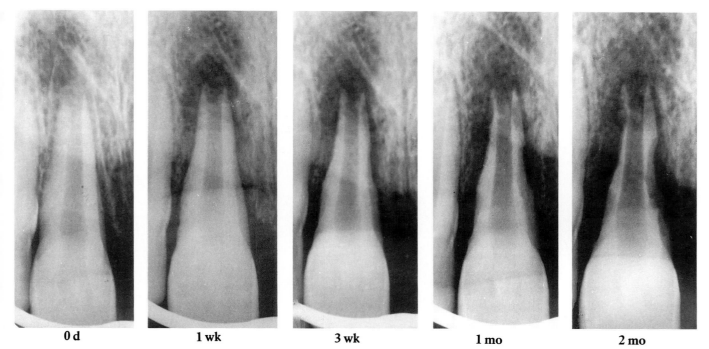

| 0 d | 1 wk | 3 wk | 1 mo | 2 mo |

Fig. 10.21.
Inflammatory resorption of a replanted right central incisor. Note the excavating nature of the resorption process on the root and a corresponding marked resorption of the lamina dura. From ANDREASEN & HJØRTING-HANSEN (6) 1966.

Treatment of the Avulsed Tooth

The case history should include exact information on the time interval between injury and replantation as well as the conditions under which the tooth has been stored (e.g. saline, saliva, milk, tap water, or dry).

In this regard a commercial tissue culture medium (Viaspan®) could be used for extraoral storage. *In vitro* experiments have shown it to be effective even for several days of storage (238). However, *in vivo* studies are still lacking that demonstrate its effectiveness.

The avulsed tooth is examined for obvious contamination. The alveolus is also examined. As prognosis is significantly related to the length of the extra-alveolar period, pre-treatment radiographs can serve to extend this period and should, therefore, be taken prior to treatment only if there is suspicion of comminution or fracture of the socket wall.

Careful planning is of utmost importance for the success of replantation of avulsed teeth.

The following conditions should be considered before replanting a permanent tooth:
1. The avulsed tooth should be without advanced periodontal disease.
2. The alveolar socket should be reasonably intact in order to provide a seat for the avulsed tooth.
3. The extra-alveolar period should be considered, i.e. dry extraoral periods exceeding 1 hour are usually associated with marked root resorption.

While certain conditions, such as those listed above, might appear to contraindicate replantation of an avulsed incisor, it should be borne in mind that the time of injury is often not the time to make such decisions. Definitive treatment planning (e.g. orthodontic evaluation of a crowded dentition) can seldom be made in the heat of acute treatment. Furthermore, an extended extraoral period - even dry storage - is not an absolute contraindication to replantation, as the root surface can be treated chemically to protract the resorption process in mature teeth (see later). In most situations, replantation of the avulsed tooth, even with a dubious prognosis, can be performed and the tooth considered as a temporary restoration until such time as definitive treatment planning, often following specialist consultation, can be carried out.

If replantation is decided upon, the following procedures are recommended (Fig. 10.22). The tooth is placed in saline. If visibly contaminated, the root surface is rinsed with a stream of saline from a syringe until visible contaminants have been washed away – including around the apical foramen. The alveolus is also rinsed with a flow of saline to remove the contaminated coagulum. No effort should be made to sterilize the root surface, as such procedures will damage or destroy vital periodontal tissue and cementum (202).

The socket is then examined. If there is evidence of fracture, it is essential to reposition the fractured bone by inserting an instrument in the socket and then modelling the bone. Local anesthesia is usually not necessary unless gingival lacerations require suturing or the alveolar socket requires remodelling. The tooth is replanted using light digital pressure. It is important that only light pressure is used during the replantation procedure, as this will permit detection of resistance from displaced alveolar bone fragments that impede replantation. If resistance is met, the tooth should again be placed in saline while the alveolus is reexamined and any displaced bone fragments repositioned. Repositioning can then be completed. The replanted incisor should fit loosely in the alveolus in order to prevent further damage to the root surface.

Recent studies have shown that rigid splinting of replanted mature and auto-transplanted immature teeth increases the extent of root resorption (147, 148, 173, 239-241). Replanted teeth should, therefore, only be splinted for a minimal period of time. One week is normally sufficient to ensure adequate periodontal support, as gingival fibers are already healed by this time.

Proper repositioning can now be evaluated by the occlusion and the tooth splinted to adjacent incisors. An acid etch/resin splint is usually the method of choice. Finally, a radiograph is taken once the splint has been applied, to verify that the normal position of the tooth has been achieved.

When the splint is to be removed, it is important to remember that the replanted tooth is still rather loose. It is therefore important to remove the splinting material carefully, with finger support on the replanted tooth. Furthermore, if endodontic treatment is indicated, it should be carried out prior to splint removal (see suggestions in Chapter 14, p. 608).

In some instances, a telephone call at the time of injury will precede the office visit. In these cases, the patient or an available adult should be instructed to replant the tooth immediately. In this way, the extra-alveolar period is decreased and the prognosis improved significantly. Replantation can be accomplished in the following manner.

The tooth can be cleaned if dirty, by simply rinsing it under cold tap water for 10 seconds and placing it immediately in its socket. If the replantation procedure cannot be performed at this time, the tooth can be stored in the patient's buccal vestibule. Animal experiments have shown that storage in milk or saliva has almost the same effect as storage in saline. However, long-term storage in tap water (i.e. more than 20 minutes) has an adverse effect on periodontal healing (146, 202). After replantation and en route to the dental office, the patient should be instructed to keep the tooth in place with either finger pressure or by biting on a handkerchief.

Tetanus prophylaxis is important, as most teeth have been in contact with soil, or the wound itself is soil-contaminated.

The value of antibiotic therapy is at this time questionable. Thus, experimental studies in monkeys have shown that systemic antibiotics may lessen the resorption attack on the root surface. However, pulpal healing is apparently not affected (226,242). In a recent clinical study, no effect could be demonstrated in the frequency of pulpal or periodontal healing (200, 202).

In case of a closed apical foramen, endodontic treatment should always be performed prophylactically, as pulp necrosis can be anticipated. A long-debated question has been whether root canal treatment of incisors with mature root development (i.e. with the diameter of the apical foramen of less than 1.0 mm) should be performed before or after replantation, if survival of the pulp cannot be expected. Recent experimental studies in monkeys have shown that extraoral root filling procedures as well as the root filling materials themselves apparently injure the periodontal ligament. This could be a result of seepage through the apical foramen or mechanical preparation of the root canal, resulting in increased ankylosis apically when compared to non-endodontically treated teeth (149, 152). Thus, endodontic treatment should be delayed for 1 week after replantation in order to prevent development of ankylosis and inflammatory

Fig. 10.22. Replantation of a tooth with completed root formation

Replantation of an avulsed maxillary right central incisor in a 19-year-old man. Radiographic examination shows no sign of fracture or contusion of the alveolar socket. The tooth was retrieved immediately after injury and kept moist in the oral cavity. Upon admission to the emergency service, the avulsed incisor was placed in physiologic saline.

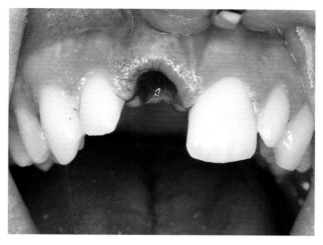 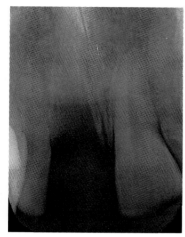

Rinsing the tooth

The tooth is examined for fractures, position of the level of periodontal attachment and signs of contamination. The tooth is then rinsed with a stream of saline until all visible signs of contamination have been removed. If this is not effective, dirt is carefully removed using a gauze sponge soaked in saline. The coagulum in the alveolar socket is flushed out using a stream of saline.

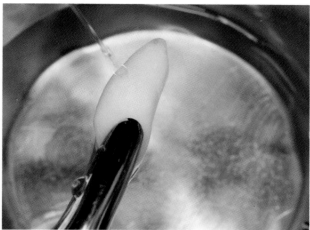 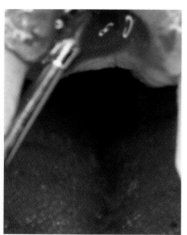

Replanting the tooth

The tooth is grasped by the crown with forceps and partially replanted in its socket. Replantation is completed using gentle finger pressure. If any resistance is met, the tooth should be removed, placed again in saline and the socket inspected. A straight elevator is then inserted in the socket and an index finger is placed labially. Using lateral pressure, counterbalanced by the finger pressure, the socket wall is repositioned. Replantation can then proceed as described.

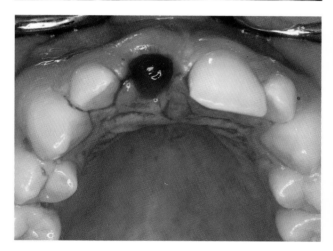 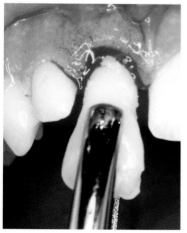

Splinting

An acid-etch retained splint is applied. As soon after injury as possible, antibiotic therapy should be instituted. Suggested dosage: penicillin 1 million units immediately, thereafter 2-4 million units daily for 4 days. Good oral hygiene is absolutely necessary in the healing period. This includes brushing with a soft tooth brush and a 0.1 % chlorhexidine mouth rinse.

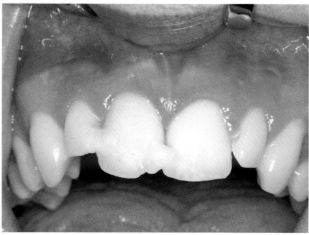 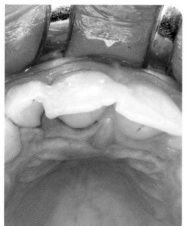

AVULSION

resorption, as well as to allow splicing of periodontal ligament fibers which limits seepage of potentially harmful root filling materials into the traumatized periodontal ligament.

Where the apical foramen is wide open and replantation has taken place within 3 hours after injury, it is justifiable to await revascularization of the pulp (200, 243). Radiographic controls should be made 2 and 3 weeks after replantation, as the first evidence of root resorption and periapical osteitis can usually be seen at this time. If this occurs, endodontic therapy should be initiated immediately and calcium hydroxide introduced into the root canal to eliminate periapical inflammation and arrest root resorption (6, 45, 174, 244) (see Chapter 14, p. 543). The timing of the endodontic procedure when pulpal revascularization is absent is critical, as root resorption can proceed very rapidly in teeth with incomplete root formation (i.e. with a speed of up to 0.1 mm root substance loss per day) (Fig. 10.22).

In teeth with prolonged extra-alveolar periods, where the periodontal ligament can be assumed to be necrotic, it has been suggested that the root surface be treated with various substances, such as sodium flouride (175), tetracycline, stannous flouride (245, 246), citric acid (247, 248), hypochloric acid (161), calcium hydroxide (178), formalin (179), alcohol (180), diphosphonates (181), and indomethacin (249) in order to inhibit root resorption. However, apart from sodium flouride, long-term resorption inhibition has not been proven.

The incorporation of fluoride ions in the cementum layer has been found to yield a root surface resistant to resorption (175). Thus, in experiments with monkeys, a significant reduction in the amount of radiographically evident root resorption was seen in teeth treated with a fluoride solution (176). Based on these experiments, it has been suggested that mature teeth with prolonged dry extra-alveolar periods (i.e greater than 1 hour) be placed in a fluoride solution (2.4% sodium fluoride phosphate acidulated at pH 5.5) for 20 minutes prior to replantation (Fig. 10.23). Thereafter the root surface is rinsed with saline and the tooth replanted and splinted for 6 weeks (177). The effect of this treatment seems to be a 50% reduction of the progression of root resorption of replanted human teeth (250).

Several attempts have been made to overcome the problem of ankylosis by placing different materials between the tooth and the socket, such as silicone grease and methyl methacrylate (methyl-2-cyanoacrylate) (178, 182, 183), absorbable surgical sponge (Gelfoam®, The Upjohn Co., Kalamazoo, USA) (184), venous tissue (160), fascia and cutaneous connective tissue (156). The general outcome of these experiments was that root resorption was either not prevented or that the teeth were exfoliated.

To overcome the resorption problem, a number of procedures have been developed, e.g. replacement of the apical part of the root with a cast vitallium implant (68, 73, 78, 190). However, the results of these procedures have not been convincing. Lately, an attempt has been made to prolong the lifetime of replanted teeth by a replacement of the root tip with a ceramic implant (dense sintered aluminum oxide) (251-262) (Fig. 10.24). Before replantation, the apical half of the root is resected, the root canal enlarged with special burs, whereafter a corresponding ceramic implant is cemented in. Preliminary studies indicate that this procedure, as expected, does not prevent root resorption, but does tend to prolong the survival time of the replant (261, 262).

Replantation of avulsed primary teeth has been reported by some investigators (58-61, 185). However, in the authors' opinion, replantation of primary teeth is not justified, due to the risk of pulp necrosis and possible interference with the development of the permanent successors.

Fig. 10.23. Replanting a tooth with an avital periodontal ligament

In this 21-year-old man, the tooth has been kept dry for 24 hours. Total and irreversible damage to the PDL and pulp can be expected. Furthermore, there is severe contusion of the alveolar socket. In this situation, delayed replantation (to allow healing of the socket), treatment of the root surface (to make it resistant to ankylosis) and endodontic therapy (to prevent inflammatory resorption) is the treatment of choice.

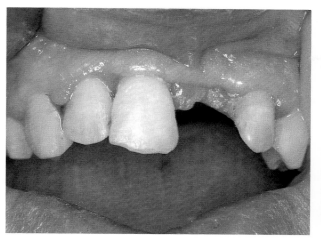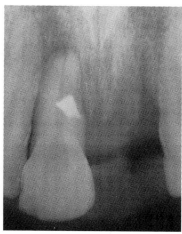

Treatment of the root surface

The avulsed tooth in this case was kept dry in a refrigerator until healing of the contused socket has taken place. Prior to sodium fluoride treatment, the root surface is rinsed and scraped clean of the dead PDL and the pulp extirpated. The goal of therapy is to incorporate fluoride ions into the dentin and cementum in order to protract the resorption process.

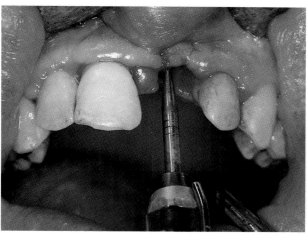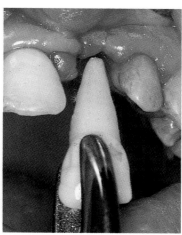

Fluoride treatment of cementum and dentin

The pulp is extirpated and the root canal enlarged to provide access for the fluoride solution along the entire root canal. The tooth is then placed in a 2.4% solution of sodium fluoride (acidulated to pH = 5.5) for 20 min.

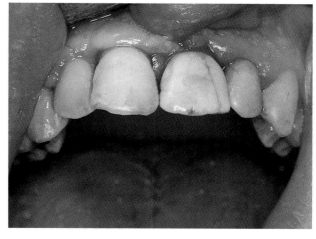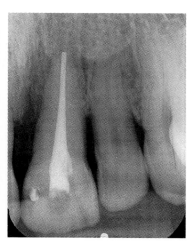

Endodontic treatment

After rinsing in saline, the root canal is obturated with gutta-percha and a sealer.

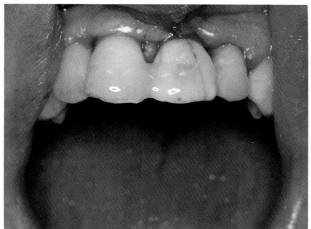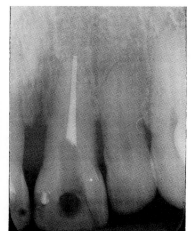

AVULSION

403

Condition of the socket
After 3 weeks, the socket area and the contused gingiva are healed.

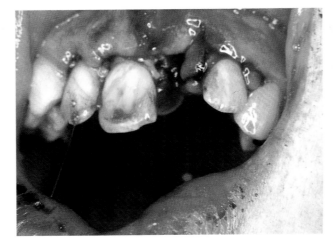 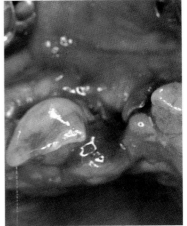

Replanting the tooth
The socket is evacuated with excavators and a surgical bur. The tooth is replanted after cleansing with saline to remove excess fluoride solution.

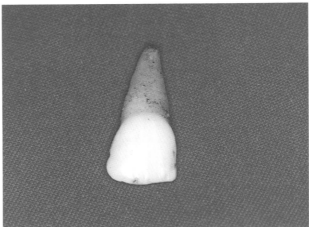 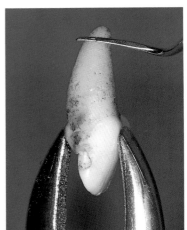

Splinting
The tooth is splinted for 6 weeks in order to create a solid ankylosis. In these cases, where no periodontal ligament exists, ankylosis is the only possible healing modality.

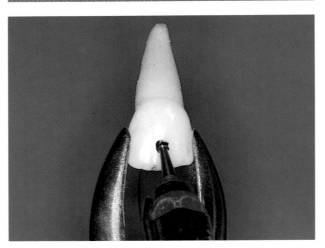 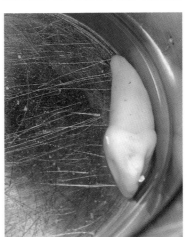

Follow-up
Radiographic follow-up over a 3-year period shows no progression of the ankylosis process.

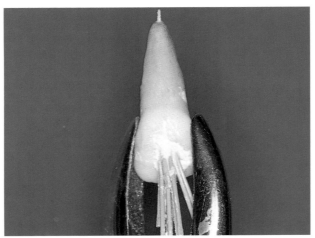 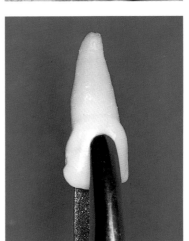

Fig. 10.24. Apical resection and root extension with a ceramic implant.
Pulp necrosis and arrested root formation in a 10-year-old child subsequent to trauma. The tooth is extracted with forceps having diamond grips. It is important that the forceps does not touch cementum after incision of the gingival fibers with a scalpel.
From KIRCHNER (253), 1981

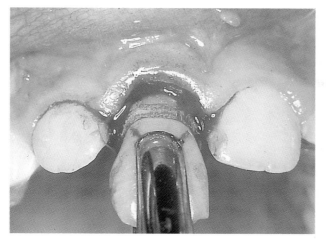 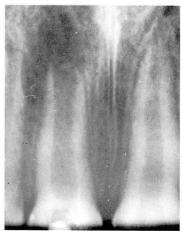

Preparing the root for the implant
The apex is resected with a diamond disc to a level where there is no obvious resorption. The root canal is enlarged with a bur which matches the ceramic implant. The root canal is enlarged with a bur with internal cooling. During all tooth preparation the root is kept moist with saline.

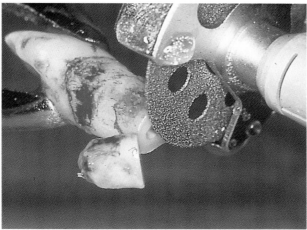 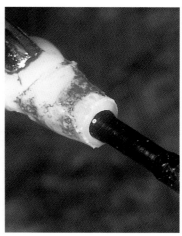

Cementing the implant
After drying the cavity with a sterile pipe cleaner, the aluminimum oxide implant (Biolox®) which matches the dimension of the drill is cemented with Diaket®.

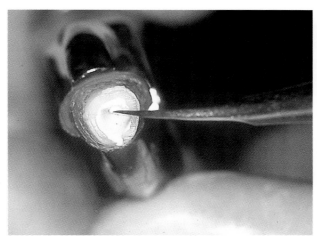 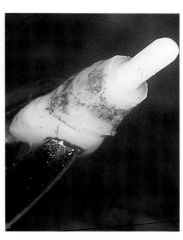

Replanting the tooth
The base of the alveolus is enlarged with a drill to accommodate the root extension. After replantation, the tooth is splinted for 2 to 4 weeks. Subsequently, the crown should be opened palatally and filled to the level of the implant. The radiographic condition is shown 2 years after implantation.

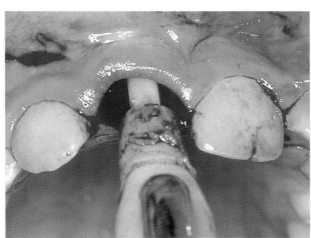 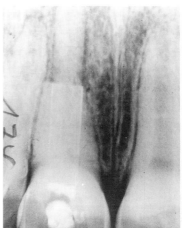

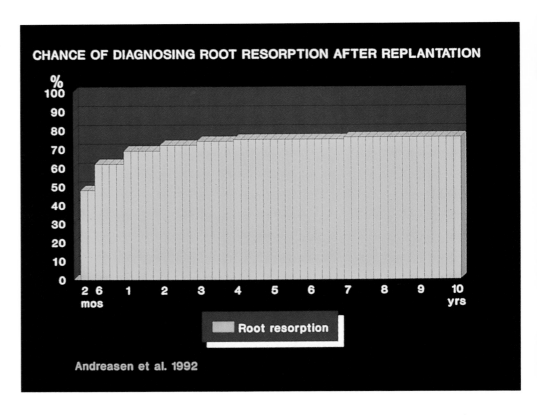

Follow-up Procedures

Successive radiographic controls should be performed in the follow-up period in order to disclose root resorption (199) (see Appendix 4. p. 750). If not present within the first 2 years after injury, the risk of root resorption is significantly reduced (202) (Fig. 10.25).

Prognosis

Replantation of teeth has been considered a temporary measure as many teeth succumb to root resorption. However, a number of cases have been reported where replanted teeth have been in service for 20 to 40 years with a normal periodontium, as revealed clinically (positive pulpal sensibility) and radiographically (6, 63-68, 186) (Fig. 10.26 and Table 10.1). Such reports demonstrate that replanted teeth, under certain conditions, can maintain their integrity and function.

Tooth Survival

Several studies have shown that teeth can function for 20 years or more after replantation (263, 267).

In one long-term study, it was shown that tooth survival was significantly related to the stage of root development at the time of injury, being more favorable with increasing developmental maturity (199) (Table 10.1 and Fig. 10.27).

Pulpal Healing and Pulp Necrosis

In rare cases, revascularization of the pulp will occur in replanted teeth with *completed* root formation, provided that replantation is carried out immediately (6, 43). Pulps of teeth with *incomplete* root formation can become revascularized if replantation is carried out within 3 hours (6, 8, 9, 43, 63, 66, 79-85, 191-196, 200, 243, 268-270). Pulpal sensibility tests are unreliable immediately after replantation. Functional repair of pulpal nerve fibers in human teeth is established approximately 35 days after replantation. At this time electrical stimuli can elicit sensibility responses. With longer observation periods, an increasing number of teeth will respond (43, 200). In the absence of a reaction to electrical stimulation, it should be borne in mind that a decrease in the size of the coronal part of the pulp chamber or root canal on the radiograph is a more reliable sign of vital pulp tissue

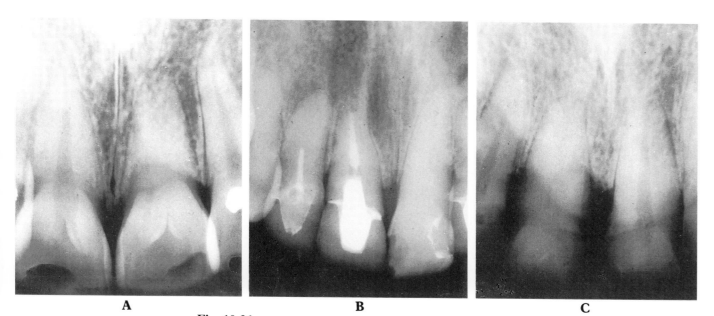

Fig. 10.26.
Cases demonstrating periodontal healing after replantation. A. Left central incisor replanted 13 years previously. B. Right central incisor replanted 37 years previously. C. Two central incisors replanted 40 years previously. From ANDREASEN & HJØRTING-HANSEN (6) 1966.

Table 10.1 Long-term results of replantation of avulsed permanent teeth

Examiner	Observa-tion period years (mean)	Age of patients years (mean)	No. of teeth	Tooth sur-vival %	PDL heal-ing %	Pulp heal-ing %	Gingi-val heal-ing %
Lenstrup & Skieller (7,8) 1957, 1959	0.2-5	5-18	47	57	9	4	
Andreasen & Hjörting-Hansen (6) 1966	0.2-15	6-24	110	54	20	4	95
Ravn & Helbo (69)1966		5-15	28		4	4	
Gröndahl et al. (181) 1974	2-5		45	69	23	7	67
Cvek et al. (188) 1974	2-6.5	6-17 (11)	38		50		
Hörster et al. (128)1976			38		26		
Kemp & Phillips (127)1977	0.1-10	10-15	71	61	30		
Ravn (129) 1977		7-16	20		20	5	
Kock & Ullbro (263)1982	1-9	7-17	55	65	27	4	
Herforth (264)1982	1-8 (4.5)	7-15	79	51	11	4	
Jacobsen (265)1986	1-14 (5)		59	39	29	15	
Gonda et al. (266) 1990	0.6-6.5	(16)	27	70	41	15	
Mackie & Worthington (267) 1992	1-7	6-14 (9)	46	89	46		
Andreasen et al. (199-203) 1992	0.2-20 (5.1)	5-52 (13.4)	400	70	36	8	93

Fig. 10.27.
Tooth survival related to stage of root development at time of injury. From ANDREASEN ET AL. (199) 1991.

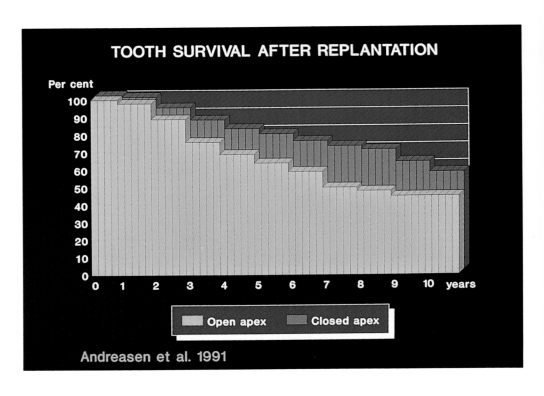

than thermal or electrical pulp testing (43) (Fig. 10.28).

The most significant predictors of pulpal healing appear to be the *width* and *length* of the root canal as well as the *duration* and *type* of *extra-alveolar storage* (200).

THE WIDTH AND LENGTH OF THE ROOT CANAL

The relationship between the diameter of the apical foramen and the chance of pulpal revascularization apparently is an expression of the size of the contact area at the pulpo-periodontal interface (Fig. 10.29), whereas the length of the root canal probably reflects the time necessary to repopulate the ischemic pulp (200) (Fig. 10.30). With a favorable ratio (i.e. broad apical foramen and short root canal versus a narrow apical foramen and long root canal) the odds for an intervening pulpal infection are reduced. A limiting factor in pulpal revascularization after replantation appears to be an apical diameter of under 1.0 mm (200, 243). This size, however, is to a certain degree arbitrary, as pulps in teeth

with constricted apical foramina are usually extirpated prophylactically.

STORAGE PERIOD AND STORAGE MEDIA

Another significant relationship which could be demonstrated in a large clinical study was the strong dependence between storage period and media and pulpal healing (200). This is possibly due to the detrimental effect of cellular dehydration during dry storage on the apical portion of the pulp or by damage incurred by nonphysiologic storage (e.g. prolonged tap water storage, chloramine, chlorhexidine and alcohol). The net result appears to be the following:

With nonphysiologic storage, the chances of pulpal revascularization are minimal. With storage in physiological media (e.g. saline, saliva or milk), there is only a weak relationship between the duration of storage and chances of pulpal revascularization (200) (Fig. 10.31). In contrast, dry storage yields a constant and, with time, increasingly harmful effect on pulpal healing (Fig. 10.32). However,

408

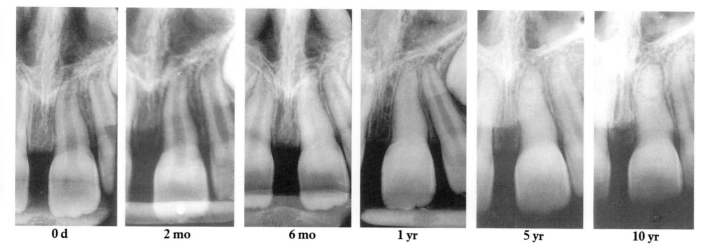

| 0 d | 2 mo | 6 mo | 1 yr | 5 yr | 10 yr |

Fig. 10.28.
Pulp canal obliteration after replantation of a left central incisor. The canal obliteration becomes apparent after 6 months. From ANDREASEN & AL. (200) 1991

Fig. 10.29.
Relationship between size of foramen and pulp revascularization after replantation. From ANDREASEN ET AL. (200) 1992.

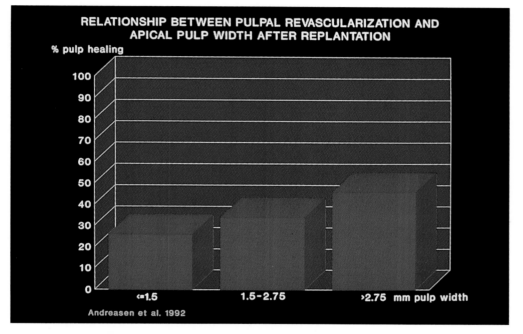

RELATIONSHIP BETWEEN PULPAL REVASCULARIZATION AND
APICAL PULP WIDTH AFTER REPLANTATION

% pulp healing

Andreasen et al. 1992

<=1.5   1.5-2.75   >2.75 mm pulp width

Fig. 10.30.
Relationship between length of the pulp canal and pulp revascularization after replantation. From ANDREASEN ET AL. (200) 1992.

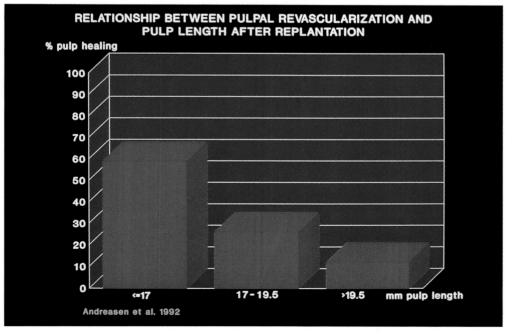

RELATIONSHIP BETWEEN PULPAL REVASCULARIZATION AND
PULP LENGTH AFTER REPLANTATION

% pulp healing

Andreasen et al. 1992

<=17   17-19.5   >19.5   mm pulp length

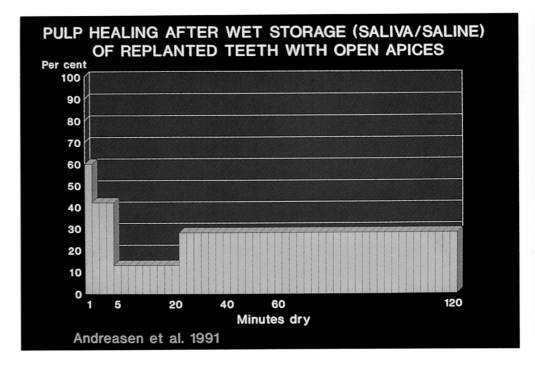

when compared to periodontal healing, this effect is less noticeable (200, 202) (see p 411).

Periodontal Healing and Root Resorption

Most replanted teeth demonstrate root resorption after a certain period of time. In the literature, the frequency of periodontal healing is usually around 20% (Table 10.1). However, a recent study following a series of public information campaigns showed a success rate of up to 36% after replantation (199).

A number of clinical factors have been shown to be associated with root resorption after replantation. Among these, the length of the *dry* extra-alveolar period seems to be the most crucial (6, 128, 171, 188, 189, 202, 271-274) (Fig. 10.33). In a follow-up study of 400 teeth replanted after traumatic injury, 73% of the teeth replanted within 5 min demonstrated PDL healing; in contrast, PDL healing occurred in only 18% when the teeth were stored prior to

Fig. 10.32.
Relationship between pulpal healing of teeth with incomplete root formation and type and length of extra-alveolar dry storage. From ANDREASEN ET AL. (200) 1993.

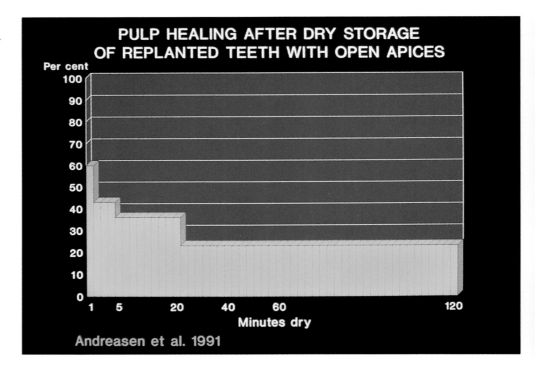

CHAPTER 10

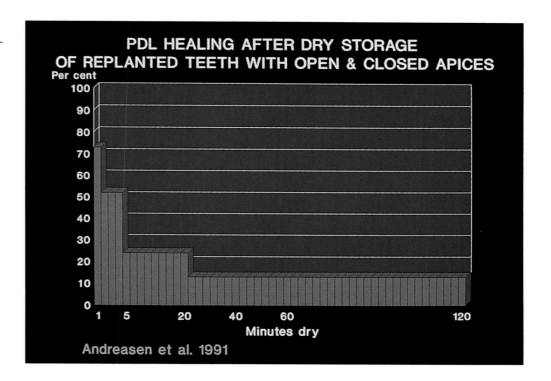

replantation (202). These findings are in agreement with animal experiments (16, 28, 33, 70, 130, 146) assessing PDL vitality of extracted teeth allowed to dry out for varying periods (275-277).

In most clinical cases, avulsed teeth have been stored either in the oral cavity or in other media, such as physiologic saline or tap water, before replantation. Recent experimental studies have indicated that the storage media more than the length of the extra-alveolar period determine prognosis.

Thus, storage in saline or saliva did not significantly impair periodontal healing, while even short dry storage periods had an adverse effect (146, 272). Although the above-mentioned experimental studies seem to stress the significance of the extra-alveolar period with these media, a less pronounced effect has been found in a larger clinical study (Fig. 10.34). It should also be mentioned that successful cases have been reported after extra-alveolar periods of several hours (71, 72, 202).

Fig. 10.34.
Relationship between PDL healing and length of extra-alveolar wet storage. From ANDREASEN *ET AL.* (202) *1993.*

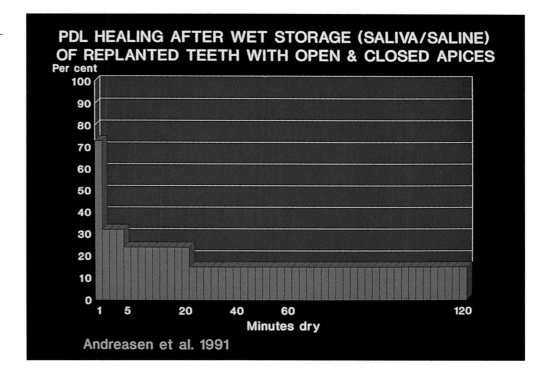

STAGE OF ROOT DEVELOPMENT

In a clinical avulsion situation, the layer of PDL on the root can vary in thickness from a single cell layer to the full thickness of a periodontal ligament. Thus, the more mature the root formation the thinner is the PDL tissue layer. This could possibly explain the influence of root formation upon development of root resorption found in a recent clinical study (202). Thus, a thick periodontal ligament, which supposedly can tolerate a certain dry period before evaporation has killed the critical cell layers next to the cementum, showed less dependence upon dry storage (222).

Among other factors influencing root resorption, experimental and human data have shown that the removal of the periodontal ligament prior to replantation is followed by extensive replacement resorption (25, 33, 48, 143). Consequently, this procedure, unless performed in relation to sodium fluoride treatment of the root surface is contraindicated. (See page. 403)

REPLACEMENT RESORPTION (ANKYLOSIS)

Ankylosis can usually be diagnosed clinically by a percussion test after 4-8 weeks, whereas radiographic evidence of root resorption usually requires a year (202). Recently, a mechanical device (Periotest®) which registers tooth mobility has also been shown to provide an early diagnosis of ankylosis (278).

A marked difference in the rate of progression of ankylosis is often seen in cases with similar extra-alveolar periods. This phenomenon might be related to differences in the initial damage to the root surface (6, 202, 273), as well as the age of the patient and the type of endodontic treatment performed (Fig. 10.35). Thus, if a tooth is replanted shortly after avulsion, the periodontal ligament is either re-established completely, or a few areas of ankylosis can arise (274). In the latter case, a long period will elapse before the process of replacement resorption results in total resorption of the root. Conversely, in teeth replanted with a long extra-alveolar period, an extensive ankylosis is formed which leads to rapid resorption of the root.

If an ankylosis is established, its progression is also dependent upon the age of the patient, or rather the turnover rate of bone. Thus, replacement resorption is usually very aggressive in young individuals and runs a very protracted course in older patients (202, 203, 273).

A factor to be considered in young patients is that ankylosis can anchor the tooth in its position and thus disturb normal growth of the alveolar process. The result is a marked infraocclusion of the replanted tooth with migration and malocclusion of adjacent teeth (6, 55, 69, 129) (Fig. 10.36). The treatment of choice in these cases is either extraction or luxation with subsequent orthodontic extrusion (see Chapter 15, p. 621). Otherwise, later restorative procedures may be unnecessarily complicated by tooth migration and decreased height of the alveolar process (69).

In planning the extraction of an ankylosed incisor, it is important to consider that ankylosed roots will ultimately be transformed to bone during the remodelling process. It is, therefore, not indicated to remove the entire root surgically, as this will lead to a marked reduction in the height of the alveolar process. The treatment of choice is to fracture the crown from the ankylosed and resorbed root and then remove the root filling with a barbed broach or a bur. This technique is described in Chapter 15, p. 624.

In older patients an ankylosed tooth can be retained; the life-span of such a tooth can vary from 10 to 20 years, due to the slow remodelling rate of bone in older age groups.

INFLAMMATORY ROOT RESORPTION

Unless treated, inflammatory resorption can result in rapid loss of the replanted tooth, even as early as 3 months after replantation (6) (Fig. 10.21). This type of resorption is, as mentioned before, related to the presence of an infected pulp. Thus, human and experimental data indicate that arrest of the resorptive processes can be achieved by appropriate endodontic therapy (6, 45, 149, 188, 202) (see Chapter 14, p. 557).

Replanted teeth can demonstrate simultaneous inflammatory and replacement resorption, a phenomenon possibly explained by superimposition of inflammatory resorption when replacement resorption exposes infected dentinal tubules or tubules leading to an infected necrotic pulp (Fig. 10.37).

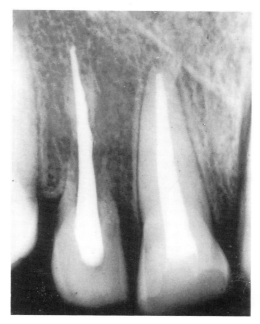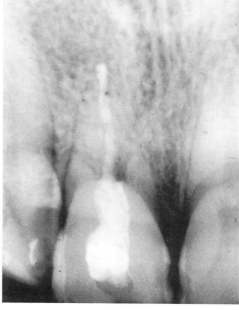

Fig. 10.35.

Difference in progression of replacement resorption after replantation. A. Marked replacement resorption of replanted right lateral incisor after 1 1/2 years. B. Same degree of replacement resorption 9½ years after replantation of right central incisor. From ANDREASEN & HJØRTING-HANSEN (6) 1966.

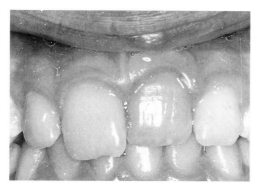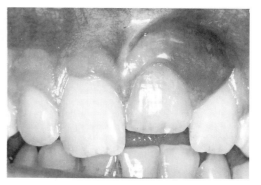

Fig. 10.36.

Progressive infraocclusion of an ankylosed replanted left central incisor. A. Condition 4 years after replantation. B. 6 years after replantation. Courtesy of J. J. RAVN, Department of Pedodontics, Royal Dental College, Copenhagen.

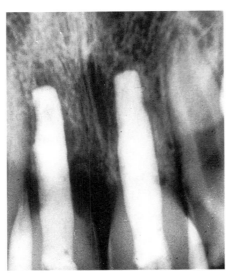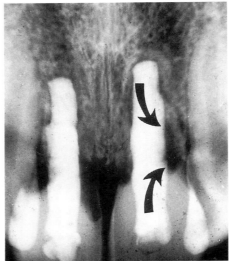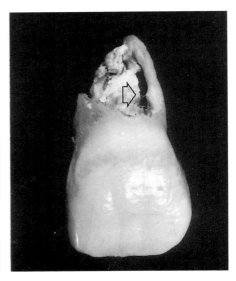

Fig. 10.37.
Continued root formation after replantation of a left central incisor. From ANDREASEN ET AL. (201) 1993.

RESORPTION BY ERUPTING TEETH

A special resorption phenomenon is encountered when a replanted tooth comes into contact with an erupting tooth, as when a lateral incisor lies close to the path of an erupting canine. Apparently, the pressure exerted by the follicle of the erupting tooth initiates or accelerates root resorption (202) (Fig. 10.38). A method to minimize the risk of resorption from the erupting tooth could be early removal of the primary predecessor in order to facili-

Fig. 10.38.
Continued root formation after partial pulp necrosis in a replanted left central incisor. From AN-DREASEN ET AL. (201) 1993.

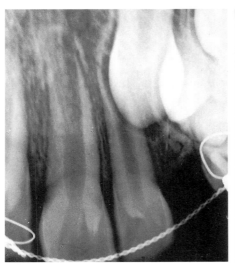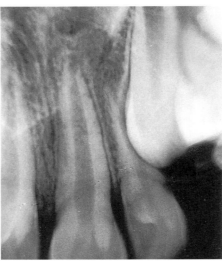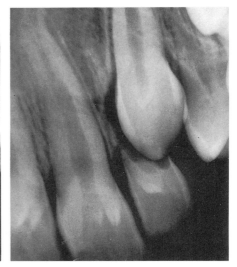

CHAPTER 10

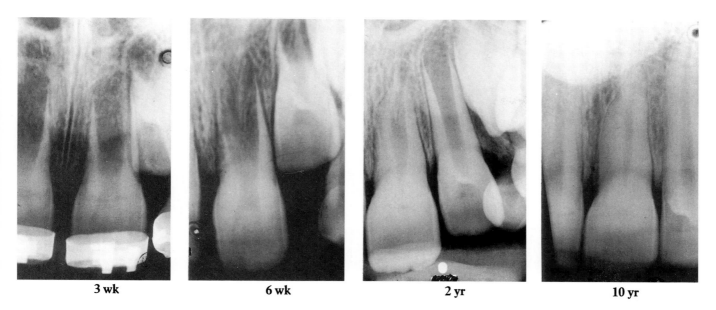

| 3 wk | 6 wk | 2 yr | 10 yr |

Fig. 10.39.
Left central incisor with simultaneous replacement and inflammatory resorption. A. Condition 2 years after replantation. Marked replacement resorption is evident. B. Three years after replantation. Replacement resorption has advanced to the root canal filling and inflammatory resorption is superimposed (arrows). C. The extracted tooth shows tunneling resorption along root canal filling (arrow).

tate eruption, possibly in a direction away from the replanted tooth.

Root Development and Disturbances in Root Growth

ROOT GROWTH

Continued root development can occur, especially if the pulp has become totally revascularized (Fig. 10.39). However, root development can continue despite pulp necrosis (201) (Fig. 10.40). Most often, however, root development is partially or completely arrested and the root canal becomes obliterated or bone and PDL can invade the pulp chamber which

Fig. 10.40.
Replantation of a left lateral incisor after extra-alveolar period of 90 minutes. A. Radiograph immediately after replantation. B and C. Condition after 10 months and 1½ years, respectively. Note marked root resorption apparently provoked by the erupting canine. The obliteration of the root canal, especially evident in B, shows that the pulp has survived replantation.

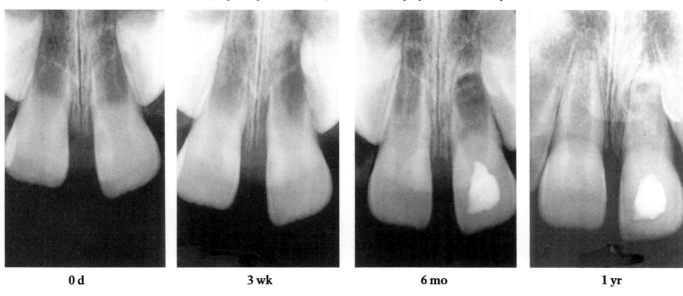

| 0 d | 3 wk | 6 mo | 1 yr |

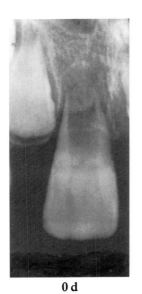 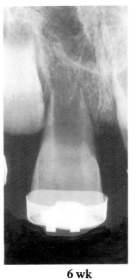 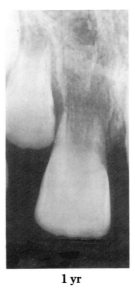 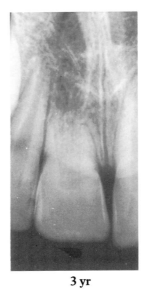 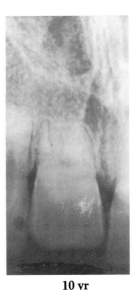

| 0 d | 6 wk | 1 yr | 3 yr | 10 yr |

Fig. 10.41.
Arrested root formation. Bone invasion in the root canal and formation of an internal PDL in a replanted right central incisor. After 12 years infraocclusion was found apparently due to an internal ankylosis process. From AN-DREASEN ET AL. (201) 1993.

in some cases can lead to an ankylosis (Fig. 10.41).

PHANTOM ROOTS

A rare complication to avulsion of immature permanent teeth is the formation of an abnormal root structure at the site of tooth loss (118-120, 194, 197, 198). The explanation for this appears to be that pulp tissue and Hertwig's epithelial root sheath remain in the alveolar socket after avulsion. These tissues resume their formative function after injury. New dentin is formed by the odontoblasts, and the Hertwig's epithelial root sheath initiates root development (118) (Fig. 10.42). A parallel to this is the tooth-like structures occasionally formed when natal or neonatal teeth are extracted and the dental papilla is left *in situ* (121, 122).

Gingival Healing and Loss of Marginal Attachment

Gingival healing is a common finding after replantation, irrespective of storage conditions (202). In cases where the trauma has elicited extensive alveolar damage, loss of marginal bone support may occur.

Complications Due to Early Loss of Teeth

MALFORMATION IN THE DEVELOPING DENTITION

A frequent complication to avulsion of

primary teeth is disturbance in the development of permanent successors (123, 124). This subject is further discussed in Chapter 12.

If it is decided *not* to replant an avulsed permanent tooth, problems arise with regard to further treatment. The same applies to cases where extraction of the replanted tooth is necessary due to root resorption. If no treatment is instituted, a marked degree of spontaneous tooth migration is often seen (90-92, 129). Unfortunately, this drifting is often esthetically undesirable due to midline deviation. Therapy should therefore consist of either orthodontic space closure, prosthetic tooth replacement or autotransplantation or implantation to the site. These treatment solutions are described in Chapters 15 to 20.

SPACE LOSS

With premature loss of *primary* incisors, there are seemingly no major space problems in the permanent dentition (113); however, eruption often occurs in labioversion (114, 115) (Fig. 10.43). A delay in eruption of the succeeding incisors of approximately 1 year is generally found if the loss has occurred at an early stage of development (114, 115). Unless the time of loss is close to the normal time of shedding, premature eruption of permanent successors is rare (116, 117).

Fig. 10.42.
New formation of a root structure after avulsion of a permanent central incisor at the age of 7 years. A. Radiographic condition immediately after injury. B. At follow-up 3½ years later a root structure is found at the site of the avulsed tooth. C. The root is surgically removed. D. Low-power view of sectioned incisor. x 5. E. Fragment of dentin (arrows) representing the apical area at time of injury which together with the pulp tissue and the Hertwig's epithelial root sheath has been left in the tooth socket after avulsion. x 75. F. Normal dentin and odontoblastic layer in the coronal part of the root structure. x 195. From RAVN (118) 1970.

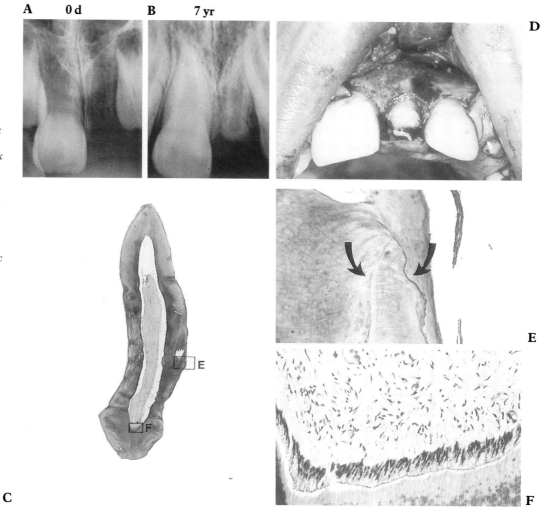

Fig. 10.43.
Eruption disturbances of a right central incisor due to avulsion of its primary predecessor at the age of 2 years. A and B. Clinical and radiographic condition at the age of 7 years. Eruption of the involved permanent tooth is delayed. C. At follow-up 1 year later the right central incisor has erupted in labio-version.

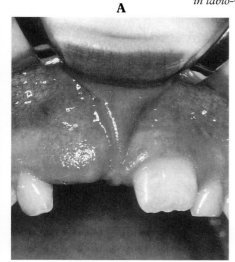
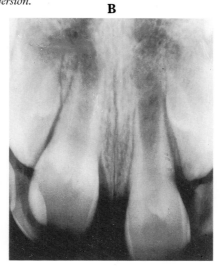
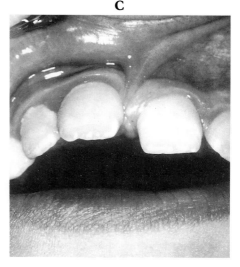

Essentials

Terminology

Complete avulsion (exarticulation)

Frequency

Permanent dentition: 0.5 to 16% dental injuries
Primary dentition: 7 to 13% dental injuries

Etiology

Fall injuries
Sports injuries
Fight injuries

History

Extra-alveolar period
Condition under which the tooth has been preserved

Clinical Examination

Condition of the exarticulated tooth
Condition of the alveolus

Radiographic Examination

Associated bone fractures

Pathology

Repair of pulpal and periodontal structures
Root resorption, external:
a. *Surface resorption*, related to minor areas of damage to the periodontal ligament upon the avulsed tooth.
b. *Replacement resorption*, permanent or transient depending upon the initial extent of damage to the periodontal ligament upon the avulsed tooth.
c. *Inflammatory resorption*, related to the presence of infected necrotic pulp tissue.

Treatment of Permanent Teeth

INDICATIONS FOR REPLANTATION

a. The avulsed tooth should be without advanced periodontal disease.
b. The alveolar socket should be reasonably intact in order to provide a seat for the avulsed tooth.

PROCEDURE FOR REPLANTATION (FIG. 10.22)

Short extra-alveolar storage

a. Immediate replantation by the patient should be encouraged. Otherwise the tooth should be stored in saline, saliva or milk.
b. If obviously contaminated, cleanse the root surface and the apical foramen with a stream of saline (from a syringe). No attempt should be made to sterilize the root surface.
c. Flush the coagulum from the socket with a flow of saline. Examine the alveolar socket. If there is a fracture of the socket wall, reposition the fracture with an instrument.
d. Replant the tooth in its socket using light digital pressure.
e. Suture gingival lacerations.
f. Apply a splint and maintain it for 1 week.
g. Verify normal position of the replanted tooth radiographically.
h. Provide tetanus prophylaxis and antibiotic therapy.
i. In case of mature teeth with a narrow apical foramen, endodontic therapy should be instituted 1 week after replantation and prior to splint removal (see Chapter 14, p. 543).
j. When the apical foramen is wide open and the tooth replanted within 3 hours, revascularization of the pulp is possible.
k. Control the tooth radiographically. If signs of inflammatory resorption appear, institute root canal treatment immediately (see Chapter 14, p. 557).

LONG EXTRA-ALVEOLAR STORAGE

In cases with an extra-oral dry period of 60 min or more, treatment of the tooth with sodium fluoride should be considered.

a. Remove the PDL and extirpate the pulp.
b. Place the tooth for 20 min in a 2.4% sodium fluoride solution.
c. Root fill the tooth extra-orally.
d. Remove the coagulum from the socket.
e. Replant the tooth.
f. Splint the tooth for 2 weeks.

Follow-up: minimum 1 year.

TREATMENT OF ROOT RESORPTION

Surface resorption:
No treatment indicated.

Replacement resorption
a. Extraction in cases with progressive infraocclusion of the ankylosed tooth.
b. Otherwise, preservation of the tooth in the interim before final treatment .

Inflammatory resorption:
Institute root canal therapy (see Chapter 14, p. 557).

Prognosis

Tooth survival: 51 to 89%
PDL healing: 9 to 50%
Pulp healing: 4 to 15%

Complications after premature loss of permanent teeth
a. Close the space orthodontically (see Chapter 15, p 608).
b. Maintain the space by means of auto-transplantation, prosthetics or orthodontic closure (see Chapters 15-20).

Treatment of Primary Teeth

Replantation of avulsed primary teeth is not indicated

Complications after premature loss of primary teeth
a. Space maintenance by prosthetic measures is generally not indicated (see Chapter 15, p. 587).
b. Risk of secondary injuries to developing successors (see Chapter 12, p. 459).

Bibliography

1. ANDREASEN JO. Etiology and pathogenesis of traumatic dental injuries. A clinical study of 1.298 cases. *Scand J Dent Res* 1970;**78:**329-42.

2. DOWN CH. The treatment of permanent incisor teeth of children following traumatic injury. *Aust Dent J* 1957;**2:**9-24.

3. SUNDVALL-HAGLAND I. Olycksfallsskador på tänder och parodontium under barnaåren. In: Holst JJ, Nygaard Østby B, Osvald O. *Nordisk Klinisk Odontologi.* Copenhagen: A/S Forlaget for Faglitteratur, Chapter 11, III:1-40.

4. GELBIER S. Injured anterior teeth in children. A preliminary discussion. *Br Dent J* 1967;**123:**331-5.

5. RAVN JJ, ROSSEN I. Hyppighed og fordeling af traumatiske beskadigelser af tænderne hos københavnske skolebørn 1967/68. *Tandlægebladet* 1969;**73:**1-9.

6. ANDREASEN JO, HJØRTING-HANSEN E. Replantation of teeth. I. Radiographic and clinical study of 110 human teeth replanted after accidental loss. *Acta Odontol Scand* 1966;**24:**263-86.

7. LENSTRUP K, SKIELLER V. Efterundersøgelse af tænder replanteret efter exartikulation. *Tandlægebladet* 1957;**61:**570-83.

8. LENSTRUP K, SKIELLER V. A follow-up study of teeth replanted after accidental loss. *Acta Odontol Scand* 1959;**17:**503-9.

9. SANDERS E. Replantatie van tanden. *T Tandheelk* 1934;**41:**254-66.

10. SCHEFF J. Die Re-, Trans- und Implantation der Zähne. In: Scheff J. *Handbuch der Zahnheilkunde.* Vol. II, No. 2. Wien: Alfred Hölder, 1892:99-128.

11. LUNDQUIST GR. Histo-pathological studies of planted teeth in dogs. In: Black AD. *Operative Dentistry.* Vol. 4. Chicago: Medico-Dental Publishing Company, 1936:200-2.

12. SKILLEN WG, LUNDQUIST GR. A study of the replanted tooth in the dog. *J Dent Res* 1929;**9:**275-6.

13. SKILLEN WG, LUNDQUIST GR. Replanting dog teeth. *J Dent Res* 1934;**14:**177-8.

14. HATTYASY D. Replantationsversuche mit Zahnkeimen. *Dtsch Zahn Mund Kieferheilk* 1940;**9:**535-51.

15. WAITE DE. Animal studies on dental transplants. *Oral Surg Oral Med Oral Pathol* 1956;**9:**40-5.

16. KAQUELER JC, MASSLER M. Healing following tooth replantation. *J Dent Child* 1969;**36:**303-14.

17. SHERMAN P. Intentional replantation of teeth in dogs and monkeys. *J Dent Res* 1968;**47:**1066-71.

18. ROTHSCHILD DL, GOODMAN AA, BLAKEY KR. A histologic study of replanted and transplanted endodontically and nonendodontically treated teeth in dogs. *Oral Surg Oral Med Oral Pathol* 1969;**28:**871-6.

19. MITSCHERLICH A. Die Replantation und die Transplantation der Zähne. *Arch Klin Chir* 1863;**4:**375-417.

20. MENDEL-JOSEPH M, DASSONVILLE M. Recherches expérimentales sur le mécanisme de la consolidation dans la greffe dentaire. *Odontologie* 1906;**36:**99-112.

21. RÖMER KR. Ueber die Replantation von Zähnen. *Dtsch Monatschr Zahnheilk* 1901;**19:**297-306.

22. BÖDECKER CF, LEFKOWITZ W. Replantation of teeth. *Dent Items* 1935;**57:**675-92.

23. KNIGHT MK, GANS BJ, CALANDRA JC. The effect of root canal therapy on replanted teeth of dogs. A gross, roentgenographic, and histologic study. *Oral Surg Oral Med Oral Pathol* 1964;**18:**227-42.

24. HAMMER H. Der histologische Vorgang bei der Zahnreplantation. *Dtsch Zahn Mund Kieferheilk* 1934;**1:**115-36.

25. HAMMER H. Der histologische Vorgang bei der Zahnreplantation nach Vernichtung der Wurzelhaut. *Dtsch Zahn Mund Kieferheilk* 1937;**4:**179-87.

26. HAMMER H. Il reimpianto biologico dei denti. *Mondo Odontostomatol* 1967;**9:**291-302.

27. HOVINGA J. *Replantatie en transplantatie van tanden. Een experimenteel en klinisch onderzoek.* Amsterdam: Oosterbaan & Le Cointre N. V.-Goes, 1968.

28. ANDERSON AW, SHARAV Y, MASSLER M. Periodontal reattachment after tooth replantation. *Periodontics* 1968;**6:**161-7.

29. ANDERSON AW, SHARAV Y, MASSLER M. Reparative dentine formation and pulp morphology. *Oral Surg Oral Med Oral Pathol* 1968;**26:**837-47.

30. HOPPE W, BREMER H. Experimenteller Beitrag zur enossalen Implantation alloplastischen Materials im Kieferbereich. *Dtsch Zahnärztl Z* 1956;**11:**551-61.

31. WILKINSON FC. Some observations on the replantation and transplantation of teeth, with special reference to the pathohistology of the tissues of attachment. *Br Dent J* 1917;**38:**929-39.

32. ROSS WS. Apicectomy in the treatment of dead teeth. *Br Dent J* 1935;**58:**473-86.

33. LÖE H, WAERHAUG J. Experimental replantation of teeth in dogs and monkeys. *Arch Oral Biol* 1961;**3:**176-84.

34. SHULMAN LB, KALIS P, GOLDHABER P. Fluoride inhibition of tooth-replant root resorption in cebus monkeys. *J Oral Ther* 1968;**4:**331-7.

35. GREWE JM, FELTS WJL. Autoradiographic investigation of tritiated thymidine incorporation into replanted and transplanted mouse mandibular incisors. *J Dent Res* 1968;**47:**108-14.

36. MEYERS H, NASSIMBENE L, ALLEY J, GEHRIG J, FLANAGAN VD. Replantation of teeth in the hamster. *Oral Surg Oral Med Oral Pathol* 1954;**7:**1116-29.

37. MEYERS HI, FLANAGAN VD. A comparison of results obtained from transplantation and replantation experiments using Syrian hamster teeth. *Anat Rec* 1958;**130:**497-513.

38. FLANAGAN VD, MEYERS HI. Long-range postoperative evaluation of survival of hamster second molars. *J Dent Res* 1958;**37:**37.

39. FLANAGAN VD, MEYERS HI. The use of a semiliquid postoperative diet following reimplantation of hamster second molars. *J Dent Res* 1959;**38:**667.

40. FLANAGAN VD, MEYERS HI. Postoperative antibiotic therapy used in association with hamster replantation procedures. *J Dent Res* 1960;**39:**726-7.

41. SORG WR. Nerve regeneration in replanted hamster teeth. *J Dent Res* 1960;**39:**1222-31.

42. COSTICH ER, HOEK RB, HAYWARD JR. Replantation of molar teeth in the Syrian hamster. II. *J Dent Res* 1958;**37:**36-7.

43. ÖHMAN A. Healing and sensitivity to pain in young replanted human teeth. An experimental, clinical and histological study. *Odontologisk Tidsskrift* 1965;**73:**165-228.

44. ANDREASEN JO, HJØRTING-HANSEN E. Replantation of teeth. II. Histological study of 22 replanted anterior teeth in humans. *Acta Odontol Scand* 1966;**24:**287-306.

45. ANDREASEN JO. Treatment of fractured and avulsed teeth. *ASDC J Dent Child* 1971;**38:**29-48.

46. HESS W. Zur Frage der Replantation von Zahnkeimen. *Schweiz Monatschr Zahnheilk* 1943;**53:**672-7.

47. SILVA IA, LIMA ACP. Reimplantaçao dentária com preservaçao do periodonto. *An Fac Farm Odontol Sao Paulo* 1954;**12:**309-31.

48. KRØMER H. Tannreplantasjon. En kirurgisk rotbehandlingsmetode. *Norske Tannlægeforenings Tidende* 1952;**62:**147-57.

49. HENRY JL, WEINMANN JP. The pattern of resorption and repair of human cementum. *J Am Dent Assoc* 1951;**42:**270-90.

50. CIRIELLO G. Impianti acrilici ed innesti dentarii nei tessuti mascellari a sostegno di protesi. *Riv Ital Stomatol* 1954;**9:**1087-143.

51. LANGELAND K. Om rotresorpsjoner i permanente tenner. *Norske Tannlægeforenings Tidende* 1958;**68**:237-47.

52. MESSING JJ. Reimplantation of teeth. *Dent Practit Dent Rec* 1968;**18**:241-8.

53. PINDBORG JJ, HANSEN J. A case of replantation of an upper lateral incisor: A histologic study. *Oral Surg Oral Med Oral Pathol* 1951;**4**:661-7.

54. LOVEL RW, HOPPER FE. Tooth replantation: A case report with serial radiographs and histological examination. *Br Dent J* 1954;**97**:205-8.

55. HERBERT WE. A case of complete dislocation of a tooth. *Br Dent J* 1958;**105**:137-8.

56. DEEB E, PRIETTO PP, McKENNA RC. Reimplantation of luxated teeth in humans. *J South Calif Dent Assoc* 1965;**33**:194-206.

57. RIVAS LA. Ergebnisse der Replantation nach Trauma im Frontzahnbereich bei Jugendlichen. *Dtsch Zahnärztl Z* 1968;**23**:484-9.

58. DUNKER L. Über die Behandlung unfallgeschädigter Milchzähne. (Unter besonderer Berücksichtigung der Replantation). *Dtsch Zahnärztebl* 1967;**21**:174-80.

59. SAKELLARIOU PL. Replantation of infected deciduous teeth: A contribution to the problem of their preservation until normal shedding. *Oral Surg Oral Med Oral Pathol* 1963;**16**:645-53.

60. EISENBERG MD. Reimplantation of a deciduous tooth. *Oral Surg Oral Med Oral Pathol* 1965;**19**:588-90.

61. SMELLHAUS S. Über die Replantation der Milchzähne. *Z Stomatol* 1925;**23**:52-7.

62. CASSARDELLI H. Zur Möglichkeit der Erhaltung unfallintrudierter Milchzähne. *Dtsch Stomatol* 1961;**11**:362-8.

63. HERBERT WE. Three successful cases of replacement of teeth immediately following dislocation. *Br Dent J* 1953;**94**:182-3.

64. AXHAUSEN G. Ein Beitrag zur Zahnreplantation. *Zahnärztl Welt* 1948;**3**:130-2.

65. JLG VK. Zur Theorie und Praxis der Replantation. *Dtsch Zahnärztl Z* 1951;**6**:585-94, 653-63.

66. MILLER HM. Reimplanting human teeth. *Dent Surv* 1953;**29**:1439-42.

67. KLUGE R. Indikation und Erfolgsaussichten bei Zahnrückpflanzung. *Zahnärztl Prax* 1957;**23**:1-2.

68. SOMMER RF, OSTRANDER FD, CROWLEY MC. *Clinical endodontics. A manual of scientific endodontics.* 3 edn. Philadelphia: WB Saunders Company, 1966:445-88.

69. RAVN JJ, HELBO M. Replantation af akcidentelt eksarticulerede tænder. *Tandlægebladet* 1966;**70**:805-15.

70. FLANAGAN VD, MEYERS HI. Delayed reimplantation of second molars in the Syrian hamster. *Oral Surg Oral Med Oral Pathol* 1958;**11**:1179-88.

71. McCAGIE JNW. A case of re-implantation of teeth after five days. *Dent Practit Dent Rec* 1958;**8**:320-1.

72. JONCK LM. An investigation into certain aspects of transplantation and reimplantation of teeth in man. *Br J Oral Surg* 1966;**4**:137-46.

73. OGUS WI. Research report on the replant-implant of individual teeth. *Dent Dig* 1954;**60**:358-61.

74. HAMMER H. Replantation and implantation of teeth. *Int Dent J* 1955;**5**:439-57.

75. THONNER KE. Vitalliumstift vid reimplantation av totalluxerade tänder. *Sverig Tandläkar Förbund Tidning* 1956;**48**:216-7.

76. WEISKOPF J, GEHRE G, GRAICHEN K-H. Ein Beitrag zur Behandlung von Luxationen und Wurzelfrakturen im Frontzahngebiet. *Stoma (Heidelberg)* 1961;**14**:100-13.

77. CIRIELLO G. Alcune considerazioni sulla tecnica del reimpianto dentario. *Riv Ital Stomatol* 1953;**8**:764-99.

78. ORLAY HG. Befestigung von lockeren Zähnen mit endodontischen Implantaten. *Schweiz Monatschr Zahnheilk* 1968;**78**:580-98.

79. ARCHER WH. Replantation of an accidentally extracted erupted partially formed mandibular second premolar. *Oral Surg Oral Med Oral Pathol* 1952;**5**:256-8.

80. LINDAHL B, MÅRTENSSON K. Replantation of a tooth. A case report. *Odontologisk Revy* 1960;**11**:325-30.

81. LJUNGDAHL L, MÅRTENSSON K. Ett fall av multipla tandreplantationer. *Odontologisk Revy* 1955;**6**:222-32.

82. PÅLSSON F. Zur Frage der Replantation von Zahnkeimen. *Acta Odontol Scand* 1944;**5**:63-78.

83. HENNING FR. Reimplantation of luxated teeth. *Aust Dent J* 1965;**10**:306-12.

84. SWEDBERG Y. Replantation av accidentellt luxerade tandanlag. *Svensk Tannläkar Tidning* 1966;**59**:649-54.

85. COOKE C, ROWBOTHAM TC. Treatment of injuries to anterior teeth. *Br Dent J* 1951;**91**:146-52.

86. ELLIS RG, DAVEY KV. *The classification and treatment of injuries to the teeth of children.* 5 edn. Chicago: Year Book Publishers Inc., 1970.

87. BENNET DT. Traumatised anterior teeth. VI. The class V injury. *Br Dent J* 1964;**116**:7-9.

88. ENGELHARDT JP. Die prothetische Versorgung des traumatisch geschädigten Jugendgebisses aus klinischer Sicht. *Zahnärztl Welt* 1968;**69**:264-70.

89. SEIPEL CM. Ortodontiska synpunkter beträffande terapien vid kronfraktur på framtänder hos barn i skolåldern. *Svensk Tannläkars Tidning* 1940;**33**:14-27.

90. PERSSON B. Bettortopediska synpunkter på behandlingen särskilt valet mellam konserverande terapi och extraktion i incisivområdet. In: Holst JJ, Nygaard Østby B, Osvald O. *Nordisk Klinisk Odontologi.* Copenhagen: A/S Forlaget for Faglitteratur, 1964, Chapter 11, III:35-8.

91. PERSSON B. The traumatised front tooth. Orthodontic aspects. *Eur Orthodont Soc Trans* 1965;**41**:329-45.

92. BRUTSZT P. Die Selbstregelung der Zahnreihe nach dem Verlust des oberen mittleren Schneidezahnes im Wechselgebiss. *Schweiz Monatschr Zahnheilk* 1956;**66**:926-31.

93. HOTZ R. Die Bedeutung, Beurteilung und Behandlung beim Trauma im Frontzahngebiet vom Standpunkt des Kieferorthopäden. *Dtsch Zahnärztl Z* 1958;**13**:42-51, 401-16.

94. SCHMUTH GPF. Die Behandlung des traumatischen Zahnverlustes durch kieferorthopädische Massnahmen. *Zahnärztl Welt* 1967;**68**:15-9.

95. VETTER H. Zwei Fälle von frühzeitigem Frontzahnverlust durch Trauma und ihre Versorgung. *Fortschr Kieferorthop* 1954;**15**:90-101.

96. VOSS R. Problematik, Möglichkeiten und Grenzen des prothetischen Lückenschlusses im Frontzahnbereich bei Jugendlichen. *Fortschr Kieferorthop* 1969;**30**:89-101.

97. RINDERER L. Deux cas de traitement orthodontique après perte traumatique des deux incisives centrales. *Rev Stomatol (Paris)*;**61**:627-32.

98. REICHENBACH E. Unfallverletzungen im Kindesalter. *Dtsch Stomatol* 1954;**4**:33-42.

99. SCHULZE C. Über die Folgen des Verlustes oberer mittlerer Schneidezähne während der Gebissentwicklung. *Zahnärztl Rdsch* 1967;**76**:156-69.

100. ESCHLER J, SCHILLI W, WITT E. *Die traumatischen Verletzungen der Frontzähne bei Jugendlichen.* 3 edn. Heidelberg: Alfred Hüthig Verlag, 1972.

101. KIPP H. Traumatischer Zahnverlust bei kieferorthopädischen Krankheitsbildern. *Fortschr Kieferorthop* 1958;**19**:165-70.

102. RAVN JJ. *Ulykkesskadede fortænder på børn. Klassifikation og behandling.* Copenhagen: Odontologisk Forening, 1966.

103. LJUNGDAHL L. Ett fall av korrektion efter trauma på överkäksincisiverna. *Odontologisk Revy* 1954;**5**:212-7.

104. MAIER-MOHR I. Über kieferorthopädische Massnahmen beim Verlust eines mittleren oberen Schneidezahnes. *Fortschr Kieferorthop* 1955;**16**:357-61.

105. FREUNTHALLER P. Möglichkeiten des Lückenschlusses durch orthodontische Massnahmen bei Frontzahnverlust. *Österr Z Stomatol* 1964;**61**:467-74.

106. HEDEGÅRD B. The traumatised front tooth. Some prosthetic aspects of therapeutic procedures. *Eur Orthod Soc Trans* 1965;**41**:347-51.

107. HECKMANN U. Die kieferorthopädische Therapie beim Frontzahnverlust im jugendlichen Alter. *Dtsch Zahnärztl Z* 1960;**15**:43-7.

108. ROSE JS. Early loss of teeth in children. *Br Dent J* 1966;**120**:275-80.

109. GRANATH L-E. Några synpunkter på behandlingen av traumatiserade incisiver på barn. *Odontologisk Revy* 1959;**10**:272-86.

110. BROGLIA ML, GUASTA G. Il problema terapeutico della lussazione totale traumatica degli incisivi permanenti nei pazienti di età pediatrica. *Minerva Stomatol* 1968;**17**:549-56.

111. BIOURGE A. Traumatismes violents des incisives supérieures dans le jeune age. *Rev Stomatol (Paris)* 1968;**69**:30-43.

112. HAUSSER E, BACKHAUS I, PELAEZ H, GREVE MR. Traitement orthodontique après traumatismes dento-alvéolaires. *Orthod Fr* 1967;**38**:382-3.

113. DAUSCH-NEUMANN D. Über die Lücken bei fehlenden Milchfrontzähnen. *Fortschr Kieferorthop* 1969;**30**:82-8.

114. ASH AS. Orthodontic significance of anomalies of tooth eruption. *Am J Orthod* 1957;**43**:559-76.

115. KORF SR. The eruption of permanent central incisors following premature loss of their antecedents. *ASDC J Dent Child* 1965;**32**:39-44.

116. BROGLIA ML, DANA F. Manifestazioni cliniche delle lesioni traumatiche accidentali della dentatura decidua. *Minerva Stomatol* 1967;**16**:623-35.

117. GYSEL C. Traumatologie et orthodontie. *Rev Fr Odontostomatol* 1962;**9**:1091-113.

118. RAVN JJ. Partiel roddannelse efter eksartikulation af permanent incisiv hos en 7-årig dreng. *Tandlægebladet* 1970;**74**:906-10.

119. LYSELL G, LYSELL L. A unique case of dilaceration. *Odontologisk Revy* 1969;**20**:43-6.

120. GIBSON ACL. Continued root development after traumatic avulsion of partly-formed permanent incisor. *Br Dent J* 1969;**126**:356-7.

121. SOUTHAM JC. Retained dentine papillae in the newborn. A clinical and histopathological study. *Br Dent J* 1968;**125**:534-8.

122. RYBA GE, KRAMER IRH. Continued growth of human dentine papillae following removal of the crowns of partly formed deciduous teeth. *Oral Surg Oral Med Oral Pathol* 1962;**15**:867-75.

123. ANDREASEN JO, SUNDSTRÖM B, RAVN JJ. The effect of traumatic injuries to primary teeth on their permanent successors. I. A clinical and histologic study of 117 injured permanent teeth. *Scand J Dent Res* 1971;**79**:219-83.

124. ANDREASEN JO, RAVN JJ. The effect of traumatic injuries to primary teeth on their permanent successors. II. A clinical and radiographic follow-up study of 213 teeth. *Scand J Dent Res* 1971;**79**:284-94.

125. HEDEGÅRD B, STÅLHANE I. A study of traumatized permanent teeth in children aged 7-15 years. Part I. *Swed Dent J* 1973;**66**:431-50.

126. RAVN JJ. Dental injuries in Copenhagen schoolchildren, school years 1967-1972. *Community Dent Oral Epidemiol* 1974;**2**:231-45.

127. KEMP WB, GROSSMAN LI, PHILLIPS J. Evaluation of 71 replanted teeth. *J Endod* 1977;**3**:30-5.

128. HÖRSTER W, ALTFELD F, PLANKO D. Behandlungsergebnisse nach Replantation total luxierter Frontzähne. *Fortsch Kiefer Gesichtschir* 1976;**20**:127-9.

129. RAVN JJ. En redegørelse for behandlingen efter exarticulation af permanente incisiver i en skolebarnspopulation. *Tandlægebladet* 1977;**81**:563-9.

130. GROPER JN, BERNICK S. Histological study of the periodontium following replantation of teeth in the dog. *ASDC J Dent Child* 1970;**37**:25-35.

131. ANDERSON AW, MASSLER M. Periapical tissue reactions following root amputation in immediate tooth replants. *Israel J Dent Med* 1970;**19**:1-8.

132. MONSOUR FNT. Pulpal changes following the reimplantation of teeth in dogs. A histologic study. *Aust Dent J* 1971;**16**:227-31.

133. GOMBOS F, BUONAIUTO C, CARUSO F. Nuovi orientamenti sui reimpianti dentari studio clinico e sperimentale. *Mondo Odontostomatol* 1972;**4**:589-610.

134. SCHMID F, TRIADAN H, KÜPPER W. Tierexperimentelle Untersuchungen zur Elektrostimulation der Pulpa nach Replantation. *Fortschrit Kiefer Gesichtschir* 1976;**20**:132-4.

135. WOEHRLE RR. Cementum regeneration in replanted teeth with differing pulp treatment. *J Dent Res* 1976;**55**:235-8.

136. SKOGLUND A, TRONSTAD L. A morphologic and enzyme histochemical study on the pulp of replanted and autotransplanted teeth in young dogs. *J Dent Res* 1978;**57**:IADR Abstract no. 478.

137. SKOGLUND A, TRONSTAD L, WALLENIUS K. A microangiographic study of vascular changes in replanted and autotransplanted teeth of young dogs. *Oral Surg Oral Med Oral Pathol* 1978;**45**:17-28.

138. ANDREASEN JO. A time-related study of root resorption activity after replantation of mature permanent incisors in monkeys. *Swed Dent J* 1980;**4**:101-10.

139. ANDREASEN JO. Relationship between surface- and inflammatory root resorption and changes in the pulp after replantation of permanent incisors in monkeys. *J Endod* 1981;**7**:294-301.

140. ANDREASEN JO. Analysis of topography of surface- and inflammatory root resorption after replantation of mature permanent incisors in monkeys. *Swed Dent J* 1980;**4**:135-44.

141. ANDREASEN JO, SCHWARTZ O, ANDREASEN FM. The effect of apicoectomy before replantation on periodontal and pulpal healing in monkeys. *Int J Oral Surg* 1985; **14**:176-83

142. ANDREASEN JO. Relationship between cell damage in the periodontal ligament after replant or removal of the periodontal ligament. Periodontal healing after replantation of mature permanent incisors in monkeys. *Acta Odontol Scand* 1981;**39**:15-25.

143. ANDREASEN JO. Periodontal healing after replantation and autotransplantation of permanent incisors. Effect of injury to the alveolar or cemental part of the periodontal ligament in monkeys. *Int J Oral Surg* 1981;**10**:54-61.

144. ANDREASEN JO, KRISTERSON L. The effect of limited drying or removal of the periodontal ligament. Perodontal healing after replantation of mature permanent incisors in monkeys. *Acta Odontol Scand* 1981;**39**:1-13.

145. ANDREASEN JO, KRISTERSON L. Repair processes in the cervical region of replanted and transplanted teeth in monkeys. *Int J Oral Surg* 1981;**10**:128-36.

146. ANDREASEN JO. Effect of extra-alveolar period and storage media upon periodontal and pulpal healing after replantation of mature permanent incisors in monkeys. *Int J Oral Surg* 1981;**10**:43-53.

147. ANDREASEN JO. The effect of splinting upon periodontal healing after replantation of permanent incisors in monkeys. *Acta Odontol Scand* 1975;**33**:313-23.

148. ANDREASEN JO. The effect of excessive occlusal trauma upon periodontal healing after replantation of mature permanent incisors in monkeys. *Swed Dent J* 1981;**5**:115-22.

149. ANDREASEN JO. The effect of pulp extirpation or root canal treatment on periodontal healing after replantation of mature permanent incisors in monkeys. *J Endod* 1981;7:245-52.

150. ANDREASEN JO. The effect of removal of the coagulum in the alveolus before replantation upon periodontal and pulpal healing of mature permanent incisors in monkeys. *Int J Oral Surg* 1980;9:458-61.

151. ANDREASEN JO. Interrelation between alveolar bone and periodontal ligament repair after replantation of mature permanent incisors in monkeys. *J Periodontal Res* 1981;16:228-35.

152. ANDREASEN JO, KRISTERSON L. The effect of extra-alveolar root filling with calcium hydroxide on periodontal healing after replantation of permanent incisors in monkeys. *J Endod* 1981;7:349-54.

153. TRONSTAD L, ANDREASEN JO, HASSELGREN G, KRISTERSON L, RIIS I. pH changes in dental tissues after root canal filling with calcium hydroxide. *J Endod* 1981;7:17-22.

154. ANDREASEN JO, REINHOLDT J, RIIS I, DYBDAHL R, SÖDER P-Ö, OTTESKOG P. Periodontal and pulpal healing of monkey incisors preserved in tissue culture before replantation. *Int J Oral Surg* 1978;7:104-12.

155. ANDREASEN JO. Delayed replantation after submucosal storage in order to prevent root resorption after replantation. An experimental study in monkeys. *Int J Oral Surg* 1980;9:394-403.

156. ANDREASEN JO, KRISTERSON L. Evaluation of different types of autotransplanted connective tissues as potential periodontal ligament substitutes. An experimental replantation study in monkeys. *Int J Oral Surg* 198;10:189-201.

157. HAMNER JE, REED OM, STANLEY HR. Reimplantation of teeth in the baboon. *J Am Dent Assoc* 1970;81:662-70.

158. CASTELLI WA, NASJLETI CE, HUELKE DR, DIAZ-PEREZ R. Revascularization of the periodontium after tooth grafting in monkeys. *J Dent Res* 1971;50:414-21.

159. HURST RVV. Regeneration of periodontal and transseptal fibres after autografts in Rhesus monkeys. A qualitative approach. *J Dent Res* 1972;51:1183-92.

160. KELLER EB, HAYWARD JR, NASJLETI CE, CASTELLI WA. Venous tissue replanted on roots of teeth in monkeys. *Oral Surg Oral Med Oral Pathol* 1972;34:352-63.

161. NORDENRAM Å, BANG G, ANNEROTH G. A histologic study of replanted teeth with superficially demineralised root surfaces in Java monkeys. *Scand J Dent Res* 1973;81:294-302.

162. NASJLETI CE, CAFFESSI RG, CASTELLI WA, HOKE JA. Healing after tooth reimplantation in monkeys. A radioautographic study. *Oral Surg Oral Med Oral Pathol* 1975;39:361-75.

163. NASJLETI CE, CASTELLI WA, BLANKENSHIP JR. The storage of teeth before reimplantation in monkeys. *Oral Surg Oral Med Oral Pathol* 1975;39:20-9.

164. BARBAKOW FH, AUSTIN JC, CLEATON-JONES PE. Experimental replantation of root-canal-filled and untreated teeth in the vervet monkey. *J Endod* 1977;3:89-93.

165. CAFFESSI RG, NASJLETI CE, CASTELLI WA. Long-term results after intentional tooth reimplantation in monkeys. *Oral Surg Oral Med Oral Pathol* 1977;44:666-78.

166. NASJLETI CE, CAFFESSI RG, CASTELLI WA. Replantation of mature teeth without endodontics in monkeys. *J Dent Res* 1978;57:650-8.

167. MANDELL ML, BERTRAM U. Calcitonin treatment for root resorption. *J Dent Res* 1970;49:182.

168. BJORVATN K, MASSLER M. Effect of fluorides on root resorption in replanted rat molars. *Acta Odontol Scand* 1971;29:17-29.

169. BJORVATN K, WEISS MB. Effect of topical application of fluoride, cortisone and tetracycline on replanted rat molars. *Fasset* 1971;1:27-31.

170. JOHANSEN JR. Reimplantation of mandibular incisors in the guinea pig: a histologic and autoradiographic study. *Acta Odontol Scand* 1970;28:633-60.

171. ANDREASEN JO. Periodontal healing after replantation of traumatically avulsed human teeth. Assessment by mobility testing and radiography. *Acta Odontol Scand* 1975;33:325-35.

172. LINE SE, POLSON AM, ZANDER HA. Relationship between periodontal injury, selective cell repopulation and ankylosis. *J Periodontol* 1974;45:725-30.

173. KRISTERSON L, ANDREASEN JO. The effect of splinting upon periodontal and pulpal healing after autotransplantation of mature and immature permanent incisors in monkeys. *Int J Oral Surg* 1983;12:239-49.

174. CVEK M. Treatment of non-vital permanent incisors with calcium hydroxide. II. Effect on external root resorption in luxated teeth compared with effect of root filling with gutta percha. A follow-up. *Odontologisk Revy* 1973;24:343-54.

175. SHULMAN LB, GEDALIA I, FEINGOLD RM. Fluoride concentration in the root surfaces and alveolar bone of fluoride-immersed monkey incisors three weeks after replantation. *J Dent Res* 1973;52:1314-6.

176. SHULMAN LB, KALIS P, GOLDHABER P. Fluoride inhibition of tooth-replant root resorption in cebus monkeys. *J Oral Ther Pharm* 1968;4:331-7.

177. SHULMAN LB. Allogenic tooth transplantation. *J Oral Surg* 1972;30:395-409.

178. MINK JR, VAN SCHAIK M. Intentional avulsion and replantation of dog teeth with varied root surface treatment. *J Dent Res* 1968;43:48.

179. REEVE CM, SATHER AH, PARKER JA. Resorption pattern of replanted formalin-fixed teeth in dogs. *J Dent Res* 1964;43:825.

180. BUTCHER EO, VIDAIR RV. Periodontal fiber reattachment in replanted incisors of the monkey. *J Dent Res* 1955;34:569-76.

181. ROBINSON PJ, SHAPIRO IM. Effect of diphosphates on root resorption. *J Dent Res* 1976;55:166.

182. HODOSH M, POVAR M, SHKLAR G. The dental polymer implant concept. *J Prosthet Dent* 1969;22:371-80.

183. HUEBSCH RF. Implanting teeth with methyl-2-cyanoacrylate adhesive. *J Dent Res* 1967;46:337-9.

184. SHERMAN P. Intentional replantation of teeth in dogs and monkeys. *J Dent Res* 1968;47:1066-71.

185. MUELLER BH, WHITSETT BD. Management of an avulsed deciduous incisor. Report of a case. *Oral Surg Oral Med Oral Pathol* 1978;46:442-6.

186. BARRY GN. Replanted teeth still functioning after 42 years: report of a case. *J Am Dent Assoc* 1976;92:412-3.

187. GRÖNDAHL H-G, KAHNBERG K-E, OLSSON G. Traumatiserade tänder. En klinisk och röntgenologisk efterundersökning. *Göteborg Tandläkar-Sällskabs Artikelserie* no 384 Årsbok 1974:37-50.

188. CVEK M, GRANATH LE, HOLLENDER L. Treatment of non-vital permanent incisors with calcium hydroxide. III. Variation of occurrence of ankylosis of reimplanted teeth with duration of extra-alveolar period and storage environment. *Odontologisk Revy* 1974;25:43-56.

189. WEPNER F. Die Replantation der Frontzähne nach traumatischen Zahnverlust. *Österr Z Stomatol* 1976;73:275-82

190. HARNDT R, HOEFIG W. Replantation of traumatically avulsed teeth. *Quintessense Int* 1972;3:19-22.

191. TOSTI A. Reimplantation: report of a case. *Dent Dig* 1970;76:98-100.

192. ADATIA AK. Odontogenesis following replantation of erupted maxillary central incisor. *Dent Pract* 1971;21:153-5.

193. PORTEOUS JR. Vital reimplantation of a maxillary central incisor tooth: report of a case. *ASDC J Dent Child* 1972;39:429-31.

194. BARKER BCW, MAYNE JR. Some unusual cases of apexification subsequent to trauma. *Oral Surg Oral Med Oral Pathol* 1975;39:144-50.

195. ECKSTEIN A. Reimplantation of permanent front teeth with incomplete root growth. *Fortschr Kiefer Gesichtschir* 1976;**20**:125-7.

196. MEYER-BARDOWICKS J. Eine Zahnreplantation mit Erhaltung der Pulpavitalität. *Quintessenz* 1977;**28**:39-42.

197. BURLEY MA, REECE RD. Root formation following traumatic loss of an immature incisor: a case report. *Br Dent J* 1976;**141**:315-6.

198. OLIET S. Apexogenesis associated with replantation. A case history. *Dent Clin North Am* 1974;**18**:457-64.

199. ANDREASEN JO, BORUM M, JACOBSEN HL, ANDREASEN FM. Replantation of 400 traumatically avulsed permanent incisors. I. Diagnosis of healing complications. *Endod Dent Traumatol* 1993, to be submitted.

200. ANDREASEN JO, BORUM M, JACOBSEN HL, ANDREASEN FM. Replantation of 400 avulsed permanent incisors. II. Factors related to pulp healing. *Endod Dent Traumatol* 1993. To be submitted.

201. ANDREASEN JO, BORUM M, ANDREASEN FM. Replantation of 400 avulsed permanent incisors. III. Factors related to root growth after replantation. *Endod Dent Traumatol* 1993, To be submitted.

202. ANDREASEN JO, BORUM M, JACOBSEN HL, ANDREASEN FM. Replantation of 400 avulsed permanent incisors. IV. Factors related to periodontal ligament healing. *Endod Dent Traumatol* 1993, To be submitted.

203. ANDREASEN JO, BORUM M, JACOBSEN HL, ANDREASEN FM. Replantation of 400 avulsed permanent incisors. V. Factors related to the progression of root resorption. *Endod Dent Traumatol* 1993, To be submitted.

204. KVINNSLAND I, HEYERAAS KJ. Dentin and osteodentin matrix formation in apicoectomized replanted incisors in cats. *Acta Odontol Scand* 1989;**47**:41-52.

205. KVINNSLAND I, HEYERAAS KJ. Cell renewal and ground substance formation in replanted cat teeth. *Acta Odontol Scand* 1990;**48**:203-15.

206. HOLLAND GR, ROBINSON PP. Pulp re-innervation in re-implanted canine teeth of the cat. *Arch Oral Biol* 1987;**32**:593-7.

207. LOESCHER AR, ROBINSON PP. Characteristics of periodontal mechanoreceptors supplying reimplanted canine teeth in cats. *Arch Oral Biol* 1991;**36**:33-40.

208. ROBINSON PP. An electrophysiological study of the reinnervation of reimplanted and autotransplanted teeth in the cat. *Arch Oral Biol* 1983;**28**:1139-47.

209. SKOGLUND A, TRONSTAD L, WALLENIUS K. A microangiographic study of vascular changes in replanted and autotransplanted teeth of young dogs. *Oral Surg Oral Med Oral Patol* 1978;**45**:17-28.

210. SKOGLUND A. Vascular changes in replanted and autotransplanted apicoectomized mature teeth of dogs. *Int J Oral Surg* 1981;**10**:100-10.

211. SKOGLUND A. Pulpal changes in replanted and autotransplanted apicectomized mature teeth of dogs. *Int J Oral Surg* 1981;**10**:111-121.

212. SKOGLUND A, HASSELGREN G, TRONSTAD L. Oxidoreductase activity in the pulp of replanted and autotransplanted teeth in young dogs. *Oral Surg Oral Med Oral Pathol* 1981;**52**:205-9.

213. KIRSCHNER H, MICHEL G. Mikromorphologische Untersuchungen der Nervregeneration im heilenden Desmodont bei Java-Makaken (Cynomolgus). *Dtsch Zahnärztl Z* 1982;**37**:929-36.

214. DURR DP, SVEEN OB. Influence of apicoectomy on the pulps of replanted monkey teeth. *Pediatr Dent* 1986;**8**:129-33.

215. LINDSKOG S, BLOMLÖF L, HAMMERSTRÖM L. Mitoses and microorganisms in the periodontal membrane after storage in milk or saliva. *Scand J Dent Res* 1983;**91**:465-72.

216. LINDSKOG S, PIERCE A, BLOMLÖF L, HAMMARSTRÖM L. The role of the necrotic periodontal membrane in cementum resorption and ankylosis. *Endod Dent Traumatol* 1985;**1**:96-101.

217. LINDSKOG S, BLOMLÖF L, HAMMARSTRÖM L. Cellular colonization of denuded root surfaces in vivo: cell morphology in dentin resorption and cementum repair. *Clin Periodontol* 1987;**14**:390-5.

218. LINDSKOG S, BLOMLÖF L, HAMMARSTRÖM L. Dentin resorption in replanted monkey incisors. Morphology of dentinoclast spreading in vivo. *J Clin Periodontol* 1988;**15**:365-70.

219. ANNEROTH G, LUNDQUIST G, NORDENRAM Å, SÖDER P-Ö. Re- and allotransplantation of teeth - an experimental study in monkeys. *Int J Oral Maxillofac Surg* 1988;**17**:54-7.

220. NASJLETI CE. Effect of fibronectin on healing of replanted teeth in monkeys: A histologic and autoradiographic study. *Oral Surg Oral Med Oral Pathol* 1987;**63**:291-9.

221. ANDREASEN JO. Experimental dental traumatology: development of a model for external root resoption. *Endod Dent Traumatol* 1987;**3**:269-87.

222. ANDERSSON L, JONSSON BG, HAMMARSTRÖM L, BLOMLÖF L, ANDREASEN JO, LINDSKOG S. Evaluation of statistics and desirable experimental design of a histomorphometrical method for studies of root resorption. *Endod Dent Traumatol* 1987;**3**:288-95.

223. KRISTERSON L, ANDREASEN JO. Influence of root development on periodontal and pulpal healing after replantation of incisors in monkeys. *Int J Oral Surg* 1984;**13**:313-23.

224. KRISTERSON L, ANDREASEN JO. Autotransplantation and replantation of tooth germs in monkeys. Effect of damage to the dental follicle and position of transplant in the alveolus. *Int J Oral Surg* 1984;**13**:324-33.

225. CVEK M, CLEATON-JONES P, AUSTIN J, LOWNIE J, KLING M, FATTI P. Pulp revascularization in reimplanted immature monkey incisors -predictability and the effect of antibiotic systemic prophylaxis. *Endod Dent Traumatol* 1990,**6**:157-69.

226. CVEK M, CLEATON-JONES P, AUSTIN J, KLING M, LOWNIE J, FATTI P. Effect of topical application of doxycycline on pulp revascularization and peridontal healing in reimplanted monkey incisors. *Endod Dent Traumatol* 1990;**6**:170-6.

227. BREIVIK M, KVAM E. Evaluation of histological criteria applied for description of reactions in replanted human premolars. *Scand J Dent Res* 1977;**85**:392-5.

228. BREIVIK M. Human odontoblast response to teeth replantation. *Eur J Orthod* 1981;**3**:95-108.

229. BREIVIK M, KVAM E. Secondary dentin in replanted teeth - a histometric study. *Endod Dent Traumatol* 1990;**6**:150-2.

230. BREIVIK M, KVAM E. Histometric study of root resorption on human premolars following experimental replantation. *Scand J Dent Res* 1987;**95**:273-80.

231. ANDREASEN JO, ANDREASEN FM. Root resoption following traumatic dental injuries. *Proc Finn Dent Soc* 1991; **88**:95-114.

232. HACKER W, FISCHBACH H. Spätergebnisse nach 35 Zahnreplantationen im Frontzahnbereich. *Dtsch Zahnärztl Z* 1983;**38**:466-9.

233. MANDEL U, VIIDIK A. Effect of splinting on the mechanical and histological properties of the healing periodontal ligament after experimental extrusive luxation in the vervet monkey (Cercopithecus aethiops). *Arch Oral Biol* 1989;**34**:209-17.

234. HAMMARSTRÖM L, BLOMLÖF L, LINDSKOG S. Dynamics of dentoalveolar ankylosis and associated root resorption. *Endod Dent Traumatol* 1989;**5**:163-75.

235. ANDERSSON L, BLOMLÖF L, LINDSKOG S, FEIGLIN B, HAMMARSTRÖM L. Tooth ankylosis. Clinical, radiographic and histological assessments. *Int J Oral Surg* 1984;**13**:423-31.

236. STENVIK A, BEYER-OLSEN EMS, ÅBYHOLM F, HAANÆS HR, GERNER NW. Validity of the radiographic assessment of ankylosis. Evaluation of long-term reactions in 10 monkey incisors. *Acta Odontol Scand* 1990;**48**:265-69.

237. SCHMITZ R, DONATH K. Morphologische Veränderungen an traumatisierten Zähnen. Eine klinische und patho-histologische Studie. *Dtsch Zahnärztl Z* 1983;**38**:462-5.

238. Hiltz J, Trope M. Vitality of human lip fibroblasts in milk, Hanks balanced salt solution and Viaspan storage media. *Endod Dent Traumatol* 1991;7:69-72.

239. Morley RS, Malloy R, Hurst RVV, James R. Analysis of functional splinting upon autologously reimplanted teeth. *J Dent Res* 1978;57:IADR Abstract no.593.

240. Nasjleti CE, Castelli WA, Caffesse RG. The effects of different splinting times on replantation of teeth in monkeys. *Oral Surg Oral Med Oral Pathol* 1982;53:557-66.

241. Andersson L, Lindskog S, Blomlöf L, Hedström K-G, Hammarström L. Effect of masticatory stimulation on dentoalveolar ankylosis after experimental tooth replantation. *Endod Dent Traumatol* 1985;1:13-6.

242. Hammarström L, Blomlöf L, Feiglin B, Andersson L, Lindskog S. Replantation of teeth and antibiotic treatment. *Endod Dent Traumatol* 1986;2:51-7.

243. Kling M, Cvek M, Mejare I. Rate and predictability of pulp revascularization in therapeutically reimplanted permanent incisors. *Endod Dent Traumatol* 1986;2:83-9.

244. Hammarström L, Blomlöf L, Feiglin B, Lindskog S. Effect of calcium hydroxide treatment on periodontal repair and root resorption. *Endod Dent Traumatol* 1986b;2:184-9.

245. Bjorvatn K, Selvig KA, Klinge B, Effect of tetracycline and SnF on root resorption in replanted incisors in dogs. *Scand J Dent Res* 1989;97:477-82.

246. Selvig KA, Bjorvatn K, Claffey N. Effect of stannous flouride and tetracycline on repair after delayed replantation of root-planed teth in dogs. *Acta Odontol Scand* 1990;48:107-12.

247. Klinge B, Nilvéus R, Selvig KA. The effect of citric acid on repair after delayed tooth replantation in dogs. *Acta Odontol Scand* 1984;42:351-9.

248. Zervas P, Lambrianidis T, Karabouta-Vulgaropuolou I. The effect of citric acid treatment on periodontal healing after replantation of permanent teeth. *Int Endod J* 1991;24:317-25.

249. Walsh JS, Fey MR, Omnell LM. The effects of indomethacin on resorption and ankylosis in replanted teeth. *ASDC J Dent Child* 1987;54:261-6.

250. Coccia CT. A clinical investigation of root resorption rates in reimplanted young permanent incisors: A five-year study. *J Endod* 1980;6:413-20.

251. Kirschner H, Bolz U, Enomoto S, Hüttemann RW, Meinel W, Sturm J. Eine neue Methode kombinierter auto-alloplastischer Zahnreplantation mit partieller Al2 O3 -Keramikwurzel. *Dtsch Zahnärztl Z* 1978;33:549.

252. Bolz U, Hüttemann RW, Kirschner H, Sturm J. Indications for the clinical use of combined auto-alloplastic tooth reimplantation with aluminium oxide (Al2 O3) ceramic. In: Heimke G, ed. *Dental Implants. Materials and Systems.* München, Wien: Carl Hanser Verlag 1980:81-8.

253. Kirschner H, Bolz U, Hüttemann RW, Sturm J. Autoplastic tooth reimplantation with partial ceramic roots made of Al2 O3 . In: Heimke G, ed. *Dental Implants. Materials and Systems. München,* Wien: Carl Hanser Verlag 1980:55-62.

254. Burk W, Brinkmann E. Indikation und Anwendung des auto-alloplastischen Replantationsverfahrens nach Kirschner. Vorläufiger Bericht. *Zahnärztl Prax* 1980;31:347-55.

255. Kirschner H. Chirurgische Zahnerhaltung. Experimente mit Aluminiumoxid-Keramik. *Dtsch Zahnärztl Z* 1981;36:274-85.

256. Brinkmann E. Indikation und Anwendung der chirurgischen Zahnerhaltung. *Zahnärztl Mitt* 1982;72:1-12.

257. Brinkmann E. Die Einzelzahnlücke aus implantologischer Sicht. *Zahnärztl Prax* 1982;7:286-91.

258. Herforth A. Zur Stabilisierung gelockerter Zähne durch transdentale Fixation. *Dtsch Zahnärztl Z* 1983;38:129-30.

259. Kirschner H. Chirurgische Zahnerhaltung. Experimente mit Aluminiumoxid-Keramik. *Dtsch Zahnärztl Z* 1981;36:274-85.

260. Kirschner H. *Atlas der chirurgischen Zahnerhaltung.* München: Hanser Verlag, 1987.

261. Nentwig GH. Geschlossene keramische Implantate zur Reintegration traumatisch geschädigter bleibender Zähne. *Fortschr Zahnärztl Implantol* 1985;1:272-6.

262. Nentwig GH, Berbecariu C, Saller S. Zur Prognose des replantierten Zahnes nach schweren Luxationsverletzungen. *Dtsch Zahnärztl Z* 1987;42:205-7.

263. Koch G, Ullbro C. Klinisk funktionstid hos 55 exartikulerade och replanterade tänder. *Tannläkartidningen* 1982;74:18-25.

264. Herforth A. *Traumatische Schädigungen der Frontzähne bei Kindern und Jugendlichen im Alter von 7 bis 15 Jahren.* Berlin: Quintessenz Verlag GmbH, 1982.

265. Jacobsen I. Long term evaluation, prognosis and subsequent management of traumatic tooth injuries. In: Gutmann JL, Harrison JW, eds. *Proceedings of the International Conference on Oral Trauma.* Chicago: American Association of Endodontists Endowment & Memorial Foundation, 1986;129-34.

266. Gonda F, Nagase M, Chen R-B, Yakata H, Nakajima T. Replantation: An analysis of 29 teeth. *Oral Surg Oral Med Oral Pathol* 1990;70:650-5.

267. Mackie IC, Worthington HV. An investigation of replantation of traumatically avulsed permanent incisor teeth. *Br Dent J* 1992;172:17-20.

268. Fuss Z. Successful self-replantation of avulsed tooth with 42-year follow-up. *Endod Dent Traumatol* 1985;1:120-2.

269. Johnson WT, Goodrich JL, James GA. Replantation of avulsed teeth with immature root develpment. *Oral Surg Oral Med Oral Pathol* 1985;60:420-7.

270. Krenkel C, Grunert I. Replantierte nicht endodontisch behandelte Frontzähne mit offenem Foramen Apicale. *Zahnärztl Prax* 1986;37:290-8.

271. Andreasen JO, Schwartz O. The effect of saline storage before replantation upon dry damage of the periodontal ligament. *Endod Dent Traumatol* 1986;2:67-70.

272. Matsson L, Andreasen JO, Cvek M, Granath L. Ankylosis of experimentally reimplanted teeth related to extra-alveolar period and storage environment. *Pediatr Dent* 1982;4:327-9.

273. Andersson L, Bodin I, Sörensen S. Progression of root resorption following replantation of human teeth after extended extraoral storage. *Endod Dent Traumatol* 1989;5:38-47.

274. Andersson L, Bodin I. Avulsed human teeth replanted within 15 minutes - a long-term clinical follow-up study. *Endod Dent Traumatol* 1990;6:37-42.

275. Hammarström L, Pierce A, Blomlöf L, Feiglin B, Lindskog S. Tooth avulsion and replantation - A review. *Endod Dent Traumatol* 1986;2:1-8.

276. Modéer T, Dahllöf G, Otteskog P. Effect of drying on human periodontal ligament repair in vitro. *J Int Assoc Dent Child* 1984;15:15-20.

277. Zimmermann M, Nentwig G-H. Überlebensrate desmodontaler Zellen in Abhängigkeit von der ektraoralen Austrocknung. *Schweiz Monatsschr Zahnmed* 1989;99:1007-10.

278. Cornelius CP, Ehrenfeld M, Umbach T. Replantationsergebnisse nach traumatischer Zahneluxation. *Dtsch Zahnärztl Z* 1987;42:211-5.

CHAPTER 11

Injuries to the Supporting Bone

J. O. ANDREASEN

Terminology, Frequency and Etiology

Injuries to the supporting bone can be divided into the following types (Fig. 11.1):

1. COMMINUTION OF THE ALVEOLAR SOCKET:
Crushing of the alveolar socket, associated with intrusive or lateral luxation (Fig. 11.1, A).

2. FRACTURE OF THE ALVEOLAR SOCKET WALL:
A fracture confined to the facial or lingual socket wall (Fig. 11.1, B).

3. FRACTURE OF THE ALVEOLAR PROCESS:
A fracture of the alveolar process which may or may not involve the alveolar socket (Fig. 11.1, C and D).

4. FRACTURE OF MANDIBLE OR MAXILLA (JAW FRACTURE):
A fracture involving the base of the mandible or maxilla and often the alveolar process. The fracture may or may not involve the alveolar socket (Fig. 11.1, E and F).

The primary etiologic factors are fights and automobile accidents (1, 2). Thus, alveolar fractures from automobile accidents result from direct impact against the steering wheel or other interior structures (2, 3, 76).

In infants, where only the incisors have erupted, lack of support in the lateral regions can imply that violent occlusion resulting from impact to the chin can lead to fracture of the anterior portion of the alveolar process (Fig. 11.2).

Clinical Findings

Clinical features and treatment of *comminution of the alveolar socket* have already been described in connection with luxation injuries (see Chapter 9, p. 322).

Fractures of the alveolar socket wall are predominantly seen in the upper incisor region, where the fracture usually affects several teeth (1). Among associated dental injuries, luxation with dislocation and avulsion are the most common (Fig. 11.3). Palpation usually discloses the fracture site. Abnormal mobility of the socket wall is demonstrated when the mobility of involved teeth is tested.

Fractures of the alveolar process are predominantly found in older age groups. A common location is the anterior region, but the canine and premolar regions can also be involved. The fracture line may be positioned beyond the apices, but in most

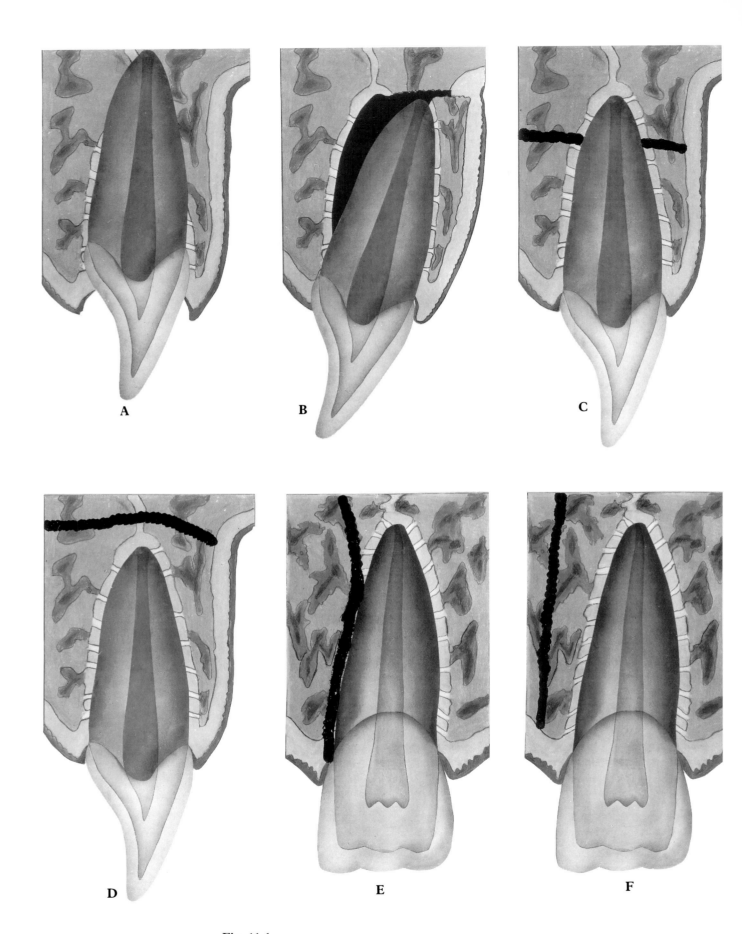

Fig. 11.1.
Injuries to the supporting bone. A. Comminution of alveolar socket. B. Fractures of the facial or lingual alveolar socket wall. C and D. Fractures of the alveolar process with and without involvement of the socket. E and F. Fractures of the mandible or maxilla with and without involvement of the socket.

CHAPTER 11

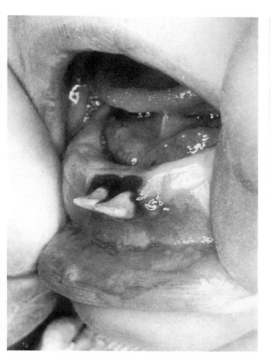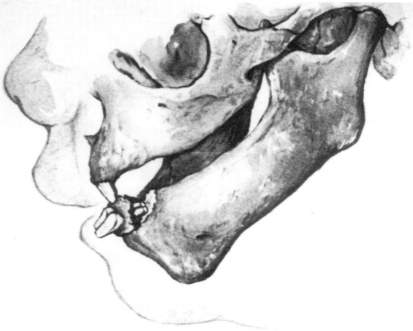

Fig. 11.2.
Pathogenesis of fractures of the mandibular alveolar process in infants.
The energy from impact to the chin area is transmitted exclusively to the incisor region due to the lack of lateral tooth support. From MÜLLER (4) 1969.

cases involves the alveolar socket. In these cases concomitant dental injuries, such as extrusive or lateral luxations as well as root fractures, are common findings (1-6).

Fracture of the alveolar process is usually easy to diagnose due to displacement and the mobility of the fragment (Fig. 11.4). Typically, when mobility of a single tooth is tested, adjacent teeth move with it. Furthermore, the percussion tone of the teeth in the fragment differs clearly from adjacent teeth in that the former yield a dull sound.

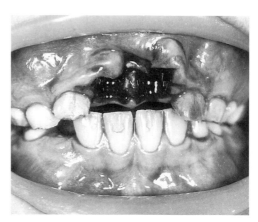

Fig. 11.3.
Gingival laceration and fracture of the facial socket wall following avulsion of both central incisors.

Fig. 11.4.
Facial displacement of alveolar fracture affecting left incisors in a 2-year-old boy.
Lingual displacement of alveolar fracture, involving right incisors in a 1½-year-old child.

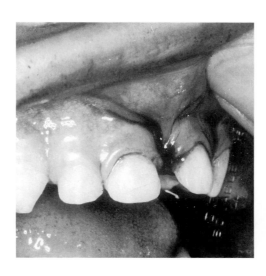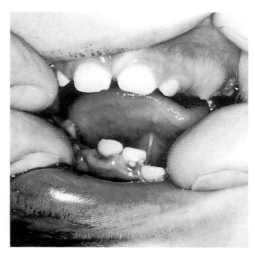

INJURIES TO THE SUPPORTING BONE

Fig. 11.5.
*Marked displacement of frag-
ments in a patient with jaw fracture in the right molar region. B.
Jaw fracture in right canine region. Note gingival laceration
and slight displacement of fragments.*

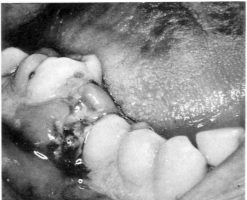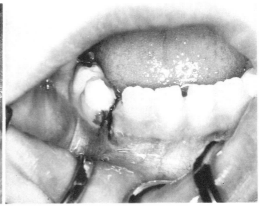

Approximately one-half of the *fractures
of the mandible or maxilla* involve teeth in
the fracture line (Fig. 11.5), and most of
these are found in the mandible (8).

The location of jaw fractures is significantly related to the state of the dentition
(11). Of the tooth-bearing areas, the lower
third molar region is most often involved;
the mandibular canine, incisor and premolar regions follow with decreasing frequency
(12, 13). The presence of a marginal periodontal bone defect also appears to be related
to the location of a fracture line (85). In
children, developing permanent teeth in the
line of fracture are usually seen in the
mandibular canine and incisor regions (14,
15).

Clinically, there is displacement of fragments and disturbance of occlusion (Fig.
11.5). Palpation with a finger placed over
the alveolar process can disclose a step in
the bony contours. In the absence of dislocation, bimanual manipulation of the
jaws will usually reveal mobility between
the fragments, often with accompanying
crepitus. Pain provoked by movement of
the mandible or maxilla, or upon palpation, is also a positive sign of fracture.

Fig. 11.6.
*Lateral luxation of a maxillary
central incisor with associated
fracture of the facial socket wall.
A. Clinical condition. B. No fracture visible on an intraoral radiograph. C. A fracture of the facial
socket wall is evident on a lateral
extraoral radiograph.*

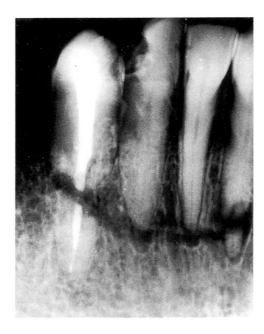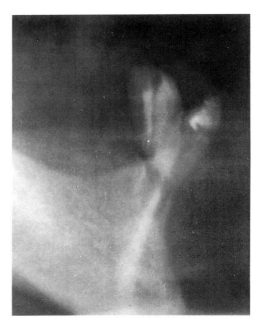

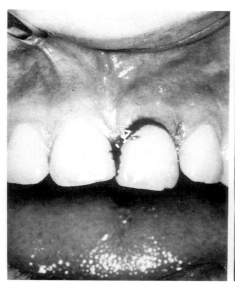
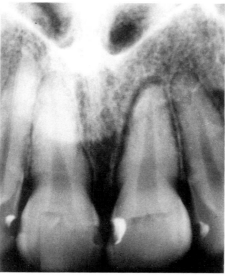
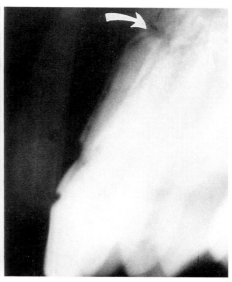

Fig. 11.7.
Dislocation of mandibular alveolar fragment clearly demonstrated by the extraoral lateral radiographic technique. (arrow).

Radiographic Findings

Intraoral radiographs of the *socket wall* seldom reveal the line of fracture; but a laterally exposed extraoral radiograph will usually disclose the fracture's location (Fig. 11.6). In contrast, in fractures involving the *alveolar process*, a distinct fracture line is usually visible in intraoral as well as extraoral radiographs (Figs. 11.6 to 11.8). Fracture lines may be positioned at all levels, from the marginal bone to the root apex (Fig. 11.8). Despite strong clinical evidence of a fracture, they are often very difficult to visualize radiographically (Fig. 11.9). When fracture lines traverse interdental sep-

Fig. 11.8.
Various locations of alveolar fractures. A. Fracture line passing through the marginal part of the interdental septum (arrow). B. Alveolar fracture traversing the septal bone close to the midportion of the root (arrow). Note the marked extrusive luxation of involved teeth. C. Alveolar fracture located close to the apices (arrow).

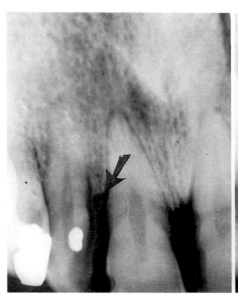
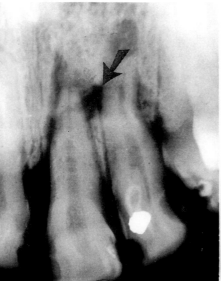
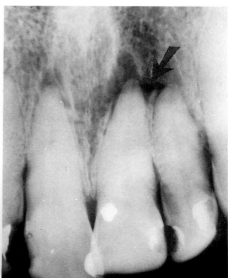

INJURIES TO THE SUPPORTING BONE

Fig. 11.9.
Alveolar fracture confined to the central incisor region. Although clinically obvious at the time of injury, there is no clear radiographic evidence of bone fracture.

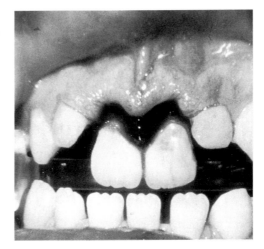 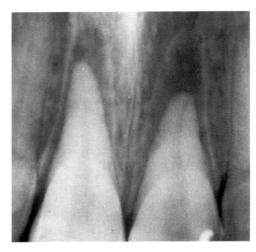

Fig. 11.10.
Fracture of the right maxillary alveolar process. Radiograph after reduction reveals the fracture line. Note the associated root fracture of upper first premolar. The alveolar fracture mimics a root fracture in the canine region.

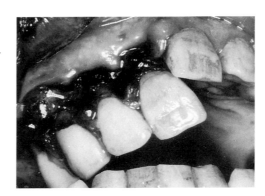 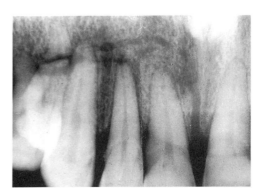

Fig. 11.11.
Alveolar fracture in the canine and premolar regions. A. In the canine region the fracture line simulates a root fracture. B. By altering angulation of the central beam, the superimposed fracture line changes position, thus ruling out a root fracture.

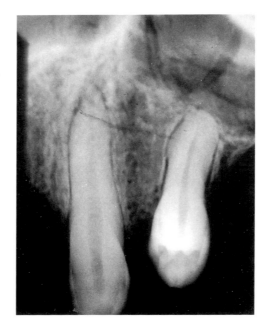 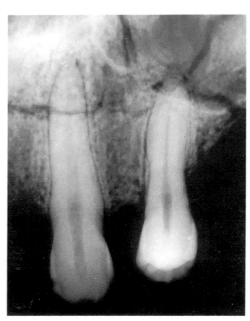

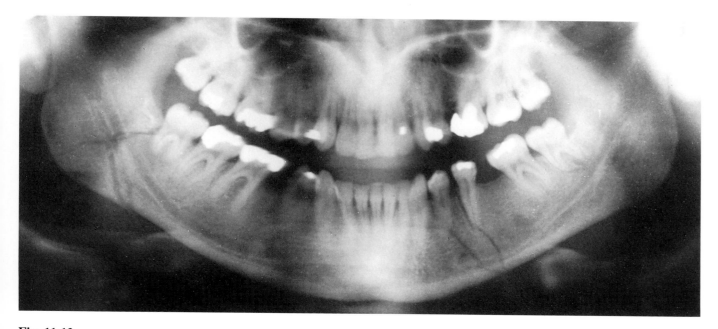

Fig. 11.12.
Fracture lines in the premolar and third molar regions as revealed by the panoramic technique.

ta, extrusive luxation and root fractures are often concomitant findings. Fractures involving the most apical portion of the root are quite common, but are often overlooked, especially in the lower anterior region. On the other hand, alveolar fracture lines transversing the apices may simulate root fractures. Careful examination of the radiographs (e.g. continuity of root surfaces and root canals) will usually reveal a superimposed fracture line and intact teeth (Fig. 11.10). Moreover, superimposed alveolar fracture lines will change position in relation to height along the root surface when the angulation of the central beam is altered (Fig. 11.11).

Radiographic examination of *mandibular* or *maxillary fractures* with dental involvement should include extraoral as well as intraoral exposures. Generally, extraoral radiographs, especially the panoramic technique, are of great help in determining the course and position of fracture lines (84, 85) (Fig. 11.12), while intraoral radiographs can reveal the relationship between involved teeth and the fracture line. This is especially important in cases of maxillary fractures, which are occasionally difficult to diagnose from extraoral radiographs due to superimposition of many anatomical structures (Fig. 11.13).

The fracture usually follows the midline of the septum or the contours of the alveolar

Fig. 11.13.
Fracture of the maxilla involving incisors, premolars, and molars. A. Only few details are depicted on extraoral radiograph. B. and C. Intraoral radiographs reveal the relationship between involved teeth and fracture lines.

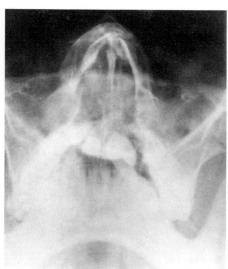
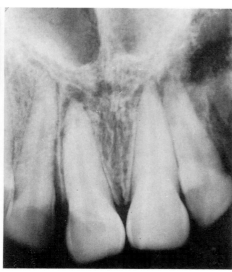
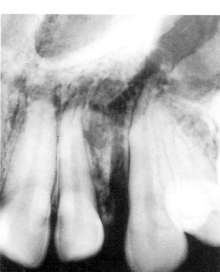

INJURIES TO THE SUPPORTING BONE

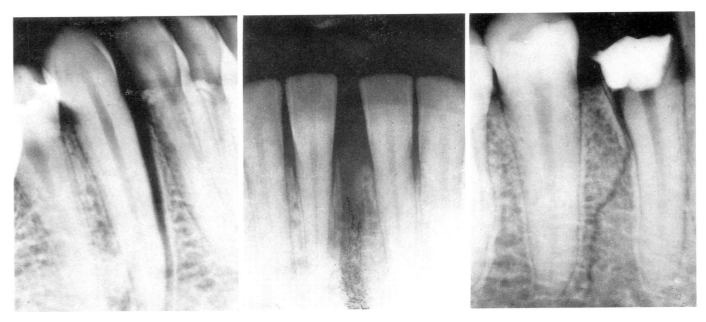

Fig. 11.14.
Different courses of jaw fracture line following the periodontal space. A. Jaw fracture passing through the periodontal ligament. B. Jaw fracture passing through the middle of the interdental septum. C. Combination of periodontal and septal involvement.

socket; but a combination of these routes can sometimes be seen (Fig. 11.14). Fractures of the *body of the mandible* do not always run parallel with the long axis of the teeth, but obliquely downwards and posteriorly towards the base of the mandible (13, 16) (Fig. 11.14).

Fractures generally follow the path of least resistance (Figs. 11.14 and 11.15).

Thus, at the angle of the mandible, the position of the lower third molar generally determines the course of the fracture line.

It should be remembered that two lines will be seen radiographically if the central beam is not parallel to the plane of the fracture, as the fracture lines of both outer and inner cortical bones plates will be depicted (84) (Figs. 11.16 to 11.18).

Fig. 11.15.
Location and course of fracture lines in 225 patients with mandibular fractures due to fights. The course of the fracture lines was determined from panoramic radiographs. Note that the majority of the fracture lines are situated in the so-called weak areas of the mandible, the subcondylar, third molar, and canine regions. Fractures of the body of the mandible usually run obliquely downwards and backwards to the base of the mandible. From OIKARINEN & MALMSTRÖM (13), 1969.

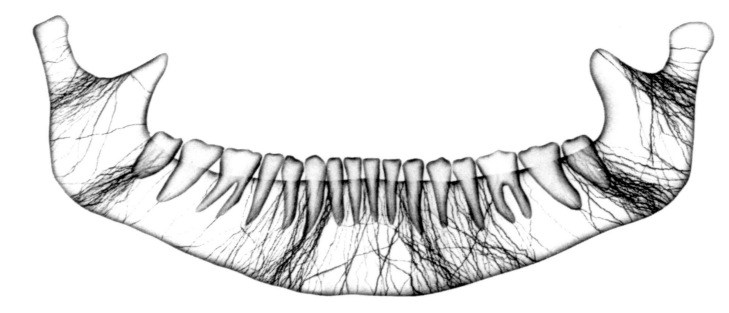

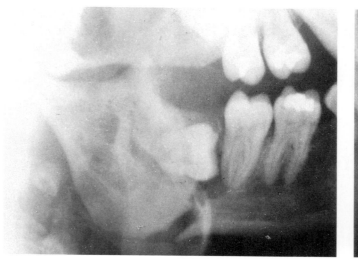
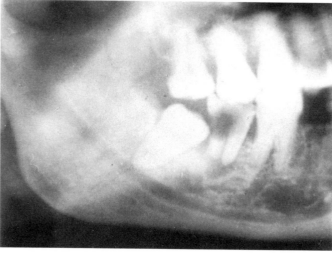

Fig. 11.16.
Fracture lines in the lower third molar region following the line of least resistance as determined by impacted third molars.

Fig. 11.17.
Diagrams illustrating the difference in the radiographic appearance of a single fracture line depending on the angle of the central beam. A and B. Central beam parallel to the fracture plane results in a single fracture line. C and D. A more posterior exposure results in projection of the fracture of the outer and inner cortical bone plate as separate lines.

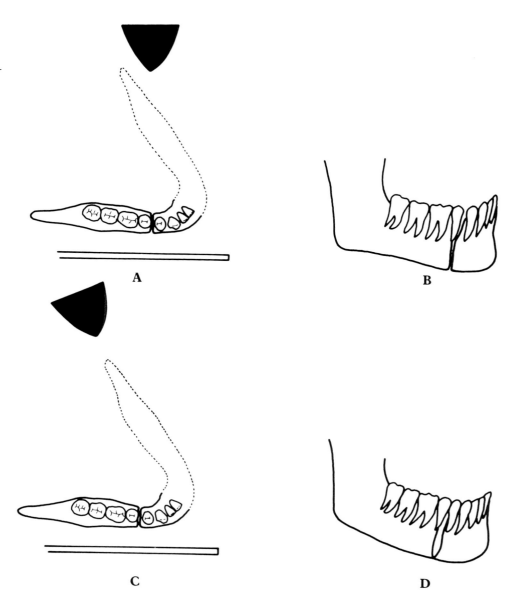

A

B

C

D

INJURIES TO THE SUPPORTING BONE

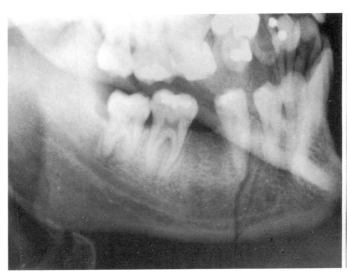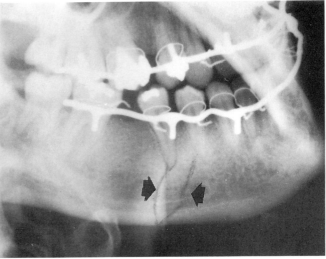

Fig. 11.18.
Radiographs illustrating change in position of the fracture lines when the angle of the central beam is altered. A. Central ray almost parallel to the fracture plane. B. A change in the projection angle results in two distinct fracture lines (arrows).

Pathology

Most fractures of the supporting bone represent a complex injury where damage has happened not only to supporting bone but also to the pulp, periodontal ligament and the gingiva (Fig. 11.19). Due to this multiplicity of tissues involved, various types of healing complications can occur, such as loss of supporting bone, root resorption and pulp necrosis.

Adequate knowledge of bony repair after fracture is necessary in order to appreciate the role teeth play in these events. As relatively little information exists on the healing events after jaw fractures, most of our present knowledge is derived from clinical and experimental findings from fractures of the shaft of long bones (18, 19, 20-44). The following description of fracture healing is therefore based upon the latter material. Special implications for bone healing in the jaws will be discussed later in this chapter.

The events immediately following fracture are extravasation and clotting of blood exuding from injured vessels. The normal vascular supply to the fracture site is compromised by the fracture; and necrosis of osteocytes is found in adjacent areas. The organization of the blood clot by formation of granulation tissue begins within the first 24 hours after fracture. The primary function of this tissue is removal of necrotic or damaged tissue components. The granulation tissue becomes dense connective tissue in which cartilage and fibrocartilage develop, forming a fibrocartilagenous callus which forms a cuff around the fracture site and thereby closes the gap between the ends of the fracture.

New bone originating from the deeper layers of the periosteum and endosteum is formed some distance from the fracture line. Immature bone then invades the fibrocartilagenous callus and ultimately unites the two fragments, whereupon mineralization of the callus takes place. At the same time, resorptive and remodelling processes make the bone structure on either side of the fracture less dense, a change often observed in follow-up radiographs (26). Subsequently, reorganization of the bony callus occurs, and the immature fibrillar bone is replaced by mature lamellated bone. Eventually, functional reconstruction takes place, i.e. internal reconstruction and resorption of excess bone.

It is presumed that the above-mentioned healing processes also apply to jaw fractures. The presence of a cartilagenous callus has, however, been questioned. In a study of experimental jaw fractures in dogs, no evidence of cartilage formation was found (22), whereas other investigators have found occasional islands of cartilage in animal experiments (23-25, 33, 35) and in human material (26). Moreover, it has been shown that mobility of the jaw fragments influences the rate of bony callus formation. When fragments are mobile, more time elapses before bony bridging is seen than in immobilized fractures (24).

CHAPTER 11

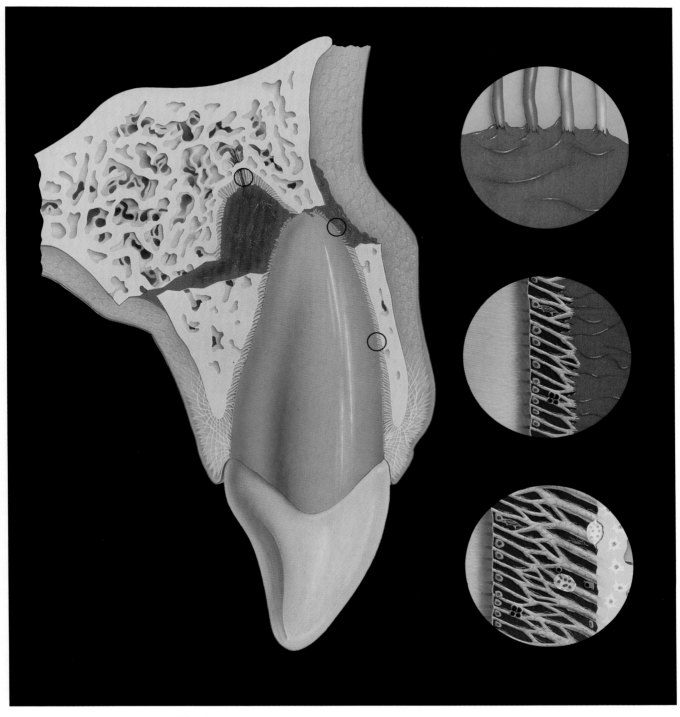

Fig. 11.19.
Fracture of the alveolar process. Both the PDL and the neurovascular supply to the pulp are severed.

The influence of the presence of teeth upon fracture healing has been elucidated primarily by animal experiments (22, 28-31). Experimental jaw fractures in dogs, with teeth present along the fracture line, have revealed formation of granulation tissue resorbing the interdental bone and adjacent root surfaces (22). Examination of human teeth located along the fracture line, however, has shown evidence of repair of resorption areas (45, 46).

Figs. 11.20 and 11.21 show the early

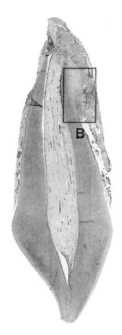
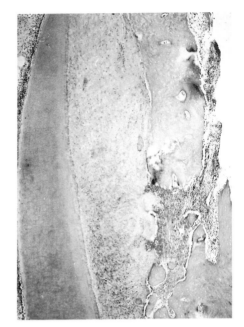
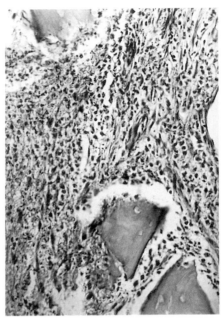

Fig. 11.20.
Early histologic changes following fracture of the facial socket wall in a 1½-year-old child. A. Low-power view of sectioned incisor, removed 5 days after injury. x 5. B and C. Higher magnification of the fracture area. The blood clot has been organized by granulation tissue. x 30 and x 195.

histologic healing events following fracture of the vestibular socket wall and alveolar process.

Treatment

Fractures of the Socket Wall

Fractures of the socket wall are usually associated with dislocation of teeth. Thus, the first step after administration of local anesthesia is to reposition the displaced teeth. Reduction in these cases is similar to that after lateral luxation (see Chapter 9, p. 336); that is, by disengaging the apices from the vestibular bone plate. This is done by simultaneous digital pressure in an incisal direction over the apical area and in a buccal direction at the lingual aspect of the crown. This maneuver will usually free the apices and permit repositioning of the fragment. The socket wall is repositioned at the same time. In case of open comminuted fractures, it may be necessary to remove loose fragments which are not adherent to the periosteum. Clinical experience has shown that, despite removal of the entire vestibular bone plate, there is still enough structural support to ensure adequate stability of the teeth. After reduction of displaced teeth and bone fractures, lacerations of soft tissues should be sutured. Although it is tempting to suture immediately, suturing of soft tissue wounds should be left to last, as suturing early in the treatment procedure limits access for repositioning procedures. Splinting is carried out according to the principles outlined in Chapter 9, p. 347.

Due to rapid bony healing in children, most fractures of the alveolar socket wall involving the primary dentition do not require splinting. In these cases, the parents should be instructed to restrict nourishment to a soft diet during the first 2 weeks after injury.

Fractures of the Alveolar Process

Treatment of *fractures of the alveolar process* includes reduction and immobilization (4, 6, 47-50, 76-77) (Fig. 11.22). After administration of local anesthesia, the alveolar fragment is repositioned with digital pressure (Fig. 11.22). In this type of fracture, apices of involved teeth can often be locked in position by the vestibular bone plate. Reduction in these cases follows the principles mentioned under fractures of the alveolar socket wall.

Splinting of alveolar fractures can be achieved by means of an acid-etch/resin splint or arch bars. Intermaxillary fixation

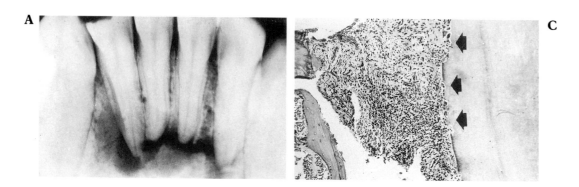

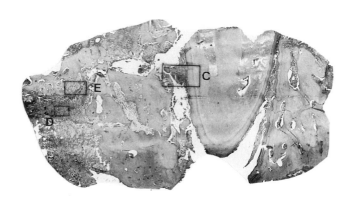

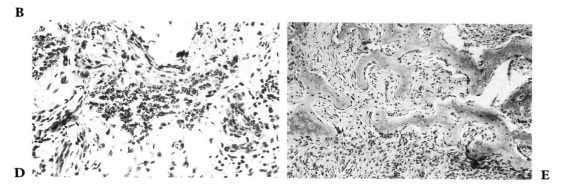

Fig. 11.21.
Healing events following a fracture of the alveolar process in the mandibular incisor region. A. Radiograph taken at time of injury. B. Surgical specimen including apex of left lateral incisor removed 18 days after trauma. x 10. C. Superficial resorption of the mesial aspect of the root (arrows). x 30. D. Remnants of coagulum. x 195. E. Developing young immature bone bridging the fracture line. x 75.

is generally not required provided that a stable splint is used (Fig. 11.22). A fixation period of 4 weeks is usually advocated. However, due to more rapid healing in children, this period can be reduced to 3 weeks.

Teeth in a loose alveolar fragment might be doomed to extraction due to marginal or

Fig. 11.22. Treatment of an alveolar fracture
This 21-year-old woman suffered a fracture of the maxillary alveolar process including the lateral and central incisors.

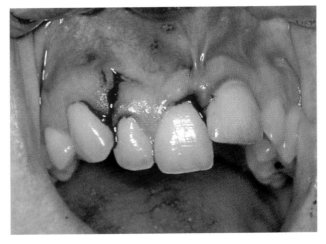 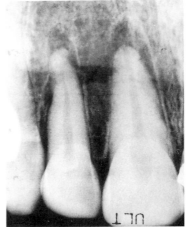

Anesthetizing the traumatized region
An infraorbital block and infiltration to the incisive canal are necessary prior to repositioning.

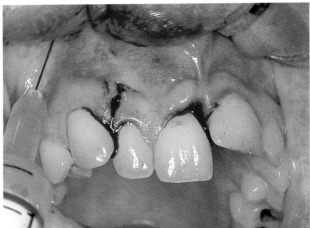 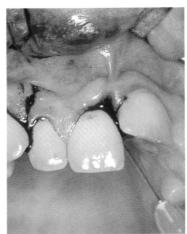

Repositioning
With firm finger pressure to the apical region, the apices are disengaged. If this is not possible, the fragment must be moved in a coronal and palatal direction with the help of a forceps.

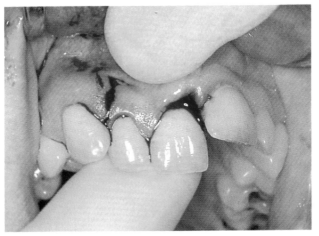 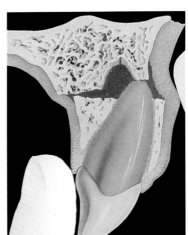

Verifying repositioning
Occlusion is checked and a radiograph taken to verify adequate repositioning.

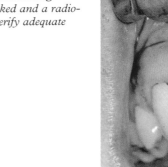 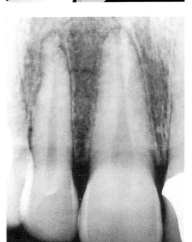

Splinting
The incisal one third of the labial aspect of injured and adjacent teeth are acid-etched (30 seconds) with phosphoric acid gel. The etchant is removed with a 20 second water spray. The labial enamel is dried with compressed air, revealing the mat, etched surface whereafter the splinting material is applied. During polymerization of the splinting material, the patient occludes in order to ensure correct repositioning of the alveolar segment.

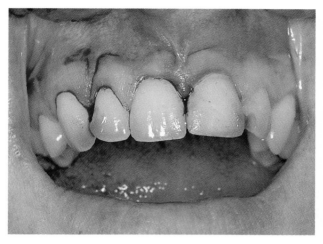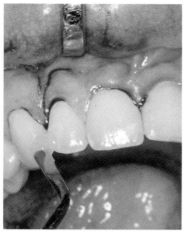

Finished splint
The splint does not contact the gingiva whereby optimal oral hygiene can be maintained

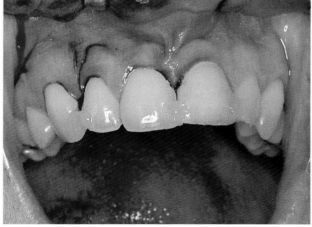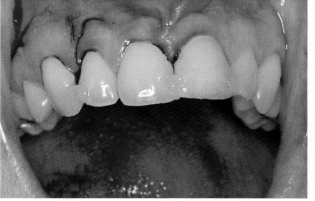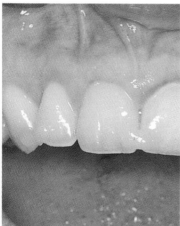

Removing the splint
After 4 weeks the splint is removed with sealer or a fissure bur.

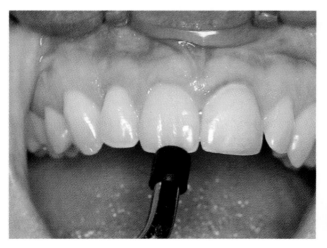

Controlling pulp sensibility
Pulp revascularization is controlled after 3 months. Due to a lack of response as well as a slight apical radiolucency, pulp necrosis is suspected.

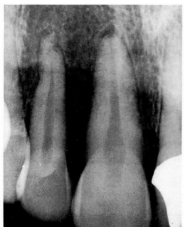

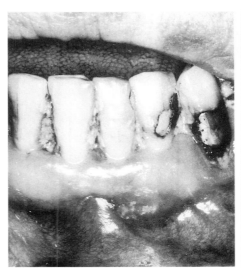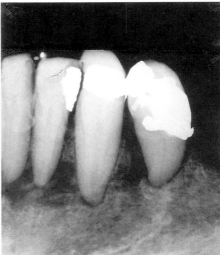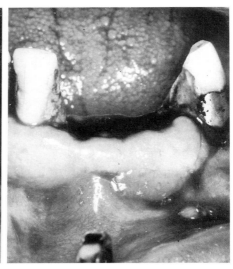

Fig. 11.23.
A and B. Alveolar fracture in left incisor and canine region associated with advanced marginal periodontitis. It was decided to splint the fracture and postpone extraction of lower incisors for 6 weeks.
C. Lower incisors extracted without damage to the alveolar process.

periapical inflammation. However, these extractions should generally be postponed until osseous healing has stabilized the fragment (Fig. 11.23), otherwise the entire alveolar fragment might be inadvertently removed with the teeth. Again, regarding treatment sequence, associated soft tissue lacerations should be sutured last in order to allow access for intraoral manipulation.

Treatment of alveolar fractures in children offers special problems due to lack of sufficient teeth for splinting procedures. In most cases where the fragment can be reduced into a stable position, one can omit the splinting procedure. In such cases, nourishment should be restricted to soft or liquid foods.

Fractures of the Mandible or Maxilla

The management of fractures of the mandible or maxilla involves many procedures beyond the scope of this book. In this regard, only teeth involved in the fracture area will be considered. The reader is otherwise referred to standard textbooks on this subject (53, 86, 87).

Treatment of jaw fractures in *children* with developing teeth in the line of fracture follows the given general principles, i.e. exact repositioning and usually intermaxillary fixation. It is important that de-

veloping permanent teeth in the fracture line be preserved. The only exception would be in cases of infection along the fracture line being maintained by infected tooth germs (54, 55).

Treatment of jaw fractures in *adults* with teeth in the fracture line is a controversial issue (68) and has recently been the subject of a review article (88). Earlier, especially before the antibiotic era, it was customary to extract all teeth in the fracture line. However, recent studies have revealed that this does not reduce the frequency of complications. These observations have gradually led to a more conservative approach.

Teeth in the Line of Fracture

In the past, a number of clinical studies have appeared concerning the effect of various factors related to healing complications when teeth were involved in the line of fracture (56-63, 68-74, 78-82). However, all of these studies are retrospective, implying a possible bias in the evaluation of extraction therapy and the use of antibiotics. The resultant conclusions should therefore be regarded with extreme caution. In the following, a survey of factors related to fracture healing complications is presented.

The presence of teeth in the fracture line apparently represents an increased risk for infection compared to a fracture where no teeth are involved (68, 89).

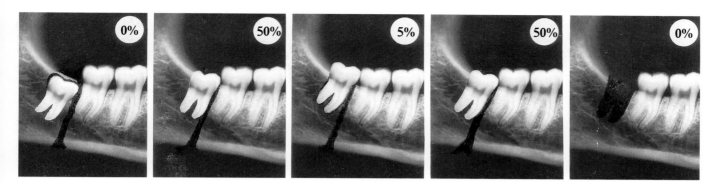

Fig. 11.24.
The infection risk in the fracture bone is strongly related to the eruption status of the third molar. The frequency is indicated according to RINK & STOEHR (91) 1978.

TYPE OF TEETH INVOLVED

The type of tooth involved also appears to be of importance. Thus, multirooted teeth appear to enhance the risk of complication compared to single-rooted teeth (68, 70) (Table 11.1).

ERUPTION STATUS

The most frequent tooth involved in jaw fractures appears to be the third molar. The eruption status of this tooth (especially semi-erupted) appears to be significantly related to the occurrence of healing complications. Thus, complications are usually only seen with semi-erupted mandibular third molars; whereas fully erup-

ted or impacted third molars rarely develop complications along the line of fracture (91) (Fig. 11.24).

EXTRACTION OF TEETH

In general, no beneficial effect has been demonstrated following the extraction of teeth in the line of fracture. In fact, recent studies have shown an increased morbidity (57-59, 79) or no effect after extraction (56, 77, 78, 89, 90, 92, 113). Only two out of 11 studies have reported the opposite (60, 68). However, none of the cited studies has been designed as randomized investigations in respect to extraction of teeth in the line of fracture.

Table 11.1 Frequency of complicated fracture healing in adults with teeth preserved along the fracture line

Examiner	No. of cases	No. of complications (inflammation)
Götte (57) 1959	178★★	30 (17%)
Andrä & Sonnenburg (56) 1966	264★★	40 (15%)
Andrä & Sonnenburg (56) 1966	139★+	7 (5%)
Müller (68) 1968	118++	23 (19%)
Neal et al. (79) 1978	132★	39 (29%)
Rink & Stoehr (91) 1978	99★	13 (13%)
Kahnberg & Ridell (81) 1979	132★	10 (8%)
Choung et al. (89) 1983	152★★	4 (3%)
Amaratunga (98) 1987	124★★	6 (5%)

  ★ antibiotics given in all cases.
  ★★ antibiotics given in some cases.
  ★+ single-rooted teeth.
  ++ multi-rooted teeth.

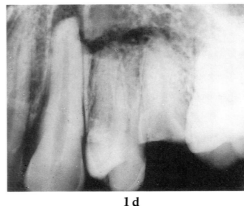
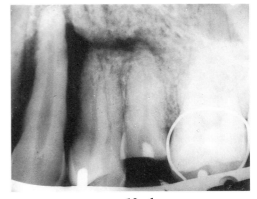

1 d

10 wk

Fig. 11.25.
Persistent infection in the fracture line of an alveolar fracture involving canine and premolars. A. Condition immediately after injury. B. Radiograph 10 weeks later reveals marked bone destruction in the fracture area.

EFFECT OF ANTIBIOTICS

In cases of conservatively or surgically treated mandibular fractures, prospective randomized studies have shown that antibiotic treatment given 30 min before surgery and 1 day afterwards significantly decreased the frequency of infection (93-95). However an extension of the antibiotic cover for more than 1 day did not decrease the rate of infection (94, 95).

The effect of antibiotics on infection in the line of fracture in dentulous parts of the jaws is presently very controversial. If teeth are *present* in the line of fracture, there is an uncertain (56, 57) or no value of antibiotic therapy (91), whereas one study showed a positive effect (60).

If teeth were *extracted*, the rate of infection was unaffected by antibiotic therapy in one investigation (91) and found to be reduced in another (56). In one study, it was found that a positive effect was only related to multirooted teeth (68).

DELAY IN TREATMENT

Delay in initial treatment seems to play a role in the frequency of healing complications. Thus, treatment delayed more than 2 - 4 days appears to be accompanied by an increased frequency of infection (10,56,62, 68-71, 79, 96), whereas one study could not find any difference in healing rate following delayed treatment (97).

TYPE OF SPLINTING

Finally, an increase in the rate of infection was found following rigid internal fixation (i.e. surgical osteosynthesis using wire or plates) in fractures with teeth in the fracture line compared to similar fractures treated with conventional intermaxillary splinting (98-100).

Another factor which influences fracture healing is *rigid arch bar fixation* compared to a *flexible wire splint*. By eliminating movement of the fragments, seepage of saliva along the fracture line is prevented, which thus decreases the possibility of secondary infection (57).

In conclusion, teeth present in the line of fracture should generally be maintained, as they can later serve as functional units. More-

Table 11.2 Frequency of late dental complications following fractures of the alveolar process. From ANDREASEN (6) *1970*

	No. of cases	No. of involved teeth	Frequency of pulp necrosis	Frequency of pulp canal obliteration	Frequency of progressive root resorption	Frequency of loss of marginal supporting bone
Alveolar fractures	29	71	75%	15%	11%	13%

Fig. 11.26. Pulpal healing after alveolar fracture in the permanent dentition. *From ANDREASEN (6) 1970.*

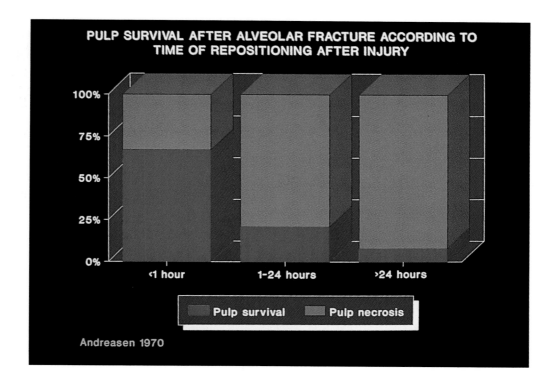

PULP SURVIVAL AFTER ALVEOLAR FRACTURE ACCORDING TO TIME OF REPOSITIONING AFTER INJURY

Andreasen 1970

over, their removal may further traumatize the fracture site and lead to dislocation of the fragment (59, 101). Exceptions to this approach would be teeth with crown-root fractures, semi erupted third molars and teeth with severe marginal or apical breakdown whose fate is already compromised. Teeth with pulp necrosis and apical breakdown can possibly be saved by endodontic therapy. This also applies to teeth with complicated crown and root fractures. Treatment of these injuries follows principles outlined in previous chapters. However, root canal treatment must necessarily be postponed until the intermaxillary fixation has been removed. When pulp exposures due to crown fractures are present, pulp extirpation should be carried out and the root canal provisionally sealed until removal of the intermaxillary fixation allows completion of therapy. Root fractured teeth are stabilized with splints.

If inflammation occurs, the treatment of choice is antibiotic therapy, possibly together with extraction of teeth involved in the inflammatory process, or endodontic therapy if pulp necrosis has developed.

Prognosis

Fractures of the Socket Wall

The immediate course of healing after fracture of the socket wall is usually uneventful; however, later follow-ups can reveal resorption of roots of involved teeth.

Fractures of the Alveolar Process

The healing events of alveolar fractures in the permanent dentition are in most cases uneventful; however, in rare cases, sequestration of bone and/or involved teeth can occur (Fig. 11.25). Careful follow-up is mandatory in order to register later pulp necrosis and periapical inflammation (5, 6). Such complications are rather frequent and apparently related to the time interval between injury and fixation (Fig. 11.26). Thus, teeth splinted within 1 hour after injury develop pulp necrosis less frequently than teeth splinted after longer intervals (6).

Fig. 11.27. Periodontal healing after alveolar fracture in the permanent dentition. *From ANDREASEN (6) 1970.*

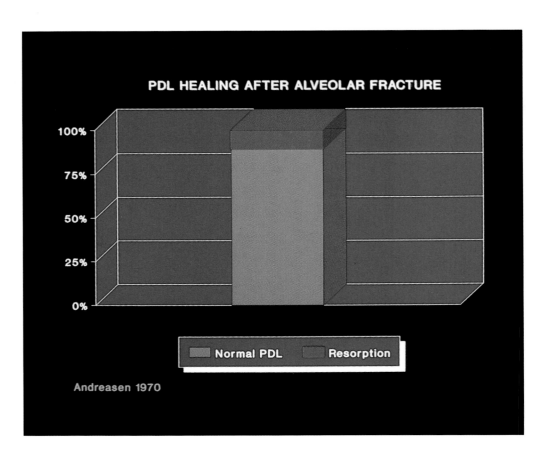

Fig. 11.27. Periodontal healing after alveolar fracture in the permanent dentition. *From ANDREASEN (6) 1970.*

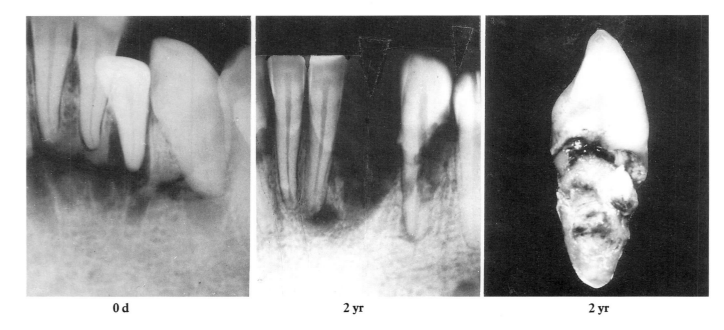

| 0 d | 2 yr | 2 yr |

Fig. 11.28.
Root resorption and periapical inflammation after an alveolar fracture involving incisors and left canine. A. Condition after injury. B. Re-examination 3 years after injury reveals periapical inflammation as well as inflammatory root resorption. C. Clinical view of extracted canine. Marked resorption areas present on root surface. From ANDREASEN (6) 1970.

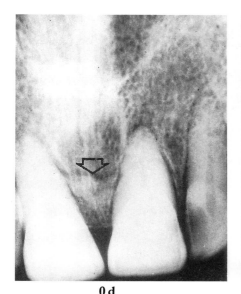 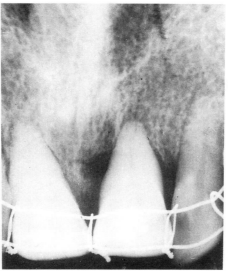 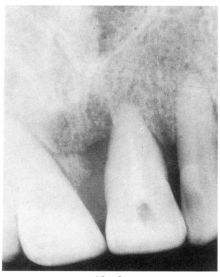

| 0 d | 6 wk | 10 wk |

Fig. 11.29.
Loss of marginal supporting bone following alveolar fracture in the central incisor region. Horizontal fracture line is evident on radiograph taken at time of injury (arrow). At follow-up, loss of marginal supporting bone is evident around left central incisor. From ANDREASEN (6) 1970.

Apart from pulp necrosis, pulp canal obliteration, root resorption (Table 11.2 and Figs. 11.27 and 11.28) and loss of supporting bone (Fig. 11.29) are common complications (6).

Concerning the prognosis of alveolar fractures in *the primary dentition,* it has been found that root development of preserved primary teeth is often arrested (51).

Fractures of the Mandible or Maxilla in Children

Inflammation at the Line of Fracture

Fractures of the mandible or maxilla in *children* with developing teeth along the fracture line are seldom complicated by inflammation. It appears from the studies listed in Table 11.3 that frequencies of complications were found to range from 10 to 18%. The clinical picture of inflam-

mation in the fracture area is characterized by swelling and abscess formation. Draining fistulae may also develop, as well as immediate or protracted sequestration of involved tooth germs (65).

When inflammation does occur, antibiotic therapy is the treatment of choice. Surgical removal of involved teeth may be indicated if radiographs reveal infected tooth germs in the fracture area (64-67). In such cases, osteolytic changes will be found in the fracture area, with disappearance of distinct outlines of the dental crypts of the involved teeth. It is conjectured from animal experiments (27) and human data (65) that infected tooth germs in these cases are responsible for protracted inflammation.

Disturbances in the Developing Dentition

Another problem which should be considered when treating jaw fractures in children is odontogenic disturbances in involved developing teeth (see Chapter 12, p 461).

Table 11.3 Frequency of complicated fracture healing in children *with developing permanent teeth involved in the fracture line*

Examiner	No. of cases	No. of complications (inflammation)
Lenstrup (14) 1955	22	4(18%)
Taatz (64) 1962	29	3(10%)

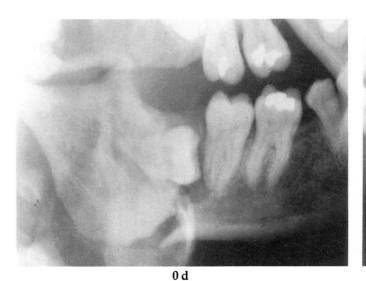

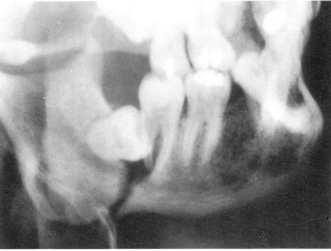

0 d   6 mo

Fig. 11.30.
Radiograph illustrating delayed fracture healing due to inflammation maintained by an impacted third molar. A. Condition at time of injury. B. Six months later, bone healing has not occurred.

Fractures of the Mandible or Maxilla in Adults

Inflammation at the Line of Fracture

Studies of jaw fractures in adults have shown that the frequency of inflammatory complications along the line of fracture when teeth are preserved ranges from 3 to 29% (Table 11.1, Fig. 11.30). A tooth positioned along the fracture line can be the source of inflammation due to pulp necrosis from compromised circulation to the pulpal tissues or already established infection in the pulp which can spread to the fracture site. This finding is supported by the finding that pulp necrosis in involved teeth is common when a fracture directly involves the apical region (69, 82). Infection can also occur along the denuded root surface when a fracture directly involves the alveolar socket (26).

Pulpal Healing and Pulp Necrosis

Teeth preserved along a fracture line should be carefully followed in order to detect later

Table 11.4 Frequency of late dental complications following jaw fractures

Examiner	No. of cases	No. of involved teeth	Frequency of pulp necrosis	Frequency of pulp canal obliteration	Frequency of progressive root resorption	Frequency of loss of marginal supporting bone
Roed-Petersen & Andreasen (69) 1969	68	110	25%	5%	0%	12%
Ridell & Åstrand (87) 1971	84	142	5%	2%	1%	11%
Kahnberg & Ridell (81) 1979	132	185	14%	-	3%	12%
Oikarinen et al. (192) 1991	45	47	38%	24%	4%	18%

Fig. 11.31.

Fig. 11.31.
Pulp necrosis and incomplete healing of marginal periodontium following jaw fracture in the canine region. Note that the fracture line involves the apex of the canine. Follow-up examination after 6 months revealed incomplete healing of the marginal periodontium as well as pulp necrosis with periapical involvement. From ROED-PETERSEN & ANDREASEN (69) 1970.

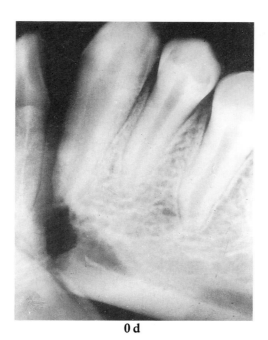

0 d

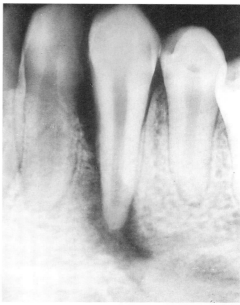

6 mo

pulp necrosis (58, 69, 74, 81, 102) (Table 11.4). In interpreting pulpal sensibility of involved teeth, one should remember that reactions may be temporarily decreased and later return to normal (75, 81, 103). It has been found that pulp necrosis is primarily associated with the relationship of the apices of involved teeth to the fracture line (69, 82, 83, 102). Thus, if the apex is exposed by the fracture line, the risk of pulp necrosis is increased (81) (Fig. 11.31) (102). Moreover, fractures treated more than 48 hours after injury show an increased incidence of later pulp necrosis (69, 82).

In the follow-up period, obliteration of the root canal is often seen in teeth involved in the fracture, and especially in individuals below 20 years of age (102) (Figs. 11.32 and 11.33).

PDL Healing and Root Resorption

Root resorption following jaw fractures is a rare finding and has been found to affect up to 4% of the teeth involved in the fracture line (69, 81, 82, 102) (Table 11.4).

Gingival Healing and Loss of Marginal Attachment

In case of arch bar fixation (i.e. Sauer's, Schuchardt's or Erich's arch bar), no significant difference in periodontal health after splinting has been found in a clinical situation (105). Experimentally, a mild periodontitis has been observed during the splinting period (106-108). However, these inflamma-

Fig. 11.32.
Obliteration of pulp canal in a second premolar following jaw fracture. The fracture line involves the apical area. At follow-up a marked pulp canal obliteration is evident. From ROED-PETERSEN & ANDREASEN (69) 1970.

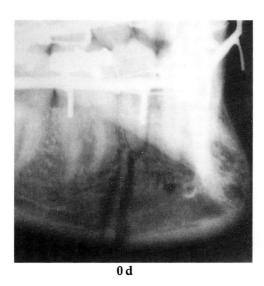

0 d

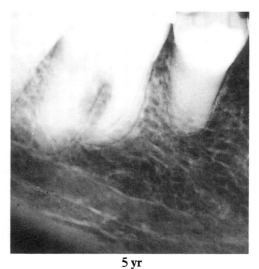

5 yr

Fig. 11.33.
Obliteration of the pulp canal secondary to a jaw fracture. A. Time of injury - the jaw fracture involves the third molar region. B. Six years later, marked pulp canal obliteration of the third molar is evident. C. Low-power view of sectioned molar. x D. Coronal part of the pulp completely occluded with hard tissue. x 30. E. Islands of bone in the middle of the pulp. x 75. F. Apposition of hard tissue following initial resorption of the canal walls (arrows). x 75. G. Normal dentin appositioned after formation of atubular dentin immediately after injury (arrows). x 75.

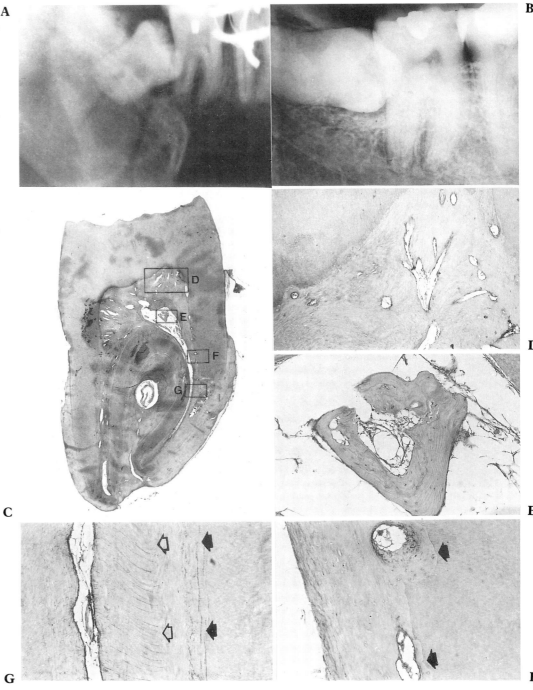

tory changes appear to be reversible following splint removal (109, 110).

The dental septum and gingiva involved in *jaw fractures* appear to possess a good healing potential. Complications, such as loss of interdental bone and pocketing, are rare (111).

Loss of marginal bone can be recorded at later follow-up examinations (69, 82, 102).

This is found especially among involved canines. Incomplete reduction of displaced fragments appears to be the main cause of loss of marginal bone support (Fig. 11.34), while optimal repositioning will ensure complete periodontal repair (69, 81) (Fig. 11.35). However, a slight long-term increase in mobility of teeth along the line of fracture has been reported (102, 112).

Fig. 11.34.
Incomplete healing of marginal periodontium following jaw fracture in the canine region. 4 years later - deep pocket formation and loss of supporting bone is found.
From ROED-PETERSEN & AN-DREASEN (69) *1970.*

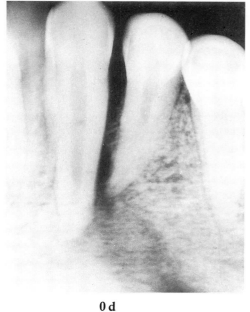 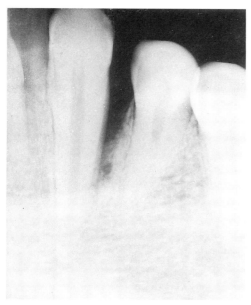

0 d   4 yr

Fig. 11.35.
Complete healing of the periodontium despite extensive dislocation of fragments and exposed cementum of a lower right canine.
From ROED-PETERSEN & AN-DREASEN (69) *1970.*

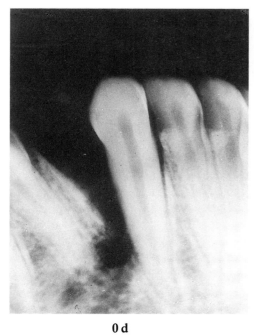 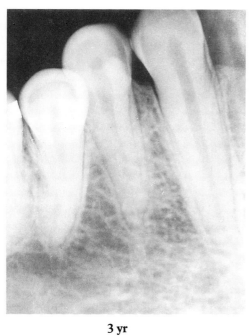

0 d   3 yr

INJURIES TO THE SUPPORTING BONE

Essentials

Terminology (Fig. 11.1)

Comminution of alveolar socket
Fracture of alveolar socket wall
Fracture of alveolar process
Fracture of mandible or maxilla (jaw fracture)

Frequency

Permanent dentition: 16% of dental injuries
Primary dentition: 7% of dental injuries

Etiology

Fight injuries
Automobile accidents

History

Symptoms

Clinical Examination

Palpation of Facial Skeleton

Mobility of fragments
Dislocation of fragments
Reaction to vitality tests

Radiographic Examination

Dislocation of fragments
Relation between bone fracture and marginal and apical periodontium

Pathology

Fracture healing
Superficial root resorption

Treatment (Fig. 11.22)

a. Administer local or general anesthesia
b. Reposition displaced fragments
c. Teeth in jaw fracture lines should generally be preserved unless severe inflammatory changes of marginal or apical origin are present. Teeth with periapical inflammation can be maintained if antibacterial medication is placed in the root canal. Semierupted third molars should, as a rule, be removed.
d. Apply rigid fixation (i.e. orthodontic band/resin splint, acid-etch/resin splint. In the primary dentition, a direct splinting method with acrylic may be used. In cases where the fragment can be reduced into a stable position, one may refrain from splinting. In such cases, the patient should be instructed to restrict nourishment to soft food.
e. Check reduction radiographically
f. Antibiotic therapy may be indicated in the treatment of jaw fractures
g. Control the involved teeth radiographically and with sensibility tests
h. Immobilize for 3 to 6 weeks
i. Follow-up period minimum one year

Prognosis for Permanent Teeth involved in Fractures of the Alveolar process

Pulp necrosis: 75%
Pulp canal obliteration: 15%
Progressive root resorption: 11%
Loss of marginal bone support: 13%

Prognosis for Permanent Teeth involved in Fractures of the Maxilla or the Mandible

Infection in the fracture line: 5 to 29%
Pulp necrosis: 5 to 38%
Pulp canal obliteration: 2 to 24%
Progressive root resorption: 0 to 4%
Loss of marginal bone support: 11 to 18%

TREATMENT OF PULP NECROSIS: SEE CHAPTER 14, p. 543

TREATMENT OF ROOT RESORPTION: SEE CHAPTER 14, p. 547

TREATMENT OF INFLAMMATION IN THE FRACTURE LINE IN THE PERMANENT DENTITION
a. Antibiotic therapy
b. Extraction or endodontic therapy of involved permanent teeth if they sustain inflammation

TREATMENT OF INFLAMMATION IN THE FRACTURE LINE IN THE PRIMARY DENTITION
a. Antibiotic therapy
b. Removal of involved permanent tooth germs is indicated only if they develop inflammation

Bibliography

1. ANDREASEN JO. Etiology and pathogenesis of traumatic dental injuries. A clinical study of 1298 cases. *Scand J Dent Res* 1970;7:329-42.

2. HUELKE DF, HARGER JH. Maxillofacial injuries: their nature and mechanisms of production. *J Oral Surg* 1969;27:451-60.

3. HAGAN EH, HUELKE DF. An analysis of 319 case reports of mandibular fractures. *J Oral Surg* 1961;19:93-104.

4. MÜLLER W. Diagnostik und Therapie der Alveolarfortsatzfrakturen in der zahnärzlichen Praxis. *Dtsch Zahnärztekalender* 1969;28;20-34.

5. FREIHOFER HPM. Ergebnisse der Behandlung vom Alveolarfortsatzfrakturen. *Schweiz Monatsschr Zahnheilkd* 1969;79:623-9.

6. ANDREASEN JO. Fractures of the alveolar process of the jaw. A clinical and radiographic follow-up study. *Scand J Dent Res* 1970;78:263-72.

7. GEHRE G. Ein Beitrag zur Therapie der Alveolarfortsatzfrakturen unter besonderer Berücksichtigung des Krankengutes der Leipziger Universitätsklinik der Jahre 1955-1966. *Dtsch Stomatol* 1962;12:97-104.

8. ENGHOFF A, SIEMSSEN SO. Kæbefrakturer gennem 10 år. *Tandlægebladet* 1956;60:851-84.

9. GISCHLER E, LÜCHE R. Beitrag zur Häufigkeit der Frakturen im Bereich der Kiefer- und Gesichtsschädelknochen. *Dtsch Zahnärztl Z* 1962;17:649-55.

10. NEUNER O. Zur Entstehung und Verhütung der Bruchspaltostitis bei Unterkieferfrakturen. *Zahnärztl Welt* 1963;64:667-8.

11. HUELKE DF, BURDI AR, EYMAN CE. Mandibular fractures as related to the site of trauma and the state of dentition. *J Dent Res* 1961;40:1262-74.

12. FUHR K, SETZ D. Nachuntersuchungen über Zähne, die zum Bruchspalt in Beziehung stehen. *Dtsch Zahnärztl Z* 1963;18:638-43.

13. OIKARINEN VJ, MALMSTRÖM M. Jaw fractures. A roentgenological and statistical analysis of 1284 cases including a special study of the fracture lines in the mandible drawn from orthopantomograms in 660 cases. *Suomi Hammaslääk Toim* 1969;65:95-111.

14. LENSTRUP K. On injury by fractures of the jaws to teeth in course of formation. *Acta Odontol Scand* 1955;13:181-202.

15. VELGOS S, STANKO V, PREVRATILOVA D. Kieferfrakturen bei Kindern. *Dtsch Stomatol* 1969;19:481-6.

16. UENO T, OKA T, MIYAGAWA Y, KOBAYASHI Y. Clinical and experimental studies of the location and lines of mandibular fractures. *Bull Tokyo Med Dent Univ* 1957;4:245-51.

17. OLECH E. Fracture lines in mandible. Comparison of radiographic and anatomic findings. *Oral Surg Oral Med Oral Pathol* 1955;8:582-90.

18. URIST MR, JOHNSON RW. Calcification and ossification IV. The healing of fractures in man under clinical conditions. *J Bone Joint Surg* 1943;25:375-426.

19. McLEAN FC, URIST MR. *Bone. An introduction to the physiology of skeletal tissue.* Chicago: The University of Chicago Press, 1961:200-14.

20. SPRINTZ R. Healing of subcondylar fracture of the mandible after ablation of the lateral pterygoid in rats. *J Dent Res* 1969;48:1097-8.

21. MESSER EJ, HAYES DE, BOYNE PJ. Use of intraosseous metal appliances in fixation of mandibular fractures. *J Oral Surg* 1967;25:493-502.

22. GREVE K. Der Heilverlauf von einfachen und komplizierten Unterkieferfrakturen mit besonderer Berücksichtigung des Mandibularkanals und der Zähne. Eine tierexperimentelle und histologische Studie. *Deutsche Zahnheilkunde* No. 67. Leipzig, Georg Thieme Verlag, 1927:1-64.

23. GRIMSON KS. Healing of fractures of the mandible and zygoma. *J Am Dent Assoc* 1937;24:1458-69.

24. RICHMAN PT, LASKIN DM. The healing of experimentally produced fractures of the zygomaticomaxillary complex. *Oral Surg Oral Med Oral Pathol* 1964;17:701-11.

25. HORNOVA J, MALY F. Die Heilung der durch verschieden Mechanismen und in verschiedenen Bedingungen entstandenen Knochendefekte. *Schr Med Fac Med Brun* 1967;40:177-85.

26. KRAMER IRH. The structure of bone and the processes of bone repair. In: ROWE NL, KILLEY HC, eds. *Fractures of the facial skeleton.* London: E & S Livingstone Ltd., 1968:615-25.

27. PASCHKE H. Experimentelle Untersuchungen über den Heilverlauf von Unterkieferfrakturen. *Zahnärztl Rdsch* 1931;40:2172-5.

28. SARNAT BG, SCHOUR I. Effect of experimental fracture on bone, dentin, and enamel. Study of the mandible and the incisor in the rat. *Arch Surg* 1944;49:23-38.

29. BENCZE J. Zahnkeimläsionen infolge Kieferfrakturen im Tierversuch. *Stoma* 1967;20:165-73.

30. SCHÄFER H. Über die Kallusbildung nach Unterkieferfrakturen. *Schweiz Monatsschr Zahnheilkd* 1923;33:567-624.

31. SKLANS S, TAYLOR RG, SHKLAR G. Effect of diphenylhydantoin sodium on healing of experimentally produced fractures in rabbit mandibles. *J Oral Surg* 1967;25:310-9.

32. FRY WK, WARD T. *The dental treatment of maxillo-facial injuries.* Oxford: Blackwell Scientific Publications, 1956:72-92.

33. BONNETTE GH. Experimental fractures of the mandible. *J Oral Surg* 1969;27:568-71.

34. HOFFER O. Indagine sperimentale sul processo evolutivo di guarigione delle ferite ossee (Con particulare reguardo alla traumatologia del condilo). *Minerva Stomatol* 1969;18:1-6.

35. KANEKO Y. Experimental studies on vascular changes in fracture and osteomyelitis. Part I. Vascular changes in mandibular fracture and healing. *Bull Tokyo Dent Coll* 1968;9:123-46.

36. SZABÓ C, TARSOLY E. Kompressziós osteosynthesis gyógyeredményei a kutya mandibuláján. *Fogorv Szle* 1967;60:91-5.

37. GILHUUS-MOE O. Fractures of the mandibular condyle in the growth period. Thesis. Oslo: Universitetsforlaget, 1969.

38. BOYNE PJ. Osseous healing after oblique osteotomy of the mandibular ramus. *J Oral Surg* 1966;24:125-33.

39. BOYNE PJ. Osseous repair and mandibular growth after subcondylar fractures. *J Oral Surg* 1967;25:300-9.

40. YRASTORZA JA, KRUGER GO. Polyurethane polymer in the healing of experimentally fractured mandibles. *Oral Surg Oral Med Oral Surg* 1963;16:978-84.

41. CLARK HB Jr., HAYES PA. A study of the comparative effects of "rigid" and "semirigid" fixation on the healing of fractures of the mandible in dogs. *J Bone Joint Surg* 1963;45-A:731-41.

42. LIGHTERMAN I, FARRELL J. Mandibular fractures treated with plastic polymers. *Arch Surg* 1963;87:868-76.

43. FRIES R. Die stabile Osteosynthese von Unterkieferfrakturen unter besonderer Berücksichtigung der offenen axialer Markdrahtung. II Teil. *Öst Z Stomatol* 1969;66:298-319.

44. HUNSUCK EE. Vascular changes in bone repair. *Oral Surg Oral Med Oral Pathol* 1969;27:572-4.

45. WANNENMACHER E. Ein Beitrag zur pathologischen Histologie der Pulpa. (Die Veränderungen der Pulpen von Zähnen, welche im Bereiche von Kieferfrakturen standen). *Dtsch Monatsschr Zahnheilk* 1927;45:12-38.

46. REICHARDT P. *Untersuchungen an Zähnen, welche im Bereich von Kieferfrakturen standen, mit besonderer Berücksichtigung des Zementmantels.* Thesis. Tübingen: Verlag Franz Pietzcker, 1933.

47. BATAILLE R, KOLF J. Les fractures alvéolaires de la région incisive et leur traitement. *Actual Odontostomatol (Paris)* 1957;40:543-59.

48. ALEXANDRE E, MARIE J-L. A propos du traitement des traumatismes dentaires antérieurs avec fracture du rebord alvéolaire. *Rev Stomatol* 1967;**68:**399-406.

49. KUPFER SR. Fracture of the maxillary alveolus. *Oral Surg Oral Med Oral Pathol* 1954;**7:**830-6.

50. FLIEGE H, HEUSER H, WARNKE M. Beitrag zur Behandlung stark dislozierter Alveolarfortsatzbrücke. *Dtsch Zahn Mund Kieferheilk* 1937;**4:**545-52.

51. MÜLLER W, TAATZ H. Therapie und Spätergebnisse der Alveolarfortsatzfrakturen des Unterkiefers im Säuglings- und Kleinkindesalter. *Dtsch Zahnärztl Z* 1965;**20:**1190-6.

52. PFEIFER G. Freihändige Kunststoffschienung bei Alveolarfortsatzfrakturen und Luxationen im Milchgebiss. *Fortschr Kiefer Gesichtschir* 1959;**5:**328-32.

53. ROWE NL, KILLEY HC. *Fractures of the facial skeleton.* London: E & S Livingstone Ltd., 1968.

54. BENCZE J. Zahnkeimschäden imfolge Kieferfrakturen in der Jugend. *Stoma* 1964;**17:**330-5.

55. BENCZE J. Spätergebnisse nach im Kindesalter erlittenen Unterkieferbrüchen. *Acta Chir Acad Sci Hung* 1964;**5:**95-104.

56. ANDRÄ A, SONNENBURG I. Die Bruchspaltostitis als Komplikation bei Unterkieferbrüchen in Beziehung zum primär vitalen Zahn am oder im Bruchspalt. *Dtsch Stomatol* 1966;**16:**336-44.

57. GÖTTE H. Die Belassung von Zähnen im Bruchspalt in Abhängigkeit von der Art des Kieferbruchverbandes. *Fortschr Kiefer Gesichtschir* 1959;**5:**333-8.

58. SCHÖNBERGER A. Behandlung der Zähne im Bruchspalt. *Fortschr Kiefer Gesishtschir* 1956;**2:**108-11.

59. WILKIE CA, DIECIDUE AA, SIMSES RJ. Management of teeth in the line of mandibular fracture. *J Oral Surg* 1953;**11:**227-30.

60. HEIDSIECK C. Über die Behandlungsergebnisse bei Unterkieferfrakturen. *Dtsch Stomatol* 1954;**4:**271-4.

61. DECHAUME M, CRÉPY C, RÉGNIER J-M. Conduite a tenir au sujet des dents en rapport avec les foyers de fracture des maxillaires. *Rev Stomatol* 1957;**58:**512-9.

62. KRØMER H. Teeth in the line of fracture: A conception of the problem based on a review of 690 jaw fractures. *Br Dent J* 1953;**95:**43-6.

63. HERRMANN M, GRASSER H-H, BEISIEGEL I. Die Kieferbrücke und der Zahn-, Mund- und Kieferklinik in Mainz von 1949-1959. *Dtsch Zahnärztl Z* 1960;**15:**657-64.

64. TAATZ H. Untersuchungen über Ursachen und Häufigkeit exogener Zahnkeimschäden. *Dtsch Zahn Mund Kieferheilk* 1962;**37:**468-84.

65. TAATZ H. Spätschäden nach Kieferbrüchen im Kindersalter. *Fortschr Kieferorthop* 1954;**15:**174-84.

66. FISCHER H-G. Traumata im jugendlichen Kieferbereich, Heilergebnisse und ihr Einfluss auf die Keime der bleibenden Zähne. *Thesis. Lepzig* 1951.

67. FRIEDERICHS W. Kieferbrücke im Kindesalter und seltene Zysten. *Dtsch Zahnärztl Wschr* 1940;**43:**508-10.

68. MÜLLER W. Häufigkeit und Prophylaxe der Bruchspaltostitiden im Zeitalter der Antibiotika. *Stomatol* 1968;**31:**110-7.

69. ROED-PETERSEN B, ANDREASEN JO. Prognosis of permanent teeth involved in jaw fractures. A clinical and radiographic follow-up study. *Scand J Dent Res* 1970;**78:**343-52.

70. MÜLLER W. Zur Frage des Versuchs der Erhaltung der im Bruchspalt stehenden Zähne unter antibiotischem Schutz. *Dtsch Zahn Mund Kieferheilk* 1964;**41:**360-70.

71. WEISKOPF J. Zahnärztlich-orthopädische Methoden der Frakturversorgung. *Dtsch Stomatol* 1961;**11:**682-97.

72. BRACHMANN F. Penicillinbehandlung bei der Kieferbruchversorgung. *Zahnärztl Welt* 1951;**6:**231.

73. SCHÖNBERGER A. Über das Schicksal im Bruchspalt belassener Zähne. *Dtsch Stomatol* 1955;**5:**19-29.

74. ROTTKE B, KARK U. Zur Frage der Extraktion in Bruchspalt stehender Zähne. *Öst Z Stomatol* 1969;**66:**465-9.

75. KOLAROW D, SISKOVA S, DARVODELSKA M. The problem of electrical excitability of teeth in mandibular fractures. *Stomatologiya (Sofia)* 1966;**48:**238-44.

76. MÜLLER W. Die Frakturen des Alveolarfortsatzes. *Dtsch Stomatol* 1972;**22:**135-48.

77. BERNSTEIN L, KEYES KS. Dental and alveolar fractures. *Otolaryngol. Clin North Am* 1972;**5:**273-81.

78. HAMILL JP, OWSLEY JQ, KAUFFMAN RR, BLACKFIELD HM. The treatment of fractures of the mandible. *Calif Med J* 1964;**101:**184-7.

79. NEAL DC, WAGNER WF, ALPERT B. Morbidity associated with teeth in the line of mandibular fractures. *J Oral Surg* 1978;**36:**859-62.

80. SCHNEIDER SS, STERN M. Teeth in the line of mandibular fractures. *J Oral Surg* 1971;**29:**107-9.

81. KAHNBERG K-E, RIDELL A. Prognosis of teeth involved in the line of mandibular fractures. *Int J Oral Surg* 1979;**8:**163-172.

82. RIDELL A, ÅSTRAND P. Conservative treatment of teeth involved by mandibular fractures. *Swed Dent J* 1971;**64:**623-32.

83. JIRAVA E. Contribution to diagnostics of teeth in fragile fissures in fractures of body of the lower jaw. *Ceskoslovenska Stomatol* 1973;**73:**102-6.

84. MATTESON SR, TYNDALL DA. Pantomographic radiology. Part II. Pantomography of trauma and inflammation of the jaws. *Dent Radiography Photography* 1983;**56:**21-48.

85. KREKELER G, PETSCH K, FLESCH-GORLAS M. Der Frakturverlauf im parodontalen Bereich. *Dtsch Zahnärztl Z* 1983;**38:**355-7.

86. ROWE NL, WILLIAMS JL. *Maxillofacial Injuries.* Edinburgh: Churchill Livingstone, 1985: Volume 1 and 2.

87. FONSECA RJ, WALKER RV, eds. *Oral and Maxillofacial Trauma.* Philadelphia: WB Saunders Company, 1991: Volume 1 and 2.

88. SHETTY V, FREYMILLER E. Teeth in the line of fracture: a review. *J Oral Maxillofac Surg* 1989;**47:**1303-6.

89. CHOUNG R, DONOFF RB, GURALNICK WC. A retrospective analysis of 327 mandibular fractures. *J Oral Maxillofac Surg* 1983;**41:**305-9.

90. GÜNTER M, GUNDLACH KKH, SCHWIPPER V. Der Zahn im Bruchspalt. *Dtsch Zahnärztl Z* 1983;**38:**346-8.

91. RINK B, STOEHR K. Weisheitzähne im Bruchspalt. *Stomatol DDR* 1978;**28:**307-10.

92. DE AMARATUNGA NA. The effect of teeth in the line of mandibular fractures on healing. *J Oral Maxillofac Surg* 1987;**45:**312-4.

93. ZALLEN RD, CURRY JT. A study of antibiotic usage in compound mandibular fractures. *J Oral Surg* 1975;**33:**431-4.

94. ADERHOLD L, JUNG H, FRENKEL G. Untersuchungen über den Wert einer Antibiotika-Prophylaxe bei Kiefer-Gesichtsverletzungen - eine prospektive Studie. *Dtsch Zahnärztl Z* 1983;**38:**402-6.

95. GERLACH KL, PAPE HD. Untersuchungen zur Antibiotikaprophylaxe bei der operativen Behandlung von Unterkieferfrakturen. *Dtsch Z Mund Kiefer Gesichtschir* 1988;**12:**497-500.

96. EICHE H, SELLE G. Zur Problematik des Zahnes am Bruchspalt. Eine retrospektive Untersuchung. *Dtsch Zahnärztl Z* 1983;**38:**352-4.

97. WAGNER WF, NEAL DC, ALPERT B. Morbidity associated with extraoral open reduction of mandibular fractures. *J Oral Surg* 1979;**37:**97-100.

98. HÖLTJE W-J, LUHR H-G, HOLTFRETER M. Untersuchungen über infektionsbedingte Komplikationen nach konservativer oder operativer Versorgung von Unterkieferfrakturen. *Fortschr Kiefer Gesichtschir* 1975;**19:**122-5.

99. JOOS U, SCHILLI W, NIEDERDELLMANN H, SCHEIBE B. Komplikationen und verzögerte Bruchheilung bei Kieferfrakturen. *Dtsch Zahnärztl Z* 1983;**38:**387-8.

100. STOLL P, NIEDERDELLMANN H, SAUTER R. Zahnbeteiligung bei Unterkieferfrakturen. *Dtsch Zahnärztl Z* 1983;**38**:349-51.

101. KAHNBERG K-E. Extraction of teeth involved in the line of mandibular fractures. I. Indications for extraction based on a follow-up study of 185 mandibular fractures. *Swed Dent J* 1979;**3**:27-32.

102. OIKARINEN K, LAHTI J, RAUSTIA AM. Prognosis of permanent teeth in the line of mandibular fractures. *Endod Dent Traumatol* 1990;**6**:177-82.

103. PÖLLMANN L. Längsschnittuntersuchungen der Sensibilität nach Kieferwinkelfrakturen. *Dtsch Zahnärztl Z* 1093;**38**:482-5.

104. ROED-PETERSEN B, MORTENSEN H. Periodontal status after fixation with Sauer's and Schuchardt's arch bars in jaw fractures. *Int J Oral Surg* 1972;**1**:43-7.

105. ROED-PETERSEN B, MORTENSEN H. Arch bar fixation of fractures in dentulous jaws: a comparative study of Sauer's and Erich's bar. *Danish Med Bull* 1973;**20**:164-8.

106. BIENENGRÄBER V, SONNENBURG I, WILKEN J. Klinische und tierexperimentelle Untersuchungen über den Einfluss von Drahtschienenverbänden auf das marginale Parodontium. *Dtsch Stomatol* 1973;**23**:86-84.

107. NGASSAPA DN, FREIHOFER H-PM, MALTHA JC. The reaction of the periodontium to different types of splints. (I). Clinical aspects. *Int J Oral Maxillofac Surg* 1986;**15**:240-9.

108. NGASSAPA DN, MALTHA JC, FREIHOFER H-PM. The reaction of the periodontium to different types of splints. (II). Histological aspects. *Int J Oral Maxillofac Surg* 1986;**15**:250-8.

109. HÄRLE F, KREKELER G. Die Reaktion des Parodontiums auf die Drahtligaturenschiene (Stout-Obwegeser). *Dtsch Zahnärztl Z* 1977;**32**:814-6.

110. FRÖHLICH M, GÄBLER K. Der Einfluss von Kieferbruchshienenverbänden auf das Parodont. *Stomatol DDR* 1981;**31**:238-47.

111. SCHMITZ R, HÖLTJE W, CORDES V. Vergleichende Untersuchungen über die Regeneration des parodontalen Gewebes nach Unfallverletzungen und Osteotomien des Alveolarfortsatzes. *Dtsch Zahnärztl Z* 1973;**28**:219-23.

112. HOFFMEISTER B. Die parodontale Reaktion im Bruchspalt stehender Zähne bei Unterkieferfrakturen. *Dtsch Zahnärztl Z* 1985;**40**:32-6.

113. BERGGREN RB, LEHR HB. Mandibular fractures: a review of 185 fractures in 111 patients. *J Trauma* 1967;**7**:357-66.

CHAPTER 12

Injuries to Developing Teeth

J. O. ANDREASEN

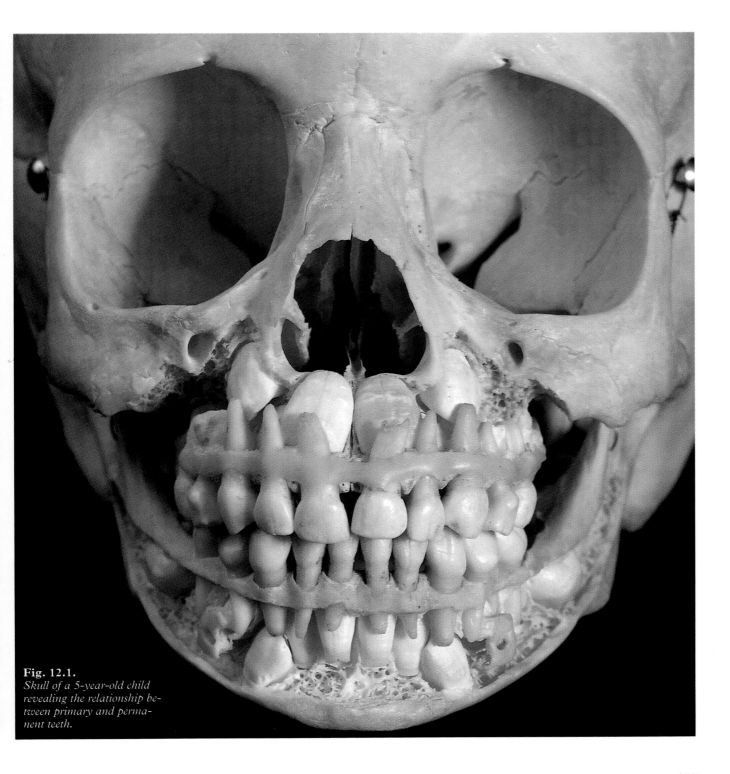

Fig. 12.1.
Skull of a 5-year-old child revealing the relationship between primary and permanent teeth.

Fig. 12.2. Anatomic relationship between the primary incisor and its permanent successor in a human skull
Note that both central and lateral primary incisors are in close relation to the permanent central incisor.

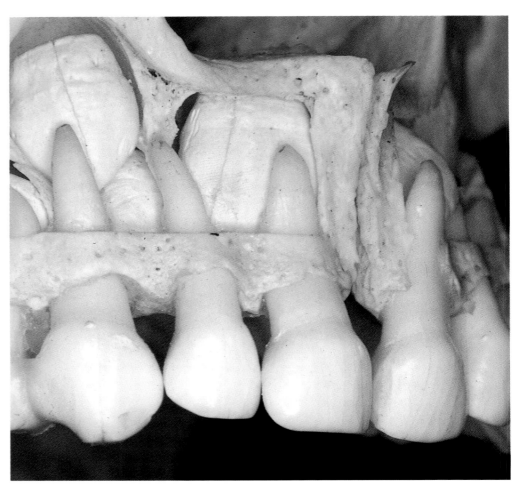

Histologic relationship between a primary incisor and its permanent successor
Note that most of the resorbing primary root is separated from the permanent tooth germ by only a thin layer of soft tissue. From AN-DREASEN (127) 1976.

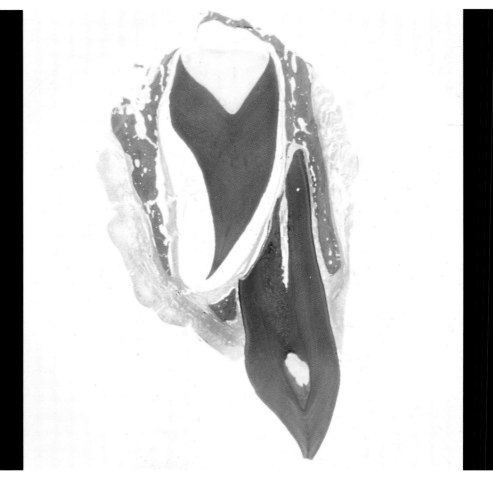

CHAPTER 12

Terminology, Frequency and Etiology

Traumatic injuries to developing teeth can influence their further growth and maturation, usually leaving a child with a permanent and often readily visible deformity. Especially when the injury occurs during initial stages of development, enamel formation can be seriously disturbed due to interference with a number of stages in ameloblastic development, i.e., the morphogenetic, organizing, formative and maturation stages (1, 2).

The close relationship between the apices of primary teeth and the developing permanent successors explains why injuries to primary teeth are easily transmitted to the permanent dentition (Figs. 12.1 and 12.2). Likewise, bone fractures located in areas containing developing tooth germs can interfere with further odontogenesis.

The nature of these injuries has been studied clinically in humans (1, 2, 120-123, 130, 131, 157-62) and experimentally in animals (3-12, 124-129). Thus, anatomic and histological deviations due to injuries to developing teeth can be classified as follows (1):

1. White or yellow-brown discoloration of enamel;
2. White or yellow-brown discoloration of enamel with circular enamel hypoplasia;
3. Crown dilaceration;
4. Odontoma-like malformation;
5. Root duplication;
6. Vestibular root angulation;
7. Lateral root angulation or dilaceration;
8. Partial or complete arrest of root formation;
9. Sequestration of permanent tooth germs;
10. Disturbance in eruption.

In this classification, the term *dilaceration* describes an abrupt deviation of the long axis of the crown or root portion of the tooth. This deviation originates from a traumatic non-axial displacement of already formed hard tissue in relation to the developing soft tissue (1).

The term *angulation* denotes a curvature of the root resulting from a gradual change in the direction of root development without evidence of abrupt displacement of the tooth germ during odontogenesis (1).

The prevalence of such disturbances, secondary to dental injuries in the primary dentition, ranges from 12 to 69%, accord-

Table 12.1. Frequency of disturbances in development of permanent teeth after traumatic injuries to the primary dentition

Examiner	No. of teeth involved	No. of teeth with developmental disturbances
Zelnner (13) 1956	26	3 (12%)
Schreiber (14) 1959	42	8 (19%)
Taatz (15) 1962	33	7 (21%)
Ravn (17) 1968	90	51 (57%)
Lind et al. (120) 1970	72	36 (50%)
Selliseth (16) 1970	128	88 (69%)
Andreasen & Ravn (2) 1971	213	88 (41%)
Andreasen & Ravn (121) 1973	147	85 (58%)
Mehnert (122) 1974	28	10 (36%)
Watzek & Skoda (123) 1976	77	39 (51%)
Brin et al. (157) 1984	56	72 (47%)
Morgantini et al. (160) 1986	60	15 (25%)
Ben-Bassat et al. (159) 1989	414	190 (46%)
Arx (162) 1991	144	33 (23%)

Table 12.2.Frequency of disturbances in development of permanent teeth according to type of injury to the primary dentition. From ANDREASEN & RAVN (2) 1971

Type of injury	No. of teeth	No. of teeth with disturbances in development
Subluxation	45	12 (27%)
Extrusive luxation	76	26 (34%)
Avulsion	27	14 (52%)
Intrusive luxation	36	25 (69%)

ing to the studies listed in Table 12.1. Considering the frequency of traumatic injuries to primary teeth (see Chapter 3, p. 171), it is apparent that enamel hypoplasia of traumatic origin must be rather common. In a recent clinical study, it was estimated that 10% of all enamel hypoplasias affecting anterior teeth in schoolchildren in Copenhagen were related to trauma in the primary dentition (121). The type of trauma sustained apparently determines the type and degree of developmental disturbance. Avulsion and intrusive luxation represent injuries with very high frequencies of developmental disturbance, while subluxation and extrusion represent low-risk groups (Table 12.2) (2, 16, 123, 130, 131, 158, 162). Furthermore, the age at the time of injury is of major importance; thus, fewer complications are seen in individuals over 4 years of age than in individuals in the younger age groups (Table 12.3).

According to the studies listed in Table 12.4, the frequency of developmental disturbances due to jaw fractures ranges from 19 to 68%. Furthermore, the frequency of developmental disturbances has been found to be related to fragment displacement at the time of injury (132). Treatment of jaw fractures by osteosynthesis has also

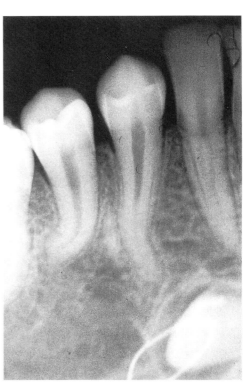

Fig. 12.3.
A 14-year-old patient with an impacted mandibular permanent canine due to osteosynthesis at the age of 5. From PERKO & PEPERSACK (135) 1975.

been shown to increase damage to developing teeth (135) (Fig. 12.3).

Table 12.3.Frequency of developmental disturbances of permanent teeth related to the age at which injury to the primary dentition occurred. From ANDREASEN & RAVN (2) 1971

Age (years)	No. of teeth	No. of teeth with disturbances in development
0-2	62	39 (63%)
3-4	43	23 (53%)
5-6	88	21 (24%)
7-9	20	5 (25%)

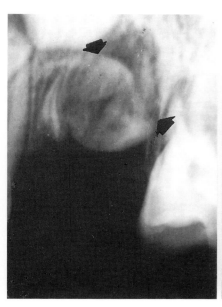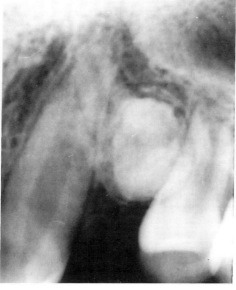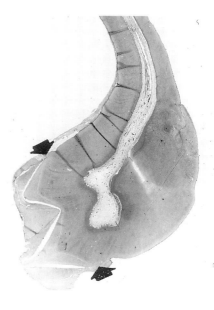

Fig. 12.4.
Crown dilaceration and impaction of a first premolar following extraction of the first primary molar. A. Radiograph taken immediately after extraction of the primary molar at the age of 4 years. The permanent tooth germ appears to be dislocated (arrows). B. Radiograph at the age of 14 years. As the first premolar was impacted, it was decided the tooth be removed. C. Low-power view of sectioned premolar. Slight crown dilaceration is seen (arrows). x 5.

Oral surgical procedures can also induce dental malformations. Thus, patients operated for cleft palate show a very high frequency of enamel defects in the primary as well as the permanent dentitions. Histologic findings in these cases indicate that the surgical trauma could be a contributing factor [22, 23]. Exodontia has also been recorded among surgical etiologic factors. Due to the close relationship between the developing crowns of the permanent premolars and the roots of their primary predecessors, developing premolars are especially prone to disturbances in enamel and dentin formation resulting from extraction of primary molars [24] (Fig. 12.4).

Evaluation of the full extent of complications following injuries sustained in early childhood must await complete eruption of all involved permanent teeth, a problem which should be considered in the case of legal action or insurance claims. However, most serious sequelae (i.e. disturbances in tooth morphology) can usually be diagnosed radiographically within the 1st year after trauma [2].

Injuries which occur very early can also interfere with the development of the primary dentition. Thus, examination of intubated prematurely born infants revealed enamel hypoplasias affecting the primary dentition in 18-80% of the children (163-

Table 12.4. Frequency of developmental disturbances among permanent teeth involved in jaw fractures

Examiner	No. of teeth involved	No. of teeth with developmental disturbances
Fischer [18] 1971	12	7 (58%)
Lenstrup [19] 1959	22	15 (68%)
Taatz [15] 1962	29	14 (48%)
Bencze [20,21] 1964	10	5 (50%)
Ideberg & Persson [132] 1971	100	19 (19%)
Ridell & Åstrand [133] 1971	170	6 (35%)
Ranta & Ylipaavalniemi [134] 1973	37	19 (51%)
Perko & Pepersack [135] 1975	35	16 (46%)

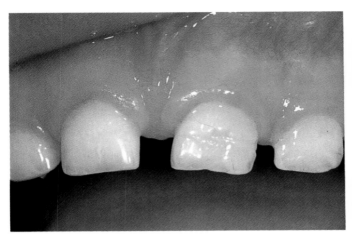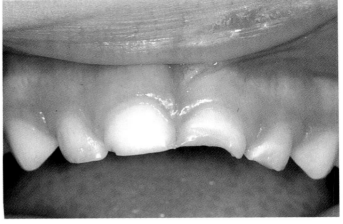

Fig. 12.5.
Enamel hypoplasias caused by a laryngoscopy and/or prolonged endotracheal intubation. The enamel defects are usually located on the left side of the maxilla due to the selective pressure in this area by the laryngoscope. From SEOW ET AL. (164) 1984.

165), usually on the left side of the maxilla corresponding to the customary placement of the tube (164, 165) (Fig. 12.5). A later autopsy study has supported the theory that compression of the alveolar process during endotracheal intubation in neonates is the causative factor which can elicit these disturbances in primary tooth development (166, 167) (Fig. 12.6).

Finally, it should be borne in mind that a number of other pathological conditions may result in enamel hypoplasia (e.g. fluorine, rickets, hypoparathyroidism, exan-

thematous fevers, severe infections and metabolic disturbances such as celiac disease and acidosis). However, these are unfortunately not entirely pathognomonic, but often overlapping in their expression. A classification system for developmental defects of enamel (DDE index) has been developed (168) which, to a certain degree, incorporates some of the pathological features for various developmental disturbances and has recently been used in multifactorial analysis of enamel defects (169-171).

Fig. 12.6.
Dilaceration of primary tooth germ due to endotracheal intubation. This 3-day-old child was intubated post partum due to respiratory distress but died after 3 days. A. At necropsy the unaffected part of the alveolar process shows a normal primary incisor tooth germ. B. Sections from the deformed alveolar ridge where the tube has rested shows disruption of the tooth germ with deviation of the long axis and a resultant cystic space around the enamel matrix. From BOICE ET AL. (166) 1976.

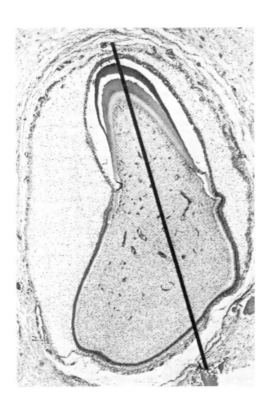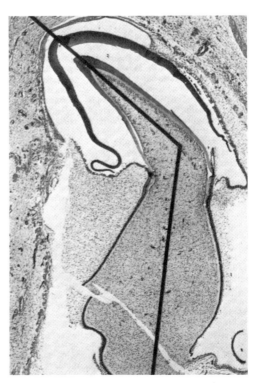

Fig. 12.7.
Discoloration and morphologic changes secondary to injuries to the primary dentition. A. Slight white enamel discolorations involving both central incisors. B. Slight white and yellow-brown staining of the enamel of both central incisors. C. Marked color changes of permanent left central and lateral incisors associated with distal inclination of the crown of the central incisor. D. Yellow-brown enamel changes of central incisor associated with a cavity in the enamel surface. E. Slight circular enamel hypoplasia apical to a yellow-brown discoloration of enamel with an external cavity in a central incisor (arrow). F. Same changes as in E, note the same positional relationship between hypoplasia and area of discoloration (arrows). G and H. Severe disturbances in development of three permanent incisors. Right central incisor is partly impacted due to malformation, left central incisor shows marked color changes. A horizontal enamel hypoplasia is especially evident in Fig. H (see also Figs. 12.14 and 12.22 which show the condition after orthodontic realignment of the right central incisor). From AN-DREASEN ET AL. (1) 1971.

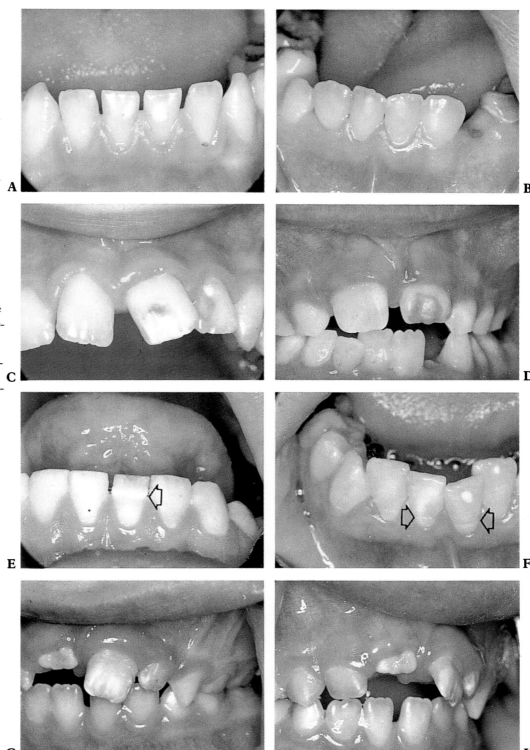

Clinical, Radiographic and Pathologic Findings

Pathologic changes in permanent tooth germs have been studied experimentally in intrusions of primary teeth in monkeys (127). Immediate changes consisted of contusion and displacement of the reduced enamel epithelium and slight displacement of the hard dental tissue in relation to the Hertwig's epithelial root sheath (see Chapter 2, p.88). After 6 weeks, metaplasia of the reduced enamel epithelium into a thin stratified squamous epithelium took place. In most cases, changes in morphology of the dentin and/or enamel matrices were seen (see Chapter 2, p. 79).

Developmental disturbances of human

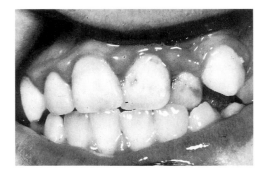
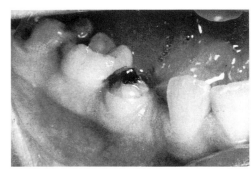

Fig. 12.8.
A. Enamel discolorations affecting left central and lateral incisors following a fracture of the maxilla at the age of 4 years. B. Disturbed enamel formation following a jaw fracture at the age of 3 years. Defective enamel covering the occlusal surface of the lower first premolar. From LENSTRUP (19) 1955.

teeth caused by trauma can be divided into the following types:

White or Yellow-Brown Discolorations of Enamel

These lesions appear as sharply demarcated, stained enamel opacities, most often located on the facial surface of the crown; their extent varies from small spots to large fields (1, 2, 13, 14, 17, 25-38, 121, 136, 159) (Fig. 12.7 A to C). These color changes are usually not associated with clinically detectable defects in the enamel surface. However, some cases can present such defects (1) (Fig. 12.7 D). In this context, it should be mentioned that white enamel discolorations with a diameter of less than 0.5 mm are frequent in teeth without a history of trauma (121, 169, 172).

The frequency of these lesions has been reported to be 23% following injuries to the primary dentition (2), commonly affecting maxillary incisors, with the age of patients at the time of injury ranging from 2 to 7 years. The stage of development of

Fig. 12.9.
A. Maxillary right permanent central monkey incisor 6 weeks after traumatic intrusion of the primary incisor. Note the circumscribed white discoloration of the enamel (arrows). B. Scanning electron micrograph of the adjacent nonaffected enamel. The pits indicate arrest of matrix formation. x 3300. C. General view of white enamel discoloration showing rupture of the enamel surface. x 110. The enclosed area is shown at a higher magnification in D. x 2400. From THYLSTRUP & ANDREASEN (129) 1977.

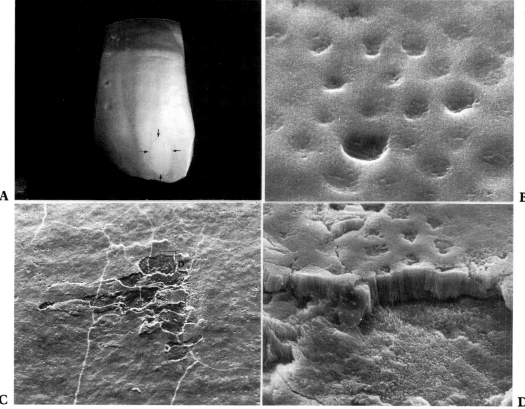

Fig. 12.10.

White enamel discoloration affecting the left central permanent incisor secondary to a dental injury at the age of 1 1/2 years. A. Macroscopic frontal view of specimen consisting of the incisal part of the crown. B. Axial view of the fracture surface; note the extension of the white lesion (arrows). C. Ground section of the specimen photographed in incident light. x 15. D. A microradiograph of the same section reveals that the clinical white area is less mineralized (arrows) than surrounding non-involved enamel. x 15. E. Electron micrographs of decalcified non-involved enamel. The black areas represent organic material. x 8,000. F. Electron micrograph of clinical white area; note that this area contains an increased amount of organic stroma. x 8,000. From ANDREASEN ET AL. (1) 1971.

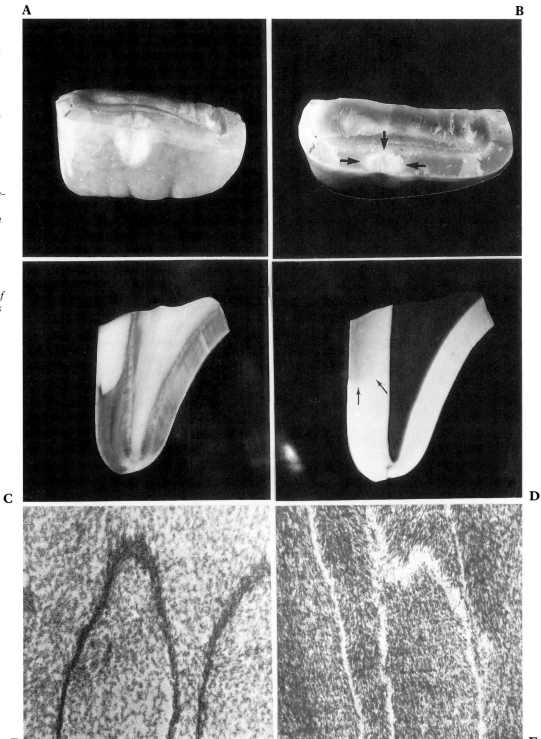

the permanent tooth germ at the time of injury may vary (159). No specific type of injury is especially related to this group of lesions.

Similar disturbances in enamel formation may be seen in developing teeth involved in jaw fractures (19, 39) (Fig. 12.8). For the sake of completeness, it should be mentioned that color changes with or without a defect in the enamel surface may occur as a sequel to periapical inflammation of primary teeth, (15, 40-45, 137-141) giving rise to so-called Turner teeth.

The nature of white enamel discolorations has been studied by means of microradiography and polarized light microscopy, as well as transmission and scanning electron microscopy (Fig. 12.9 and 12.10). Findings from these investigations indicate that the trauma interferes with

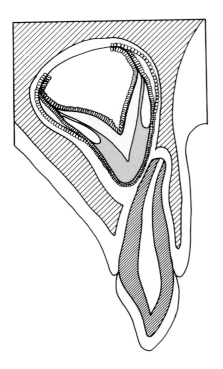 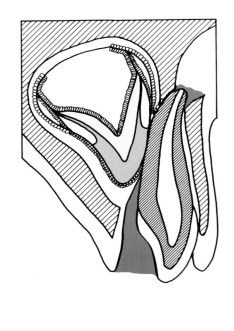 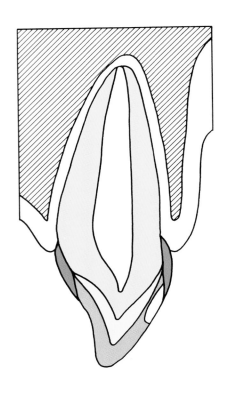

Fig. 12.11.
Schematic drawing illustrating the mechanism of white or yellow-brown discolorations of enamel. A. Condition before injury. B. Primary incisor intruded through the labial socket wall resulting in moderate damage to the reduced enamel epithelium of the permanent successor. C. As a result, enamel maturation is arrested in the area with affected enamel epithelium, creating a white or yellow-brown enamel discoloration.

enamel mineralization, while matrix formation is apparently not involved (1, 129) (Fig. 12.10). An experimental study in monkeys indicates that these areas develop corresponding to areas where trauma has altered the reduced enamel epithelium into a flattened stratified squamous epithelium (see Chapter 2, p 86) (127).

Radiographic examination prior to tooth eruption will usually not reveal defective mineralization. Consequently, these disturbances can only be diagnosed clinically after complete eruption (2).

White or Yellow-Brown Discoloration of Enamel with Circular Enamel Hypoplasia

These lesions are a more severe manifestation of trauma sustained during the formative stages of the permanent tooth germ (1, 2, 29, 46-48, 121, 128). The typical finding in this group, which distinguishes these lesions from those in the first group, is a narrow horizontal groove which encircles the crown cervically to the discolored areas (Fig. 12.7 E to H). In some cases, an

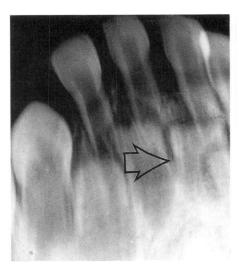 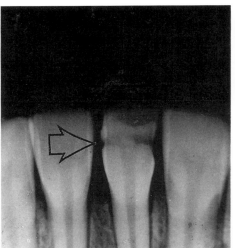 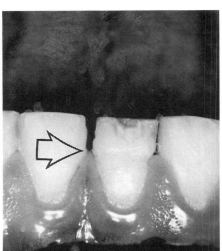

Fig. 12.13.
Microradiographic and electron microscopic findings in a permanent central incisor with crown dilaceration and a yellow-brown enamel discoloration. The patient sustained intrusion of the primary incisor at the age of 2 years. A. Microradiograph of ground section. B. Higher magnification of the enamel defect. Note the radiolucency in this area, indicating a decrease in mineral content. C. Note angulation of enamel prisms (arrows), possibly the result of a direct trauma sustained during matrix formation. The scalloped external surface possibly indicates resorption before deposition of new hard tissue. D. Electron micrograph showing transition between the injured enamel in the cavity (e) and cementum-like tissue (c) deposited in the defect. x 10,000. Insert, in upper right corner, a higher magnification of the cementum-like tissue showing cross-banded fibers (collagen). x 20,000. From ANDREASEN ET AL. (1) 1971.

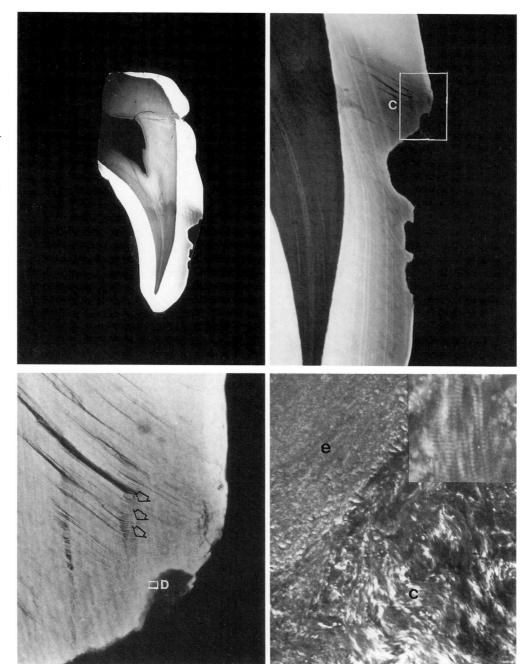

←
Fig. 12.12.
Discoloration and circular enamel hypoplasia of a permanent incisor following injury to the primary dentition. A. Slight intrusive luxation of left central primary incisor at the age of 1 year. Note the degree of mineralization of the permanent incisor (arrow). B. and C. Radiographic and clinical condition at the age of 12 years. Note mineralization disturbances of the incisal edge as well as the circular hypoplasia related to the part of the tooth formed at time injury (arrow), From ANDREASEN ET AL. (1) 1971.

external defect is found centrally in the coronally placed white or yellow-brown lesions (Fig. 12.7 E).

The frequency of this type of change has been reported to be 12% following injuries to the primary dentition (2). Maxillary central incisors are usually involved; the age at the time of injury is usually 2 years. The stage of development of the permanent tooth germ varies from half to complete crown formation at the time of injury. As a rule, the injury to the primary tooth is either avulsion, extrusive or intrusive luxation (1).

Radiographic examination of these teeth

reveals a transverse radiolucent line at the level of indentation and usually a radiolucent area corresponding to the coronally placed enamel defect (Fig. 12.12). This type of developmental disturbance can usually be diagnosed before eruption (2).

It should be noted that the enamel changes are confined to the site of coronal mineralization at the time of injury (Fig. 12.13). Although the pathogenesis of color changes in enamel has not yet been completely clarified, it is assumed that the displaced primary tooth traumatizes tissue adjacent to the permanent tooth germ and possibly the odontogenic epithelium,

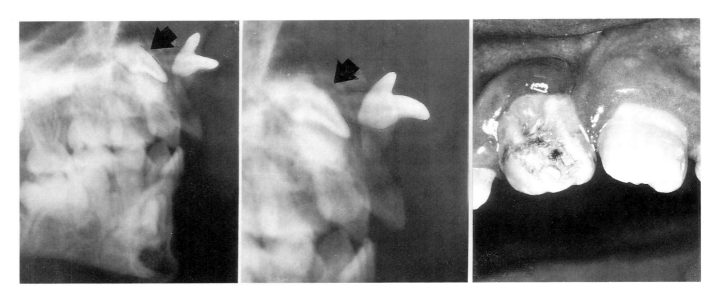

Fig. 12.14.
Severe disturbances in tooth development caused by intrusive luxation of both central incisors at the age of 3 years. A. Lateral projection showing displaced primary incisors (arrow). B. Enlarged view of A. Note that one of the displaced teeth (the right central incisor) faces the facial surface of the permanent tooth germ (arrow). C. Clinical view after surgical exposure and orthodontic realignment of right permanent central incisor. Note the hypoplastic enamel corresponding to previous trauma region (see also Fig. 12.7, G and H, and Fig. 12.22). From ANDREASEN ET AL. (1) 1971.

Fig. 12.15.
Schematic drawing illustrating the possible mechanism of enamel discoloration and circular enamel hypoplasia. A. Condition before injury. B. Slight axial dislocation of the already formed part of the tooth in relation to the remaining tooth germ. C. While enamel formation is resumed apical to the site of dislocation from the intact cervical loops, no further enamel formation occurs coronal to this level. Thus, a horizontal indentation is created between enamel formed before and after injury. From ANDREASEN ET AL. (1) 1971.

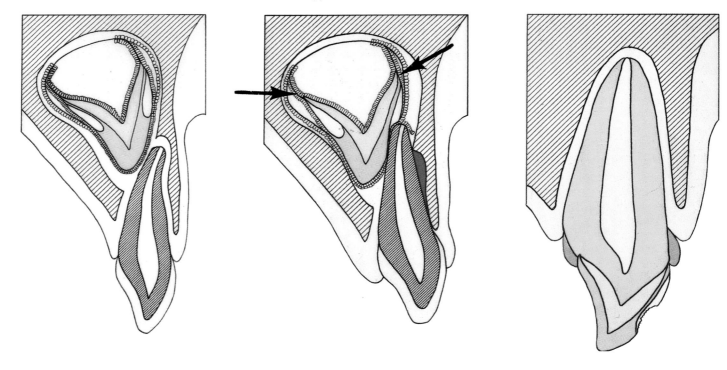

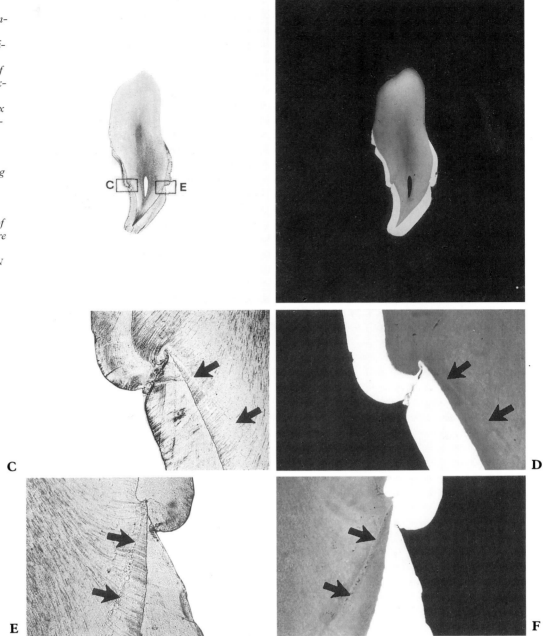

Fig. 12.16.
Yellow-brown discoloration of enamel and circular enamel hypoplasia of a maxillary lateral incisor as a result of avulsion of the primary predecessor at the age of 3 years. A. Ground section of extracted incisor. x 3. B. Microradiograph of the same section. x 3. C. and D. Higher magnification of lingual surface of the crown. Note a slight axial displacement and the calcio-traumatic line in the dentin revealing disturbance in dentin formation immediately after injury (arrows). x 30. E. and F. Higher magnification of facial surface of the crown. The same findings are present in this area as described above. x 30. From ANDREASEN ET AL. (1) 1971.

thereby interfering with final mineralization of enamel (1). The configuration of the resulting hypomineralized area closely coincides with the outline of normal progressive "secondary" mineralization. The lesions are usually white; however, blood breakdown products in the traumatized area can seep into areas of mineralization during further enamel formation. This could explain why yellow-brown areas are located exclusively apical to the white lesions (1) (Fig. 12.7 B). Surface defects in

the enamel most probably reflect direct injury to the enamel matrix before mineralization has been completed (Figs. 12.13 and 12.14).

Experiments in monkeys have shown that circular enamel hypoplasia represents localized damage to the ameloblasts in their formative stages due to traumatic displacement of already formed hard tissue in relation to the developing soft tissues (127) (Figs. 12.15 and 12.16).

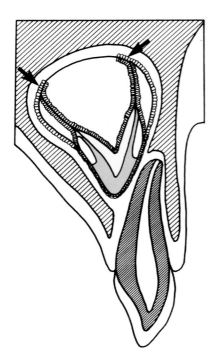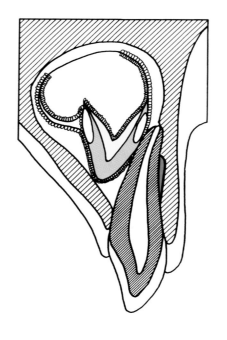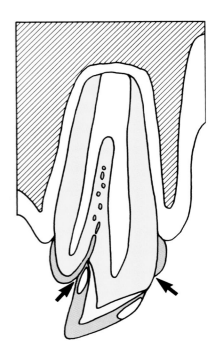

Fig. 12.17.
Schematic drawing illustrating the possible mechanism of crown dilaceration. A. Condition before injury (arrows indicate the cervical loops). B and C. Non-axial dislocation of the already formed part of the tooth in relation to the dental papilla, inner and outer dental epithelium and the cervical loops. Facially, the stretched inner enamel epithelium is able to induce differentiation of new odontoblasts, but its enamel-forming capacity is not expressed. Consequently, a horizontal band of dentin will be left without enamel facially. The facial cervical loop has either not been injured or has been completely regenerated, thus explaining normal amelogenesis apical to the trauma site (arrow). On the lingual aspect of the crown, the displaced inner enamel epithelium and ameloblasts form a cone of hard tissue projecting into the pulp canal. Presumably the ameloblasts stripped from their matrix proliferate and induce dentin as well as enamel matrix formation. The presumably intact lingual cervical loop forms an enamel-covered cusp (arrow). From ANDREASEN ET AL. (1) 1971.

Crown Dilaceration

These malformations are due to traumatic non-axial displacement of already formed hard tissue in relation to the developing soft tissues (1, 2, 17, 27, 31, 49-77, 142-145, 161, 162, 178). Three per cent of the injuries to primary teeth result in this type of malformation (2).

Due to their close contact to the primary incisors, crown-dilacerated teeth are usually maxillary or mandibular central incisors. Approximately half of these teeth become impacted; whereas the remaining erupt normally or in facio- or linguo-version. Injury to the primary dentition usually occurs at the age of 2 years, with a range of from less than 1 year to 5 years. Most often the injury occurs at a time when up to half the crown has been formed, a finding possibly related to the anatomy of the developing tooth germ which allows tilting of the tooth germ within its socket. The trauma to the primary dentition which can result in crown dilaceration is usually avulsion or intrusion (1).

The pathology of crown-dilacerated teeth supports the theory of displacement of the enamel epithelium and the mineralized portion of the tooth in relation to the dental papilla and cervical loops (1, 73-77) (Figs. 12.17 to 12.19). This results in the loss of enamel on a part of the facial surface of the crown. On the lingual aspect, a cone of hard tissue is formed which projects into the root canal, while the lingual cervical loop forms an enamel-covered cusp (1). A pathogenesis of displacement of the non-mineralized portion of the tooth in the socket is supported by radiographic findings immediately after injury where a tilting of the tooth germ can be seen (see Chapter 9, p. 323).

The deviation of the coronal portion varies according to the tooth's location. Maxillary incisors usually show lingual deviation, while lower incisors are usually inclined facially (1).

Radiographically, unerupted crown-dilacerated teeth are seen as foreshortened coronally.

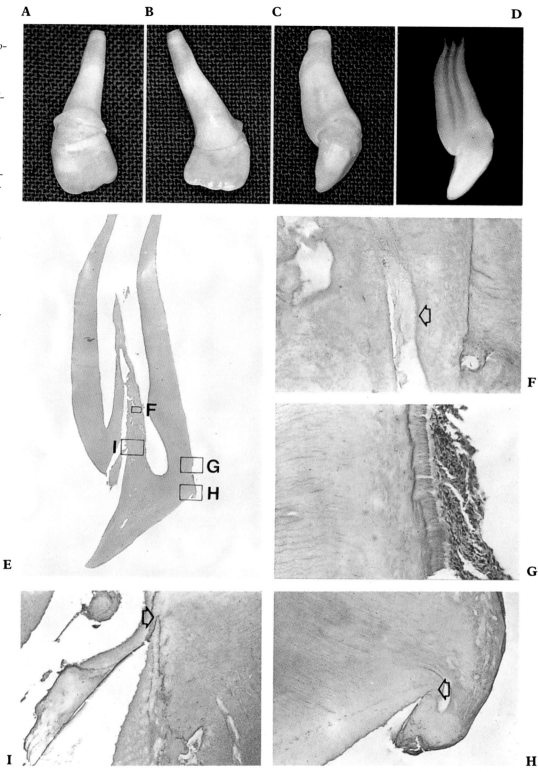

Fig. 12.18.
Clinical, radiographic, and histologic features of a crown dilacerated maxillary central incisor. The patient sustained intrusive luxation of the corresponding primary incisor at the age of 2 1/2-years. A to C. Clinical appearance of extracted incisor. Note area on the facial surface of the crown without enamel and the white and yellow-brown discoloration of the enamel. D. A radiograph discloses an internal cone of hard tissue. E. Low-power view of sectioned incisor. x 4. F. Internal hard tissue cone consisting of enamel matrix (arrow) and dentin. x 195. G. Enamel-free crown area covered with cementum. x 195. H and I. Dilaceration area facially and lingually. Arrows indicate the margins of hard tissue formed at the time of injury. x 75. From AN-DREASEN ET AL. (1) 1971.

Fig. 12.19.
Microradiographic features of crown-dilacerated tooth shown in Fig. 12.18. A. Ground section. x 5. B. Microradiograph. x 5. C. Enamel covers the lingual cusp (arrows). x 30. D. Irregular dentin formed immediately after injury (arrows). x 30. From AN-DREASEN ET AL. (1) 1971.

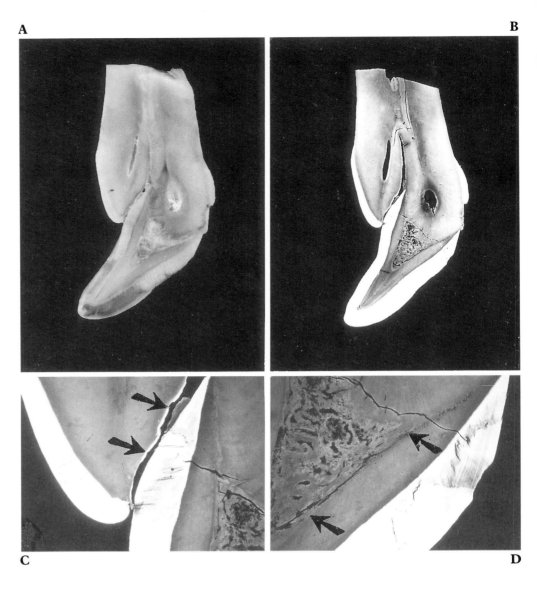

Fig. 12.20.
Odontoma-like malformation of permanent tooth germ due to intrusive luxation of primary left central incisor at the age of 2 years. A. Condition at time of injury. Note the outline of the calcified portion of the permanent tooth germ (arrows). B. Radiograph taken at the age of 8 years. An odontoma-like malformation is found at the site of the central incisor. From ANDREASEN ET AL. (1) 1971.

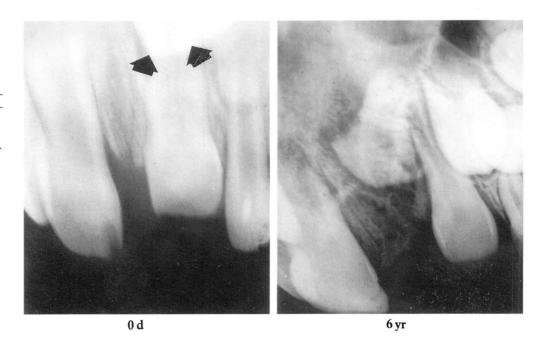

0 d   6 yr

CHAPTER 12

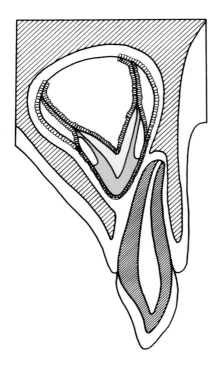
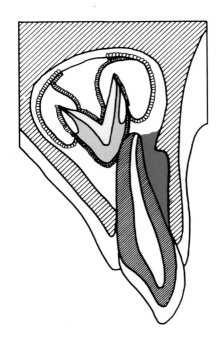
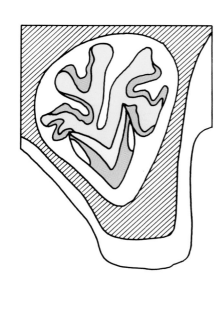

Fig. 12.21.
Schematic drawing illustrating possible mechanism for odontoma-like malformation. A. Condition before injury. B. Axial dislocation of the primary incisor with extensive damage to the permanent tooth germ. C. Formation of an odontoma-like malformation.

Odontoma-like Malformations

These malformations are rare sequelae to injuries in the primary dentition. Reported cases are confined primarily to maxillary incisors (1, 29, 35, 51, 55, 68, 78-81, 161, 162). The age at the time of injury ranges from less than 1 year to 3 years. The type of injury affecting the primary dentition appears to be intrusive luxation or avulsion (1) (Fig. 12.20). The histology and radiology of these cases show a conglomerate of hard tissue, having the morphology of a complex odontoma or separate tooth elements (Figs. 12.21 and 12.22).

Experimental evidence supports the the-

Fig. 12.22.
Development of a separate tooth element following intrusive luxation of primary incisors at the age of 3 years (see also Fig. 12.7, G to H, and Fig. 12.14). A. Radiographic condition at the age of 8 years. Note the small tooth element in the central incisor region (arrow). B. Lateral view of removed odontoma. C. Microradiograph reveals an enamel layer covering part of the tooth element. From AN-DREASEN ET AL. (1) 1971.

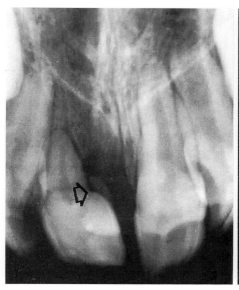
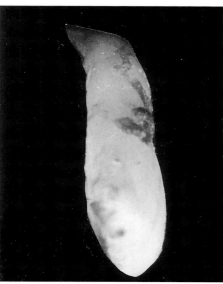
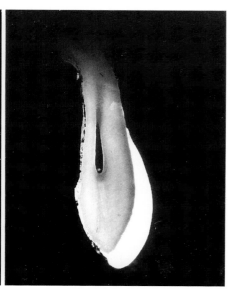

Fig. 12.23.
Odontoma-like malformation of a permanent lateral incisor following avulsion of the primary lateral incisor at the age of 2 years. A. Left central incisor shows a marked crown dilaceration (arrow). B. Radiograph revealing odontoma-like malformation of left lateral incisor (arrow). C. Low-power view of sectioned lateral incisor. x 7. D. Apical part of the odontoma bears similarities to a normal root. Note intact odontoblast layer. x 75. E. Odontoma-like enamel inclusions - most of the enamel was lost during demineralization. x 75. F. Reduced enamel epithelium. x 195. G and H. Preserved enamel matrix. x 75. From ANDREASEN ET AL. (1) *1971.*

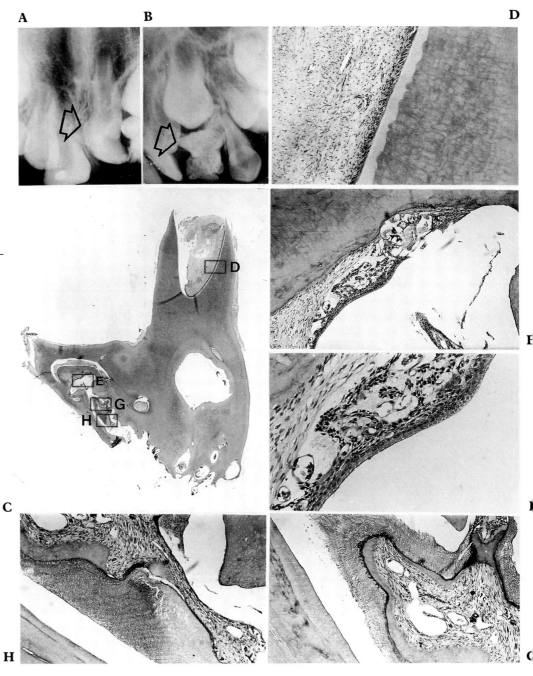

474

Fig. 12.24.
*Malformation of permanent teeth
following ritual extractions of
lower primary canines in an Afri-
can population. A. In place of
the left canine, two apparently
separate tooth elements have
erupted. B. Severe crown malformation of lower right permanent
canine. From PINDBORG (83),
1969.*

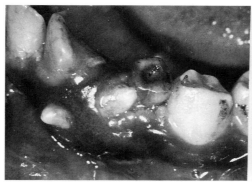
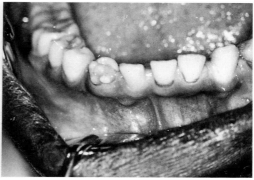

ory that these malformations occur during early phases of odontogenesis and affect the morphogenetic stages of ameloblastic development (4, 5, 10, 82) (Figs. 12.23 and 12.24). The traumatic origin of these malformations is further supported by the observation that similar changes have been reported after ritual extractions of primary canines in peoples in Africa (83) (Fig. 12.24), as well as sequelae to extraction of primary molars due to pulpal complications (24).

Radiographically there is a radiopaque mass with little resemblance to a tooth germ. Sometimes, however, a relatively normal root may be seen (Fig. 12.22).

Root Duplication

This is a rare occurrence, seen following intrusive luxation of primary teeth (1, 84, 85, 173). This complication is usually the result of an injury at the time when half or less than half of the crown is formed (1) (Fig. 12.25). The pathology of these cases indicates that a traumatic division of the cervical loop occurs at the time of injury, resulting in the formation of two separate roots (84) (Fig. 12.26).

Radiographically, a mesial and distal root can be demonstrated which extends from a partially formed crown (Figs. 12.25 and 12.26).

Fig. 12.25.
*Root duplication of 2 central incisors following intrusive luxation of both primary incisors at the age
of 2 years. A. Lateral radiograph at time of injury. Note the displaced primary incisors (arrow). B.
Radiograph taken at the age of 9 years. The root is divided into a mesial and distal portion in both
incisors (arrows). C. After surgical exposure, abnormal root development is evident as well as vertical fractures of the crown of both central incisors (arrows), presumably a result of the previous injury.*

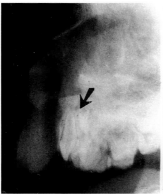
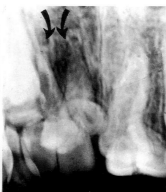
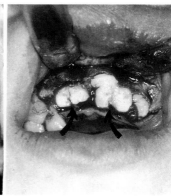

INJURIES TO DEVELOPING TEETH

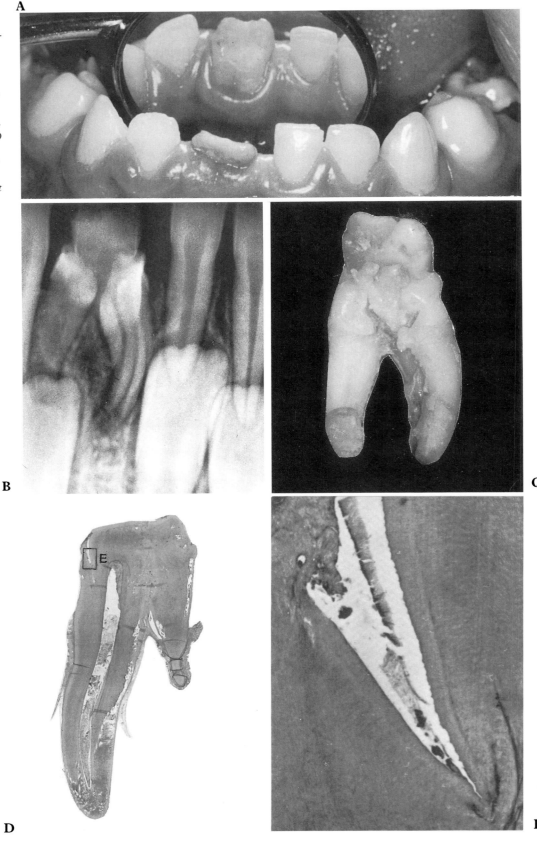

Fig. 12.26.
Histologic features of root duplication of a right permanent central incisor due to an injury sustained at the age of 6 months. A. Clinical appearance. B. Radiograph showing root division. C. Frontal aspect of the extracted tooth. D. Low-power view of sectioned incisor. E. Higher magnification of D indicates that the incisal part of the crown has been intruded. The cleft is lined with enamel. The dentinal tubules are compressed at the bottom of the cleft. From ED-LUND (84) 1964.

Fig. 12.27.
Facial root angulation of a central incisor secondary to extrusive luxation of a primary central incisor at the age of 4 years. A. Lateral radiograph showing facial orientation of the crown (arrow). B. Intraoral radiograph of malformed incisor. C. Low-power view of sectioned incisor. x 9. D. The normally structured dentin indicates that no acute dental trauma has been inflicted on the tooth. x 30. E and F. Slight increase in thickness of the facial cementum compared to the lingual. x 75. From AN-DREASEN ET AL. (1) 1971.

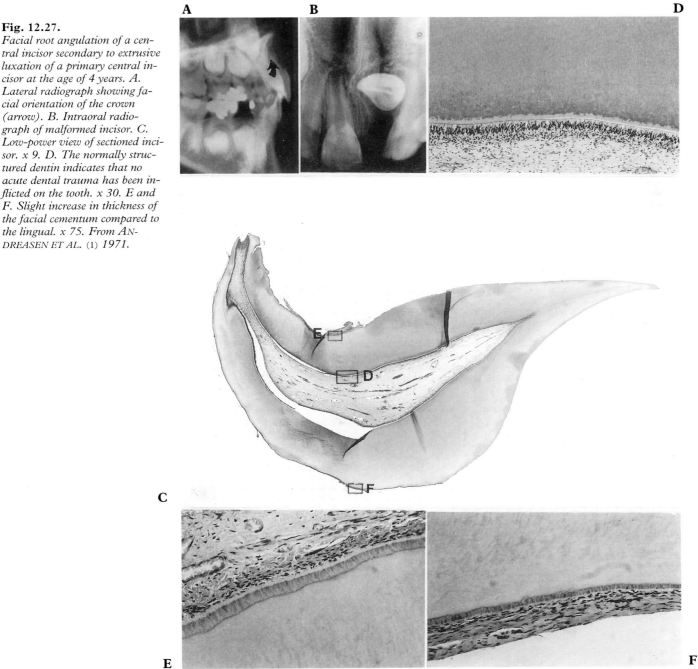

Vestibular Root Angulation

This developmental disturbance appears as a marked curvature confined to the root as a result of an injury sustained at the age of 2 to 5 years (1, 25, 30, 31, 71, 75, 86-96, 137). The malformed tooth is usually impacted and the crown palpable in the labial sulcus. The only teeth demonstrating this malformation are maxillary central incisors. The injuries to the primary dentition consist of intrusive luxation and avulsion (1).

The histopathologic findings in these cases consist of a thickening of cementum in the area of angulation, but with no sign of acute traumatic changes in the hard tissue formed (1, 75, 87) (Fig. 12.27). The loss of a primary incisor can present an obstacle in the eruption of the developing

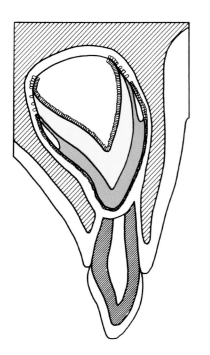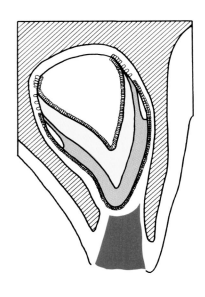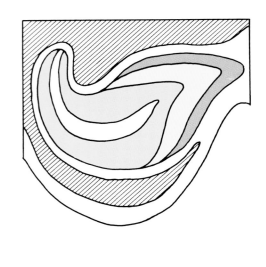

Fig. 12.28.
Schematic drawing illustrating possible mechanism of facial root angulation. A. Condition before injury. B. Primary incisor lost at an early age. C. Possibly due to formation of scar tissue along the path of eruption, the developing tooth changes its position facially.

Fig. 12.29.
Lateral root angulation as a result of avulsion of left primary lateral and central incisors at the age of 5 years. A. Condition after injury. Note that root development of the central incisors has just started. B. Radiograph taken at the age of 7 years reveals angulation between the root and crown portion. From ANDREASEN ET AL. (1) 1971.

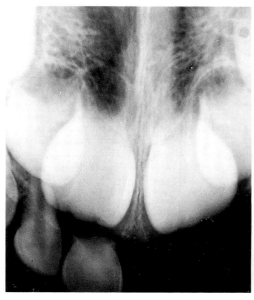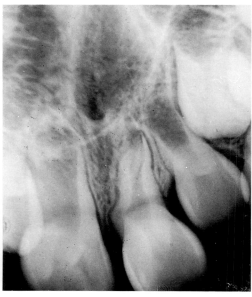

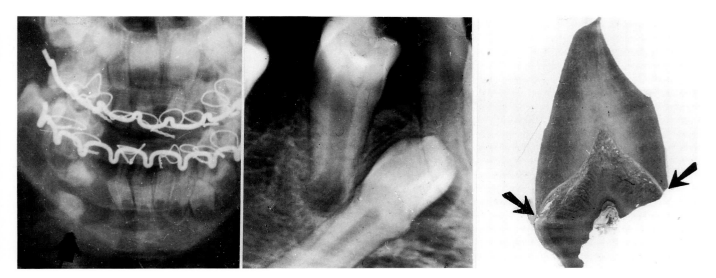

Fig. 12.30.
Impaction and slight root dilaceration of a right canine after jaw fracture sustained at the age of 5 years. A. Radiograph taken 5 days after the injury. Note displacement of the developing canine (arrow). B. Condition 9 years later. Note that the impacted and dislocated canine shows slight root dilaceration. C. Histologic examination of the coronal part of the canine. The dilaceration is clearly visible (arrows). From LENSTRUP (19) 1955.

tooth, forcing it to change its path of eruption in a labial direction (Fig. 12.28). Presumably Hertwig's epithelial root sheath remains in position despite the impact and thereby creates a curvature of the root (1). It should be mentioned, however, that the traumatic origin of this malformation has been questioned. Thus, in a study of 29 teeth, STEWART (146) found no history of trauma. Moreover, this type of malformation was 6 times more frequent in girls than in boys. According to STEWART, the most likely explanation for facial root angulation was ectopic development of the tooth germ (146).

Radiographically a root-angulated tooth appears foreshortened. Lateral projections can more precisely localize the position of the tooth within the jaw (Fig. 12.27).

Lateral Root Angulation or Dilaceration

These changes appear as a mesial or distal bending confined to the root of the tooth (29, 30, 52, 55, 71, 77, 78, 86, 94, 98, 147, 161) (Fig. 12.29). They are seen in 1% of cases with injury to the primary dentition, usually avulsion. The injury usually occurs at age 2 to 7 years and usually affects the maxillary incisors. In contrast to vestibular angulation, most teeth with lateral root angulation or dilaceration erupt spontaneously (1). Similar malformations have been seen in developing teeth involved in jaw fractures (15, 18-21, 99, 100, 148) (Fig. 12.30).

The pathogenesis of these lesions is not fully understood, but histologic studies have shown that displacement apparently occurs between the mineralized root portion and the developing soft tissues (19, 77) (Fig. 12.30).

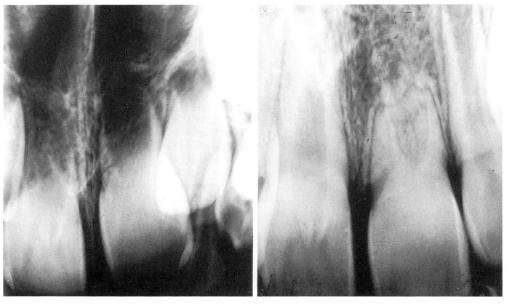

Fig. 12.31.
Complete arrest of root formation following avulsion of a left primary central incisor at the age of 5 years. A. Radiograph at time of injury. B. Condition at the age of 7 years. Note complete arrest of root development, invasion of bone into the root canal and development of an internal periodontal ligament. From ANDREASEN ET AL. (1) *1971.*

Fig. 12.32.
Partial arrest of root formation of a right central incisor. The patient sustained luxation injury of both primary central incisors at the age of 5 years. A and B. Frontal and lateral views of extracted incisor. A small resorption cavity is evident cervically (arrows) possibly inflicted by previous surgical exposure of the impacted tooth. C. Low-power view of sectioned incisor. Apart from peripheral root resorption there is no evidence of acute injury. x 5. From ANDREASEN ET AL. (1) *1971.*

Partial or Complete Arrest of Root Formation

This is a rare complication among injuries in the primary dentition, affecting 2% of involved permanent teeth (1, 2, 29, 69, 71, 86, 101-107, 161, 162) (Figs. 12.31 to 12.36). The injury to the primary dentition usually occurs between 5 and 7 years of age and normally affects maxillary incisors. The injury sustained is usually avulsion of the primary incisors (1). A number of teeth with this type of root malformation remain impacted, while others erupt precociously and are often exfoliated due to inadequate periodontal support. Similar root abnor-

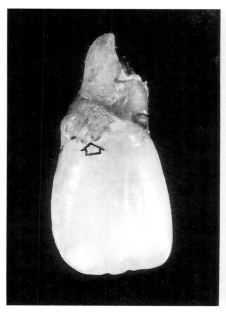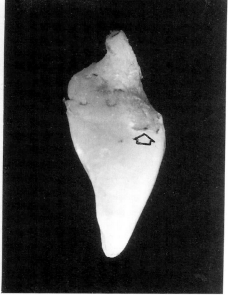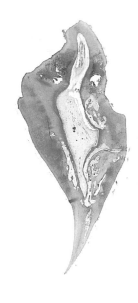

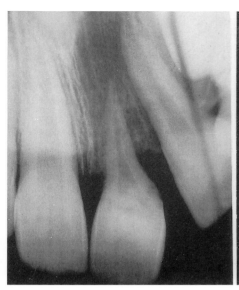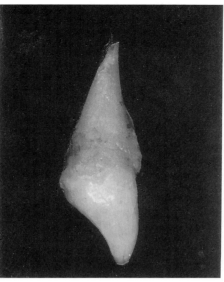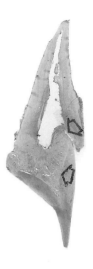

Fig. 12.33.
Partial arrest of root formation of an upper left central incisor. The patient sustained an injury to the primary dentition at the age of 5 years. A. Radiographic examination at the age of 8 years shows a secondary pulp necrosis and a periapical radiolucency. Pulp necrosis was possibly induced by bacterial invasion through the poorly mineralized tissue formed immediately following injury. B. Mesial view of extracted incisor. C. Low-power view of sectioned incisor. A slight dilaceration and a marked calcio-traumatic line with poorly mineralized tissue (arrows) indicate that an acute injury has occurred during odontogenesis. x 3. From ANDREASEN ET AL. (1) *1971.*

Fig. 12.34.
Partial arrest of root development after jaw fracture affecting the right side of the mandible in an 8-year-old patient. A. Condition immediately after injury. B. Six years later. The canine is impacted with a partial arrest of root development. C. Histologic examination of the removed canine. Note sharp demarcation between pre- and post-traumatic hard tissue formation. x 8. From LENSTRUP (19) *1955.*

malities have been found in developing teeth involved in jaw fractures (15, 18, 19, 99, 108-111).

The histopathology of root malformation varies. Some cases show diminutive

root development without evidence of a previous acute traumatic episode during hard tissue deposition (1, 106, 107) (Fig. 12.32). Scar tissue developing after premature loss of the primary predecessor has

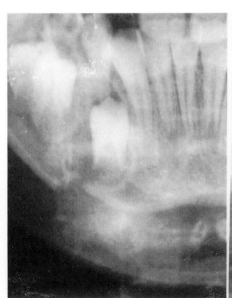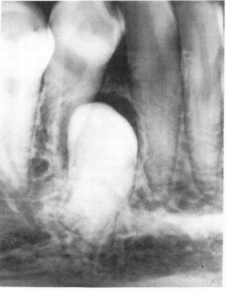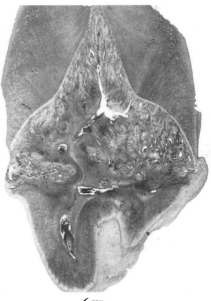

0 d **6 yr** **6 yr**

INJURIES TO DEVELOPING TEETH

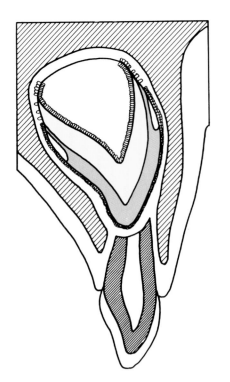 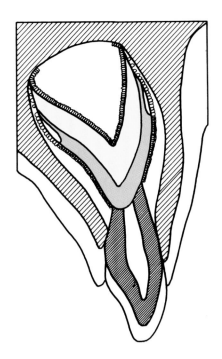 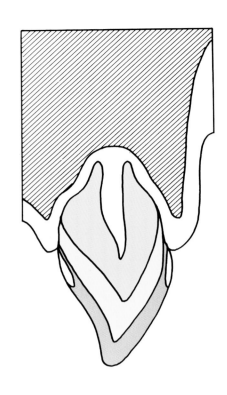

Fig. 12.35.
Schematic drawing illustrating mechanism of partial arrest of root formation. A. Condition before injury. B. The impact from the intruded primary incisor is transmitted to the permanent incisor with subsequent damage to the Hertwig's epithelial root sheath. C. Partial arrest of root formation.

been thought to prevent normal eruption and also to interfere with root formation (1). In other instances, a typical calcio-traumatic line, separating hard tissue formed before and after injury, is seen (1, 19, 103, 112) (Figs. 12.33 and 12.34). In these cases, the trauma has apparently directly injured Hertwig's epithelial root sheath, thus compromising normal root development (Fig. 12.35).

Radiographic examination reveals typical foreshortening of the root. Root resorption may also be seen with this type of root abnormality (19, 108, 111) (Fig. 12.36).

Fig. 12.36.
Complete arrest of root development and root resorption after jaw fracture in the second molar region of a 9-year-old child. A and B. Condition immediately after trauma. The developing second molar is displaced. C. Condition 7 years later. The second molar has erupted; however, there is a complete arrest of root development and root resorption. From LENSTRUP (19) 1955.

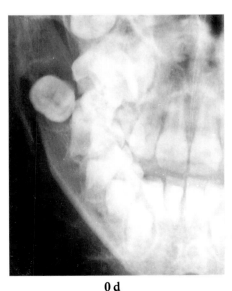 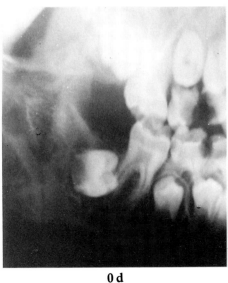 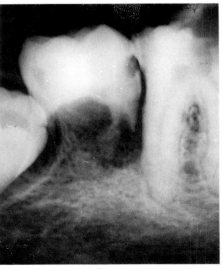

| 0 d | 0 d | 7 yr |

CHAPTER 12

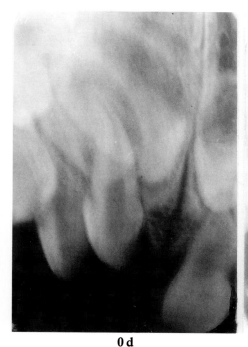

0 d

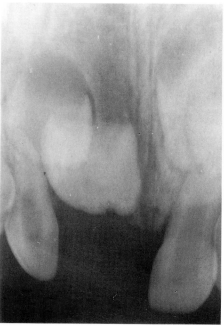

2 mo

6 mo

Fig. 12.37.
Sequestration of a permanent central incisor tooth germ in a 1 1/2-year-old child. A. Radiographic examination at the time of injury reveals intrusion of the right primary central incisor. The primary incisor was removed 2 weeks later due to acute inflammation and a labial abscess. B. A chronic fistula appeared in the region 2 months later. Antibiotic therapy was instituted and the fistula disappeared. However, upon withdrawal of antibiotics, the fistula returned. C. Radiographic condition after 6 months. Note the osteolytic changes around the permanent tooth germ. At this time, the tooth germ was removed. Courtesy of Dr. H. ECHERBOM, Luleå, Sweden.

Sequestration of Permanent Tooth Germs

This is exceedingly rare after injuries to the primary dentition (71, 92, 161) (Fig. 12.37).

Infection can complicate healing of jaw fractures. In these instances, swelling, suppuration and fistula formation are typical clinical features, sometimes leading to spontaneous sequestration of involved tooth germs (18, 100, 111, 113) (Fig. 12.36).

Radiographic examination discloses osteolytic changes around the tooth germ, including disappearance of the outline of the dental crypt.

Disturbances in Eruption

Disturbances in permanent tooth eruption may occur after trauma to the primary dentition and it is suggested that this is related to abnormal changes in the connective tissue overlying the tooth germ (149). The eruption of succeeding permanent incisors is generally delayed for about 1 year after premature loss of primary incisors (114, 115), whereas premature eruption of permanent successors is rare (69, 71). Early loss of primary incisors (avulsion or extraction) leads to space loss only in rare instances (158, 162). However, ectopic eruption of permanent successors has been

seen, possibly due to lack of eruption guidance otherwise offered by the primary dentition (158). These teeth often erupt labially (162). Impaction is very common among teeth with malformations confined to either the crown or root (1, 116). When the permanent tooth does erupt, it is often in facio- or linguoversion (114, 115, 150).

Treatment

Minor *white or yellow-brown discolorations of enamel* seldom require treatment. However, if the enamel changes are esthetically disturbing, recently developed techniques for enamel microabrasion have been suggested (174-176) (Fig. 12.38). This implies application of an 18% hydrochloric acid-pumice paste to the isolated enamel surfaces for a series of, e.g., 6-8 sequential 5-sec rubbing applications with 10-sec interim water rinsings. This treatment is followed by a 4-min application of 2% sodium fluoride gel and polishing with abrasives when necessary.

It has been found experimentally on extracted teeth with intact enamel surfaces, that such a procedure removes 12μm enamel initially and 26μm with successive applications (177), but that the amount of enamel which was lost was clinically undetectable (175). Unfortunately most ena-

Fig. 12.38. Microabrasion of a tooth with superficial enamel discoloration
A central incisor with multicolored superficial enamel defects is shown on the left. Immediately after enamel microabrasion (right), the discoloration is eliminated. Courtesy of Dr. TP CROLL, Doyletown, USA.

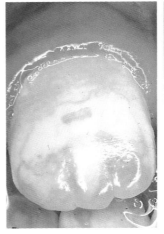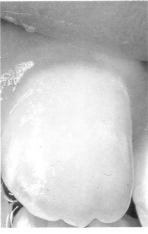

Microabrasion of trauma-induced enamel discolorations
The enamel changes consist of opaque white and yellow color changes.

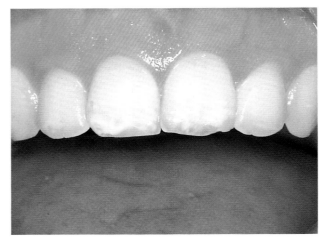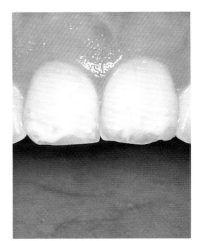

Enamel abrasion
Both central incisors are isolated with a rubber-dam and enamel abrasion carried out with hydrochloric acid-pumice mixture, a mandrel tip and a hand applicator.

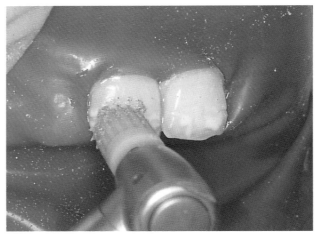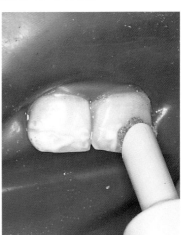

Condition after enamel abrasion
The enamel changes are markedly accentuated compared to the status before enamel abrasion.

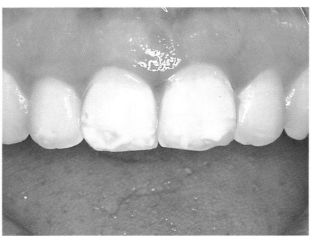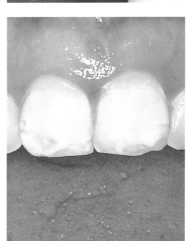

Fig. 12.39.
Restoration of a right central inci-sor with yellow-brown discolored enamel with a composite resin. A. Clinical condition. B. Cleans-ing the enamel with pumice fol-lowed by a bur. C. Etching the enamel. D and E. A celluloid crown form is used as a matrix for the composite resin. F. The finished restoration.

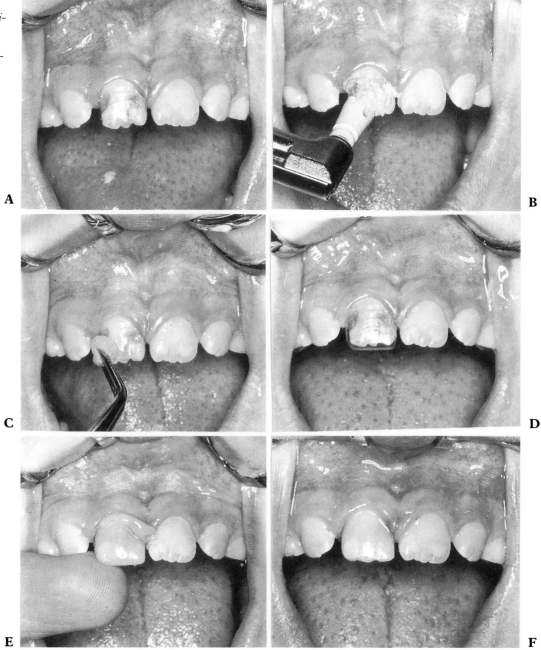

mel discolorations due to trauma pene-trate the entire enamel thickness (1)(Figs. 12.10, 12.13 and 12.19). This fact ex-plains why this technique does not work satisfactorily in trauma-related enamel discoloration and may sometimes even ac-centuate these discolorations (Fig. 12.38).

Treatment of *white or yellow-brown disco-loration of enamel* with circular enamel hyp-poplasia implies removal of the discolored enamel with a bur, etching with an acid conditioner and restoration with a compo-site resin (151-156) (Fig. 12.39).

When discoloration and enamel defects

occupy most of the labial surface, a porce-lain jacket crown or laminate veneer can be indicated (117,118).

Crown dilacerated teeth often erupt spon-taneously into normal position. In some cases, surgical exposure of the crown is necessary (Fig. 12.40). Because of the se-verity of the malposition, surgical expo-sure sometimes has to be supplemented with orthodontic realignment (178,179). (Chapter 15, p. 6.17).

When the tooth has erupted to the level such that the dilacerated area is free of the gingiva, restorative therapy should be in-

Fig. 12.40. Surgical and restorative treatment of a crown-dilacerated incisor
The patient sustained an intrusion injury of both right primary incisors at the age of 1 year. These teeth were later removed due to pulp necrosis. The radiographic examination shows crown dilaceration of the right central incisor and enamel hypoplasia of the right lateral incisor.

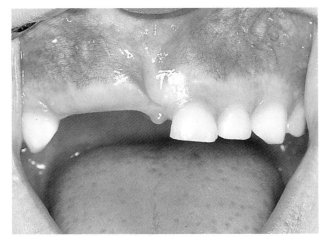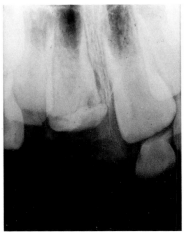

Clinical and radiographic condition at the age of 7 years
Eruption has not taken place of the right central incisor. Surgical exposure was therefore planned.

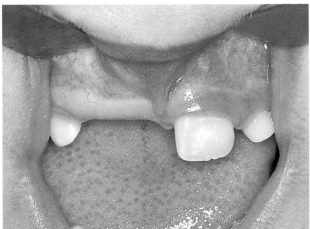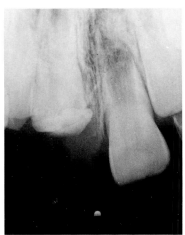

Surgical exposure of the malformed incisors
After administration of a local anesthesia both incisors were surgical exposed.

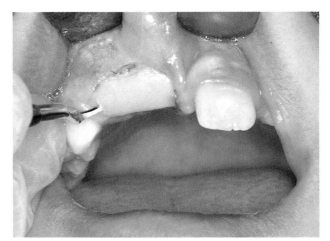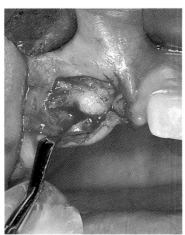

Condition after exposure
Two weeks after surgical exposure a new gingival collar has been formed

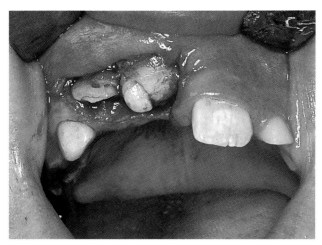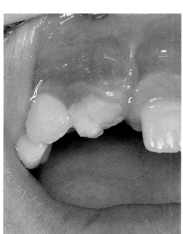

Condition 4 months later
The incisors have further erupted and are now ready for restoration.

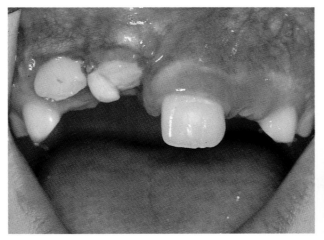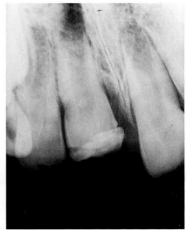

Removing the dilacerated crown portion
After a local anesthesia the dilacerated crown portion is removed and the exposed dentin is covered with a hard-setting calcium hydroxide cement.

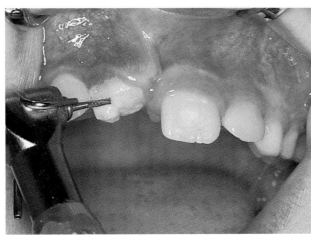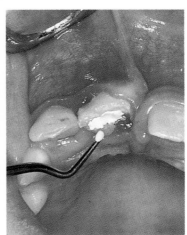

Temporary restoration
The incisor is temporarily restored. Due to problems with moisture control the tooth was initially restored with a steel crown and later with a temporary bridge material.

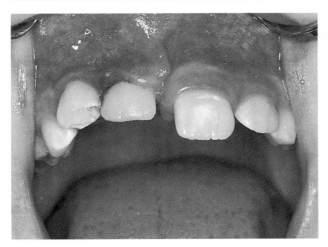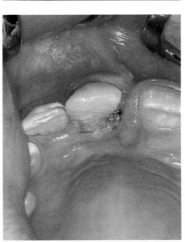

Restoration with composite resin
As an interim restoration both incisors were restored with composite resin.

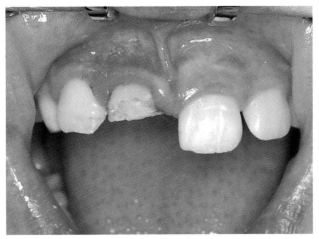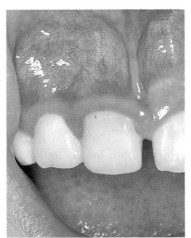

INJURIES TO DEVELOPING TEETH

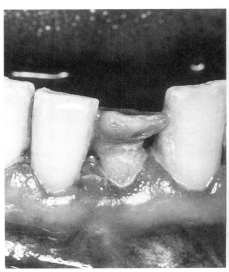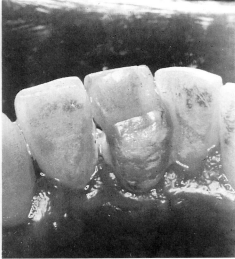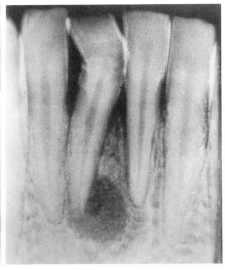

Fig. 12.41.
Pulp necrosis and periapical inflammation following crown dilaceration of a central incisor. A and B. Frontal and lingual view of involved incisor. C. Radiographic demonstration of pulp necrosis and periapical inflammation.

stituted, as the central lumen of the "internal root" constitutes a pathway for bacteria into the pulp. Thus, a number of these teeth have been found to develop pulp necrosis and periapical inflammation after eruption without any evidence of decay (1, 74, 76, 136) (Fig. 12.41). It is therefore important to remove the dilacerated part of the crown as soon as possible. A temporary crown can then be placed until eruption is complete, when an acid-etch/composite resin restoration, a veneer or a cast restoration can be made (Figs. 12.40).

Malformed impacted teeth, e.g., *odontoma-like malformations*, teeth with *root duplication, root dilaceration* or *angulation* should generally be removed. However, future treatment needs (i.e. dental implants) might indicate their preservation in order to maintain the alveolar ridge at an acceptable height. A possible exception is *vestibular root angulation*. Provided there is adequate space, such teeth can be realigned by surgical exposure followed by orthodontic intervention (29, 86, 91, 119, 136) (see Chapter 15, p. 617).

Infection of tooth germs usually leeds to spontaneous *sequestration of the tooth germ*, if not, they should be removed surgically (137).

In some cases, premature loss of primary teeth can lead to *disturbance in eruption*. Apparently the tooth germ is not able to penetrate the mucosa covering the alveolar process. In these cases, excision of the tissue overlying the incisal edge will result in rapid eruption of the impacted tooth (149, 180) (Fig. 12.42). If the teeth are impacted with their crowns inclined facially and above the mucogingival junction, it is important to know that a wide incision of nonfunctional mucosa can give rise to retraction of the gingiva. Furthermore, the gingiva is nonkeratinized and prone to periodontal disease (149) (Figs. 12.43). While this finding has been questioned in a recent case report (180), It is recommended that a smaller incision be made, preferably only in the functional gingivae.

Fig. 12.42. Surgical exposure of impacted permanent incisors
This 1-year-old girl suffered avulsion of all primary incisors due to a fall.

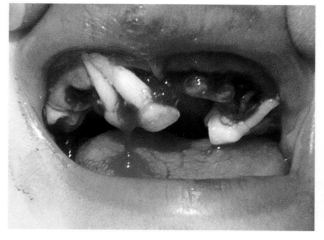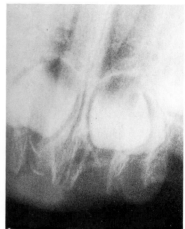

Condition at the age of 10
There is no sign of eruption in spite of advanced root development. The incisal edges of the impacted incicors can be palpated.

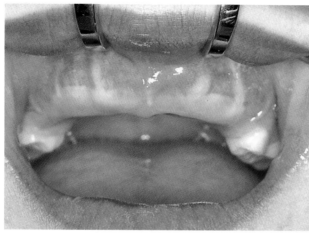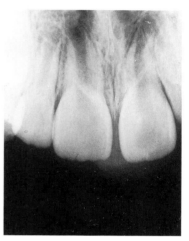

Exposing the incisors
After administration of a local anesthesia the mucosa overlaying the incisal edges is removed with a surgical blade.

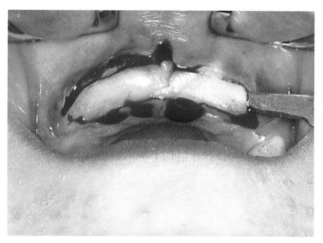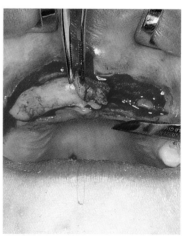

Condition 6 months after exposure
The incisiors are now fully erupted.

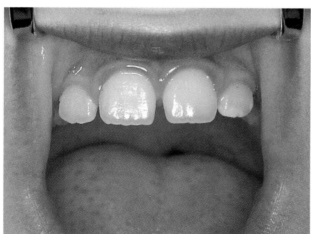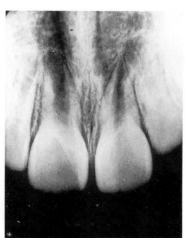

INJURIES TO DEVELOPING TEETH

Fig. 12.43.
Gingival retraction and enlarged gingival cuffs in a patient where both central incisors were exposed above the muco-gingival junction. From DiBiase (149) 1971.

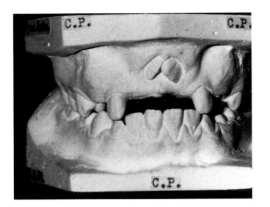 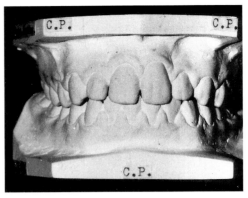

Essentials

Terminology

White or yellow-brown discoloration of enamel

White or yellow-brown discoloration of enamel and circular enamel hypoplasia

Crown dilaceration

Odontoma-like malformation

Root duplication

Vestibular root angulation

Lateral root angulation or dilaceration

Partial or complete arrest of root formation

Sequestration of permanent tooth germ

Disturbance in eruption

Frequency

Injuries to primary teeth: 12 to 69% of involved permanent teeth

Jaw fractures: 19 to 68% of involved permanent teeth

Pathology

Disturbances in mineralization and morphology

Treatment

YELLOW-BROWN DISCOLORATION OF ENAMEL WITH OR WITHOUT ENAMEL HYPOPLASIA

a. Enamel micro abrasion (Fig. 12.38)

b. Composite resin restoration (Fig. 12.39)

c. Porcelain-fused-to-gold restoration

d. Porcelain jacket crown

CROWN DILACERATION (FIG. 12.40)

a. Surgical exposure and possibly orthodontic realignment

b. Removal of dilacerated part of the Crown

c. Temporary crown until root formation is completed

d. Semi- or permanent restoration

VESTIBULAR ROOT ANGULATION

a. Combined surgical and orthodontic realignment

OTHER MALFORMATIONS

a. Extraction is usually the treatment of choice

DISTURBANCE IN ERUPTION (FIG. 12.41)

a. Surgical exposure

Bibliography

1. ANDREASEN JO, SUNDSTRÖM B, RAVN JJ. The effect of traumatic injuries to primary teeth on their permanent successors. I. A clinical and histologic study of 117 injured permanent teeth. *Scand J Dent Res* 1971;**79**:219-83.

2. ANDREASEN JO, RAVN JJ. The effect of traumatic injuries to primary teeth on their permanent successors. II. A clinical and radiographic follow-up study of 213 injured teeth. *Scand J Dent Res* 1971;**79**:284-94.

3. SARNAT BG, SCHOUR I. Effect of experimental fracture on bone, dentin and enamel. Study of the mandible and the incisor in the rat. *Arch Surg* 1944;**49**:23-38.

4. SANTONÉ P. Über die Folgen von umschriebenen, traumatischen Verletzungen in Geweben der Zahnanlage. *Dtsch Zahn Mund Kieferheilk* 1937;**4**:323-37, 602-14.

5. LEVY BA. Effects of experimental trauma on developing first molar teeth in rats. *J Dent Res* 1968;**47**:323-7.

6. SCHOUR I. The effect of tooth injury on other teeth. I. The effect of a fracture confined to one or two incisors and their investing tissues upon the other incisors in the rat. *J Physiol Zool* 1934;**7**:304-29.

7. ADLOFF P. Experimentelle Untersuchungen zur Regeneration des Gebisses. *Dtsch Monatschr Zahnheilk* 1920;**38**:385-412.

8. SHAPIRO HH, LEFKOWITZ W, BODECKER CF. Role of the dental papilla in early tooth formation. Part I - Roentgenographic study. *J Dent Res* 1942;**21**:391-34.

9. LEFKOWITZ W, BODECKER CF, SHAPIRO HH. Experimental papillectomy. Part II: Histological study. (Preliminary report). *J Dent Res* 1944;**23**:345-61.

10. BRAUER W. Mechanisch erzeugte Entwicklungsstörungen des Zahnkeimes. ("Experimentelle Zahnkeimmissbildungen".) *Dtsch Monatschr Zahnheilk* 1928;**46**:737-51.

11. BENCZE J. Zahnkeimläsionen infolge Kieferfrakturen im Tierversuch. *Stoma (Heidelberg)* 1967;**20**:165-73.

12. GREWE JM, FELTS WJL. The consequences of mandibular incisor extraction in the young mouse I. Histologic aspects. *J Dent Res* 1969;**48**:583-9.

13. ZELLNER R. Schmelzmissbildungen am permanenten Gebiss nach Milchzahnluxation. *Zahnärztl Prax* 1956;**7**:1-2.

14. SCHREIBER CK. The effect of trauma on the anterior deciduous teeth. *Br Dent J* 1959;**106**:340-3.

15. TAATZ H. Untersuchungen über Ursachen und Häufigkeit exogener Zahnkeimschäden. *Dtsch Zahn Mund Kieferheilk* 1962;**37**:468-84.

16. SELLISETH N-E. The significance of traumatised primary incisors on the development and eruption of permanent teeth. *Eur Orthodont Dent Soc* 1970;**46**:443-59.

17. RAVN JJ. Sequelae of acute mechanical traumata in the primary dentition. *ASDC J Dent Child* 1968;**35**:281-9.

18. FISCHER H-G. *Traumata im jugendlichen Kieferbereich - Heilergebnisse und ihr Einfluss auf die Keime der bleibenden Zähne.* Thesis, Leipzig 1951.

19. LENSTRUP K. On injury by fractures of the jaws to teeth in course of formation. *Acta Odontol Scand* 1955;**13**:181-202.

20. BENCZE J. Spätergebnisse nach im Kindesalter erlittenen Unterkieferbrücken. *Acta Chir Acad Sci Hung* 1964;**5**:95-104.

21. BENCZE J. Zahnkeimschäden infolge Kieferfrakturen in der Jugend. *Stoma (Heidelberg)* 1964;**17**:330-5.

22. DIXON DA. Defects of structure and formation of the teeth in persons with cleft palate and the effect of reparative surgery on the dental tissues. *Oral Surg Oral Med Oral Pathol* 1968;**25**:435-46.

23. MINK JR. Relationship of hypoplastic teeth and surgical trauma in cleft repair. *J Dent Res* 1959;**38**:652-3.

24. WILLIAMSON JJ. Trauma during exodontia. An aetiologic factor in hypoplastic premolars. *Br Dent J* 1966;**121**:284-9.

25. ELLIS RG, DAVEY KV. *The classification and treatment of injuries to the teeth of children.* 5th edn. Chicago: Year Book Publishers Inc., 1970.

26. RADKOVEC F. Les dents de Turner. *8 congrés dentaire international*, Section 3. Paris 1931:210-21.

27. BENNET DT. Traumatised anterior teeth. *Br Dent J* 1964;**116**:52-5.

28. SZYMANSKA-JACHIMCZAK I. Wplyw ostrych mechanicznych urazów zebów mlecznych na znieksztalcenia koron zebow stalych w okresie ich wczesnego rozwoju. *Czas Stomatol* 1960;**13**:9-21.

29. HOTZ R. Die Bedeutung, Beurteilung und Behandlung beim Trauma im Frontzahngebiet vom Standpunkt des Kieferorthopäden. *Dtsch Zahnärztl Z* 1958;**13**:42-51.

30. BJÖRK A. Störningar i tandutvecklingen som följd av trauma. *Svensk Tandläkaras Tidning* 1943;**36**:470-85.

31. MacGREGOR SA. Management of injuries to deciduous incisors. *J Canad Dent Assoc* 1969;**35**:26-34.

32. BRUSZT P. Die Beeinflussbarkeit der Schmelzoberfläche bleibender Zähne durch Traumen der Milchzähne in frühester Jugend. *Dtsch Zahnärztl Z* 1956;**11**:190-2.

33. PAPILLON-LÉAGE, VILLENEUVE. Dystrophie de cause locale. *Rev Stomatol (Paris)* 1951;**52**:320-5.

34. MONICA WS. Anaplasia. Report of a case. *Oral Surg Oral Med Oral Pathol* 1960;**13**:581-3.

35. SCHINDLER J. Über traumatische Schädigungen des Zahnkeimes und ihre Folgen. *Schweiz Monatschr Zahnheilk* 1943;**53**:697-702.

36. SCHEUER O. Ein Beitrag zur Kenntnis von Infraktionen der Zähne. *Österr Ung Vjschr Zahnheilk* 1914;**30**:303-7.

37. DECHAUME M. Dystrophies et malpositions dentaires et maxillaires d'origine traumatique. *Rev Stomatol (Paris)* 1935;**37**:87-102.

38. ANDERSON BG. Developmental enamel defects. Clinical descriptions and classification. *Am J Dis Child* 1942;**63**:154-63.

39. PERINT EJ. A case of local hypoplasia of the second upper premolar due to trauma. *Dent Practit Dent Rec* 1951-52;**2**:51.

40. BAUER WH. Effect of periapical processes of deciduous teeth on the buds of permanent teeth. Pathological-clinical study. *Am J Orthod* 1946;**32**:232-41.

41. BINNS WH, ESCOBAR A. Defects in permanent teeth following pulp exposure of primary teeth. *ASDC J Dent Child* 1967;**34**:4-14.

42. McCORMICK J, FILOSTRAT DJ. Injury to the teeth of succession by abscess of the temporary teeth. *ASDC J Dent Child* 1967;**34**:501-4.

43. MORNINGSTAR CH. Effect of infection of the deciduous molar on the permanent tooth germ. *J Am Dent Assoc* 1937;**24**:786-91.

44. KAPLAN NL, ZACH L, GOLDSMITH ED. Effects of pulpal exposure in the primary dentition of the succedaneous teeth. *ASDC J Dent Child* 1967;**34**:237-42.

45. MATSUMIYA S. Experimental pathological study on the effect of treatment of infected root canals in the deciduous tooth on growth of the permanent tooth germ. *Int Dent J* 1968;**18**:546-59.

46. VIA WF. Enamel defects induced by trauma during tooth formation. *Oral Surg Oral Med Oral Pathol* 1968;**25**:49-54.

47. FECHNER F. Frühkindliche Frontzahntraumen und ihre Folgen. *Zahnärztl Prax* 1965;**16**:221.

48. POWERS DF. Enamel dysplasia due to trauma. *Dent Surv* 1962;**38**:43-6.

49. WEDL C. Ueber Knickungen und Drehungen an den Kronen und Wurzeln der Zähne. *Dtsch Vjschr Zahnheilk* 1867;**7**:247-53.

50. M'QUILLEN JH. Dilaceration, or flexion of the crown of a left superior central incisor. *Dent Cosmos* 1874;**16**:80-3.

51. PECKERT. Ein Fall von Zahnmissbildung durch Trauma. *Korresp Bl Zahnärzte* 1912;**41**:58-61.

52. DECHAUME M. Dystrophies dentaires d'origine traumatique. *Presse Med* 1933;**41**:1832.

53. KOWARSKY M. Zur Kauistik der traumatischen Affektion der Zähne. *Z Stomatol* 1934;**32**:1082-7.

54. MERLE-BÉRAL J. Malformation et anomalie dentaires. *Rev Stomatol (Paris)* 1936;**38**:844-8.

55. ASCHER F. Unfallfolgen während der Kleinkinderzeit in der Betrachtung als kieferorthopädisches Problem. *Zahnärztl Welt* 1949;**4**:283-8.

56. ASCHER F. Folgen nach Unfällen während der Kleinkinderzeit. *Zahn- Mund- und Kieferheilkunde in Vorträgen*. No. 9. München: Carl Hanser Verlag, 1952:107-16.

57. GUSTAFSON G, SUNDBERG S. Dens in dente. *Br Dent J* 1950;**88**:111-22.

58. CHEMIN. Anomalie de forme par traumatisme. *Rev Stomatol (Paris)* 1951;**52**:325-7.

59. BOYLE PE. *Kronfeld's histopathology of the teeth and their surrounding structures*. 4th edn. Philadelphia 1956: Lea & Febiger, 1956:452-3.

60. JACHNO R, LISKA K. Pri1spvek k traumatickému poskozeni zubnick zárodku. *Cs Stomatol* 1967;**67**:285-92.

61. PFEIFER H. Erhaltung traumatisch geschädigter Zähne. *Dtsch Zahnärztl Z* 1969;**24**:263-7.

62. GLENN FB, STANLEY HR. Dilaceration of a mandibular permanent incisor. Report of a case. *Oral Surg Oral Med Oral Pathol* 1952;**13**:1249-52.

63. BODENHOFF J. Dilaceratio dentis. *Tandlægebladet* 1963;**67**:710-7.

64. MICHANOWICZ AE. Somatopsychic trauma as a result of a dilacerated crown. *ASDC J Dent Child* 1963;**30**:150-2.

65. BOHÁTKA L. Dilaceratio dentis. *Fogorv Szle* 1969;**62**:43-8.

66. KLUGE R. Auswirkung einer zweimaligen Traumatisierung auf einen unteren Frontzahn. *Dtsch Zahnärztl Z* 1964;**19**:800-8.

67. GERLING K. Ein Fall von Pfählungsverletzung bleibender Frontzahnkeime. *Dtsch Stomatol* 1965;**15**:273-7.

68. GAGLIANI N. Malposizioni e malformazioni dentarie conseguenti a trauma in dentatura decidua. *Dent Cadm (Milano)* 1967;**35**:1393-1409.

69. GYSEL C. Traumatologie et orthodontie. *Rev Fr Odontostomatol* 1962;**9**:1091-113.

70. SCHROETER. Formanomalie und Retention eines Zahnes, bedingt durch Trauma im Entwicklungsstadium. *Zahnärztl Rdsch* 1925;**34**:175.

71. BROGLIA ML, DANA F. Manifestazioni cliniche delle lesioni traumatiche accidentali della dentatura decidua. *Minerva Stomatol* 1967;**16**:623-35.

72. TOMES JA. *System of dental surgery*. London: John Churchill, 1859:240-1.

73. RUSHTON MA. Partial duplication following injury to developing incisors. *Br Dent J* 1958;**104**:9-12.

74. ZILKENS K. Beiträge zur traumatischen Zahnschädigung. In: Wannenmacher E. *Ein Querschnitt der deutschen Wissenschaftlichen Zahnheilkunde*. No. 33. Leipzig: Verlag von Hermann Meusser, 1938:43-70.

75. ARWILL T. Histopathologic studies of traumatized teeth. *Odontologisk Tidsskrift* 1962;**70**:91-117.

76. CASTALDI CR. Traumatic injury to unerupted incisors following a blow to the primary teeth. *J Canad Dent Assoc* 1959;**25**:752-62.

77. TAATZ H, TAATZ H. Feingewebliche Studien an permanenten Frontzähnen nach traumatischer Schädigung während der Keimentwicklung. *Dtsch Zahnärztl Z* 1961;**16**:995-1002.

78. BRUSZT P. Durch Traumen verursachte Entwicklungsstörungen bei Schneidezähnen. *Z Stomatol* 1936;**34**:1056-77.

79. RODDA JC. Gross maldevelopment of a permanent tooth caused by trauma to its deciduous predecessor. *N Z Dent J* 1960;**56**:24-5.

80. GIUSTINA C. Su di un caso di malformazione dentaria d'origine traumatica. *Minerva Stomatol* 1954;**3**:190-5.

81. HITCHIN AD. Traumatic odontome. *Br Dent J* 1969;**126**:260-5.

82. GLASSTONE S. The development of halved tooth germs. A study of experimental embryology. *J Anat* 1952;**86**:12-5.

83. PINDBORG JJ. Dental mutilation and associated abnormalities in Uganda. *Am J Physiol Anthrop* 1969;**31**:383-9.

84. EDLUND K. Complete root duplication of a lower permanent incisor caused by traumatic injury. Case report. *Odontologisk Revy* 1964;**15**:299-306.

85. ARWILL T, ÅSTRAND P. Dilaceration av 2+. Ett intressant fall. *Odontologisk Tidskrift* 1968;**76**:427-49.

86. ESCHLER J. *Die traumatischen Verletzungen der Frontzähne bei Jugendlichen*. 2nd edn. Heidelberg: Alfred Hüthig Verlag, 1966.

87. TRIEBSCH E. Durchbruchsstörungen nach Zahnkeimschädigung und traumatischem Milchzahnverlust. *Fortschr Kieferorthop* 1958;**19**:170-9.

88. WUNSCHHEIM GV. Frakturen, Infraktionen und Knickungen der Zähne. *Österr Ung Vjschr Zahnheilk* 1904;**20**:45-102.

89. GRADY R. An everted crown. *Dent Cosmos* 1889;**31**:911-2.

90. SMITH JM. A case of dilaceration. *Dent Cosmos* 1930;**72**:667.

91. HEHRING H, KRUSE H. Über die Dilaceration von Zähnen. *Zahnärztl Welt* 1961;**62**:33-7.

92. ALEYT G. Milchzahnintrusionen und mögliche Folgen an den oberen permanenten Schneidezähnen. *Dtsch Stomatol* 1969;**19**:459-64.

93. BROGLIA ML, RE G. Malformazioni dentarie secondarie a traumatismo dei germi permanenti. *Minerva Stomatol* 1959;**8**:520-6.

94. RECKOW JF v. Das intraorale Röntgenbild und seine klinische Auswertung. *Zahn-, Mund- und Kieferheilkunde in Vorträgen*. No. 16. Zahnärztliche Röntgenologie in diagnostischer und therapeutischer Anwendung. München: Carl Hanser Verlag, 1955:9-30.

95. BORGMANN H. Das akute Trauma im Milchgebiss. *Dtsch Zahnärztl Z* 1959;**14**:325-31.

96. EULER H. *Die Anomalien, Fehlbildungen und Verstümmelungen der menschlichen Zähne*. München-Berlin: JF Lehmanns Verlag, 1939:125-41.

97. MEYER W. Der verbogene obere mittlere Schneidezahn. *Zahnärztl Welt* 1955;**10**:406-7.

98. TAATZ H. Verletzungen der Milchzähne und ihre Behandlung. In Reichenbach, E. *Zahnärztliche Fortbildung*. No. 16. Kinderzahnheilkunde im Vorschulalter. Leipzig: Johan Ambrosius Barth, 1967:363-86.

99. FUHR K, SETZ D. Über die Folgen von Zahnkeimschädigungen durch Kieferfrakturen. *Dtsch Zahnärztl Z* 1963;**18**:482-6.

100. TAATZ H. Spätschäden nach Kieferbrüchen im Kindesalter. *Fortschr Kieferorthop* 1954;**15**:174-84.

101. BECKMANN K, BECKMANN P. Wurzelverkümmerung durch Trauma. *Quintessenz Zahnärztl Lit* 1967;**18**:79.

102. BALL JS. A sequel to trauma involving the deciduous incisors. *Br Dent J* 1965;**118**:394-5.

103. FIELD GS. Case of repair after injury to developing permanent incisors. *N Z Dent J* 1931;**24**:125.

104. SCHMELZ H. Über die Bedeutung traumatisch geschädigter Zahnkeime für den kieferorthopädischen Behandlungsplan. *Zahnärztl Welt* 1957;**58**:327-30.

105. FREY JS. Dilaceration. *Oral Surg Oral Med Oral Pathol* 1966;**21**:321-2.

106. MEYER W. Ein Beitrag zur traumatischen Schädigung von Zahnkeimen. *Dtsch Monatschr Zahnheilk* 1924;**42**:497-510.

107. WALLENIUS B, GRÄNSE KA. Eruption disturbances: Two cases with different etiology. *Odontologisk Revy* 1954;**5**:297-310.

108. CARMICHAEL AF, NIXON GS. Two interesting cases of root resorption. *Dent Rec* 1954;**74**:258-60.

109. PARFITT GJ. Maxillofacial injuries in children and their sequelae. *Dent Rec* 1946;**66**:159-68.

110. HALL SR, IRANPOUR B. The effect of trauma on normal tooth development. Report of two cases. *ASDC J Dent Child* 1968;**35**:291-5.

111. FRANKL Z. Über die Folgen von Zahnkeimschädigungen durch Kieferfrakturen. *Dtsch Zahnärztl Z* 1963;**18**:1225-7.

112. BERGER B, Fischer C-H. Frontzahntrauma und Zahnentwicklung. *Dtsch Zahn Mund Kieferheilk* 1967;**49**:319-27.

113. FRIEDERICHS W. Kieferbrüche im Kindesalter und seltene Zysten. Dtsch Zahnärztl Wochenschr 1940;43:508-10.

114. ASH AS. Orthodontic significance of anomalies of tooth eruption. *Am J Orthod* 1957;**43**:559-76.

115. KORF SR. The eruption of permanent central incisors following premature loss of their antecedents. *ASDC J Dent Child* 1965;**32**:39-44.

116. BROGLIA ML. Considerazioni su un caso di intrusione traumatica di un dente deciduo causa di ritenzione del corrispondente permanente. *Minerva Stomatol* 1959;**8**:811-3.

117. FADDEN LE. The restoration of hypoplastic young anterior teeth. *ASDC J Dent Child* 1951;**18**:21-30.

118. MAGNUSSON B. Några synpunkter på unga permanenta tänder med emaljhypoplasier. *Svensk Tandläkare Tidskrift* 1960;**53**:53-72.

119. SCHULZE C. Über die Folgen des Verlustes oberer mittlerer Schneidezähne während der Gebissentwicklung. *Zahnärztl Rdsch* 1967;**76**:156-69.

120. LIND V, WALLIN H, EGERMARK-ERIKSSON I, BERNHOLD M. Indirekta traumaskador. Kliniska skador på permanenta incisiver som följd av trauma mot temporära incisiver. *Sverig Tandläkar Förbund Tidning* 1970;**62**:738-56.

121. ANDREASEN JO, RAVN JJ. Enamel changes in permanent teeth after trauma to their primary predecessors. *Scand J Dent Res* 1973;**81**:203-9.

122. MEHNERT H. Untersuchungen über die Auswirkungen von Milschzahnverletzungen auf das bleibende Gebiss. *Österr Z Stomatol* 1974;**71**:407-13.

123. WATZEK G, SKODA J. Milchzahntraumen und ihre Bedeutung für die bleibenden Zähne. *Zahn Mund Kieferheilk* 1976;**64**:126-33.

124. BIENENGRÄBER V, SOBKOWIAK E-M. Tierexperimentelle Untersuchungen zur Frage des indirekten Milschzahntraumas. *Z Exper Chir* 1971;**4**:174-80.

125. CUTRIGHT DE. The reaction of permanent tooth buds to injury. *Oral Surg Oral Med Oral Pathol* 1971;**32**:832-9.

126. FREDÉN H, HEYDEN G, INGERVALL B. Traumatic injuries to enamel formation in rat incisors. *Scand J Dent Res* 1975;**83**:135-44.

127. ANDREASEN JO. The influence of traumatic intrusion of primary teeth on their permanent successors. A radiographic and histologic study in monkeys. *Int J Oral Surg* 1976;**5**:207-19.

128. SUCKLING GW, CUTRESS TW. Traumatically induced defects of enamel in permanent teeth in sheep. *J Dent Res* 1977;**56**:1429.

129. THYLSTRUP A, ANDREASEN JO. The influence of traumatic intrusion of primary teeth on their permanent successors in monkeys. A macroscopic, polarized light and scanning electron microscopic study. *J Oral Pathol* 1977;**6**:296-306.

130. RAVN JJ. Developmental disturbances in permanent teeth after exarticulation of their primary predecessors. *Scand J Dent Res* 1976;**83**:131-41.

131. RAVN JJ. Developmental disturbances in permanent teeth after intrusion of their primary predecessors. *Scand J Dent Res* 1976;**84**:137-46.

132. IDEBERG M, PERSSON B. Development of permanent tooth germs involved in mandibular fractures in children. *J Dent Res* 1971;**50**:721.

133. RIDELL A, ÅSTRAND P. Conservative treatment of teeth involved by mandibular fractures. *Swed Dent J* 1971;**64**:623-32.

134. RANTA R, YLIPAAVALNIEMI P. The effect of jaw fractures in children on the development of permanent teeth and the occlusion. *Proc Finn Dent Soc* 1973;**69**:99-104.

135. PERKO M, PEPERSACK W. Spätergebnisse der Osteosynthesebehandlung bei Kieferfrakturen im Kindesalter. *Fortschr Kiefer Gesichtschir* 1975;**19**:206-8.

136. VAN GOOL AV. Injury to the permanent tooth germ after trauma to the deciduous predecessor. *Oral Surg Oral Med Oral Pathol* 1973;**35**:2-12.

137. ANDO S, SANKA Y, NAKASHIMA T, SHINBO K, KIYOKAWA K, OSHIMA S, AIZAWA K. Studies on the consecutive survey of succedaneous and permanent dentition in the Japanese children. Part 3. Effects of periapical osteitis in the deciduous predecessors on the surface malformation of their permanent successors. *J Nihon Univ Sch Dent* 1966;**8**:21-41.

138. WINTER GB, KRAMER IRH. Changes in periodontal membrane, bone and permanent teeth following experimental pulpal injury in deciduous molar teeth of monkeys (Macaca irus). *Arch Oral Biol* 1972;**17**:1771-9.

139. VALDERHAUG J. A histologic study of experimentally induced periapical inflammation in primary teeth in monkeys. *Int J Oral Surg* 1974;**3**:111-23.

140. VALDERHAUG J. Periapical inflammation in primary teeth and its effect on the permanent successors. *Int J Oral Surg* 1974;**3**:171-82.

141. MØLLER E. En efterundersøgelse af patienter med paradentale ostitter i mælketandsættet med henblik på mineralisationsforstyrrelser i det blivende tandsæt.3 (Autoreferat) *Tandlægebladet* 1957;**61**:135-7.

142. TAYLOR RMS. Dilaceration of incisor tooth crowns. Report of two cases. *N Z Dent J* 1970;**66**:71-9.

143. VAN DEN HUL H. Het gevolg van trauma op een tandkiem. *Ned T Tandhelk* 1972;**79**:75-80.

144. EDLER R. Dilaceration of upper central and lateral incisors. A case report. *Br Dent J* 1973;**134**:331-2.

145. EDMONSON HD, CRABB JJ. Dilaceration of both upper central incisor teeth: a case report. *J Dent* 1975;**3**:223-4.

146. STEWART DJ. Dilacerate unerupted maxillary central incisors. *Br Dent J* 1978;**145**:229-33.

147. KVAM E. Et tilfelle av misdannelse av roten på den maxillære lateral. *Norske Tannlægeforenings Tidende* 1971;**81**:289-92.

148. LORBER CG. Einige Untersuchungen zur Pathobiologie unfallgeschädigter Zähne. *Schweiz Monatschr Zahnheilk* 1973;**83**:989-1014.

149. DIBIASE DD. Mucous membrane and delayed eruption. *Dent Practit* 1971;**21**:241-50.

150. HAAVIKKO K, RANTANEN L. A follow-up study of injuries to permanent and primary teeth in children. *Proc Finn Dent Soc* 1976;**72**:152-62.

151. ULVESTAD M, KEREKES K, DANMO C. Kompositkronen. En ny type semipermanent krone. *Norske Tannlægeforenings Tidende* 1973;**83**:281-4.

152. OPPENHEIM MN, WARD GT. The restoration of fractured incisors using a pit and fissure sealant and composite material. *J Am Dent Assoc* 1974;**89**:365-8.

153. CRABB JJ. The restoration of hypoplastic anterior teeth using an acid-etched technique. *J Dent* 1975;**3**:121-4.

154. KOCH G, PAULANDER J. Klinisk uppföljning av compositrestaureringar utförda med emaljetsningsmetodik. *Swed Dent J* 1976;**69**:191-6.

155. Jordan RE, Suzuki M, Gwinnett AJ, Hunter JK. Restoration of fractured and hypoplastic incisors by the acid etch resin technique; a three-year report. *J Am Dent Assoc* 1977;**95**:795-803.

156. Mink JR, McEvoy SA. Acid etch and enamel bond composite restoration of permanent anterior teeth affected by enamel hypoplasia. *J Am Dent Assoc* 1977;**94**:305-7.

157. Brin I, Ben-Bassat Y, Fuks A, Zilberman Y. Trauma to the primary incisors and its effect on the permanent successors. *Pediatr Dent* 1984;**6**:78-82.

158. Brin I, Ben Bassat Y, Zilberman Y, Fuks A. Effect of trauma to the primary incisors on the alignment of their permanent successors in Israelis. *Community Dent Oral Epidemiol* 1988;**16**:104-6.

159. Ben Bassat Y, Brin I, Fuks A, Zilberman Y. Effect of trauma to the primary incisors on permanent successors in different developmental stages. *Pediatr Dent* 1985;**7**:37-40.

160. Morgantini J, Maréchaux SC, Joho JP. Traumatismes dentaires chez l'enfant en âge prèscolaire et répercussions sur les dents permanentes. *Schweiz Monatsschr Zahnmed* 1986;**96**:432-40.

161. Zilberman Y, Ben Bassat Y, Lustmann J. Effect of trauma to primary incisors on root development of their permanent successors. *Pediatr Dent* 1986;**8**:289-93.

162. von Arx T. Traumatologie im Milchgebiss (II). Langzeitergebnisse sowie Auswirkungen auf das Milchgebiss und die bleibende Dentition. *Schweiz Monatsschr Zahnmed* 1991;**101**:57-69.

163. Moylan FMB, Seldin EB, Shannon DC, Todres ID. Defective primary dentition in survivors of neonatal mechanical ventilation. *J Pediatr* 1980;**96**:106-8.

164. Seow WK, Brown JP, Tudehope DI, O'Callaghan M. Developmental defects in the primary dentition of low birth-weight infants: adverse effects of laryngoscopy and prolonged endotracheal intubation. *Pediatric Dent* 1984;**6**:28-31.

165. Angelos GM, Smith DR, Jorgenson R, Sweeney EA. Oral complications associated with neonatal oral tracheal intubation: a critical review. *Pediatr Dent* 1989;**11**:133-140.

166. Boice JB, Krous HF, Foley JM. Gingival and dental complications of orotracheal intubation. *J Am Med Assoc* 1976;**236**:957-5

167. Wetzel RC. Defective dentition following mechanical ventilation. *J Pediatr* 1980;**96**:334.

168. Ainamo J, Cutress TW. An epidemiological index of developmental defects of dental enamel (DDE Index). *Int Dent J* 1982;**3**:159-67.

169. Suckling GW, Brown RH, Herbison GP. The prevalence of developmental defects of enamel in 696 nine-year-old New Zealand children participating in a health and development study. *Community Dent Health* 1985;**2**:303-13.

170. Dummer PHM, Kingdon A, Kingdon R. Prevalence of enamel developmental defects in a group of 11- and 12-year-old children in South Wales. *Community Dent Oral Epidemiol* 1986;**14**:119-22.

171. Clarkson J, O'Mullane D. A modified DDE Index for use in epidemiological studies of enamel defects. *J Dent Res* 1989;**68**:445-50.

172. Holm A-K, Andersson R. Enamel mineralization disturbances in 12-year-old children with known early exposure to fluorides. *Community Dent Oral Epidemiol* 1982;**10**:335-9.

173. Kaufman AY, Keila S, Wasersprung D, Dayan D. Developmental anomaly of permanent teeth related to traumatic injury. *Endod Dent Traumatol* 1990;**6**:183-8.

174. Croll TP, Cavanaugh RR. Enamel color modification by controlled hydrochloric acid-pumice abrasion. I. Technique and examples. *Quintessence Int* 1986;**17**:81-87.

175. Croll TP, Cavanaugh RR. Enamel color modification by controlled hydrochloric acid-pumice abrasion. II. Further examples. *Quintessence Int* 1986;**17**:157-64.

176. Croll TP, Cavanaugh RR. Hydrochloric acid-pumice enamel surface abrasion for color modification: results after six months. *Quintessence Int* 1986;**17**:335-41.

177. Waggoner WF, Johnston WM, Schumann S, Schikowski E. Microabrasion of human enamel in vitro using hydrochloric acid and pumice. *Pediatric Dentistry* 1989;**11**:319-23.

178. van Gool AV. Lésions des germes définitifs suite à des traumatismes de la dentition de lait. *Rev Belge Med Dent* 1986;**41**:96-9.

179. Ben-Bassat Y, Brin I, Zilberman Y. Effects of trauma to the primary incisors on their permanent successors: multidisciplinary treatment. *ASDC J Dent Child* 1989;**56**:112-6.

180. Lundberg M, Wennström JL. Development of gingiva following surgical exposure of a facially positioned unerupted incisor. *J Periodontol* 1988;**59**:652-5.

CHAPTER 13

Soft Tissue Injuries

J. O. ANDREASEN

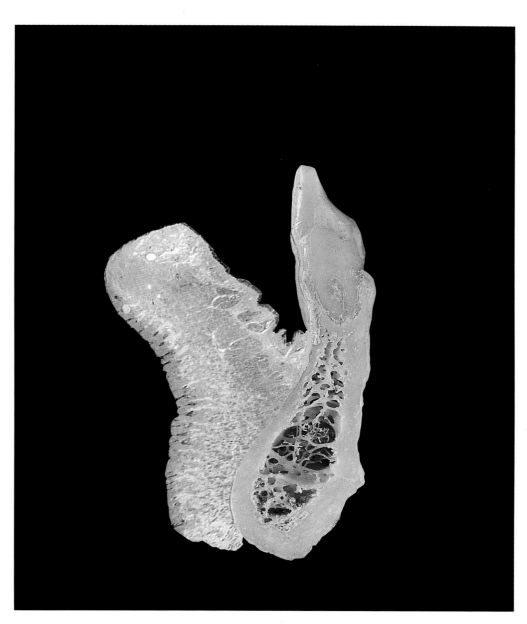

Fig.13.1. Section through a human lower lip in the midline

Note the composite structure of the lip, with musculature, salivary glands and hair follicles. Most of the musculature is oriented parallel to the vermilion border.

Terminology, Frequency and Etiology

The more or less complete labial cover which shields the dentition is the reason for the large number of dental traumas being associated with injuries to the lip, gingiva and oral mucosa. Thus, more than half of all patients treated in a hospital emergency setting showed associated soft tissue injury (1-3).

Management of oral and facial soft tissue wounds presents very complex treatment problems. In this chapter, a survey of treatment principles will be presented. For a more detailed presentation, the reader is referred to recent textbooks on maxillofacial trauma (4-13) and wound healing (14-18).

In the following, the diagnosis and treatment of soft tissue injuries will be presented. The tissues usually involved are the gingiva, alveolar mucosa and the lips. The lips present specific healing problems after injury due to their complex anatomy that includes skin, mucosa, musculature and salivary glands (Fig 13.1). Thus contusion of salivary glands may lead to a prolonged course of healing with subsequent scarring (Fig. 13.2).

The treatment approach for soft tissue lesions includes a *diagnostic phase*, where the nature, extent and contamination of the lesion is examined (19).

The *nature* of the injury can be abrasion, laceration, contusion or tissue loss. Ascertainment of the *extent* of tissue damage demands thorough exploration after administration of local anesthesia.

Possible *contamination* of the wound requires inspection for foreign bodies. In deeper wounds, clinical inspection should be supplemented with a radiographic examination which can reveal at least some of the contaminating foreign bodies (see later). The sequence of treatment in the case of soft tissue wounds and acute dental trauma implies:

EVALUATION OF ANTIBIOTIC COVERAGE

and

INITIAL TREATMENT OF DENTAL INJURIES PRIOR TO SOFT TISSUE MANAGEMENT

If reversed, the treatment of dental injuries (i.e. reposition and application of splints) may represent a hazard to the sutured soft tissue wounds. Moreover, sutured soft tissue wounds limit access to the injured teeth and supporting structures and thereby impede repositioning and other treatment procedures. Thereafter, the treatment approach for soft tissue lesions implies the following stages:

WOUND DEBRIDEMENT AND CLEANSING

This implies removal of all foreign bodies and contused tissues as well as rinsing the lesion with saline.

REPOSITIONING AND SUTURING OF DISPLACED TISSUES

In the following, the implications of the various steps in the treatment of soft tissue injuries will be discussed.

Table. 13.1. Effect of systematic antibiotic treatment subsequent to various combinations of cutaneous and oral mucosal wounds. After GOLDBERG (21) 1965

Type of lesion	Antibiotic treatment	No. of cases	Frequency of infection	Probability level*
Mucosal wounds	-	32	4 (13%)	0.66
	+	17	2 (12%)	
Mucosal and cutaneous wounds	-	33	11 (33%)	0.16
(Penetrating lesions)	+	24	4 (17%)	

*Probability level based on a Fisher's exact test.

Fig.13.2. Scarring subsequent to a penetrating wound in the lower lip
A 3-cm wide laceration of the cutaneous and mucosal aspects of the lower lip in a 9-year-old girl. Suturing of the cutaneous aspect of the wound was the only treatment provided.

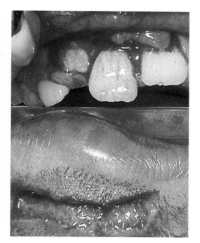

Condition after 1 week
Note saliva seepage and non-closure of the wound.

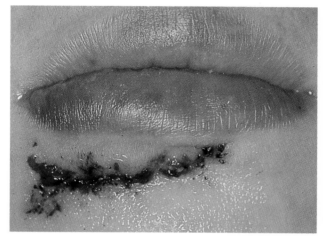
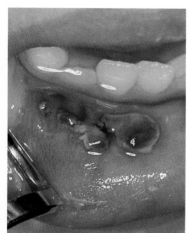

Follow-up
Healing has resulted in extreme scarring of the skin; whereas the previous wound in the mucosa is hardly noticeable.

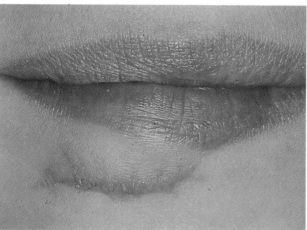
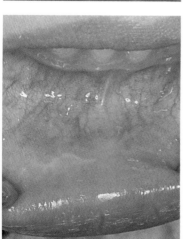

Antibiotic Prophylaxis

It is surprising that the benefit of antibiotic therapy in oral soft tissue injuries has only been sparsely documented. Due to their pathogenesis, almost all of these injuries can be considered contaminated with microorganisms and sometimes with foreign bodies. Based on this assumption, it has been proposed that the surgical treatment of mucosal and cutaneous wounds should always be supported by prophylactic antibiotic coverage (20). However, clinical evidence for the benefit of this treatment is presently tenuous (21-23) (Tables 13.1 and 13.2). Thus, no effect of antibiotic therapy could be shown on the rate of infection in cutaneous and/or mucosal wounds. In penetrating wounds to the oral cavity, conflicting results were found in the two studies cited (see Tables 13.1 and 13.2). It should, however, be mentioned that neither of the two studies had a randomized strategy for antibiotic administration.

Based on these findings it seems reasonable – until further studies are presented – to restrict the prophylactic use of antibiotics in soft tissue wounds to the following situations:

1. When the wound is heavily contaminated and wound debridement is not optimal (e.g. impacted foreign bodies or otherwise compromised wound cleansing).
2. When wound debridement has been delayed (i.e. more than 24 hours) [21].
3. When open reduction of jaw fractures is part of the treatment. In these situations, the benefit of short-term antibiotic coverage preceding and following osteosynthesis has been documented [20,24-26].(see also Chapter 11, p. 444). This relationship is in contrast to the lack of effect of antibiotic treatment in relation to "clean" orthognathic surgery [27-31].
4. When the general defense system of the patient is compromised (e.g. diabetes, alcohol abuse, immunocompromised patients, patients with prosthetic heart valves or patients suffering from endocarditis).
5. Human or animal bite wounds.

In Table 13.3, factors increasing the risk of infection are listed [32,33]. If prophylactic antibiotic coverage is decided upon, early institution is very important. Thus, experimental studies have shown that the first 3 hours after trauma are critical; i.e. to obtain an optimal effect from the antibiotics, they should be administered within this period (see Chapter 1 p. 59). If delayed, contaminating bacteria may multiply and invade the wound [33-36]. Antibiotics should therefore be administered before surgery and maintained for 24 hours [37]. Prolonged administration does not optimize healing [32,38,39], and has a serious effect upon the ecology of the oral microflora. The antibiotic of choice is Penicillin (Phenoxymethyl penicillin). The dosage (adults) should be: 2 million units (=1.2 g) p.o. at once followed by 2 million units (1.2 g) b.i.d. for 1 day. For children the dosage is 1 million units (0.6 g) p.o. at once followed by 1 million units (0.6 g) b.i.d. for 1 day.

In case of Penicillin allergy, Erythromycin should be administered. The dosage (adults) should be: 1 g p.o. at once followed by 1 g b.i.d. for 1 day. For children, the dosage is 0.5 g p.o. at once followed by 0.5 g b.i.d. for 1 day.

Tetanus prophylaxis should always be considered in the case of contaminated wounds. In case of a previously immunized patient (i.e. longer than 10 years previous to injury), a dose of 0.5 ml tetanus toxoid should be used (booster injection). In unimmunized patients, passive immunization should be provided.

Wound Cleansing and Debridement

Whereas a surgical wound in the skin of the face can be considered clean, all oral wounds can be considered contaminated.

One of the aims of wound cleansing is to remove or neutralize microorganisms which contaminate the wound surface in order to prevent infection. However, the fact remains that almost all common wound disinfectants have been shown to have a detrimental effect upon wound healing [41]. Thus, at present only physiologic saline or a Ringers lactated solution appear to be without a harmful effect upon cells in the wound. It has also been claimed that a nonionic surfactant (Pluronic F68 ®) has no detrimental effect upon cells in the wound [34,36].

The adjacent intact cutaneous surface should also be cleansed with a wound detergent. However, it is surprising that a "clean" surgical wound has not been shown experimentally to lower the incidence of wound infections [40,41].

Foreign Bodies

The presence of foreign bodies in the wound significantly increases the risk of infection [34] and retards healing, even in wounds free of infection [44]. (see Chapter 1, p. 60). This finding emphasizes the importance of adequate cleansing of the wound prior to suturing.

The removal of foreign bodies in facial and oral tissues after trauma is known to be a difficult and time-consuming procedure [45]. A syringe with saline under high pressure, a scrub brush or gauze swabs soaked in saline can be used to remove foreign bodies. If this is not effective, a surgical blade (no. 11 or 15) or a small

Table. 13.2. Effect of systemic antibiotic treatment subsequent to various combinations of facial cutaneous and oral mucosal wounds. After PATERSON ET AL. (22) 1970

Type of lesion	Antibiotic treatment	No. of cases	Frequency of infection	Probability level*
Mucosal wounds	-	23	0 (0%)	1.0
	+	12	0 (0%)	
Cutaneous wounds	-	85	2 (2%)	0.06
	+	51	6 (12%)	
Mucosal and cutaneous wounds	-	21	0 (0%)	1.0
	+	23	0 (0%)	
Mucosal and cutaneous wounds (Penetrating lesions)	-	24	3 (13%)	0.08
	+	48	15 (31%)	

*Probability level based on a Fisher's exact test.

spoon excavator may be used. Complete removal of all foreign bodies is important, to prevent infection and also to prevent disfiguring scarring or tattooing.

Devitalized soft tissue serves to enhance infection by at least three mechanisms: First, as a culture medium that can promote bacterial growth; second, by inhibiting leukocyte migration, phagocytosis and subsequent bacterial kill; and third, by limiting leukocyte function due to the anaerobic environment within devitalized tissue (i.e. low oxygen tension impairs killing of bacteria) (34-36) (see Chapter 1, p. 60).

For these reasons severely contused and/or ischemic tissue should be removed in order to facilitate healing (33,46).

Suturing

A general principle in wound treatment is the approximation of wound edges in order to reduce the distance for the wound healing module and thereby increase the speed of healing. This principle has, unfortunately, not been supported by animal experiments in which sutures were used to approximate wound edges (44,47-52). The explanation for these findings could be that, as well as approximating the wound edges, suturing also induces ischemia of wound edges and acts as a wick, leading bacteria into the wound. Thus, the placement of just a single suture significantly decreases the number of bacteria needed

Table 13.3. Factors increasing the risk of surgical wound infection. After BURKE (33) 1979

	Approximate increase
Age over 60 years	3x
Malnutrition	3x
Active infection elsewhere	2-3x
Obesity	2x
Steroid therapy	2x
Diabetes	2-3x
Prolonged preoperative hospitalization:	
1-2 wk	2x
over 2 wk	4x
Night-time or emergency operation	2-3x
Duration of operation over 3 h	2-3x
Preoperative shaving operative site	2x
Use of electrosurgical knife	2x
Penrose wound drain	2x

Fig.13.3 A. Clinical reaction to sutures

The clinical responce to PGA, silk, chromic gut and plain gut sutures placed in human oral mucosa. After WALLACE ET AL. (59) 1970.

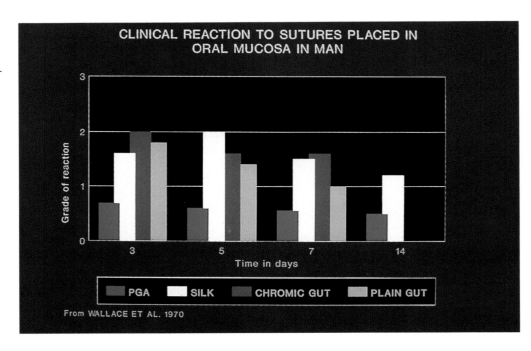

to cause wound infection (49).(see Chapter 1, p. 61).

The tissue response to various types of sutures in the oral mucosa has been studied extensively in animals (53-59) and in humans (60,61), whereby a vigorous inflammatory reaction around the sutures could be demonstrated.

The general findings in these experimental studies have been that silk and catgut sutures (plain or chromic) elicited a very intense clinical and histological inflammatory reaction after 3, 5 and 7 days; whereas polyglycol acid (Dexon®) showed considerably less clinical and histological reaction (59) (Figs. 13.3 A and B).

The greatest part of the inflammatory reaction is probably related to the presence of bacteria within the interstices of multifilament suture materials (51,54-57). Thus the impregnation of multifilament sutures with antibiotics has been shown to decrease the resultant tissue response (57). A further finding has been that monofilament sutures (e.g. nylon and Prolene®) display a significant reduction of adverse reactions compared to multifilament sutures, a finding possibly related to a reduced wick effect of monofilament sutures (10,58).

Finally, it should be borne in mind that it has been shown experimentally that

Fig.13.3 B. Histologic reaction to sutures

The histologic reaction to PGA, silk, chromic gut and plain gut sutures placed in human oral mucosa. After WALLACE ET AL. (59) 1970.

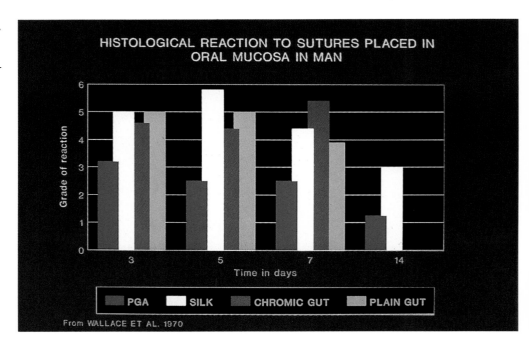

Fig.13.4. Treatment of horizontal gingival laceration with tissue displacement in the permanent dentition
Due to an impact the gingiva has been lacerated and displaced whereas the central incisors are left intact.

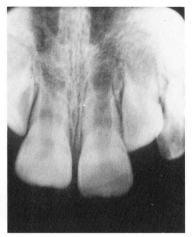

Treatment
The displaced attached gingiva is repositioned and sutured.

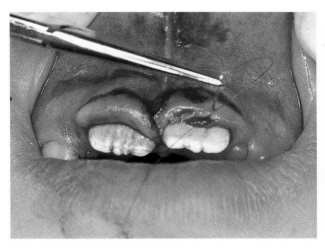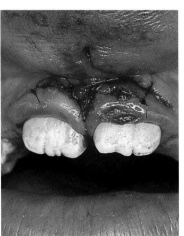

there is an increased risk of infection with both increased suture diameter and sub-mucosal/subcutaneous suture length (34).

Recently a new monofilament suture material has been developed of a very inert and tissue compatible biomaterial made of polytetrafluoroethylene (PTFE). A comparison between the tissue response in oral mucosa between this material and silk sutures shows definitively less tissue response in the former (36).

The essential lesson of all these experiments in suturing and subsequent wound healing is therefore: use *a minimal number* of sutures with *a small diameter*, preferably *monofilament* and, finally, institute *early suture removal* (i.e. after 3-4 days in oral tissues), eventually in two stages, i.e. 3 and 6 days.

Treatment of Oral Soft Tissue Injuries

Gingival Wounds

The gingiva can present a variety of sequelae to frontal and horizontal impacts, such as abrasion, contusion or separation from the neck of the tooth.

ABRASION OF THE GINGIVA
Treatment can be limited to removal of any possible foreign bodies.

LACERATION OF THE GINGIVA
After administration of a local anesthetic, the wound is cleansed with saline, and foreign bodies removed. The lacerated gingiva is brought back into normal position, implying that displaced teeth have been repositioned. After repositioning of the gingiva, the necessary number of thin sutures (e.g. 5.0 or 6.0 silk or Prolene®) are placed to prevent displacement of tissue. In that regard, a minimum number of sutures should be used (Fig. 13.4). The patient is then placed on an oral hygiene regimen using 0.1% chlorhexidine for 4-5 days, whereafter the sutures are removed.

In case of trauma to the primary dentition, an impact often occurs parallel to the front of the maxilla or the mandible, which can result in complete displacement of the

Fig. 13.5. Treatment of a gingival laceration with exposure of bone in the primary dentition
Due to a fall against an object, the gingiva has been displaced into the labial sulcus and bone is exposed whereas the incisors are left intact.

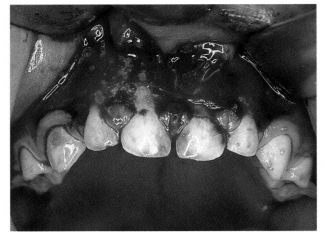 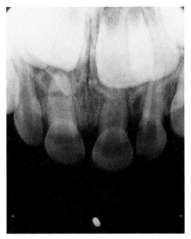

Repositioning and suturing of the gingiva
The condition immediately after gingival repositioning and suturing. The labial bone has been removed.

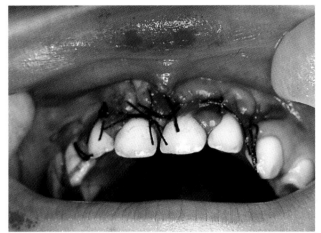 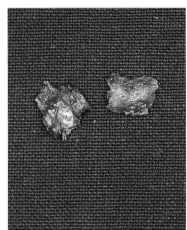

Fig. 13.6. Treatment of a vertical gingival laceration with tissue displacement in the permanent dentition
Due to an impact parallel to the front of the maxilla, the gingiva has been lacerated and displaced apically, whereas the incisors are left intact.

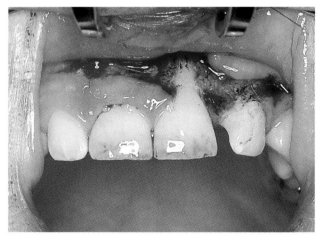 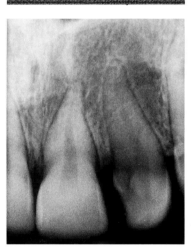

Treatment and follow-up
The displaced attached gingiva is repositioned and sutured.

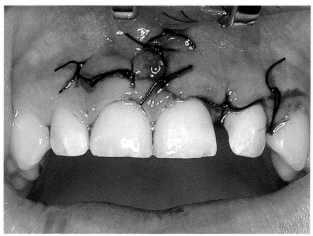 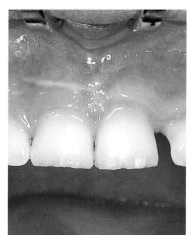

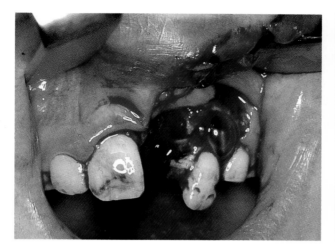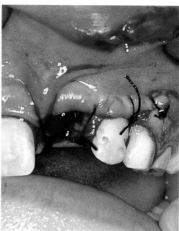

Fig.13.7.Gingival tissue loss
The central incisor has been avulsed and lost. There is tissue loss with exposure of labial bone. A flap is raised and the periosteum incised, whereby it is possible to cover the denuded bone.

labial mucosa into the sulcus area (Fig 13.5). In these cases, it is necessary to reposition the gingiva, as exposure of the labial bone leads to protracted healing with subsequent gingival retraction and sometimes sequestration of the denuded labial bone. The same type of gingival displacement may also occur in the permanent dentition (Fig. 13.6).

In case of loss of gingival tissue, a gingi-

voplasty should be performed whereby flaps are elongated by the placement of periosteal incisions (Fig. 13.7). If tissue loss has occurred in the region of erupting teeth, it is important to consider whether tissue loss has exposed the cemento-enamel junction. If this is not the case, further eruption and physiologic gingival retraction will normalize the clinical appearance with time (Fig. 13.8). With minor dis-

Fig.13.8.Gingival loss in an erupting permanent central incisor
In erupting teeth, gingival displacement or tissue loss should be assessed in relation to the position of the cemento-enamel junction. In this case of a 12-year-old boy, trauma resulted in tissue loss not extending beyond the cemento-enamel junction of the left central incisor. At a follow-up examination 5 years later, there is almost complete gingival symmetry.

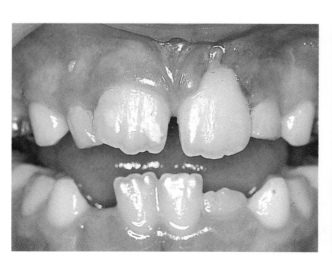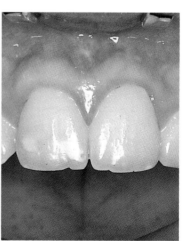

SOFT TISSUE INJURIES

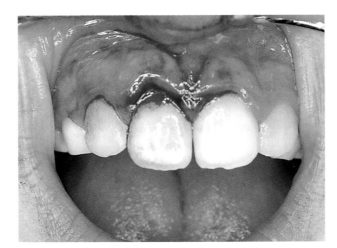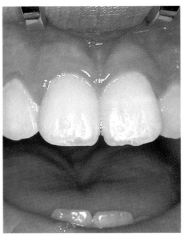

Fig.13.9.Gingival laceration with spontaneous regeneration
The marginal gingiva in this 9-year-old girl was displaced apically and not repositioned. At the 1-month follow-up examination, normal gingival relations could be observed.

placement or loss, gingival regeneration amounting to approximately 1 mm will usually occur (62) (Fig. 13.9).

CONTUSION OF GINGIVA

In these cases, it is essential that optimal oral hygiene is maintained during the healing period. Due to the excellent vascularity in the area, revacularization of ischemic gingiva is often possible.

Lip Wounds

HORIZONTAL PENETRATING LESIONS

These injuries are the result of a localized impact to the lips. Depending upon the angulation of impact, different types of lesion will occur. In case of a frontal impact, the labial surfaces of protruding incisors may act as a bayonet, resulting in a sagittal split of the lip (Fig. 13.10). Due to the circumferential orientation of the orbicularis oris muscles, these wounds will usually gape, with initally intense arterial bleeding due to the rich vasculature in the region. Hemorrhage, however, is soon arrested due to vasoconstriction and coagulation.

If the direction of impact is more parallel to the axis of either the maxillary or mandibular incisors, the incisal edges may penetrate the entire thickness of the lip (Fig. 13.11). When the incisal edges hit the impacting object, fracture of the crown usually occurs. Upon retraction of the lip,

Fig.13.10.Split lip due to a frontal impact
This patient was hit in the face with a bottle, resulting in a split lip and lateral luxation of the right central incisor. The vermilion border is sutured first, whereafter the rest of the laceration is closed with interrupted sutures (e.g. Prolene ® 6.0).

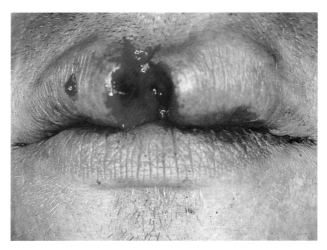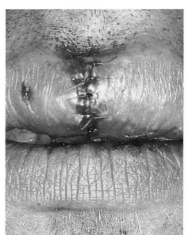

Fig.13.11. Penetrating lip lesion with embedded foreign body

This 8-year-old girl fell against a staircase, whereby the maxillary incisors penetrated the prolabium of the lower lip. Parallel lesions are found corresponding to each penetrating incisor.

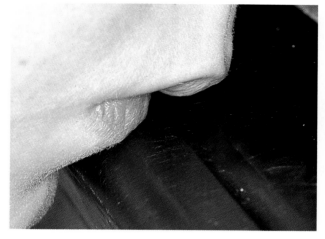
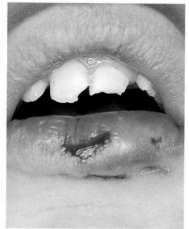

Radiographic demonstration of foreign bodies

A dental film was placed between the lip and the dental arch. Exposure time is 1/4 of that for conventional dental radiographs. A large occlusal film is placed on the cheek and a lateral exposure taken using half the normal exposure time.

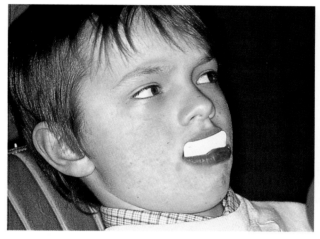
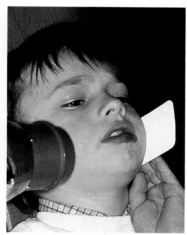

Radiographic demonstration of multiple foreign bodies in the lower lip

Orthoradial and lateral exposures show multiple fragments in lower lip. The lateral exposure could demonstrate that the fragments are equally distributed from the cutaneous to the mucosal aspect of the lip.

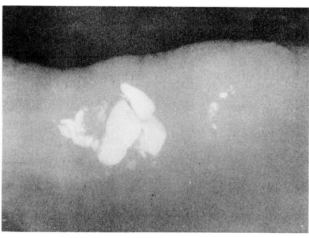
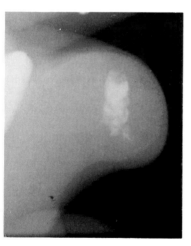

Retrieved dental fragments

The lip lesion is sutured after removal of tooth fragments.

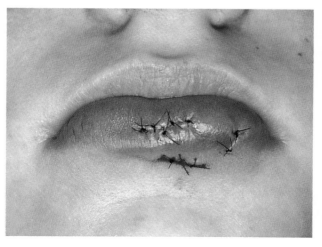
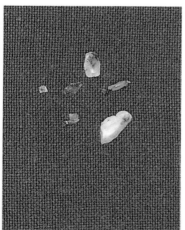

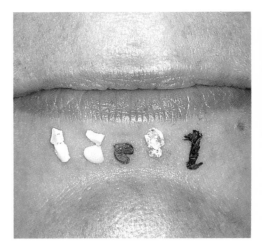 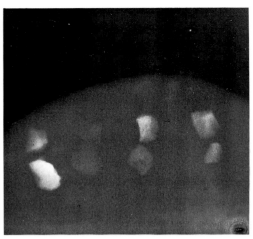

foreign bodies such as tooth fragments, plaque, calculus and fragments from the impacting object usually become trapped within the lip.

DIAGNOSIS AND TREATMENT

Diagnosis consists of determining the extent of the wound and verifying the presence of foreign bodies. In that regard, a radiographic examination will be able to demonstrate a variety of typical foreign bodies, such as tooth fragments, calculus, gravel, glass and fragments of paint (Fig. 13.12). However, other typical foreign bodies such as cloth and wood cannot be seen.

The radiographic technique consists of placing a dental film between the lip and the alveolar process. In case of a wide lesion, orientation of images is facilitated by placing a small metal indicator (e.g. a piece of lead foil) in the midline of the vermillion border in order to locate possible foreign bodies. The exposure should be made at a low kilovoltage (to increase contrast), and the exposure time should be kept to approximately 25% of a usual dental exposure.

If the intraoral film discloses foreign bodies, a lateral exposure at 50% of the usual exposure time should be made in order to verify their position in a sagittal plane (Fig. 13.11).

Treatment of lip lesions should await completion of treatment of dental injuries (Fig. 13.13). A regional block anesthesia is administered (infiltration anesthesia of the wound may increase the risk of infection (34)). Treatment starts by cleansing the wound and surrounding tissue with a wound detergent. The wound edges are elevated and foreign bodies are found and retrieved. It is essential to consider that foreign bodies are usually contained within small cul de sacs within the wound. When all fragments that have been registered radiographically have been retrieved, the wound is debrided for contused muscle and salivary gland tissue. Thereafter the wound is carefully rinsed with saline; and a check is made to ensure that bleeding has been arrested. The mucosal side of the wound is then sutured tightly so that no saliva can enter the wound. Thereafter, the cutaneous part of the wound is closed with fine sutures (e.g. 6.0 silk or Prolene®). Normally it is not necessary to use deep sutures, as the muscles along the wound edges will adapt to each other. Sutures placed in the musculature will induce scar formation because of their slow resorption and concomitant inflammation. Magnifying lenses, e.g. ordinary spectacles with 4 x loupes can be used to ensure meticulous suturing. The anatomy of the wound should be respected. Never excise wounds to make long straight scars which invariably are more visible.

Fig.13.13. Treatment of a broad penetrating lip lesion
Penetrating lesion of the upper lip in a 66-year-old woman due to a fall. Clinical appearance 4 hours after injury.

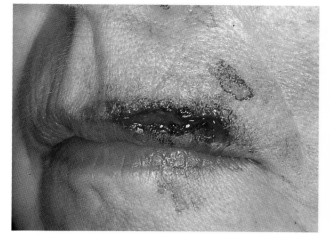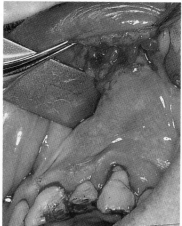

Dental injuries
The crown of the left central and lateral incisors and canine have been fractured while the lateral incisor and canine have been intruded. Soft tissue radiographs demonstrate 2 foreign bodies in the upper lip.

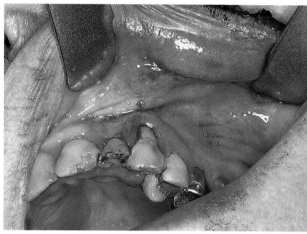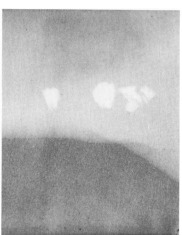

Wound cleansing
The cutaneous and mucosal aspects of the wounds are cleansed with a surgical detergent followed by saline.

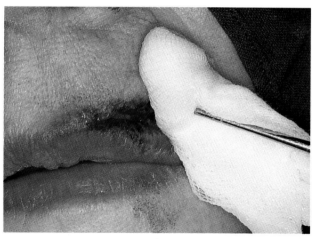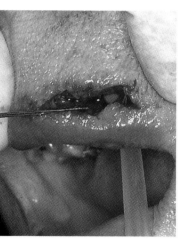

Removal of foreign bodies
All radiographically demonstrated tooth fragments are located and removed.

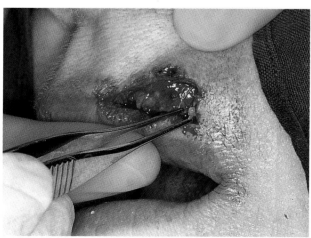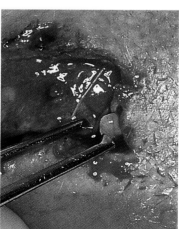

SOFT TISSUE INJURIES

Wound debridement

Traumatized salivary glands are excised in order to promote rapid healing.

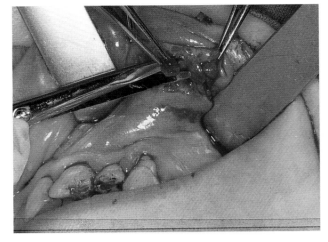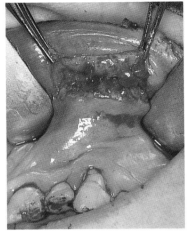

Wound closure

The oral wound is closed with interrupted 4.0 silk sutures.

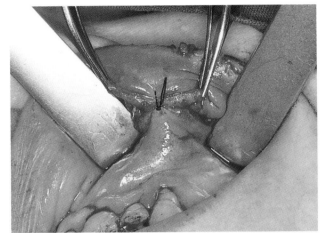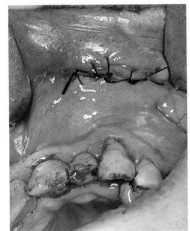

Repeated cleansing of the cutaneous wound

The cutaneous aspect of the wound is cleansed with saline to minimize contamination from closure of the mucosal wound.

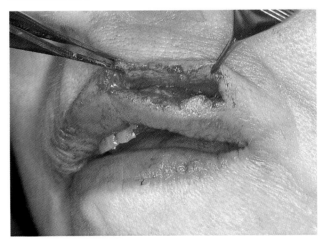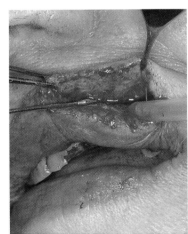

Buried sutures

As a matter of principle, buried sutures should be kept to a minimum; and, when indicated, be resorbed over a short period of time (e.g. Vicryl ® sutures). The point of entry of the needle should be remote from the oral and cutaneous wound surfaces in order to place the knot (i.e. the most infection-prone part of the suture) far from the wound edges; that is, at approximately one-half the total thickness of the lip.

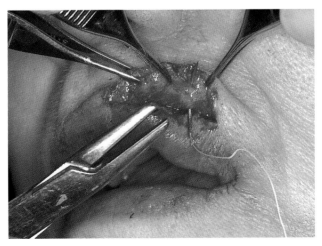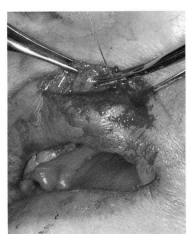

CHAPTER 13

Assessing cutaneous wound closure

After closing the muscular tissue, the cutaneous part of the wound is evaluated. It is important that after muscular approximation, the wound edges can be approximated without tension. If this is not possible, approximation of the muscular part of the wound must be revised.

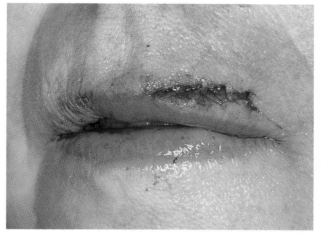 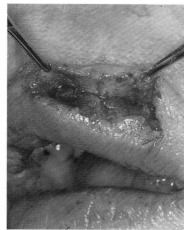

Suturing the cutaneous wound

Wound closure is principally begun at the vermilion border. In cases where the wound is parallel to the vermilion border, the first suture is placed at a site where irregularities of the wound edge ensure an anatomically correct closure. The wound is closed with fine, monofilament interrupted sutures (Prolene® 6.0), under magnification (i.e. using spectacles with a 2 or 4 x magnification).

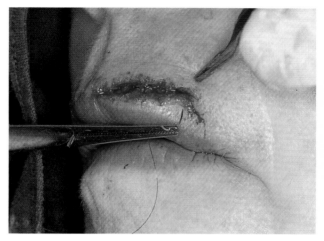 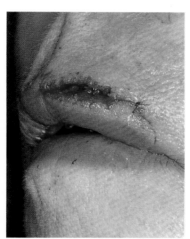

Suturing completed

The wound is now fully closed and antibiotics administered (i.e. penicillin, 1 million Units x 4, for 2 days).

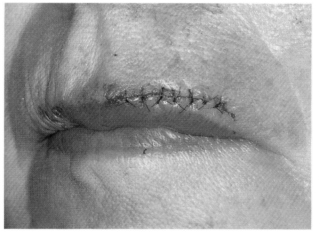 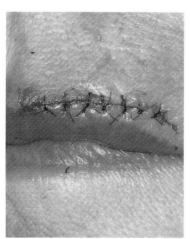

Healing 6 weeks after injury

There is a minimum of scarring.

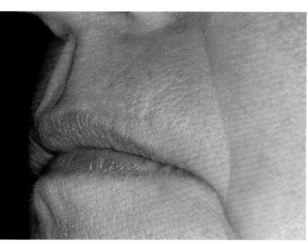 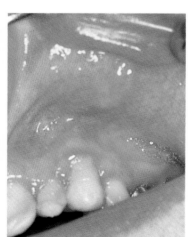

SOFT TISSUE INJURIES

Fig.13.14. Treatment of narrow penetrating lip lesion
This 27-year-old man fell, whereby the right central incisor penetrated the lower lip and fractured. Multiple tooth fragments are buried in the lip.

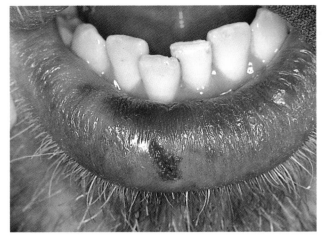 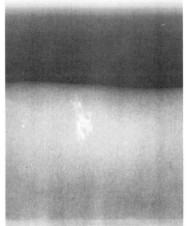

Removing foreign bodies from the lip
After administration of local anesthesia the narrow penetrating wound is opened using a pincette. When the pincette is open, a rectangular wound is formed whereby two sides of the wound become clearly visible. Foreign bodies are removed and the wound cleansed with saline.

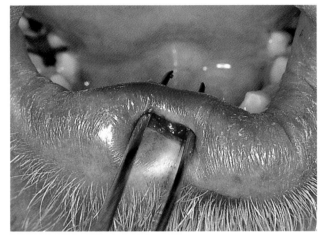 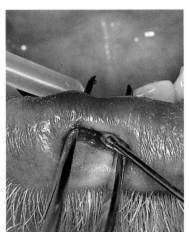

Repeating the cleansing procedure
The pincette is turned 90° and the procedure is repeated.

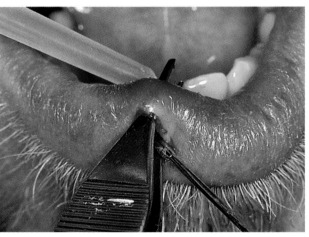 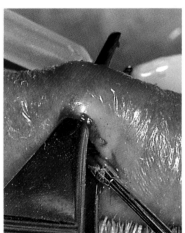

Suturing the wound
The wound is sutured with interrupted 6.0 silk sutures. A radiograph shows that all fragments have been removed.

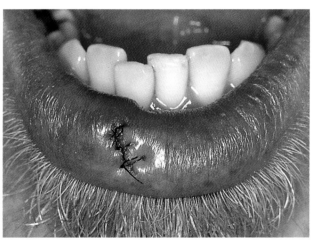 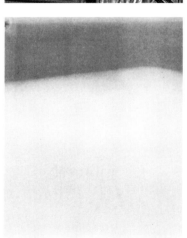

CHAPTER 13

Fig.13.15.Extensive asphalt tattoo
The patient suffered an injury years earlier. Inadequate wound debridement resulted in extensive asphalt tattooing. Courtesy of Dr. S. BOLUND, University Hospital, Copenhagen

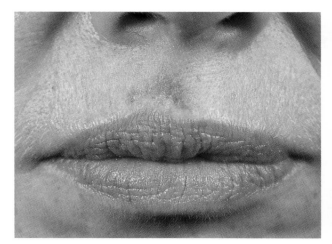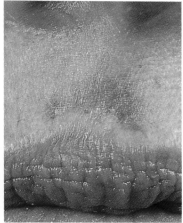

In case of narrow penetrating wounds, a special technique of opening up the wound as illustrated in Fig. 13.14 is recommended.

Concerning the use of antibiotics, see p. 498

VERTICAL MUCOCUTANEOUS WOUNDS

DIAGNOSIS AND TREATMENT
These lesions are open lesions which lend themselves well to inspection for foreign bodies (Fig. 13.10). After administration of a local anesthetic, the wound and surroundings are cleansed with a wound detergent, whereafter foreign bodies and contused tissue are removed. Following these procedures, a few resorbable sutures are placed in the musculature (e.g. 5.0 Dexon®) to reduce tension on the cutaneous sutures. A minimum of sutures should be used, as deep sutures in contaminated wounds have been shown to increase the risk of infection (34).

The wound is then closed. The vermilion border is approximated and sutured first, as any inaccuracy in wound closure will be very apparent. Thereafter, mucosal and cutaneous sutures are placed. As it can be difficult to visualize the vermilion border once local anesthetic has been administered, Bonnies blue or methylene blue in a 27-gauge syringe can be applied to "tattoo" the lip prior to suturing.

Finally, the patient is placed under prophylactic antibiotic cover as previously described.

SKIN OR MUCOSAL ABRASION
If the direction of impact is parallel to the lip, the surface layer of the skin or the mucosa are peeled off and foreign bodies are often impressed into the wound. These foreign bodies are usually gravel or asphalt. Any failure to remove foreign bodies may lead to seriously disfiguring scarring and discoloring (asphalt tattoo) (Fig. 13.15).

After administration of local anesthesia, the wound and surroundings are washed with a wound detergent (Fig. 13.17). Thereafter, all foreign bodies are removed with a small excavator or a surgical blade which is placed perpendicular to the cutaneous surface in order to prevent it from cutting into the tissue. The wound is either left open or covered with a bandage.

Tongue Wounds

Other than in patients suffering from epilepsy, tongue lesions due to trauma are rare. In the former instance, bite lesions may occur along the lateral part of the tongue during seizures. Furthermore, following an impact to the chin with the tongue protruding, a wound may be caused by incisor penetration through the apex of the tongue.

DIAGNOSIS AND TREATMENT
A wound located on the dorsal surface of the tongue should always be examined for a ventral counterpart (Fig. 13.18). If there are concomitant crown fractures, frag-

Fig.13.16.Cleansing of a skin wound containing asphalt particles

In order to adequately cleanse the abrasions, a topical anesthetic is necessary. In this case, a lidocain spray was used. Note that the nostrils are held closed to reduce discomfort from the spray entering the nose.

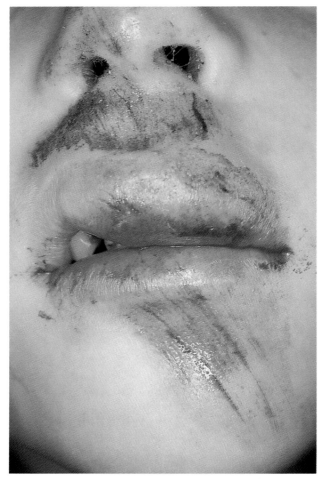

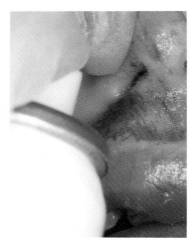

Washing the wounds

The lips are washed with surgical sponges or gauze swabs soaked in a wound detergent.

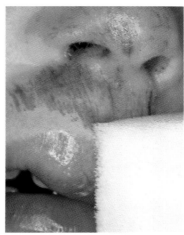

Removing asphalt particles

The impacted foreign bodies cannot be adequately removed by scrubbing or washing; but should be removed with a small excavator or a surgical blade held perpendicular to the direction of the abrasions.

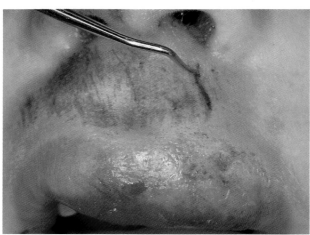

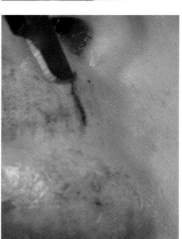

Follow-up examination

Two weeks after injury, the soft tissue wounds have healed without scarring.

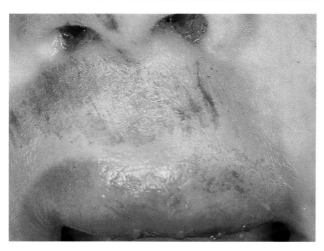

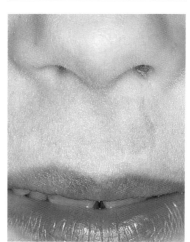

Fig.13.17. Treatment of a penetrating tongue lesion
This 10-year-old girl suffered a penetrating tongue lesion. Note the parallel lacerations on the dorsal and ventral surfaces of the tongue.

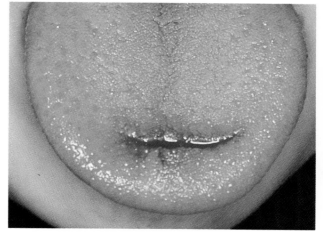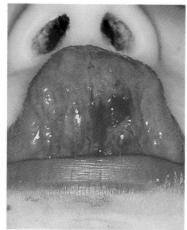

Radiographic examination
A dental film is placed under the extended tongue and exposed at 1/4 the normal exposure time. The exposure demonstrated several tooth fragments embedded within the tongue.

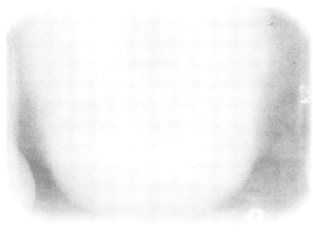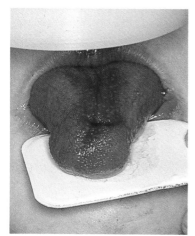

Removal of tooth fragments
After administration of regional anesthestic, all tooth fragments were retrieved. It is important that all fragments radiographically demonstrated are also retrieved in order to prevent infection and/or scar formation.

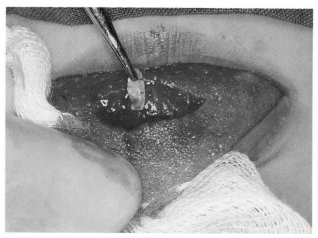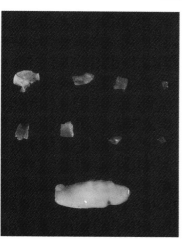

Suturing the tongue wound
After all foreign bodies have been removed, the wound is cleansed and sutured on the dorsal and ventral surfaces.

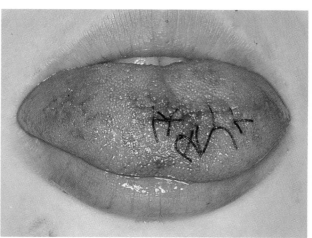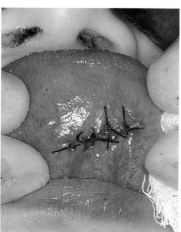

SOFT TISSUE INJURIES

ments may be located within the wound. These fragments can be revealed by a radiographic examination (see above).

Treatment principles include cleansing of the wound, removal of foreign bodies and suturing of the dorsal and ventral aspects of the lesion. After administration of anesthesia (local, regional or general), foreign bodies are retrieved, the wound cleansed with saline, and the wound entrances sutured tightly (Fig. 13.17).

Essentials

Type of Soft Tissue Lesion

The type of lesion can be abrasion, laceration, contusion (including hematoma) or tissue loss (avulsion).

Treatment Principles

Cleansing of the wound with a detergent, repositioning of displaced tissues and immobilization of the tissue, usually with sutures.

Gingival Wounds (Figs. 13.4 to 13.6)

a. Rinse the wound and surroundinngs with a wound detergent.
b. Reposition displaced gingiva.
c. Place a few fine sutures.
d. Instruct in good oral hygiene including daily mouth rinse with 0.1% chlorhexidine.
e. Remove sutures after 4-5 days.

Lip Wounds

Examine whether the injury is a penetrating wound of the lip or a laceration of the vermilion border (split-lip lesion).

PENETRATING LIP WOUNDS (FIGS. 13.11 TO 13.14)

a. Administer antibiotics if indicated. (See Table 13.3).
b. Take a radiograph of the lip. (Use 25% of the normal exposure time).
c. Use a regional anesthesia.
d. Rinse the wound and surroundinngs with a wound detergent.

e. Remove foreign bodies and contused muscle and salivary gland tissue.
f. Suture the labial mucosa first.
g. Rinse the wound again with saline.
h. Suture the cutaneous wound with fine sutures (6.0 nylon or Prolene®).
i. Remove sutures after 4-5 days.

SPLIT LIP WOUNDS (FIG. 13.10)

Use the same procedure as for penetrating lip lesions. However, in this case a few buried resorbable sutures are indicated (e.g. Dexon® 4.0/5.0).

Tongue Wounds

Examine whether the injury is a penetrating wound or a lesion of the lateral border.

PENETRATING TONGUE WOUNDS (FIG. 13.17)

a. Administer antibiotics if indicated (see Table 13.3)
b. Take a radiograph of the tongue (exposure time 25% of normal exposure time).
c. Use a regional or general anesthesia.
d. Rinse the wound with saline.
e. Remove foreign bodies.
f. Rinse the wound again with saline.
g. Suture the mucosal wound.
h. Remove sutures after 4-5 days.

LATERAL BORDER WOUNDS

After administration of a regional anesthetic the wound is rinsed and sutured. Buried resorbable sutures are sometimes indicated in order to approximate the wound edges and relieve tension on the mucosal sutures.

Bibliography

1. ANDREASEN JO. Etiology and pathogenesis of traumatic dental injuries. *Scand J Dent Res* 1970;**78**:329-42.

2. GALEA H. An investigation of dental injuries treated in an acute care general hospital. *J Am Dent Assoc* 1984;**109**:434-8.

3. O'NEIL DW, CLARK MV, LOWE JW, HARRINGTON MS. Oral trauma in children: A hospital survey. *Oral Surg Oral Med Oral Pathol* 1989;**68**:691-6.

4. LIEBLICH S, TOPAZIAN RG. Infection in the patient with maxillofacial trauma. In: FONSECA RL, WALKER RV, eds. *Oral and Maxillofacial trauma.* Philadelphia: WB Saunders Company, 1991:1150-71.

5. STARK RB, ed. *Plastic Surgery of the Head and Neck.* New York: Churchill-Livingstone, 1987.

6. HUGHES NC. Basic techniques of excision and wound closure. In: *Operative Surgery: Plastic Surgery.* 4th edn. London: Butterworths, 1986.

7. LYNCH JB. Trauma to the facial skin. Part 1. Lacerations. In: STARK RB, ed. *Plastic surgery of the head and neck.* New York: Churchill Livingstone, 1987:271-5.

8. SCHULTZ TC. *Facial injuries.* 3rd edn. Chicago: Year Book Medical Publishers, 1988.

9. Zook EG. *The primary care of facial injuries.* Littleton: PSG Publishing Company, 1980.

10. POWERS MP, BERTZ JB, FONSECA RJ. Management of soft tissue injuries. In: FONSECA RL, WALKER RV, eds. *Oral and Maxillofacial trauma.* Philadelphia: WB Saunders Company, 1991:616-50.

11. LYNCH J. Trauma to the facial skin. In: STARK RB, ed. *Plastic Surgery of the Head and Neck.* New York: Churchill-Livingstone, 1987.

12. HUGHES NC. Basic techniques of excision and wound closure. In: *Operative Surgery: Plastic Surgery.* 4th edn. London: Butterworths, 1986.

13. SCHULTZ TC. *Facial injuries.* 3rd edn. Chicago: Year Book Medical Publishers, 1988.

14. HUNT TK, DUNPHY JE, eds. *Fundamentals of wound management.* New York: Appleton-Century-Crofts, 1979.

15. HUNT TK, ed. *Wound healing and wound infection. Theory and surgical practice.* New York: Appleton-Century-Crofts, 1980.

16. DINEEN P, HILDICK-SMITH G, eds. *The surgical wound.* Philadelphia: Lea & Febiger, 1981.

17. PEACOCK EE. *Wound repair.* Philadelphia: W.B. Saunders Company, 1984.

18. Hunt TK, Heppenstall R, Pines E, Rovee D, eds. *Soft and hard tissue repair.* New York: Praeger, 1984.

19. ANDREASEN JO. Management of soft tissue trauma and alveolar fractures. In: GUTMANN JL, HARRISON JW, eds. *Proceedings of the International Conference on Oral Trauma.* Illinois: American Association of Endodontists Endowment & Memorial Foundation, 1986:147-54.

20. ZALLEN RD, BLACK SL. Antibiotic therapy in oral and maxillofacial surgery. *J Oral Surg* 1976;**34**:349-51.

21. GOLDBERG MH. Antibiotics and oral and oral-cutaneous lacerations. *J Oral Surg* 1965;**23**:117-22.

22. PATERSON JA, CARDO VA, STRATIGOS GT. An examination of antibiotic prophylaxis in oral and maxillofacial surgery. *J Oral Surg* 1970;**28**:753-9.

23. GUGLIELMO BJ, HOHN DC, KOO PJ, HUNT TK, SWEET RL, CONTE JE. Antibiotic prophylaxis in surgical procedures. A critical analysis of the literature. *Arch Surg* 1983;**118**:943-55.

24. ZALLEN RD. A study of antibiotic usage in compound mandibular fractures. *J Oral Surg* 1975;**33**:431-4.

25. ADERHOLD L, JUNG H, FRENKEL G. Untersuchungen über den Wert einer Antibiotika-prophylaxe bei Kiefer-Gesichtsverletzungen eine prospektive Studie. *Dtsch Zahnärztl Z* 1983;**38**:402-6.

26. GERLACH KL, PAPE HD. Untersuchungen zur Antibiotikaprophylaxe bei der operativen Behandlung von Unterkieferfrakturen. *Dtsch Z Mund Kiefer Gesichtschir* 1988;**12**:497-500.

27. ZALLEN RD, STRADER RJ. The use of prophylactic antibiotics in extraoral procedures for mandibular prognathism. *J Oral Surg* 1971;**29**:178-9.

28. YRASTORZA JA. Indications for antibiotics in orthognathic surgery. *J Oral Surg* 1976;**34**:514-6.

29. PETERSON LJ, BOOTH DF. Efficacy of antibiotic prophylaxis in intraoral orthognathic surgery. *J Oral Surg* 1976;**34**:1088-91.

30. MARTIS C, KARABOUTA I. Infection after orthognathic surgery, with and without preventive antibiotics. *Int J Oral Surg* 1984;**13**:490-4.

31. EPPLEY BL, DELFINO JJ. Use of prophylactic antibiotics in temporomandibular joint surgery. *J Oral Maxillofac Surg* 1985;**43**:675-9.

32. BURKE JF. Preventive antibiotics in surgery. *Postgrad Med J* 1975;**58**:65-8.

33. BURKE JF. Infection. In: HUNT TK, DUNPHY JE, eds. *Fundamentals of wound management.* New York: Appleton-Century-Crofts, 1979:171-240.

34. EDLICH RF, RODEHEAVER G, THACKER JG, EDGERTON MT. Technical factors in wound management. In: HUNT TK, DUNPHY JE, eds. *Fundamentals of Wound Management.* New York: Appleton-Century-Crofts, 1979:364-454.

35. EDLICH RF, KENNEY JG, MORGAN RE, et al. Antimicrobial treatment of minor soft tissue lacerations: A critical review. *Emerg Med Clin North Am* 1986;**4**:561-80.

36. EDLICH R, RODEHEAVER GT, THACKER JC. Technical factors in the prevention of wound infections. In: HOWARD RJ, SIMMONS RL, eds. *Surgical Infectious Diseases.* New York: Appleton-Century-Croft, 1982:449-72.

37. BECKERS H, KÜHNLE T, DIETRICH H-G. Einfluss prophylaktischer Antibiose auf infektiöse Komplikationen nach Dysgnathieoperationen. *Fortschr Kiefer Gesichtchir* 1984;**29**:118-9.

38. CONOVER MA, KABAN LB, MULLIKEN JB. Antibiotic prophylaxis for major maxillocraniofacial surgery. *J Oral Maxillofac Surg* 1985;**43**:865-70.

39. RUGGLES JE. Antibiotic prophylaxis in intraoral orthognathic surgery. *J Oral Maxillofac Surg* 1984;**42**:797-801.

40. BYSTEDT H, JOSEFSSON K, NORD CE. Ecological effects of penicillin prophylaxis in orthognatic surgery. *Int J Oral Maxillofac Surg* 1987;**16**:559-65.

41. BRÅNEMARK P-I, EKHOLM R, ALBREKTSSON B, LINDSTRÖM J, LUNDBORG G, LUNDSKOG J. Tissue injury caused by wound disinfectants. *J Bone Joint Surg* 1967;**49A**:48-62.

42. DAVIES J, BABB JR, AYLIFFE GAJ. The effect on the skin flora of bathing with antiseptic solutions. *J Antimicrob Chemother* 1977;**3**:473-81.

43. MAIBACH HI, ALY R. *Skin microbiology: relevance to clinical infection.* New York: Springer-Verlag, 1981:88-102.

44. FORRESTER JC. Sutures and wound repair. In: HUNT TK, ed. *Wound healing and wound infection. Theory and surgical practice.* New York: Appleton-Century-Crofts, 1980:194-207.

45. OSBON DB. Early treatment of soft tissue injuries of the face. *J Oral Surg* 1969;**27**:480-7.

46. HAURY B, RODEHEAVER G, VENSKO J, EDGERTON MT, EDLICH RF. Debridement: An essential component of traumatic wound care. In: HUNT TK, ed. *Wound healing and wound infection. Theory and surgical practice.* New York: Appleton-Century-Crofts, 1980:229-41.

47. ORDMAN LJ, GILLMAN T. Studies in the healing of cutaneous wounds. *Arch Surg* 1966;**93**:883-928.

48. BRUNIUS U. Wound healing impairment from sutures. *Acta Chir Scand* 1968;Supplement 395.

49. FORRESTER JC, ZEDERFELDT BH, HUNT TK. The tape-closed wound - a bioengineering analysis. *J Surg Res* 1969;**9:**537-42.

50. CONOLLY WB, HUNT TK, ZEDERFELDT B, CAFFERATA HT, DUNPHY JE. Clinical comparison of surgical wounds closed by suture and adhesive tapes. *Am J Surg* 1969;**117:**318-22.

51. ELEK SD. Experimental staphylococcal infections in the skin of man. *Ann NY Acad Science* 1956;**65:**85-90.

52. EDLICH RF, RODEHAVER G, GOLDEN GT, EDGERTON MT. The biology of infections: Sutures, tapes, and bacteria. In: HUNT TK, ed. *Wound healing and wound infection. Theory and surgical practice.* New York: Appleton-Century-Crofts 1980:214-28.

53. BERGENHOLZ A, ISAKSSON B. Tissue reactions in the oral mucosa to catgut, silk, and mersilene sutures. *Odontologisk Revy* 1967;**18:**237-50.

54. LILLY GE. Reaction of oral tissues to suture materials. *Oral Surg Oral Med Oral Pathol* 1968;**26:**128-33.

55. LILLY GE, ARMSTRONG JH, SALEM JE, CUTCHER JL. Reaction of oral tissues to suture materials. Part II. *Oral Surg Oral Med Oral Pathol* 1968;**26:**592-9.

56. LILLY GE, SALEM JE, ARMSTRONG JH, CUTCHER JL. Reaction of oral tissues to suture materials. Part III. *Oral Surg Oral Med Oral Pathol* 1969;**28:**432-8.

57. LILLY GE, CUTCHER JL, JONES JC, ARMSTRONG JH. Reaction of oral tissues to suture materials. Part IV. *Oral Surg Oral Med Oral Pathol* 1972;**33:**152-7.

58. KÁCLOVÁ J, JANOÚSKOVÁ M. Etude expérimentale sur la réaction des tissus de la cavité buccale aux différents matériaux de suture en chirurgie. *Med Hyg (Geneve)* 1965;**23:**1239.

59. CASTELLI WA, NASJLETI CE, CAFFESSE RE, DIAZ-PEREZ R. Gingival response to silk, cotton, and nylon suture materials. *Oral Surg Oral Med Oral Pathol* 1978;**45:**179-85.

60. WALLACE WR, MAXWELL GR, CAVALARIS CJ. Comparison of polyglycolic acid suture to black silk, chromic, and plain catgut in human oral tissues. *J Oral Surg* 1970;**28:**739-46.

61. RACEY GL, WALLACE WR, CAVALARIS CJ, MARQUARD J V. Comparison of a polyglycolic-polyactic acid suture to black silk and plain catgut in human oral tissues. *J Oral Surg* 1978;**36:**766-70.

62. MONEFELDT I, ZACHRISSON BU. Adjustment of clinical crown height by gingivectomy following orthodontic space closure. *Angle Orthod* 1977;**47:**256-64.

63. RIVERA-HIDALGO F, CUNDIFF EJ, WILLIAMS FE, McQUADE MG. Tissue reaction to silk and Goretex sutures in dogs. *J Dent Res* 1991;**71**(Special Issue):508.

CHAPTER 14

Endodontic Management of Traumatized Teeth

M. CVEK

The majority of accidents affect children, often at an age when root development of the injured teeth is not completed. In the following, the treatment of young permanent teeth has therefore beeen emphasized and an attempt made to give a clinically oriented description, including conservative clinical procedures.

Crown Fractures with Dentin Exposure

Pathology

Crown fractures involving dentin result in exposure of dentinal tubules to the oral environment. Exposure of dentin, as such, causes only insignificant changes in the pulp, which may resolve, with the exposed dentinal tubules being sealed off by the secondary dentin [1]. However, if deeply exposed dentin is left unprotected, bacteria and their components in dental plaque on the fracture surface may penetrate the tubules and cause inflammation in the underlying pulp [3,4] (Figs. 14.1 and 14.2). Judging from experimental studies, the subsequent reparative or degenerative changes depend on the time that has elapse since injury and the distance between the fracture surface and pulp. In young permanent teeth, the wide dentinal tubules may be an additional factor [5]. If the irritation is eliminated by treatment of the exposed dentin, localized inflammation in the pulp may resolve, with damaged tissue being replaced by reparative dentin [6,141,142]. When deeply exposed dentin is left unprotected over a longer period of time, the pulp may in some cases

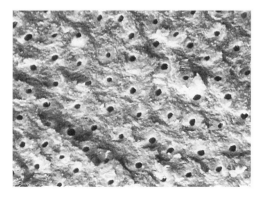
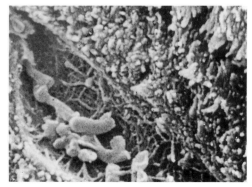

Fig. 14.1.
Surface of fractured dentin. A. There are 36,000 exposed tubules per mm^2, x 1,200. From GARBEROGLIO & BRÄNNSTRÖM *(2) 1976. B. Invasion of bacteria into the tubules of acid-etched dentin, after exposure for 1 week, x 400.*
From OLGART ET AL.(3) *1974.*

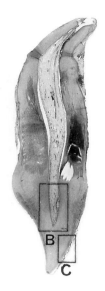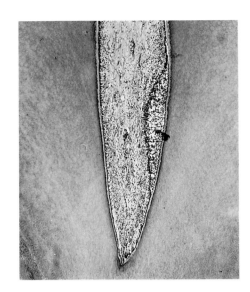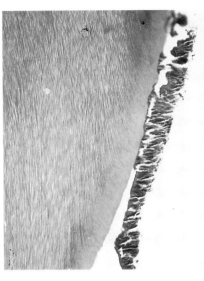

Fig. 14.2.
Early changes in the pulp of a primary incisor 3 days after an uncomplicated crown fracture. A. Low power view, x 3. B. Displacement of odontoblasts and slight infiltration of leukocytes corresponding to the fracture surface, x 30. C. Bacterial accumulation along the fracture surface, x 75.

Fig. 14.3.
Late pulpal changes in an untreated uncomplicated fracture of a primary incisor 4 months after injury. A. Necrosis of the pulp tissue subjacent to the fracture surface, x 32. B. Formation of reparative dentin at a distance from the fracture surface, x 60. C. Penetration of bacteria from fracture surface towards the pulp, Brown & Brenn bacterial stain, x 200

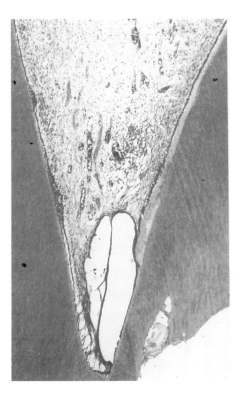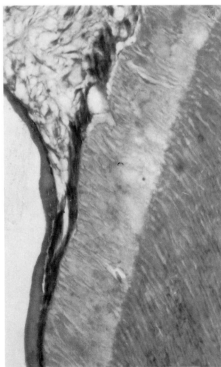

Fig. 14.4.
Treatment of exposed dentin and affected pulp. A. Appearance of fracture after the crown-root fragment has been removed and the surface cleansed 3 days after injury. A hyperemic pulp can be seen through the thin dentin, probably due to irritation from plaque between the fragments. B. Four weeks after treatment with calcium hydroxide; the red discoloration has disappeared.

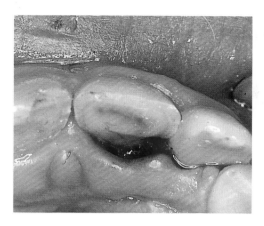
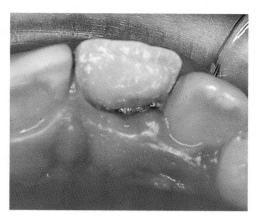

become necrotic and the crown discolored. However, a more frequent cause of pulp necrosis in crown-fractured teeth is probably impaired blood circulation in the pulp due to a concomitant luxation injury (see Chapter 9, p. 350).

Treatment

A crown fracture occurs mostly as a single injury and the crown can be restored during the first visit, normally with a composite material using an enamel acid-etch technique. The exposed dentin is either covered with a liner, or a dentin-bonding agent can be used in order to improve retention. The treatment procedures are described in detail in Chapter 16.

Modern dentin bonding systems have been reported to increase the bonding strength of composite restorations, reduce microleakage, decrease permeability of dentin and to possess an antibacterial effect (143-156). At present, however, it is difficult to form an opinion about the biocompatibility of these agents. Some systems appear more promising than others, but the number of animal or human studies is limited and the results are either uncertain or controversial (145-156). The occurrence of pulp inflammation has been explained by the cytotoxicity of materials, thickness of remaining dentin and poor bonding that allows microleakage and bacterial ingrowth, or a combination of these. It has therefore been recommended that in deep cavities the pulp should be protected, e.g. by lining of the deepest part of the cavity before a dentin bonding agent is placed over the rest of the dentin (151,156). This should also be valid for crown-frac-

tured teeth with a deeply exposed dentin. Furthermore, in cases where the color of the pulp can be seen through a very thin dentin layer or when a deep fracture is left untreated over a couple of days, it may be advisable that the dentin be initially treated with calcium hydroxide and the crown temporarily restored for about 2-3 weeks (Fig. 14.4). In such teeth, treatment with calcium hydroxide may remove bacteria from the fracture surface and give an eventually inflamed pulp a chance to recover and seal off the exposed dentinal tubules by deposition of reparative dentin (6,141,142). Moreover, calcium hydroxide significantly decreases the permeability of dentin to penetration by bacterial components towards the pulp, which may provide additional pulp protection under a subsequent restoration (7,157,158).

If, for some reason, the crown restoration cannot be immediately performed, e.g. due to incorporation in a splint, the pulpo-dentinal complex should be protected. Before the splint is adapted, the exposed dentin may be covered with a hard-setting calcium hydroxide compound or a glass ionomer cement (see Chapter 6, p. 231).

Prognosis

Restoration of a fractured crown with composites and acid-etch techniques can be regarded as an effective tooth repair, although bacterial leakage has been demonstrated in the gaps between composites and dentinal walls in experimental cervical cavities (159). However, most clinical restorations of uncomplicated fractures do not involve the cervical area and, according to clinical studies, the risk of

Fig. 14.5. Clinical appearance of pulp exposures at various observation periods
Four hours after injury hemorrhage is the predominant finding. After 2 days (right), granulation tissue is formed at the exposure site.

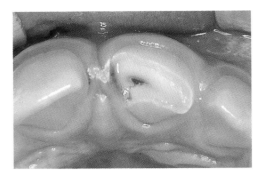 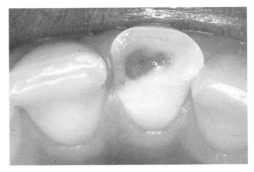

Clinical appearance after 1 week and 3 months
One week after injury: hyperplasia of the pulp. Three months after injury: a polyp is covered with plaque.

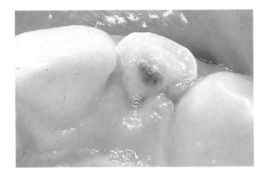 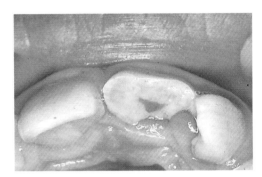

Histologic appearance after 2 days and 1 week
Pulp reactions to experimental exposure in monkey incisors. After 2 days (left), the exposed surface is covered with fibrin, under which a limited pulp proliferation can be seen with moderate infiltration of inflammatory cells to a depth of 1.4 mm, x 90. After 1 week (right), there is proliferation of the pulp through the exposure and moderate inflammation in the proliferated tissue and a mild infiltration of inflammatory cells in the pulp to a depth of 0.4 mm, x 32. From CVEK ET AL.(14) 1982.

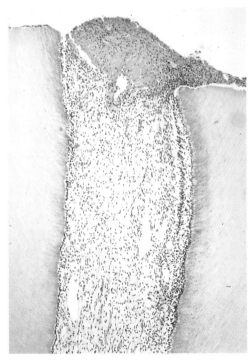 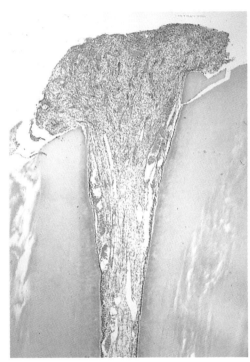

later pulpal damage seems to be minimal (160,161) (see Chapter 6, p. 245).

PRIMARY TEETH

Exposed dentin in primary teeth does not usually require treatment, apart from reducing sharp edges to avoid laceration of the lips and tongue. If dentin remains sensitive, it can be treated with a fluoride-containing varnish to increase mineral deposition onto the fractured dentin (8). However, if requested and if the child is

Fig. 14.6.
Necrosis of the pulp at the exposure site. A. Necrosis of the pulp tissue in a tooth in which the exposure was only covered with a surgical packing for 2 weeks. B. Necrosis of the pulp at the exposure site 4 weeks after injury. The tooth was restored with a temporary crown, seated with a temporary cement and lost after 3 weeks.

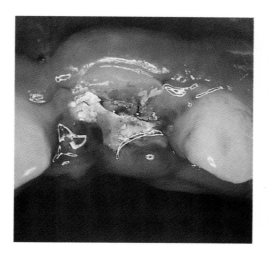
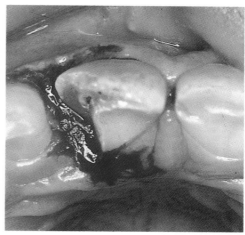

cooperative, the fractured crown can be restored with a composite material in the same manner as a permanent incisor.

Crown Fractures with Pulp Exposure

Pathology

A crown fracture through the pulp chamber causes laceration and exposure of the pulp to the oral environment. Healing does not occur spontaneously and untreated exposures ultimately lead to pulp necrosis, a process in which bacteria are the dominant factor (9). The early changes in the pulp are hemorrhage and local inflammation caused by breakdown products from lacerated tissue and bacterial toxins (10,11). The fibrin clot that forms over the wound surface resolves after a couple of days. The subsequent changes can either be proliferative or destructive, such as abscess formation or necrosis.

During the first days after injury a fresh wound or proliferative changes, i.e. formation of granulation tissue at the exposure site, seem to be most common (Fig. 14.5). In studies of patients aged 7 to 16 years, seen 12 hours or more after injury, hyperplasia was a typical pulpal reaction seen in crown-fractured incisors, regardless of the extent of the exposure (12,162). Similar observations have been made in multirooted human teeth when the pulp was exposed by removal of the crown and left untreated for 2 weeks (13). These findings have also

been supported by experimental studies in which pulps of monkey incisors were exposed by either crown fracture or grinding. In these experiments, pulpal changes were characterized by a proliferative response, invariably associated with only superficial inflammation, extending not more than 2 millimeters from the exposure site (14,15) (Fig. 14.5).

A proliferative response of the pulp is probably favored by an exposure which permits salivary rinsing and prevents impaction of contaminated debris, as occurs in caries or experimentally made cavities (14,163).

Necrosis of an exposed pulp occurs rarely. A common etiological factor seems to be plaque and contaminated debris that is permitted to accumulate over the exposed pulp, or microleakage of inadequate temporary restorations which may neutralize calcium hydroxide and allow bacteria to settle into necrotized pulp tissue (Fig. 14.6). Thus, in pulpotomized monkey incisors in which the coronal cavities were left open for 7 days, impaction of contaminated food debris caused deep abscesses in the underlying pulp (14).

Treatment

The aim of treatment should be the preservation of a vital, non-inflamed pulp, biologically walled off by a continuous hard tissue barrier. In most cases, this can be achieved by pulp capping or pulpotomy. When these treatment alternatives are not possible, the pulp must be extirpated and

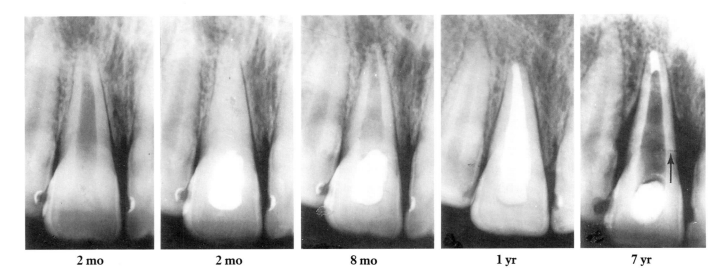

| 2 mo | 2 mo | 8 mo | 1 yr | 7 yr |

Fig. 14.7.
Spontaneous root fracture due to thin dentinal walls following pulp necrosis at an early stage of root development. Permanent incisor treated with calcium hydroxide and root filled with gutta-percha. Cervical fracture of the thin dentinal walls (arrow) occurred during chewing 6 years later.

the root canal obturated with a filling material. Indications for these forms of treatment are discussed later in connection with endodontic procedures. Some factors, however, such as maturity of the tooth, concomitant luxation injury, age of the patient as well as the effect of surgical procedures and choice of wound dressing, should also be discussed here.

The maturity of the tooth is of utmost importance in the choice of treatment. It is generally agreed that the exposed vital pulp should be maintained in young teeth with incomplete root formation while it can be removed in mature teeth where constriction of the apical foramen allows adequate obturation of the root canal.

However, maturation of a tooth is not complete with constriction of the apical foramen. Removal of the pulp in children and adolescents deprives the tooth of physiologic dentin apposition, leaving thin dentinal walls, which increases the risk of later cervical root fractures, a problem that should be considered in treatment planning[16,17] (Fig. 14.7).

A concomitant luxation injury compromises the nutritional supply to the pulp and, in principle, contraindicates conservative treatment. However, in immature luxated teeth the chance of pulp survival is considerable and conservative treatment may allow further root development [18,19] (Fig. 14.8). Treatment should

Fig. 14.8.
Treatment of pulp exposure in a slightly dislocated immature incisor. Formation of a hard tissue barrier in the pulp and closure of the apical foramen, subsequent to partial pulpotomy.

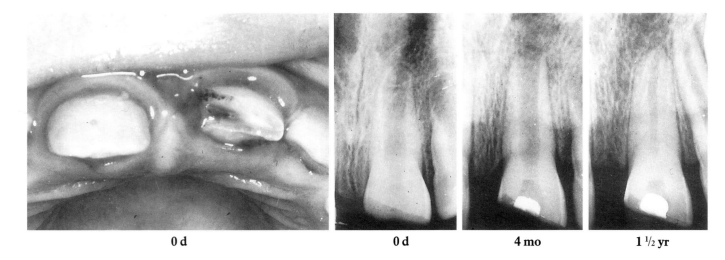

| 0 d | 0 d | 4 mo | 1 ½ yr |

Fig. 14.9. Effect of pulp amputation technique upon the pulp

The effect of cutting with an abrasive diamond instrument in a high speed contra-angle hand piece; no tissue damage below the wound surface x 25 and 100. From GRANATH & HAGMAN (32) 1971

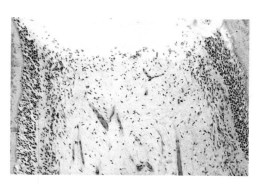

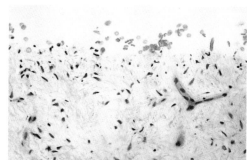

Effect of calcium hydroxide on the pulp

Left: Formation of liquefaction necrosis (L) close to calcium hydroxide. Coagulation necrosis (C) close to the vital pulp is colored yellow, x 75. Right: formation of hard tissue 17 days after capping; layer of necrotic tissue (N) and dark stained band of necrotic and later calcified tissue (C) and osteoid-like tissue (O) with lining cells x 75. From SCHRÖDER & GRANATH (36) 1971.

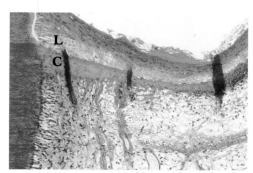

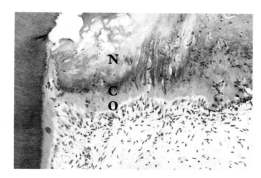

Formation of a hard tissue barrier

A completely formed hard tissue barrier after capping with calcium hydroxide paste (Calasept®), x 25. Right: formation of hard tissue barrier without visible intermediate layer of necrosis after capping with a hard-setting calcium hydroxide compound (Dycal ®), x 25. From BRÄNNSTRÖM ET AL.(40) 1979.

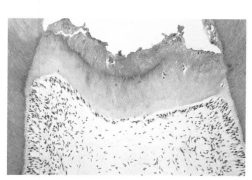

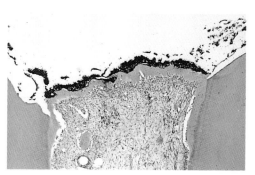

therefore be determined according to the severity of the periodontal injury and the maturity of the tooth.

The effect of age is controversial. Experimentally, an inferior response to injury and treatment has been observed in pulps of old rats compared to young ones (10,11). Yet, successful treatment of pulp exposure due to either trauma or caries in older patients has repeatedly been reported (20-23). For various reasons, degenerative changes in the pulp undoubtedly increase with age. Thus, removal of the pulp could be a more successful procedure, although no age limit can be set for either pulp preservation or removal. However, conservative treatment, i.e. capping or pulpotomy, should not be performed if degenerative or inflammatory changes are anticipated, such as in teeth with reduced pulpal lumen due to trauma

or age, or in periodontally involved teeth in adults (24-27).

Surgical procedures invariably cause further injury to the remaining pulp and should be kept to a minimum. Various instruments have been recommended for pulpal amputation, such as spoon excavators, slowly rotating round burs and high-speed abrasive diamonds. Of these, the spoon excavator, successfully used in molars (28), has proven unsuitable in young incisors. Slowly rotating instruments are known to inflict significant injury to the remaining pulp, limiting the chance of survival (29-31). However, it has been shown that injury to the underlying tissue is minimal when abrasive diamond is used at high speed to remove part of the pulp, provided that the bur and tissues are adequately cooled (32) (Fig. 14.9). If effective cooling is not possible, e.g. when the am-

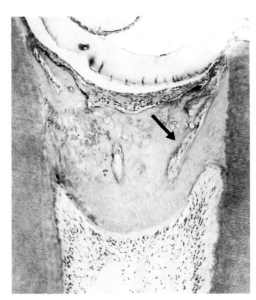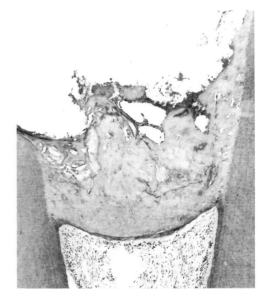

Fig. 14.10.
Response of monkey incisor to capping with cyanoacrylate or short-term dressing with calcium hydroxide. A. Formation of hard tissue barrier 3 months after the pulp was treated temporarily with calcium hydroxide for 10 minutes and, after it was washed away, covered with several sterile teflon discs sealed in place with IRM ® , x 50.
B. Formation of hard tissue barrier 3 months after the pulp was covered with cyanoacrylate, x 40. Note that hard tissue barriers are not continuous and include etunnels (arrow). From CVEK ET AL.(166) 1987.

putation site is deep in the root canal, a round bur at low speed should be used in order to avoid overheating the pulp.

The most common wound dressing is calcium hydroxide. This material has been widely used for the treatment of accidentally exposed pulps since the first histological studies appeared decades ago (33,34,164). Calcium hydroxide has been the subject of extensive experimental research and several explanations have been offered for its effect on the vital pulp (165).

When placed over a vital pulp, pure calcium hydroxide causes a superficial tissue necrosis, approximately 1-1.5 mm in depth (35). This necrosis consists of several layers, including a layer of firm coagulation necrosis in close contact with vital tissue which seems not to be appreciably affected (36). Based on observation in experiments with sound human teeth, it has been suggested that it is neither calcium hydroxide nor its components, but the low-grade irritation from coagulation necrosis that induces defensive reactions in the pulp, resulting in formation of a demarcating hard-tissue barrier (36,37). To this irritation, the underlying tissue seems to react by producing collagen that is subsequently mineralized, while the coagulated tissue is calcified, which is later fol-

lowed by differentiation of dentin (Fig. 14.9). This hypothesis of a low-grade irritation that is not strong enough to destroy the pulp tissue but is sufficient to elicit defensive reactions was strongly supported by findings of the formation of hard tissue barriers after only 10 minutes' treatment with calcium hydroxide or capping with cyanoacrylate, a material possessing none of the calcium or hydroxyl ions that are thought to be responsible for induction of hard tissue (166) (Fig. 14.10). Cyanoacrylate is degradable in a biological environment and it is probable that some released substance(s) may exert just enough irritation to elicit defensive reactions in the pulp leading to formation of a hard tissue barrier (167). Similar results have been reported in experiments with light-cured composite, zinc phosphate and silicate cements (168). On the other hand, when a biologically inert material, such as teflon, has been brought into contact with pulpal tissue no hard tissue formation could be found in relation to this material1(66,169). Thus, the role of calcium hydroxide appears to be limited to its chemical effect that is able to elicit defensive processes in the pulp by exerting a low-grade irritation, either through the induction of coagulation necrosis or directly on the pulp tissue without a visible necrosis when hard-setting compounds are used (38,170-173) (Fig. 14.9). Accordingly, formation of the hard tissue barrier itself can be regarded as a defensive, probably stereotypic, reaction of the pulp to a non-specific low-grade irritant (174).

During the course of time, various materials have been tested for pulp dressing (167,175). Indeed, in absence of bacteria, healing of the pulp with or without formation of hard tissue was observed after capping with various materials, such as cyanoacrylate, zinc-phosphate, tricalcium phosphate or silicate cements and composite materials but, so far, none of these materials can be recommended for routine clinical use (166,168,176-178).

Calcium hydroxide seems to be a suitable and well-tested pulp dressing which repeatedly gives predictable results in the form of a non-inflamed pulp under a well-formed hard-tisssue barrier. However, it should be stressed that calcium hydroxide has no beneficial effect on healing of a chronically inflamed pulp and it should therefore only be brought into contact with a non-inflamed pulp tissue (39). In clinical terms, this means that the compound should be placed against vital pulp tissue with intact vascularity in teeth which respond to sensibility testing. Internal dentin resorption and dystrophic calcifications, reported to occur after dressing of the pulp with calcium hydroxide, seem to be related to the presence of an extrapulpal blood clot or to the damage caused by operative procedures (30,41-45). Thus, when an extrapulpal blood clot was not allowed to form and a gentle amputation technique was used for amputation, these changes were not observed clinically nor histologically (12,37,162,179-181).

Pulp Capping

Capping of the pulp is indicated when a small exposure can be treated shortly after injury which, according to experimental studies, seems to mean within 24 hours (173,182,183). Pulp capping implies that the pulpal wound caused by the injury is covered with calcium hydroxide. It is thought that, in small exposures treated soon after injury, the mechanical damage and inflammation in the pulp cannot be deeper than the necrotizing effect of calcium hydroxide. Thus, the effect actually is exerterted on healthy pulp tissue, while bacteria on the dentin fracture and the wound surfaces are eliminated by the action of calcium hydroxide. Accordingly, the primary contamination of the pulp should not be critical for healing. However, pulp healing may be threatened by later contamination due to microleakage of defective restorations, since all calcium hydroxide compounds gradually lose their antibacterial property. Futhermore, the hard tissue barriers formed after treatment may include structural defects which may increase their permeability and, in the case of "tunnel" formation due to vascular inclusions, offer a direct contact with underlying pulp tissue (166,168,184-189) (Fig.14.10).

TREATMENT

The fracture surface and pulpal wound are washed with saline. When bleeding has ceased, the exposed pulp is covered with a soft- or a hard-setting calcium hydroxide compound. If the pulp is covered with a soft calcium hydroxide compound, the exposed dentin should be protected with a glass ionomer cement or a hard-setting calcium hydroxide liner before the crown is restored (Fig. 14.11). If the definitive restoration of the crown must be postponed, a temporary crown restoration should be placed with a material that does not allow microleakage, e.g. zinc-oxide eugenol or polycarboxylate cement (190,191).

Pulpotomy

Pulpotomy involves removal of damaged and inflamed tissue to the level of a clinically healthy pulp, followed by a calcium hydroxide dressing. Depending on the size of the exposure and time elapsed since injury, different levels of pulpal amputation have been recommended, i.e. partial or cervical pulpotomy (46). It has been shown, however, that neither exposure size nor time interval between injury and treatment are critical for healing when only superficial layers of the pulp are removed (12,162,179). Thus, in teeth showing vital and/or hyperplastic pulp tissue at the exposure, only superficial layers of the pulp and surrounding dentin should be removed; i.e. a partial pulpotomy can be performed in immature as well as mature teeth.

Fig. 14.11. Treatment of a complicated crown fracture with pulp capping
A fractured incisor with a small pulp exposure 4 hours after injury. Note the good vascularity of the exposed pulp.

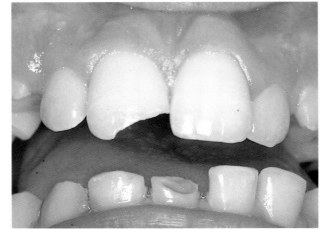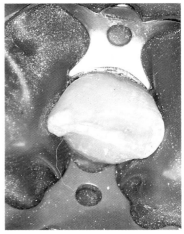

Pulp capping
After isolation with a rubber dam, the exposed pulp is covered with a soft calcium hydroxide compound (Calasept ®) which together with the remaining dentin is covered with a hard-setting calcium hydroxide cement, whereafter the tooth is restored with a composite.

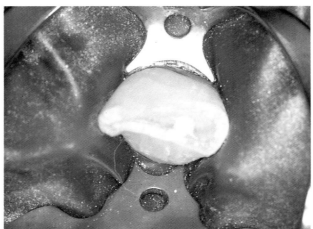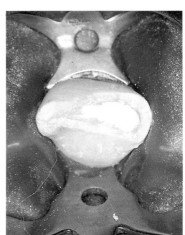

TREATMENT

Pulpotomy should be performed with a diamond bur, of a size corresponding to the exposure, in a high speed contra-angle handpiece (Fig. 14.12). Effective cooling is essential and to avoid injury to the pulp due to insufficient cooling, the tooth and cutting instrument should be flushed continuously with water or saline by means of a syringe or the turbine spray. Furthermore cutting should be performed intermittently for brief periods and without unnecessary pressure.

The level of amputation should be about 2 mm below the exposure site. This level is deep enough to remove inflamed tissue and provide an adequate cavity for both the dressing and the sealing material. The pulpal wound is then rinsed with saline until bleeding has ceased. The wound surface is covered with calcium hydroxide and adapted with cotton pellets using light pressure, whereby the water from the paste is also removed. The surplus of calcium hydroxide is then easily removed with an excavator. The coronal cavity is closed with a tight-sealing material, e.g. zinc oxide-eugenol cement. However, as eugenol may interfere with polymerization of composites, it should be covered with a liner or glassionomer cement before restoration with composites, especially if the crown is restored immediately after pulpotomy. Another choice is to seal the cavity with Prader's zinc-sulphate cement (192). This material does not interfere with polymerization but possesses sealing properties equal to those of zinc oxide-eugenol cement (190).

The advantage of partial pulpotomy lies in the minor injury to the pulp and undisturbed physiologic apposition of dentin, especially in the critical cervical area of the tooth. The limited loss of crown substance offers continuing opportunities for sensitivity testing and, in most cases, a post in the root canal will not be required for crown restoration. Compared with pulp capping, it implies better wound control and, by sealing off the cavity with a material which does not allow microleakage, provides effective protection for

Fig. 14.12. Treatment of a complicated crown fracture with partial pulpotomy
A complicated crown fracture of an immature incisor 2 days after injury.

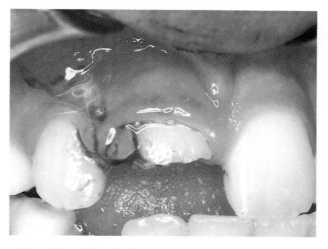
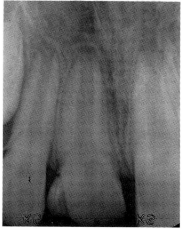

Clinical condition
After the crown fragments were removed a large pulp exposure is found.

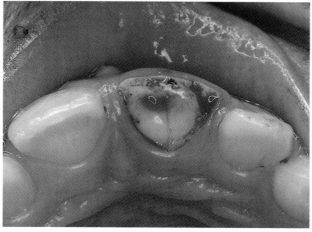
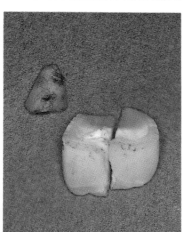

Isolation with a rubber dam
After administration of a local anesthesia, the tooth is isolated with a rubber dam and washed with saline. A suitable diamond bur is chosen for the pulpotomy.

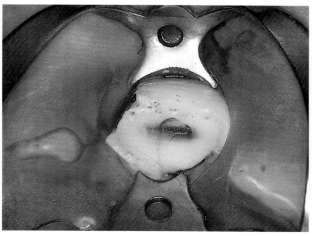
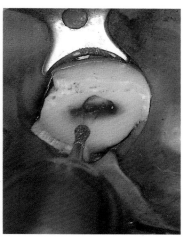

Pulpotomy
The pulpotomy is carried out to a depth of 2.0 mm. The cutting of the pulp and surrounding dentin is performed using a high-speed turbine. This is done intermittently, with brief cutting periods and continuous flushing with the water spray from the turbine, eventually supplemented with extra saline from a syringe.

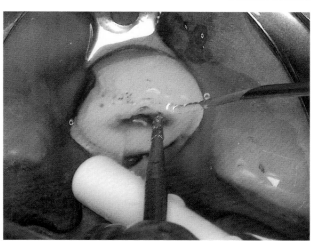
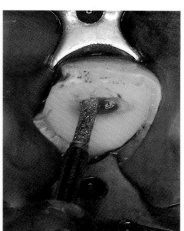

ENDODONTIC MANAGEMENT OF TRAUMATIZED TEETH

Cavity preparation
The cavity should be boxlike, with a slight undercut in dentin.

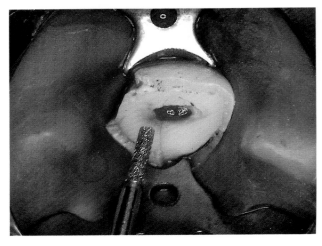

Applying the dressing material
Hemostasis is awaited, and usually takes place within a couple of minutes. Otherwise a slight pressure can be applied with a cotton pellet soaked in saline or an anesthetic solution with vaso-constrictor. After complete arrest of bleeding, calcium hydroxide paste (e.g. Calasept ®) is placed over the pulpal wound.

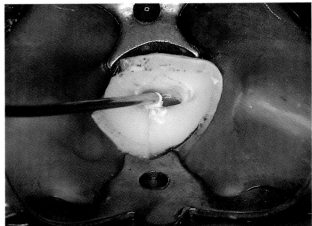
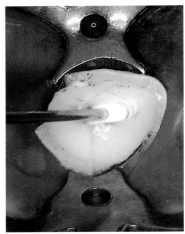

Compressing the dressing material
The material is compressed slightly with a dry cotton pellet to adapt the material to the wound surface. After surplus dressing material is removed, the amputation cavity is sealed with a zinc-euge-nol cement. In cases where the tooth is immediately restored, the cavity is sealed with a hard-set-ting calcium hydroxide com-pound, or zinc phosphate cement can be used.

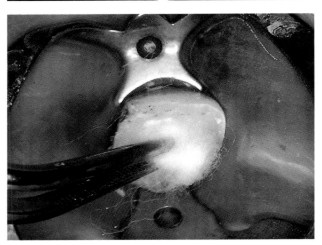
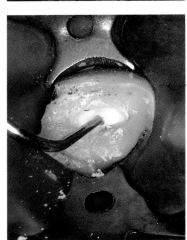

Restoration
The tooth has been restored dur-ing the same sitting, using a com-posite resin and a dentin bonding agent.

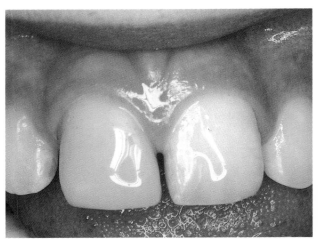
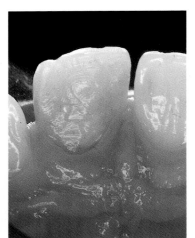

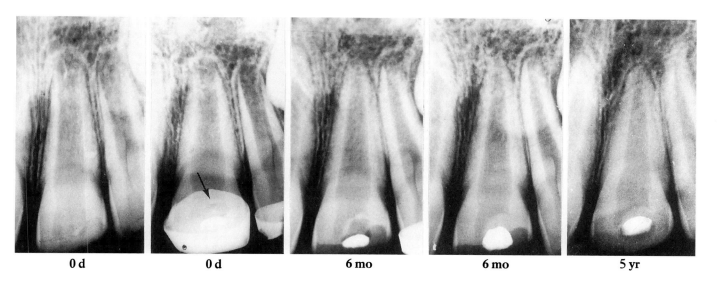

| 0 d | 0 d | 6 mo | 6 mo | 5 yr |

Fig. 14.13.
Radiographic demonstration of healing after partial pulpotomy in an incisor with immature root formation. The tooth was treated 3 hours after injury. Note initial formation of hard tissue after 3 weeks (arrow) and completed barrier after 6 months. A control after 5 years shows healing and completed root developmnet.

the pulp. Most probably, this is one of the reasons for the high rate of healing reported after this type of treatment (12,162,179) (Figs. 14.13 and 14.14).

It has been suggested that, after capping of pulp exposures in the coronal or cervical area of anterior teeth, formation of hard tissue sometimes may compromise the blood supply to the coronal part of the

pulp tissue, causing it to degenerate (24). However, this phenomenon appears to be rare (193). Thus, in a comprehensive clinical study, no adverse effects could be observed after partial pulpotomy treatment of proximal exposures in crown-root fractured teeth (162) (Fig. 14.15).

When necrotic tissue or obviously impaired vascularity is present at the expo-

Fig. 14.14.
Radiographic demonstration of healing after partial pulpotomy in an incisor with completed root formation, treated 12 hours after injury. Formation of a hard tissue barrier is present after 6 months and healing is evident 7 years after treatment.

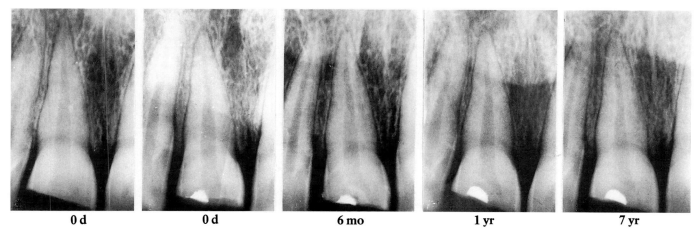

| 0 d | 0 d | 6 mo | 1 yr | 7 yr |

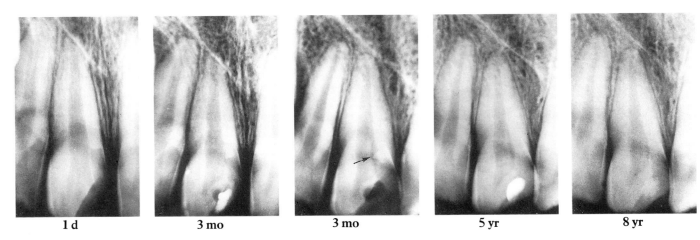

| 1 d | 3 mo | 3 mo | 5 yr | 8 yr |

Fig. 14.15.
A crown-root fractured incisor with a proximal exposure of the pulp, treated 24 hours after injury with a partial pulpotomy. A loose fragment (arrow) was removed 3 months later. There is formation of a hard tissue barrier but no further constriction of the coronal pulp.

sure site of immature teeth, the pulp should be amputated to a level at which fresh bleeding tissue is found, i.e. a cervical or deep pulpotomy should be performed (Fig. 14.16). Due to problems with adequate cooling of the diamond at high speed at that level, a round carbide bur at low speed should be used. In mature teeth, a pulpectomy is the treatment of choice.

Pulpectomy

Pulpectomy, i.e. removal of the entire pulp to the level of 1-2 mm from the apical foramen, is performed in mature teeth when conservative pulp treatment is not indicated (47,48). After removal of the pulp, the root canal is cleansed chemomechanically and obturated with guttapercha points and a suitable sealer. There are, however, instances when interim dressing with calcium hydroxide is the treatment of choice, i.e. when periapical healing and closure of the apical foramen with hard tissue is desired before obturation, or when adequate treatment is not possible due to the presence of splints (49,50). In the latter instance, it is difficult to adapt a rubber dam and access to the root canal can be limited. In such cases, calcium hydroxide can be used as an interim dressing and treatment continued once the splint has been removed.

CLINICAL EVALUATION OF PULP HEALING

Only histological techniques can verify pulpal healing, i.e. a non-inflamed pulp walled off by a continuous hard tissue barrier. However, a fairly adequate evaluation can be made according to the following criteria: 1. no clinical symptoms; 2. no radiographically demonstrable intraradicular or periradicular pathological changes; 3. continued root development in immature teeth; 4. radiographically observed (and clinically verified) continuous hard tissue barrier; 5. sensitivity to electrical stimulation; and 6. a follow-up for at least 3 years. These criteria apply both to pulp capping and pulpotomy, with the exception of sensitivity testing which usually is not possible after cervical or deep pulpotomy. In the pulps of teeth treated with partial pulpotomy and judged to be healed according to these criteria, no or only insignificant pathological changes were found in histologically examined pulps (180,181).

A hard tissue barrier that appears continuous in radiographs may be discontinuous when examined histologically. On the the other hand, it has been found that teeth which demonstrate a clinically continuous barrier usually contain non-inflamed pulps (31,51). Clinical exploration by probing can therefore be used as a criterion when pulp healing is evaluated,

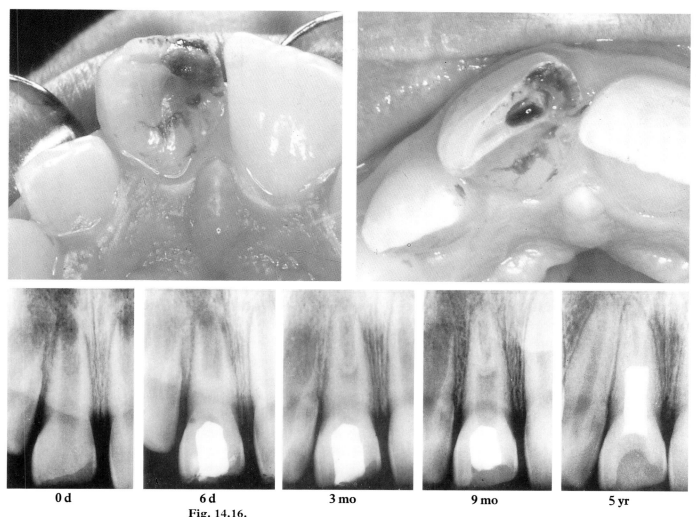

| 0 d | 6 d | 3 mo | 9 mo | 5 yr |

Fig. 14.16.
Deep pulpotomy in an incisor with crown fracture and impaired pulpal vascularity. Vital and bleeding pulp tissue was found in the middle of the root canal. Three and 9 months after a deep pulpotomy, formation of a hard-tissue barrier can be seen deep in the root canal. A 5-year control of the subsequent root canal filling with gutta-percha shows completed root development.

but this is not compulsory in clinical practice (162). It is important to consider that a continuous hard tissue barrier and positive sensitivity do not exclude chronic pulpal inflammation which may persist in an asymptomatic tooth. Thus, the follow-up period should be extended. In a comprehensive long-term clinical study of permanent incisors treated with partial pulpotomy, all failures occurred within 26 months after treatment. The teeth that were judged as healed at the 3-years control remained healed 10-15 years thereafter; indicating that a 3-year follow-up should be considered adequate (162).

Because pulp canal obliteration and pulp necrosis are rather frequent long-term complications after cervical pulpotomy, this procedure is regarded as a temporary treatment to be followed by pulpectomy once root formation is complete (175). Furthermore, the treatment may cause a loss of tooth substance in the cervical area to such an extent that a full crown restoration with anchorage in the root canal is required to prevent a root fracture.

Prognosis

The frequency of success after pulp capping or pulpotomy treatments varies from 72 to 96 % (12,51-54,162,163,179,194-196). Results in more comprehensive clinical studies are shown in Table 14.1. The reported frequency of healing after pulpectomy followed by root filling with various materials varies from 80 to 96 % (55-58,197)

PRIMARY TEETH

The exposed pulps in primary teeth may be treated by capping or pulpotomy according to the same criteria as permanent teeth, provided that physiologic resorption is only limited. This requirement, however, restricts the treatment to such an early age that cooperation from the patient in an acute situation is seldom achieved and thus the treatment can rarely be adequately performed. In practice, extraction of the tooth is most often the treatment of choice.

Root Fractures

Pathology

Pulp necrosis with subsequent periradicular involvement occurs with a relatively low frequency, that is in about 25 % of root-fractured teeth. It is a characteristic of a root fracture that only the coronal fragment is dislocated and that pulpal circulation in the apical fragment is not severely disturbed. Thus, when pulp necrosis does occur, it normally takes place only in the coronal fragment, while in the apical fragment the pulp remains vital (59,60,198-200). However, if the coronal fragment is left untreated, the bacteria from its necrotic pulp may spread and cause inflammation and necrosis of the pulp in the apical fragment as well.

Diagnosis

Clinical symptoms such as changes in crown color and pulp sensibility are interpreted in the same way as in other traumatically injured teeth. The first radiographic sign of pulpal necrosis is often a progressive widening of the space between the two fragments, later followed by pathologic changes in the periradicular bone, seen as a widened and diffusely outlined periodontal space or radiolucency, usually present within 3 months after injury (198,199) (Fig. 14.17). If the tooth is not splinted, these changes can make the coronal fragment loose and tender to percussion.

Internal surface or tunnelling resorption seem to be a part of healing processes and normally do not require endodontic intervention (199) (see Chapter 8, p. 291). On the other hand, external inflammatory root resorption indicates necrotic and infected pulp tissue (61,201).

Treatment

Conservative endodontic treatment of root-fractured teeth can be divided into treatment of the coronal fragment alone, or both fragments. If these treatments are unsuccessful, surgical removal of the apical fragment can be indicated.

The choice of treatment depends on radiographic findings, such as periradicular changes, width of the pulpal lumen and separation between the two fragments, as well as on the clinical finding of pulp vitality in the apical fragment at the time

Table 14.1. Healing frequencies after treatment of the exposed pulp in crown-fractured teeth

Examiner	No of teeth	Healing
Pulp capping		
Kozlowska (52) 1980	53	38 (72 %)
Ravn (53) 1982	84	4 (88 %)
Fuks et al. (194)1982	38	31 (81 %)
Partial pulpotomy		
Cvek (12) 1978	60	58 (96 %)
Fuks et al. (179) 1987	63	59 (94 %)
Cvek (162) 1992	178	169 (95 %)
Cervical pulpotomy		
Hallet & Porteous (54) 1963	93	67 (72 %)
Gelbier & Winter (195)1988	175	139 (79 %)

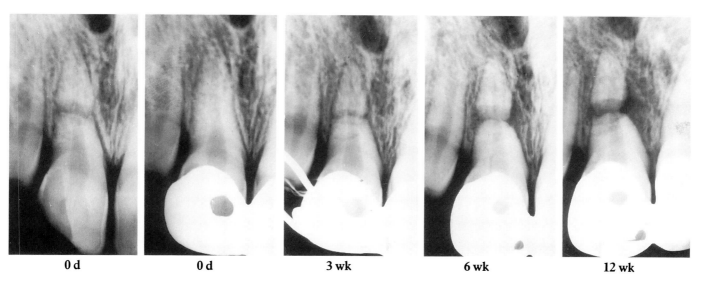

| 0 d | 0 d | 3 wk | 6 wk | 12 wk |

Fig. 14.17.
Radiographic signs of pulp necrosis after root fracture. Note progressive widening of the space between fragments and appearance of a radiolucency in the adjacent alveolar bone.

of treatment. The location of the fracture on the root does not affect the choice of treatment unless it is located in the cervical third. For treatment of these teeth (see Chapter 15. p. 606).

Root canal treatment of the coronal fragment is indicated for teeth which do not show pathologic changes periapically and in which bleeding and/or sensitivity to probing at the fracture site indicate a vital pulp in the apical fragment. This is the case in the majority of root fractured teeth

Fig. 14.18.
Endodontic treatment of the coronal fragment of a root-fractured incisor with gutta-percha. Condition is shown before and after repositioning of the coronal fragment at the time of injury. After 6 weeks, a slightly widened space between the fragments and a radiolucency in the adjacent alveolar bone indicate pulp necrosis in the coronal fragment. The tapered root canal in the fragment permitted an adequate filling with gutta-percha.

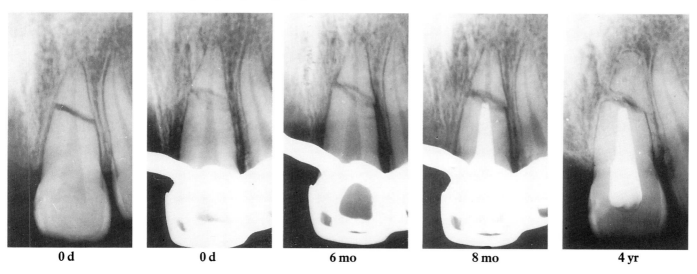

| 0 d | 0 d | 6 mo | 8 mo | 4 yr |

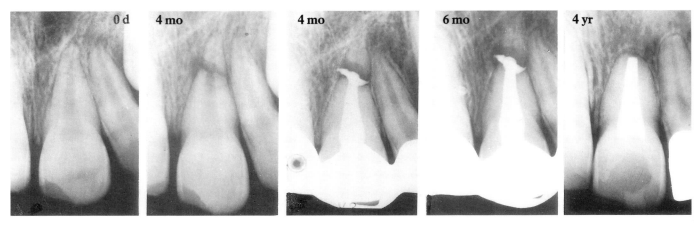

Fig. 14.19.
Difficulties in root canal obturation of the coronal fragment after root fracture. After 4 months there is a widening of the space between the fragments and a radiolucency adjacent to the fracture. After antibacterial treatment, the coronal root canal was obturated and gutta-percha became extruded into the fracture site. Six months later the space between the fragments as well as the adjacent radiolucency have increased whereafter the apical fragment was removed. At the 4-year control, periapical healing is evident.

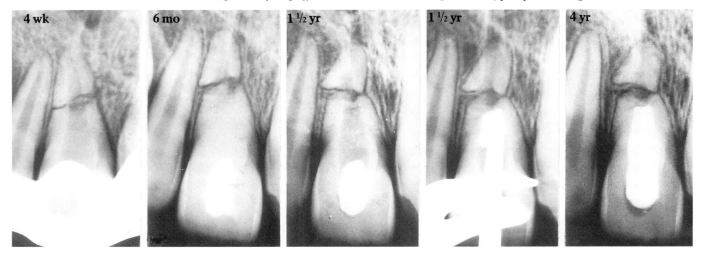

Fig. 14.20.
Treatment of the coronal fragment of a root-fractured incisor with a wide pulpal lumen 4 weeks after injury with calcium hydroxide. After 18 months, periradicular healing has taken place and a hard tissue barrier has formed apically in the coronal fragment, against which an adequate root filling with gutta-percha can be performed.

Fig. 14.21.
Root canal treatment of both fragments of a root-fractured incisor. Note the widening of the space between fragments and the adjacent radiolucency 4 months after injury. The root canal in both fragments was filled with gutta-percha which extruded into the space between the two fragments. After 3 months, the space between the fragments and adjacent radiolucency have increased and the apical fragment was therefore removed. Periradicular healing can be seen 4 years later.

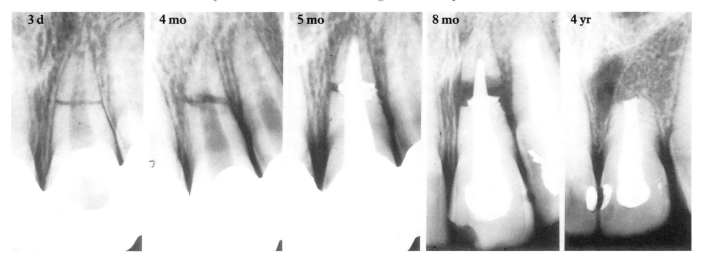

CHAPTER 14

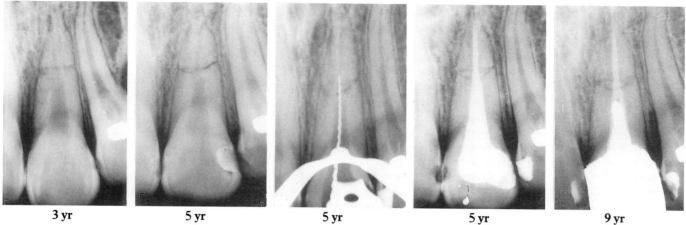

3 yr   5 yr   5 yr   5 yr   9 yr

Fig. 14.22.

Treatment of a tooth with a healed root fracture and subsequent pulpitis due to a carious lesion. Three years after injury the root fracture appears healed. Two years later, a deep carious lesion was filled temporarily. Due to symptoms of pulpitis endodontic treatment was instituted. Note that there was no gutta-percha pressed between fragments at the time of filling and no periradicular changes 4 years later (i.e. 9 years after injury).

with pulpal complications. The coronal fragment may be filled with gutta-percha immediately after root canal treatment if the anatomy of the root canal permits adequate obturation (Fig. 14.18). However, achieving satisfactory cleansing and obturation with gutta-percha is difficult, especially in teeth with a wide pulpal lumen (Fig. 14.19). The coronal fragment can instead be treated initially with calcium hydroxide and obturated with gutta-percha after a hard tissue barrier has formed apically in the coronal fragment and periradicular healing has taken place (Fig. 14.20). Clinical procedures and the effect of calcium hydroxide are discussed later in connection with treatment of non-vital immature teeth.

Root canal treatment of both fragments can be performed when the entire pulp is necrotic. The treatment is complicated as it is difficult to avoid impacting necrotic tissue and filling debris between the fragments during mechanical cleansing as well as overfilling with gutta-percha (Fig. 14.21). This could explain the poor prognosis of this type of treatment. However, once the root fracture has healed, leaving no empty space between the fragments, this type of treatment may have a better prognosis, in the case of a late secondary pulp necrosis (Fig. 14.22).

Root canal treatment of the coronal fragment and surgical removal of the apical fragment is indicated in teeth in which the apical fragment with necrotic pulp is not accessible for treatment or when prognosis is poor due to a wide space between the two fragments (Figs. 14.21 and 14.23), as well as in teeth in which either of the first two treatments has not been successful (Figs. 14.19 and 14.21).

In the case of a concomitant crown fracture, the exposed dentin is covered with

Fig. 14.23.

Endodontic treatment of the coronal fragment and simultaneous surgical removal of the apical fragment. Displacement of the apical fragment made endodontic treatment of both fragments impossible.

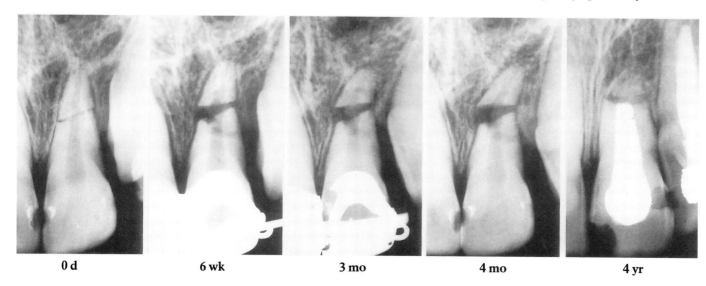

0 d   6 wk   3 mo   4 mo   4 yr

ENDODONTIC MANAGEMENT OF TRAUMATIZED TEETH

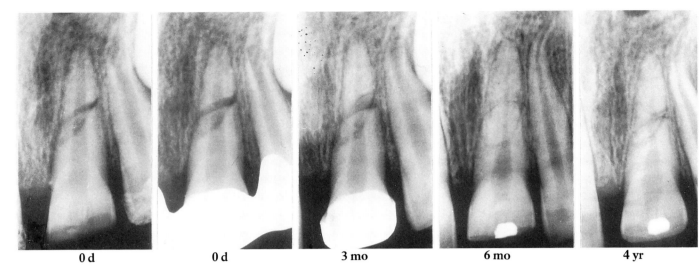

| 0 d | 0 d | 3 mo | 6 mo | 4 yr |

Fig. 14.24.

Treatment of an incisor with concomitant complicated crown and root fracture. A partial pulpotomy was performed and the tooth splinted. At the final control, a hard tissue barrier is seen in the coronal fragment as well as a connective tissue healing of the root fracture.

a hard-setting calcium hydroxide or glass ionomer cement, followed by a layer of composite material. The final restoration of the crown is performed after an immobilization splint is removed, i.e. periodontal healing has taken place.

An exposed pulp is treated by pulp capping or partial pulpotomy, provided that vital and fresh bleeding tissue is found at the exposure site (Fig. 14.24). Root canal treatment is instituted later in the event of pulp necrosis.

Prognosis

Successful conservative treatment of root-fractured teeth with partial or total pulp necrosis has been reported in a number of publications (62-67,197), but little information is available on healing frequencies after the various types of treatment. However, in clinical studies of root-fractured teeth with necrosis of the coronal pulp alone, periodontal healing and formation of a hard-tissue barrier apically in the coronal fragment was seen in all teeth treated with calcium hydroxide and subsequently filled with gutta-percha. Furthermore the root canal in the apical fragment became obliterated (66,198) (Fig. 14.20).

PRIMARY TEETH

Primary root-fractured teeth with pulpal complications are not treated endodontically. In the case of total pulp necrosis the whole tooth should be ex-

Fig. 14.25.

Continued root development after replantation of an immature incisor. The tooth was replanted after 30 min dry storage. From KLING ET AL.(209) 1986.

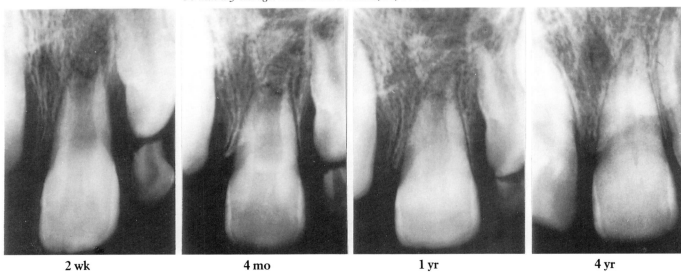

| 2 wk | 4 mo | 1 yr | 4 yr |

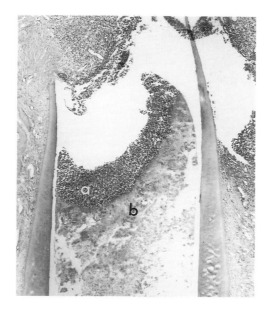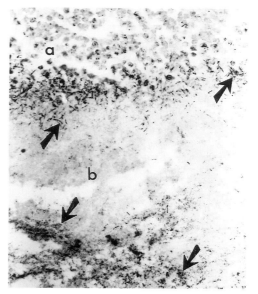

Fig. 14.26.

Presence of a contaminated blood clot in the pulpal lumen of a replanted immature monkey incisor. A. Apical area of the tooth; abscess formation at the apical foramen (a) and beneath it a blood clot (b), x 15. B. Enlarged view of the area between dense accumulation of leukocytes (a) and blood clot (b) shows heavy contamination of the blood clot with microorganisms (arrows), Brown & Brenn bacterial stain, x 140. From CVEK ET AL. (207) 1990.

tracted. However, the pulp in the apical fragment normally remains vital so that only the coronal fragment must be removed and the apical fragment allowed to resorb spontaneously (see Chapter 8, p. 303).

Luxated or Avulsed and Replanted Teeth

Pathology

When a tooth is forcefully displaced in its alveolus, vessels at the apical foramen can be compressed, lacerated or severed. Subsequent reactions in the pulp depend on the degree and duration of circulatory disturbances, the stage of root development and eventual bacterial contamination of the affected tissues. In general, the risk of pulp necrosis increases with increasing stages of root development and severity of the luxation injury (68-70,202-206).

A sudden, complete break in pulpal circulation leads to infarction and coagulation necrosis of the pulp. In mature teeth and in the absence of bacteria, such tissue may persist without clinical symptoms or obvious radiographic change for long periods of time. However, the pulp often becomes contaminated by microorgan-

isms from the oral cavity, with subsequent periapical involvement (71-75,207).

In immature teeth, the infarcted tissue can be revascularized, i.e. replaced by ingrowth of mesenchymal tissues. This is followed by deposition of hard tissue along the canal walls and, sometimes, continued root development (Fig. 14.25). These processes are described in detail in Chapter 2, p. 104.

In clinical and experimental studies of immature replanted teeth, the frequency of complete pulp revascularization was found to be rather low (76,201,207-209). In all teeth in which revascularization did not occur, a periapical radiolucency and/or inflammatory root resorption developed, i.e. changes known to be related to the presence of microorganisms in the pulpal lumen.

In experimental studies designed to imitate clinical conditions, the presence of microorganisms was the predominant reason for the absence of complete revascularization (201,207). Two particular sources of contamination were demonstrated. One was the presence of blood clots harboring bacteria in the apical area of the pulpal lumen, most probably contaminated during the extra-alveolar period (Fig. 14.26). The other source of contamination was mechanically damaged cervical root surfaces through which bacteria from dental

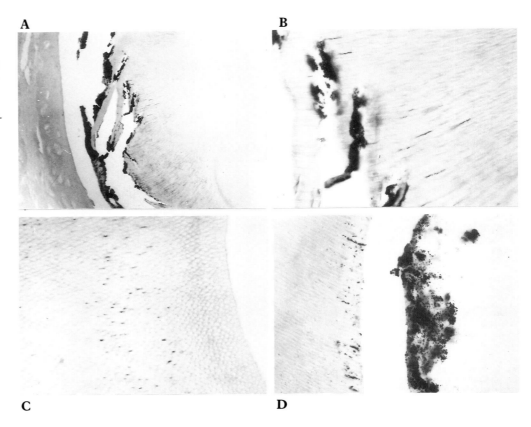

Fig. 14.27.
Pathway of microorganisms via cervical root damage to the pulpal lumen. A and B. Crushed cementum and dentin in the cervical area of the tooth, formation of plaque and penetration of microorganisms into dentinal tubules, which could be followed in serial sections through the dentinal wall into the pulpal lumen, x 30 and 140. C and D. Microorganisms in the dentinal wall close to the pulpal lumen and formation of colonies in the necrotic pulp.
From CVEK ET AL.(207) 1990.

A

B

C

D

plaque could penetrate into the necrotic pulp tissue (Fig. 14.27).

Systemic treatment with doxycycline had no effect on the frequency of pulp revascularization or presence of bacteria in the pulpal lumen (207,209). On the other hand, the frequency of revascularization was significantly increased and the presence of bacteria decreased when the teeth were treated topically with doxycycline for 5 minutes before replantation (201). This effect seemed to be due to elimination of bacteria from the root surface, while the contamination via dentinal tubules from mechanical damage to the root surface cervically was not affected. How-

Fig. 14.28.
Effect of the impact of marginal bone on the root surface of an intruded incisor. The arrow points to the area of impact. Three weeks later there is resorption of the root surface and periapical radiolucency. After calcium hydroxide treatment and filling of the root canal with gutta-percha, root resorption is arrested and periapical healing is evident 5 years after injury.

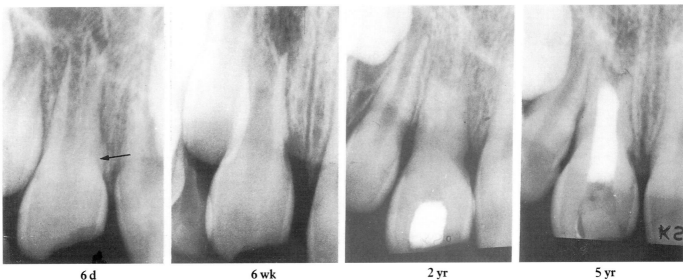

6 d **6 wk** **2 yr** **5 yr**

CHAPTER 14

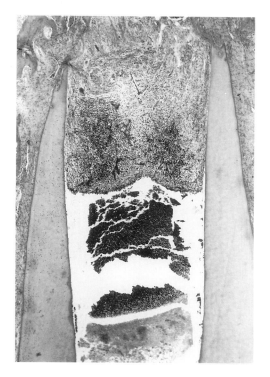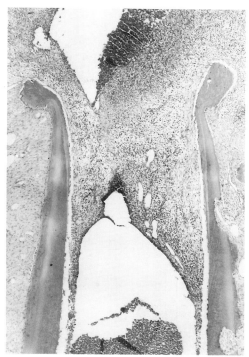

Fig. 14.29.
Presence of vital tissue in the apical portion of the pulpal lumen in replanted immature incisors, despite presence of intra-radicular and periapical abscesses, x 20.

ever, before a general recommendation for similar use of antibiotics in patients, the toxic effects of various antibiotics and antibiotics in varying concentrations on the periodontal cells should be tested.

Regarding luxated teeth, the pathways for bacterial invasion to the damaged pulp tissue are still obscure. One pathway that appears reliable is the invasion of bacteria from mechanical damage on the cervical root surface that can be inflicted by the fulcrum effect of marginal bone at the time of luxation (Fig. 14.28). It is also conceivable that bacteria may originate from a contaminated blood clot along the root surface. Anachoretic contamination of the pulp by blood-borne bacteria appears less likely in healthy individuals, although it cannot be excluded. Thus it has been shown that the damaged dental tissues can be contaminated when severe septicemia is experimentally introduced by repeated intravenous injections of a bacterial suspension [210].

In most experimentally replanted immature teeth with necrotic and contaminated pulps, formation of new hard tissues can be seen in the apical portion of the pulpal lumen, despite adjacent inflammation and abscess formation either in the root canal or periapically [207] (Fig. 14.29). In some teeth, formation of dentin can even be seen, indicating that a part of the original pulp has survived, probably due

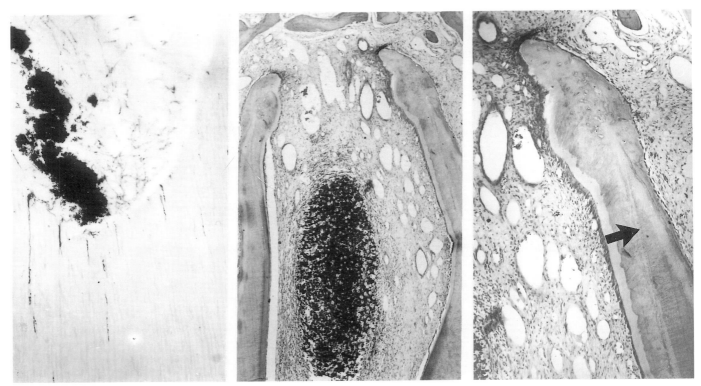

Fig. 14.30.
Immature monkey incisor replanted after 30 min storage in saliva. Inflammation stimulates forma-tion of dentin close to the apical foramen. A. Penetration of microorganisms through dentinal tubules of coronal dentin into the pulpal lumen; bacterial colonies are seen in the necrotized pulp, Brown & Brenn bacterial stain, x 100. B. Abscess formation in apical area, x 15. C. Formation of dentin is seen. The arrow indicates the line between pre- and post-traumatically formed dentin, x 33. From CVEK ET AL.(207) 1990.

to the diffusion of nutrients from periapical tissues (211) (Fig. 14.30).

The presence of vital tissue in the apical part of the pulpal lumen is important from a therapeutic point of view, as this may ensure formation of a hard-tissue barrier and sometimes continued root development after treatment of non-vital immature teeth with calcium hydroxide (77-79).

Diagnosis

Acute clinical symptoms, such as pain or swelling, are seldom present in the early post-traumatic period. However, the tooth may become loose and tender to percussion (206). Clinical diagnosis of pulpal status and decision on endodontic treatment should be based on evaluation of coronal color changes, sensibility testing and radiographic findings including disturbances in root development of immature teeth. Regarding clinical decision-making, there is no difference between the various types of injuries, with the exception of severely intruded or replanted mature teeth. In these teeth no healing of the pulp can be expected and the root canal

treatment should therefore be instituted, irrespective of clinical findings, 1-2 weeks after injury in order to prevent inflammatory root resorption.

Discoloration of the crown subsequent to trauma has been described as pink, yellow, brown and grey or a combination of these (69). A color change to pink or reddish seen within 2-3 days after injury indicates intrapulpal bleeding, which may resolve and the crown may regain its natural color 2-3 weeks later (80,81,212,213). Persistent discoloration, especially with a shift to grey, indicates necrosis and probably bacterial contamination of the pulp (82,214) (see also Chapter 9, p. 355).

Sensibility of the pulp can be checked in different ways but the usual method is electrical stimulation (see Chapter 5, p.204). There is, however, no correlation between the sensibility threshold and the histological condition of the pulp (83,84).

Erupting non-injured teeth, for example, may not respond to electrical stimulation and the injured teeth which do not respond to testing immediately after injury may regain their sensitivity, sometimes months or years after injury (85-87,212-215). Furthermore, a negative response is sometimes

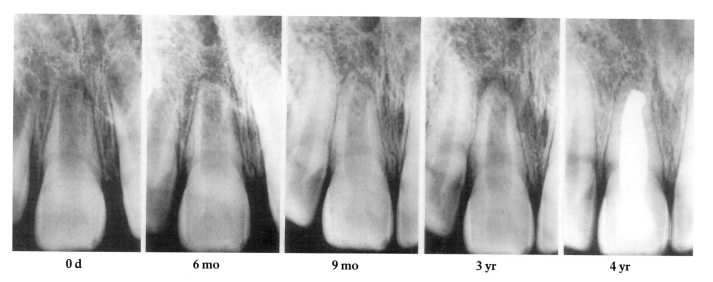

| 0 d | 6 mo | 9 mo | 3 yr | 4 yr |

Fig. 14.31.
Arrested root development after a luxation injury. There is formation of hard tissue apically but none in the rest of pulpal lumen, indicating necrosis of the underlying pulp. A periapical radiolucency is seen 3 years after injury. Periapical healing is evident 4 years after endodontic treatment.

found in teeth in which the pulpal lumen has been reduced by hard tissue formation (88,89,214). Sensibility testing should therefore be regarded only as a diagnostic aid; a negative response alone should not be considered the sole indication for endodontic treatment, whereas a positive response is a relatively safe sign of pulpal innervation. However, the test should be adequately performed as a positive response may be elicited by contact of the electrode with gingiva or a moist crown surface (216). (see Chapter 5, p. 204).

Recently, a new test of pulp vascularity by the use of laser Doppler flowmetry has

been reported (217,218). However, the prototype must be refined for clinical use (see Chapter 5, p. 206).

Radiographic findings, such as a widened and diffusely outlined periodontal space, radiolucency and/or external inflammatory root resorption can normally be seen within 2-8 weeks after injury. However, periapical radiolucency may appear later (212,213) (Figs. 14.31 to 14.33).

Inflammatory changes of periradicular tissues are clearly related to the presence of bacteria in the pulpal lumen (61,75,201,219). However, it has been reported recently that in about 10% of extruded or laterally lux-

Fig. 14.32.
A minor disturbance in root development of a luxated incisor. There is formation of irregular hard tissue in the apical area, followed by further root development. Note the absence of hard tissue formation in the rest of pulpal lumen, indicating pulp necrosis. A periapical radiolucency was noted 1 year after injury. Periradicular healing is evident 5 years after root canal treatment with calcium hydroxide and subsequent filling with gutta-percha.

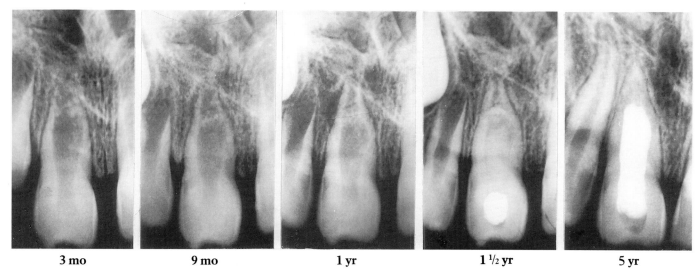

| 3 mo | 9 mo | 1 yr | 1 ½ yr | 5 yr |

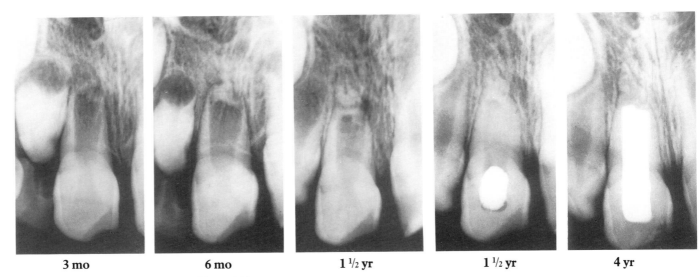

| 3 mo | 6 mo | 1 ½ yr | 1 ½ yr | 4 yr |

Fig. 14.33.

Disturbance in root development and formation of a root tip. There is formation of hard tissue apically but none in the rest of pulpal lumen, indicating necrosis of the remaining pulp. Formation of a separate root tip as well as a periradicular radiolucency was noted 1 ½ years after injury. Healing is evident at a control 4 years after root canal treatment with calcium hydroxide and subsequent filling with gutta-percha.

ated mature permanent teeth a periapical radiolucency may spontaneously heal and be followed by pulp canal obliteration (212,214). This finding points out the intricacy of healing processes after traumatic injuries which still are not understood in full detail and stresses the need for further research. Clinical implications, however, seem to be minor. Considering the low frequency of this phenomenon and maturity of the involved teeth, the risk of a false diagnosis or a negative consequence of the root canal treatment in these teeth appears minimal. On the other hand, expectation that healing will occur may neglect a risk of inflammatory root resorption. However, guidelines for a more conservative approach are presented in Chapter 9, p. 359.

Disturbed or arrested root development is frequently seen after luxation injuries to immature teeth and is usually followed by obliteration of the pulpal lumen, indicating the presence of vital pulp tissue (Figs. 14.34 and 14.35). However, formation of hard tissue apically, with or without continued root development, may also occur when the coronal pulp is necrotic. Sooner or later it becomes bacterially contaminated with acute or chronic periapical inflammation as a result. Thus absence of any hard tissue formation in the rest of the pulp cavity in these teeth, indicating no cell activity, is a strong indication of a coronal pulp necrosis (Figs. 14.31 to 14.33). In these teeth, endodontic intervention should therefore be considered before the appearance of radiographic periapical changes.

In general, the decision to perform endodontic treatment should be based on an evaluation of clinical and radiographic findings as well as history and information gained from a comparison between radiographs at the time of injury and subsequent controls.

In replanted mature teeth it is advisable to postpone endodontic treatment until 1-2 weeks after replantation to avoid further damage to the periodontal ligament by the endodontic procedures. During early stages of periodontal healing it is easy to expel drugs and filling materials into the periodontal space and, for example, if calcium hydroxide is used it may cause necrosis of living cells on the root surface with ankylosis as a result (220).

Immature teeth, in which revascularization can be expected to occur, should not be endodontically treated until signs of periapical lesions or external inflammatory root resorption are observed. This implies close radiographic follow-up, as root resorption in immature teeth may progress very rapidly. Controls at 3, 6 and 12 weeks after injury will normally disclose these changes.

CHAPTER 14

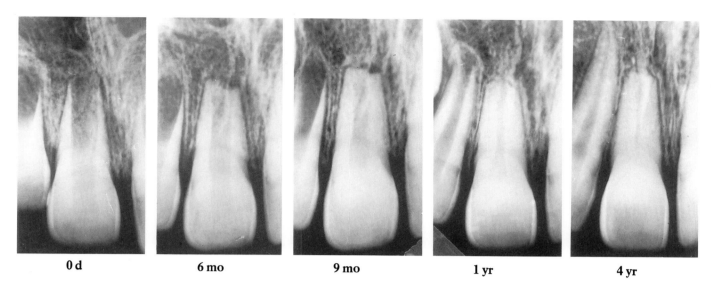

| 0 d | 6 mo | 9 mo | 1 yr | 4 yr |

Fig. 14.34.
Arrested root development after a luxation injury. The pulpal lumen is successively diminished by formation of hard tissue, indicating presence of vital tissue.

TREATMENT OF IMMATURE TEETH

Wide or funnel-shaped root canals make endodontic treatment in immature teeth difficult. The difficulties lie in removing all necrotic tissue from the dentinal walls and achieving adequate obturation of the root canal. A number of treatment solutions have been described, but it was not until calcium hydroxide was introduced that favorable results could be obtained. Since then, numerous clinical and histologic investigations have been carried out and calcium hydroxide is today the most commonly used root canal dressing for the treatment of immature non-vital teeth [90-93,221].

THE EFFECT OF CALCIUM HYDROXIDE

The purpose of calcium hydroxide treatment is to achieve healing of periradicular tissues, including arrest of inflammatory root resorption, and formation of a hard tissue barrier apically, against which an adequate root filling can be placed (Fig. 14.36). In clinical and experimental studies, this has been shown to occur with a high predictability [94-103,222-228] (Table 14.2).

These favorable results depend on several of the properties of calcium hydroxide, related to its high pH (12.5) [229]. One property is a strong antibacterial effect [104-106,230-236]. Thus, 99.9 % of bacteria from the common root canal flora are killed within a few minutes upon direct contact with calcium hydroxide [230], *Enterococcus faecalis* apparently being the only resistant strain. In contact with calcium hydroxide, bacteria are killed at pH 12.5 but not at pH 11.5. Resistance of *E. faecalis* to short exposure to calcium hydroxide has been confirmed in *in vitro* experiments with contaminated dentin, but findings as to its resistance to a longer exposure have not been unanimous. In one study, the bacte-

Table 14.2. Frequency of periapical healing in non-vital teeth after root canal treatment with calcium hydroxide

Examiner	No of teeth	Healing
Immature teeth:		
Kerekes et al. [95] 1980	66	62 (94%)
Mackie et al.[223] 1988	112	108 (96%)
Cvek [227] 1992	328	314 (96%)
Mature teeth:		
Vernieks et al.[107] 1978	78	62 (79%)
Kerekes et al.[95] 1980	27	26 (96%)
Cvek [227] 1992	441	414 (94%)

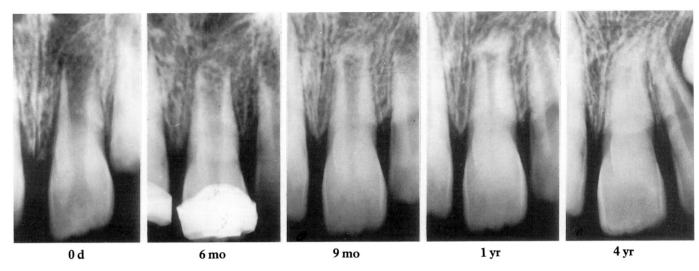

| 0 d | 6 mo | 9 mo | 1 yr | 4 yr |

Fig. 14.35.
Disturbance in root development of an immature incisor after a luxation injury. Note successive diminution of the pulpal lumen by formation of hard tissue.

ria survived a 10-day exposure while in another they were killed after 24 hours (235,236). In clinical studies, however, *E. faecalis* do not seem to cause endodontic problems. Thus, from infected root canals very few bacteria could be cultivated after 1-4 weeks' dressing with calcium hydroxide and, among these, the presence of *E. faecalis* was rare (106,230,233).

Another property of calcium hydroxide is its capacity to dissolve necrotic pulp remnants, rendering root canal walls clean (237,238). Hence, no difference in the debridement effect was found when the root canal dressing with calcium hydroxide was compared with ultrasonic instrumentation (239). This is important for the treatment of immature teeth, in which

Fig. 14.36.
Treatment of a non-vital immature tooth with calcium hydroxide. Periapical healing and apical closure with hard tissue was present after 18 months and the tooth was permanently filled with guttapercha. A master point with a heat-softened tip was placed against the hard tissue barrier and, thereafter, the root canal was obturated with additional points, using lateral condensation.

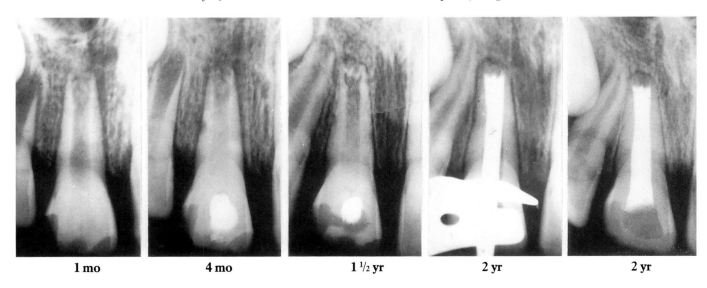

| 1 mo | 4 mo | 1 ½ yr | 2 yr | 2 yr |

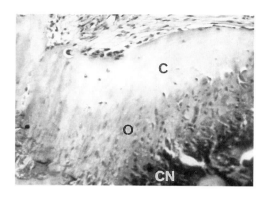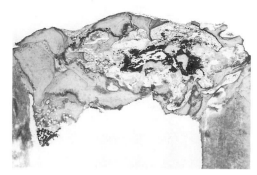

Fig. 14.37.

Layers of the apical hard tissue barrier. A. Necrotic and calcified tissue (CN), followed by irregular, less organized tissue (O) and, apically, of cementum-like tissue (C), x 65. B. Irregular arrangement of hard tissue layers in the apical barrier; gutta-percha (stained black) was pressed into the barrier, x 20.

the thin dentinal walls do not permit intensive reaming.

Findings regarding the ability of calcium hydroxide to induce ectopic bone have not been convincing (240-242). However, elimination of bacteria from the root canal makes healing of the surrounding vital tissue and the formation of an apical hard tissue barrier possible. When in contact with vital tissue in the apical area, calcium hydroxide seems to cause tissue reactions similar to those in the coronal pulp. Thus, layers of the hard tissue in an apical barrier are similar to those formed after pulpotomy or pulp capping, the only difference being that a cementum-like tissue is formed instead of dentin, indicating involvement of periodontal tissues in the barrier formation (96-103,228).

The apical barrier typically consists of a layer of coagulated and later calcified tissue, adjacent to which are layers of first less then more organized cementum-like tissue (Fig. 14.37, A). These layers can be arranged very irregularly and often include islands of soft connective tissue, probably a result of placing calcium hydroxide against lacerated tissue (Fig. 14.37, B).

An apical barrier can be formed around the apex of the tooth, over the apical foramen or in the root canal. The location of the barrier seems to depend on the level at

Fig. 14.38.
Different levels of formation of the hard tissue barrier after treatment with calcium hydroxide. Radiographs were taken before treatment and after completed apical closure. The teeth were extracted because of cervical root fractures. A. Formation of hard tissue in the periapical area as a result of overfilling with calcium hydroxide, x 10. B and C. Barriers formed across the apical foramen, x 20. D. Formation of hard tissue barrier within the root canal, x 20. In all cases, newly formed hard tissue was found to be cementum-like.

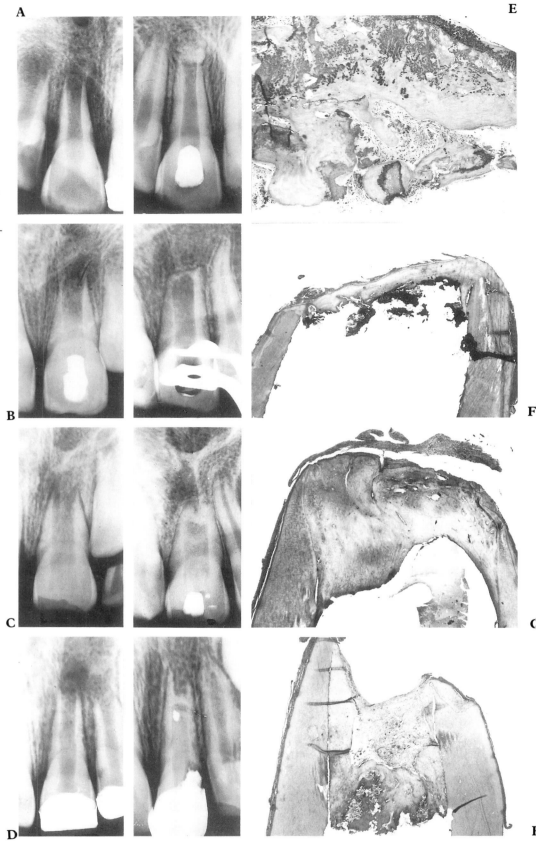

which calcium hydroxide has been brought into contact with vital tissue (Fig. 14.38).

The ability of periodontal tissues to respond with hard-tissue formation in contact with calcium hydroxide does not seem to be related to the maturity of the tooth, the time of treatment after injury, or the location on the root surface. Thus, after repeated dressings, formation of the hard tissue can be seen apically in mature teeth (107) (Fig. 14.39), in root perforations (91,108,109,243-245) (Fig.14.40), at the fracture site in the coronal fragment of

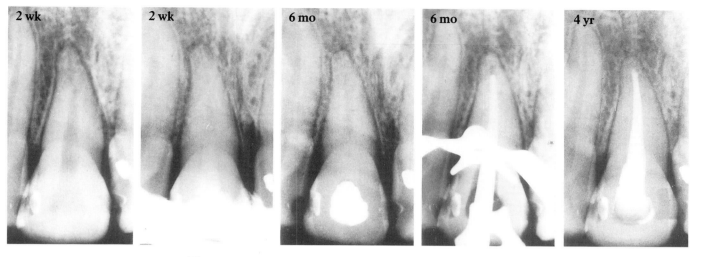

Fig. 14.39.

Treatment of a mature permanent incisor with calcium hydroxide. Periapical healing and apical closure with hard tissue was found after 9 months and the root canal was filled with gutta-percha. Periapical healing is seen at a 4-year control.

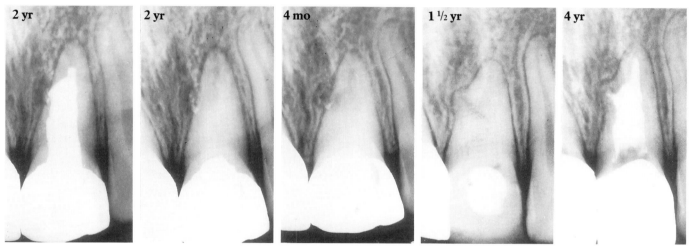

Fig. 14.40.

Treatment of accidental root perforation with calcium hydroxide. A radiolucency adjacent to perforation was found 2 years after gutta-percha filling. The tooth was initially treated by a cervical pulpotomy because of a pulp exposure and a root perforation occurred at the time of removing the hard tissue barrier in connection with pulpectomy. The root canal was treated with calcium hydroxide; the initial formation of hard tissue was seen after 4 months and the perforation was completely sealed with hard tissue 1 ½ years later. The control 4 years after subsequent filling with gutta-percha shows periodontal healing.

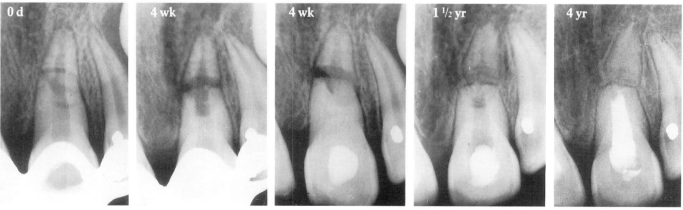

Fig. 14.41.

Root fracture and treatment of the non-vital coronal fragment with calcium hydroxide. Four weeks after injury there is widening of the space between fragments and adjacent radiolucency. The coronal fragment was treated with calcium hydroxide and 1 ½ years later, periradicular healing and apical closure with hard tissue of the coronal fragment was observed. Four years after filling with gutta-percha, periradicular healing is evident. From CVEK (66) 1974.

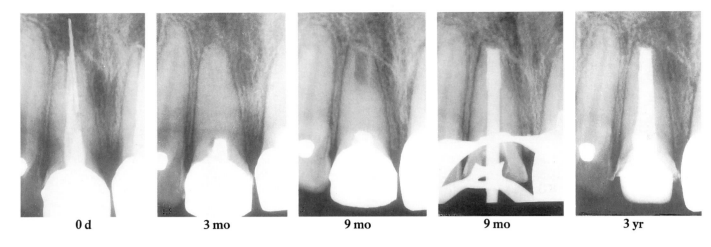

| 0 d | 3 mo | 9 mo | 9 mo | 3 yr |

Fig. 14.42.

Late endodontic treatment of an incisor with arrested root development. Control 4 years after previous treatment shows incomplete root canal obturation and a broken file left in the canal with associated periapical radiolucency. After removal of the root filling and the file, the root canal was filled with calcium hydroxide. Nine months later, periapical healing and formation of apical hard tissue barrier was found, against which adequate obturation with gutta-percha was performed. Periapical healing is evident 3 years later.

Fig. 14.43.

Continued root development after treatment of an incisor with partial pulp necrosis. Note the level of calcium hydroxide in the root canal, indicating the presence of some vital tissue in the apical portion. Formation of a hard-tissue barrier and continued root development can be seen at controls 6 and 12 months after initial treatment. A and B. Histologic section of a similarly treated tooth which was extracted due to a cervical root fracture. Close to the calcium hydroxide is a darkly stained area of necrotic and later calcified tissue (CN), followed by a layer of bone-like tissue (O), and above it dentin and predentin with lining odontoblasts (D), x 20 and 40.

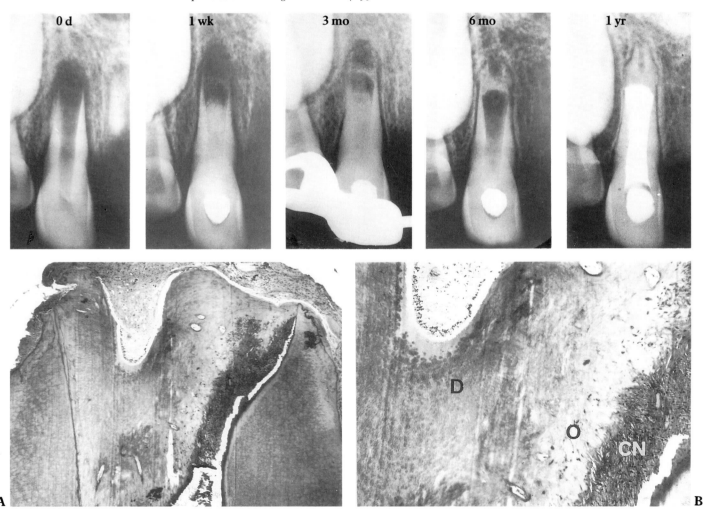

| 0 d | 1 wk | 3 mo | 6 mo | 1 yr |

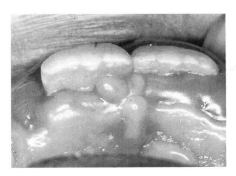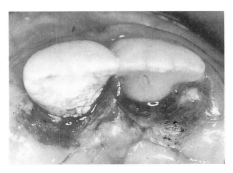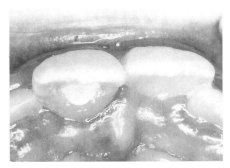

Fig. 14.44.
Surgical pretreatment of a partially erupted incisor in order to allow endodontic treatment. A. Condition before treatment. B. A palatal gingivectomy and root canal treatment were performed at the same visit. C. Condition 6 weeks later.

root fractured teeth (66,198) (Fig. 14.41), after unsuccessful apicoectomy or periapical curretage (109,246) and in teeth in which the root development ceased years prior to treatment (Fig. 14.42).

In immature teeth, continued root development or formation of a separate part of the root may occasionally occur, probably due to the survival of a part of pulp tissue and/or the Hertwig's epithelial root sheath (77-79) (Figs. 14.33 and 14.43).

TECHNICAL PROCEDURES

Permanent teeth can be injured before they have erupted completely, with subsequent development of pulp necrosis. In such cases, a palatal gingivectomy may be necessary to allow adaptation of a rubber dam and provide accesss into the root canal (Fig. 14.44).

In partially erupted or splinted teeth, adaptation of a rubber dam can be diffi-

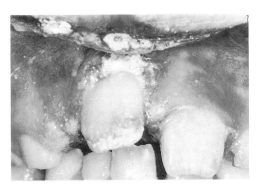

Fig. 14.45.
Damage of the soft tissues due to the leakage of 30% hydrogen peroxide, used for disinfection of a poorly adapted rubber dam on an infrapositioned incisor.

cult. As leakage may occur, solutions that can damage oral tissues should not be used for disinfection (Fig. 14.45). A satisfactory effect can be achieved if the crown is cleaned with water-mixed pumice using a rubber cup and, after a rubber dam is adapted, the crown is washed with a mild disinfectant, e.g. a solution of chlorhexidine in 96 % ethyl alcohol (110).

When access to the root canal has been gained and necrotic pulp tissue removed, an effective chemo-mechanical cleansing of the root canal is necessary because necrotic tissue remants always remain along the dentinal walls. In immature teeth, this is a difficult procedure because of wide root canals and inadequacy of files or reamers (111,112). Canal cleansing should be performed by careful, methodical filing of the dentinal walls, using lateral pressure and vertical movements. Only moderate pressure should be used, in order to avoid weakening of the root canal walls in the cervical area, as well as to avoid fracture of the fragile dentinal walls in the apical region, which may impair periapical healing (113). It is important to consider that the vital tissue present in the apical part of the pulpal lumen should not be removed, as this tissue may improve the quality and speed of apical bridging or provide further root development, depending on the type and differentiation of the cells involved. During cleansing, the canal should be repeatedly flushed with 0.5 % sodium hypochlorite (114,115,247,248).

After cleansing, the root canal is filled with calcium hydroxide with a spiral. In immature teeth with wide root canals, a syringe with a special cannula may be used

Fig. 14.46. Filling of the root canal with calcium hydroxide
A palatal opening is made wide enough to allow adequate mechanical cleansing of the root canal.

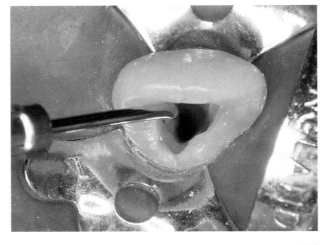 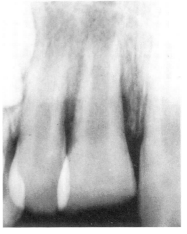

Filling the root canal
After completed cleansing, the cannula is introduced in the root canal close to the apical area and then slowly withdrawn while pressing calcium hydroxide out of the syringe.

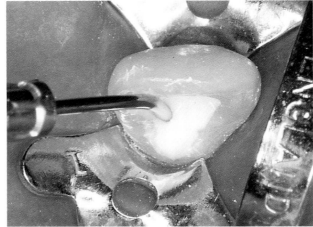 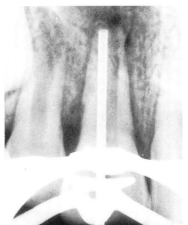

Compressing calcium hydroxide
The paste is then pressed lightly towards the apex with a dry cotton pellet to ensure apical contact with vital tissue. Filling and condensing of calcium hydroxide is repeated until the root canal assumes same radiodensity as surrounding dentin.

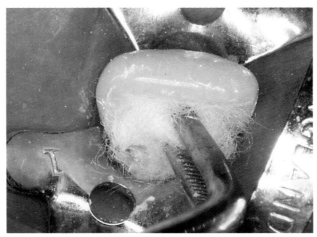 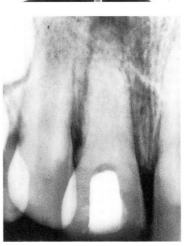

Sealing the access cavity
After the excess of the paste is removed, the coronal cavity is sealed of with a zinc oxide-eugenol cement (e.g IRM®).
One year after root canal treatment periapical healing and formation of the apical hard tissue barrier is seen.

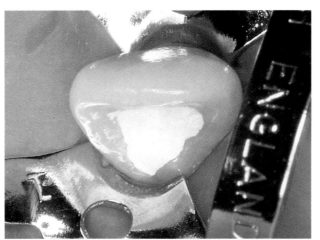 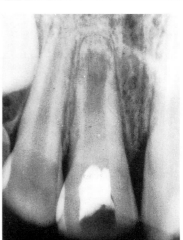

Fig. 14.47. Effect of over in-strumentation.

Over ambitious cleansing in an immature incisor resulting in exacerbation of periapical inflammation 3 days after treatment.

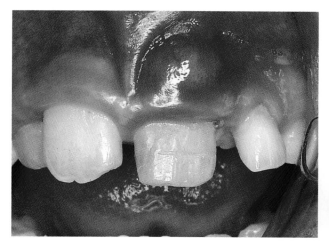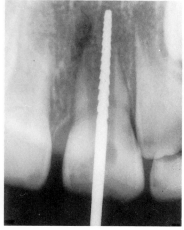

Fig. 14.47. Effect of over in-strumentation.

Over ambitious cleansing in an immature incisor resulting in exacerbation of periapical inflammation 3 days after treatment.

(Fig. 14.46). After filling, the calcium hydroxide dressing is compressed slightly towards the apex with a cotton pellet in order to ensure contact with the vital tissue apically, whereafter the access cavity is sealed with a zinc oxide-eugenol cement.

The root canal can be filled with calcium hydroxide immediately after chemomechanical cleansing (106,230-232). Calcium hydroxide that is eventually pressed through the apical foramen during filling is readily resorbed by periapical tissues (116). However, necrotic and infected pulp tissue remnants pressed into the periapical space may cause an acute exacerbation of a chronic periapical inflammation (117) (Fig. 14.47).

The addition to calcium hydroxide of toxic antibacterial drugs such as camphorated parachlorophenol does not seem to be justified (112,115,118,230). Nor does the mixing of calcium hydroxide with corticosteroids or antibiotics (249).

After being filled with calcium hydroxide, the teeth should be controlled at 3- to 6-month intervals. If periapical healing does not occur, the root canal should be retreated. In the root canal, calcium hydroxide is dissolved and eventually forms compounds with different ions available from the vital tissue present at the apical foramen, resulting in the fall of the calcium hydroxide level in the root canal. In immature teeth, this appears to be an ongoing process that continues until the apical foramen is closed with a hard-tissue barrier.

When left empty, the root canal can be reinfected and a new periapical radiolucency can occur, most probably due to leakage from an inadequate coronal seal

Fig. 14.48.

Recurrence of periapical inflammation. Periapical radiolucency and inflammatory root resorption were evident 6 weeks after injury. The root canal was treated with calcium hydroxide and a complete apical closure was observed 12 months later. Note the absence of calcium hydroxide above sealing material, pressed into the root canal at a previous treatment. Thereafter, the patient was not available for control and when seen again after 2 years, a new periapical radiolucency has developed.

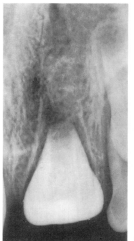 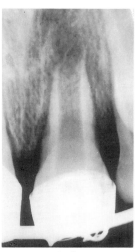 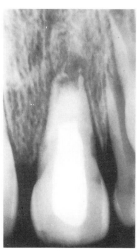 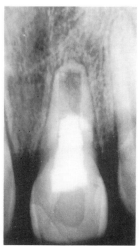 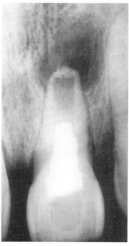

| 0 d | 6 wk | 3 mo | 1 yr | 2 yr |

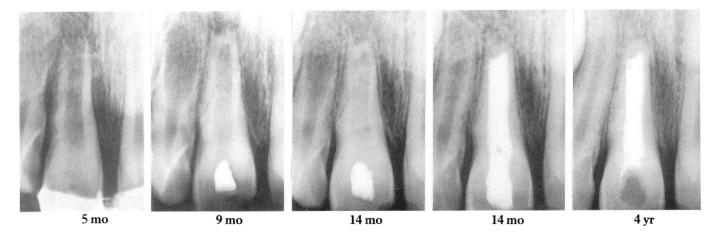

| 5 mo | 9 mo | 14 mo | 14 mo | 4 yr |

Fig. 14.49.

Retreatment of periapical inflammation. Five weeks after injury there is a widened and diffusely out-lined periodontal space periapically and inflammatory root resorption. Nine months after treatment with calcium hydroxide, there is arrest of inflammatory resorption, hard tissue formation apically and periapically a radiolucency. Note the inadequate coronal seal. Periapical healing was found 5 months after retreatment with calcium hydroxide. Condition 4 years after obturation of the root canal with gutta-percha. From CVEK (227) 1992.

Fig. 14.50.

Disruption of the apical hard tissue barrier due to forceful obturation of the root canal. During filling of the canal with gutta-percha, an attempt was made to fill a void in the root canal (arrow). The pressure applied resulted in the rupture of the apical hard tissue barrier and overfilling.

(Fig. 14.48). These teeth can sometimes be successfully retreated with calcium hydroxide (Fig. 14.49). However, if bacteria have settled in the newly-formed hard tissue apically, this may be difficult and apical surgery may be neccessary. Thus, when the level of calcium hydroxide falls in the cervical part of the root canal, it should be refilled in order to promote further formation of the hard-tissue barrier.

Permanent obturation with gutta-percha, and a sealer is performed when radiographic and clinical examination demonstrate periapical healing and the root canal is closed apically with a hard-tissue barrier. Depending on the width of apical foramen and size of the periapical lesion, this may take 12 to 18 months after initial treatment (65,94,107,222-225). The apical barriers have proven in clinical and histological investigations to be quite resistant to pressure exerted during condensation of gutta-percha (94,96,227). However, a thin barrier can be damaged or broken and gutta-percha expelled into the periapical space if too much pressure is used (Fig. 14.50). A gentle obturation technique is therefore recommended (119). Experience has shown that the following procedure gives satisfactory results. The tip of a gutta-percha master point, i.e. the largest point that can easily reach the apical barrier, is warmed by passing it once through an alcohol flame. The point is then immediately introduced into the root canal and gently but steadily pressed against the apical barrier. To achieve the desired results, i.e. the apical

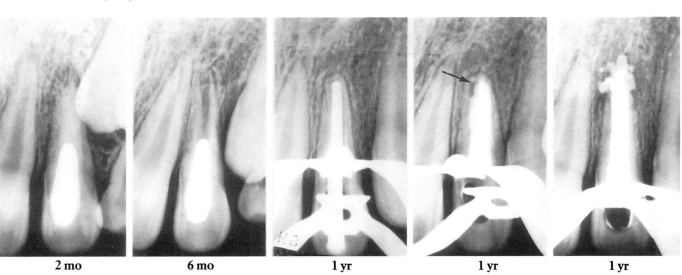

| 2 mo | 6 mo | 1 yr | 1 yr | 1 yr |

Fig. 14.51. Clinical procedures for filling the canal with partially heated gutta-percha.
A. Selection of a suitable master point. B. The tip of the point is softened by passing it once through an alcohol flame and is then introduced into the root canal and pressed against the apical barrier. C. Subsequent filling using lateral condensation. D. Completed filling. E. The tip of the point is softened by passing it once through alcohol flame. Only the tip of the point should be softened and the rest should remain stiff if the desired effect is to be achieved. F. The effect of pressing a partially softened point against a firm surface. G to J. Obturation of the root canal in a non-vital immature incisor after treatment with calcium hydroxide. The softened tip of a master point was pressed against the hard tissue barrier and the root canal completely obturated by additional points, dipped in resin-chloroform, and using lateral condensation.

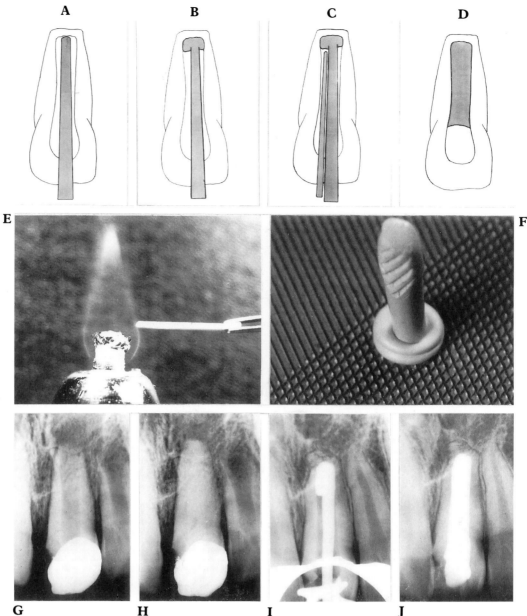

part of the root canal filled and the gutta-percha point well-adapted to the barrier, only the tip of the gutta-percha point should be softened and the rest of it should remain stiff (Fig. 14.51). Once the gutta-percha has cooled in the root canal and a control radiograph is taken, the root canal can be obturated by lateral condensation of additional points which have been dipped into resin-chloroform, or by using an endodontic sealer. The other promising possibilities for wide root canal obturation are the modern methods, using thermoplasticized gutta-percha and vertical condensation.

Prognosis

Successful treatment with calcium hydroxide, i.e. periapical healing and formation of a hard-tissue barrier, has been reported to occur in 79 to 96 % of the treated teeth (93-95,222-228). The results obtained in

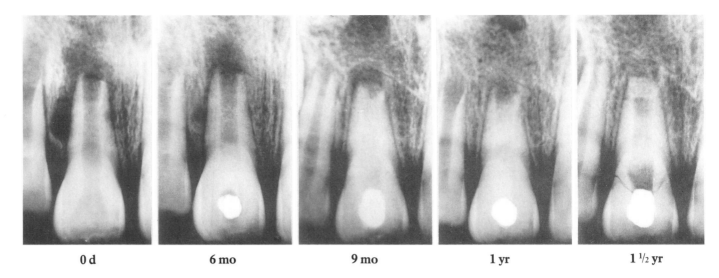

| 0 d | 6 mo | 9 mo | 1 yr | 1 ½ yr |

Fig. 14.52.
Cervical root fracture after successful endodontic treatment of an incisor with immature root development. A minor trauma caused the cervical root fracture 18 months after initial treatment.

more comprehensive studies are shown in Table 14.2, p. 543.

In a long-term study of calcium hydroxide treated incisors, periapical healing was observed in 92 % of 589 teeth, 4 years after permanent filling of the root canal with gutta-percha (228). No difference was found between immature and mature teeth, indicating that the prognosis of root filling in immature teeth was not impaired by their wide root canals and often irregular hard tissue barriers containing inclusions of soft tissue. On the other hand, long-term tooth survival of immature teeth was seriously threatened by the occurrence of cervical root fractures (Fig. 14.52). As a rule, these fractures were caused by only weak forces and were clearly related to the stage of root development at the start of treatment, indicating that the thin dentinal walls left behind after the pulpal death in young immature teeth were the reason for their occurrence (Figs. 14.52 and 14.53).

A significant relationship to accidental fractures was also found in the teeth in which dentinal walls in the cervical area were weakened by root defects after arrest of inflammatory root resorption (see p. 559).

Finally, it should be mentioned that reappearance of periapical changes in teeth filled with gutta-percha can often be resolved by the retreatment with calcium hydroxide (Fig. 14.54).

Treatment of Mature Teeth

Treatment of non-vital traumatized mature teeth is the same as for the teeth with pulp necrosis of other etiology. Commonly accepted endodontic procedures, drugs and filling materials can be used (250,251). However, high frequencies of healing have been reported if the root canals have been dressed with calcium hydroxide prior to filling with gutta-percha (95,107,227,230). Dressing with calcium hydroxide for 1-6 months before obturation with gutta-percha can therefore be recommended for routine use in infected root canals.

Prognosis

Periapical healing after treatment and obturation of the root canal with various filling materials has been reported in

Fig. 14.53. Frequency of
cervical root fractures
*Fractures in 759 luxated, non-
vital maxillary incisors, following initial calcium hydroxide
treatment and a 4 years observation period after filling with
gutta-percha, distributed according to the stage of root development. From* CVEK (227) *1992.*

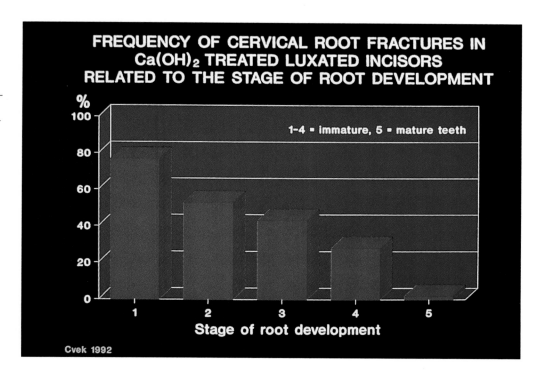

FREQUENCY OF CERVICAL ROOT FRACTURES IN
Ca(OH)$_2$ TREATED LUXATED INCISORS
RELATED TO THE STAGE OF ROOT DEVELOPMENT

1-4 = immature, 5 = mature teeth

Stage of root development

Cvek 1992

various clinical studies to range from 76 to
91 % (55-58,251). Periapical healing, after
initial dressing with calcium hydroxide
and subsequent filling with gutta-percha,
was found in 92 to 96% of treated teeth
(95,107,227).

Primary Teeth

Traumatized primary teeth can become
discolored and their pulps necrotic. Periapical osteitis occurs in about 80 % of
discolored primary teeth during the first
months after injury and in about 50 % of
the remaining teeth within 2 years (82).

Opinions differ as to whether non-vital
primary incisors should be treated
endodontically. Traumatized incisors
have been said to be well-suited for root
canal treatment and filling with a resorbable pastes, such as formocresol, iodoform
or calcium hydroxide (120-122). However,
when the advantages, mostly esthetic, are
weighed against the potential risk of disturbances in enamel formation of the
permanent successor caused by toxic filling materials or a persistent periapical
lesion, endodontic treatment of these
teeth does not appear justified (123-125) (see
also Chapter 9, p. 361)

Fig. 14.54.
Treatment of secondary periapical inflammation with calcium hydroxide.
*A periapical radiolucency has developed 18 months after filling with gutta-percha. Six months after
retreatment with calcium hydroxide, there is formation of a new hard tissue barrier at the apical foramen and a diminished radiolucency. Periapical healing is seen at the 4-year control of retreatment
with gutta-percha.*

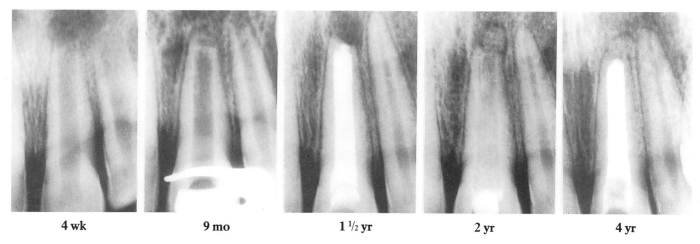

| 4 wk | 9 mo | 1 ½ yr | 2 yr | 4 yr |

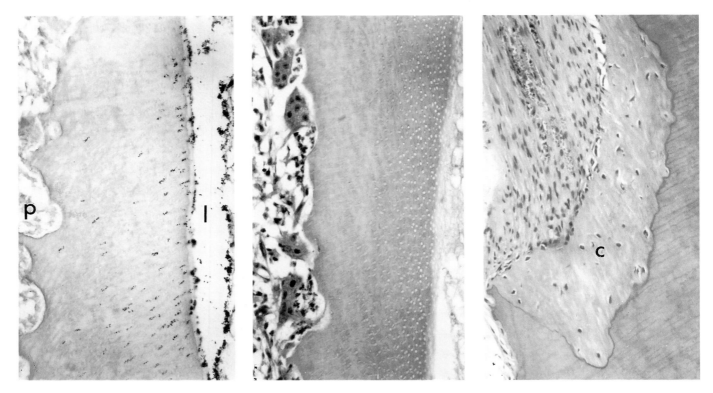

Fig. 14.55.
Histologic appearance of inflammatory root resorption. A. Penetration of bacteria through dentinal tubules, from the contaminated pulpal lumen towards the periodontium, Brown and Brenn bacterial stain, x 100. B. Bacteria and their toxins cause accumulation of leukocytes. As these cannot reach bacteria in the tubules, osteoclasts are stimulated to resorb dentin, x 100. C. If bacteria are removed from the root canal, resorption lesions can be repaired by cementum-like tissue, x 80.

External Inflammatory Root Resorption

Pathology

External root resorption after luxation injuries has been described as surface, inflammatory or replacement resorption, of which only inflammatory resorption is related to a necrotic and infected pulp (61,126,201,207). Thus, when dentinal tubules are exposed by the resorption of damaged tissues on the root surface, bacteria and toxins from the root canal may cause inflammation in the adjacent periodontal tissues and lead to progressive resorption of the root via dentinal tubules (Fig. 14.55). This resorption seems to be more frequent and rapid in immature teeth, most probably due to the thin dentinal walls and wide tubules (5,86).

Fig. 14.56.
Radiographic appearance of external inflammatory root resorption. There is a progressive loss of root substance associated with increasing radiolucency in the adjacent alveolar bone.

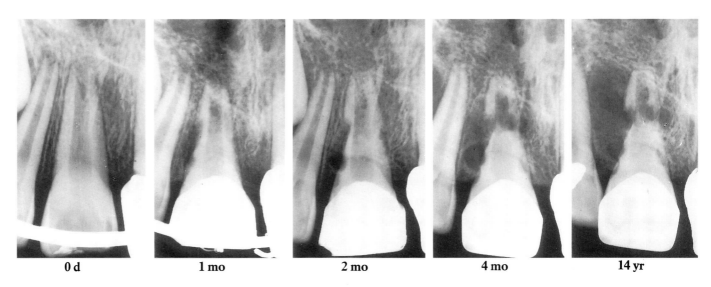

| 0 d | 1 mo | 2 mo | 4 mo | 14 yr |

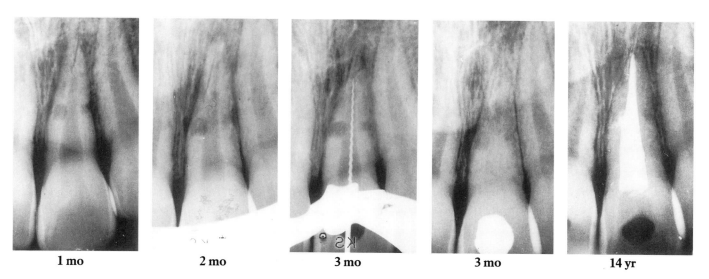

| 1 mo | 2 mo | 3 mo | 3 mo | 14 yr |

Fig. 14.57.

Treatment of inflammatory root resorption which has perforated to the root canal. Three months after injury, the root canal was treated with calcium hydroxide and after 1 year, a gutta-percha filling was inserted. Note that the filling material has been forced into the resorption defect, but not into the periodontal space.

Diagnosis and Treatment

Radiographically, inflammatory resorption is characterized by a progressive loss of tooth substance associated with a persistent or progressive radiolucency in the adjacent alveolar bone (Fig. 14.56). The critical period for onset of these changes seems to be 2 to 12 weeks after injury, but they may occur earlier (see also Chapters 2, p. 100 and Chapter 10, p.398). It is also important that endodontic therapy be instituted as soon as clinical and radiographic signs of pulp necrosis and inflammatory resorption are evident.

Endodontic treatment of teeth with inflammatory root resorption is identical to treatment of other non-vital traumatized teeth. In principle, the choice of antibacterial drugs or filling materials should be of minor importance, as the effect on healing depends upon removal of the necrotic pulp and bacteria from the pulpal lumen (127). However, dressing of the root canal with calcium hydroxide has been shown to give a high frequency of healing (127,227). It should therefore be used before filling with gutta-percha, especially in immature teeth and in teeth in which the resorptive process has perforated the root canal walls, i.e. the teeth in which formation of hard tissue may prevent overfilling (Figs. 14.36 and 14.57).

Fig. 14.58.

Treatment of inflammatory root resorption. Six months after luxation extensive inflammatory resorption cavities are seen and, in some places, only very thin dentinal walls seem to remain. The root canal was filled with calcium hydroxide. After 9 months, there is arrest of resorption and periodontal healing. At the 1 year control of the gutta-percha filling, deposition of hard tissue into the resorption cavities is evident.

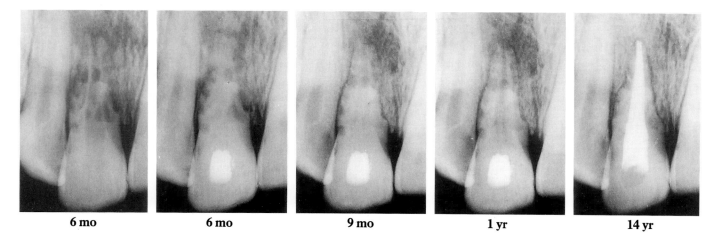

| 6 mo | 6 mo | 9 mo | 1 yr | 14 yr |

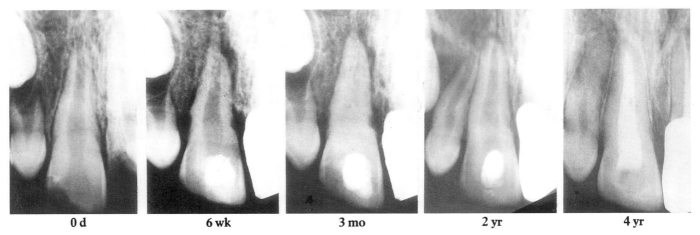

| 0 d | 6 wk | 3 mo | 2 yr | 4 yr |

Fig. 14.59.
Treatment of inflammatory root resorption apparent 6 weeks after replantation. Two years after filling with calcium hydroxide, there is periradicular healing and arrest of root resorption. At a 4-year control, there is repair of all resorption lesions.

The effect of calcium hydroxide upon the arrest and healing of inflammatory root resorption is not clearly understood. Elimination of bacteria from the root canal and dentinal tubules appears to be the main factor. It has also been reported that calcium hydroxide from the root canal may raise the pH at the root surface to such a level that the tissue along the resorption cavity, including the resorbing cells, can be damaged (252). This effect, however, appears to be of short duration and the repair of the experimental lesions in the root surface by deposition of new hard tissue has been observed within a short period (253,254). It is conceivable that hydroxyl ions passing through the dentinal tubules also denaturate its protein contents, whereby further release of hydroxyl ions towards the periodontium is prevented or reduced to harmless concentrations.

Follow-up and Prognosis

Radiographically, healing is characterized by the arrest of the resorption process and a reestablishment of the periodontal space, bordered by a lamina dura. Healing may occur irrespective of the extent of resorption and the amount of root substance lost (Figs. 14.57 to 14.61). Arrest

Fig. 14.60.
Arrest of inflammatory root resorption after calcium hydroxide treatment.
After 18 months there is periapical healing and arrest of root resorption. Three months later, a cervical root fracture has occurred through the resorption defect. From CVEK (227) *1992.*

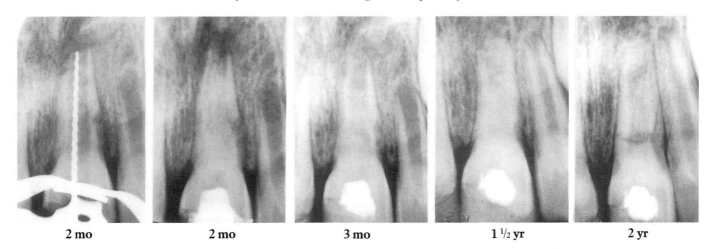

| 2 mo | 2 mo | 3 mo | 1 ½ yr | 2 yr |

**Fig 14.61. Healing of in-
flammatory root resorption
after luxation injuries**
*The frequency of periodontal
healing as well as the occurrence
of ankylosis was analyzed in
187 luxated permanent teeth.
From CVEK (227) 1992*

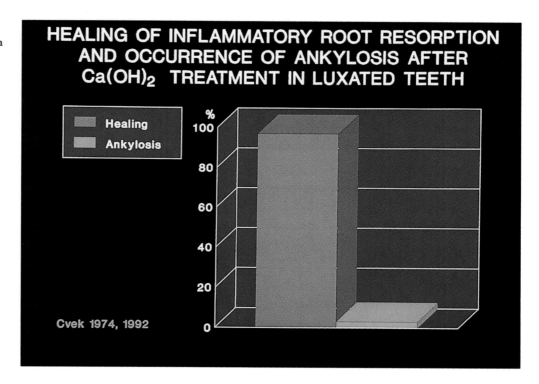

of inflammatory resorption usually leaves
a defect on the root surface which, however, is usually diminished by the successive apposition of new hard tissue (Fig.
14.59). In the cervical area of the root,
such a defect may become a site of least
resistance leading to a cervical root fracture, especially in teeth with immature
stages of root development (227) (Figs.
14.60 and 14.62).

In replanted teeth, ankylosis can often
develop at sites of previously arrested
inflammatory resorption (Fig. 14.63). It
has been suggested that release of calcium

**Fig. 14.62. Relationship be-
tween cervical root frac-
tures and presence of de-
fects after inflammatory
root resorption**
*Fractures in 397 non-vital im-
mature incisors, following calcium hydroxide treatment and
an observation period of 4 years
after filling with gutta-percha.
The material is distributed according to the presence of resorption defects in the cervical area of
the root as well as the stage of
root development. From CVEK
(227) 1992*

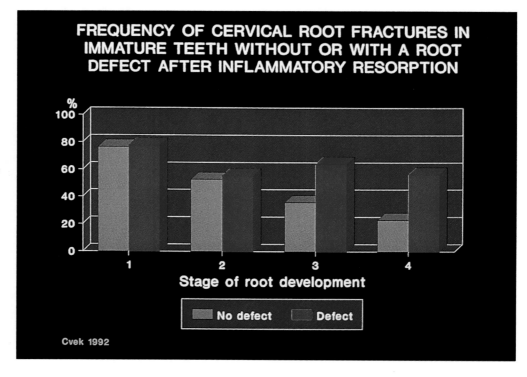

ENDODONTIC MANAGEMENT OF TRAUMATIZED TEETH

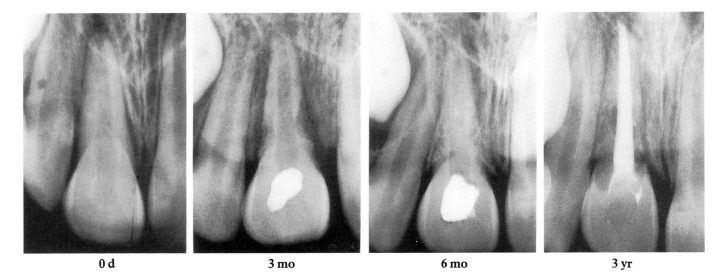

| 0 d | 3 mo | 6 mo | 3 yr |

Fig. 14.63.
Change of inflammatory root resorption into ankylosis. The tooth was replanted after 60 min dry storage. Three months after replantation there is inflammatory root resorption with associated radiolucency in the adjacent alveolar bone and the tooth was treated with calcium hydroxide. Six months after treatment there is periradicular healing with dento-alveolar ankylosis.

hydroxide from the root canal may contribute to its occurrence by damaging periodontal cells (253-256). This assumption, however, is in conflict with clinical studies of luxated teeth in which very high frequencies of healing of inflammatory root resorption were found after treatment with calcium hydroxide (127,227). In these studies, ankylosis was rare and was found only after severe intrusive luxations. This seems to indicate that initial periodontal injury rather than calcium hydroxide should be blamed for the occurrence of ankylosis, subsequent to healing of inflammatory resorption (Fig. 14.61).

PRIMARY TEETH
Primary teeth with inflammatory root resorption should be extracted.

Late External Root Resorptions

Pathology

Progressive external resorption associated with inflammatory changes in surrounding tissues, may occur years after injury and is, as a rule, located near the cemento-enamel junction (257,258). It is primarily found in replanted and ankylosed teeth in infraposition but may also occur in luxated teeth. In its advanced stages, resorption

Fig. 14.64.
Progression of late external root resorption. Three years after replantation there is progressive replacement resorption. At the 6-year control, a marked inflammatory root resorption is found cervically. Clinically, a pink discoloration of the crown and perforating granulation tissue is seen close to the gingival margin.

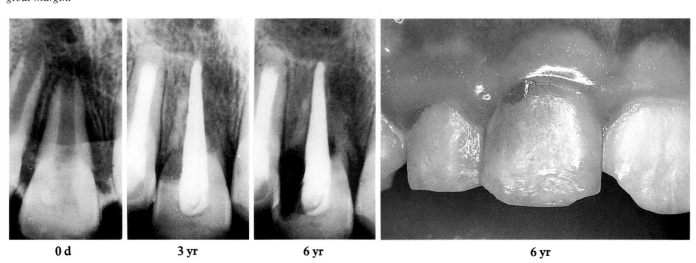

| 0 d | 3 yr | 6 yr | 6 yr |

CHAPTER 14

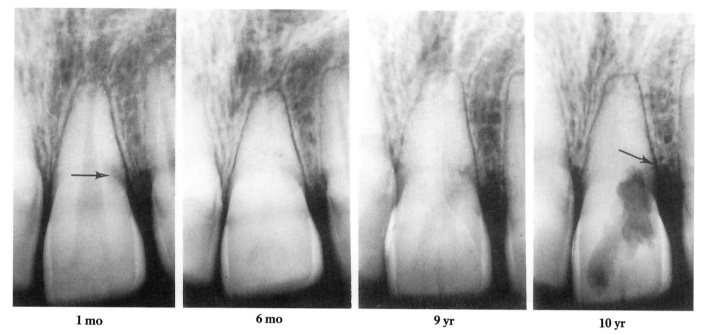

1 mo **6 mo** **9 yr** **10 yr**

Fig. 14.65.
Late progression of external root resorption. A small external root resorption cavity (arrow) is seen 1 month after a luxation injury. At the 6-year control, the pulpal lumen has been diminished by hard tissue and the external resorption apparently arrested. Controls 9 and 10 years after injury show a rapid progression of external root resorption and the reduced level of marginal bone (arrow).

may undermine the crown and become clinically evident as a pink spot below the cervical enamel, in both vital or root-filled teeth (Fig. 14.64). The etiology is obscure. One conceivable factor could be the presence of bacteria in the gingival crevice causing inflammation in the area and penetration into dentinal tubules, exposed by active or poorly repaired resorption (259). This may elicit a progressive root resorption and interfere with ankylosing processes (Figs. 14.64 and 14.65).

Fig. 14.66.
Treatment of a late external root resorption in a vital incisor. A and B. Cervical resorption 6 years after subluxation. C. Appearance of resorption after elevation of a flap. D. Preparation of the resorption cavity disclosed no connection with the pulpal lumen. Dentin was covered with calcium hydroxide and the cavity restored.
E and F. Radiographic and clinical status 10 years after treatment.

A **B** **C**

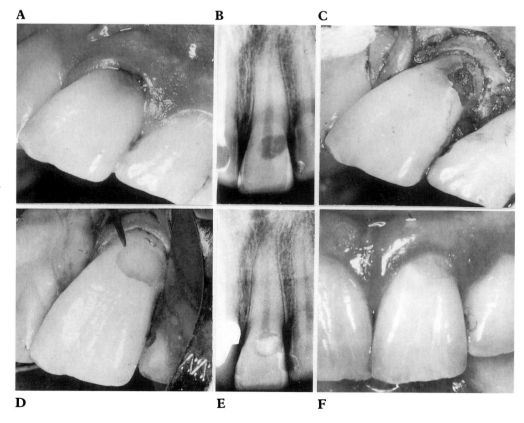

D **E** **F**

ENDODONTIC MANAGEMENT OF TRAUMATIZED TEETH

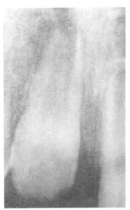 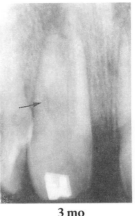 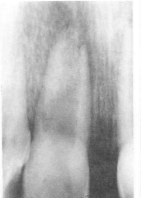 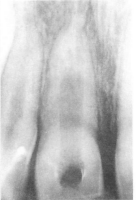 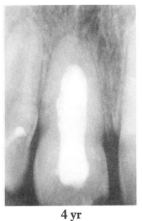

| 0 d | 3 mo | 4 mo | 1 ½ yr | 4 yr |

Fig. 14.67.
Internal inflammatory root canal resorption after an intrusive luxation of a central incisor. Three and 4 months after injury, an inflammatory internal resorption with communication to the periodontium has developed cervically (arrow). After 18 months' treatment with calcium hydroxide, there is apical closure with hard tissue and communication with periodontium was no longer found. A control 2 years after filling of the root canal with guttapercha shows periradicular healing.

Treatment

Cervical root resorption can be treated in several ways. If esthetic considerations are of minor importance and the resorption cavity does not extend below the cervical bone margin, a gingivectomy with subsequent filling of the resorption cavity with a dentin bonded composite or a glass ionomer cement is the method of choice (260). If esthetic considerations are important, a gingival flap can be raised and the same restoration as above performed (128,261). In cases where the cervical resorption defect extends below the alveolar crest, an orthodontic or surgical extrusion can be considered before cavity restoration (262-265). In cases where the cervical resorption is related to ankylosis, the choice is either to accept the condition or to remove the crown and leave the ankylosed root to bony replacement (266). (see Chapter 15, p.623)

Root Canal Resorption

Pathology

Root canal resorption is often seen in root fractures, but seldom in luxated teeth (200,214). The processes have been described as transient surface or tunnelling resorption, or as progressive. *Surface resorption* is seen radiographically as a limited loss of hard tissue, usually at the fracture site or near the apical foramen in luxated teeth. *Tunnelling resorption* is characterized by the loss of root substance behind the predentin border which slowly progresses in a coronal direction, followed by obliteration of both resorption lesions and the pulpal lumen (200). Although the triggering mechanisms have not been assessed, these changes can possibly be looked upon as a part of healing processes

Fig. 14.68.
Treatment of internal inflammatory root canal resorption in a dilacerated incisor with calcium hydroxide. Repeated filling with calcium hydroxide was done at 3-week intervals. Note that the calcium hydroxide has finally obliterated the entire resorption cavity, indicating absence of soft tissue in the lesion. At the control 4 years after filling with gutta-percha there are normal periradicular conditions.

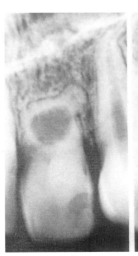 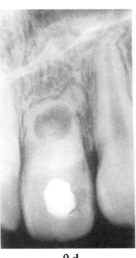 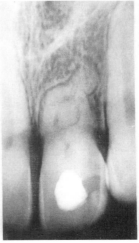 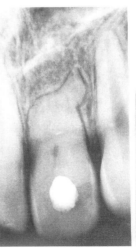 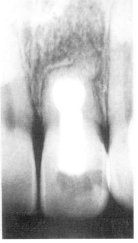

| 0 d | 0 d | 6 wk | 3 mo | 4 yr |

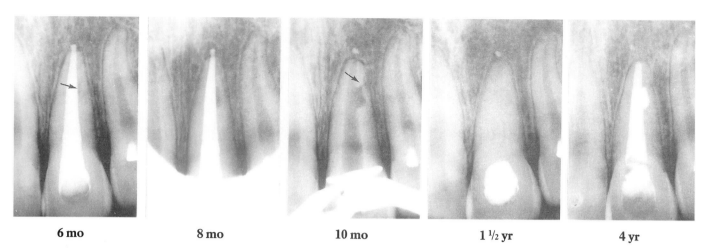

| 6 mo | 8 mo | 10 mo | 1 ½ yr | 4 yr |

Fig. 14.69.
Internal root canal resorption in a luxated and root-filled central incisor. At controls 6, 8 and 10 months after filling of the root canal with gutta-percha, a progressive internal root canal is seen in relation to an accessory root canal in the apical area of the tooth (arrow). The root canal was treated with calcium hydroxide and after 18 months filled with gutta-percha. There is no extrusion of the filling material into the periodontal space through the previous accessory canal.

in which resorption of damaged or altered tissue is necessary before repair can take place (see Chapter 8, p. 285). Thus, endodontic treatment is not indicated unless other changes occur, such as periradicular inflammatory changes.

Internal inflammatory resorption is a late and rare complication that usually occurs in the cervical area of the root canal in luxated teeth (Fig. 10.67 and 14.68). It is characterized radiographically by the progressive loss of root substance with no hard tissue formation in the resorption cavity. The process seems to be elicited by irritation from bacteria or its components in dentinal tubules, originating from a mechanical damage, dilaceration or cracks in the cervical area of the root (266-269).

Occasionally, a progressive dentin resorption may also occur in root-filled teeth. A conceivable reason for this could be presence of bacteria in the root canal and communication with the periodontium via an accessory canal, from which soft tissue may proliferate into the root canal and resorb contaminated dentin (Fig. 14.69).

Treatment

Endodontic treatment of teeth with internal root resorption is complicated by the difficulty in removing tissue from a resorp-

tion cavity. Soft tissue remnants may impede healing if communication exists with the periodontium. However, soft tissue in the lesion can be dissolved by means of repeated filling with calcium hydroxide at 2- to 3-week intervals. If treatment with calcium hydroxide is maintained for a couple of months, communication with the periodontium may be closed by apposition of hard tissue and thus overfilling with gutta-percha can be avoided (Figs. 14.67 to 14.69).

PRIMARY TEETH

Primary teeth with progressing dentin resorption should be removed, because in advanced stages of internal root resorption a root fracture may occur and complicate extraction.

Pulp Necrosis following Pulp Canal Obliteration

Pathology

Pulp canal obliteration by progressive hard tissue formation is relatively common after luxation injuries. The hard tissue varies histologically depending on the origin and differentiation of cells involved in its production (see Chapter 2, p. 104). Formation of hard tissue can be followed radiographically

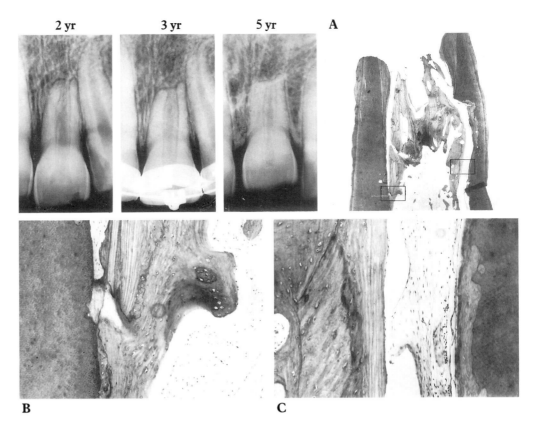

2 yr **3 yr** **5 yr** **A**

B **C**

Fig. 14.70.
Radiographic appearance of bony ingrowth into the pulpal lumen. There is increasing infraposition of the tooth at 2 and 5 year controls after injury. Histologic appearance of bone ingrowth into pulpal lumen of an intruded and subsequently infrapositioned incisor, 3 years after injury. A. Low power view of the extracted tooth. Note ingrowth of the bone into the root canal, x 3. B. Internal ankylosis, x 40. C. Internal periodontal ligament, x 40.

as it assumes typical morphologic patterns. There may be ingrowth of bone and PDL into the root canal, usually after pulp revascularization in replanted or luxated teeth (Fig. 14.70) or the pulpal lumen may be diminished by excessive, irregular hard tissue formation (Fig. 14.71). These changes are only seen in young teeth with incomplete root formation, resulting in cessation of further root development. In these teeth neither prophylactic nor therapeutic endodontic treatment can be recommended because of apparent problems of a mechanical nature. Thus the irregular arrangement of hard tissue prevents effective canal debridements.

In most canal obliterated teeth, the new hard tissue is deposited regularly along dentinal walls and the pulpal lumen diminishes gradually until only a narrow root canal remains which may or may not be seen in the radiographs (Fig. 14.72). In these instances a periapical radiolucency has been reported to occur in 13 to 16 % of teeth with traumatically-induced pulp canal obliteration, during observation periods of up to 20 years (89,129). According to clinical experience, occurrence of periapical lesions can in most cases be related to caries, inadequate crown restorations or new trauma (Figs. 14.73 and 14.74). In other teeth with apparently intact crowns the pathogenesis can be difficult to define. An additional minor injury may cause ischemic necrosis of a pulp due to rupture

Fig. 14.71.
Irregular hard tissue formation in the pulpal lumen of a luxated immature incisor. Six years after injury, a deep carious lesion (arrow) and a periapical radiolucency is seen. A. Low power view of the extracted tooth. Note arrested root development and irregular formation of hard tissue in the pulpal lumen containing islands of soft, inflamed and necrotic tissue, x 7. B. Connection between necrotic pulp and periodontal space where chronic inflammation can be seen, x 10. C. Areas of dystrophically calcified tissue (arrows) surrounded by irregularly formed dentin, x 50.

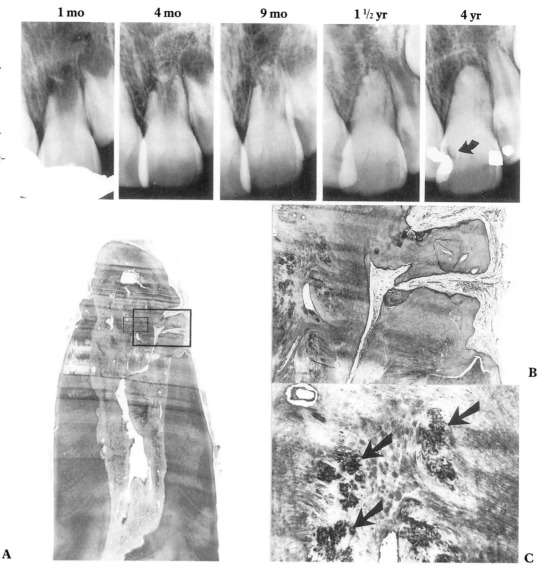

| 1 mo | 4 mo | 9 mo | 1 ½ yr | 4 yr |

A   B   C

Fig. 14.72.
Radiographic appearance of the gradual diminishing of the pulpal by hard tissue apposition on the dentinal walls. A luxated incisor at the time of injury and 1, 2, 3 and 4 years afterwards.

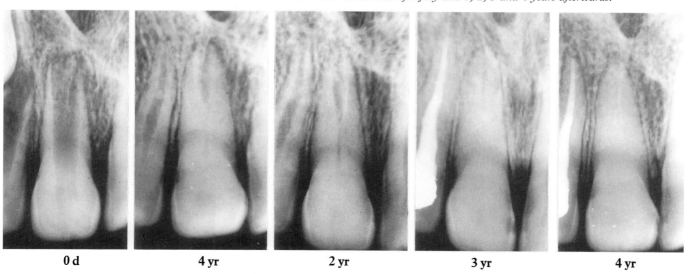

| 0 d | 4 yr | 2 yr | 3 yr | 4 yr |

ENDODONTIC MANAGEMENT OF TRAUMATIZED TEETH

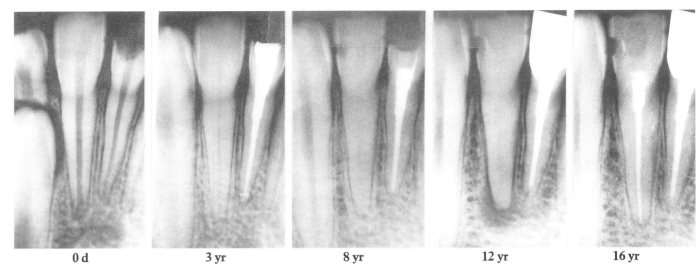

| 0 d | 3 yr | 8 yr | 12 yr | 16 yr |

Fig. 14.73.
An incisor with reduced pulpal lumen and pulp necrosis due to a deep carious lesion. Periapical healing can be seen 4 years after root canal treatment. From CVEK ET AL.(134) 1982.

of the few existing blood vessels. However, the access of bacteria to the pulpal lumen remains to be explained.

Opinions vary as to whether a prophylactic endodontic treatment should be instituted as soon as the onset of pulp canal obliteration has been diagnosed (130-132,270,271). In teeth with normal periradicular conditions, there seem to be only two logical justifications for endodontic intervention. One is on the premise of ongoing degenerative changes leading to necrosis of the pulp, and the second is on the premise that ongoing obliteration will make the root canal inaccessible for a later endodontic treatment. However,

when the pulps from prophylactically treated teeth with reduced pulpal lumen were examined histologically, changes were characterized by an increase of collagen content and a varying decrease in the number of cells, i.e. changes which do not seem to warrant endodontic intervention (133).

In another study, the accessibility for mechanical treatment was investigated in 54 obliterated incisors treated for periapical lesions (134). The root canal could be found in all teeth but one, although no or only a hairline canal was visible in preoperative radiographs. During treatment, fracture of a file or perforation of the root

Fig. 14.74.
Endodontic treatment of an incisor with reduced pulpal lumen and pulp necrosis due to a secondary trauma. The tooth was crown-fractured in a new injury. Five months later, a periapical radiolucency has developed. At the 4-year control after root canal treatment periapical healing is evident.

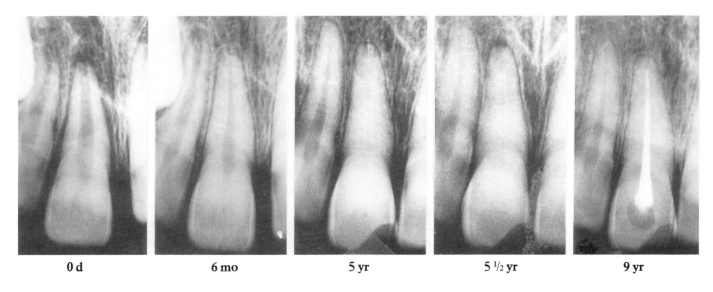

| 0 d | 6 mo | 5 yr | 5 ½ yr | 9 yr |

CHAPTER 14

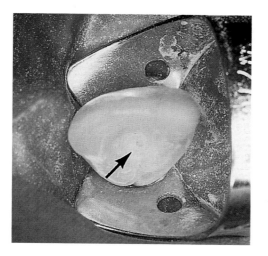

Fig. 14.75.
Preparation for root canal treatment of an incisor with an obliterated pulpal lumen. An area of discolored dentin (arrow) indicates the location of the obliterated root canal.

occurred in 10 teeth. In only 5 instances, however, did these complications have consequences for periapical healing, which was seen seen in 80% of teeth 4 years after treatment. Thus, considering the low frequency of late periapical osteitis

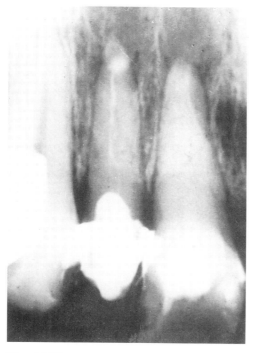

Fig. 14.76.
Use of 10% potassium iodide as contrast medium for disclosing the root canal. In a lateral incisor, the contrast is seen in the root canal that was not visible radiographically prior to treatment. From HASSELGREN & STRÖMBERG (135) 1976.

and accessibility of these teeth for endodontic treatment (including surgical retrograde filling techniques), routine endodontic intervention in teeth with ongoing obliteration of the root canal does not seem justified. However, such prophylactic endodontic treatment intervention could be considered in crown-fractured teeth in which a post in the root canal is necessary for future restoration.

Treatment

Mechanical preparation of an obliterated root canal requires patience and cannot be forced. Just locating the root canal may take more than one appointment. A cavity is prepared through the oral surface to the level of the cervical part of the root. Control radiographs taken after injury may be of help with respect to the level in the root at which the canal can be expected. After the access cavity has been rinsed, the canal is patiently sought after with the thinnest file. If the canal cannot be found, the cavity is prepared a step further and the search continued. Sometimes, a change in the color of dentin in the center of the root will indicate the position of the canal (Fig. 14.75). The use of a contrast medium, e.g. 10 % potassium iodide, can sometimes disclose a root canal which could not be seen in earlier radiographs (135). A cotton pellet is soaked in the contrast medium and placed in the cavity, which is then sealed with zinc oxide-eugenol cement, supplied with firm pressure for 10 seconds to faciliate penetration of the contrast medium into the root canal (Fig. 14.76). Thereafter, at least two radiographs are taken at different angulations in order to establish the position of the root canal. An operating microscope, which can magnify the base of the cavity, may also help in locating the root canal (272).

When the entrance to the canal has been found, further reaming should be performed step by step, carefully and without unneccessary pressure, in order to avoid fracture of the file. It is important that the thinnest file be used to track the root canal all the way to the apical foramen (Fig. 14.77). Too early a change to a larger file may lead to a false route or may complicate further treatment by pressing dentin debris in the root canal. To avoid obturation of the canal with dissolved dentin,

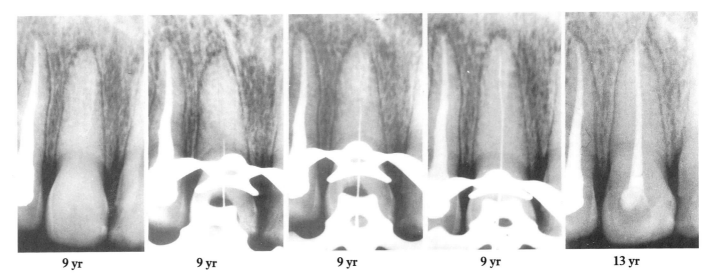

9 yr **9 yr** **9 yr** **9 yr** **13 yr**

Fig. 14.77.
Endodontic treatment of a central incisor with complete pulp canal obliteration. Note progressive diminution of the pulpal lumen by hard tissue after a luxation injury. A periapical radiolucency developed 9 years after injury. The root canal was found and carefully reamed using the finest files. Periapical healing is evident 4 years after root canal filling with gutta-percha. From CVEK ET AL. (134) *1982.*

solutions capable of dissolving hard tissue should not be used at an early stage of treatment. However after the root canal has been reamed to the apical area, EDTA (ethylene diamine tetraacetic acid) can be used to facilitate widening of the canal. It is not neccessary to remove all hard tissue formed after injury, just enough to assure an adequate root canal filling with gutta-percha and a sealer (Fig. 14.77).

Prognosis

The prognosis for successful endodontic treatment of incisors with pulp canal obliteration, pulp necrosis and periapical involvement has been found to be 80 % (134).

Pʀɪᴍᴀʀʏ ᴛᴇᴇᴛʜ
Primary teeth demonstrating obliteration of the pulpal lumen and associated periapical osteitis should be extracted (273).

Fig. 14.78.
Periapical radiolucency in a crown-dilacerated incisor 18 months after eruption. A histologic section of the extracted tooth shows a pathway via the dilaceration for bacterial penetration to the pulp canal resulting in a pulp necrosis (P), x 2.5 and 15.

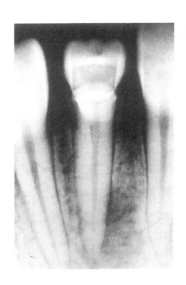
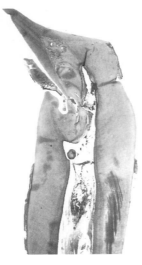
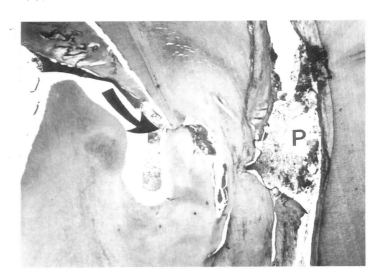

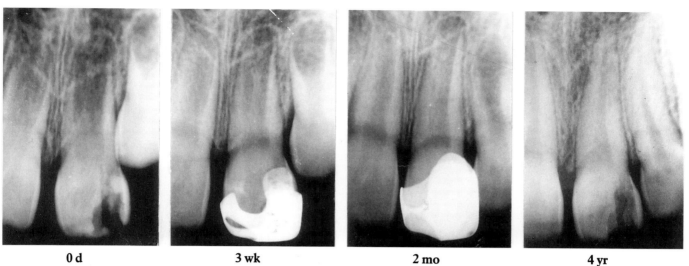

| 0 d | 3 wk | 2 mo | 4 yr |

Fig. 14.79.

Treatment of a permanent tooth with external enamel and dentin hypoplasia caused by impact from the luxated predecessor. Large hypomineralized area in the crown of a newly erupted incisor. The external hypoplasia was treated with calcium hydroxide and temporarily restored with a stainless steel crown. Four years after subsequent restoration with a composite material, root formation is complete.

Crown Malformations

Pathology

Impact from a displaced primary incisor can be the cause of mineralization disturbances in developing permanent successors, which later may assume various morphologic deviations (136-138) (Figs. 14.79 and 14.80, see also Chapter 12, p. 459). Soft tissue inclusions in hypomineralized dentin and malformations in dilacerated teeth may serve as pathways for rapid bacterial penetration, from plaque or a carious lesion, towards the pulp (Fig.14.78).

Inflammation and subsequent necrosis of the pulp may occur already during or soon after eruption, when hypomineralized dentin or the dilacerated part of

the crown or root comes into contact with the oral environment (139,140) (Fig. 14.78).

Treatment

To avoid involvement of the pulp and ensure further root development, it is important that defects in the crown, especially those in which hypomineralized dentin is not covered with enamel, are treated as soon as possible after eruption. Hypoplastic lesions should be cleaned, eventually treated with calcium hydroxide and thereafter restored, e.g., with glass ionomer cement and/or composite resin (Fig. 14.79).

In crown-dilacerated teeth, there is always a fissure present, according to the site of dilaceration, through which bacteria can enter the invaginated part of the tooth. This fissure should be enlarged, the bot-

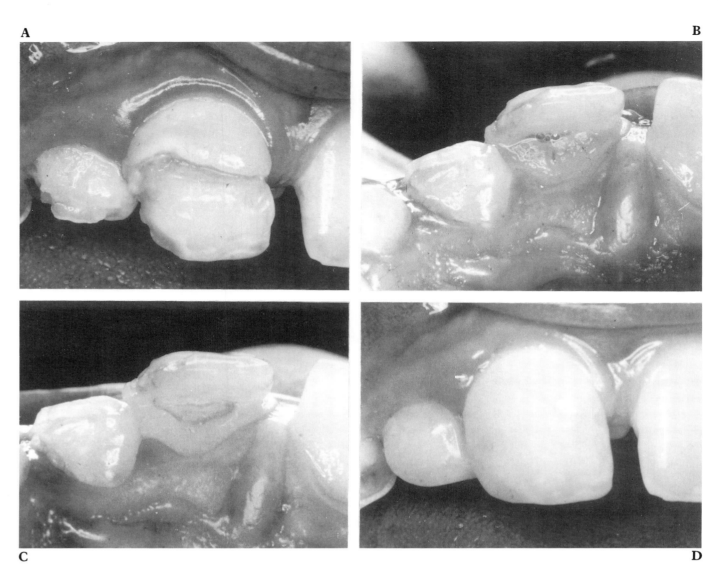

A **B**

C **D**

Fig. 14.80.
Restoration of malformed crowns of 2 permanent incisors. A and B. Dilacerated crown of central incisor and hypoplastic crown of the lateral incisor. C. Preparation of the palatal fissure. D. The hypoplastic areas and the base of the palatal cavity were covered with calcium hydroxide and the crowns restored with a composite using an acid-etch technique.

tom carefully cleaned and thereafter the cavity restored with a composite material (Fig. 14.80).

Non-vital teeth can be treated by conventional endodontic procedures if the root canal is accessible for treatment and the root sufficiently developed to support an eventual crown restoration (Fig. 14.81).

Discoloration and Bleaching of Non-Vital Teeth

Discoloration of the crown caused by intrapulpal bleeding is a relatively common sequel to luxation injuries. A pink discoloration that occurs shortly after the injury, i.e. within 2-3 days, can be reversible (87,88,212). Extravasated blood can be resorbed, tissue damage repaired and the crown can regain its natural color. On the other hand, a persistent or later appearing discoloration, especially with a shade of grey, indicates irreversible changes, i.e. necrosis of the pulp. Discoloration of the crown may occur and persist without radiographic changes. However, for esthetic reasons, a severe discoloration can *per se* be considered an indication for endodontic treatment, in order to make bleaching of the crown or other treatment solutions possible (274).

Pathology

In traumatized teeth, a persistent discoloration of the clinical crown has been ascribed to hemorrhage and/or decomposition of pulp tissue and presence of bacteria in the pulpal chamber. After lysis of extravasated erythrocytes in a necrotic pulp, the released hemoglobin breaks down to variously colored substances, such as hematoidin, hematoporphyrin and hemosiderin which, after diffusion into the dentinal tubules, cause discoloration

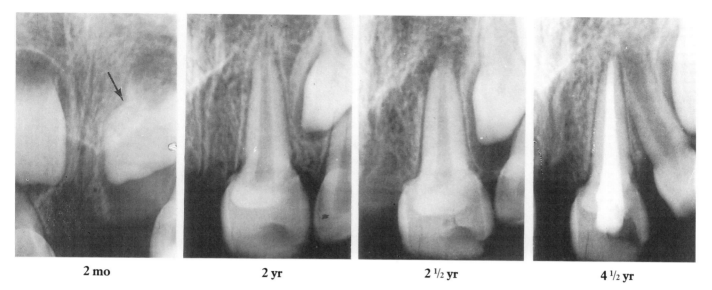

| 2 mo | 2 yr | 2 ½ yr | 4 ½ yr |

Fig. 14.81.
Endodontic treatment of a malformed permanent incisor with secondary pulp necrosis. Cervical dilaceration of the tooth (arrow) was noted 2 months after intrusive luxation of the primary incisor which was later removed. Six months after eruption a periapical radiolucency was observed. After root canal treatment, periapical healing has taken place.

Fig. 14.82.
Inflammatory root resorption after bleaching of a discolored crown with 30% hydrogen peroxide and a light beam from a heat-producing lamp. The tooth had previously suffered a luxation injury with subsequent pulp necrosis and root filling. Extensive cervical inflammatory root resorption is seen 1 year after bleaching. From CVEK & LINDWALL (283) 1985.

of dentin. In the event of infection, bacteria produce hydrogen sulphide which may combine with iron from hemoglobin and form iron sulphide, a black compound that further enhances discoloration (274-277).

BLEACHING PROCEDURES
Bleaching of non-vital discolored teeth has been practiced since the end of the 18th century, using various drugs and methods (278,279). More recently, the most commonly recommended drugs for bleaching have included 30 % hydrogen peroxide and sodium perborate, to be used alone or in combination (274-279).

The bleaching effect of these compounds is based on the release of nascent oxygen which oxidizes the colored substances in dentinal tubules. However, it has been reported that the use of 30 % hydrogen peroxide, especially when activated by heat, may cause ankylosis and/or a progressive root resorption in the cervical area of the tooth (280-284) (Figs. 14.82 and 14.83). It appears that hydrogen peroxide may penetrate dentin and cementum and cause damage to tissues on the root surface with inflammatory root resorption or a dento-alveolar ankylosis as a result (285-289).

The cause of progressive inflammatory root resorption has not been determined. It has been speculated that, after seepage of hydrogen peroxide and its initial damaging effect on the periodontium

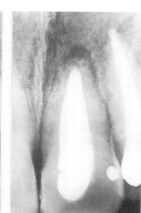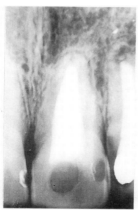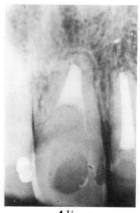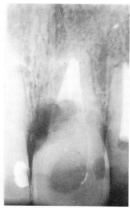

| 0 d | 2 mo | 4 ½ yr | 4 ½ yr | 5 ½ yr |

ENDODONTIC MANAGEMENT OF TRAUMATIZED TEETH

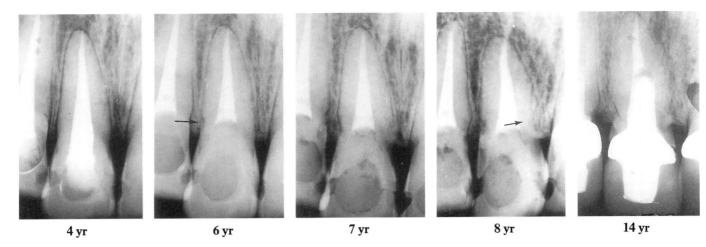

| 4 yr | 6 yr | 7 yr | 8 yr | 14 yr |

Fig. 14.83.
Ankylosis after bleaching of a discolored crown with 30% hydrogen peroxide. After the first bleaching a cavity with arrested resorption was seen cervically (arrow). After the second series of bleaching 2 years later, a slowly progressing root resorption associated with ankylosis developed in the cervical part of the root. From CVEK & LINDWALL (283) 1985.

leading to osteoclast activation (see Chapter 2, p. 112), bacteria may colonize dentinal tubules and cause inflammation in and progressive root resorption (283). Because these changes may lead to tooth loss, the use of 30 % hydrogen peroxide should be avoided. Bleaching with water-moistened sodium perborate appears to give equally good results without adverse effects such as root resorption (290-295).

Bleaching with sodium perborate is simple and easy to perform. The tooth should be checked radiographically and a poorly condensed root canal filling should be revised before treatment. At the time of bleaching, the crown is cleaned with a water-pumice slurry in a rubber cup to remove any extrinsic debris. At this stage, as well as after completed bleaching, it is advisable to take a color photograph for future comparison. Inadequate restorations are removed and the cavities restored temporarily; final restorations are postponed until bleaching is completed. A rubber dam is adapted and all material in the coronal access cavity as well as 2-3 mm of the coronal part of the root filling are removed. For this purpose, a round bur with a long shank can be used at low speed. Care should be taken not to remove dentin in the cervical area, as this could weaken the root and lead to a cervical fracture, especially in young teeth with thin dentinal walls. It is also important that the incisal part of the pulpal chamber is checked and eventual

necrotic pulp remnants removed (Fig. 14.84). In the coronal cavity only a thin, superficial layer of dentin should be removed in order to facilitate penetration of the bleaching agent into the tubules. Etching of coronal dentin for the same purpose has not been found to have any effect on the results of bleaching (288). Thereafter, the root filling is sealed cervically with an approximately 2-mm thick zinc oxide-eugenol cement. The coronal chamber is then rinsed with water and chloroform, dried with air and filled with a paste made of sodium perborate and water. The paste is condensed with a dry cotton pellet, the surplus removed and the cavity sealed with a 2-3 mm thick layer of, e.g., zinc-oxide eugenol or glass ionomer cement.

Bleaching is repeated at 1-week intervals until the desired effect is achieved, usually after 1 to 4 treatments. After completed bleaching, remnants of bleaching material are removed from the coronal cavity with either sodium hypochlorite or chloroform. Thereafter, the cavity is air-dried and filled with a light-activated glass ionomer cement. After the surplus cement has been removed and the enamel thoroughly cleaned, the cavity is sealed with a composite resin material using an acid-etch technique (279). Alternatively, the entire cavity can be acid-etched and filled with the lightest shade of composite resin available using a dentin bonding technique (296).

Fig. 14.84. Bleaching with sodium perborate.

The necessary depth for the removal of filling material from the cervical part of the root canal can be estimated by measuring the distance between the incisal edge of the tooth to a level about 3-4 mm below the buccal gingival margin. A rubber dam is adapted and contents in the pulpal chamber and cervical parts of the root filling material are removed as well as the necrotic remnants in the pulp horns. A 2-3 mm thick seal of a suitable base material (e.g. zinc oxide-eugenol or zinc phosphate cement) is placed cervically over the root filling material and the pulp chamber is filled with a paste of sodium perborate moistened with water or saline. The paste is condensed, surplus removed and the cavity is temporarily sealed, e.g. with zinc oxide-eugenol cement.

The coronal cavity can be filled, e.g., with a light-activated glass ionomer cement and sealed with a composite material using an acid-etch technique.

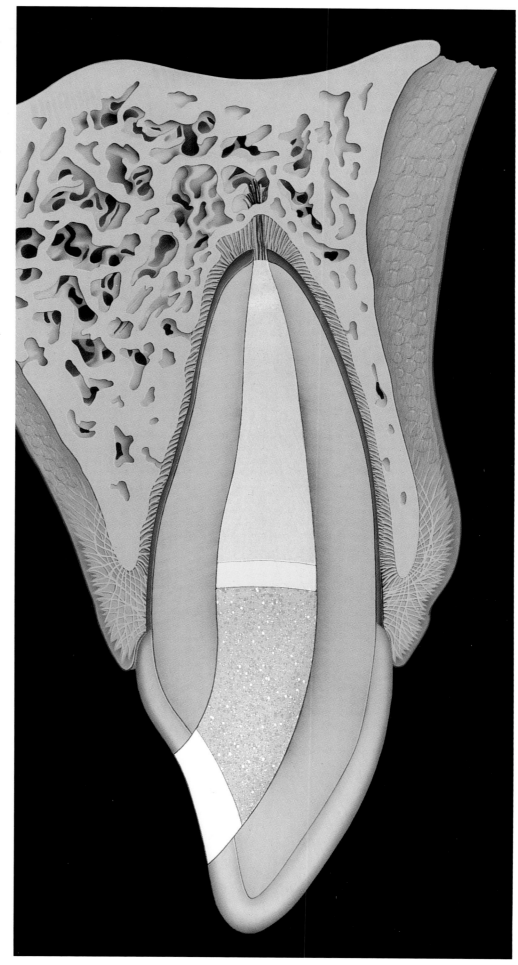

ENDODONTIC MANAGEMENT OF TRAUMATIZED TEETH

573

Fig. 14.85. Result of bleaching with sodium perborate
Condition before and 3 years after bleaching: Good esthetic result.

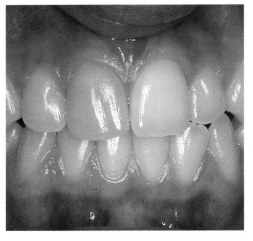

Fig. 14.86. Result of bleaching with sodium perborate
Condition before and 3 years after bleaching: Acceptable esthetic result.

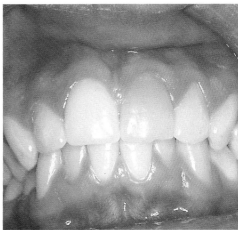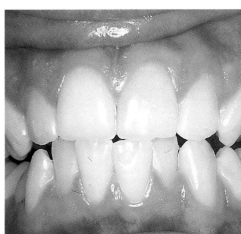

Fig. 14.87. Result of bleaching with sodium perborate
Condition before and 3 years after bleaching: Unacceptable esthetic result.

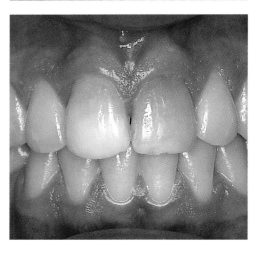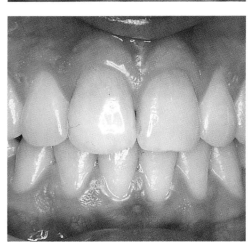

Prognosis

The results of bleaching can be classified as good, when the tooth has regained its natural color (Fig. 14.85); acceptable (Fig 14.86), when slight discoloration remains but is accepted by the patient; or unacceptable, when severe discoloration persists (Figs. 14.87).

In recent studies of sodium perborate bleaching, the immediate results were found to be good or acceptable in about 80 % of treated teeth. However, following 5 years' observation, discoloration recurred in about 30 % of the controlled teeth (292,294).

The cause for rediscoloration is not known; but microleakage around an inadequate seal, causing reduction of oxidized compounds, has been suggested (291).

Essentials

Crown Fractures with Pulp Exposure

PERMANENT TEETH
The exposed pulp can be treated with capping, partial pulpotomy, cervical pulpotomy or pulpectomy.

PULP CAPPING (FIG. 14.11)
Indicated in mature and immature teeth when exposure is minimal and can be treated soon after injury; i.e. within 24 hours.

a. Isolate with rubber dam and wash with saline.
b. Cover the exposed pulp with calcium hydroxide and the exposed dentin with a liner. When using a hard-setting calcium hydroxide, both pulp and dentin are covered with the compound.
c. Restore the crown with a composite using acid-etch technique or another type of restoration, e.g., porcelain laminate veneer.
d. If immediate restoration is not possible, restore the crown temporarily, e.g., with a prefabricated steel crown cemented with a zinc oxide-eugenol cement. If the tooth is incorporated in a splint, cover fracture surface with a glass ionomer cement or a hard-setting calcium hydroxide cement before the splint is adapted.
e. Follow-up: Clinical and radiographic controls after 6 months, 1 year and annually for a minimum of 3 years.

PROGNOSIS
PULP HEALING: 71 - 88 %.

Partial Pulpotomy (Fig. 14.12)

Indicated in mature and immature teeth showing vital pulp tissue at the exposure site, irrespective of its size and interval between injury and treatment. When the pulp is necrotic or demonstrates impaired vascularity, consider cervical pulpotomy in immature or pulpectomy in mature teeth.

a. Administer local anesthesia.
b. Isolate with a rubber dam and wash with a mild disinfectant.
c. Amputate the pulp together with surrounding dentin to a depth of about 2 mm below the exposure site with a diamond bur in high-speed contra-angle handpiece, using a continuous water spray. Cut intermittently, for brief periods and without unnecessary pressure.
d. Await hemostasis.
e. Cover the wound with calcium hydroxide and seal the cavity. If the crown is to be immediately restored with a composite material, seal the coronal cavity with zinc-sulphate cement according to Prader (193) (Consists of two parts: part a.: zinc oxide 300 g; part b.: zinc sulphate 150 g, boric acid 1 g and distilled water 120 ml; mix parts a. and b. to a paste consistency). If the crown is restored temporarily, seal the cavity with a zinc oxide-eugenol cement.
f. Follow-up: Clinical and radiographic controls after 6 months, 1 year and annually for at least 3 years.

Prognosis
Pulp healing: 94 - 96 %.

CERVICAL PULPOTOMY (FIG.14.16)
Indicated for immature teeth when necrotic tissue or obviously impaired vascularity is seen at the exposure site.

a. Administer local anesthesia.
b. Isolate with a rubber dam and wash with a mild disinfectant.
c. Amputate the pulp to a level at which fresh bleeding is encountered, usually in the cervical region. Due to problems of inadequate cooling of a diamond bur run at high speed, a round bur at low speed should be used.
d. Await hemostasis.
e. Cover the pulp with calcium hydroxide and seal the coronal cavity. If the crown is restored immediately with a composite resin, seal the cavity with Prader's sulphate cement, otherwise with zinc oxide-eugenol cement.
f. Follow-up: Clinical and radiographic controls after 6 months, 1 year and annually to completion of root development. Consider then eventual further endodontic or prosthetic treatment.

Prognosis
*Pulp healing:*72 - 79 %.

PULPECTOMY

Indicated in mature teeth when necrotic tissue or impaired pulp vascularity is seen at the exposure site, or when extensive loss of crown substance indicates restoration with a post in the root canal.

a. Administer local anesthesia.
b. Isolate with a rubber dam and wash with a mild disinfectant.
c. Amputate the pulp 1-2 mm from the apical foramen.
d. Clean the root canal mechanically while constantly flushing with saline or 0.5 % sodium hypochlorite solution.
e. Obturate the root canal with gutta-percha, using resin-chloroform, chloropercha or another sealer.
f. Follow-up: Clinical and radiographic controls after 6 months, 1 year and annually for a minimum of 4 years.

Prognosis
Periapical healing: 90 %.

PRIMARY TEETH

Primary teeth can be treated according to the general principles for treatment of permanent teeth, provided:

a. Physiologic root resorption is negligible.
b. The child is cooperative.

Otherwise, the treatment of choice is extraction.

Root-Fractured Teeth

PERMANENT TEETH

Root canal treatment of *coronal fragment:*
Is performed when the pulp in the apical fragment is vital.

a. When the anatomy of the root canal permits adequate obturation, i.e. a narrow or tapering canal, it may be treated and filled conventionally with gutta-percha and a sealer.
b. When the root canal and/or the space between the fragments is wide, the initial treatment is with calcium hydroxide in order to induce formation of a hard tissue barrier at the fracture site before filling with gutta-percha. (For more specific procedures, see treatment of non-vital immature teeth).

Root canal treatment of *both fragments:*
Is performed when the pulp is necrotic in both fragments and the space between the fragments is narrow.

Root canal treatment of *coronal fragment and surgical removal of apical fragment:*
Is performed when the root canal in a non-vital apical fragment is not accessible for treatment.

Prognosis
Not known

Primary Teeth

Endodontic treatment of root-fractured primary teeth with pulp necrosis is generally not indicated. In the case of total pulp necrosis the whole tooth should be extracted. When the pulp in the apical fragment is vital, only the coronal fragment is extracted and the apical fragment left to physiologic resorption.

Luxated or Replanted Teeth with Pulp Necrosis

IMMATURE PERMANENT TEETH
(FIG. 14.46)

a. Isolate with a rubber dam and wash with a disinfectant.
b. Establish access to the root canal.
c. Remove necrotic pulp with a barbed broach; clean the walls of the root canal using large files and a copious flow of 0.5 % sodium hypochlorite solution.
d. Fill the root canal with calcium hydroxide using a lentulo spiral or a syringe with a special cannula. Seal the coronal cavity with zinc oxide-eugenol cement.
e. In case of acute periapical osteitis and swelling, treat the root canal with, e.g., 2 % iodine potassium iodide, eventually administer antibiotics for 7 days before filling with calcium hydroxide.
f. Control radiographically at 3- to 6-month intervals. If radiographic signs of healing are not present, the root canal should be retreated and refilled with calcium hydroxide. Furthermore, when the level of calcium hydroxide in the root canal retracts to the cervical part of the canal, it should be refilled with calcium hydroxide.
g. Permanent filling with gutta-percha is completed when follow-up exami-

nation shows periradicular healing, including arrested inflammatory root resorption, and an apical hard-tissue barrier which clinically is found to be continuous.

h. Choose the thickest gutta-percha point that can easily fit to the apical barrier.

i. Warm the tip of the gutta-percha point by passing it once through an alcohol flame; introduce it immediately into the root canal and press it steadily but not too hard against the apical barrier (Fig. 14.51).

j. Verify the position with a control radiograph.

k. Fill the root canal completely with additional guttapercha points using lateral condensation.

l. Follow-up: Clinical and radiographic controls after 6 months, 1 year and annually for at least 4 years.

Prognosis
Periapical healing and formation of an apical hard tissue barrier: 75 - 96 %.

Mature permanent teeth

a. Isolate with a rubber dam and wash with a disinfectant.

b. Establish access to the root canal.

c. Remove necrotic pulp with a barbed broach and clean the canal mechanically with files and a copious flow of 0.5 % sodium hypochlorite solution.

d. After antibacterial treatment with 2 % iodine potassium iodide, fill the root canal with gutta-percha, using resin-chloroform or a sealer. If periapical healing is desired before filling with gutta-percha, or if inflammatory root resorption is present, the tooth should be treated initially with calcium hydroxide. Permanent filling with gutta-percha is carried out when follow-up examination shows periradicular healing and arrest of the inflammatory processes.

e. Follow-up: Clinical and radiographic controls after 6 months, 1 year and annually for at least 4 years.

Prognosis
Periapical healing: 79 - 95 %.

PRIMARY TEETH

Luxated primary teeth with pulp necrosis should generally be extracted.

Luxated or Replanted Teeth with Inflammatory Resorption
Teeth with external inflammatory root resorption are treated by removal of the necrotic and infected pulp tissue and interim root canal dressing with calcium hydroxide. (See procedures described for root canal treatment of permanent immature teeth with pulp necrosis).

Prognosis
Luxated teeth: arrest of resorption and periapical healing: 97 %.

Late External Cervical Root Resorption
According to location and esthetic demands, one of the following treatment procedures can be chosen:

a. Gingivectomy and removal of soft tissue from the resorption cavity followed by insertion of a dentin-bonded composite resin or a glass ionomer cement;

b. A gingival flap is raised, a dentin bonded composite placed in the resorption cavity, and the flap replaced (Fig. 14.66).

c. The tooth is surgically or orthodontically extruded whereafter the resorption defect is repaired with a dentin-bonded composite restoration.

Prognosis
Not known.

Internal Resorption
Teeth with progressive internal root resorption are treated according to common endodontic principles. In case of a large resorption area, and in order to remove inflamed tissue in the lesion, the following procedure can be employed. (Fig. 14.67).

a. Clean the root canal mechanically, flush constantly with sodium hypochlorite and fill with calcium hydroxide.

b. Flush the canal with sodium hypochlorite and re-fill with calcium hydroxide at 2- to 3-week intervals until all pulp tissue in the lesion has been dissolved, i.e. when calcium hydroxide is radiographically seen to fill the entire resorption cavity.

c. Obturate the canal with gutta-percha and lateral condensation.

Prognosis
Not known.

Pulp Canal Obliteration with Subsequent Pulp Necrosis

PERMANENT TEETH

Endodontic treatment is performed in teeth in which a periapical radiolucency has developed.

a. Isolate with a rubber dam and wash with a disinfectant.
b. Establish access through the crown to the cervical part of the root.
c. Search for the canal with the finest file.
d. If the canal is not found, prepare the cavity a step deeper and continue the search.
e. Clean the disclosed canal without unnecessary pressure, using the thinnest file until the apex is reached (Fig. 14.77). Do not use solutions capable of dissolving dentin.
f. Enlarge the root canal mechanically.
g. Fill the root canal with gutta-percha and a sealer.
h. Follow-up: Clinical and radiographic controls after 6 months, 1 year and annually for at least 4 years.

Prognosis
Periapical healing: 80 %.

PRIMARY TEETH

Primary teeth demonstrating pulp canal obliteration and pulp necrosis should be extracted.

Crown Malformation with Pulp Necrosis

a. To prevent infection of the pulp through hypomineralized parts of the dentin, the tooth should be restored as soon as possible.
b. Non-vital teeth are treated by conventional endodontic therapy.

Bleaching of Discolored Teeth with Sodium Perborate (Fig. 14.84)

a. Measure the distance between the incisal edge of the tooth and a level about 3-4 mm from the gingival margin buccally, to define the access cavity to the root canal and the extent of removal of the coronal part of the root filling.
b. Clean the crown with a pumice-water slurry in a rubber cup; remove inadequate fillings and restore the cavities with a temporary filling (eventually take a color photograph).
c. Adapt a rubber dam and remove all material from the coronal pulp chamber and the coronal part of the root filling to the previously defined level, using round burs run at a low speed.
d. Remove only a thin, superficial layer of dentin in the coronal cavity to facilitate penetration of bleaching agent into dentinal tubules; search for and remove eventual pulpal remnants.
e. Seal the root filling cervically with a 2-3 mm thick barrier of a suitable base material, e.g., zinc oxide eugenol or glass ionomer cement; therafter wash, e.g., with water and chloroform, and dry with air.
f. Fill the coronal cavity with a paste made of sodium perborate mixed with water and compress with a dry cotton pellet.
g. Remove excess sodium perborate and seal the cavity with a 2-3 mm thick layer of zinc oxide-eugenol cement. If neccessary, repeat the treatment with sodium perborate (f and g) at 1-week intervals.
h. After completed bleaching, clean the coronal cavity with water and sodium hypochlorite or chloroform, dry with air and fill the cavity, e.g., with light-activated glass ionomer cement. Remove 2-3 mm of glass ionomer to prepare a cavity for the coronal seal. Clean the enamel carefully of glass ionomer remnants, acid-etch and seal the cavity with a composite resin.

Prognosis
Good or acceptable esthetics:
> 3 YEARS: 80 %
> 5 YEARS: 70%

Bibliography

1. STEWART JK. The immediate response of odontoblasts to injury. *Odont T* 1965;**73**:417-23.

2. GARBEROGLIO R, BRÄNNSTRÖM M. Scanning electron microscopic investigation of human dentinal tubules. *Arch Oral Biol* 1976;**21**:355-62.

3. OLGART L, BRÄNNSTRÖM M, JOHNSSON G. Invasion of bacteria into dentinal tubules. Experiments in vivo and in vitro. *Acta Odontol Scand* 1974;**32**:61-70.

4. BRÄNNSTRÖM M. Observations on exposed dentine and corresponding pulp tissue. A preliminary study with replica and routine histology. *Odont Revy* 1952;**13**:253-45.

5. DARLING AI. Response of pulpodentinal complex to injury. In: Gorlin RJ, Goldman H, eds. *Thoma's Oral Pathology.* 6th edn. St. Louis: CV Mosby Co, 1970:308-34.

6. MJÖR IA, TRONSTAD L. The healing of experimentally induced pulpitis. *Oral Surg Oral Med Oral Pathol* 1974:**38**:115-21.

7. BERGENHOLTZ G, REIT C. Pulp reactions on microbial provocation of calcium hydroxide treated dentin. *Scand J Dent Res* 1980:**88**:187-92.

8. GRANATH L-E. Traumatologi. In: Holst JJ, Nygaard Östby B, Osvald O, eds. *Nordisk Klinisk Odontologi.* Copenhagen: A/S Forlaget for Faglitteratur, 1978:79-100.

9. KAKEHASHI S, STANLEY HR, FITZGERALD RJ. The effect of surgical exposures on dental pulps in germ-free and conventional laboratory rats. *Oral Surg Oral Med Oral Pathol* 1965;**20**:340-9.

10. SHEININ A, POHTO M, LUOSTARINEN V. Defense reactions of the pulp with special reference to circulation. An experimental study in rats. *Int Dent J* 1967;**17**:461-75.

11. LUOSTARINEN V, POHTO M, SHEININ A. Dynamics of repair in the pulp. *J Dent Res* 1966;**45**:519-25.

12. CVEK M. A clinical report on partial pulpotomy and capping with calcium hydroxide in permanent incisors with complicated crown fracture. *J Endod* 1978;**4**:232-7.

13. SMUKLER H, TAGGER N. Vital root amputation. A clinical and histologic study. *J Periodontol* 1976;**47**:324-30.

14. CVEK M, CLEATON-JONES P, AUSTIN J, ANDREASEN JO. Pulp reactions to exposure after experimental crown fractures or grinding in adult monkeys. *J Endod* 1982;**8**:391-7.

15. HEIDE S, MJÖR IA. Pulp reactions to experimental exposures in young permanent monkey teeth. *Int Endod J* 1983;**16**:11-19.

16. FUSAYAMA T, MAEDA T. Effect of pulpectomy on dentin hardness. *J Dent Res* 1969;48:452-60.

17. TRABERT KC, CAPUT AA, ABOU-RASS M. Tooth fracture - a comparison of endodontic and restorative treatments. *J Endod* 1978;**4**:341-5.

18. ANDREASEN JO. Luxation of permanent teeth due to trauma. A clinical and radiographic follow-up of 189 injured teeth. *Scand J Dent Res* 1970;**78**:273-86.

19. EKLUND G, STÅLHANE I, HEDEGÅRD B. A study of traumatized permanent teeth in children aged 7 - 15. Part III. A multivariate analysis of post-traumatic complications of subluxated and luxated teeth. *Svensk Tandläk T* 1976;**69**:179-89.

20. MASTERTON JB. The healing of wounds of the dental pulp of man. A clinical and histological study. *Br Dent J* 1966;**120**:213-24.

21. WEISS M. Pulp capping in older patients. *NY State Dent J* 1966;**32**:451-7.

22. HASKELL EW, STANLEY HR, CHELLEMI J, STRINGFELLOW H. Direct pulp capping treatment: a long-term follow-up. *J Am Dent Assoc* 1978;**97**:607-12.

23. HEYDUCK G, WEGNER H. Klinische, röntgenologische und histologische Ergebnisse nach Vitalbehandlung der freigelegten Pulpa. *Stomat DDR* 1978;**28**:614-19.

24. SELTZER S, BENDER IB. *The dental pulp.* 2nd edn. Philadelphia: JB Lippincott Co, 1975:356.

25. BERNICK S, ADELMAN C. Effect of aging on the human pulp. *J Endod* 1975;**1**:88-94.

26. STANLEY HR. Management of the aging patient and the aging pulp. *J Calif Dent Assoc* 1978;**57**:25-8.

27. TOTO PD, STAFFILENO H, WEINE FS, DAS S. Age change effects on the pulp in periodontitis. *Ann Dent* 1977;**36**:13-20.

28. KRAKOW AA, BERK H, GRÖN P. Therapeutic induction of root formation in the exposed incompletely formed tooth with a vital pulp. *Oral Surg Oral Med Oral Pathol* 1977,**43**:755-65.

29. BERG C, MÅRTENSSON K. Pulpabehandling av mjölktänder. En efterundersökning av pulpaamputationer och överkappningar. *Odontol Revy* 1965;**6**:135-62.

30. PATTERSON SS. Pulp calcification due to operative procedures - pulpotomy. *Int Dent J* 1967;**17**:490-505.

31. MASTERTON JB. The healing of wounds of the dental pulp. An investigation of the nature of the scar tissue and of the phenomena leading to its formation. *Dent Pract* 1966;**16**:325-39.

32. GRANATH L-E, HAGMAN G. Experimental pulpotomy in human bicuspids with reference to cutting technique. *Acta Odontol Scand* 1971;**29**:155-63.

33. ZANDER HA. Reaction of the pulp to calcium hydroxide. *J Dent Res* 1939;**18**:373-9.

34. GLASS RL, ZANDER HA. Pulp healing. *J Dent Res* 1949;**28**:97-107.

35. MEJÁRE I, HASSELGREN G, HAMMARSTRÖM LE. Effect of formaldehyde-containing drugs on human dental pulp evaluated by enzyme histochemical technique. *Scand J Dent Res* 1976;**84**:29-36.

36. SCHRÖDER U, GRANATH L-E. Early reaction of intact human teeth to calcium hydroxide following experimental pulpotomy and its significance to the development of hard tissue barrier. *Odont Revy* 1971;**22**:379-96.

37. SCHRÖDER U. Reaction of human dental pulp to experimental pulpotomy and capping with calcium hydroxide (Thesis). *Odont Revy* 1973;**24** (Suppl. 25):97 p.

38. STANLEY HR, LUNDI T. Dycal therapy for pulp exposures. *Oral Surg Oral Med Oral Pathol* 1972;**34**:818-27.

39. TRONSTAD L, MJÖR IA. Capping of the inflamed pulp. *Oral Surg Oral Med Oral Pathol* 1972;**34**:477-85.

40. BRÄNNSTRÖM M, NYBORG H, STRÖMBERG T. Experiments with pulp capping. *Oral Surg Oral Med Oral Pathol* 1979;**48**:347-52.

41. SCHRÖDER U. Effect of extra-pulpal blood clot on healing following experimental pulpotomy and capping with calcium hydroxide. *Odont Revy* 1973;**24**:257-68.

42. CABRINI RI, MAISTO OA, MANFREDI EE. Internal resorption of dentine. Histopathologic control of eight cases after pulp amputation and capping with calcium hydroxide. *Oral Surg Oral Med Oral Pathol* 1957;**10**:90-96.

43. JAMES VE, ENGLANDER HR, MASSLER M. Histologic response of amputated pulps to calcium compounds and antibiotics. *Oral Surg Oral Med Oral Pathol* 1957;**10**:975-86.

44. MASTERTON JB. Internal resorption of dentine. A complication arising from unhealed pulp wounds. *Br Dent J* 1965;**118**:241-9.

45. SCHRÖDER U, GRANATH L-E. On internal dentin resorption in deciduous molars treated by pulpotomy and capped with calcium hydroxide. *Odont Revy* 1971;**22**:179-88.

46. MALONE AJ, MASSLER M. Fractured anterior teeth - diagnosis, treatment and prognosis. *Dent Dig* 1952;**58**:442-7.

47. NYGAARD ÖSTBY B. Über die Gewebsveränderungen im apikalen Paradentium des Menschen und verschidenartigen Eingriffen in den Wurzelkanälen. *Det Norske Videnskaps-Akademi Oslo,* 1939 no.4.

48. KUTTLER Y. Analysis and comparison of root canal filling techniques. *Oral Surg Oral Med Oral Pathol* 1967;**48**:153-9.

49. ENGSTRÖM B, SPÅNGBERG L. Wound healing after partial pulpectomy. A histologic study performed on contralateral tooth pairs. *Odont T* 1967;**75**:5-18.

50. HOLLAND R, DE MELLO MJ, NERY MJ, BERNABE PFE, de SOUZA V. Reaction of human periapical tissues to pulp extirpation and immediate root canal filling with calcium hydroxide. *J Endod* 1977;**3**:63-7.

51. NYBORG H. Pulpaöverkappning och vitalamputation in permanenta tänder.In: Holst JJ, Nygaard Østby O, Osvald O, eds. Copenhagen: *Nordisk Klinisk Odontologi*, A/S Forlaget for Faglitteratur, Copenhagen: 1965 (Chapter 10-11):1-18.

52. KOZLOWSKA I. Pokrycie bezposrednie miazgi preparatem krajowej produkcji.*Czas Stomat* 1960;**13**:375-88.

53. RAVN JJ. Follow-up study of permanent incisors with complicated crown fractures after acute trauma. *Scand J Dent Res* 1982;**90**:363-72.

54. HALLET GE, PORTEOUS JR. Fractured incisors treated by vital pulpotomy. A report on 100 consecutive cases. *Br Dent J* 1963;**115**:279-87.

55. STRINBERG L-Z. The dependence of the results of pulp therapy on certain factors. An analytic study based on radiographic and clinical follow-up examinations. *Acta Odont Scand* 1956 14:(Suppl 21).

56. GROSSMAN LI, SHEPPARD LI, PEARSON LA. Roentgenologic and clinical evaluation of endodontically treated teeth. *Oral Surg Oral Med Oral Pathol* 1964;**17**:368-74.

57. ADENUBI JO, RULE DC. Success rate for root fillings in young patients. A retrospective analysis of treated cases. *Br Dent J* 1976;**141**:237-41.

58. GRAHNEN H, HANSSON L. The prognosis of pulp and root canal therapy. A clinical and radiographic follow-up examination. *Odont Revy* 1961;**12**:146-65.

59. ANDREASEN JO, HJØRTING-HANSEN E. Intraalveolar root fractures: Radiographic and histologic study of 50 cases. *J Oral Surg* 1967;**25**:414-26.

60. LINDAHL B. Transverse intra-alveolar root fractures: Roentgen diagnosis and prognosis. *Odont Revy* 1963;**9**:10-24.

61. ANDREASEN JO. Relationship between surface and inflammatory root resorption and pathologic changes in the pulp after replantation of mature incisors in monkeys. *J Endod* 1981;**7**:194-301.

62. MICHANOWICZ AE. Root fractures. A report of radiographic healing after endodontic treatment. *Oral Surg Oral Med Oral Pathol* 1963;**16**:1242-8.

63. FELDMAN G, SOLOMON G, NOTARO PJ. Endodontic treatment of traumatized tooth. *Oral Surg Oral Med Oral Pathol* 1966;**21**:100-12.

64. MICHANOWICZ AE, MICHANOWICZ JP, ABOU-RASS M. Cementogenic repair of root fractures. *J Am Dent Assoc* 1971;**82**:569-79.

65. ANDREASEN JO. Treatment of fractured and avulsed teeth. *ASDC J Dent Child* 1971;**38**:29-48.

66. CVEK M. Treatment of non-vital permanent incisors with calcium hydroxide. IV. Periodontal healing and closure of the root canal in the coronal fragment of teeth with intra-alveolar fracture and vital apical fragment. *Odont Revy* 1974;**25**:239-45.

67. RAVN JJ. En klinisk og radiologisk undersogelse af 55 rodfrakturer i unge permanente incisiver. *Tandlaegebladet* 1976;**80**:391-96.

68. ARWILL T. Histopathologic studies of traumatized teeth. *Odont T* 1962;**70**:91-117.

69. ARWILL T, HENSCHEN B, SUNDWALL-HAGLAND I. The pulpal reaction in traumatized permanent incisors in children aged 9-18. *Odont T* 1967;**75**:130-47.

70. STANLEY HR, WEISMANN MI, MICHANOWICZ AE, BELLIZZI R. Ischemic infarction of the pulp: Sequential degenerative changes of the pulp after traumatic injury. *J Endod* 1978;**4**:325-35.

71. HASSELGREN G, LARSSON Å, RUNDQUIST L. Pulpal status after autogenuous transplantation of fully developed maxillary canines. *Oral Surg Oral Med Oral Pathol* 1977;**44**:106-12.

72. MAKKES PCH, THODEN VAN VELZEN SK, VAN DEN HOOFF A. Response of the living organism to dead and fixed dead, enclosed isologous tissue. *Oral Surg Oral Med Oral Pathol* 1978;**46**:131-44.

73. GROSSMAN LI. Origin of micro-organisms in traumatized, pulpless, sound teeth. *J Dent Res* 1967;**46**:551-3.

74. BERGENHOLTZ G. Micro-organisms from necrotic pulps of traumatized teeth. *Odont Revy* 1974;**25**:347-58.

75. SUNDQVIST G. *Bacteriological studies of necrotic dental pulps.* Umeå: Umeå University Odontological Dissertations, No 7, 1976:94 p.

76. RAVN JJ, HELBO M. Replantation af akcidentelt exartikulerede tænder. *Tandlægebladet* 1966;**70**:805-15.

77. FRANK AL. Therapy for the divergent pulpless tooth by continued apical formation. *J Am Dent Assoc* 1966;**72**:87-93.

78. RULE DC, WINTER GB. Root growth and apical repair subsequent to pulpal necrosis in children. *Br Dent J* 1966;**120**:586-90.

79. HEITHERSAY GS. Stimulation of root formation incompletely developed pulpless teeth. *Oral Surg Oral Med Oral Pathol* 1970;**29**:620-30.

80. MCDONALD RE, AVERY DR. *Dentistry for the child and adolescent.* 3rd edn. St. Louis: CV Mosby Co, 1878:640.

81. HOTZ R. Die Bedeutung, Beurteilung und Behandlung beim Trauma in Frontzahngebiet vom Standpunkt des Kieferorthopäden. *Dtsch Zahnartzl Z* 1958;**13**:42-51.

82. SCHRÖDER U, WENNBERG E, GRANATH L-E, MÖLLER H. Traumatized primary incisors follow-up program based on frequency of periapical osteitis related to tooth color. *Swed Dent J* 1977;**1**:95-8.

83. SELTZER S, BENDER IB, ZIONZ M. The dynamics of pulp inflammation: correlations between diagnostic data and actual histologic findings in the pulp. *Oral Surg Oral Med Oral Pathol* 1963;**16**:846-71.

84. MUMFORD JM. Pain reception threshold in stimulating human teeth and histologic condition of the pulp. *Br Dent J* 1967;**123**:427-33.

85. STENBERG S. Vitalitetsprövning med elektrisk ström av incisiver i olika genombrottsstadier. *Svensk Tandläkare Tidskrift* 1950;**43**:83-6.

86. SKIELLER V. The prognosis of young loosened teeth after mechanical injuries. *Acta Odont Scand* 1960;**18**:181-8.

87. MAGNUSSON B, HOLM A-K. Traumatized permanent teeth in children - a follow-up. I. Pulpal complications and root resorption. *Svensk Tandläkare Tidskrift* 1969;**62**:61-70.

88. ÖHMAN A. Healing and sensivity to pain in young replanted teeth. An experimental, clinical and histological study. *Odont T* 1965;**73**:165-228.

89. JACOBSEN I, KEREKES K. Long-term prognosis of traumatized permanent anterior teeth showing calcifying processes in the pulp cavity. *Scand J Dent Res* 1977;**85**:588-98.

90. ROHNER A. Calxyl als Wurzelfüllungsmaterial nach Pulpaextirpation. *Schweiz Monatschr Zahnheil* 1940;**50**:903-48.

91. HEITHERSAY GS. Calcium hydroxide in the treatment of pulpless teeth with associated pathology. *J Br Endod Soc* 1962;**8**:74-93.

92. MARTIN DM, CRABB HSM. Calcium hydroxide in root canal therapy. A review. *Br Dent J* 1977;**142**:277-83.

93. HERFORTH A, STRASSBURG M. Zur Therapie der chronischapikalen Paradontitis bei traumatisch beschädigten Frontzähnen mit nicht abgeschlossenem Wurzelwachstum. *Dtsch Zahnärtzl Z* 1977;**32**:453-9.

CHAPTER 14

94. CVEK M. Treatment of non-vital permanent incisors with calcium hydroxide. I. Follow-up of periapical repair and apical closure of immature roots. *Odont Revy* 1972;**23**:27-44.

95. KEREKES K, HEIDE S, JACOBSEN I. Follow-up examination of endodontic treatment in traumatized juvenile incisors. *J Endod* 1980;**6**:744-8.

96. CVEK M, SUNDSTRÖM B. Treatment of non-vital permanent incisors with calcium hydroxide. V. Histologic appearance of roentgenologically demonstrable apical closure of immature roots. *Odont Revy* 1974;**25**:379-92.

97. HEIDE S, KEREKES K. Endodontisk behandling av rotåpne permanente incisiver. En histologisk undersökelse over hårdvevsdannelse etter rotfylling med kalsiumhydroxid. *Norske Tandlægeforen Tid* 1977;**87**:426-30.

98. HOLLAND R, DE SOUZA V, TAGLIAVINI RT, MILANEZI LA. Healing processes of teeth with open apices: histologic study. *Bull Tokyo Dent Coll* 1971;**12**:333-8.

99. DYLEWSKI JJ. Apical closure of non-vital teeth. *Oral Surg Oral Med Oral Pathol* 1971;**32**:82-9.

100. STEINER JC, VAN HASSEL HJ. Experimental root apexification in primates. *Oral Surg Oral Med Oral Pathol* 1971;**31**:409-15.

101. HAM JW, PATTERSON SS, MITCHELL DF. Induced apical closure of immature pulpless teeth in monkeys. *Oral Surg Oral Med Oral Pathol* 1972;**33**:438-49.

102. HOLLAND R, DE SOUZA V, DE CAMPOS RUSSO M. Healing processes after root canal therapy in immature human teeth. *Rev Fac Odont Aracatuba* 1973;**2**:269-79.

103. BINNIE WH, ROWE AHR. A histological study of the periapical tissues of incompletely formed pulpless teeth filled with calcium hydroxide. *J Dent Res* 1973;**52**:1110-6.

104. CASTAGNOLA L. *Die Lebenderhaltung der Pulpa in der konservierenden Zahnheilkunde.* Munchen: Carl Hanser Verlag, 1953:127.

105. MATSUMIYA S, KITAMURA K. Histopathological and histobacteriological studies of the relation between the condition of sterilisation of the interior of the root canal and the healing process of periapical tissues in experimentally infected root canal treatment. *Bull Tokyo Dent Coll* 1960;**1**:1-19.

106. CVEK M, HOLLENDER L, NORD C-E. Treatment of non-vital permanent incisors with calcium hydroxide. VI. A clinical, microbiological and radiological evaluation of treatment on one sitting of teeth with mature and immature roots. *Odont Revy* 1976;**27**:93-108.

107. VERNIEKS AA, MASSER LB. Calcium hydroxide induced healing of periapical lesions. A study of 78 non-vital teeth. *J Br Endod Soc* 1978;**11**:61-9.

108. FRANK AL, WEINE FS. Non-surgical therapy for the perforative defect of internal resorption. *J Am Dent Assoc* 1973;**87**:863-8.

109. STEWART GG. Calcium hydroxide-induced root healing. *J Am Dent Assoc* 1975;**90**:793-800, 1975.

110. LAMBJERG-HANSEN L, LEVIN A. Kofferdam. *Tannlægebladet* 1967;**81**:714-16.

111. FRIEND A. The treatment of immature teeth with non-vital pulps. *J Br Endod Soc* 1967;**1**:28-33.

112. TORNECK CD, SMITH JS, GRINDAHL P. Biologic effects of endodontic procedures on developing incisor teeth. III. Effect of debridement and disinfection procedures in treatment of experimentally induced pulp and periapical disease. *Oral Surg Oral Med Oral Pathol* 1973;**35**:532-40.

113. TORNECK CD, SMITH JS, GRINDAHL P. Biologic effects of endodontic procedures on developing incisors teeth. II. Effect of pulp injury and oral contamination. *Oral Surg Oral Med Oral Pathol* 1973;**35**:378-88.

114. CVEK M, NORD C-E, HOLLENDER L. Antimicrobial effect of root canal debridement in teeth with immature root. *Odont Revy* 1976;**27**:1-10.

115. SPÅNGBERG L, RUTBERG M, RYDINGE E. Biologic effects of endodontic antimicrobial agents. *J Endod* 1979;**5**:166-75.

116. HOLLAND R, NERY MJ, DE MELLO W, DE SOUZA V, BERNABÉ PFE, OTOBONI FILHO JA. Root canal treatment with calcium hydroxide. I. Effect of overfilling and refilling. *Oral Surg Oral Med Oral Pathol* 1979;**47**:87-92.

117. HOLLAND R, NERY MJ, DE MELLO W, DE SOUZA V, BERNABÉ PFE, OTOBONI FILHO JA. Root canal treatment with calcium hydroxide. III. Effect of debris and pressure filling. *Oral Surg Oral Med Oral Pathol* 1979;**47**:185-8.

118. TORNECK CD, SMITH JS, GRINDAHL P. Biologic effects of endodontic procedures in developing incisor teeth. IV. Effect of parachlorophenol paste in the treatment of experimentally induced pulp and periapical disease. *Oral Surg Oral Med Oral Pathol* 1973;**35**:541-4.

119. SIMPSON TH, NATKIN E. Guttapercha techniques for filling canals of young permanent teeth after induction of apical root formation. *J Br Endod Soc* 1972;**5**:35-9.

120. RAVN JJ. Konserverende behandling af nekrotiske primære tænder belyst ud fra litteraturen. *Tandlægebladet* 1977;**81**:456-9.

121. RØLLING I, POULSEN S. Formocresol pulpotomy of primary teeth and occurrence of enamel defects on the permanent successors. *Acta Odont Scand* 1978;**36**:243-77.

122. WEINLANDER GHG. Clinical effects of formaldehyde preparations in pulpotomy of primary molars. *J Can Dent Assoc* 1971;**37**:154-9.

123. PRUHS RJ, OLEN GA, SHARMA PS. Relationship between formocresol pulpotomies in primary teeth and enamel defects on their permanent successors. *J Am Dent Assoc* 1977;**94**:698-700.

124. MATSUMIYA S. Experimental pathological study on the effect of treatment of infected root canals in the deciduous tooth on root growth of the permanent tooth germ. *Int Dent J* 1968;**18**:546-59.

125. VALDERHAUG J. Periapical inflammation in primary teeth and its effect on the permanent successors. *Int J Oral Surg* 1974;**3**:171-82.

126. ANDREASEN JO, HJØRTING-HANSEN E. Replantation of teeth. II. Histological study of 22 replanted anterior teeth in humans. *Acta Odont Scand* 1966;**24**:287-306.

127. CVEK M. Treatment on non-vital permanent incisors with calcium hydroxide. II. Effect on external root resorption in luxated teeth compared with effect of root filling with guttapercha. *Odont Revy* 1973;**24**:343-54.

128. LUSTMAN J, EHRLICH J. Deep external resorption: treatment by combined endodontic and surgical approach. A report of 2 cases. *Int J Dent* 1974;**2**:203-6.

129. STÅLHANE I. Permanenta tänder med reducerat pulpalumen som följd av olycksfallsskada. *Svensk Tandläkare Tidskrift* 1971;**64**:311-16.

130. PATTERSON SS, MITCHELL DF. Calcific metamorphosis of the dental pulp. *Oral Surg Oral Med Oral Pathol* 1965;**20**:94-101.

131. FISCHER C-H. Hard tissue formation of the pulp in relation to treatment of traumatic injuries. *Int Dent J* 1974;**24**:387-96.

132. HOLCOMB JB, GREGORY WB JR. Calcific metamorphosis of the pulp: its incidence and treatment. *Oral Surg Oral Med Oral Pathol* 1967;**24**:825-30.

133. LUNDBERG M, CVEK M. A light microscopy study of pulps from traumatized permanent incisors with reduced pulpal lumen. *Acta Odont Scand* 1980;**38**:89-94.

134. CVEK M, GRANATH L-E, LUNDBERG M. Failures and healing in endodontically treated non-vital anterior teeth with posttraumatically reduced pulpal lumen. *Acta Odont Scand* 1982;**40**:223-8.

135. HASSELGREN G, STRÖMBERG T. The use of iodine as a contrast medium in endodontic therapy. *Oral Surg Oral Med Oral Pathol* 1976;**41**:785-8.

136. CASTALDI CR. Traumatic injury to unerupted incisors following a blow to the primary teeth. *J Can Dent Assoc* 1959;**25**:752-62.

137. CUTRIGHT DE. The reaction of permanent tooth buds to injury. *Oral Surg Oral Med Oral Pathol* 1971;**32**:832-9.

138. ANDREASEN JO, SUNDSTRÖM B, RAVN JJ. The effect of traumatic injuries to primary teeth on their permanent successors. I. A clinical and histologic study of 117 injured permanent teeth. *Acta Odont Scand* 1971;**79**:219-83.

139. VAN GOOL AV. Injury to the permanent tooth germ after trauma to the deciduous predecessor. *Oral Surg Oral Med Oral Pathol* 1973;**35**:2-12.

140. SZPRINGER M. Pourazowe znieksztalcenie przednich zebów stalych i zwiazane z tym trudnosci lecznieze. *Czas Stomat* 1973;**26**:855-60.

141. WARFVINGE J, BERGENHOLTZ G. Healing capacity of human and monkey dental pulps following experimentally-induced pulpitis. *Endod Dent Traumatol* 1986;**2**:256-62.

142. BERGENHOLZ G. Relationship between bacterial contamination of dentin and restorative success. In: Rowe NH, ed. *Proceedings of Symposium: Dental pulp - reactions of restorative materials in presence or absence of infection.* Michigan: School of Dentistry, University of Michigan 1982:93-107.

143. SETCOS JC. Dentin bonding in perspective. *Am J Dent* 1988;**6** (Spec Iss):173-175.

144. REES JS, JACOBSEN PH, KOLINIOTOU-KUBIA E. The current status of composite materials and adhesive systems. Part 4.: Some clinically related research. *Rest Dent* 1990;**6**:4-8.

145. HÖRSTED-BINDSLEV P. Monkey pulp reactions to cavities treated with Gluma dentin and restored with a microfilled composite. *Scand J Dent Res* 1987;**95**:347-55.

146. COX CG, FELTON D, BERGENHOLTZ G. Histopathological response of infected cavities treated with Gluma and Scotchbond dentine bonding agents. *Am J Dent* 1988;**6** (Spec Iss):189-94.

147. STANLEY HR, BOWEN RL, COBB EN. Pulp responses to a dentin and enamel adhesive bonding procedures. *Oper Dent* 1988;**13**:107-13.

148. CHOHAYEB AA, BOWEN RL, ADRIAN J. Pulpal response to a dentin and enamel bonding system. *Dent Mater* 1988;**4**:144-6.

149. FRANQUIN C, BROUILLET JL. Biocompatibility of an enamel and dentin adhesive under different conditions of applications. *Quintessenz Int* 1988;**19**:813-26.

150. FELTON D, BERGENHOLTZ G, COX C. Inhibition of bacterial growth under composite restorations following Gluma pretreatment. *J Dent Res* 1989;**68**:1-5.

151. VIRGILLITO A, HOLZ J. Produits adhésifs dentinaires et de scellement soumis au contrôle biologique in vivo. *J Biol Buccale* 1989;**17**:209-24.

152. BOWEN RL, ROPP NW, EICHMILLER FC, STANLEY HR. Clinical biocompatibility of an experimental dentine-enamel adhesive for composites. *Int Dent J* 1989;**39**:247-52.

153. BLOSSER RL, RUPP NW, STANLEY HR, BOWEN RL. Pulpal and micro-organism response to two experimental dental bonding systems. *Dent Mat* 1989;**5**:140-4.

154. LUNDIN S-Å, NOREN JG, WARFVINGE J. Marginal bacterial leakage and pulp reactions in Class II composite resin restorations in vivo. *Swed Dent J* 1990;**14**:185-92.

155. GRIEVE AR, ALANI A, SAUNDERS WP. The effects on the dental pulp of a composite resin and two dentin bonding agents and associated bacterial microleakage. *Int Endod J* 1991;**24**:108-18.

156. ELBAUM R, PIGNOLI C, BROUILLET J. A histologic study of the biocompatiliblity of a dentinal bonding system. *Quintessenz Int* 1991;**22**:901-10.

157. WARFVINGE J, ROZELL B, HEDSTRÖM K-G. Effect of calcium hydroxide treated dentin on pulpal responses. *Int Endod J* 1987;**20**:183-93.

158. PASHLEY DH, KALATHOR S, BURHAM D. The effects of calcium hydroxide dentin permeability. *J Dent Res* 1986;**65**:417-20.

159. MEJÁRE B, MEJÁRE I, EDWARDSSON S. Acid etching and composite resin restorations. A culturing and histologic study on bacterial penetration. *Endod Dent Traumatol* 1987; **3**:1-5.

160. ANDREASEN FM, BROHOLM FAHRNER A, BORUM M, ANDREASEN JO. Long-term prognosis of crown fractures treated by reattachment of the original fragment using the Gluma dentin bonding system. 1993. Manuscript in preparation.

161. ANDREASEN FM, BROHOLM FAHRNER A, BORUM M, ANDREASEN JO. Long-term prognosis of crown fractures: pulp survival after injury. 1993: Manuscript in preparation.

162. CVEK M. Results after partial pulpotomy in crown fractured teeth 3-15 years after treatment. *Acta Stomatol Croat* (in press).

163. COX CF, BERGENHOLTZ G, FITZGERALD M, HEYS DR, AVERY JK, BAKER JA. Capping of the dental pulp mechanically exposed to the oral microflora - a 5 week observation of wound healing in monkey. *J Oral Pathol* 1982;**11**:327-39.

164. HERMANN BW. *Biologische Wurzelbehandlung.* Frankfurt am Main: von Kramer Co, 1936:272.

165. FOREMAN PC, BARNES IE. A review of calcium hydroxide. *Int Endod J* 1990;**23**:83-97.

166. CVEK M, GRANATH L, CLEATON-JONES P, AUSTIN J. Hard tissue barrier formation on pulpotomized monkey teeth capped with cyanoacrylate or calcium hydroxide for 10 and 60 minutes. *J Dent Res* 1987;**66**:1166-74.

167. GRANATH L. Pulp capping materials. In: Smith DC, Williams DF. eds. *Biocompatibility of dental materials* Vol. II. Boca Raton, FL: CRC Press Inc.1982:253-67.

168. COX CF, KEALL HJ, OSTRO E, BERGENHOLTZ G. Biocompatibility of surface-sealed dental materials against exposed pulps. *Prosthet Dent* 1987;**57**:1-8.

169. HEYS DR, FITZGERALD RJ, HEYS RJ, CHIEGO DJ. Healing of primate dental pulps capped with teflon. *Oral Surg Oral Med Oral Pathol* 1990;**69**:227-37.

170. GORDON TM, RANDLY DM, BOYAN BD. The effects of calcium hydroxide on bovine pulp tissue: Variations in pH and calcium concentration. *J Endod* 1985;**11**:156-60.

171. TRONSTAD L. Reaction of the exposed pulp to Dycal treatment. *Oral Surg Oral Med Oral Pathol* 1974;**34**:477-85.

172. HEYS DR, HEYS RJ, COX CF, AVERY JK. The response of four calcium hydroxides on monkey pulp. *J Oral Pathol* 1989;**9**:372-9.

173. COX CF, BERGENHOLTZ G, HEYS DR, SYED SA, FITZGERALD M, HEYS RJ. Pulp capping of dental pulp mechanically exposed to oral microflora: a 1-2 year observation of wound healing in the monkey. *J Oral Pathol* 1985;**14**:156-68.

174. SCHRÖDER U. Effects of calcium hydroxide-containing pulp-capping agents on pulp cell migration, proliferation and differentiation. *J Dent Res* 1985;**64** (Spec Iss):541-48.

175. SELTZER S, BENDER IB. *The dental pulp. Biologic considerations in dental procedures.* 3rd edn. Philadelphia: JB Lippincott Co, 1984:356.

176. BERKMAN D, CUCOLO FA, LEVIN MP, BRUNELLE LJ. Pulpal response to isobutyl cyanoacrylate in human teeth. *J Am Dent Assoc* 1971;**83**:140-5.

177. HEYS DR, COX CF, HEYS RJ, AVERY JK. Histological considerations of direct pulp capping agents. *J Dent Res* 1981;**60**:1371-9.

178. HELLER AL, KOENINGS JF, BRILLIANT JD, MELFI RC, DRISKELL TD. Direct pulp capping of permanent teeth in primates using resorbable form of tricalcium phosphate ceramics. *J Endod* 1975;**1**:95-101.

179. FUKS A, CHOSAK A, EIDELMAN E. Partial pulpotomy as an alternative treatment alternative for exposed pulps in crown-fractured permanent incisors. *Endod Dent Traumatol* 1987;**3**:100-2.

180. CVEK M, LUNDBERG M. Histological appearance of pulps after exposure by a crown fracture, partial pulpotomy and clinical diagnosis of healing. *J Endod* 1983;**9**:8-11.

CHAPTER 14

181. MESIC-PAR N, PECINA-HRNCEVIC A, STIPETIC S. Clinical and histological examination of young permanent teeth after vital amputation of the pulp (English summary). *Acta Stomatol Croat* 1990;**24**:253-62.

182. HEIDE S, KEREKES K. Delayed direct pulp capping in permanent incisors of monkeys. *Int Endod J* 1987;**20**:65-74.

183. PITT FORD TR, ROBERTS GJ. Immediate and delayed direct pulp capping with the use of a new visible light-cured calcium hydroxide preparation. *Oral Surg Oral Med Oral Pathol* 1991;**71**:388-42.

184. BERGENHOLTZ G, COX CF, LOESHE WJ, SYED SA. Bacterial leakage around dental restorations: its effect on the dental pulp. *J Oral Pathol* 1982;**11**:439-50.

185. BERGENHOLTZ G. Bacterial leakage around dental restorations-impact on the pulp. In: Anusavice KJ, ed. *Quality evaluation of dental restorations,* Lombard IL: Quintessence Publishing Co, 1989:243-54.

186. PASHLEY DH. Clinical considerations of microleakage. *J Endod* 1990;**16**:70-7.

187. SCHRÖDER U, GRANATH L-E. Scanning electron microscopy of hard tissue barrier following experimental pulpotomy of intact human teeth and capping with calcium hydroxide. *Odont Revy* 1974;**25**:57-67.

188. ULMANSKY M, SELA J, SELA M. Scanning electron microscopy of calcium hydroxide induced bridges. *J Oral Pathol* 1972;**1**:244-8.

189. GOLDBERG F, NASSONE EJ, SPIELBERG C. Evaluation of the dentinal bridge after pulpotomy and calcium hydroxide dressing. *J Endod* 1984;**10**:318-20.

190. MÖLLER ÅJR. *Microbiologic examination of root canals and periapical tissues of human teeth* (Thesis). Gothenburg: Akademiförlaget 1966:380 p.

191. PLANT CG. The effect of polycarboxylate cement on the dental pulp. A study. *Br Dent J* 1970;**129**:424-6.

192. PRADER F. *Diagnose und Therapie des infizierten Wurzelkanales.* Basel: Beno Schwabe Co, 1949:224.

193. PEREIRA JC, STANLEY HR. Pulp capping: influence of the exposure site on pulp healing - histologic and radiographic study. *J Endod* 1981;**7**:213-23.

194. FUKS AB, BIELAK S, CHOSAK A. Clinical and radiographic assessment of direct pulp capping and pulpotomy in young permanent teeth. *Pediatr Dent* 1982;**4**:240-4.

195. GELBIER MJ, WINTER GB. Traumatized incisors treated by vital pulpotomy: a retrospective study. *Br Dent J* 1988;**164**:319-23.

196. HÖRSTED P, SØNDERGAARD B, THYLSTRUP A, EL ATTAR K, FEJERSKOV O. A retrospective study of direct pulp capping with calcium hydroxide. *Endod Dent Traumatol* 1985;**1**:29-34.

197. DELESSERT Y, HOLZ J, BAUME L-J. Contrôle radiologique a court et à long terms du traitement radiculaire de la catégorie III de pulpopathies. *Schweiz Monatschr Zahnheil* 1980;**90**:585-607.

198. JACOBSEN I, KEREKES K. Diagnosis and treatment of pulp necrosis in permanent anterior teeth with root fracture. *Scand J Dent Res* 1980;**88**:370-6.

199. ANDREASEN FM, ANDREASEN JO, BAYER T. Prognosis of root-fractured permanent incisors - prediction of healing modalities. *Endod Dent Traumatol* 1989;**5**:11-22.

200. ANDREASEN FM, ANDREASEN JO. Resorption and mineralization processes following root fracture of permanent incisors. *Endod Dent Traumatol* 1988;**4**:202-14.

201. CVEK M, CLEATON-JONES P, AUSTIN J, KLING M, LOWNIE J, FATTI P. Effect of topical application of doxycycline on pulp revascularization and periodontal healing in reimplanted monkey incisors. *Endod Dent Traumatol* 1990;**6**:170-6.

202. ANDREASEN FM, VESTERGAARD PEDERSEN B. Prognosis of luxated permanent teeth - the development of pulp necrosis. *Endod Dent Traumatol* 1985;**1**:207-20.

203. CIPRIANO TJ, WALTON RE. The ishemic infarct pulp of traumatized teeth: A light and electron microscopic study. *Endod Dent Traumatol* 1986;**2**:196-204.

204. TZIAFAS D. Pulpal reactions following experimental acute trauma of concussion type on immature dog teeth. *Endod Dent Traumatol* 1988;**4**:27-31.

205. OIKARINEN K, GUNDLACH KKH, PFEIFER G. Late complications of luxation injuries to teeth. *Endod Dent Traumatol* 1987;**3**:296-303.

206. ANDREASEN FM. A histological and bacteriological investigation of pulps extirpated following luxation injuries. *Endod Dent Traumatol* 1988;**4**:170-81.

207. CVEK M, CLEATON-JONES P, AUSTIN J, LOWNIE J, KLING M, FATTI P. Pulp revascularization in reimplanted monkey incisors - predictability and the effect of antibiotic systemic prophylaxis. *Endod Dent Traumatol* 1990;**6**:1567-69.

208. KOCH G, ULLBRO C. Klinisk funktionstid hos 55 exartikulerade och replanterade tänder. *Tandläkartidningen* 1982;**74**:18-25.

209. KLING M, CVEK M, MEJÁRE I. Rate and predictability of pulp revascularization in therapeutically reimplanted permanent incisors. *Endod Dent Traumatol* 1986;**2**:83-9.

210. DELIVANIS PD, FAN VSC. The localization of blood-borne bacteria in instrumented and overinstrumented canals. *J Endod* 1984;**10**:521-4.

211. BARRET AP, READE PC. Revascularization of mouse tooth isographs and allographs using autoradiography and carbonperfusion. *Arch Oral Biol* 1981;**26**:541-5.

212. ANDRESEN FM. Transient apical breakdown and its relation to color and sensitivity changes after luxation injuries to teeth. *Endod Dent Traumatol* 1986;**2**:9-19.

213. JACOBSEN I. Criteria for diagnosis of pulp necrosis in traumatized permanent incisors. *Scand J Dent Res* 1980;**88**:306-12.

214. ANDREASEN FM. Pulpal healing after luxation injuries and root fracture in the permanent dentition. *Endod Dent Traumatol* 1989;**5**:11-31.

215. FULLING H-J, ANDREASEN JO. Influence of maturation status and tooth type of permanent teeth upon electrometric and thermal pulp testing. *Scand J Dent Res* 1976;**84**:286-90.

216. FULLING H-J, ANDREASEN JO. Influence of splints and temporary crowns upon electric and thermal pulp-testing procedures. *Scand J Dent Res* 1976;**84**:291-6.

217. GAZELIUS B, OLGART L, EDWALL B. Restored vitality in luxated teeth assessed by Laser Doppler flowmeter. *Endod Dent Traumatol* 1988;**4**:265-8.

218. OLGART L, GAZELIUS B, LLINDH-STRÖMBERG U. Laser Doppler flowmetry in assessing vitality in luxated permanent teeth. *Int Endod J* 1988;**21**:300-6.

219. MÖLLER ÅJR, FABRICIUS L, DAHLEN G, ÖHMAN AE, HEYDEN G. Influence on periapical tissues of indigenous oral bacteria and necrotic pulp tissue in monkeys. *Scand J Dent Res* 1981;**89**:475-84.

220. ANDREASEN JO. The effect of pulp extirpation or root canal treatment on periodontal healing after replantation of permanent incisors in monkeys. *J Endod* 1981;**7**:245-52.

221. NICHOLLS E. Endodontic treatment during root formation. *Int Dent J* 1981;**31**:49-59.

222. GHOSE LJ, BAGHDADY VS, HIKMAT BYM. Apexification of immature apices of pulpless permanent anterior teeth with calcium hydroxide. *J Endod* 1987;**13**:285-90.

223. MACKIE IC, BENTLEY EM, WORTHINGTON HV. The closure of open apices in non-vital immature incisor teeth. *Br Dent J* 1988;**165**:169-73.

224. YATES JA. Barrier formation time in non-vital teeth with open apices. *Int Endod J* 1988;**21**:313-19.

225. CHAWLA HS. Apical closure in a non-vital permanent tooth using one Ca(OH)$_2$ dressing. *ASDC J Dent Child* 1986;**53**:44-7.

226. KLEIER DJ, BARR ES. A study of endodontically apexified teeth. *Endod Dent Traumatol* 1991;**7**:112-7.

227. CVEK M. Prognosis of luxated non-vital maxillary incisors treated with calcium hydroxide and filled with guttapercha. *Endod Dent Traumatol* 1992;**8**:45-55.

228. HERFORTH A, SEICHTER U. Die apikale Hartsubstanzbarriere nach temporären Wurzelkanalfüllungen mit Kalziumhydroxid. *Dtsch Zahnärtzl Z* 1980;**35**:1053-7.

229. JAVELET J, TORABINEJAD M, BAKLAND L. Comparison of two pH levels for the induction of apical barriers in immature teeth of monkeys. *J Endod* 1985;**11**:375-8.

230. BYSTRÖM A, CLAESSON R, SUNDQVIST G. The antibacterial effect of camphorated paramonochlorophenol, camphorated phenol and calcium hydroxide in the treatment of infected root canals. *Endod Dent Traumatol* 1985;**1**:170-5.

231. SAFAVI KE, DOWDEN WE, INTROCASO JH, LANGELAND K. A comparison of antimicrobial effects of calcium hydroxide and iodine-potassium iodide. *J Endod* 1985;**11**:454-6.

232. ALLARD U, STRÖMBERG U, STRÖMBERG T. Endodontic treatment of experimentally induced apical periodontitis in dogs. *Endod Dent Traumatol* 1987;**3**:240-4.

233. SJÖGREN U, FIDGOR D, SPÅNGBERG L, SUNDQVIST G. The antibacterial effect of calcium hydroxide as a short-term intracanal dressing. *Int Endod J* 1991;**24**:119-25.

234. ØRSTAVIK D, KEREKES K, MOLVEN O. Effects of extensive apical reaming and calcium hydroxide dressing on bacterial infection during treatment of apical periodontitis. *Int Endod J* 1991;**24**:1-7.

235. HAAPASALO M, ØRSTAVIK D. In vitro infection and disinfection of dentinal tubules. *J Dent Res* 1987;**66**:1375-9.

236. SAFAVI KE, SPÅNGBERG LSW, LANGELAND K. Root canal dentinal tubule disinfection. *J Endod* 1990;**16**:207-10.

237. HASSELGREN G, OLSSON B, CVEK M. Effects of calcium hydroxide and sodium hypochlorite on the dissolution of necrotic porcine muscle tissue. *J Endod* 1988;**14**:125-7.

238. ANDERSEN M, LUND J, ANDREASEN JO, ANDREASEN FM. In vitro solubility of human pulp tissue in calcium hydroxide and sodium hypochlorite. *Endod Dent Traumatol* 1992;**8**:104-8.

239. METZLER RS, MONTGOMERY S. The effectiveness of ultrasonic and calcium hydroxide for the debridement of human mandibular molars. *J Endod* 1989;**15**:373-8.

240. MITCHELL DF, SHANKWALKER GB. Osteogenetic potential of calcium hydroxide and other materials in soft tissue and bone wounds. *J Dent Res* 1958;**37**:1157-63.

241. RASMUSSEN P, MJÖR IA. Calcium hydroxide as an ectopic bone inductor in rats. *Scand J Dent Res* 1971;**79**:24-30.

242. RÖNNING O, KOSKI AK. The fate of anorganic implants in the subcutaneous tissue in rat. *Plast Reconstr Surg* 1966;**37**:121-4.

243. TROPE M, TRONSTAD L. Long-term calcium hydroxide treatment of a tooth with iatrogenic root perforation and lateral periodontitis. *Endod Dent Traumatol* 1985;**1**:35-8.

244. PETTERSSON K, HASSELGREN G, TRONSTAD L. Endodontic treatment of experimental root perforations in dog teeth. *Endod Dent Traumatol* 1985;**1**:22-8.

245. NORDENWALL K-J, HOLM K. Management of cervical root perforation: report of a case. *ASDC J Dent Child* 1990;**57**:454-8.

246. OHARA PK, TORABINEJAD M. Apical closure of an immature root subsequent to apical curretage. *Endod Dent Traumatol* 1992;**8**:134-7.

247. BYSTRÖM A, SUNDQVIST G. The antibacterial action of sodium hypochlorite and EDTA in 60 cases of endodontic therapy. *Int Endod J* 1985;**18**:35-40.

248. BYSTRÖM A, HAPPONEN R-P, SJÖGREN U, SUNDQVIST G. Healing of periapical lesions of pulpless teeth after endodontic treatment with controlled asepsis. *Endod Dent Traumatol* 1987;**3**:58-63.

249. CHONG BS, PITT FORD TR. The role of intracanal medication in root canal treatment. *Int Endod J* 1992;**25**:97-106.

250. ØRSTAVIK D. Endodontic materials. *Adv Dent Res* 1988;**2**:12-24.

251. KEREKES K, TRONSTAD L. Long-term results of endodontic treatment performed with a standardized technique. *J Endod* 1979;**5**:83-90.

252. TRONSTAD L, ANDREASEN JO, HASSELGREN G, KRISTERSON L, RIIS I. pH changes in dental tissues after root canal filling with calcium hydroxide. *J Endod* 1981;**7**:17-21.

253. HAMMARTSTRÖM LE, BLOMLÖF LB, FEIGLIN B, LINDSKOG S. Effect of calcium hydroxide treatment on periodontal repair and root resorption. *Endod Dent Traumatol* 1986;**2**:184-9.

254. BLOMLÖF L, LINDSKOG S, HAMMARSTRÖM L. Influence of pulpal treatments on cell and tissue reactions in the marginal periodontium. *J Periodontol* 1988;**59**:577-83.

255. LENGHEDEN A, BLOMLÖF L, LINDSKOG S. Effect of immediate calcium hydroxide treatment and permanent root-filling on periodontal healing in contaminated replanted teeth. *Scand J Dent Res* 1991;**99**:139-146.

256. LENGHEDEN A, BLOMLÖF L, LINDSKOG S. Effect of delayed calcium hydroxide treatment on periodontal healing in contaminated replanted teeth. *Scand J Dent Res* 1991;**99**:147-53.

257. MAKKES PG, THODEN VAN VELZEN SK. Cervical external root resorption. *J Dent Res* 1975;**3**:217-22.

258. TRONSTAD L. Pulp reactions in traumatized teeth. In: Guttman, JI, Harrison JW, eds. *Proceedings of the International Conference on Oral Trauma.* Chicago: American Association of Endodontists Endowment and Memorial Foundation 1984:55-77.

259. TRONSTAD L. Root resorption - etiology, terminology and clinical manifestations. *Endod Dent Traumatol* 1988;**4**:241-52.

260. RUD J, RUD V, MUNKSGAARD EC. Retrograd rodfyldning med plast og dentinbinder: Indikation og anvendelsesmuligheder. (Retrograde root filling with resin and a dentin bonding agent: indication and applications). *Tandlægebladet* 1989;**93**:223-29

261. FRANK AL, BAKLAND LK. Non-endodontic therapy for supraosseous extracanal invasive resorption. *J Endod* 1987;**13**:348-55.

262. HEITHERSAY GS. Combined endodontic-orthodontic treatment of transverse root fractures in the region of the cervical alveolar crest. *Oral Surg Oral Med Oral Pathol* 1973;**36**:404-15.

263. MALMGREN O, MALMGREN B, FRYKHOLM A. Rapid orthodontic extrusion of crown-root and cervical root fractured teeth. *Endod Dent Traumatol* 1991;**7**:49-54.

264. TEGSJÖ U, VALERIUS-OLSSON H, OLGART K. Intra-alveolar transplantation of teeth with cervical root fractures. *Swed Dent J* 1978;**2**:73-82.

265. KAHNBERG K-E. Intraalveolar transplantation of teeth with crown-root fractures. *J Oral Maxillofac Surg* 1985;**43**:38-42.

266. MALMGREN B, CVEK M, LUNDBERG M, FRYKHOLM A. Surgical treatment of ankylosed and infrapositioned reimplanted incisors in adolescents. *Scand J Dent Res* 1984;**92**:391-9.

267. WEDENBERG C, ZETTERQVIST L. Internal resorption in human teeth - a histological, scanning electron microscopic and enzyme histochemical study. *J Endod* 1987;**13**:255-9.

268. WEDENBERG C, LINDSKOG S. Experimental internal resorption in monkey teeth. *Endod Dent Traumatol* 1985;**1**:221-7.

269. WALTON RE, LEONARD LE. Cracked tooth: an etiology for "idiopathic" internal resorption ? *J Endod* 1986;**12**:167-9.

270. SMITH JW. Calcific metamorphosis: a treatment dilemma. *Oral Surg Oral Med Oral Pathol* 1982;**54**:441-4.

271. SCHINDLER WG, GULLICKSON DC. Rationale for the management of calcific metamorphosis secondary to traumatic injuries. *J Endod* 1988;**14**:408-12.

272. SELDEN HS. The role of a dental operating microscope in improved non-surgical treatment of "calcified" canals. *Oral Surg Oral Med Oral Pathol* 1989;**68**:93-8.

273. JACOBSEN I, SANGNES G. Traumatized primary anterior teeth. Prognosis related to calcific reactions in the pulp cavity. *Acta Odont Scand* 1978;**36**:199-204.

274. FRANK AL. Bleaching of vital and non-vital teeth. In: Cohen S, Burns RC, eds. *Pathways of the pulp*, 2nd edn. St. Louis: C.V. Mosby Co 1980:568-75.

275. NUTTING EB, POE GS. A new combination for bleaching teeth. *J South Calif Dent Assoc* 1963;**31**:289-291.

276. GROSSMAN LI. *Endodontic practice*. 9nd edn. Philadelphia: Lea & Febiger, 1978:440.

277. VAN DER BURGT T. *Tooth color and tooth discoloration. In vitro studies on tooth color and tooth discoloration related to endodontic procedures* (Thesis). Nijmegen: Catholic University of Nijmegen 1985.

278. STEWART GG. Bleaching discolored pulpless teeth. *J Am Dent Assoc* 1965;**70**:325-8.

279. LEMON RR. Bleaching and restoring endodontically treated teeth. *Current Opinion in Dentistry* 1991;**1**:754-59.

280. HARRINGTON GW, NATKIN E. External resorption associated with bleaching of pulpless teeth. *J Endod* 1979;**5**:344-8.

281. LADO AE, STANLEY HR, WEISMAN MI. Cervical resorption in bleached teeth. *Oral Surg Oral Med Oral Pathol* 1983;**55**:78-80.

282. MONTGOMERY S. External cervical resorption after bleaching a pulpless tooth. *Oral Surg Oral Med Oral Pathol* 1984;**57**:203-6.

283. CVEK M, LINDWALL A-M. External root resorption following bleaching of pulpless teeth with oxygen peroxide. *Endod Dent Traumatol* 1985;**1**:56-60.

284. FRIEDMAN S, ROTSTEIN I, LIBFELD H, STABHOLTZ A, HELING I. Incidence of external root resorption and esthetic results in 58 bleached pulpless teeth. *Endod Dent Traumatol* 1988;**4**:23-26.

285. FUSS Z, SZAJKIS S, TAGGER M. Tubular permeability to calcium hydroxide and to bleaching agents. *J Endod* 1989;**15**:362-4.

286. MADISON S, WALTON R. Cervical root resorption following bleaching of endodontically treated teeth. *J Endod* 1990;**16**:570-4.

287. ROTSTEIN I, FRIEDMAN S, MOR C, KATZNELSON J, SOMMER M, BAB I. Histological characterization of bleaching-induced external root resorption in dogs. *J Endod* 1991;**17**:436-41.

288. ROTSTEIN I, TOREK Y, LEWINSTEIN I. Effect of bleaching time and temperature on the radicular penetration of hydrogen peroxide. *Endod Dent Traumatol* 1991;**7**:196-8.

289. ROTSTEIN I, TOREK Y, MISGAV R. Effect of cementum defects on radicular penetration of 30 % H_2O_2 during intracoronal bleaching. *J Endod* 1991;**17**:230-3.

290. SPASSER HF. A simple bleaching technique using sodium perborate. *NY State Dent J* 1961;**27**:332-4.

291. SARP OP. Blegning af rodfyldte, misfarvede taender. *Tandlægebladet* 1978;**82**:73-7.

292. HOLMSTRUP G, PALM AM, LAMBJERG-HANSEN H. Bleaching of discoloured root-filled teeth. *Endod Dent Traumatol* 1988;**4**:197-201.

293. HO S, GOERIG A. An in vitro comparison of different bleaching agents in the discoloured tooth. *J Endod* 1989;**15**:106-11.

294. HOLMSTRUP G, PALM AM, LAMBJERG-HANSEN H. Blegning af misfarvede rodfyldte tænder. Resultater efter 3 og 5 års observationstid. *Tandlægebladet* 1989;**93**:445-9.

295. ROTSTEIN I, ZALKIND M, MOR C, TAREBAH A, FRIEDMAN S. In vitro efficacy of sodium perborate preparations used for intracoronal bleaching of discoloured non-vital teeth. *Endod Dent Traumatol* 1991;**7**:177-80.

296. SCHRÖDER U, HEIDE S, HÖSKULDSSON O, RØLLING I. Endodontics. In: Koch G, Modeer TH, Poulsen S, Rasmussen P, eds. *Pedodontics - a clinical approach*. Copenhagen: Munksgaard 1991:185-210.

CHAPTER 15

Orthodontic Management of the Traumatized Dentition

O. MALMGREN, B. MALMGREN & L. GOLDSON

Treatment planning for patients with traumatized teeth involves a detailed evaluation of both the prognosis for the injured teeth and treatment of an eventual malocclusion. A coordinated treatment plan, incorporating clinical and radiographic findings of healing and of complications must be established before orthodontic treatment is initiated. This plan should be based on a realistic evaluation of the prognosis for the injured teeth.

Diagnosis and Treatment Planning

Preventive Orthodontics

Dental injuries in the mixed and permanent dentitions are most frequent in children from 8 to 9 years of age and most injuries involve the upper incisors. Boys are injured twice as often as girls. Patients with an increased overjet are at significantly greater risk of dental injury (1-22). One study has shown that an increase of the overjet from 0 - 3 mm to 3 - 6 mm doubles the extent of traumatic dental injuries. With an overjet exceeding 6 mm, the severity is tripled (20). An additional trauma factor is insufficient lip closure, which often leaves the upper incisors unprotected (10,11,14,137,138). Patients treated for dental injuries often sustain repeated trauma to the teeth (13).

Considering the frequency of traumatic dental injuries in school-age children, it is apparent that the majority of children with increased maxillary overjet will have sustained a traumatic dental injury prior to school-leaving age (13,20,23-25). The treatment of increased maxillary overjet should therefore begin early, as a precaution against traumatic dental injuries (81,82). If this is not possible, the child should be provided with a mouthguard during contact sports. Such a mouthguard can even be combined with a fixed orthodontic appliance (see Chapter 21, p.731).

Primary Dentition

Avulsion or extraction of primary incisors can lead to drifting of adjacent teeth as well as disturbances in eruption of the permanent successors. Early loss of primary teeth sometimes leads to delayed eruption of the permanent successors often in a more labial position (26-28). Conversely, loss of primary teeth at a later stage of development can lead to premature eruption of permanent teeth (27). However, these disturbances do not usually lead to loss of space and consequently do not require space maintenance or other orthodontic treatment (29).

Mixed Dentition

To minimize the risk of injuries in patients with proclined incisors, orthodontic treatment should be planned at the mixed dentition stage. Treatment of skeletal and dento-alveolar deviations, particularly in patients with Angle Class II, division 1 and 2 malocclusions, should be based on individual growth rate (30).

In the case of accidental loss of 1 or more incisors, it should be decided at the mixed dentition stage whether to partially or completely close the space or to maintain it.

In patients with skeletal deviations, extraoral forces can be used. But in some Class II division 1 cases with accidental loss of one or more permanent incisors, it may be better to leave the molars in their disto-occlusion and close the space anteriorly.

In patients with normal skeletal sagittal relations without crowding, it is usually better to delay orthodontic therapy until the permanent dentition stage. Meanwhile it is important to avoid tooth migrations and midline shift (Fig. 15.1).

Permanent Dentition

If trauma occurs in the permanent dentition, it must be determined whether any growth potential remains. Especially in cases with skeletal deviations, it is essential to coordinate the remaining growth potential with the proposed orthodontic treatment.

Factors in Treatment Planning

A treatment plan which involves the various dental specialities (i.e. pedodontics, endodontics, oral surgery, orthodontics and general dentistry) must be based on a realistic evaluation of orthodontic treatment possibilities and optimal treatment of the traumatized dentition. Before orthodontic treatment of a traumatized dentition is initiated, a number of factors should be considered.

Treatment Sequence and Timing

Sequence and timing of treatment is essential in all dentitions. Dental injuries to the primary teeth most often occur at 2 to 4 years of age. There is a close relationship between the apices of the primary incisors and the permanent successors. Thus a trauma to the primary dentition may cause disturbances in development and eruption of the permanent successors.

In general, orthodontic treatment should be initiated in the mixed dentition. In cases of trauma at an early age, treatment can be shorter and performed with less complicated appliances if the age of the patient as well as the dental and skeletal development and maturity are considered.

Observation Periods Prior to Orthodontic Treatment

CROWN AND CROWN-ROOT FRACTURES

Crown fractures and crown-root fractures without pulpal involvement have a good prognosis if properly treated. An observation period of about 3 months prior to initiation of treatment is sufficient.

A crown and crown-root fracture with pulpal involvement can be treated orthodontically after partial pulpectomy, once a hard tissue barrier has been established. As a rule, such a barrier can be diagnosed radiographically 3 months after treatment.

ROOT FRACTURES

While an observation period of 2 years has been recommended before orthodontic movement of root-fractured teeth (31), recent clinical experience indicates that most complications (e.g. pulp necrosis) occur during the 1st year after the trauma (83,84). Thus the observation period may be shortened if no complications occur.

LUXATED TEETH

After luxation of teeth, a number of complications (e.g. pulp necrosis, root resorption and loss of marginal bone) may occur.

Clinical experience indicates an observation period of at least 3 months after a mild injury (e.g. concussion and subluxation).

If endodontic treatment is to be performed, orthodontic movement should be postponed until there is radiographic evidence of healing (Fig. 15.2).

Pulp canal obliteration as a consequence of trauma indicates repair of the traumatized pulp. However, a repeated trauma or a heavy orthodontic force may cause further damage to the pulp.

Fig. 15.1. The use of a space maintainer in the mixed dentition

This is an 8-year-old boy. Due to a trauma in the primary dentition, the right upper incisor was malformed, and adjacent teeth were tilting towards the area of the impacted incisor. The radiograph shows the condition at 8 years of age. Due to the immature root development of the lateral incisor, surgery was postponed for 2 years.

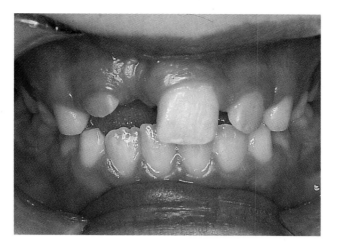

Inserting a space maintainer and timing of surgical removal of the malformed central incisor

A removable plate with Adam's clasps and fingersprings was inserted for uprighting the tilted incisors. Due to large difference in incisor width and wide apical base conditions, space closure was not indicated.

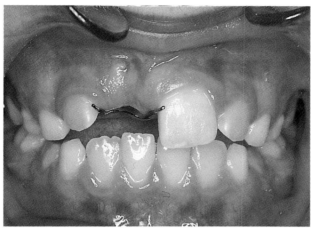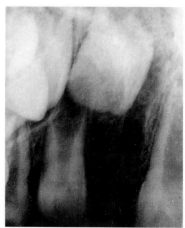

Inserting a removable appliance with a prosthetic tooth

When the teeth had been uprighted, a prosthetic tooth was fitted to the plate.

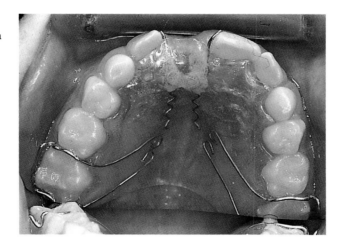

Fixed space maintainer in the late mixed dentition

After eruption of the first bicuspids, and during eruption of the canines, a lingual arch was soldered to molar bands. Occlusal stops on the first bicuspids and stops on both sides of a prosthetic tooth were used. When the upper canines were fully erupted, an acid-etch bridge was constructed.

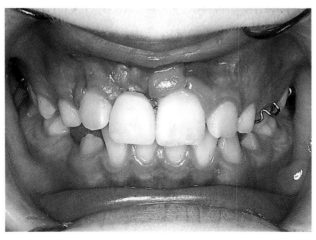

ORTHODONTIC MANAGEMENT OF THE TRAUMATIZED DENTITION

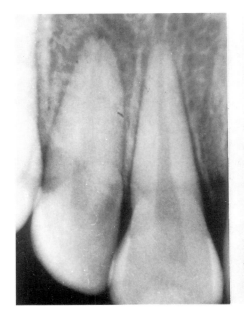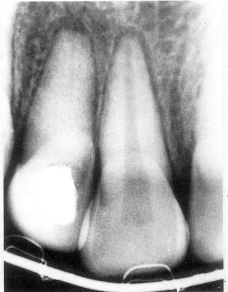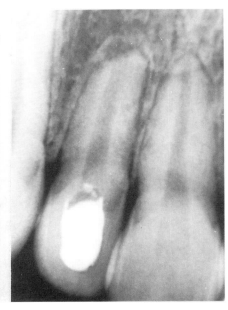

Fig. 15.2. Endodontic problems arising when orthodontic movement is initiated prior to completion of endodontic therapy of the right lateral incisor
A. Radiographic examination at the time of injury. B. As a result of orthodontic movement, apical root resorption is seen 3 months after initiation of orthodontic therapy. Moreover, a hard tissue barrier at the apical foramen has failed to appear despite repeated filling with calcium hydroxide. C. One year after initiation of orthodontic therapy and 3 years after the initial radiograph, there is still no sign of hard tissue formation.

After a moderate or severe luxation injury (e.g. extrusion, lateral luxation, intrusion and avulsion followed by replantation) the observation period should be at least 1 year. Concerning intruded teeth, see page 617.

Endodontically-Treated Teeth

A slightly greater frequency of root resorption after orthodontic treatment has been reported in endodontically-treated compared with vital teeth (32), but it has also been found that root-filled teeth sometimes resorb less than their vital antimeres (85, 86) (Fig. 15.3). A few root-filled teeth, however, resorb for unknown reasons (Fig. 15.4). Another experimental study has shown no difference in the frequency of root resorption after orthodontic movement when comparing vital and endodontically-treated teeth (138). This is in agreement with the authors' observations that root-filled teeth without signs of already existing root resorption can normally be moved without extensive root resorption.

In order to minimize the risk of root resorption, or its exacerbation, in teeth requiring endodontic therapy during orthodontic movement, clinical experience indicates that the final gutta-percha root filling should be postponed until completion of orthodontic tooth movement. An interim dressing of calcium hydroxide should therefore be maintained during active orthodontic treatment. This is not to say, however, that a successful gutta percha root filling should be removed when already in place.

Root Surface Resorption (External Root Resorption)

Damage to the periodontal ligament after a trauma can result in three types of external root resorption: surface resorption, inflammatory resorption and replacement resorption. (see Chapter 10, p. 391).

Surface resorption implies a self-limiting resorption process which is repaired with new cementum. Teeth with minor surface resorptions can be moved orthodontically with a prognosis similar to that of uninjured teeth.

Inflammatory resorption implies a rapid resorption of both cementum and dentin with inflammation of adjacent periodontal tissue. This type of resorption is related to an infected and necrotic pulp and can usually be seen 3 to 6 weeks after injury. It is essential that proper endodontic treatment is initiated immediately. Arrest of the inflammatory resorption can be seen in about 96% of cases (87) (see Chapter 14, p. 558). Orthodontic treatment should be postponed until radiographic healing is seen and at least 1 year should elapse before orthodontic treatment is instituted.

Teeth with evidence of root resorption

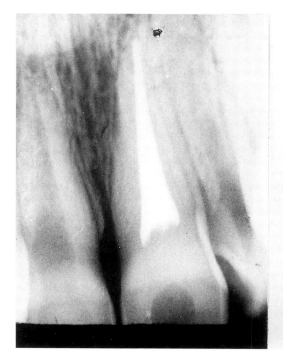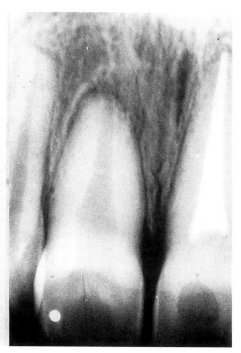

Fig. 15.3.

Response of a vital and a root-filled tooth to orthodontic movement. The patient had a Class II div. 1 malocclusion and was treated with fixed appliances for 18 months A. Condition before orthodontic treatment. Both central incisors sustained traumatic dental injury. As a result, the left central incisor was treated endodontically due to pulp necrosis. B. After orthodontic treatment, the left central incisor demonstrates slight apical root resorption and the right central incisor, with a vital pulp, severe root resorption. Both teeth were moved orthodontically in the same manner.

Fig. 15.4.

Different responses to orthodontic movement of 2 endodontically treated teeth. Both teeth were moved in the same manner
The patient had a Class II div. 1 malocclusion and was treated with fixed appliances for 19 months. A. Before orthodontic treatment. Both central incisors were traumatically injured and root filled. B. After orthodontic treatment, the right central incisor demonstrates slight root resorption, while the left central incisor demonstrates unusually extensive root resorption.

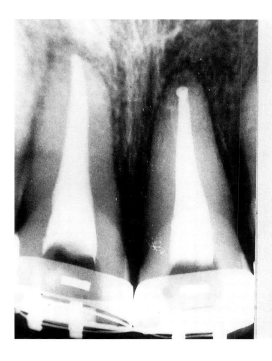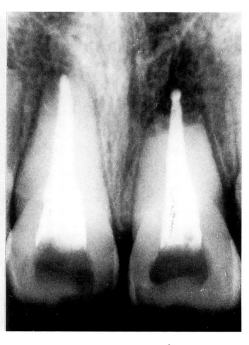

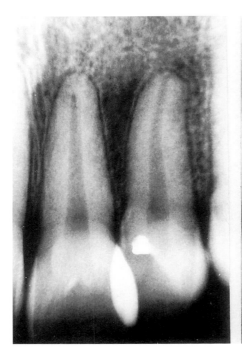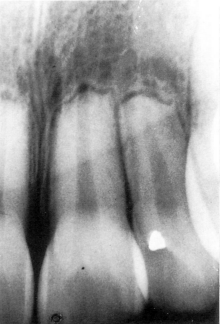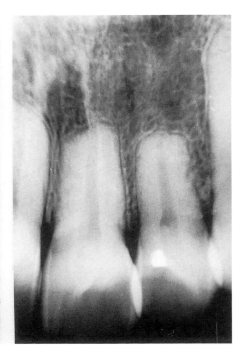

Fig. 15.5.
Vital teeth with signs of root resorption before orthodontic treatment. A. The lateral incisor shows an irregular root contour due to root resorption prior to initiation of orthodontic treatment. B. Conditions after orthodontic treatment with fixed appliances for 20 months. Extensive root resorption of the incisors has taken place. C. At a 10-year follow-up, slight rounding of the resorbed root surface can be seen. Otherwise, there has been no progression of the root resorption.

appear to be more liable to further resorption during orthodontic movement (32-35,88) (Fig. 15.5). This does not necessarily contraindicate orthodontic treatment; but special care should be taken to avoid excessive pressure during movement (Fig. 15.6).

Replacement resorption or *ankylosis* implies fusion of the alveolar bone and root substance and disappearance of the periodontal ligament space. This type of resorption is progressive, eventually involving the entire root. The rate of the resorption varies with age and growth rate. In many cases the root can be used as a space maintainer for several years (89).

Ankylosed teeth do not respond to orthodontic movement. This resorption entity can be recognized clinically during the first 2 months after injury and most often within 1 year after a severe trauma. The tooth becomes immobile and percussion produces a high tone compared with adjacent uninjured teeth.

In children and adolescents, the ankylosed tooth prevents growth of the jaw segment. The ankylosed tooth may thus become infraoccluded, permitting the ad-

jacent teeth to tilt towards the affected tooth. If the patient is in a period of rapid growth and the degree of infraocclusion is more than 1/4 of the crown length, the tooth should be removed. A special extraction technique is then needed to avoid excessive loss of alveolar bone (90) (see page 623).

General Treatment Principles

As seen from the foregoing section, teeth which have sustained traumatic injuries are possibly more liable to root resorption than non-injured teeth (91,92). During orthodontic treatment, special care should therefore be taken to avoid excessive pressure on such teeth. The following procedures can be of value in reducing the risk of root surface resorption.

It is necessary to carefully study the anatomy of the roots before treatment (Fig. 15.7). An assessment of the radiographic outline of the apex provides useful information regarding the risk of root re-

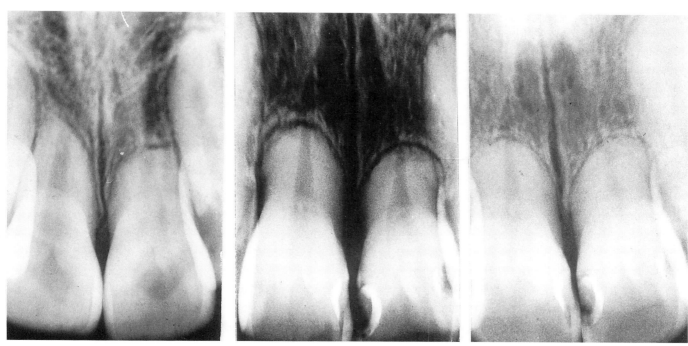

Fig. 15.6.
Patient with Class II div 1 malocclusion and severe root resorption of both central incisors due to trauma. Orthodontic treatment is possible if it is performed carefully. A. Condition before orthodontic treatment. Activator treatment was carried out for 2 years. B. Seven years later, slight rounding of the root surfaces is seen. Secondary crowding developed later, and 4 first premolars were extracted. Fixed appliances were then used for 18 months. C. Control after 20 years. There has been no progression of the resorptive process.

Fig. 15.7.
Root anatomy differing from normal. These roots are probably prone to resorption. Special care must be taken in these cases to avoid excessive forces during tooth movement. A. Incisors with slightly irregular apical root contour. B. Concavity along the distal surface of the root (surface resorption). C. Root malformation.

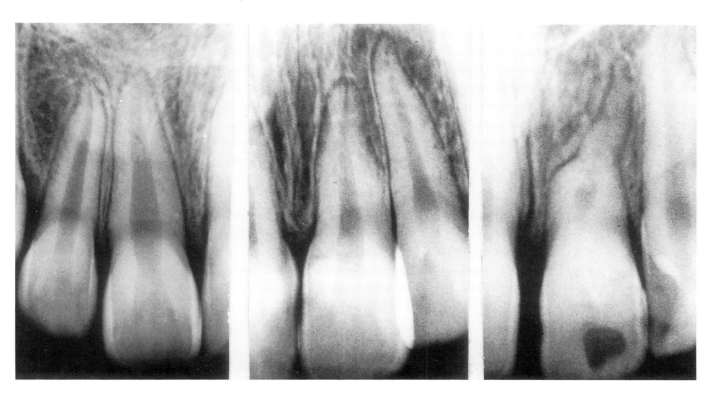

ORTHODONTIC MANAGEMENT OF THE TRAUMATIZED DENTITION

593

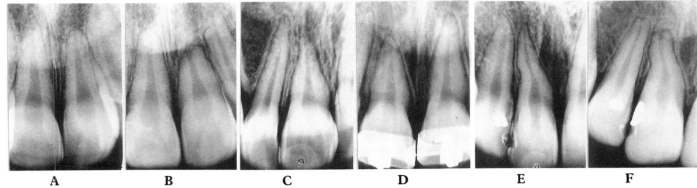

Fig. 15.8.
Root resorption developing during orthodontic treatment in teeth with abnormal root anatomy
A. Slightly irregular apical contour of a left central incisor. B. Marked root resorption after treatment. C. Right central incisor with a concavity along the distal root surface. D. Root resorption seen after treatment. E. Malformed root of a right central incisor. F. Marked root resorption is evident after treatment. All patients were treated with fixed appliances for 18-21 months.

Fig. 15.9.
Root resorption index used for quantitative assessment of root resorption
Score description:
1. *Irregular root contour.*
2. *Root resorption apically amounting to less than 2 mm of the original root length.*
3. *Root resorption apically amounting to from 2 mm to one-third of the original root length.*
4. *Root resorption exceeding one-third of the original root length.*
5. *Lateral root resorption.*

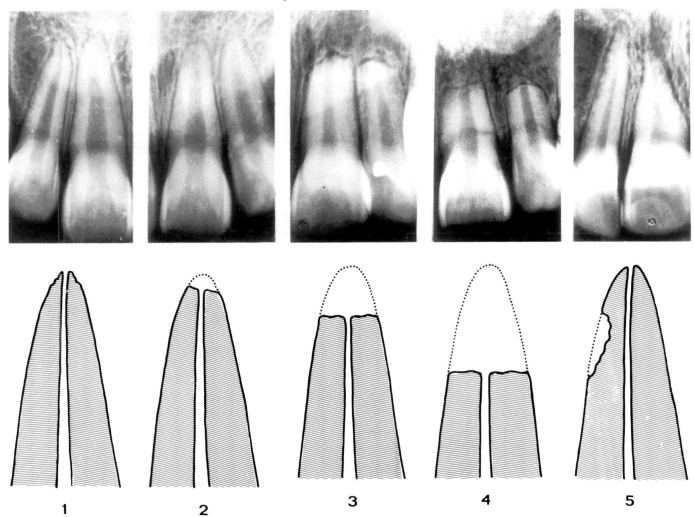

Fig. 15.10. Deviating root forms
1. Short root.
2. Blunt root.
3. Root with apical bend.
4. Root with apical pipette shape.

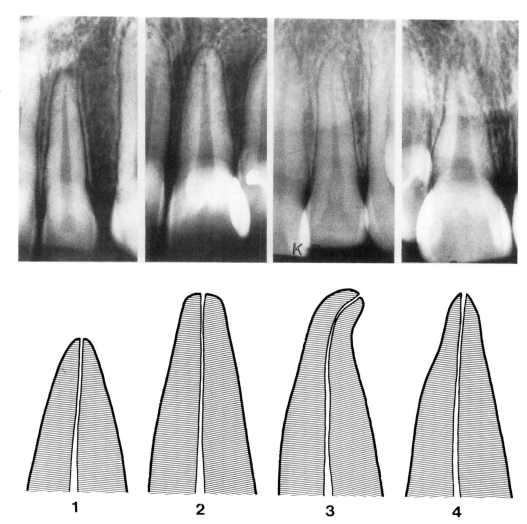

sorption during orthodontic treatment [88] (Fig. 15.8). A root resorption index permits quantitative assessment of root conditions prior to treatment and can be used for evaluation of further resorption [35] (Fig. 15.9).

A study involving 610 incisors in pa-tients consecutively treated with fixed appliances has shown that the risk of root resorption is related to the form of the root [88]. The root form was described as nor-mal, short, blunt, with an apical bend or pipette-shaped (Fig. 15.10). The incisors were evaluated before and after treatment.

Fig. 15.11. Frequency of
root resorption after orthodontic treatment in relation
to root morphology
*The index scores presented in Fig.
15.9 were used. The degree of root
resorption in teeth with blunt and
pipette shaped roots was significantly higher than in roots with
normal root form. (After LEVAN-
DER & MALMGREN 1988) (85).*

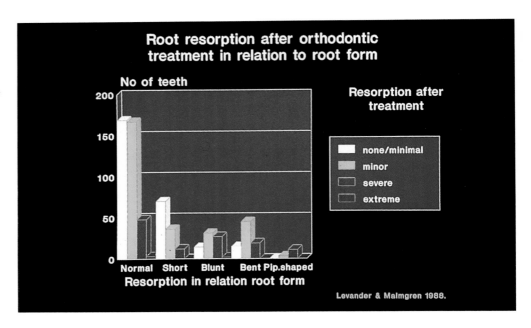

The extent of root resorption in teeth with blunt and pipette-shaped roots was significantly greater than in teeth with a normal root form (Figs. 15.11 and 15.13).

As it has been shown that movement into labial or lingual cortical bone can initiate extensive root resorption, it is imperative to establish the borders of the cortical bone, based on profile radiographs, prior to initiation of orthodontic therapy (37,38,93) (Fig. 15.12). Particularly if the alveolar crest is narrow, resorption can easily occur (Fig. 15.12 B). During retraction of the maxillary incisors, it is therefore necessary to avoid juxtaposition with the palatal or buccal cortical plates (Fig. 15.12 C,D). In many situations, the incisors are protrusive and require palatal root torque during retraction. It is then advisable to perform this root movement in the roomier cancellous bone than in the compact cortical bone of the maxillary alveolus (Fig. 15.12 E). It is therefore desirable to use a treatment approach that can intrude the anterior segment at the onset of orthodontic therapy (39).

The etiology of root resorption during orthodontic treatment is complicated.

Fig. 15.12. Schematic drawing illustrating the importance of examining the relation between the position of the root and cortical bone prior to orthodontic treatment
A. An alveolar crest with a wide cancellous bone area.
B. An alveolar crest with a narrow cancellous bone area.
C. Lingual tipping of the crown moves the root into juxtaposition with the buccal cortical plate, which can initiate root resorption.
D. Lingual root torque during retraction can move the root into juxtaposition with the palatal cortical bone, which can initiate root resorption.
E. Intrusion of an incisor into the roomier cancellous part of the bone area is probably the best procedure.

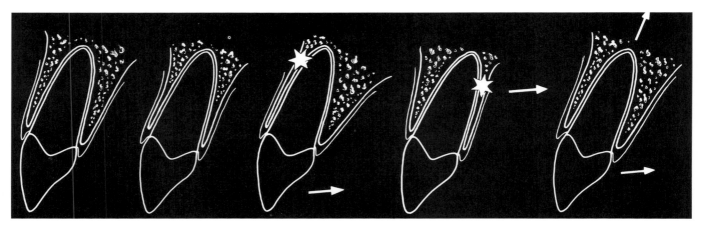

Fig. 15.13. **Typical effect of root resorption**

Fig. 15.13. Typical effect of root resorption
A. A pipette-shaped root (1) before and (2) after treatment.
B. A blunt root (1) before and (2) after treatment.
C. A root with an apical bend (1) before and (2) after treatment.

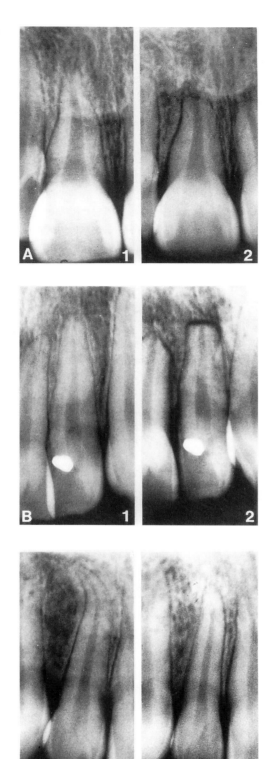

There are some factors which, alone or in combination, can contribute to the development of root resorption. The importance of forces has been discussed for years. Most authors consider only heavy forces to be responsible for root resorption (33,34,40,41). Intensity and duration of forces are, however, also of great importance (94).

Continuous heavy forces could cause resorption (42). Prolonged tipping can also cause resorption of a tooth as well as resorption of the alveolar crest, especially in adult patients (42,95). Thus, there is no single explanation as to why certain teeth resorb severely; but one factor often mentioned in the literature is an earlier trauma (226).

Fig. 15.14. A.Degree of root resorption after orthodontic treatment
Root resorption in 55 traumatized teeth. After MALMGREN ET AL. (91) *1982.*

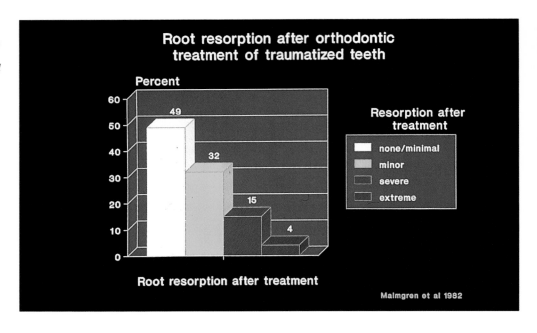

Fig. 15.14. B.Degree of root resorption after orthodontic treatment
Root resorption in 264 incisors without trauma, treated with edgewise *technique. After MALMGREN ET AL.* (91) *1982*

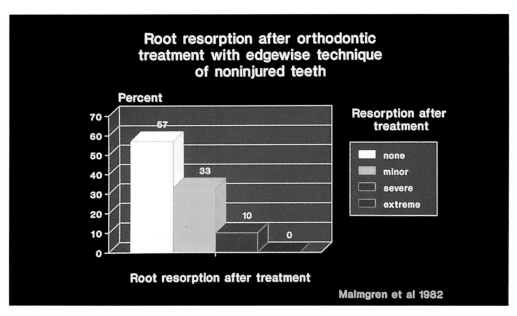

Fig. 15.14. C.Degree of root resorption after orthodontic treatment
Root resorption in 176 incisors without trauma, treated with Begg *technique. After MALMGREN ET AL.* (91) *1982.*

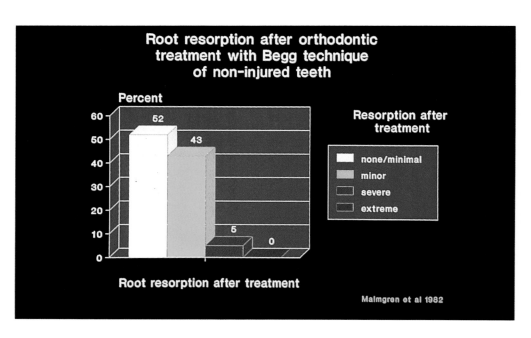

**Fig. 15.15. Frequency of
root resorption after orthodontic treatment with fixed
appliances in a study of 390
incisors**
*The radiographic examinations
were performed before treatment,
after 6 to 9 months and finally
after completion of treatment.
The index scores presented in
Fig. 15.9 were used. After
MALMGREN ET AL.* (91) *1982*

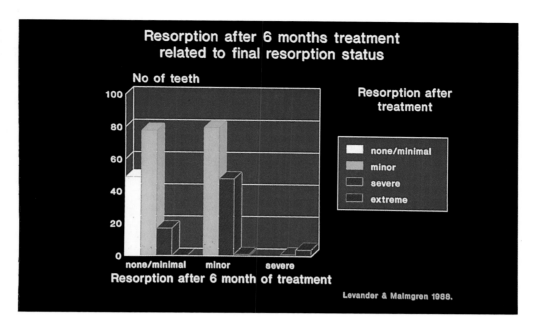

In a study of root resorption after orthodontic treatment of traumatized teeth, 55
traumatized incisors were analyzed (91).
All teeth had been examined at the time of
injury by experienced pedodontists at the
Eastman Institute in Stockholm according
to standardized procedures. The types of
injury were: crown fracture in 18 teeth and
periodontal injury in 37 (i.e., concussion,
subluxation or luxation). Signs of root
resorption before and after treatment were
registered with scores from 0 to 4 (Fig.
15.9).

After orthodontic treatment, 9% of the
traumatized incisors showed an irregular
root contour, 32% minor resorption, 15%
moderate root resorption and only 4% (2
teeth) showed severe resorption. The resorptions were more frequent in teeth with
periodontal injuries, but the difference
was not significant. The extent of root
resorption was the same in the traumatized and in the contralateral control uninjured teeth in the same individual (Fig.
15.14 A).

The extent of root resorption in the
traumatized teeth was also compared with
that of uninjured incisors in a group of 55
consecutive patients treated with fixed appliances (edgewise and Begg technique)
and extraction of 4 first bicuspids. Also
this part of the study showed no significant
difference in the tendency towards root
resorption of traumatized and uninjured
teeth (Fig. 15.14 B,C). However, a few
teeth that exhibited resorption before orthodontic treatment were severely resorbed during treatment.

The risk of root resorption during orthodontic treatment with fixed appliances
was studied in relation to initial resorption
6 to 9 months after start of treatment in 98
consecutive patients (88). The mean treatment time was 19 months. A total of 390
incisors were examined (Fig. 15.15). The
same type of index (scale 0 to 4) as illustrated in Fig. 15.9 was used. The results
are illustrated in Figs. 15.15 and 15.16.
Minor resorption was found in 33% of the
teeth and severe resorption in 1%. No
severe resorption after treatment was
found in any teeth without resorption after
initial treatment (i.e. 6 to 9 months). In
teeth with an irregular root contour, 12%
showed severe resorption at the end of
treatment. In teeth with minor resorption
after initial treatment, 38% showed severe
resorption. Extreme resorption was registered in 4 of 5 teeth with severe resorption
after initial treatment.

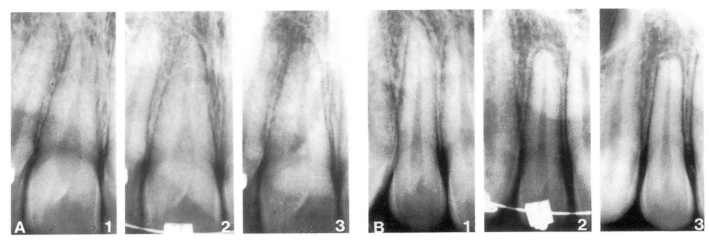

Fig. 15.16.
Root resorption after completion of treatment in relation to initial resorption status.
A. (1) Status before treatment. (2) After 6 months there is no resorption. (3) At the end of treatment, minor resorption and blunting of the apex is seen. B. (1) Before treatment. (2) After 6 months, minor resorption is seen. (3) At the end of treatment, severe resorption is seen.

The conclusions are: if a severe resorption is found after half a year of treatment with a fixed appliance, there is a high risk of extreme resorption at the end of treatment; minor resorption at that time indicates a moderate risk of severe resorption; irregular root contour indicates a limited risk of severe resorption at the end of treatment.

Therefore, regular radiographic controls are necessary in order to check if any root resorption occurs or increases during treatment. It is advisable to make the first control 6-9 months after the start of treatment. If signs of root resorption are seen, controls every 2 months are recommended. A pause in treatment for about 3 months can reduce the risk of further resorption (89) (Fig. 15.17). Marked root resorption diagnosed at this time should lead to reevaluation of the treatment goal.

Thus, in trauma patients it is imperative to start treatment with light, preferably intermittent forces, avoid prolonged tipping, aim at a limited goal and in this way achieve a shorter treatment procedure.

In the following, orthodontic treatment of various types of dental injuries will be discussed.

Specific Treatment Principles for Various Trauma Types

Crown and Crown-Root Fractures

It is essential that, even in teeth with slight injuries such as uncomplicated crown fractures, tests for sensibility and a radiographic examination are made before the start of orthodontic treatment. When in doubt as to the clinical condition of the pulp, a 3-months observation period with repeated sensibility tests is recommended before initiating orthodontic treatment.

A complicated crown fracture implies involvement of enamel, dentin and pulp. A complicated crown-root fracture also involves the root.

Capping of the pulp or partial pulpotomy on proper indications followed by a calcium hydroxide cover will in most cases preserve the vitality of the pulp (see Chapter 14, p. 525).

It is recommended that orthodontic movement of the injured immature teeth is postponed until root development is seen to resume. Clinical and radiographic controls should be carried out after 6 months, 1 year and 2 years.

Fig. 15.17. Root resorption in relation to two orthodontic treatment regimes
A material of 62 upper incisors was studied. In all teeth, a minor apical root resorption was observed after the initial 6 to 9 months of treatment with a fixed appliance. In 20 patients (group I) treatment continued according to the original plan and 20 patients had a treatment pause of 2 to 3 months (group II). There was significantly less root resorption in patients treated with a pause than in those without. From LEVANDER & MALMGREN 1992 (89).

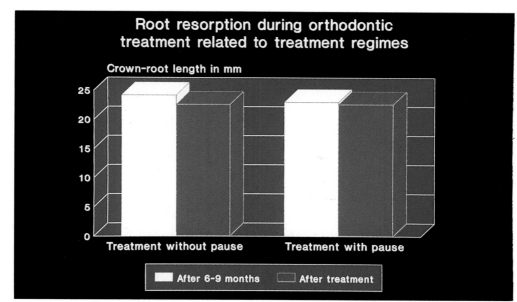

Continuous treatment
An upper lateral incisor before treatment; after 6 months when a minor resorption is seen; and at the end of treatment when the resorption is severe. Treatment was performed without pause.

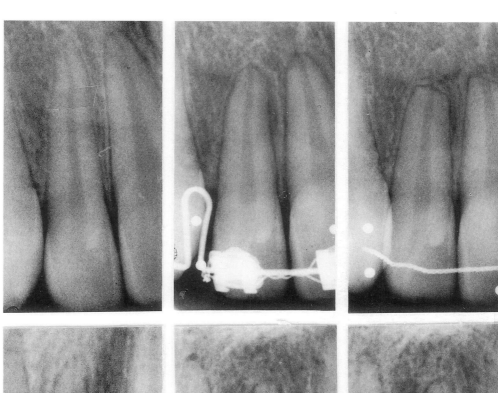

Treatment with pause
An upper incisor before treatment; after 6 months when a minor resorption is seen; and at the end of treatment, when no further resorption is observed.

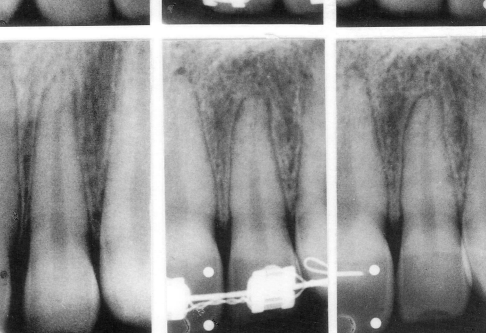

Fig. 15.18. Crown-root fractures where orthodontic extrusion can be used. Oblique crown-root fracture below the marginal bone buccally.

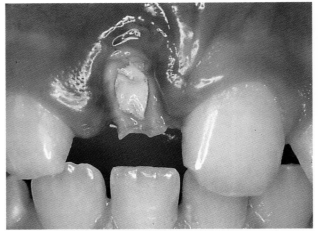 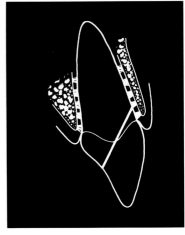

Oblique crown-root fracture below the marginal bone palatally.

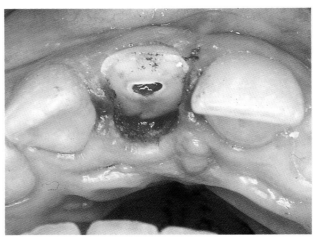 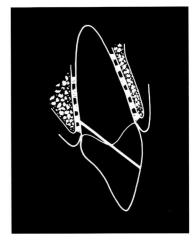

Crown-root fracture extending below marginal bone proximally.

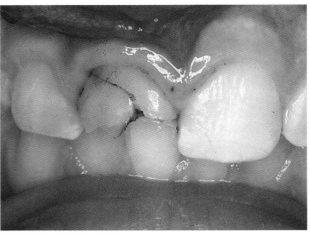 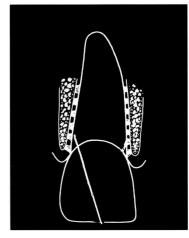

Transverse root fracture.

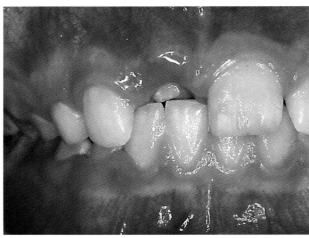 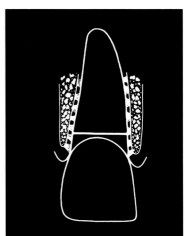

Fig. 15.19. Rapid extrusion of a crown-root fractured central incisor
A steel hook cemented in the root canal. Traction with an elastic thread is applied axially.

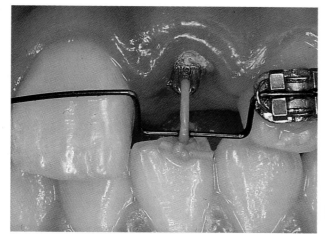 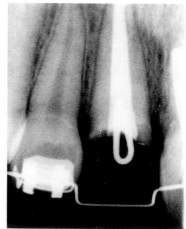

Condition after 4 weeks
The root is fully extruded and retained with a stainless steel ligature wire. A marginal flap is raised.

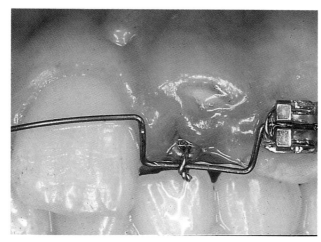

Condition after raising a mucoperiosteal flap
No coronal shift of the bone margin is found. Note the rapid remodelling of bone surrounding the apex.

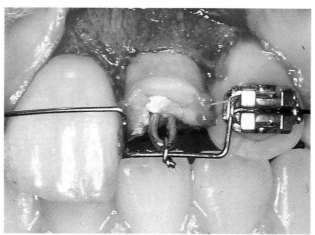 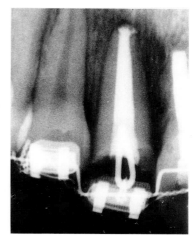

EXTRUSION OF CROWN-ROOT AND CERVICAL ROOT FRACTURES

To complete a crown restoration of a tooth with a crown-root or a cervical root fracture, it is often necessary to extrude the fractured root orthodontically (69-74, 93-103). Different types of fractures amenable to orthodontic extrusion are illustrated in Fig. 15.18.

Orthodontic extrusion can be performed with a variety of orthodontic appliances. A rapid extrusion technique to save such teeth was introduced by

HEITHERSAY in 1973 (69) and further developed by INGBER in 1976 (71). Endodontic treatment of the root portion is usually performed before the orthodontic phase of treatment.

Orthodontic extrusion normally leads to a coronal shift of the marginal gingiva (40,77). This has been shown to be caused by growth of the attached gingiva and not by coronal displacement of the muco-gingival junction (Fig. 15.19). The increase of gingival tissue may partially mask the extent of root extrusion.

Fig. 15.20. Orthodontic extrusion of a crown-root fractured central incisor
The coronal fragment has been used as a temporary crown, cemented with a screw post in the root canal.

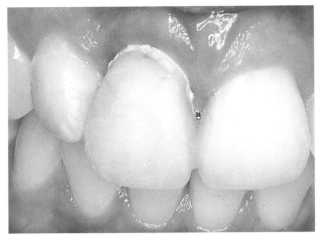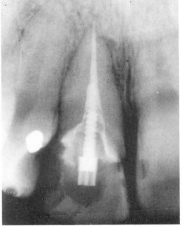

Orthodontic appliance
A heat-treated spring of Elgiloy® wire (.016 x .016 inches) with a force of approximately 60 to 70 p is used for the extrusion.

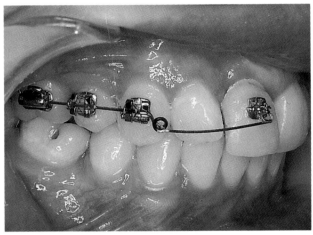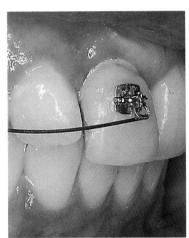

Condition after 1 week
The tooth has been extruded 1.5 mm. The crown is shortened to enable further extrusion.

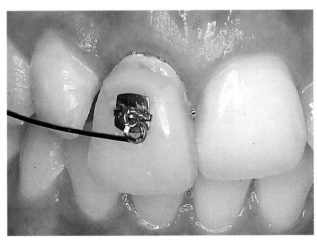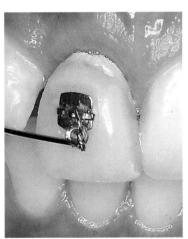

Condition after 2 weeks
The tooth has been extruded another 1.5 mm and the root is now available for preparation.

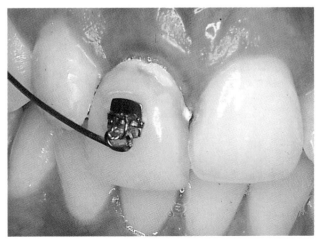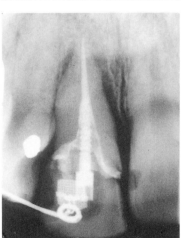

Fibrotomy
A fibrotomy extending below the level of marginal bone is performed prior to the retention period.

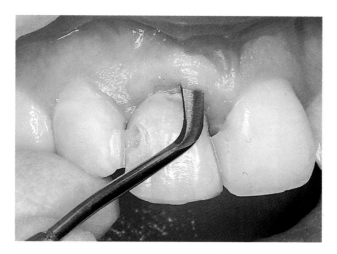

Retention
The extruded tooth is splinted to adjacent teeth.

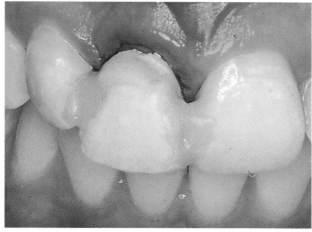

Final restoration
A post-retained crown is fabricated. Radiographically there is no sign of resorption after 2 years.

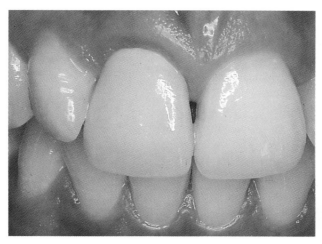
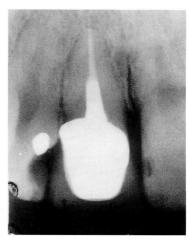

Rapid extrusion involves stretching and readjusting of the periodontal fibers, thereby avoiding marked bone remodelling by virtue of the rapid movement. It can thus be achieved without a coronal shift of marginal bone, thereby facilitating the coronal restoration as there is no need to reshape bone.

Relapse may follow orthodontic extrusion, the prime reason being the stretched state of marginal periodontal fibers (72). To avoid relapse, fibrotomy should be performed before the retention period, which should last at least 3-4 weeks (101,102) (Fig. 15.20).

A non-vital tooth can be extruded , 3-5 mm during 3-4 weeks. Rapid movement is possible because bone remodelling is accomplished by stretching and readjusting the fibers. Rapid extrusion of teeth, in comparison to conventional orthodontic extrusion, may in rare cases elicit root resorption (103). However, both histologic and clinical studies of extruded teeth indicate that root resorption after extrusion is very rare (69-75,97-102).

Fig. 15.21. Orthodontic movement of a root fractured tooth healed by a hard tissue callus

A. Models of a Class II div. 1 malocclusion with deep bite before and B. after treatment. The patient was treated with extra-oral traction and an activator for 2 years. C. The root-fractured incisor before treatment. Note internal surface resorption at the level of the root fracture, which is typical for hard tissue healing D. Immediately after active treatment. There is obliteration of only the apical part of the root canal, also an indication of continued hard tissue fracture healing. E. Condition 4 years after active treatment. Note that tooth movement was achieved without separating the fragments.

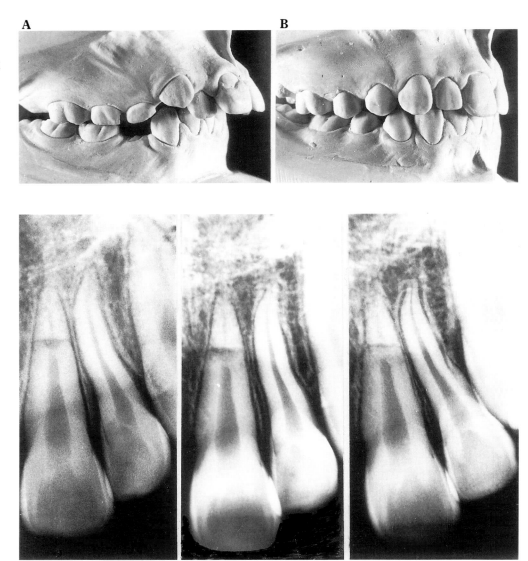

For a tooth with a complicated crown-root or cervical root fracture, two types of therapy are available: orthodontic or surgical extrusion (104-106). In teeth with thin root canal walls, i.e. teeth treated endodontically at an early stage of root formation, orthodontic extrusion seems to be less traumatic.

Root Fractures

Orthodontic management of root-fractured teeth depends on the type of healing and location of the fracture (31,107,108). Radiographic and histologic observations have shown different types of healing after root fracture: healing with calcified tissue and with interposition of connective tissue, sometimes combined with ingrowth of bone (107-109).

Healing with calcified tissue means that the fracture is healed with dentin and cementum. The bridging of the fracture may not be complete, but the fracture is consolidated. Tooth mobility is normal, as is response to pulpal sensibility testing.

Orthodontic movement of a root-fractured tooth which has healed with a hard tissue callus can be performed without breaking up the fracture site (Fig. 15.21).

Healing with interposition of connective tissue means that the fracture edges are covered with cementum and PDL.

Orthodontic movement of a root-fractured tooth where the fragments are separated by connective tissue leads to further separation of the fragments (Fig. 15.22). A common finding after treatment is rounding of fracture edges. In planning orthodontic therapy, it must therefore be realized that a fractured root with interposition of connective tissue should be looked upon as a tooth with a short root. As a result, such a tooth must be evaluated

Fig. 15.22. Orthodontic movement of a root-fractured tooth with healing by interposition of connective tissue
A. Models of a Class II div. 1 malocclusion with deep bite before and B. after treatment. The patient was treated with a fixed appliance for 19 months. C. The fractured incisor 3 years prior to treatment. Note initial obliteration of the apical and coronal aspects of the root canal. D. Condition at the start of orthodontic treatment. There is rounding of the fracture edges and obliteration of the entire root canal, indications of interposition of connective tissue between root fragments. E. Four months after the start of orthodontic treatment. F. Condition 2 years after orthodontic treatment.

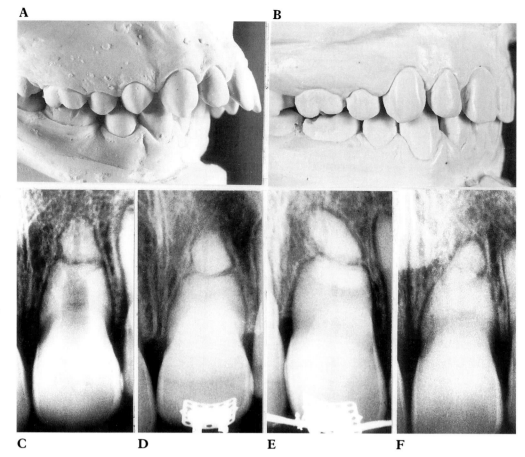

with respect to the length of the coronal fragment. This means that teeth with fractures in the apical third of the root generally have enough periodontal support to allow orthodontic movement (Fig. 15.23 A). Teeth with fractures located in the middle third of the root represent a hazard to tooth integrity because of the risk of further shortening of the very short coronal fragment (Fig. 15.23 B). Orthodontic movement of such a tooth may result in a root with very little periodontal support. In cervical root fractures, the apical fragment can sometimes be extruded with a

Fig. 15.23. Evaluation of the prognosis for orthodontic treatment of root-fractured teeth healed with interposition of connective tissue
A. Root fractures apically of line d. The coronal part of the root is so long that movement of the root is possible without impairment of the prognosis. B. Root fractures between d and c. The coronal portion of the root is long enough to withstand careful orthodontic movement. Note the thin labial part of the root (arrow) which can easily resorb during orthodontic movement and which will lead to a significant shortening of the root length. C. Root fractures between c and b. The coronal part of the root is usually too short to assure enough periodontal support and orthodontic treatment is therefore contraindicated. If the fracture line is too close to b, extrusion of the apical fragment is an alternative.

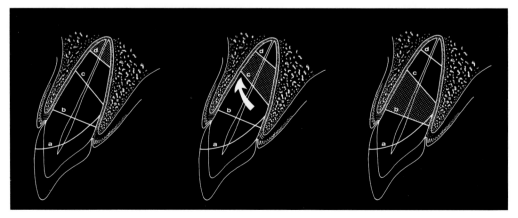

rapid extrusion technique or by surgical means (Fig. 15.23 C).

Movement of root-fractured teeth with an adequate root filling may be performed with the same prognosis as when the coronal fragment is vital.

Luxated Teeth

It has not yet been clearly established whether luxated teeth are more liable to resorb during orthodontic treatment than non-injured teeth (68). In one study, luxated teeth were reported to develop more root resorption than their non-injured antimeres (43). However, in the evaluation of the results, the different types of luxation injuries were not taken into account. With respect to the occurrence of root resorption, it has been observed clinically that luxated teeth without root resorption can be moved with the same prognosis as non-injured teeth (91). Teeth with repaired surface resorption or repaired inflammatory resorption should be followed carefully during orthodontic treatment. A radiographic assessment of the outline of the roots prior to treatment gives information of some risk factors, such as an irregular root contour, concavities along the surface of the root, or root malformation (88). Regular radiographic controls are necessary in order to disclose early root resorption. An index provides a useful tool for quantitative assessment of root conditions during treatment (85,88,89, 91).

Inflammatory and replacement resorption can be clearly related to traumatic injuries and have never been reported as a result of orthodontic treatment alone. Luxated teeth which have developed inflammatory resorption should be treated endodontically and observed for arrest of root resorption prior to initiation of orthodontic movement. Teeth with ankylosis (replacement resorption) do not respond to orthodontic treatment.

Avulsed Teeth

PRIMARY DENTITION
Traumatic loss of a primary tooth is not usually an indication for orthodontic treatment (29). A secondary effect of the traumatic episode might be malformation or impaction of the succedaneous tooth.

The orthodontic implication of this will be discussed later in this chapter.

MIXED DENTITION
After traumatic loss of permanent teeth, orthodontic treatment planning becomes relevant (46-54,110-114). The main question is whether the space should be maintained for the purpose of anterior tooth replacement by either autotransplantation, implant insertion or fixed bridgework. (A cost-benefit analysis of these treatment procedures is given in Appendix 5, p. 751).

An unfavorable development of the width and height of the alveolar crest is sometimes seen in growing individuals with missing maxillary incisors. Severe traumatic injuries can also damage the alveolar ridge. Autotransplantation of premolars to replace missing incisors can contribute to favorable development of the alveolar bone (115,116). Autotransplantation can be performed with both immature and mature teeth, but several reports conclude that autotransplantation has the best prognosis if performed when the tooth germ has developed to three-fourths of its anticipated root length or to full length with a wide open apex (117-121) (see Chapter 19, p 671). At this stage of root development, vitality of the pulp can be maintained and root development continued (Fig. 15.24). It has also been shown that transplanted teeth can be moved with only a minor loss of root length (122).

A new method using single standing implants has recently been developed. It is important to note that this procedure cannot be used until the alveolar process has been fully developed (see Chapter 20 p 692). It should be noted that implants cannot be moved orthodontically.

Space closure for a missing maxillary *lateral* incisor usually implies mesial positioning of the maxillary cuspid in the lateral incisor region. Periodontal status has been reported to be better in patients with closed lateral incisor spaces than in patients with prosthetic lateral incisors (55).

Space closure after loss of a *central* incisor seldom leads to a lasting esthetically satisfactory result. The recent development of autotransplantation techniques and prosthetic therapy has minimized the need for orthodontic closure of spaces after loss of central incisors.

Fig. 15.24. Combined orthodontic treatment and premolar autotransplantation after anterior tooth loss
Three maxillary incisors have been avulsed in a 10-year-old girl. Note the extensive loss of alveolar bone buccally. Radiographic examination revealed that the mandibular second premolars were suitable as grafts.

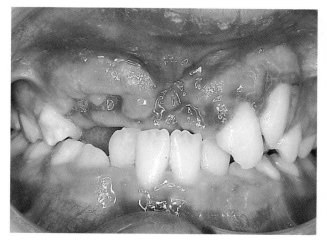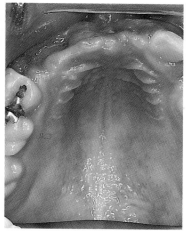

Temporary restoration
A temporary plate with 2 incisors is used as a space maintainer. After 5 months the upper right cuspid has erupted in a mesial position. The cuspid was therefore moved distally with elastics to make room for the 2 transplants.

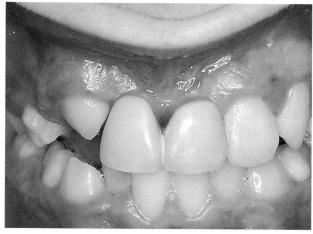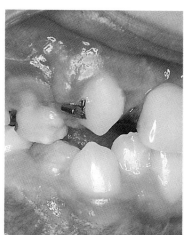

Autotransplantation of premolars
Two years after the trauma, the roots of the premolars have developed to 3/4 of anticipated root length. The premolars are then transplanted to the central incisor region. The teeth are aligned with a fixed appliance 6 months after transplantation.

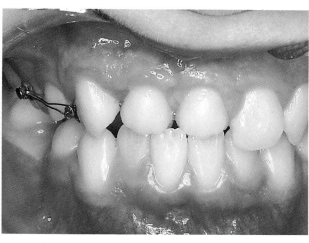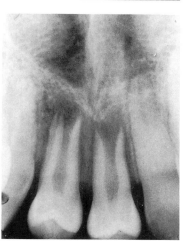

Completion of treatment
At the end of treatment the premolars and the cuspid are recontoured with composite resin. The clinical and radiographic situation is shown 4 years after trauma and 2 years after transplantation.

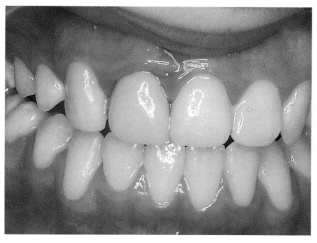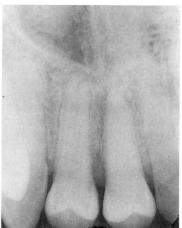

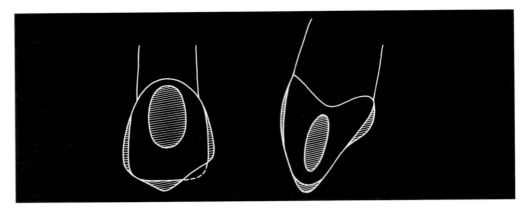

Fig. 15.25. Reduction of a canine to simulate a lateral or central incisor
The shaded areas illustrate the spots of grinding. The dotted line indicates where a corner can be enhanced by composite resin build-up.

Space closure

If space closure is indicated, treatment should start early or at least be planned in the mixed dentition. Space closure is of prime importance in patients with maxillary arch length deficiency in Class I and II malocclusions. If treatment is started in the early mixed dentition, it is possible by extraction or interproximal reduction of deciduous molars to guide molars, premolars and canines mesially. An intact dental arch without any appliance therapy can then be obtained.

Crown form, dental arch symmetry and lip seal are important factors for an acceptable end result. A satisfactory esthetic alteration of crown form can in some cases be obtained by slight reduction of canines and incisors, sometimes supplemented with gingivectomy to adjust differences in clinical crown height (57-59). Altering the crown form with composite materials or porcelain veneers can also contribute to an esthetically pleasing result (Figs. 15.25 to 15.28).

Treatment of missing maxillary lateral

Fig. 15.26. Closure of the space resulting from avulsion of a permanent central incisor
A. The lateral incisor has moved mesially and has a fairly good position, which would have been better if the tooth had been uprighted. Note the mesial drift of the central incicor. A base plate or a lingual arch wire with a stop could have prevented this. B. The lateral incisor has been recontoured by selective grinding and the crown form reshaped with composite resin.

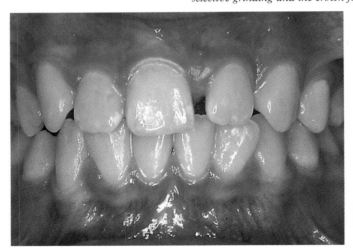
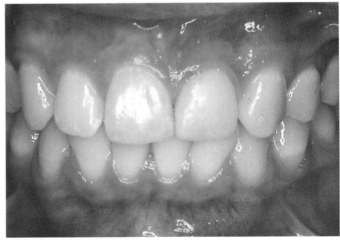

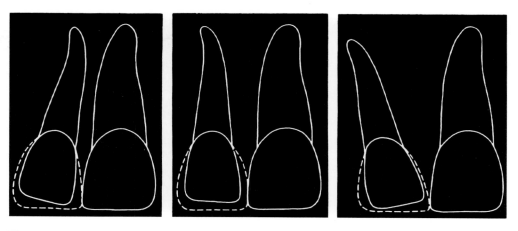

Fig. 15.27. Schematic illustration of the need for mesio-distal uprighting of a lateral incisor which has been moved mesially to replace a missing maxillary central incisor

Fig. 15.28. Schematic illustration of buccal root torque of a lateral incisor which is moved mesially to replace a missing maxillary central incisor
The solid line illustrates the inclination of a central incisor and the dotted line a lateral incisor.

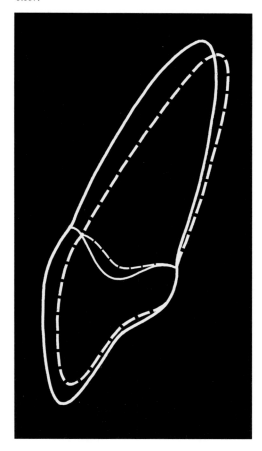

Fig. 15.29. Treatment alternatives when a lateral incisor is avulsed in a Class I malocclusion Arch length deficiency
A. Early extraction of the primary second molar facilitates mesial movement of the first permanent molar, arch length in the upper jaw is thereby reduced. B. The canine and premolars have moved mesially one tooth width and a Class II occlusion without spacing has been achieved. No arch length deficiency. C. The canine is positioned mesially. The root of the primary canine demonstrates no extensive resorption. D. The canine replaces the avulsed lateral incisor and the primary canine is used as a space maintainer as long as possible. E. A space maintainer is constructed while awaiting permanent therapy. F. The canine is used as a lateral incisor and a space is maintained between the canine and the first premolar.

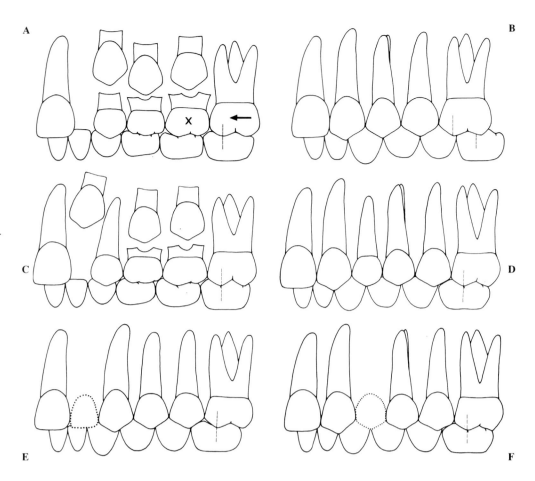

incisors in patients with Class I malocclusion is schematically illustrated in Fig.15. 29 A to F. (114). The same principles can be applied in cases with loss of central incisors. In these cases, crown form and inclination of the lateral incisors and canines must be favorable. In Class III malocclusion, space for a permanent tooth or teeth must often be maintained despite arch length deficiency because of the obvious risk of anterior crossbite. Spontaneous space closure is contraindicated in malocclusions with open bite, deep bite and anterior crossbite. This is particularly true in the lower jaw in Class II and in the upper jaw in Class III malocclusions. If space closure is desired in combination with such anomalies, it is recommended that the basic malocclusion be treated first whenever possible. After this treatment, it

Fig. 15.30. A model set-up for a patient with aplasia of the maxillary right lateral incisor and traumatic loss of left central incisor
Treatment planning involves mesial movement of the maxillary right central incisor, distal movement of left canine and alignment of the maxillary teeth. Acrylic teeth are used as space maintainers during treatment and retention (To be continued in Fig. 15.33).

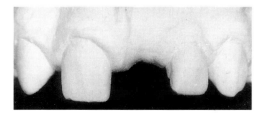 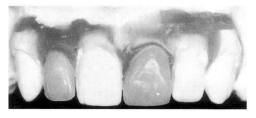

CHAPTER 15

**Fig. 15.31. Severe infraoc-
clusion of a central incisor
with mesial tipping of adjacent teeth in a 14-year-
old boy**
*To avoid these complications, the
ankylosed tooth should have been
extracted earlier.*

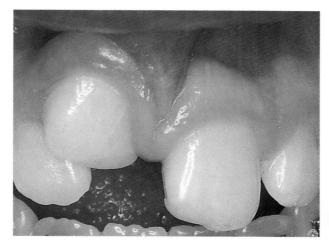
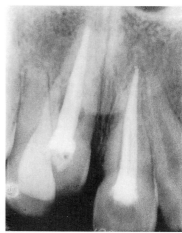

can be decided how space closure can be achieved. In cases with extreme crowding, however, it can be done at the time of initial treatment.

In cases where there is doubt about the functional or esthetic result of space closure, after insisor loss, it is advisable to wait until the patient has reached the permanent dentition stage. Meanwhile, the space can be maintained prosthetically (60-61).

When treatment is planned, arch length and form, crown form and inclination of the anterior teeth should be studied carefully on casts and radiographs. Different alternatives of tooth position and compensatory extractions can be studied on diagnostic set-up models. The set-up model also facilitates discussion with the patient, parents and colleagues (Fig. 15.30).

Space maintenance
If space closure is contraindicated, a space maintainer can be constructed. This situation arises if more than 1 incisor is lost in the same arch. It is also true in patients with good alignment of teeth and normal occlusion, and in patients with spaces between teeth. If a tooth is lost in the upper jaw in a Class II division 2 or a Class III

malocclusion, a space maintainer is often the treatment of choice.

For esthetic reasons, space closure is contraindicated if there is great discrepancy in crown form between central and lateral incisors. The crown form of cuspids sometimes also contraindicates space closure. Asymmetry of the upper incisors after space closure could be very obvious in patients with incomplete lip seal. A space maintainer followed by autotransplantation, a fixed bridge or an implant is then to be preferred.

A fixed space maintainer followed by bridge work is often the only possible treatment in an uncooperative patient who does not want appliance therapy. Various space maintainers can be used. The easiest method is to use the traumatized tooth for as long as possible, even when the prognosis is poor. It is, however, important to control such a tooth. If it becomes ankylosed, it should be extracted before severe infraocclusion and tipping of adjacent teeth has occurred (Fig. 15.31).

The most common space maintainer is a removable appliance fitted to the teeth (Fig. 15.1). An alternative is a lingual arch wire soldered to bands on the molars with a tooth fixed to the arch wire (Fig. 15.32).

**Fig. 15.32. Fixed space
maintainer in early mixed
dentition**
*A lingual arch wire is soldered to
bands on the primary second molars. Axial view, note the mesial
and distal stops around the prosthetic tooth.*

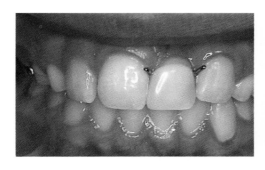
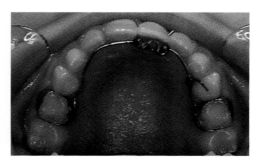

Fig. 15.33. Combination of space maintainer and orthodontic appliance
Acrylic teeth, right lateral and left central incisors, used as space maintainers during orthodontic treatment. Two acrylic teeth are replacing the missing incisors.

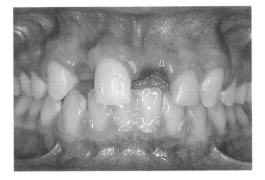 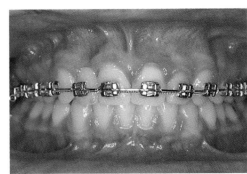

Frontal and occlusal view of retainer
After treatment the same teeth are used in the retainer. Note the occlusal stops on the retainer used to avoid excessive pressure on the alveolar ridge.

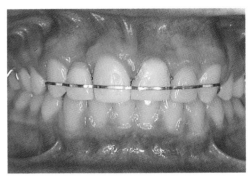

Various types of bonded appliances can also be used (129). An important factor is that the different appliances do not interfere with eruption of teeth and growth of jaws. In many cases, space maintainers can be combined with orthodontic appliances (62-67) (Fig. 15.33). The crown of the extracted incisor can also be used as a pontic.

A technique has recently been developed which consists of treating tooth loss in the anterior region by autotransplantation of premolars (Fig. 15.34). The anatomy of the transplant is subsequently altered by a composite resin restoration or a porcelain veneer (see Chapter 19, p. 680).

Autotransplantation of bicuspids to maintain the alveolar arch width and length in growing child is illustrated in Fig. 15.34. The anatomy of the transplant is

subsequently altered by a composite resin restoration. Both pre- and postsurgical treatment planning is important, to make transplantation possible at an optimal stage of root development of the bicuspids and to minimize the postsurgical movement of the transplant (66,67,115,117-121).

Another technique recently developed is the insertion of implants. In this context it is important to consider that single standing implants can only be used when alveolar growth is complete (see Chapter 20, p. 692).

PERMANENT DENTITION
Space closure
In patients with Class I malocclusion and loss of an incisor, the degree of crowding and mesiodistal width of teeth must act as

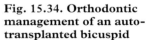

Fig. 15.34. Orthodontic management of an autotransplanted bicuspid
A 9-year-old boy with a postnormal occlusion and bimaxillary crowding. The maxillary left central incisor had to be extracted due to severe root resorption. Treatment plan was extra-oral traction and a modified activator, followed by extraction of 4 bicuspids and fixed appliance with a mandibular first bicuspid transplanted to the region of the traumatized maxillary incisor.

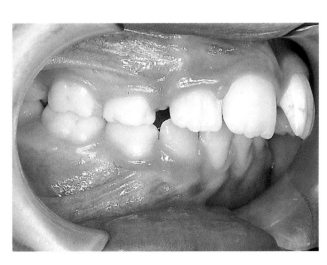 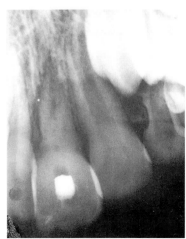

After transplantation
At the age of 12 the mandibular first bicuspid has reached an optimal stage for transplantation. Due to crowding, the transplant was placed in labial deviation.

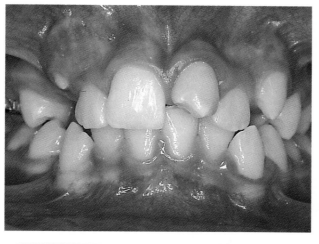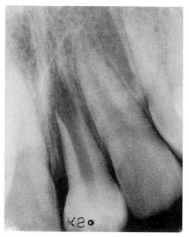

Orthodontic alignment
Orthodontic alignment of the upper arch and palatal positioning of the transplant was initiated 6 months after surgery.

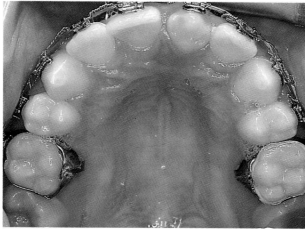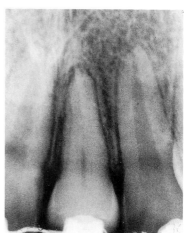

Axial view
Note the similarity between the transplant and the right central incisor.

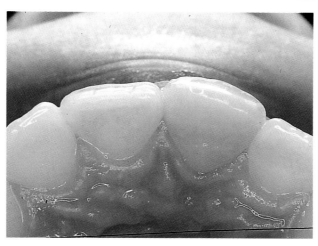

Completion of restoration
The tooth has been restored with composite resin.

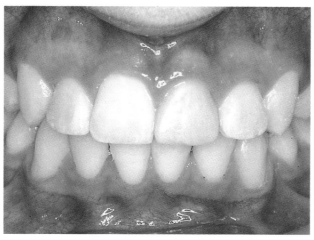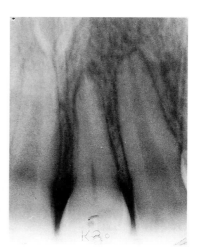

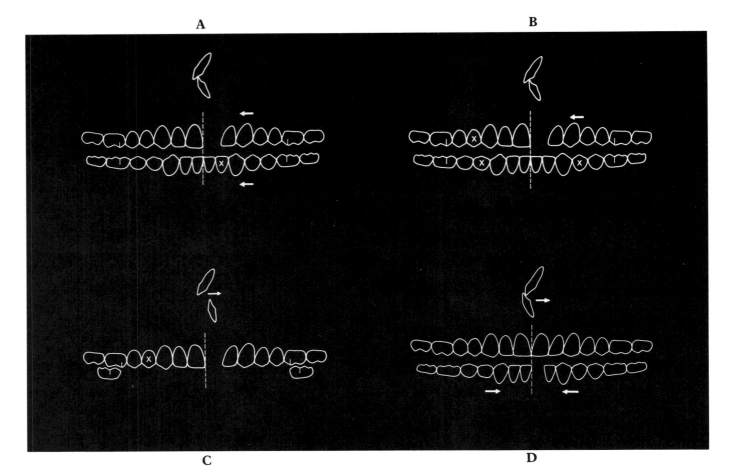

A   B

C   D

Fig. 15.35. Schematic drawing illustrating treatment alternatives of space closure in patients with avulsed incisors

Different degrees of crowding must be imagined. A. A slightly crowded Class I malocclusion. Compensatory extraction of 1 incisor in the lower jaw is suggested. After space closure, it is important to upright the teeth. B. A severely crowded Class I malocclusion. One maxillary premolar and 2 mandibular premolars are extracted. C. Class II malocclusion with overjet, good alignment of the lower arch, but without overbite. One premolar on the opposite side of the upper jaw is extracted and the molars are left in a postnormal position. D. A functional Class III malocclusion with anterior cross bite. The lower incisors are tipped lingually to decrease the mandibular arch length.

a guide to therapy. Compensatory extraction in the opposite jaw is a common solution. An alternative, if a maxillary incisor is lost, is extraction of 1 incisor in the lower jaw (Fig. 15.35 A). In patients with extensive crowding, extraction of 1 premolar in the upper jaw and 2 premolars in the lower jaw is a second alternative (Fig. 15.35 B).

A fixed appliance is required to close spaces, align, and set the teeth upright. In patients with Class II malocclusion, the prime decision is whether to maintain the disto-occlusion or to alter it. In patients with an extensive overjet and protruding incisors it is posssible to keep the lateral segments in disto-occlusion and close the space created by an avulsed incisor. This is particularly true if the patient has a tendency towards open bite. In order to keep the arch symmetrical, compensatory extractions are often necessary in the lateral segment on the opposite side of the upper jaw (Fig. 15.35 C).

When treating Class II malocclusions, it is often necessary to extract teeth in both the upper and lower jaws. If the malocclusion is combined with deep overbite, crowding in the lower jaw, or protrusion of the lower incisors, premolars are most often extracted.

If a lower incisor is lost in a functional Class III malocclusion with an anterior cross bite, space closure has a relatively good prognosis. By tipping the incisors lingually, mandibular arch length can be decreased (Fig. 15.35 D).

Space maintenance

If space closure is contraindicated, prosthetic therapy must be carried out. To facilitate treatment, preprosthetic orthodontic therapy is often necessary.

Malocclusions due to skeletal deviations, (primarily open and deep bites, cross bites and Class II malocclusions) should be treated in the early permanent dentition. Remaining growth can thereby facilitate orthodontic therapy. After this treatment, semipermanent prosthetic therapy can be provided. A schematic illustration of treatment options in Class II division 1 malocclusions is given in Fig. 15.36 A and B.

In other malocclusions, treatment can be performed in close association with definitive therapy. This facilitates both orthodontic and prosthetic treatment planning and shortens the retention period.

Fig. 15.36.
Pre-prosthetic orthodontic therapy when space closure is contraindicated. Two alternatives of Class II div. 1 treatment are illustrated. A. The prosthetic reconstruction is facilitated and the overjet reduced if the incisors are tipped back to an upright position. This is achieved by extraction of 2 premolars and ordinary orthodontic treatment with a fixed appliance. In adult patients with extensive overjet this is a common alternative. B. In young growing patients the overjet can be reduced and a normal occlusion obtained with extraoral appliances, functional orthopedics or Class II traction.

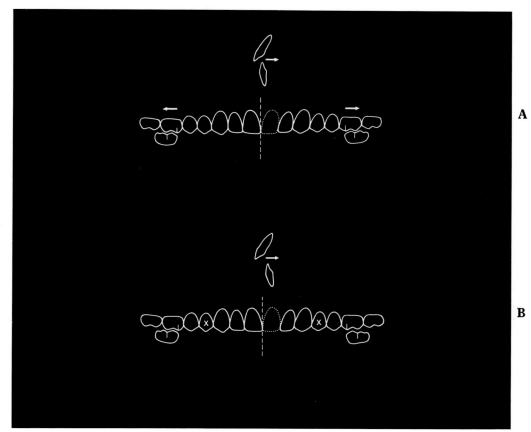

A

B

Crown- and Root-malformations

Malformations of permanent teeth due to traumatic injuries to primary predecessors often lead to impaction (28). If root development is reasonably advanced, combined surgical and orthodontic realignment is possible. Thus, teeth with crown or root dilaceration can be moved into a normal position orthodontically. Treatment, however, should be postponed until the mixed dentition stage.

Intruded Teeth

Intrusion of a permanent tooth into the alveolar bone is a severe traumatic injury. The trauma can cause pulp necrosis, root resorption and ankylosis. The risks of pulpal damage and ankylosis are important considerations in treatment planning.

Pulp canal obliteration as a consequence of intrusive luxation can be seen in immature teeth (127). Special care should be taken during orthodontic treatment of such teeth.

IMMATURE TEETH
Intruded immature teeth may be left to erupt spontaneously if the intrusion is not too severe (128,129). If the tooth has not begun erupting within 2 weeks, orthodontic extrusion with light forces must be performed. Intrusion always leads to pulpal damage. Sometimes the pulp may heal with subsequent obliteration of the pulpal lumen. Providing ankylosis does not develop, these teeth may have a good prognosis, as might teeth with pulp necrosis after adequate endodontic treatment (Figs. 15.37 and 15.38).

MATURE TEETH
Intrusion of mature teeth always leads to pulp necrosis. Prophylactic endodontic treatment is therefore recommended, as a necrotic and infected pulp can lead to rapidly progressive inflammatory root re-

Fig. 15.37. Orthodontic extrusion of an intruded incisor

An 8-year-old boy suffered intrusion of an immature maxillary right incisor. Over a period of 2 months there has been no sign of reeruption.

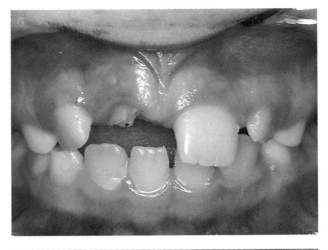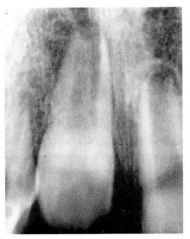

Orthodontic appliance

A removable appliance with an extrusion spring acting on a bracket bonded to the injured tooth. A light force was used to avoid damage to the pulp.

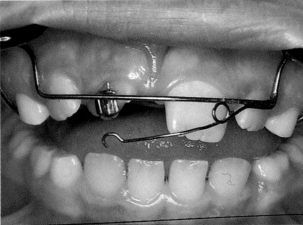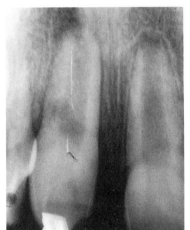

Extrusion completed

The extrusion was complete within 2 months. The clinical situation is shown after 1 year. Pulp necrosis and inflammatory resorption necessitated endodontic treatment.

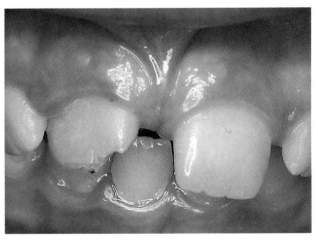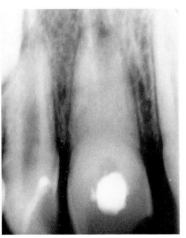

Condition after restoration

The clinical and radiographic condition is shown 4 years after trauma.

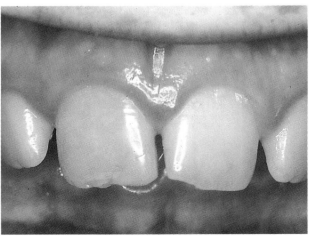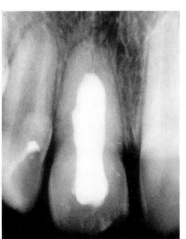

sorption. The critical period for the onset of external root resorption is 2 to 3 weeks. Therefore, in order to facilitate endodontic therapy, the intruded tooth must be repositioned within the first 3 weeks after injury. This can be accomplished either orthodontically or surgically (130-134).

Before treatment, there are some factors that must be considered. If the intrusion is severe, there is a risk that orthodontic extrusion will have little effect. The tooth might be tightly locked in bone and orthodontic forces may not be able to overcome this mechanical barrier. This may cause ankylosis and make orthodontic extrusion impossible. To avoid this complication, the intruded incisor can be slightly luxated before orthodontic extrusion (Fig. 15.38). Severe intrusion is often accompanied by fracture and displacement of the labial alveolar bone plate. Immediate surgical repositioning is then indicated, whereby the fractured labial bone plate is also repositioned.

Fig. 15.38. Orthodontic extrusion of 2 severely intruded central incisors
Preinjury condition. This 8-year-old boy suffered intrusion of both central incisors 1 week after this photo was taken.

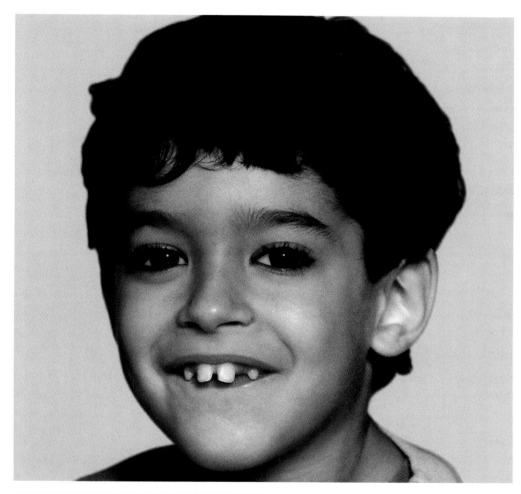

Post injury condition
The patient suffered intrusion of both central incisors.

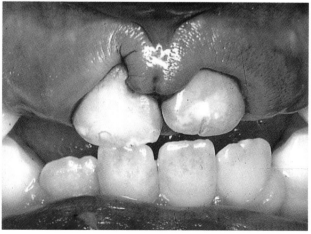
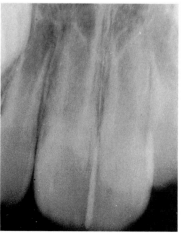

ORTHODONTIC MANAGEMENT OF THE TRAUMATIZED DENTITION

Loosening of the incisors
Both incisors were loosened with finger pressure. If this is not possible, forceps may be used.

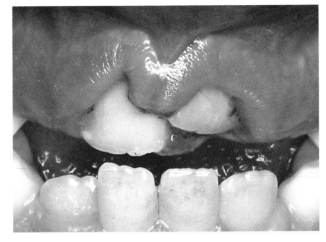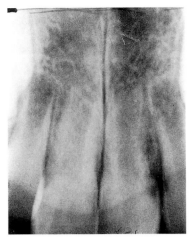

Status 2 months after injury
There was no spontaneous eruption. Orthodontic extrusion was therefore initiated. Endodontic treatment was performed in the left incisor due to pulp necrosis.

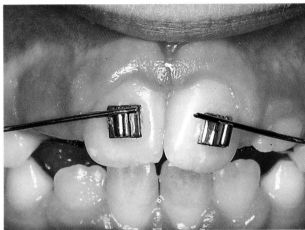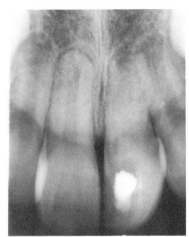

Status after 1 and 4 years
Clinical condition after 1 year and radiographic follow-up after 4 years. Note the partial pulp canal obliteration in the coronal part of the pulp chamber of the right incisor. Endodontic treatment was performed in the left incisor due to pulp necrosis.

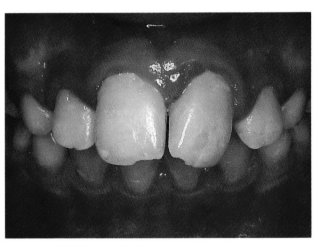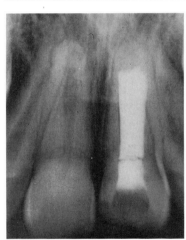

As a clinical guideline, teeth with severe intrusive luxations can be surgically repositioned if the intrusion is accompanied by fracture of the alveolar walls. Teeth with less severe intrusion might be orthodontically extruded. If the tooth is firmly locked within bone, slight luxation facilitates the orthodontic therapy. If surgical repositioning of the intruded incisor is desired, optimal healing with respect to marginal bone support and periodontal ligament is achieved if the tooth is only repositioned partially. Repositioning can then be completed either by orthodontic traction or by spontaneous reeruption.

Replanted and Transplanted Teeth

In cases where an avulsed tooth has been replanted, it may later be necessary to move the replanted tooth. The problem then arises whether orthodontic movement of the replanted tooth is possible

Fig. 15.39. Relation between general growth and infraposition of an ankylosed central incisor
The right central incisor was replanted in a boy at 14 years of age. Slight infraposition can be seen after 1 year. At 4-year control, there is a slight increase in infraposition.

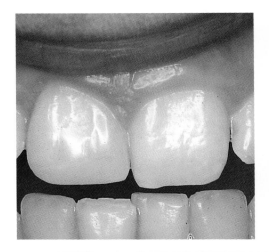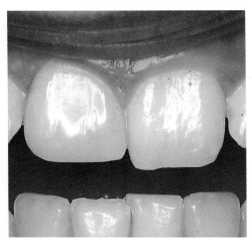

Relation between general growth and rate of infraposition
Annual body height measurements were registered for the patient and showed almost completed growth 2 years after the injury. The degree of infraposition was measured in mm.

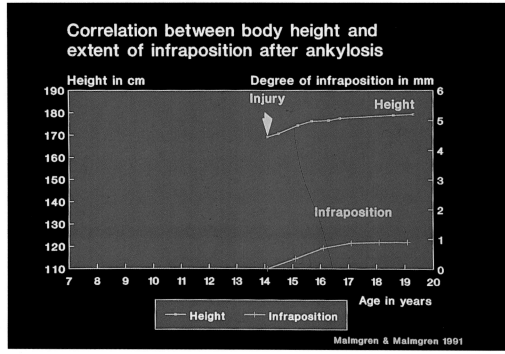

without a significant risk of root resorption.

Preliminary clinical studies (43, 45) as well as an experimental study in monkeys (44) indicate that severe root resorption can be elicited after orthodontic movement. Most root resorptions after replantation are seen during the 1st year after injury (see Chapter 10, p. 410). Thus, if no such complication is seen in this period, movement of the replanted tooth is possible. However, it must be considered that both replanted and intruded teeth may show progressive root resorption 5 or 10 years after trauma despite more optimistic evaluation earlier in the course of healing (see Chapter 9 and 10).

Ankylosis

If a tooth is ankylosed, it cannot be moved orthodontically. When ankylosis is diagnosed, it must therefore be decided whether to extract the tooth or to keep it as a space maintainer until complete resorption of the root has taken place. Providing no other changes are seen, the ankylosed tooth can be expected to be retained until the crown breaks off or is removed with forceps when most of the root substance has been replaced by bone.

In children and adolescents, however, the ankylosis is accompanied by increasing infraposition of the tooth, often with tilting of adjacent teeth. Such a tooth should

Fig. 15.40. Relation between general growth and infraposition of an ankylosed central incisor

The right central incisor was replanted in a boy at 12 ½ years of age. Slight infraposition can be seen after 1 year. At 2- and 1 1/2-year control there is a marked increase in infraposition.

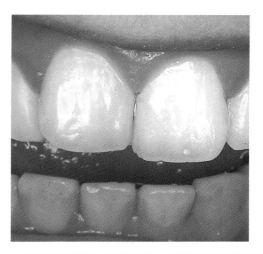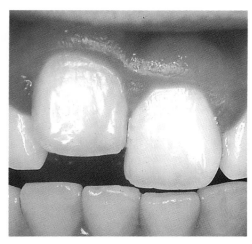

Relation between general growth and rate of infraposition

There is a marked growth spurt in this patient which correlates with the marked infraposition.

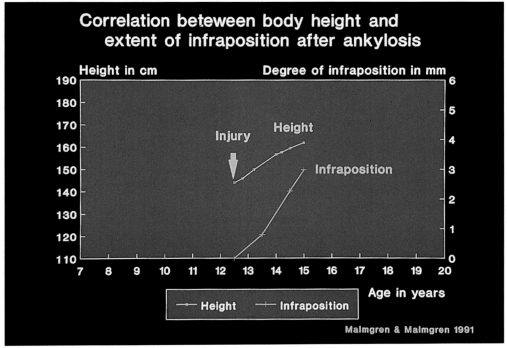

Correlation beteween body height and extent of infraposition after ankylosis

Malmgren & Malmgren 1991

Fig. 15.41.

Extraction of an ankylosed incisor where the bone plate was simultaneously removed

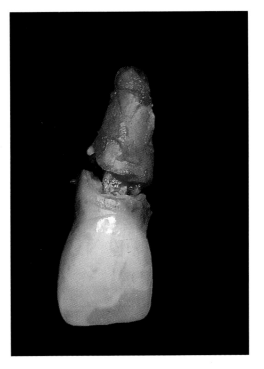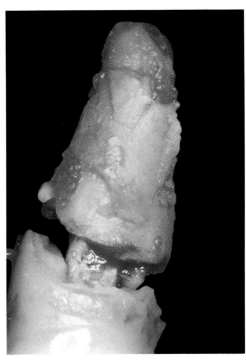

Fig. 15.42. Severe loss of alveolar bone after ankylosis of 2 incisors
An 18-year-old boy with ankylosed incisors due to a trauma 10 years earlier. Infraposition was allowed to progress.

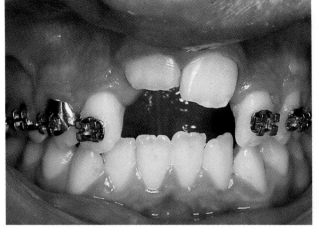 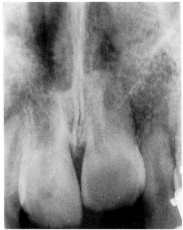

Status after extraction
An undesirable arrested development of the alveolar ridge is seen as a result of treatment neglect of the ankylosed teeth.

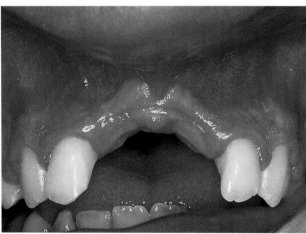 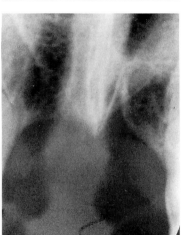

be removed before these changes become so advanced that satisfactory orthodontic or prosthetic therapy becomes difficult (Fig. 15.31).

It has been found that the progression of infraposition varies individually (Figs. 15.39 and 15.40). A recent study has shown that the risk of severe infraposition is particularly great if the ankylosis is diagnosed *before* the growth spurt (135). In these cases the ankylosed tooth must be removed within 2 to 3 years. If ankylosis develops *during* the growth spurt, the tooth must be observed at 6-month intervals. In such teeth, no active treatment is necessary as long as the adjacent teeth do not tilt and the extent of infraposition is minor and stable. In all other cases, the affected tooth must be removed and repla-

ced by autotransplantation, orthodontic closure or fixed prosthetics (135,136) (Figs. 15.39 and 15.40).

EXTRACTION OF ANKYLOSED INCISORS

Clinical experience shows that extraction of an ankylosed tooth may involve vertical and horizontal loss of alveolar bone (Fig. 15.41). If infraposition is allowed to progress, even an uncomplicated extraction of the incisor may lead to loss of the alveolar ridge (Fig. 15.42).

To avoid such bone loss, a technique for extracting ankylosed teeth has been developed (86) (Fig. 15.43). The crown of the tooth is removed and the ankylosed root is left in the alveolus to be substituted by bone (Figs. 15.44 to 15.46). In children,

Fig. 15.43. Surgical treatment of an ankylosed and infrapositioned incisor
Moderate infraposition of a right upper central incisor due to ankylosis in a 14-year-old boy.

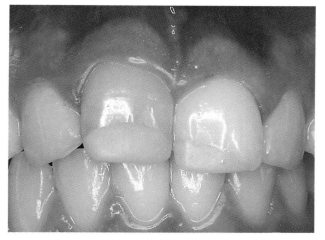 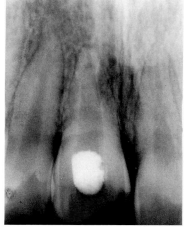

Sectioning the crown from the root
A mucoperiosteal flap is raised. The crown is removed with a diamond bur under a continuous flow of saline.

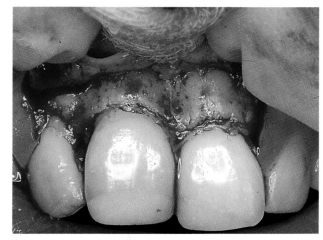 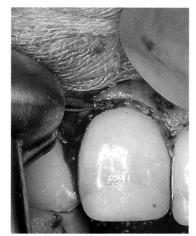

Removing of the root filling
The crown has been removed and the root filling removed with an endodontic file.

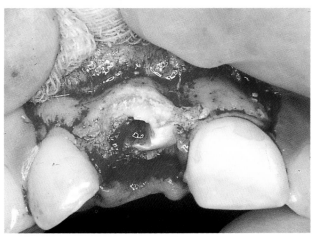 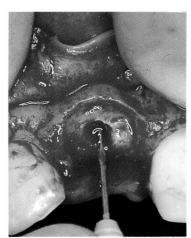

Preparation of the root
The coronal part of the root surface is reduced to a level of 2.0 mm below the marginal bone. The empty root canal is thoroughly rinsed with saline and thereafter allowed to fill with blood.

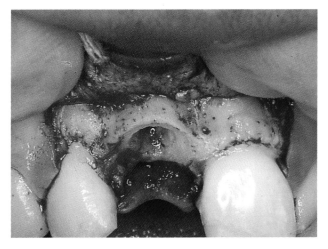 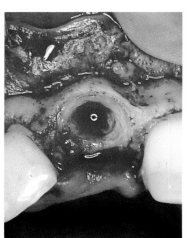

Suturing the flap
The mucoperiosteal flap is pulled over the alveolus and sutured with single sutures. A blood clot is formed in the gap between the labial and palatal mucosa.

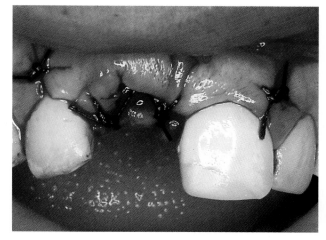
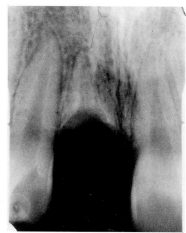

Temporary restoration
The removed crown is shaped as a pontic with composite material and splinted to the adjacent teeth with acid-etch technique and an enamel composite bond.

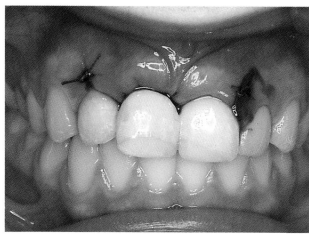

Follow-up 1 year after treatment
A resin-retained bridge has been inserted.

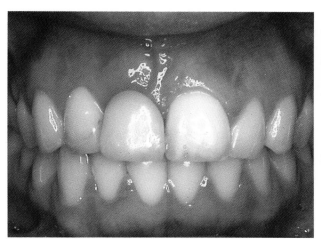
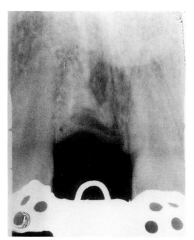

new marginal bone will then be formed coronal to the resorbing root. The height of the alveolar bone is thus improved vertically and preserved in the facio-lingual direction. The conditions for subsequent orthodontic or prosthetic therapy are thereby improved. Moreover, the possibility for placing an implant is facilitated if the alveolar bone is preserved (Figs. 15.44 to 15.46) (see Chapter 20, p 671).

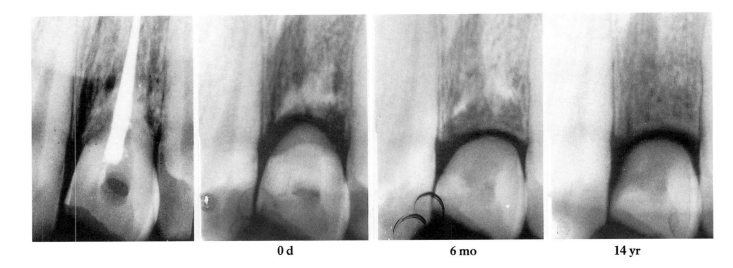

0 d   6 mo   14 yr

Fig. 15.44. Partial removal of an ankylosed maxillary incisor in infraposition
There is continous resorption of the ankylosed root and replacement with bone. Note shortened pontic and formation of new marginal bone coronal to the root remnants.

Retention

Space closure or space maintenance during treatment determines the demands for retention.

Retention planning can be divided into three categories:
1. No retention;
2. Limited retention;
3. Semipermanent or permanent retention.

The need for retention in orthodontically-treated patients with traumatic injuries depends on several factors. The following are the most important:
1. Elimination of the cause of the malocclusion;
2. Proper occlusion;
3. Reorganization of bone and soft tissues around newly positioned teeth;
4. Correction of skeletal deviations during the growth period.

In cases where all of these objectives have been met, the need for retention is limited.

Space Closure

The need for retention is reduced if the roots of the teeth are parallel after treatment. Tooth size discrepancies between the mesio-distal widths of the upper and lower teeth can be adjusted by selective grinding. This procedure might reduce the problem to one of limited retention, consisting of a removable or fixed appliance.

In cases where only a limited treatment goal can be achieved, semipermanent or permanent retention may be the only alternative. Semipermanent retention consists of a removable appliance, a lingual arch wire or a bonded appliance.

Space Maintenance

In cases where the space is maintained throughout treatment and the teeth are moved to positions best suited for a forthcoming bridge or implant, retention usually presents no problem. Permanent retention will then usually consist of a fixed prosthesis or a single standing implant.

Prognosis

Very little is known today about the prognosis of orthodontic movement of traumatized teeth. A pilot study, from the Eastman Institute in Stockholm, involving orthodontic treatment of 27 patients with

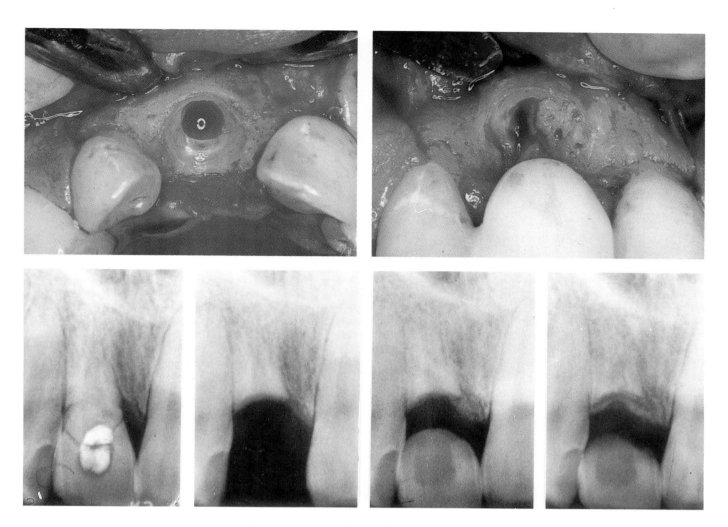

Fig. 15.45. Formation of bone after partial tooth removal
A. Condition at the time of surgery. B. A flap was raised 10 months later. New bone is seen replacing the resorbed root remnants. C. Radiographs immediately before and after surgery and at 6- and 18-month follow-ups. Note regeneration of coronal bone.

55 traumatized teeth and 60 non-traumatized teeth has been performed (85). Registration of the extent of root resorption before and after orthodontic movement showed a slight increase in the extent of root resorption in both traumatized and non-traumatized teeth, but with no significant difference between the two groups.

There is also a lack of information as to the risk of root resorption among the individual trauma entities. Empirical observations indicate that teeth with mild or moderate luxation injuries (i.e. con-

cussion or subluxation) can be moved orthodontically with limited risk of root resorption if treatment is performed carefully. This means using light orthodontic forces, avoiding contact with cortical bone and ensuring a short period of treatment. After severe luxation (i.e. extrusion, lateral luxation, intrusion and after replantation), movement of a tooth is more hazardous. However, if no ankylosis has occurred 1 year after trauma, orthodontic therapy can be performed.

It is possible to move root-fractured

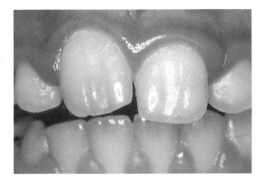
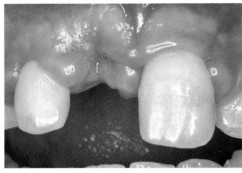

Fig. 15.46. Preserved alveolar ridge after partial removal of an ankylosed incisor
Ankylosis and subsequent infraposition of a right central incisor in a 13-year-old boy following replantation. Three weeks after surgery there is still a defect in the alveolar ridge.

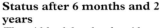

Status after 6 months and 2 years
The width of the alveolar ridge has been maintained. Note the proliferation and downgrowth of the gingiva 6 months after partial removal (left). After 2 years the width of the alveolar ridge has been maintained (right).

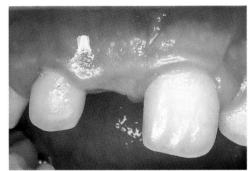
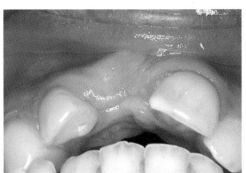

teeth, if the fracture is healed with a hard tissue callus, with almost the same prognosis as a non-injured tooth. If the fragments are separated by connective tissue, further separation can be expected and the tooth should be evaluated according to the length of the coronal segment.

The prognosis after orthodontic extrusion of crown-root fractured teeth depends upon the technique used. Relapse after orthodontic extrusion can be minimized by a cervical fibrotomy.

In treatment planning, it is essential to coordinate the prognosis for the traumatized tooth with the treatment of the malocclusion. Consequently, prognosis for the total treatment can be classified as follows:

Good prognosis for the traumatized tooth; good prognosis for the malocclusion. The treatment procedure for the malocclusion does not differ from orthodontic treatment in patients without injured teeth.

Good prognosis for the traumatized tooth; poor prognosis for the malocclusion. The orthodontic treatment is complicated, e.g. prolonged treatment time and severe anchorage problems. A limited goal must

often be accepted in order not to overload the traumatized tooth.

Poor prognosis for the traumatized tooth; good prognosis for the malocclusion. The traumatized tooth must often be extracted, but can otherwise serve as a space maintainer. The orthodontic treatment has a good prognosis and can provide optimal results. This is particularly true if the malocclusion is caused by habits and the habits are stopped. Malocclusions combined with skeletal deviations have a better prognosis if they are treated during periods of active growth. The orthodontic treatment can in most cases provide optimal results with either space closure or space maintenance.

Poor prognosis for the traumatized tooth; poor prognosis for the malocclusion. The traumatized tooth must often be extracted, but can serve as a space maintainer for some time. Prosthetic therapy, autotransplantation of a premolar or an implant to the trauma region can be indicated, depending upon the age of the patient. Orthodontic treatment in combination with orthognathic surgical correction is sometimes the treatment of choice.

Essentials

Preventive Orthodontics

Patients with increased overjet have a 2-3 times greater risk of traumatic dental injuries. Early orthodontic treatment is therefore indicated.

Diagnosis and Treatment

Based on the combined prognosis for the traumatized tooth and the malocclusion.

PRIMARY DENTITION

There is normally no need for interceptive orthodontic therapy.

MIXED DENTITION

Orthodontic treatment is indicated in patients with the following malocclusions.
a. Class II division 1 (Angle)
b. Class II division 2 (Angle)
c. Deep and open bites
d. Cross bites (labial, lingual and anterior)

PERMANENT DENTITION

Coordinate any remaining growth potential with the proposed orthodontic treatment.

Specific treatment problems for orthodontic treatment of traumatized teeth.

Observation Period after Trauma prior to Orthodontic Treatment

a. Mild injury (e.g. concussion, subluxation): 3 months
b. Moderate or severe injury (e.g. extrusion, intrusion, lateral extrusion, replantation): 6 months
c. Root-fractured teeth: 1 year
d. In endodontically treated teeth, orthodontic-treatment should be postponed until radiographic evidence of healing is seen.

General Treatment Principles for Orthodontic Treatment of Traumatized Teeth

Orthodontic treatment represents a certain extra hazard to the periodontium and pulp. In this regard, the following factors are of importance (Figs. 15.11 and 15.12).

a. The anatomy of the root.
b. Borders of cortical bone.
c. The use of light and short-acting orthodontic forces, possibly aimed at a limited goal.

ENDODONTICALLY TREATED TEETH

There is no evidence today of a greater risk of root resorption than in vital teeth.

ROOT RESORPTION SUBSEQUENT TO ORTHODONTIC TREATMENT

Regular radiographic controls are necessary in order to check if any root resorption occurs or increases during treatment.
a. The first control should be 6-9 months after initiation of treatment.
b. Signs of root resorption indicate controls every 2 months.
c. A suspension of treatment for about 3 months can reduce the risk of resorption.

Specific Treatment Principles for Orthodontic Treatment of Different Types of Trauma

AVULSION

a. *Primary dentition.* No immediate orthodontic treatment is indicated.

b. *Mixed dentition.*

Lateral incisor loss.
1. The space can be closed orthodontically.
2. The space can be maintained for later prosthetic treatment. A space maintainer can be used in the interim.
3. The space can be closed by an autotransplanted tooth.

Central incisor loss.
1. The space closure seldom leads to optimal esthetic results.
2. The space can be maintained and autotransplantation evaluated.
3. Alternatively a later fixed prosthetic therapy or an implant.

c. *Permanent dentition.*
1. The space can be closed orthodontically.

2. The space can be closed prosthetically.
3. The space can be closed by an auto-transplanted tooth or an implant.

LUXATION

Teeth with pulp necrosis and/or inflammatory root resorption should be treated endodontically prior to orthodontic treatment.

Orthodontic movement of luxated teeth with initial signs of resorption should be carefully checked for further resorption. The first observation should be made after 6 months and thereafter at 3-month intervals.

CROWN-ROOT FRACTURE

a. A non-vital tooth can be extruded over a period of 3-4 weeks (Fig. 15.19).
b. After a retention period of 4 weeks, the tooth can be restored.

ROOT FRACTURE

Orthodontic treatment possibilities are related to the type of healing and location of the fracture (Fig. 15.33).

a. Root-fractured teeth healed with a calcified tissue can be moved without breaking the callus.
b. Root-fractured teeth healed by interposition of connective tissue can be moved. They must be looked upon as teeth with short roots and further shortening can be expected. This implies shortening can be expected. This implies that fractures located in the apical third can normally be moved without difficulty, whereas fractures located in the middle third

should be evaluated for adequate periodontal support.

CROWN OR ROOT MALFORMATION

Combined surgical and orthodontic therapy can secure realignment of teeth with crown or root malformations.

INTRUDED TEETH

Orthodontic extrusion using light forces can secure repositioning (Fig. 15.37).

REPLANTED AND TRANSPLANTED TEETH

Orthodontic movement using light forces is possible.

ANKYLOSIS

If an ankylosed tooth in a growing child is accompanied by increasing infraposition, the tooth should be removed. The crown of the teeth is sectioned from the root and an eventual root filling is removed. The ankylosed root is thereafter left in the alveolus for subsequent replacement with bone (Fig. 15.43).

Retention

Follows the same principles as for non-traumatized teeth.

Prognosis

No definite values are known for the prognosis for orthodontic treatment of traumatized teeth. Preliminary figures indicate that teeth with an intact periodontal ligament prior to orthodontic treatment (e.g. without periapical inflammation, inflammatory or replacement resorption) can be moved with a prognosis, with respect to root resorption, comparable to that of non-traumatized teeth.

Bibliography

1. SCHÜTZMANNSKY G. Unfallverletzungen an jugendlichen Zähnen. *Dtsch Stomat* 1963;**13**: 919-927.

2. SCHÜTZMANNSKY G. Statistisches über Häufigkeit und Schweregrad von Unfalltraumen an der Corona Dentis im Frontzahn-bereich des kindlichen und jugendlichen Gebisses. *Z GesamteHyg* 1970;**16**: 133-135.

3. GLUCKSMANN DD. Fractured permanent anterior teeth complicating orthodontic treatment. *J Am Dent Assoc* 1941;**28**: 1941-1943.

4. HARDWICK JL, NEWMAN PP. Some observations on the incidence and emergency treatment of fractured permanent anterior teeth of children. *J Dent Res* 1954;**33**: 730.

5. LEWIS TE. Incidence of fractured anterior teeth as related to their protrusion. *Angle Orthod* 1959;**29**: 128-131.

6. HALLET GEM. Problems of common interest to the paedodontist and orthodontist with special reference to traumatized incisor cases. *Eur J Orthod Soc Trans* 1953;**29**: 266-277.

7. EICHENBAUM IW. A correlation of traumatized anterior teeth to occlusion. *J Dent Child* 1963;**30**: 229-236.

8. BÜTTNER M. Die Häufigkeit von Zahnunfällen im Schulalter. *Zahnärztl Prax* 1968;**19**: 286.

9. WALLENTIN I: Zahnfrakturen bei Kindern und Jugendlichen. *Zahnärztl Mitt* 1967;**57**: 875-877.

10. MCEWEN JD, MCHUGH WD, HITCHIN AD. Fractured maxillary central incisors and incisal relationships. *J Dent Res* 1967;**46**: 1290.(abs no. 87)

11. MCEWEN JD, MCHUGH WD. Predisposing factors associated with fractured incisor teeth. *Eur Orthod Soc Trans* 1969;**45** 343-351.

12. JOHNSON JE. Causes of accidental injuries to the teeth and jaws. *J Public Helth Dent* 1975;**35**: 123-131.

13. RAVN JJ. Dental injuries in Copenhagen school children school years 1967-1972. *Community Dent Oral Epidemiol* 1974;**2**: 231-245.

14. O'MULLANE DM. Some factors predisposing to injuries of permanent incisors in schoolchildren. *Br Dent J* 1973;**134**: 328-332.

15. BERZ H, BERZ A. Schneidezahnfrakturen und sagitale Schneidezahnstufe. *Dtsch Zahnärztl Z* 1971;**26**: 941-944.

16. WÓJCIAK L, ZIÓLKIEWICS T, ANHOLCE H. Trauma to the anterior teeth in school-children in the city of Poznan with reference to masticatory anomalies. *Czas Stomat* 1974;**27**: 1355-1361.

17. ANTOLIC I, BELIC D. Traumatic damages of teeth in the intercanine sector with respect to the occurrence with schoolchildren. *Zoboz Vestn* 1973;**28**: 113-120.

18. PATKOWSKA - INDYKA E, PLONKA K. The effect of occlusal anomalies on fractures of anterior teeth. *Protet Stomatol* 1974;**24**: 375-379.

19. DE MUNIZ BR, MUNIZ MA. Crown fractures in children.(Relationship with anterior occlusion.) *Rev Asoc Odont Argent* 1975;**63**: 153-157.

20. JÄRVINEN S. Incisal overjet and traumatic injuries to upper permanent incisors. A retrospective study. *Acta Odontol Scand* 1978;**36**: 359-362.

21. FERGUSON FS, RIPA LW. Incidence and type of traumatic injuries to the anterior teeth of preschool children. *I.A.D.R. Abstract* no. 401,1979.

22. GAUBA ML. A correlation of fractured anterior teeth to their proclination. *J Indian Dent Assoc* 1967;**39**: 105-112.

23. HELM S. Prevalence of malocclusion in relation to development of the dentition. *Acta Odontol Scand* 1970;**28**: Suppl. 58.

24. HELM S. Indikation af behov for ortodontisk behandling. En kritisk litteraturoversigt. *Tandlægebladet.* 1980;**84**: 175-185.

25. ANDREASEN JO, RAVN JJ. Epidemiology of traumatic dental injuries to primary and permanent teeth in a Danish population sample. *Int J Oral Surg* 1972;**1**: 235-239.

26. ASH AS. Orthodontic significance of anomalies of tooth eruption. *Am J Orthod* 1957;**43**: 559-576.

27. KORF SR. The eruption of permanent central incisors following premature loss of their antecedents. *ASDC J Dent Child* 1965;**32**:39-44.

28. ANDREASEN JO. SUNDSTRÖM B, RAVN JJ. The effect of traumatic injuries to primary teeth on their permanent successors. I. A clinical and histologic study of 117 injured permanent teeth. *Scand J Dent Res* 1971;**79**: 219-283.

29. DAUSCH-NEUMANN D. Uber die Lücken bei fehlenden Milchfront-zähnen. *Fortschr Kieferorthop* 1969;**30**: 82-88.

30. BJÖRK A. Käkarnas tillväxt och utveckling i relation till kraniet i dess helhet. In: HOLST JJ. NYGAARD ÖSTBY B, OSVALD O, eds. *Nordisk Klinisk Odontologi.* Copenhagen: A/S Forlaget for Faglitteratur 1973 Chapter 1-I:1-44.

31. ZACHRISSON BU, JACOBSEN I. Response to orthodontic movement of anterior teeth with root fractures. *Eur Orthod Soc Trans* 1974;**50**: 207-214.

32. WICKWIRE NA, MCNEIL MH, NORTON LA, DUELL RC. The effects of tooth movement upon endodontically treated-teeth. *Angle Orthod* 1974;**44**: 235-242.

33. PHILLIPS JR. Apical root resorption under orthodontic therapy. *Angle Orthod* 1955;**25**: 1-22.

34. DE SHIELDS RW. A study of root resorption in treated Class II Division I malocclusions. *Angle Orthod* 1969;**39**:231-245.

35. GOLDSON L, HENRIKSSON CO. Root resorption during Begg treatment: A longitudinal roentgenologic study. *Am J Orthod* 1975;**68**:55-66.

36. EPKER BN, PAULUS PJ. Surgical - orthodontic correction of adult malocclusions: single tooth dento-osseous osteotomies. *Am J Orthod* 1978;**74**: 551-563.

37. TEN HOEVE A, MULIE RM. The effect of antero-postero incisor repositioning on the palatal cortex as studied with laminagraphy. *J Clin Orthod* 1976;**10**: 804-822.

38. MULIE RM, TEN HOEVE A. The limitations of tooth movement within the symphysis studied with laminagraphy and standardized occlusal films. *J Clin Orthod* 1976;**10**: 882-899.

39. EDWARDS JG. A study of the anterior portion of the palate as it relates to orthodontic therapy. *Am J Orthod* 1976;**69**:249-273.

40. REITAN K. Initial tissue behavior during apical root resorption. *Angle Orthod* 1974;**44**: 68-82.

41. MASSLER M, MALONE AJ. Root resorption in human permanent teeth. A roentgenographic study. *Am J Orthod* 1954;**40**: 619-633.

42. REITAN K. Biomechanical principles and reactions. In: GRABER TM, SWAIN BF, eds. *Current orthodontic concepts and techniques.* Philadelphia: W. B. Saunders Company, 1975. vol I: 111-229.

43. HINES FB. Jr. A radiographic evaluation of the response of previously avulsed teeth and partially avulsed teeth to orthodontic movement. *Am J Orthod* 1979;**75**: 1-19.

44. GORDON NS. Effects of orthodontic force upon replanted teeth: a histologic study. *Am J Orthod* 1972;**62**: 544.

45. GRAUPNER JG. The effects of orthodontic force on replanted teeth: a radiographic survey. *Am J Orthod* 1972;**62**: 544-545.

46. ANTOLIC I. Functional treatment of traumatic teeth in children and youth. *Zobozdravstveni vestnik* 1973;**28**:121-127.

47. WOJTOWICZ N. Orthodontic-prosthetic management in cases of absent permanent incisors in children. *Czas Stomat* 1971;**24**: 1067-1073.

48. RAVN JJ. En redogørelse for behandlingen efter eksartikulation af permanente incisiver i en skolebarnspopulation. *Tandlægebladet.* 1977;**81**: 563-569.

49. SELMER-OLSEN R. Hvordan skal vi bedst mulig hjelpe barn som har slått ut en eller flere av sine permanente fortenner i overkjeven? *Norske Tandlægeforen Tid* 1975;**45**:41-50.

50. VAN DER LINDEN FPGM. De orthodontische behandeling van een geval met agenesie van een premolaar a verlies door trauma van een central incisief in dezelfde vobenkaakhelft. *Ned T Tandheelk* 1972;**79**: 436-443.

51. DORENBOS J. Algemeen tandheelkundige en orthodontische aspecten bij traumata van fronttanden. *Ned T Tandheelk* 1972;**79**:398-405.

52. DROSCHL H. Kieferorthopädisch-prophylaktische Massnahmnen beim Frontzahntrauma. *Öst Z Stomat* 1974;**71**: 459-464.

53. PHILIPPE J. Remplacement d'une incisive centrale et orthodontie. *Actual Odontostomatol* 1972;**99**: 389-393.

54. BRÜCKL H, BIRKE P. Zur kieferorthopädischen Behandlung des traumatischen Frontzahnverlustes. *Fortschr Kieferorthop* 1964;**25**: 289-294.

55. NORDQUIST GG, McNEIL RW. Orthodontic vs. restorative treatment of the congenitally absent lateral incisor - long term periodontal and occlusal evaluation. *J Periodontol* 1975;**46**:139-143.

56. RAMFJORD SP, ASH Jr. MM. *Occlusion.*Philadelphia: W. B. Saunders Company, 1966,333.

57. ZACHRISSON BU, MJÖR IA. Remodelling of teeth by grinding. *Am J Orthod* 1975;**68**: 545-553.

58. ZACHRISSON BU. Improving orthodontic results in cases with maxillary incisors missing. *Am J Orthod* 1978;**73**:274-289.

59. MONEFELDT I, ZACHRISSON B. Adjustment of clinical crown height by gingivectomy following orthodontic space closure. *Angle Orthod* 1977;**47**: 256-264.

60. HALLONSTEN A.-L, KOCH G, LUDVIGSSON N, OLGART K, PAULANDER J. Acid-etch technique in temporary bridgework using composite pontics in the juvenile dentition. *Swed Dent J* 1979;**3**: 213-219.

61. RAKOW B, LIGHT EI. Enamel-bonded immediate tooth replacement. *Am J Orthod* 1978;**74**: 430-434.

62. DIXON DA. Autogenous transplantation of tooth germs into the upper incisor region. *Br Dent J* 1971;**131**: 260-265.

63. KRISTERSON L. Unusual case of tooth transplantation: report of case. *J Oral Surg* 1970;**28**: 841-844.

64. SLAGSVOLD O, BJERCKE B. Applicability of autotransplantation in cases of missing upper anterior teeth. *Am J Orthod* 1978;**74**:410-421.

65. SLAGSVOLD O. Autotransplantation of premolars in cases of missing anterior teeth. *Eur Orthod Soc Trans* 1970;**46**: 473-485.

66. ANDREASEN JO. *Atlas of replantation and transplantation of teeth.* Fribourg: Mediglobe, 1992.

67. KUGELBERG R, TEGSJÖ U, MALMGREN O. Autotransplantation of 45 teeth to the upper incisor region. In preparation.

68. RÖNNERMAN A. Orthodontic movement of traumatized upper central incisors. Report of two cases. *Swed Dent J* 1973;**66**: 527-534.

69. HEITHERSAY GS. Combined endodontic-orthodontic treatment of transverse root fractures in the region of the alveolar crest. *Oral Surg Oral Med Oral Pathol* 1973;**36**: 404-415.

70. WOLFSON EM, SEIDEN L. Combined endodontic-orthodontic treatment of subgingivally fractured teeth. *J Canad Dent Assoc* 1975;**11**: 621-624.

71. INGBER JS. Forced eruption: Part II. A method of treating nonrestoreable teeth - periodontal and restorative considerations. *J Periodontol* 1976;**47**: 203-216.

72. PERSSON M, SERNEKE D. Ortodontisk framdragning av tand med cervikal rotfraktur för att möjliggöra kronersättning. *Tandläkartidningen* 1977;**69**: 1263-1269.

73. DELIVANIS P, DELIVANIS H, KUFTINEC MM. Endodontic-orthodontic management of fractured anterior teeth. *J Am Dent Assoc* 1978;**97**: 483-485.

74. SIMON JHS, KELLY WH, GORDON DG, ERICKSEN GW. Extrusion of endodontically treated teeth. *J Am Dent Assoc* 1978;**97**: 17-23.

75. BESSERMANN M. Ny behandlingsmetode af krone-rodfrakturer. *Tandlægebladet* 1978;**82**: 441-444.

76. BESSERMANN M. Personal communication.

77. OPPENHEIM A. Artificial elongation of teeth. *Am J Orthod Oral Surg* 1940;**26**: 931-940.

78. RIEDEL RA. Retention. In GRABER TM, SWAIN BF: eds. *Current orthodontic concepts and techniques.* Philadelphia:W. B. Saunders Company, 1975;Vol I: 1095-1137.

79. DAVILA JM, GWINNET AJ. Clinical and microscopic evaluation of a bridge using the acid-etch resin technique. *ASDC J Dent Child* 1978;**45**: 228-232.

80. JORDAN RE, SUZUKI M, SILLS PS, GRATTON DR, GWINNET AJ. Temporary fixed partial dentures fabricated by means of the acid-etch resin technique: a report of 86 cases followed for up to three years. *J Am Dent Assoc* 1978;**96**: 994-1001.

81. MACKIE IC, WARREN VN. Avulsion of immature incisor teeth. *Dental Update* 1988: 406-408

82. MOHLIN B. Early reduction of large overjet. *Proceedings of the Second International Conference on Dental Trauma.* Folksam IADT 1991: 88-95.

83. ANDREASEN FM, ANDREASEN JO, BAYER T. Prognosis of root-fractured permanent incisors - prediction of healing modalities. *Endod Dent Traumatol* 1989; **5**:11-22.

84. ANDREASEN FM, VESTERGAARD-PEDERSEN B. Prognosis of luxated permanent teeth - the development of pulpal necrosis. *Endod Dent Traumatol* 1985;**1**:202-220.

85. REMINGTON DN, JOONDEPH DR, ÅRTUN J, RIEDEL RA, CHAPKO MK. Long term evaluation of root resorption occurring during orthodontic treatment. *Am J Orthod Dentofacial Orthop* 1989; **98**: 43-46.

86. SPURRIER SW, HALL SH, JOONDEPH DR, SHAPIRO PA, RIEDEL RA. A comparison of apical root resorption during orthodontic treatment in endodontically treated and vital teeth. *Am J Orthod Dentofacial Orthop* 1990;**97**: 130-134.

87. CVEK M. Treatment of non-vital permanent incisors with calcium hydroxide. An effect on external root resorption in luxated teeth compared with effect of root filling with gutta-percha. A follow-up. *Odont Revy* 1973;**24**:343-354.

88. LEVANDER E, MALMGREN O. Evaluation of the risk of root resorption during orthodontic treatment. *Eur J Orthod* 1988; 30-38.

89. LEVANDER E, MALMGREN O, ELIASSON S. Evaluation of root resorption in relation to two orthodontic treatment regimes. In manus. 1992.

90. MALMGREN B, CVEK M, LUNDBERG M, FRYKHOLM A. Surgical treatment of ankylosed and infrapositioned reimplanted incisors in adolescents. *Scand J Dent Res* 1984; **92**:391-399.

91. MALMGREN O, GOLDSON L, HILL C, ORWIN A, PETRINI L, LUNDBERG M. Root resorption after orthodontic treatment of traumatized teeth. *Am J Orthod Dentofacial Orthop* 1982;**82**:487-491.

92. LINGE L, LINGE B.O. Patient characteristics and treatment variables associated with apical root resorption during orthodontic treatment. *Am J Orthod Dentofacial Orthop* 1991; **99**: 35-43.

93. WEHRBEIN H, BAUER W, SCHNEIDER B, DIETRICH P. Experimentelle körperliche Zahnbewegung durch den knöchernen Nasenboden-eine Pilotstudie. *Fortschr Kieferorthop* 1990;**51**:271-276.

94. GÖS G, RAKOSI T. Die apikale Wurzelresorption unter kieferorthopädischer Behandlung. *Fortschr Kieferorthop* 1989;**50**:196-206.

95. HIRSCHFELDER U. Nachuntersuchung zur Reaktion des marginalen und apikalen Parodontiums unter kontinuerlicher Kraftapplikation. *Fortschr Kieferorthop* 1990; **51**: 82-89.

96. STÅLHANE I, HEDEGÅRD B. Traumatized permanent teeth in children aged 7-15 years. Part II. *Swed Dent J* 1975;**68**:157-159.

97. BENENATI FW, SIMON JHS. Orthodontic root extrusion: its rationale and uses. *Gen Dent* 1986; **34**: 285-289.

98. WEISSMAN J. Orthodontic extrusion of endodontically treated anterior teeth. *Can Dent Assoc J* 1983;**11**:21-24.

99. GHAREVI N. Extrusions-Therapiemöglichleiten bei tieffrakturierten Zähnen. *Konservierende Zahnheilkunde* 1986;**4**: 671-681.

100. KING NM, SO L. A laboratory fabricated fixed appliance for extruding anterior teeth with subgingival fractures. *Pediatr Dentistry* 1988;**10**:108-110.

101. PONTORIERO R, CELENZA F, RICCI G, CARNEVALE G. Rapid extrusion with fiber resection: a combined orthodontic - periodontic treatment modality. *Int J Period Rest Dent* 1987;**5**: 31-43.

102. MALMGREN O, MALMGREN B, FRYKHOLM A. Rapid orthodontic extrusion of crown root and cervical root fractured teeth. *Endod Dent Traumatol* 1991;**7**:49-54.

103. ÅRTUN J, AAMDAL HMA. A Severe root resorption of fractured maxillary lateral incisor following endodontic treatment and orthodontic extrusion. *Endod Dent Traumatol* 1987; **3**:263-267.

104. TEGSJÖ U, VALERIUS-OLSSON H, FRYKHOLM A, OLGART K. Clinical evaluation of intra-alveolar transplantation of teeth with cervical root fractures. *Swed Dent J* 1987;**11**:235-250.

105. KAHNBERG K-E. Intra-alveolar transplantation of teeth with crown-root fractures. *J Oral Maxillofac Surg* 1985;**43**:38-42

106. KAHNBERG K-E. Surgical extrusion of root-fractured teeth - a follow-up study of two surgical methods. *Endod Dent Traumatol* 1988;**4**:85-89.

107. ANDREASEN FM, ANDREASEN JO, BAYER T. Prognosis of root-fractured permanent incisors - prediction of healing modalities. *Endod Dent Traumatol* 1989;**5**:11-22.

108. ANDREASEN FM. Pulpal healing after luxation injuries and root fracture in the permanent dentition. *Endod Dent Traumatol* 1989;**5**:111-31.

109. ZACHRISSON BU, JACOBSEN I. Long term prognosis of 66 permanent anterior teeth with root fracture. *Scand J Dent Res* 1975;**83**:345-354.

110. SCHOPF P. Frontzahntrauma/Frontzahnverlust - epidemiologische und kieferorthopädische Aspekte. *Fortschr Kieferorthop* 1989;**50**:564-598.

111. JOHO JP. Das Zahntrauma aus kieferothopädischer Sicht. *Schweiz Monatsch Zahnheilk* 1974;**84**:934-946.

112. KRAFT J, HERTRICH J, SPITZER WJ, HICKEL R, MUSSIG D. Das Frontzahntrauma bei Kindern und Jugendlichen. *ZWR* 1986; **95**: 915-921.

113. NEWSOME PRH, COOK MS. Modifying upper lateral incisors to mimic missing central incisors: New ways to overcome old problems? *Restorative Dentistry* 1987;**13**:91-99.

114. SCHRÖDER U. GRANATH L. A new interceptive treatment of cases with missing maxillary lateral incisors. *Swed Dent J* 1981 **5**:155-158.

115. KRISTERSON L, LAGERSTRÖM L. Autotransplantation of teeth in cases with agenesis or traumatic loss of maxillary incisors. *Eur J Orthod* 1991;**13**:486-492.

116. BOWDEN DEJ, PATEL HA. Autotransplantation of premolar teeth to replace missing maxillary central incisors. *Br J Orthod* 1990;**17**:21-28.

117. KRISTERSON L. Autotransplantation of human premolars. A clinical and radiographic study of 100 teeth. *J Oral Surg* 1985; **14**:200-213.

118. ANDREASEN JO, PAULSEN HU, YU Z, AHLQUIST R, BAYER T, SCHWARTZ O. A long-term study of 370 autotransplanted premolars. Part I. Surgical procedures and standardized techniques for monitoring healing. *Eur J Orthod* 1990; **12**:3-13.

119. ANDREASEN JO, PAULSEN HU, YU Z, BAYER T, SCHWARTZ O. A long-term study of 370 autotransplanted premolars. Part II. Tooth survival and pulp healing subsequent to transplantation. *Eur J Orthod* 1990;**12**:14-24.

120. ANDREASEN JO, PAULSEN HU, YU Z, SCHWARZ O. A long-term study of 370 autotransplanted premolars. Part III. Periodontal healing subsequent to transplantation. *Eur J Orthod* 1990;**12**:25-37.

121. ANDREASEN JO, PAULSEN HU, BAYER T. A long-term study of 370 autotransplanted premolars. Part IV. Root development subsequent to transplantation. *Eur J Orthod* 1990; **12**: 38-50.

122. LAGERSTRÖM L, KRISTERSON L. Influence of orthodontic treatment on root development of autotransplanted premolars. *Am J Orthod Dentofacial Orthop* 1986;**89**:146-150.

123. ÅRTUN J, ZACHRISSON U. New technique for semipermanent replacement of missing incisors. *Am J Orthod Dentofacial Orthop* 1984;**85**:367-375.

124. ADELL R, ERIKSSON B, LEKHOLM U, BRÅNEMARK P-I, JEMT T. A long term follow-up study of osseointegrated implants in treatment of totally edentulous jaw. *Int J Oral Maxillofac Implants* 1990;**5**:347-359.

125. JEMT T, LEKHOLM U, GRÖNDAHL K. A three year follow-up study of early single implant restorations ad modum Brånemark. *Int J Period and Restorative Dent* 1990;**5**: 341-349.

126. ÖDMAN J, GRÖNDAHL K, LEKHOLM U, THILANDER B. The effect of osseointegrated implants on the dento-alveolar development. A clinical and radiographic study in growing pigs. *Eur J Orthod* 1991;**13**:279-286.

127. ANDREASEN FM, YU Z, THOMSEN BL, ANDERSEN PK. Occurrence of pulp canal obliteration after luxation injuries in the permanent dentition. *Endod Dent Traumatol* 1987;**3**:103-115.

128. BRUSZT P. Secondary eruption of teeth intruded into the maxilla by blow. *Oral Surg Oral Med Oral Pathol* 1958;**11**:146-149.

129. RAVN JJ. Intrusion of permanent incisiver. *Tandlægebladet* 1975;**79**:643-646.

130. TURLEY PK, JOINER MW, HELLSTRÖM S. The effect of orthodontic extrusion on traumatically intrudeed teeth. *Am J Orthod Dentofacial Orthop* 1984;**85**:47-56.

131. VINCKIER F, LAMBRECHTS W, DECLERCK D. Intrusion de l'incisive définitive. *Rev Belge Med Dent* 1989;**44**: 99-106.

132. JACOBSEN I. Clinical follow-up study of permanent incisors with intrusive luxation after acute trauma. *J Dent Res* 1983; **62**: Abstract No 37.

133. PEREZ B, BECKER A, CHOSAK A. The repositioning of a traumatically intruded mature rooted permanent incisor with removable orthodontic appliance. *J Pedod* 1982;**6**:343-354.

134. SHAPIRA J, REGEV L, LIEBFELD H. Re-eruption of completely intruded immature permanent incisors. *Endod Dent Traumatol* 1986;**2**:113-116.

135. MALMGREN B, MALMGREN O. Infraposition of reimplanted ankylosed incisors related to growth in children and adolescents. In preparation.

136. ALBERS DD. Ankylosis of teeth in the developing dentition. *Quintessenz Int* 1986;**17**:303-308.

137. GHOSE LJ, BAGHDADY VS, ENKE H. Relation of traumatized permanent anterior teeth to occlusion and lip condition. *Community Dent Oral Epidemiol* 1980;**8**:381-384.

138. HUNTER ML, HUNTER B, KINGDON A, ADDY M, DUMMER PMH, SHAW WC. Traumatic injury to maxillary incisor teeth in a group of South Wales school children. *Endod Dent Traumatol* 1990;**6**:260-264.

CHAPTER 16

Restoration of Traumatized Teeth with Composites

R.E. JORDAN

Resin bonding is by far the most frequently utilized, most reliable, and most predictable of all bonding procedures involving composite resin materials (1). The basis for enamel bonding involves the use of phosphoric acid etching (2). The application of phosphoric acid to an enamel surface renders it self-retentive (3) owing to the fact that microporosities are thereby formed which extend between 25 and 50 microns deep into the subsurface enamel (4) (Fig. 16.1). Should a free-flow bonding resin be placed on such an enamel surface, the resin enters the enamel microporosities in the form of long projecting tags, thereby forming a deeply penetrative interlocking relationship at the resin-enamel interface which is unique in operative dentistry (Fig. 16.1). Such a relationship provides not only a conservative means of securing retention of resin material to tooth structure but also a reliable method of eliminating the marginal leakage for which resin materials have been notorious (5).

Discoloration and leakage around the margin of a resin restoration are primarily due to a contraction gap at the enamel interface resulting from polymerization shrinkage. Phosphoric acid etching of enamel surfaces prior to the introduction of

Fig. 16.1
A. Scanning electron micrograph (5000 x) of phosphoric acid-etched enamel surface. B. Scanning electron micrograph (1800 x) of resin tags. Courtesy of Dr. K D. Jørgensen Department of Dental materials, Dental College. Copenhagen.

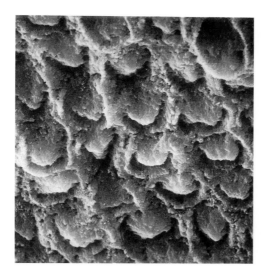
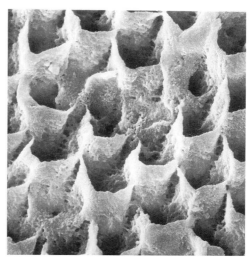

resin materials eliminates the contraction gap at the enamel boundary and thereby enhances the marginal seal of the material on a long-term basis.

Material Considerations

Conservative restoration of an extensively fractured young incisor crown may be an exceedingly demanding procedure since the primary requisites for the material of choice involve a combination of esthetic acceptability, resistance to fracture and abrasive wear, and biological acceptability (Fig. 16.2). Concerning acute treatment strategy and pulpal management, the reader is referred to Chapters 6 and 14.

Full coverage, in the form of a porcelain jacket or porcelain fused to metal crowns are options which should be carefully considered. There is no question as to their esthetic acceptability and resistance to fracture and abrasive wear; these are the major advantages of full coverage restorations. However, full coverage should be avoided in the young adolescent or early adult dentition because the pulp chambers are usually large and, accordingly, the pulp response to the combined irritants of trauma, extensive preparation, temporization, and cementation is unpredictable. Further, since the young anterior teeth have not reached the state of full eruption, the gingival response to placement of full crown margins beneath the free gingival crest is often less than positive (6).

Composite crown build-up should be seriously considered as an alternative in the young patient, since esthetics, biological acceptability, and resistance to abrasive wear are all excellent (7). Fracture resistance varies with the material selected. However, should fracture of the composite restoration occur, it is easily and reliably repaired (8).

Composite crown build-up may be carried out with microfilled, macrofilled, or hybrid materials. The microfilled materials should only be used to restore incisal fractures when the maxillo-mandibular relationship is normal and when the remaining natural teeth can serve as the primary support for centric, protrusive, and protrusive lateral functions. When the occlusion is heavy and the incisal composite restoration is expected to bear most of the occlusal load, particularly in protrusive and protrusive lateral function, macrofilled or hybrid types of "heavy filled" composite materials are specifically indicated because of their greater fracture resistance in stress-bearing situations.

The best materials for restoration of incisal fracture are as follows:
1. Highly polishable hybrids are comprised of microparticles/co/bisdalsilica) .04 microns and macroparticles 1 to 3 microns. Average filler particle size is usually 0.6 to 1 micron.
2. *Heavy filled microfilled composites* are comprised entirely of microparticles .04 microns in diameter. Filler loading is above 75% by weight.
3. Semi-polishable hybrids are comprised of microparticles and macroparticles. The average filler particle size is usually 1 to 3 microns.

The technique of composite crown build-up is identical irrespective of the materials used.

Shade Selection

Rubber dam isolation of the field is essential. However, the proper shade should be selected before the field is isolated, as dehydrated enamel whitens considerably, thus precluding the possibility of a proper shade match after rehydration. Multiple shades are an important requirement with composite materials, and it is essential that at least eight to ten shades are available.

Unfortunately, few shade guides provided by manufacturers accurately indicate the shade of the composite material. To further complicate the problem of shade selection, light-cured composite materials undergo a shade transformation when subjected to light. Accordingly, before a new composite material is used clinically, fabrication of a customized shade guide is recommended. The base shades are placed in several different transparent crown forms and cured. Subsequently, various mixtures of the base shades are placed in additional crown forms and cured. An accurate custom shade guide is thus created which greatly simplifies precise shade matching clinically.

Fig. 16.2. A. Restoration of fractured incisor with composite
This patient has suffered an uncomplicated crown fracture of a central incisor. The pulp responds to sensibility testing and there is no sign of injury to the periodontal ligament.

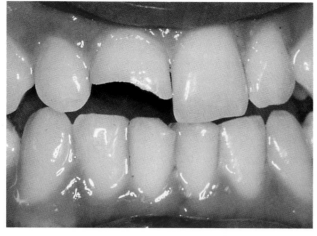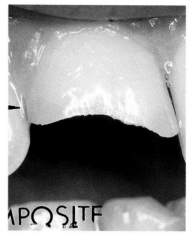

B. Pulp protection
Exposed dentin immediately over the pulp horn is covered with a light-cured glass ionomer cement.

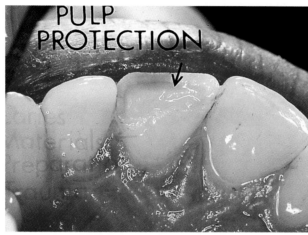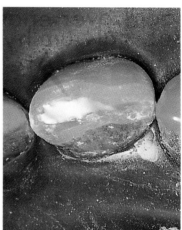

C. Preparing a circumferential chamfer-shoulder
A bullet-nosed diamond is used to prepare the shoulder labially and lingually, while a thin tapered diamond is used proximally. The chamfer extends 1-2 mm cervically and to a depth of at least half of the enamel thickness.

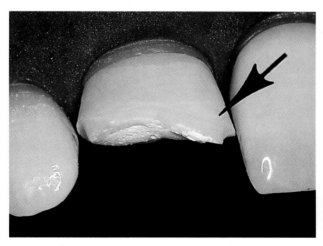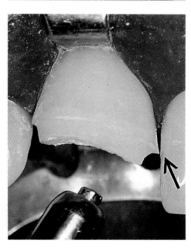

D. Selecting a matrix crown form
A crown form is selected which matches the mesio-distal dimension of the tooth and extends 1 mm apical to the chamfer margin.

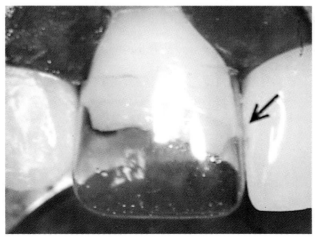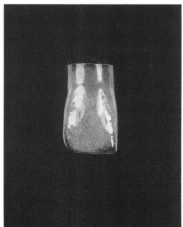

Pulp Protection

The clinical case under consideration involves a maxillary central incisor with extensive fracture exposing deep dentin in close proximity to the pulp. For details concerning exposed dentin with or without an exposed dental pulp, the reader is referred to Chapters 6 and 14 respectively.

Relative to differential choice of pulp protective materials, for deep situations in very close proximity to the pulp a hard-setting calcium hydroxide liner is recommended. Otherwise, either self-cured glass ionomer cements (Fig. 16.2B) or the various light-cured pulpal protective materials are recommended (see also Chapters 6 and 14).

Preparation

A bevel should not be used prior to crown build-up in order to avoid a "white line margin". Instead a chamfer shoulder should be prepared (Fig. 16.2C). For this purpose a bullet-nosed diamond is used around the *entire* enamel periphery. The preparation should extend cervically approximately 1 mm beyond the edge of the fractured enamel and, in depth, should involve at least half of the enamel thickness (Figure 16.2C). Ideally, the chamfer should be cut as far through the enamel thickness as possible without exposing dentin in order to allow a maximal bulk of composite material to overlie cut tooth structure. Particular care should be taken to ensure that the chamfer preparation is not too shallow, or a halo effect will occur in the final restoration. The chamfer shoulder preparation has the following functions:

a) removes the acid-resistant superficial enamel;

b) allows a "resin lap joint" which effectively masks the abrupt interface between the enamel and composite material;

c) provides a well-defined marginal finishing line to which the composite material may be precisely finished; and

d) ensures proper enamel prism orientation for effective acid etching.

Pins, particularly self-threading pins, should be avoided in crown build-up since they are associated with a high incidence of dentinal cracking with resultant subsequent discoloration (9).

Acid Etching

There is overwhelming clinical evidence that all composite resin restorations (Class III, IV, or V) are greatly enhanced by the routine utilization of enamel acid-etching techniques (7). There are four important considerations in acid etching, namely; *method, time, concentration,* and *type* of acid utilized. All may significantly affect the longevity of the restoration (10).

Method. Phosphoric acid may be brush applied or injected in viscous gel form. A brush is recommended because the fine tip confines the acid to the enamel periphery of the chamfer shoulder preparation, (i.e. a controlled etching technique), and the soft bristles prevent a heavy rubbing or scrubbing mode of acid application that would result in decreased retention due to the fracture of interstitial enamel surrounding the micropores (4).

Type of acid. Either an aqueous solution or a phosphoric acid gel may be utilized. Aqueous solutions are very easy to apply, but difficult to control because of their free-flow nature. High viscosity phosphoric acid gels are much more readily controlled clinically.

Time. The acid should be applied for a period of 15 to 20 sec, as prolonged etching does not improve the bond. The application time should be increased to 1 min for either fluorosed or deciduous enamel because both are relatively resistant to the etching procedure.

Acid concentration. Although the subject is controversial, clinical as well as laboratory observations indicate that concentrations of 30-40% are the most reliably effective in creating microporous enamel surfaces (11).

Post-etch cleaning. After acid-etching, the enamel surface should be thoroughly rinsed by means of a copious water lavage for at least 15-30 sec (12). The prolonged water lavage is necessary to remove contaminant residues, consisting mainly of soluble calcium salts, from the treated enamel surface prior to bonding. Failure to do so may inhibit effective resin bonding and constitutes a common reason for bond failure.

Drying the enamel surface. A dual air-water syringe is not recommended for drying the etched surface, as these syringes are notorious for contaminating the enamel surface with microdroplets of water.

E. Seating the crown form with composite
The crown form is seated. Contoured wooden wedges are placed interproximally.

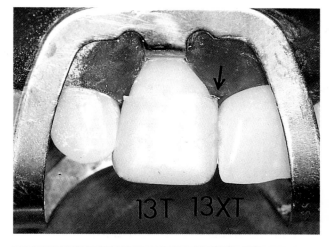

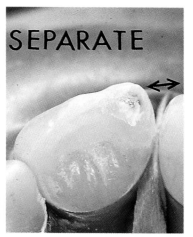

F. Removing the crown form
The crown matrix is peeled away from the composite and gross excess of composite is removed from the labial surface with a tapered carbide bur. Surplus of material is removed with a special composite knife.

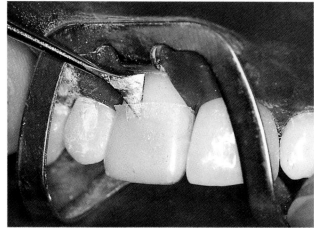

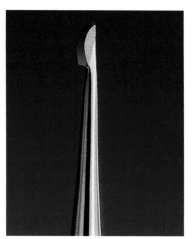

G. Finishing the labial cervical margins
A tapering carbide bur is used for labial finishing of excess composite.

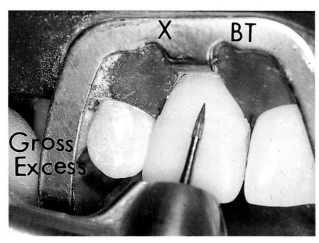

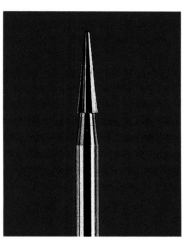

H. Completed composite restoration
Good color harmony has been achieved and no filling margins can be seen.

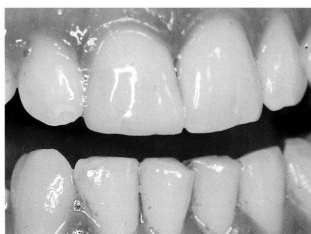

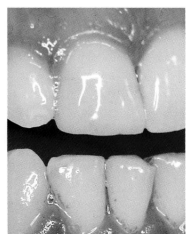

RESTORATION OF TRAUMATIZED TEETH WITH COMPOSITES

The enamel surface should be carefully dried after rinsing. Although chemical drying agents may be used, warm air-drying is preferred. After drying, the enamel surface should present a chalky white opaque appearance. At this point the enamel surface is said to be in a critical state for it is most sensitive to contamination. Should even a small quantity of saliva come in contact with the etched enamel surface, the microporous surface becomes obliterated by a firmly adherent contaminant layer composed mainly of salivary proteins, i.e. pellicle. Should this occur, the surface can only be effectively re-cleansed by the application of phosphoric acid for a 15- to 20-sec period (13). The maintenance of strictly controlled dry conditions renders this measure unnecessary.

Dentin bonding agents. Concerning the use of dentin bonding agents, the reader is referred to Chapter 6.

Bonding resins. The routine use of a bonding resin, irrespective of the particular composite material utilized, is a necessary expedient as it increases working time with the composite material and enhances marginal integrity (14, 15). Since most composite materials are highly viscous, they do not adapt well to acid-etched enamel surfaces. The problem is further complicated by the fact that the viscosity of a self-cured material rapidly increases with time after mixing, thereby compromising adaptation even further. Similarly, the viscosity of a light-cured composite material rapidly increases on extrusion from its container as room or operatory light begins the polymerization process. The use of a bonding resin gives the clinician time to properly manipulate the composite material irrespective of whether it is light- or self-cured. The mechanism by which this is brought about is the "air-inhibited" surface layer of the bond resin. The bond resins may be either visible light-cured or self-cured systems. Such materials are not only excellent dentin bonding agents, but also bond extremely well to phosphoric acid-etched enamel since they are excellent wetting agents.

The technique for applying the bonding resin should be carefully controlled. A fine-tipped, soft-bristle brush is used for this purpose. Since they are relatively weak in comparison to composite materials, bonding resins should be placed in the form of a thin controlled film; a small bead of bonding resin is picked up on the end of the brush and applied carefully to the acid-etched enamel. Care must be taken to ensure that excess material is not applied beyond the margin of the preparation. After thin spreading with the fine-tipped brush, the bonding resin surface should be carefully blown with an air syringe to further ensure the thin application of the material. Once the bonding resin has been applied, the fine-tipped brush should be cleaned of all adherent resin material by dipping it into ethyl acetate or acetone solvent. The brush may then be used for successive applications.

Irrespective of whether a self-cured or a light-cured bonding resin is utilized, it should be prepolymerized prior to the insertion of the composite material. This ensures a more easily controlled composite insertion technique and also reduces gap formation due to composite contraction during polymerization. Accordingly, if a self-cured bonding resin is utilized it should be gently warm-air-blown. In the event that a light-cured bonding resin is utilized, it should be precured by means of the application of visible light for a 20-sec period before composite insertion. After polymerization of the bonding resin, a tacky, "air-inhibited" layer is observed on the surface. This is a thin reactive surface layer of nonpolymerized bonding resin, which should neither be removed nor contaminated prior to the insertion of the composite material. It will not polymerize until it is covered with composite material. Thus the clinician has ample time to manipulate the composite material irrespective of whether it is self- or light-cured.

Manufacturers commonly recommend that the composite material be inserted over the bonding resin quickly, before the latter has set, to ensure maximum bonding between bonding and composite resin materials. This is not essential, however. If the bonding resin is allowed to set fully before placement of the composite resin and if the air-inhibited layer is left intact, there will be excellent bonding between composite and bonding resins because of the surface-reactive air-inhibited layer, which quickly polymerizes after the composite resin is placed, thereby ensuring a tight bond between the two materials.

Insertion of the Composite Material

It is well known that composites cured against a matrix have a resin-rich surface that is the smoothest attainable (16). A carefully controlled matrix technique, designed particularly to minimize the amount of labial finishing, is therefore conducive to an excellent result. A properly trimmed thin resin crown form greatly facilitates insertion of the composite, particularly in extensive incisal build-up techniques (Fig. 16.2 D). Unfortunately, most crown forms are unduly thick and have a raised proximal seam coursing down the midproximal region. Presently there are two crown matrix systems that are highly conducive to extensive crown build-up techniques, namely the Odus-Pella® and the Interberg® (IB) crown forms. Both are relatively thin and neither has a raised proximal seam. They are, accordingly, well-designed for efficient crown build-up and for effective restoration of tight proximal contacts.

The crown form should be carefully adapted to the prepared tooth with the following in mind (Fig. 16.2 E):

1. A minimum of labial finishing should be necessary after the composite material has polymerized.
2. A thin film of composite excess should extend no more than 1 mm beyond the marginal periphery of the chamfer shoulder preparation.
3. Vent holes should be placed palato-incisally in order to allow for air escape during insertion.

The crown matrix is filled with composite material and seated over the prepared tooth. An anatomically contoured wooden wedge (Hawe-Neos® Co.) is then placed into the gingival embrasure to compress the matrix form into tight adaptive contact with the proximo gingival surface and to ensure slight tooth separation to allow for the thickness of the matrix (Fig. 16.2 E). The crown form should be lightly compressed labio lingually. This expands the proximal portion of the matrix form into tight adaptive contact with the adjacent tooth, thereby ensuring tight proximal contact.

Polymerizing the Composite Material

Careful visible light curing of the composite material is essential for long-term clinical success. In effecting proper cure of a light-cured composite material, six factors must be recognized and controlled (17-19).

1. *Time* of application;
2. *Plane* of direction of the light source;
3. *Distance* from the end of the light source to the composite surface;
4. *Shade* of the composite material;
5. *Nature of the filler particle* within the composite material;
6. *Temperature* of the composite material.

Time. The more closely the time of application of the visible light source approximates 40 sec, the better will be the cure. In an incisal restoration, therefore, the application of light 20 sec labially and 20 sec lingually will result in optimal cure of the material. Although there are variations between the various types of composite materials, the average depth of cure resulting from a single-direction application of light is between 2.5 and 3 mm.

In the event that the composite thickness exceeds 2.5 to 3 mm and visible light cannot be applied from two directions (i.e. in Class II situations), the composite material must be placed in multiple increments, each of which must be sequentially light-cured before proceeding to the next addition.

Plane. The light source should be applied at right angles to the composite surface being cured.

Distance. The optimal distance from the end of the light source to the composite surface being cured should be as close as possible to zero. In any event, the maximum distance from the end of the light source to the composite surface should not exceed a few millimeters for most effective curing.

Shade. Dark shades are more difficult to cure than light shades, as pigments present in the dark shades tend to absorb visible light. In the event that a dark shade is utilized, curing time should be extended by an additional 10 sec.

Nature of the filler particles. Microfilled composites are more difficult to fully cure than other types of composites. It is essential, therefore, that the light application used with the microfilled systems be of adequate duration. It should be kept in mind that microfilled materials are shallow cure whereas hybrid materials are deep cure. That is, the maximum depth of cure of a microfilled material after light curing from one direction is approximately 2 to 2.5 mm whereas the maximum comparable depth of cure with a hybrid material is 4 to 4.5 mm.

Temperature. A cool composite material subjected to visible light will cure to only a fraction of the depth of room temperature composite. Therefore a composite material must always be allowed to assume room temperature before it is light cured.

All six factors are of crucial clinical importance in that they all singly and cumulatively affect the extent and depth of cure of the composite material. Accordingly, control must be exercised relative to each. Overcure constitutes no problem with composite materials, but the clinician must exercise extreme caution to ensure that undercure does not result. Particular care should be taken to avoid the "skin effect". If a dark microfilled material is taken directly from the refrigerator and subjected to a total of 20 sec of light application, multiple factors are compromised and the "skin effect" results. That is, the composite surface is fully cured, but the subsurface material is only partially polymerized. The result may be clinical failure of the restoration. Another important precaution in avoiding undercure is related to the light-curing unit. It should be monitored frequently (at least once a month) through the use of an appropriate instrument which effectively measures curing ability (e.g. Radiometer/Demetron® Co.).

Finishing

The crown form is removed after light curing (Fig. 16.2 F) and only minor marginal finish is required. Labial marginal finishing is conveniently accomplished by the use of a thin tapering carbide bur placed on the labial margin (Fig. 16.2 G). The bur must not break through to margin or a "white line" margin results. A carbide-tipped finishing knife can be used to shave from composite material gingivally to tooth structure in order to remove final marginal excess. A pair of carbide-tipped interproximal finishing knives are used to finish the proximogingival margin. The proximogingival region is then polished carefully using very thin abrasive strips to complete the finish in this region. In finishing the lingual concavity region, an appropriate donut-shaped white stone may be used to incorporate proper anatomic detail.

DISC CONTOURING

Final finish of the labial contour is accomplished by the use of aluminum oxide discs (medium, fine and superfine), at low speed with light intermittent contact, carefully avoiding heat generation. Application of the superfine disc to the hybrid composite surface results in a smooth surface topography (Fig. 16.2 H). Dry discing the composite in such a manner enhances the polymerization of the material and results in a hard wear-resistant surface [20].

PASTE POLISHING

Hybrid materials should finally be polished using a very fine abrasive polishing paste applied with a soft rubber cup, in order to bring out a final lustrous sheen; or impregnated abrasive points and Prisma Gloss®. Both result in a highly reflective surface gloss on the final restoration.

A good deal of care must be taken to adjust the occlusion in order to provide light group contact in centric, protrusive, and protrusive lateral positions. If the occlusion is inadvertently left slightly high, particularly during eccentric movements, cohesive fracture of the composite material can result. This point is particularly critical with the microfilled composite materials, as they are less filled than the conventional composites.

Microfilled composites show a 15% to 20% reduction in tensile strength relative to other composite materials and accordingly demonstrate less resistance to impact forces when placed in stress-bearing situations.

The final composite restoration, comparable in both surface smoothness and reflectivity to the adjacent tooth structure (Fig.16.2 H), does not require a glazing technique, as the final disced surface presents a glossy smooth, highly reflective appearance.

In the event that a light-filled on heavy-filled composite resin sandwich technique is used for the crown build up, the crown is restored using exactly the same technique as previously described with a semi-polishable hybrid material. The following procedure is then used for veneering: the composite labial surface is flattened using a bullet-nosed diamond. The ground composite surface is phosphoric acid etched for 20 sec, washed and dried. A layer of bonding resin is then applied followed by a labial veneer of microfilled composite material. The microfilled composite surface is then finished using aluminum oxide discs.

White Spot Lesions and Hypoplastic Defects

Both white spot lesions and hypoplastic defects are treated in a similar fashion (7, 21).

Materials. Since such lesions usually are encountered on the labial enamel surfaces in predominantly nonfunctional situations, light-cured, microfilled materials are normally indicated. Hypoplastic defects involving the functional incisal surfaces of anterior teeth should be restored with heavy-filled, macrofilled, or hybrid-type materials, particularly when heavy occlusal function predominates.

Technique. Whatever material is utilized, the technique is as follows:

1. A bullet-nosed diamond is used to remove all of the discolored enamel even if this necessitates exposure of the superficial labial dentin. If this occurs, the dentin should be protected by application of a dentin bonding agent (see Chapter 6). Opaquers should be avoided if possible because of the associated "shine-through" effect.
2. Using a viscous gel-type etchant, the enamel should be etched for 1 min, washed, and dried.
3. After bonding, composite is placed, cured, and finished.

Prognosis

Long-term success of composite resin restorations can be assessed by several parameters: loss of restoration, marginal integrity/discoloration, bodily discoloration, bulk fracture, surface texture, occurrence of secondary caries along the margins of the restoration. There exist numerous clinical studies which have evaluated treatment success based on types of composite materials used (22-33), preparation type (e.g. with or without a bevel, Cl. III, IV, V) (25, 30, 34-39), and cavity treatment (e.g. +/- enamel etch, +/- use of an unfilled enamel bonding resin) (27, 32, 36, 39, 40, 41). From this historical review, it would seem that WINKLER'S remarks in 1975 bear true, "that dentists and their patients have had to test clinically many of the earlier resin products which were later withdrawn from the market" (42).

Despite the variety of techniques and materials used, some general principles can be extracted from these reports.

-Enamel etching and the use of an unfilled enamel bonding resin improves composite resin adaptation to cavity margins and thereby improves long-term success with respect to marginal discoloration and leakage (24, 27, 39, 41).

-Light-cured composites have a greater color stability than self-cured materials (23, 24, 30, 33, 40).

-Improvements in physical properties (i.e. surface texture, marginal adaptation, color stability) have been achieved by alterations in filler particle size and proportion in the composite resin restorative materials (i.e. from conventional to microfilled and hybrid composites) (28-33, 43).

-Class IV restorations (i.e. crown fractures) are more susceptible to marginal and bulk fracture than Class III or V restorations, thereby challenging the physical properties of the restorative materials used (25, 30, 37, 40).

While many studies have been published

Fig. 16.3. Survival of anterior composite restorations
Life table statistics based on 1770 anterior restorations assessed over a period up to 17 years. (After SMALES ET AL.(39,41) *1991).*

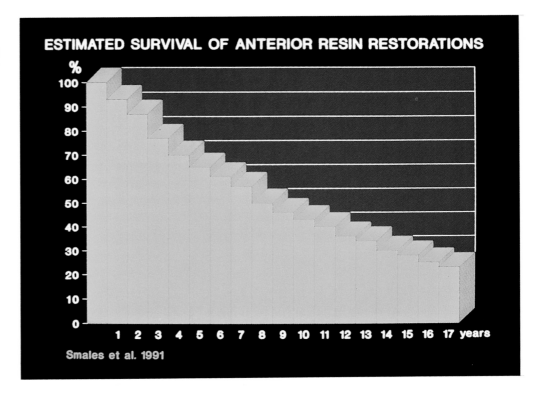

on the long-term survival of posterior and anterior restorative materials, few have comprised enough data to permit life table analysis (see Chapter 22). SMALES (39, 41) have performed such studies and have demonstrated a half-life of anterior composite restorations (i.e. replacement of 50% of placed restorations) of 8-9 years on the whole; while Class IV restorations had a half-life of only 4 years. *True failure* was defined as fractured or loosened restorations, replaced or repaired restorations and marginal caries. *Apparent failure* (i.e. loss of restoration due to endodontic access preparation, unrelated tooth extraction or restoration loss due to acute trauma) were not included in the survival analysis.

The general conclusion from these studies was that the use of an enamel bonding resin minimized color mismatch, marginal staining and marginal fracture (41).

The results of presently available studies should, however, be assessed with some caution as no clinical study on the long-term survival of anterior composite restorations exist to date where dentin bonding agents have been used. This would be especially significant with respect to failures due to gingival caries, as in Class IV restorations.

Finally it should be mentioned that pulpal response to restorative procedures appears to be minimal if appropriate treatment guidelines are respected (see Chapters 6 and 14).

Essentials

Indications

Composites offer a conservative restoration of crown-fractured teeth with a minimal risk of pulpal complication. Restoration can be performed immediately after injury if there is no associated periodontal or pulpal injury. Hybrid or microfilled composites are especially useful.

Treatment

Restoration of an enamel dentin fracture (Fig. 16.1).

a. Shade selection.
b. Select a type of composite according to functional and esthetic demands.
c. Isolate the tooth with a rubber dam.
d. Prepare a chamfer shoulder.
e. A pulp protective agent should be applied only on dentin closest to the pulp in case of deep fractures.
f. Enamel and dentin conditioning for composite retention.
g. Apply the bond resin and polymerize.
h. Adapt a matrix.
i. Insert the composite material.
j. Polymerize for 20 sec labially and 20 sec lingually.
k. Remove matrix and major excess material.
l. Trim cavity margins with burs or knives.
m. Polish the filling with abrasive discs or paste.

PROGNOSIS
Survival of composite restorations

3 years: 92%
5 years: 65%
10 years: 40%

Bibliography

1. JORDAN RE, SUZUKI M, GWINNETT AJ. Conservative applications of acid etch resin techniques. *Dent Clin North Am* 1981;**25**:307-36.

2. BUONOCORE MG. A simple method of increasing the adhesion of acrylic filling materials to enamel surfaces. *J Dent Res* 1955;**34**:849-53.

3. SILVERSTONE LM. The acid etch technique. *Proc Int Symp Acid Etch Tech*, St. Paul: North Central Publishing Co, 1975.

4. GWINNETT AJ. The scientific basis of the sealant procedure. *J Prev Dent* 1976;**3**:15-28.

5. HEMBREE JH, ANDREW JT. In vivo microleakage of several acid etch composite resins. *J Dent Res* 1976;**55**:139.

6. DELLO RUSSO NM. Replacement of crown margins in patients with altered passive eruption. *Int J Periodont Restor Dent* 1984;**4**:59.

7. JORDAN RE, SUZUKI M, GWINNETT AJ, HUNTER JK. Restoration of fractured and hypoplastic incisors by the acid etch technique. *J Am Dent Assoc* 1977;**95**:795-803.

8. CHAN RC, BOYER DB. Repair of conventional and microfilled composite resins. *J Prosthet Dent* 1983;**50**:345-50.

9. SUZUKI M, GOTO G, JORDAN RE. Pulpal response to pin placement. *J Am Dent Assoc* 1973;**87**:636-40.

10. GWINNET AJ. Bonding factors in technique which influence clinical success. *NY State Dent J* 1982;**48**:223-6.

11. ROCK WP. The effect of etching of human enamel upon bone strengths with fissure sealant resins. *Arch Oral Biol* 1974;**19**:873-7.

12. SOETEPO, BEECH DR, HARDWICK J. Mechanism of adhesion of polymers to acid etched enamel. Effect of acid concentration and washing on bond strength. *J Oral Rehabil* 1978;**5**:69-79.

13. HORMATI AA, FULLER JL, DENEHY GE. Effects of contamination and mechanical disturbance on the quality of acid etched enamel. *J Am Dent Assoc* 1980;**100**:34-8.

14. MITCHEM JC, TURNER LR. The retentive strength of acid-etched retained resins. *J Am Dent Assoc* 1974;**89**:1107-10.

15. MEURMAN JG, NEVASTE M. The intermediate effect of low-viscous fissure sealants on the retention of resin restoratives in vitro. *Proc Finn Dent Soc* 1975;**71**:96-101.

16. CHANDLER HH, BOWEN RL, PAFFENBARGER GC. Method for finishing composite restorative materials. *J Am Dent Assoc* 1971;**83**:344-48.

17. COMBE EC. Personal communication, 1983.

18. SWARTZ ML, PHILLIPS RW, RHODES B. Visible-light-activated resins - Depth of cure. *J Am Dent Assoc* 1983;**106**:634-7.

19. WATTS DC, AMER O, COMBE EC. Characteristics of visible-light-activated composite systems. *Br Dent J* 1984;**156**:209-15.

20. DAVIDSON CL, DUYSTERS PPE, DE LANGE C, BAUSCH JR. Structural changes in composite surface material after dry polishing. *J Oral Rehabil* 1981;**8**:431-9.

21. MINK JR, McEVOY SA. Acid etch and enamel bond composite restoration of permanent anterior teeth affected by enamel hypoplasia. *J Am Dent Assoc* 1977;**94**:305-7.

22. ROBERTS MW, MOFFA JP. Repair of fractured incisal angles with an ultraviolet-light-activated fissure sealant and a composite resin: two-year report of 60 cases. *J Am Dent Assoc* 1973;**87**:888-91.

23. KOCH G, PAULANDER J. Klinisk uppföljning av compositrestaureringar utförda med emaljetsningsmetodik. *Swed Dent J* 1976;**69**:191-6.

24. SMALES RJ. Composite resin restorations: A clinical assessment of two materials. *J Dent* 1977;**5**:319-26.

25. SMALES RJ. Incisal angle adhesive resins: A two-year clinical survey of three materials. *Aust Dent J* 1977;**22**:267-71.

26. WATKINS JJ, ANDLAW RJ. Restoration of fractured incisors with an ultra-violet light-polymerised composite resin. A clinical study. *Br Dent J* 1977;**142**:249-52.

27. ORAM V, LYDERS B. Marginal defects of etched and unetched composite resin restorations. A 2 years clinical investigation. *J Dent Res* 1981;*Special Issue*:Abstract no. 12.

28. CHRISTENSEN RP, CHRISTENSEN GJ. In vivo comparison of a microfilled and a composite resin: a three-year report. *J Prosthet Dent* 1982;**48**:657-63.

29. TYAS MJ. The restoration of fractured incisors in children: A comparative clinical trial of a composite and a microfine filled resin. *Australian Dent J* 1982;**27**:77-80.

30. DIJKEN JWV VAN, HÖRSTEDT P, MEURMAN JH. SEM study of surface characteristics and marginal adaptation of anterior resin restorations after 3-4 years. *Scand J Dent Res* 1985;**93**:453-62.

31. DIJKEN JWV VAN. A clinical evaluation of anterior conventional, microfiller, and hybrid composite resin fillings. A 6-year follow-up study. *Acta Odontol Scand* 1986;**44**:357-67.

32. DIJKEN JWV VAN, HÖRSTEDT P. Marginal adaptation of composite resin restorations placed with or without intermediate low-viscous resin. An SEM investigation. *Acta Odontol Scand* 1987;**45**:115-23.

33. CRUMPLER DC, HEYMANN HO, SHUGARS DA, BAYNE SC, LEINFELDER KF. Five-year clinical investigation of one conventional composite and three microfilled resins in anterior teeth. *Dent Mater* 1988;**4**:217-22.

34. HILL FJ, SOETOPO A. A simplified acid-etch technique for the restoration of fractured incisors. *J Dent* 1977;**5**:207-12.

35. ULVESTAD H. A 5-year evaluation of sempipermanent composite resin crowns. *Scand J Dent Res* 1978;**86**:163-8.

36. QVIST V, STRÖM C, THYLSTRUP A. Two-year assessment of anterior resin restorations inserted with two acid-etch restorative procedures. *Scand J Dent Res* 1985;**93**:343-50.

37. SMALES RJ, GERKE DC. Clinical study of four auto-cured resins: 3-year survivals. *J Dent Res* 1987;*Special Issue*:Abstract no. 80.

38. KULLMAN W. Das klinische Verhalten von polierbaren Komposit-Kunststoffen bei der Versorgung von Frontzahnkavitäten nach zwei Jahren. *Dtsch Zahnärztl Z* 1988;**43**:287-90.

39. SMALES RJ. Effects of enamel-bonding, type of restoration, patient age and operator on the longevity of an anterior composite resin. *Am J Dent* 1991;**4**:130-3.

40. SMALES RJ. Incisal angle adhesive resins: a 5-year clinical survey of two materials. *J Oral Rehab* 1983;**10**:19-24.

41. SMALES RJ. Long-term deterioration of composite resin and amalgam restorations. *Oper Dent* 1991;**16**:202-9.

42. WINKLER S. Symposium on resins in dentistry: Foreword. *Dent Clin N Am* 1975;**19**:209-10.

43. RAVN JJ, NIELSEN LA, JENSEN IL. Plastmaterialer til restaurering af traumebeskadigede incisiver. En foreløbig redegørelse. *Tandlægebladet* 1974;**6**:233-40.

CHAPTER 17

Resin-Retained Bridges in the Anterior Region

N.H.J. CREUGERS

Resin-retained bridges can be used both as interim and definitive treatment in the traumatized dentition. Compared to conventional fixed prostheses, there are some advantages which make this treatment especially useful following dental trauma.

Advantages of adhesive-bonded bridges compared to conventional bridges include: minimal tooth preparation, i.e. reversible procedures and no pulpal involvement; as well as short working time, thereby implying lower costs. The ultra-conservative approach makes the resin-bonded bridge a standard treatment option in the case of uncertain prognosis.

Disadvantages associated with resin-bonded bridges may be the anticipated limited length of clinical service and the need for intact or almost intact abutment teeth.

Treatment Planning

In the treatment of missing anterior teeth, the following factors must be considered (1):

- age of the patient;
- general condition of the dentition;
- occlusion;
- location and width of the edentulous space;
- quality of the teeth adjacent to the edentulous space;
- atrophy of alveolar bone.

In the case of missing anterior teeth, there are several treatment options, such as orthodontic space closure (see Chapter 15, p. 608), autotransplantation of teeth (see Chapter 19, p. 671), prosthodontic treatment including conventional fixed (see Chapter 18, p. 661) and implants (see Chapter 20, p. 692). The main advantages and disadvantages of these treatments are listed in Appendix 5, p. 751.

Based on these advantages and disadvantages, it can be concluded that possible indications for resin-bonded bridges in the replacement of lost teeth include the following situations (2):

- where orthodontic closure or autotransplantation is not indicated;
- where conventional prostheses are unwanted;
- where interim treatment is desired because of complicating prognostic factors.

The classical indication for a resin-bonded bridge is replacement of a single tooth with 2 intact abutment teeth (Fig 17.1).

In general there are only two absolute contraindications for resin-bonded bridges. The first is if the abutment teeth are in need of crowns because of the presence of large restorations or when esthetics dictate. A second contraindication for the use of resin-bonded bridges is insufficient enamel on the abutment teeth for adequate bonding. At this time the bonding capacity of adhesive

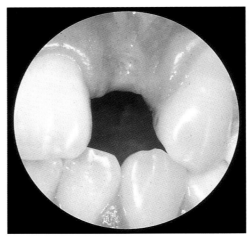

Fig. 17.1.
Classical indication for a resin-retained bridge is the replacement of a single tooth and the presence of sound adjacent abutment teeth.

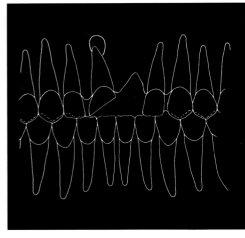

Fig. 17.2.
Schematic representation of the complicating factors which may be present in moderate or severely traumatized dentitions.

luting cements to dentin is not sufficient to withstand the forces that will be applied to the bridges (3,4).

In specific situations, such as after moderate or severe trauma to dentitions, the following complicating factors may be present displaced position of the abutment teeth: abutment teeth with crown or root fractures; pulpal involvement of the abutment teeth and atrophy of alveolar bone (Fig.17.2).

The treatment sequence and timing for resin-bonded bridges depends on the age of the patient and the presence or absence of complicating factors listed above. In many cases an observation period of several months is necessary before treatment can be initiated. If a resin-bonded bridge is to serve as definitive therapy the complicating factors should be eliminated. In these situations, because of the reversible character of the system, early application

of the resin-bonded bridge may be appropriate, and a resin-bonded bridge can serve as an interim or short-term restoration during evaluation or treatment of the complicating factors (Fig. 17.3).

Although some of the complicating factors are not absolute contraindications, they may influence the prognosis and quality of service substantially. Thus position of an abutment tooth, for instance, can make an esthetic solution impossible. Extreme loss of alveolar bone may be a good reason for alveolar ridge augmentation procedures (see Chapter 20, p. 698).

Direct Resin-bonded Bridges

Although clinical studies have indicated that cast metal resin-bonded bridges are

Table 17.1. Different types of resin-bonded bridges according to the main indications and key characteristics

Type of Bridge	Indication	Key Characteristics
Direct bridges		
All-composite	Young patients,	Time conserving,
Custom tooth	interim treatment up to	immediate application,
Natural tooth	one year	low cost, easy technique and completely reversible
Cast-metal bridge		
Rochette	Interim treatment for one year or more	Easy to adjust and remove
Maryland	Definitive treatment	Reasonably good long-term survival

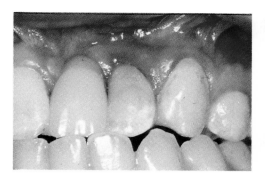
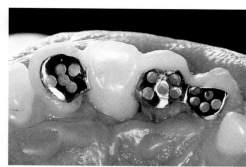

more durable than other types of resin-bonded bridges, there is still a need for directly applied resin-bonded bridges, especially in cases where the device is meant as an interim solution (11). The direct technique provides an interim restoration with relatively low cost and good esthetics and oral comfort.

The direct-pontic systems that have been described in the literature include: the acrylic tooth pontic, the all-composite pontic, and the natural tooth pontic. The reported survival from a number of clinical studies varies from 30 % to 100 % for resin- bonded bridges using direct pontics (5-9). The main disadvantage of the direct-pontic technique is the inherent lack of strength against torquing forces which may cause cohesive failure of the luting composite resin.

Table 17.1 presents a list of the different types of resin-bonded bridges according to the main areas of indication.

Clinical Procedures in Direct Resin-Bonded Bridge

Direct resin-bonded bridges can be fabricated in a single session, whereas indirect resin-bonded bridges always need two or three sessions. The clinical procedures for both types of bridges are well-described by several clinicians. Since a detailed presentation of these procedures is beyond the scope of this book, only a brief overview is presented:

All-composite resin-bonded bridge (Fig. 17.4)
-cleaning of the abutment teeth and isolation by means of cotton rolls or rubber dam
- etching of the enamel and application of bonding and a stainless steel mesh
- building up the pontic in layers
- finishing of the restoration

Acrylic denture tooth or natural tooth bridge (Fig. 17.5)
- molding, fitting and aligning of the pontic tooth into a proper position on a study model or in the mouth
- retentive preparation of the proximal surfaces of the pontic
- fabrication of a silicone matrix for orienting the pontic in the desired position
- etching of the enamel and application of bonding agent
- application of composite resin in the

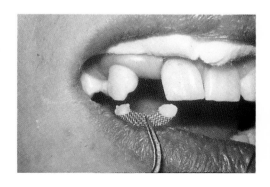
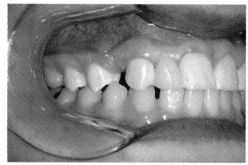

RESIN-RETAINED BRIDGES IN THE ANTERIOR REGION

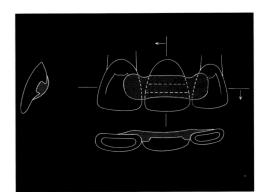

Fig. 17.5.
Schematic representation of the construction of an acrylic denture bridge.

preparations and on the proximal and palatal surfaces of the abutment teeth
- finishing of the restoration.

Cast Resin-Bonded Bridges

The cast resin-bonded bridge consists of a pontic and a cast metal framework which is fabricated individually in the dental laboratory. The design is such that forces that are applied to the pontic during function are absorbed by the metal framework (10-12). The success of the restoration is directly related to the success of the bonding system. With respect to bonding system of resin-bonded bridges, the following specific problems are defined (13) (Fig.17.6):
  - The resin-cement/tooth interface,
  - The resin-cement/metal interface,
  - The physical and chemical properties of the resin-cement,
  - The design of the resin-bonded bridge.

Resin /Tooth Interface

The bond strength of composite luting cements to present composite resin restorations is in the same order as the bond strength to tooth enamel (14,15). However, the quality of bonding at the resin-tooth interface depends on several factors. The reported bond strengths of composite resins to enamel vary from about 7 to 20 MPa (16,17). As it is not possible to assess the biological variation of the enamel surface adequately in the clinic, the quality of composite resin bond to enamel surface is always unpredictable to some extent. To achieve the best possible results, the following steps must be performed meticulously: (1) cleaning of the enamel with pure pumice and water before etching, (2) etching of the abutment teeth for about 45 sec, (3) adequate rinsing of the etched surface for at least 20 sec to remove the etchant and enamel debris, and (4) avoid any contamination to the conditioned surface, preferably by the use of a rubber dam.

The presence of restorations in the abutment teeth may be a contraindication for a resin-bonded bridge in cases where the *resistance form* of the tooth is seriously affected. However, with respect to *retention*, the presence of composite resin restorations generally presents no problem. The highest bond strength is to be expected when the restoration of the cavity and the insertion of the bridge takes place in the same session. However, in many cases this is impossible, as the restoration can interfere with the fit of the bridge.

Table 17.2. Classification of indirect resin-bonded prostheses, according to the mechanism of attachment of the resin cement to the framework

Mechanical bonding	Chemical bonding
Macromechanical	Adhesive layer
- perforated metal framework	Tin electroplated framework
- mesh retention	Silicoated framework
- retention beads	
- particle-roughened surface	
Micromechanical	Chemically active cements
- sandblasted framework	4-META resins
- electrochemically etched framework	Phosphonated monomers
- chemically etched framework	
- porous metal coated framework	

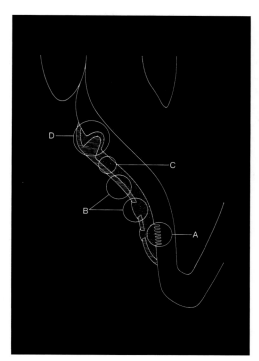

Fig. 17.6.
Schematic representation of the weak points in cast-metal resin-bonded bridges. A: the interface between resin cement and the tooth enamel, B: the resin-cement/metal interface, C: physical and chemical properties of the composite resin-cement, and D: the design of the bridge.

Resin-Cement/Metal Interface

Depending upon the system used, retention of resin-bonded bridges is a result of mechanical retention and chemical adhesion. Classifications as presented in Table 17.2 are given by several authors (18,19). However, a clear distinction is not always possible as a number of systems combine both mechanical and chemical bonding. The best known and described systems are the *Rochette bridge* (macromechanical retention) and the *Maryland bridge* (micromechanical retention by metal etching).

In general, the bond strength at the resin/metal interface is related to : (1) the type of metal alloy; (2) the surface treatment of the metal alloy; and (3) the resin luting agent.

The bond strength values reported in the literature show substantial variation, from less than 10 MPa to over 40 MPa (20-24). This variation is not only a result of differences in quality of the surface treatments (25,26), or in materials and methods of the studies, but within one experiment wide variations can be seen (13). The best clinical results were reported for etched metal resin-bonded bridges (Maryland bridges) (27,28).

Properties of the Resin-Cement

Since a resin-bonded bridge is a cast restoration, having a precise fit in the patient's mouth, the requirements for the resin luting agents resemble those formulated for conventional dental cements (13). However, there are distinct differences between the requirements for conventional dental cements and those for adhesive cements. Only recently, special resin luting agents have been made available which could satisfy the special demands made by resin-bonded bridges. Apart from the general requirements for a dental adhesive there are some additional requirements which are related to the application of the adhesive (29). For resin-bonded bridge cements the additional requirements include : (1) sufficient working time for the insertion of the bridge, preferably variable by the operator; (2) low-viscosity resulting in an acceptable film thickness; and (3) adequate bonding to metal surfaces. Furthermore it is required that the resin cement is a chemically (self-) cured or dual-cured system. The bond strength to enamel should be in the order of 15 to 20 MPa and greater than 20 MPa to metal.

In case of Rochette bridges (see later) the use of high wear-resistant composite resins, such as conventional or hybrid composites is recommended (27). The opacity of the cement should be sufficient to mask the metal framework which could result in a darkening of the abutment teeth.

Design of the Resin-Bonded Bridge

The most important criterion in the design of the bridge is the way in which it spares the weakest link and strengthens the bonding system. For this purpose, many suggestions have been made (12,19,30,31). The design principles are based on abutment tooth modifications and on the outline form of the retention wings. When a truly adhesive restoration is desired, there is the dilemma that resistance against tensile and oblique forces must be sufficient, while on the other hand only minimal tooth preparation is required.

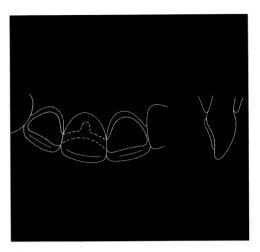

Fig. 17.7.
Schematic representation of the design of the retention wings of a resin-retained bridge.

The following factors must be taken into consideration in planning a cast resin-bonded bridge (Fig.17.7):
- the design of the retention wings
- tooth preparation
- the number of abutment teeth

The *retention wings* should occupy a maximum surface of the enamel while not compromising esthetics. Incisal translucency of the abutment teeth must also be taken into consideration. Proximal wrap around is preferable when esthetics permit. Plaque-retentive areas must be avoided, implying marginal placement at least 1 mm from the gingiva. The patients's occlusion must also be considered in the design of the retention wings in order to avoid premature contacts or excessive loading during excursions. Occlusion on the retention wings is preferable to occlusion on the abutment teeth as occlusal forces load the retention wings in the direction of the teeth, while occlusion on the abutment teeth forces the tooth away from the resin-bonded bridge (32).

With respect to *tooth preparation* there are divergent opinions. Some authors recommend extensive preparation while others advocate a more conservative design. Tooth preparation should always be included in the design of the bridge in cases of insufficient interocclusal space and increased mobility of the abutment teeth. Tooth preparation is also indicated in cases where more than 2 abutment teeth are involved in the construction or when there is an unclear seat or an unclear path of insertion (Fig.17.8).

Finally, preparation of grooves may be indicated, to increase retention. An anatomical guide for enamel reduction during preparation for resin-bonded bridges has been published by FERRARI et al. (33) 1987. The choice of the optimal *number of abutment teeth* depends on the situation. Usually 2 abutment teeth are sufficient for 3-or 4-unit bridges. In case 3 or more teeth are to be replaced, or in cases where the abutment teeth have increased mobility, more abutment teeth can be used for retaining the bridge (Fig.17.9).

Orthodontic pretreatment may be another indication for the use of extra abutment teeth and tooth preparation. Fig.17.10 presents a patient with missing cuspids and lateral incisors, who is orthodontically pretreated. A central diastema was closed with a simple orthodontic method. To prevent any relapse, the bridge was cast as a single unit crossing the midline.

Fig. 17.8.
Model set-up demonstrating the preparation form for a resin-retained bridge in the anterior region.

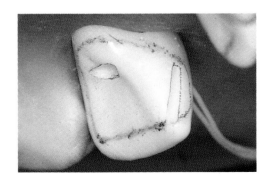

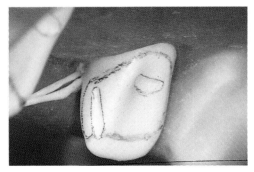

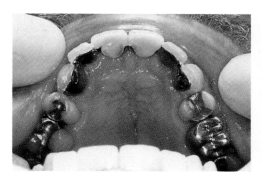

Fig. 17.9.
Palatal view of a 6-unit resin-retained bridge. More than 2 abutment teeth were used as the lateral incisors demonstrated increased mobility.

Clinical Procedures in Cast Resin-bonded Bridges

The fabrication of cast resin-bonded bridge usually takes three sessions.

The main steps during these sessions are as follows:

First session

- cleaning of the abutment teeth
- preparation (modification) of the abutment teeth (if required)
- selection of shade and color of the pontic
- taking the impressions

Second session

- cleaning of the abutment teeth
- isolation with cotton rolls
- check of the fit of the resin-bonded bridge
- application of rubber dam
- cleaning of the resin-bonded bridge
- etching of the abutment teeth for 30-45 seconds
- cementation of the bridge with resin luting cement
- check of the occlusion and occlusal adjustment if required
- removal of the excess cement

Fig. 17.11.
A method of stabilizing interdental and interocclusal relationships following abutment preparation. The interocclusal space is preserved by placing a thin layer of composite resin on the antagonist to the abutment tooth.

Third session

- re-check of outline and eventual polishing of the restoration
- re-check of the occlusion
- oral hygiene instructions

In cases where the abutment teeth are prepared in a way that occlusal stops are lost, an interim restoration might be necessary. A simple way to maintain the occlusal relationship and to prevent displacement of teeth is demonstrated in Fig.17.11.

Fig. 17.10.
Example of a six-unit resin-retained bridge after orthodontic pretreatment. A and B. Before and after placement of the restoration respectively.

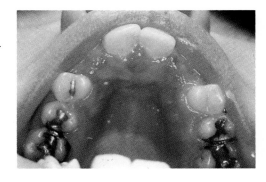

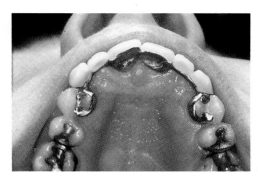

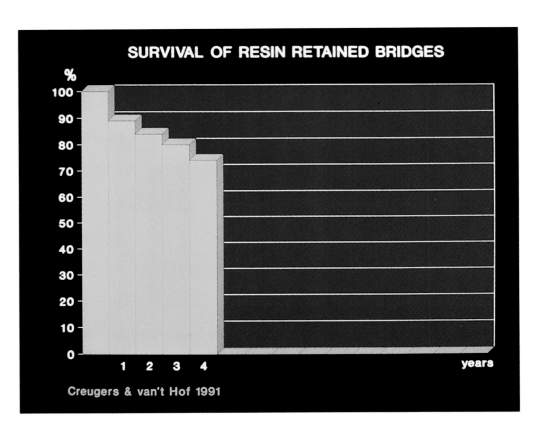

Fig. 17.12. Survival of resin-bonded bridges
Overall survival of 1598 resin-bonded bridges based on a meta-analysis. From CREUGERS & VAN'T HOF (28) *1992*

Prognosis

Clinical data on the efficacy of resin-bonded bridges include data from both retrospective clinical studies as well as from prospective trials.

The durability data reported in the literature are not especially representative for the resin-bonded bridges in the case of trauma. It is reported that resin-bonded bridges in young patients with trauma tend to fail more frequently than in "average" patients (34,35). In one study (13) the reasons for anterior tooth loss of the "average" patient was described in detail: 26% of the cases resulted from trauma, 41% were related to caries or periodontal problems. In 33% of the cases there was no real tooth loss but bridge constructions were related to aplasia (28%) and spacing (5%). Although it is not proven that the "average patient" in the described study is representative, it may be expected that the populations of other studies do not differ substantially.

The reported survivals in clinical studies vary widely, and the conclusions are sometimes conflicting. The heterogeneity of the results of the different studies indicates that interpretation of only one study may significantly mislead clinicians, especially with short-term results. The variation between survivals in different studies may be a result of variation in patient selection, materials and operator's experience. A method of combining the results of different studies with different protocols and procedures in order to draw conclusions about the effectiveness is the so-called *meta-analysis* (28) (see also Chapter 22, p. 742). Although many publications were reviewed only some of them were useful for an overall analysis of the data. The survival adapted from this type of analysis is shown in Figure 17.12.

As such, the calculated overall survival may be representative for the general practice. On the other hand the results of the different studies may be an underestimation of the results which can be achieved in case all "best" success factors are combined and unfavorable situations are excluded.

A similar type of study was done to calculate the survival of conventional fixed bridges (47). The overall survival of these bridges was calculated from the results adapted from seven clinical studies in-

Fig. 17.13. Survival rates of anterior and posterior resin-retained bridges
From CREUGERS ET AL. (28) 1992

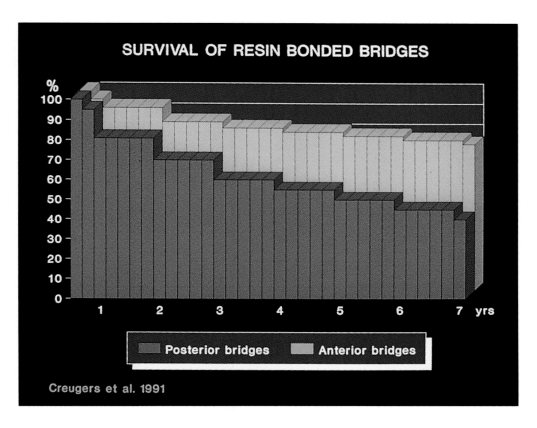

cluding a total of 4118 conventional fixed bridges (48-54). The survival rate was 74% after 15 years (in cases where the bridges were still *in situ*, the bridges were considered as not-failed). (see Chapter 18, Fig. 18.19)

Factors Influencing the Survival of Bridges

Mobility of the abutment teeth has been found to be a significant risk factor for failure (36).

Excessive occlusal loading due to prema-

Fig. 17.14. Survival rates of Maryland and Rochette bridges
From CREUGERS ET AL. (28) 1991.

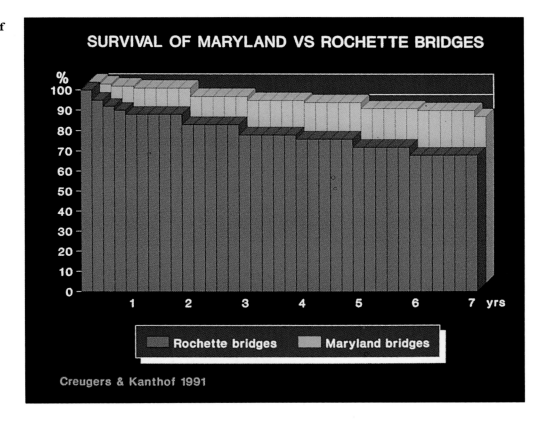

RESIN-RETAINED BRIDGES IN THE ANTERIOR REGION

ture contacts on the abutment teeth or the pontic have been recognized as an important cause of failure in several studies (36,37,38).

Silicoated resin-bonded bridges have been found to perform better than bridges using other retention systems (36).

Bridge location have been found to influence prognosis. Thus CHANG et al. reported that resin-bonded bridges in the maxilla were more durable than those in the mandible (85% success versus 45% after 4 years) (39). CREUGERS et al. (1991) found no significant patient-related risk factors except that a *posterior* location was a risk for the success of the bridge (37) (Fig.17.13).

Etched-metal bridges (Maryland bridges) has been found more retentive than Rochette bridges Fig. 17.14.

Preparation of the abutment teeth has been suggested for improving succesful retention; however, no comparative long-term studies have been performed so far (36,38-41).

Cementing agents. Conventional restorative composite resin (Clearfil F2) appeared to be the best resin cement for both macromechanical and micromechanical retainers (13).

Besides the above-mentioned risk factors, which were all adapted from longitudinal clinical studies, it is worth mentioning some contraindications which have been described, such as: (a) bruxism and parafunctional oral habits, (b) unesthetic abutment teeth, (c) deep-bite occlusion, and (d) long-span bridges.

One of the main advantages of resin-bonded bridges is the possibility of rebonding in case of loosening. However, rebonded bridges are susceptible to new failure. Hence the failure rate has been found to be higher than the failure rate of originally bonded bridges (34,36,37,42). Thus risk of failure after rebonding is estimated to be about twice the risk of failure after original bonding (43).

Before rebonding, the causes of loss of retention must be investigated carefully. In case of instability of the metal framework a revision of the resin-bonded bridge must be considered.

The *cost-effectiveness* of dental restorations depends primarily on the durability and the cost of the restoration. In one report, a method is described to compare the cost-effectiveness using the durability data of resin-bonded bridges and conventional bridges (44). This study showed that, for the situation that costs are in a ratio of 1 to 3, the break-even point for equal cost-effectiveness compared to conventional bridges is achieved when the 50 % survival for resin-bonded bridges is approximately 6.5 years. Clinical data presently indicate a higher cost-effectiveness for anterior resin-bonded bridges and a lower cost-effectiveness for posterior resin-bonded bridges.

In conclusion, resin-bonded bridges have been evaluated extensively over the past 20 years. Although there are still some important questions to be answered, it may be concluded that this type of restoration is a useful prosthetic solution for missing anterior teeth with a reasonably high survival rate in cases were 1 or 2 teeth are to be replaced. The main advantage of these procedures is that they can be carried out in individuals with no or only slight preparation of abutment teeth.

Partial Dentures

The indication for removable partial dentures in individuals with traumatized dentitions is restricted to:
- cases in which an interim treatment is needed and in which a resin-retained restoration cannot be made
- cases with severe loss of alveolar process
- very severe traumas in which it is not possible to make fixed appliances

However, also in situations as described above, it is preferable that supporting treatment (i.e. surgical preprosthetic treatment) is performed so as to allow the application of fixed prostheses as soon as possible. The application of removable partial dentures should be kept as reversible as possible.

Essentials

Indications

Individuals with intact or almost intact abutment teeth and no spacing between teeth and an intact alveolar process.

Interim solution in cases waiting for diagnosis of eventual complications.

Treatment Planning

Depends on the age of the patient and presence or absence of complicating factors.

a. A direct resin-bonded bridge or a Rochette bridge can serve very well as interim treatment and can be made almost immediately after the loss of a tooth.

b. A resin-retained bridge can serve as a definitive solution.

Clinical Procedure

ALL-COMPOSITE RESIN-BONDED BRIDGE

a. Cleaning and isolation of the abutment teeth
b. Etching of the enamel and application of bonding and a stainless steel mesh
c. Building up of the pontic in layers
d. Finishing the restoration

ACRYLIC DENTURE TOOTH OR NATURAL TOOTH BRIDGE

a. Molding, fitting and aligning of the pontic tooth into a proper position
b. Retentive preparation of the proximal surfaces of the pontic
c. Fabrication of a silicone matrix for orienting the pontic in the desired position
d. Etching of the enamel and application of composite resin in the preparations and on the proximal and palatal surfaces of the abutment teeth
e. Finishing of the restoration

CAST RESIN-BONDED BRIDGE

First session:
a. Cleaning of the abutment teeth
b. Preparation of teeth
c. Selection of shade and color taking
d. Impression taking

Second session:
a. Cleaning of the abutment teeth
b. Check of the fit
c. Application of rubber dam
d. Cleaning of the bridge
e. Etching for 30-45 seconds and cementation
f. Check of the occlusion and removal of the excess cement

Third session:
a. Re-check of the occlusion
b. Oral hygiene instruction

Follow-up

a. Checking of retention.
b. Application of normal prosthodontic maintenance program

Prognosis

4-years bridge survival: 74%

Risk factors

a. Mobility of abutment teeth
b. Excessive occlusal loading
c. Mandible versus maxilla; especially in case of posterior location
d. Posterior location (versus anterior)
e. Rochette bridges

Bibliography

1. KÄYSER AF, PLASMANS PJJM, SNOEK PA. *Kronen und Brüc kenprothetik.* Köln: Deutscher Ärzte-Verlag, 1985.

2. VRIJHOEF MMA, ESCHEN S. *De etsbrug.* Leiden: NMT-mediatheek, 1984.

3. DOUGLAS WH. Clinical status of dentine bonding agents. *J Dent* 1989; 17: 209-215.

4. PRATI C. Early marginal leakage and shear bond strength of adhesive restorative systems. *Dent Mater* 1990; 6: 195-200.

5. HALLONSTEN A-L, KOCH G, LUDVIGSSON N, et al. Acid-etch technique in temporary bridgework using composite pontics in the juvenile dentition. *Swed Dent J* 1979; 3: 213-219.

6. IBSEN RL. Fixed prosthetics with a natural crown pontic using an adhesive composite. *J S Calf Dent Assoc* 1973; 41: 100-102.

7. IBSEN RL. One-appointment technic using an adhesive composite. *Dent Survey* 1973;49:30-32.

8. JENKINS CBG. Etch retained anterior pontics, a 4-year study. *Br Dent J* 1978; 144: 206-208.

9. JORDAN RE, SUZUKI M, SILLS PS, et al. Temporary fixed partial dentures fabricated by means of the acid-etched resin technique: a report of 86 cases followed for up to three years. *J Am Dent Assoc* 1978; 96:994-1001.

10. ROCHETTE AL. Attachment of a splint to enamel of lower anterior teeth. *J Prosthet Dent* 1973; 30: 418-423.

11. HOWE DF, DENEHY GE. Anterior fixed partial dentures utilizing the acid-etch technique and a cast metal framework. *J Prosthet Dent* 1977; 37: 28-31.

12. LIVIDITIS GJ. Resin bonded cast restorations: clinical study. *Int J Periodont Rest Dent* 1981; 1: 70-79.

13. CREUGERS NHJ. *Clinical performance of adhesive bridges.* Thesis, Nijmegen, the Netherlands,1987.

14. CHAN KC, BOYER DB. Repair of conventional and micro-filled composite resin. *J Prosthet Dent* 1983; 50: 345-350.

15. CREUGERS NHJ, VRIJHOEF, MMA. Bond strength of adhesive bridges luting resins to restorative composite. *J Dent Res* 1986; 65: 258.

16. LUTZ F, LÖSCHER B, OCHSENBEIN H, et al. *Adhäsive Zahnheilkunde.* Zürich: Juris Druck und Verlag 1976.

17. BEECH DR. Bonding restorative resins to dentin. In: *Posterior composite resin dental restorative materials.* Peter Szilc Publishing Co, the Netherlands, 1985.

18. HANSSON O. The Silicoater technique for resin-bonded prostheses: clinical and laboratory procedures. *Quintessenz Int* 1989; 20: 85-99.

19. SIMONSEN R, THOMPSON VP, BARRACK G. *Etched cast restorations: clinical and laboratory techniques.* Chicago: Quintessence, 1983.

20. HILL GL, ZIDAN O, MARIN O. Bond strength of etched base metals: effects of errors in surface area estimation. *J Prosthet Dent* 1986; 56: 41-46.

21. CREUGERS NHJ, WELLE PR, VRIJHOEF MMA. Four bonding systems for resin-retained cast metal prostheses. *Dent Mater* 1988; 4: 85-88.

22. WIRZ J, BESIMO C, SCHMIDLI F. Verbundfestigkeit von Metallgerüst und Haftvermittler in der Adhäsivbrückentechnik. *Schweiz Monatsschr Zahnmed* 1989; 99:24-39.

23. ZARDIACKAS LD, CALDWELL DJ, CAUGHMAN WF, et al. Tensile fatigue of resin cements to etched metal and enamel. *Dent Mater* 1988; 4: 163-168.

24. AQUILINO SA, DIAZ-ARNOLD AM, PIOTROWSKI TJ. Tensile fatigue limits of prosthodontic adhesives. *J Dent Res* 1991; 70 : 208-210.

25. SLOAN AM, LOREY RB, MYERS GE. Evaluation of laboratory etching of cast metal resin-bonded retainers. *J Dent Res* 1983; 62: 1220.

26. HUSSEY DL, GRATTON DR, McCONNELL RJ, SANDS TD. The quality of bonded retainers from commercial dental laboratories. *J Dent Res* 1989; 68: 919.

27. SAUNDERS WP. Resin bonded bridgework: a review. *J Dent* 1989; 17:255-265.

28. CREUGERS NHJ, VAN 'T HOF MA. An analysis of clinical studies on resin-bonded bridges. *J Dent Res* 1991;70: 146-149.

29. CRAIG RG. *Restorative dental materials.* 8th edn. St Louis: CV Mosby Co, 1989.

30. LIVIDITIS GJ. Cast metal resin-bonded retainers for posterior teeth. *J Am Dent Assoc* 1980; 101: 926-929.

31. MARINELLO CP, LÜTHY H, KERSCHBAUM TH, et al. Die Flächen- und Umfangbestimmung bei Adhäsivhalteelementen: eine Möglichkeit der Langzeitprognose. *Schweiz Monatsschr Zahnmed* 1990; 100: 291-299.

32. CREUGERS NHJ, SNOEK PA, VAN 'T HOF MA, KAYSER AF. Clinical performance of resin-bonded bridges: a 5-year prospective study. part II: The influence of patient-dependent variables. *J Oral Rehabil* 1989; 16: 521-527.

33. FERRARI M, CAGIDIACO MC, BERTELLI E. Anatomic guide for reduction of enamel for acid-etched retainers. *J Prosthet Dent* 1987; 58: 106-110.

34. BERGENDAL B, HALLONSTEN AL, KOCH G, et al. Composite retained onlay bridges. *Swed Dent J* 1983;7:217-225.

35. EDWARDS GD, MITCHELL L, WELBURY RR. An evaluation of resin-bonded bridges in adolescent patients. *J Ped Dent* 1989; 5: 107-114.

36. PASZYNA CH, MAU J, KERSCHBAUM TH. Risikofactoren dreigliedriger Adhäsivbrücken. *Dtsch Zahnärztl Z* 1989; 44:328-331.

37. CREUGERS NHJ, SNOEK PA, VAN 'T HOF MA, KAYSER AF. Clinical performance of resin-bonded bridges: a 5-year prospective study. part III: failure characteristics and survival after rebonding. *J Oral Rehabil* 1990; 17: 179-186.

38. CLYDE CS, BOYD T. The etched cast metal resin-bonded (Maryland) bridge: a clinical review. *J Dent* 1988; 16:22-26.

39. CHANG HK, ZIDAN O, GOMEZ-MARIN O. Resin-bonded fixed partial dentures: a recall study. *J Prosthet Dent* 1991; 65:778-781.

40. YAMASHITA A, YAMAMI T. Adhesion bridge background and clinical procedures. In: *Adhesive prosthodontics: adhesive cements and techniques.* Nijmegen: Eurosound, 1988.

41. MARINELLO CP. *Adhäsivprothetik: Klinische und materialkundliche Aspekte.* Thesis, Quintessenz Verlags GmbH, Berlin, 1991.

42. MARINELLO CP, KERSCHBAUM TH, PFEIFFER P, et al. Success rate experience after rebonding and renewal of resin-bonded fixed partial dentures. *J Prosthet Dent* 1990; 63:8-11.

43. CREUGERS NHJ, SNOEK PA, VAN 'T HOF MA. An analysis of multiple failures of resin- bonded bridges based on a 7.5 year follow-up. *J Dent* 1992;20:348-351.

44. CREUGERS NHJ, KÄYSER AF. A method to compare cost-effectiveness of dental treatments: adhesive bridges compared to conventional bridges. *Community Dent Oral Epidemiol* 1992;20:280-283.

45. CREUGERS NHJ, SNOEK PA. 7.5 year report of a clinical trial on resin-bonded bridges. *J Dent Res* 1991; 70:284 (abstr.nr.148).

46. CREUGERS NHJ, KÄYSER AF, VAN 'T HOF MA. A seven-and-a-half-year survival study on resin-bonded bridges. *J Dent Res* 1992:71:1822-1825.

47. CREUGERS NHJ, KÄYSER AF, VAN'T Hof MA. A meta-analysis of clinical data on conventional fixed bridges, 1993; To be submitted.

48. BRUNNER T, WÄLTI D, MENGHINI G. Spätergebnisse mit fixem Zahnersatz bei Minderbemittelten Erwachsenen. *Schweiz Monatsschr Zahnmed* 1992;102:1029-1036.

49. KARLSSON S. Failures and length of service in fixed prosthodontics after long-term function. *Swed Dent J* 1989;**13**:185-192.

50. KERSCHBAUM T, PASZYNA D, KLAPP S, MAYER G. Verweilzeit- und Risicofaktorenanalyse von festsitzendem Zahnersatz. *Dtsch Zahnärztl Z* 1991;**46**:20-24.

51. LEEMPOEL PJB. *Levenduur en nabehandlingen van kronen en conventionele bruggen in de algemene praktijk 1987.* Thesis, University of Nijmegen, Netherlands; pp. 137-146.

52. RANDOW K, GLANTZ PO, ZÖGER B. Technical failures and some related clinical complications in extensive fixed prosthodontics. *Acta Odontol Scand* 1986;**44**:242-255.

53. REUTER JE, BROOSE MO. Failures in full crown retained dental bridges. *Br Dent J* 1984;**157**:61-63

54. VALDERHAUG JA. 15-years clinical evaluation of fixed prosthodontics. *Acta Odontol Scand* 1991;**49**:35-40.

CHAPTER 18

Conventional Bridges in the Anterior Region

R. R. WINTER

Replacement of lost anterior teeth must satisfy several basic needs. Form, function, phonetics and esthetics must be restored. Not only must the restorations be biologically compatible with the adjacent hard or soft tissue, they must also satisfy the patient's expectations and desires. It is important to realize that the restorations created can greatly affect the personal appearance of an individual, and subsequently affect their self image and confidence during social interactions.

The means of replacement of anterior teeth lost due to trauma is determined by the extent of trauma to the teeth and alveolar process. The extent of initial damage and the long-term residual effects will dictate which restorative procedures are necessary to repair the damaged teeth, replace the lost teeth or augment the lost gingival contours of the residual ridge. Residual ridge augmentation, either with bone or soft tissue grafts may be required to rebuild the edentulous space so that the restoration which is ultimately placed appears as if it is growing out of the gingival tissue (1-5)(see also Chapter 20). Most often, the optimal residual ridge for positioning of the fixed prosthetic pontics can be achieved if one has the opportunity to guide healing after tooth extraction. This could minimize the need for residual ridge augmentation.

There are several treatment options for replacing missing teeth. These include fixed and removable prosthetics, osseointegrated implants, autotransplantation of premolars and orthodontic space closure (see Chapter 17, 19 and 20). This chapter will focus on the fixed prosthetic replacement using conventional bridges. The basic principles which will be discussed can be applied to a wide variety of restorative situations, not only to traumatized patients.

Treatment Planning

A comprehensive study of existing conditions through clinical evaluation, radiographic evaluation and the use of diagnostic casts is essential in determining the appropriate treatment plan.

One must evaluate the abutment teeth and their supporting structure to determine if they can sustain the load which they will be subjected to. The crown to root ratio and periodontal health must be assessed. The retentive qualities of the proposed retainer must be determined as well as their esthetic qualities.

An important aspect which cannot be overlooked is the maxillo-mandibular relationship and the load which will be applied on the bridge. Ante's law should always be considered when deciding on the number of abutment teeth required (6). The fulcrum line which passes through the abutment teeth and the lever arm which is created by the pontics must be assessed.

Generally the point of greatest leverage on the bridge must be supported by an abutment, or the areas of retention must be extended in each direction away from the spaces far enough to counteract the lever arm and establish counterbalancing retention (7). In the clinical situation which is presented in this Chapter the maxillo-mandibular relationship minimizes the functioning load on the proposed maxillary bridge. Therefore, minimal stress will be applied to the abutment teeth. Other considerations in this case are the youth of the patient, the opportunity to leave the maxillary cuspids as unrestored teeth which are in function against the mandibular cuspids, and the possibilities to avoid splinting of adjacent teeth thus allowing the patient to maintain better oral hygiene (8).

Esthetic Considerations

Developing the esthetic ideas necessary for a successful outcome begins with a facial analysis. The anterior incisal plane, posterior occlusal plane, interpupillary line and smile line are evaluated individually, as are their harmony with each other.

Analysis of the smile more specifically includes the incisal edge (labiol-lingual) position, maxillary and mandibular incisal planes, harmony of the facial midline to the midline of the maxillary dentition, amount of visible maxillary tooth structure in a repose position, amount of visible maxillary tooth structure in a full smile, amount of maxillary gingival exposure in a full smile, and gingival architecture.

One must not forget to consider the psychological factor of the patient's desires and expectations.

The initial factors to consider when one must replace teeth which will be extracted include: their existing labio-lingual orientation, arch shape and maxillo-mandibular relationship, and incisal length of the teeth. Function (anterior guidance), phonetics and esthetic considerations will determine any necessary changes. An important factor which also must be considered is the position, height and form of the healing ridge after extraction. This may affect the labio-lingual position and apical (gingival) length of the pontics.

Clinical Considerations

The treatment planning and treatment will be illustrated in this chapter based on an actual clinical situation. A 25-year-old woman presented with the maxillary central incisors severely discolored and a fistulous tract apical to the left incisor (Fig. 18.1). Five years previously, the patient traumatized these teeth in a bicycle accident. Endodontic therapy was performed with placement of calcium hydroxide in an effort to retain the incisors. The radiographs, however, revealed extensive internal and external resorption and continued drainage through the fistulous tract (Fig. 18.1).

The incisal length of the maxillary anterior teeth should follow the curve of the lower lip when smiling. This patient's central incisors were previously shortened, resulting in a disharmony with the smile line. The treatment plan is, therefore, to lengthen these 2 teeth in the final restoration. The mounted diagnostic casts demonstrate that there is no anterior tooth contact when the teeth are in full intercuspation (Fig. 18.2). The mandible must move anteriorly 2 mm prior to maxillary and mandibular tooth contact and onset of anterior guidance.

In this case, changes in tooth position or morphology would be inappropriate. Positioning the central incisor pontics lingually to achieve contact with the mandibular anterior teeth would adversely affect the arch form and maxillary lip support. Increasing the labio-lingual thickness of the teeth is not consistent with maintaining natural tooth morphology

Tooth Preparation and Temporization

The lateral incisors are prepared as abutments prior to extraction of the central incisors. Ideally, a 1-mm wide shoulder is prepared to provide adequate space for the shoulder porcelain. This will ensure proper color and translucency. The preparation is positioned minimally into the gingival sulcus. One and one-half mm of tooth structure is reduced from the labial aspect in the incisal one-third. A maximum of 2.5 mm is removed from the incisal edge (Fig. 18.3).

An impression is taken before extraction so that a stone cast can be made on which the temporary bridge will be fabricated. Self-curing acrylic is used to fabricate the temporary restoration (Fig. 18.4).

Fig. 18.1. Condition 5 years after trauma

A 25-year-old female patient presents 5 years after traumatic injury to her maxillary central incisors. Both incisors show root resorption. A fistulous tract is apparent in the area of the apex of the maxillary left central incisor. Both central incisors have become discolored as a result of the trauma and subsequent endodontic treatment.

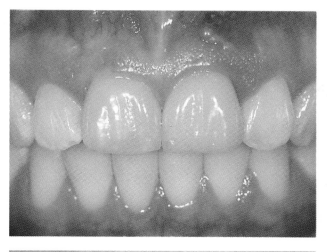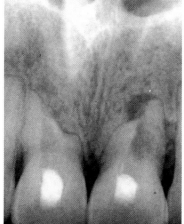

Fig. 18.2. Treatment planning

Note the disharmony of the shortened central incisors in relation to the smile line. Articulated diagnostic casts show that there is no anterior tooth contact in full intercuspidation. Due to this lack of tooth contact and minimal contact during function, a 4-unit fixed prosthesis is planned to replace the central incisors.

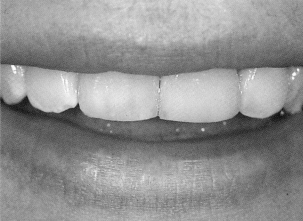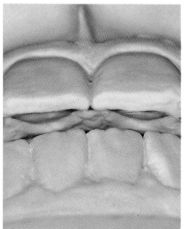

Fig. 18.3. Preparation of abutment teeth

The maxillary lateral incisors are prepared as abutment teeth prior to extraction of the central incisors.

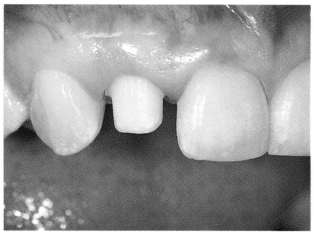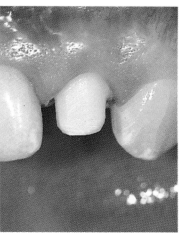

Fig. 18.4. Construction of temporary bridge

Removing the central incisors on the stone cast and extending the depression approximately 2 to 3 mm below the crest of the free gingival margin permit fabrication of pontics which can support the gingiva and control soft tissue contours during healing. The depression is concave in all directions. The mucosal surfaces of the pontics are convex in all directions and highly polished.

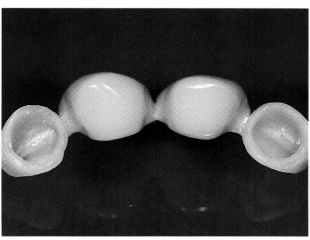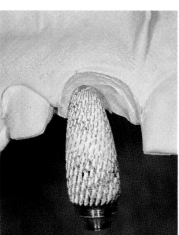

CONVENTIONAL BRIDGES IN THE ANTERIOR REGION

The extracted incisors exhibit extensive external resorption (Fig. 18.5). A temporary restoration is fabricated and inserted immediately after the extractions to maintain gingival contour and to provide labial support (Fig. 18.6).

Three weeks after extraction, a new impression is taken. A provisional bridge of heat-cured acrylic is fabricated in the same labio-lingual position as the natural teeth. This is maintained during healing (Fig. 18.7). The final impression is taken 9 months after incisor extraction and the final restoration fabricated and cemented (Fig. 18.8).

Development of Contour

There are several aspects which need to be addressed when one attempts to create natural contours in a restoration. Developing the proper contour to an abutment tooth or single crown does not begin with the ceramic but with tooth preparation. Sufficient tooth structure must be removed to make room for the restorative materials. The tooth preparation can be reviewed in Fig. 18.3.

It is essential when taking the impression to clearly impress the root structure apical to the preparation's margin. When the master die is trimmed this root area is left untouched and will clearly aid in contouring the ceramic in the gingival one-third. Visualizing the angle of the root will prevent over- or undercontouring of the restoration (Fig. 18.6).

The metal framework design will obviously dictate placement of the ceramic. There are two options in designing the framework. If a diagnostic cast of the natural teeth is available, make a silicone index of the labial and palatal aspects of the teeth. This can be transferred to the working cast to verify the labio-lingual position of the pontics, the incisal length and the position of the connector areas. If a diagnostic cast is not available, a full form wax-up of the bridge is essential. This is followed by a controlled cut-back of the wax, which allows space for the porcelain.

Analysis of Tooth Shade

Shade analysis should first begin by analyzing the natural dentition for hue (color), chroma (saturation or intensity of color), value (brightness), relative changes in opacities to translucencies, and the way light is reflected off the tooth surface, which is greatly affected by surface texture and luster. Surface texture and luster in turn will influence the perceived depth of color, value of the tooth, and translucency. One should evaluate the texture and luster of a tooth both while it is dry and wet with saliva. Surface moisture can greatly affect light reflection and the perceived surface topography. By drying the teeth, one is able to detect fine details in surface texture. Perikymata are the finest and most difficult to simulate in ceramic restorations.

When evaluating a single tooth, one notes the increasing chroma in the gingival one-third. This is due to the thinning of the enamel which allows the underlying dentin to show through more intensely. There may be zones or bands of varying hues or values. The incisal one-third exhibits increasing thickness of enamel, thereby diffusing or filtering the underlying color and increasing the translucency. As teeth age, there is typically an increase in chroma due to the increasing translucency of the enamel mineralization of dentin. The degree of translucency of the enamel layer also alters the value of the teeth. Older teeth are generally lower in value than younger "brighter" teeth. In all teeth, one should note the internal incisal effects which must be built into the ceramic restoration.

The degree and intensity of these effects vary with the age of the tooth. In young teeth one will recognize the mammelon structures. Wear in older teeth on the incisal edge exposes the dentin, which absorbs fluids and stains and which results in a more intense color.

One will also note the increasing gradation of chroma from the central incisor to the cuspid. There may also be hue or value changes from the central incisor to the cuspid.

Fig. 18.5. Extracted incisors
Both central incisors exhibit extensive external resorption.

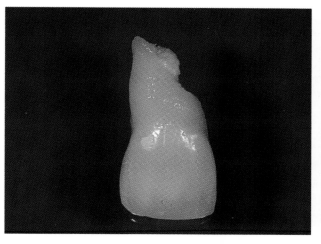 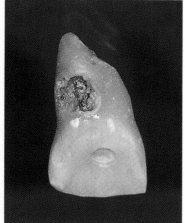

Fig. 18.6. Insertion of temporary bridge
Insertion of the temporary bridge showing how the pontics extend into the extraction sites and how the bridge supports the gingiva.

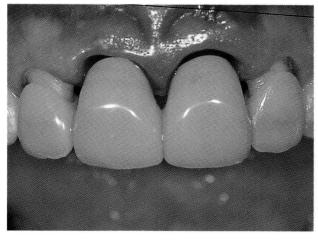 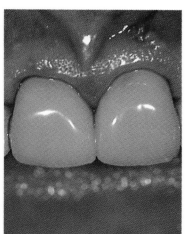

Fig. 18.7. Condition before cementation
The temporary restoration is shown 10 months after extraction of the central incisors. The patient has been maintaining the temporaries by brushing and flossing. Note the healthy pontic sites which are smooth and concave in all directions.

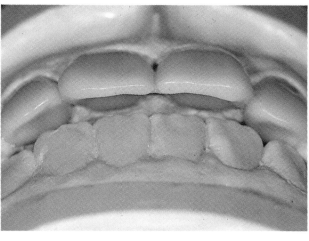 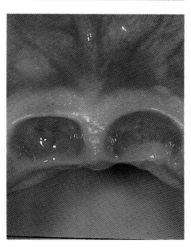

Fig. 18.8. Cementation of restoration
Different perspectives of the cemented restoration. The appearance of the surface texture, surface luster, contour and translucency change with the perspective of view. The profile shows the natural labial contour of the teeth and a smooth, gradual transition from the gingiva.

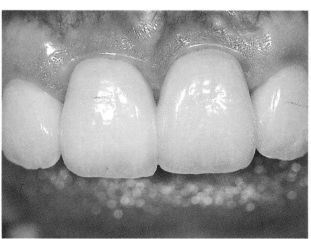 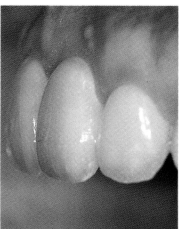

CONVENTIONAL BRIDGES IN THE ANTERIOR REGION

In accumulating information necessary to fabricate ceramic restorations one utilizes manufactured shade guides, porcelain tabs of the porcelain modifiers, custom shade guides, detailed drawings, slides and photographs.

Ceramic Application

During ceramic application, it is important to control form, position and thickness of the various layers. Varying the shade and translucency can assist in creating illusions during contouring of the restoration.

Certain areas of the restoration are predetermined and the clinician has little control. The root of an abutment tooth dictates the position of the gingival one-third of the tooth. The residual ridge (pontic site) has the same influence on the pontic. Incisal edge position is dictated by function and phonetics. Tooth contacts and function dictate the palatal aspect. The key to maintaining periodontal health is proper contouring of the interproximal areas. This is also critical in the creation of an individualized look to the teeth. Changing one's perspective changes the amount of proximal surface which is visualized. Too often there is lack of definition in this area.

The shape of the incisal edge and incisal embrasures are other important areas to develop in order to achieve a natural esthetic restoration. Here one must develop an individualized character that is not only in harmony with the surrounding dentition but must be in harmony with the patient's age and personality. The incisal one-third is visualized during speech and smiling.

Before glazing, the subtle details of surface texture are incorporated into the restoration. This will affect how the light is reflected off the surface.

After the restoration is glazed, one begins to work the surface with rubber wheels. Typically, the heights of contour are smoother and have a higher shine than concave areas.

The final luster is achieved by polishing the surface with pumice. The surface can vary from a dull or matte finish to a high shine. A polished surface appears more natural than a glazed surface.

The restoration is then inserted (Figs. 18.7 and 18.8). The esthetic goal is to create the illusion that the ceramic is natural tooth structure. Most importantly, form, function and phonetics must be achieved and the restoration must be biologically kind to the oral tissues.

Follow-up

The patient is given instructions on oral hygiene and placed on a 6-month recall schedule for professional prophylaxis. Brushing techniques are the same as with natural dentition. A flossthreader is used to thread the dental tape between the abutment tooth and pontic. The dental tape slides between the concave mucosa and the convex undersurface of the pontic, removing the plaque and deposits. Clinical signs of inflammation will not be present if there is adequate oral hygiene [11]. It has been concluded that bacterial plaque is essential for the production of inflammation of the mucosa subjacent to bridge pontics [11].

The abutment teeth will have approximately the same PI score as uncrowned teeth. The GI score will be higher when crown margins are located intracravicularly as compared to location at the gingival margin or supragingivally. WALDERHAUG also has found that there is a small increase in pocket depth, and a little more loss of attachment on those teeth where the crown margin is placed intracrevicular [12, 13]. SILNESS and others have shown that periodontal conditions around abutment teeth are significantly better when patients are instructed to practice oral hygiene [14- 16].

Prognosis

Dental bridges fail for a wide variety of reasons such as caries, periodontal disease, mobility of abutment and periapical-involvement. Mechanical problems such as uncemented crowns, defective margins, broken solder joints, etc., account for a number of failures [11-21].

In a recent metaanalysis of 4118 bridges where adequate information was available a survival analysis indicated 5-, 10- and 15- year survival of fixed bridges of 97%, 90% and 74% [21] (See Fig. 18.9).

Fig. 18.9. Survival of fixed
bridges
A metaanalysis of 4118 conven-
tional fixed bridges. From:
CREUGERS ET AL. (21, 23) 1992

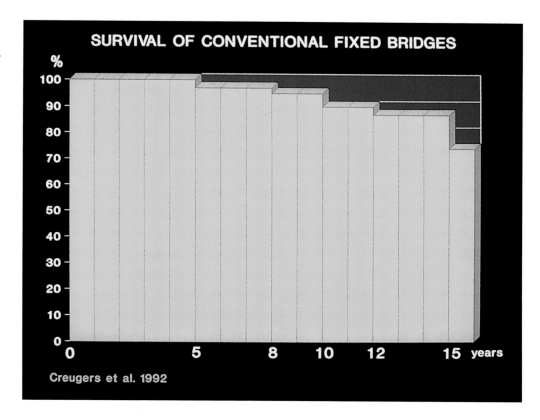

Essentials

Treatment Planning

CLINICAL EVALUATION

RADIOGRAPHIC EVALUATION

DIAGNOSTIC CASTS

EVALUATE:
- maxillo-mandibular relationship-abutment teeth and supporting structures
- crown to root ratio
- retentive qualities
- esthetic qualities

Esthetic Considerations

Facial analysis
- anterior incisal plane
- posterior occlusal plane
- interpupillary line
- smile line

Smile analysis
- incisal edge (labio-lingual) position
- maxillary and mandibular incisal planes
- harmony of facial midline to midline of the maxillary dentition
- maxillary tooth structure visible in repose
- maxillary tooth structure visible in full smile
- maxillary gingival exposure
- gingival architecture

PSYCHOLOGICAL FACTORS
- desires
- expectations

ANALYSIS OF TEETH
- shade
- contour
- surface texture and luster
- translucency

Clinical Considerations and Procedures

EVALUATION OF MAXILLO-MAN-DIBULAR RELATIONSHIP

EVALUATION OF TEETH TO BE EXTRACTED
a. Labio-lingual orientation
b. Incisal crown length

TOOTH PREPARATION
a. 2.5 mm incisal reduction
b. 1.5 mm facial reduction in incisal 1/3
c. 1.0 mm shoulder preparation with margin placement minimally into gingival sulcus

FABRICATION OF TEMPORARY RE-STORATION
a. Pre-extraction impression
b. Pontic should extend 2-3mm into extraction site in order to control shape of healing gingiva
c. Revision of temporaries 3 weeks after extraction
d. Final preparation 9 months after extraction

e. Maintenance of optimal oral hygiene during temporization

FINAL RESTORATION
a. Final impression must include root surface apical to preparation margin
b. Ceramic build-up
c. Anatomic considerations
d. Root anatomy determines contour of gingival 1/3 of abutment
e. Residual ridge determines contour of gingival 1/3 of pontic
f. Incisal edge position determined by phonetics
g. Palatal aspect determined by tooth contacts and function
h. Contour of interproximal areas for maintenance of periodontal health

Follow-up

Oral hygiene instructions
6-month recall for prophylaxis

Prognosis

5-year bridge survival: 97%
10-year bridge survival: 90%
15-year bridge survival: 74%

Bibliography

1. ABRAMS L. Augmentation of the deformed residual edentulous ridge for fixed prosthesis. *Compend Contin Educ Gen Dent* 1980;**3**:205-14.

2. LANGER B, CALAGNA LJ. The subepithelial connective tissue graft. A new approach to the enhancement of anterior cosmetics. *Int J Periodont Restor Dent* 1982;**2**:22-33.

3. SEIBERT JS. Reconstruction of deformed, partially edentulous ridges, using full thickness onlay grafts. Part I. Technique and wound healing. *Compend Contin Educ Gen Dent* 1983;**5**:437-53.

4. SEIBERT JS.Reconstruction of deformed, partially edentulous ridges, using full thickness onlay grafts. Part II. Prosthetic/periodontal interrelationships. *Compen Contin Educ Dent* 1983;**6**:549-62.

5. SEIBERT JS. Current concepts and techniques for localized ridge augmentation. Research paper Univ. of Pennsylvania School of Dental Medicine.

6. ANTE IH. The fundamental principles of abutments. *Michigan State D Soc Bul* 1926;**8**:14.

7. DYKEMA RW. Fixed partial prosthodontics. *J Tennessee Dent Assoc* 1962;**42**:309.

8. SILNESS J, OHM E. Periodontal conditions in patients treated with dental bridges, V. Effects of splinting adjacent abutment teeth. *J Periodont Res* 1974;**9**:121-6.

9. ZADIK D, CHOSACK A, EIDELMAN E. The prognosis of traumatized permanent anterior teeth with fracture of the enamel and dentin. *Oral Surg, Oral Med, Oral Pathol* 1979;**47**:173-5.

10. RAVN JJ. Follow-up study of permanent incisors with enamel-dentin fractures after acute trauma. *J Dent Res* 1981;**89**:355-65.

11. SILNESS J, GUSTAVSEN F, MANGERSNES K. The relationship between pontic hygiene and mucosal inflammation in fixed bridge recipients. *J Periodont Res* 1982;**17**:434-9.

12. VALDERHAUG J. Periodontal conditions and carious lesions following the insertion of fixed prostheses: a 10 year follow-up study. *Int Dent J* 1980;**30**:296-304.

13. VALDERHAUG J, HELÖE LA. Oral hygiene in a group of supervised patients with fixed prostheses. *J Periodont* 1970:**48**:221-24.

14. SILNESS J. Periodontal conditions in patients treated with dental bridges. *J Periodont Res* 1970;**5**:60-8.

15. SILNESS J. Periodontal conditions in patients treated with dental bridges. II. The influence of full and partial crowns on plaque accumulation, development of gingivitis and pocket formation. *J Periodont Res* 1970;**5**:219-24.

16. SILNESS J. Periodontal conditions in patients treated with dental bridges, III. The relationship between the location of the crown margin and the periodontal condition. *J Periodont Res* 1970;**5**:225-9.

17. REUTER J, BROSE M. Failures in full crown retained dental bridges. *Br Dent J* 1984;**157**:61-3.

18. MORRANT G. Bridges. *Dent Practit* 1956;**6**:!78-86.

19. SCHWARTZ N, WHITSETT LD, BERRY TG, STEWARD J L. Unserviceable crowns and fixed partial dentures: life-span and causes for loss of serviceability. *J Am Dent Assoc* 1970;**81**:1395-1401.

20. ROBERTS D. The failure of retainers in bridge prostheses. *Br Dent J* 1970;**128**:117-24.

21. CREUGERS N, KÄYSER AF, VAN'T HOF MA. A meta-analysis of clinical data on conventional fixed bridges. To be submitted.

CHAPTER 19

Autotransplantation of Teeth to the Anterior Region

J.O. ANDREASEN, L. KRISTERSON, M. TSUKIBOSHI & F.M. ANDREASEN

A new procedure, autotransplantation of teeth, has recently been developed for the treatment of anterior tooth loss (1-23). Due to the unique osteogenic capacity of the graft, this procedure offers a treatment alternative, where both the lost tooth and the atrophied alveolar process can be replaced (21-22).

Recent studies have demonstrated good long-term survival of these transplants, thus providing a realistic treatment alternative for tooth replacement in young individuals (see Appendix 5, p. 751).

The key to successful tooth transplantation has been shown clinically and experimentally to be proper selection of grafts with adequate root development as well as the design of surgical techniques for atraumatic graft removal and graft insertion. These techniques are described in detail in a recently published textbook on tooth replantation and transplantation (21).

Treatment Planning

When anterior tooth loss occurs before completion of mandibular growth, a panoramic radiograph should be made available, whereby potential grafts, such as canines, premolars and in some cases diminutive third molars, can be identified. When donor teeth are available, the cost-benefit of autotransplantation should be weighed against other treatment solutions, such as orthodontic space closure (see Chapter 15, p. 608 , fixed prosthetics (see Chapters 18, p. 661 and Chapter 19, p. 671) and implants (see Chapter 21, p. 692). As optimal prognosis depends upon teeth with incomplete root formation, the patient group best suited for this procedure is from 10 to 13 years old. At this age, alveolar growth is not yet complete, thereby contraindicating implants and fixed prosthetics (except for resin-retained bridges).

The use of teeth with incomplete root formation for grafting induces new alveolar bone formation (Fig. 19.1). Thus, only orthodontic space closure remains as a realistic treatment option. The choice between autotransplantation and orthodontic space closure depends upon an orthodontic analysis of growth and occlusion (see Chapter 15, p. 608).

Graft Selection

In the selection of donor teeth, crown and root anatomy should be considered. With respect to coronal anatomy, reduction of tooth structure should generally be limited to enamel. Dentin exposure should be limited or avoided due to the risk of exposure of soft tissue inclusions which are found in post-transplantation dentin and which can imply a risk of subsequent pulp necrosis (see later).

Concerning root anatomy, the graft should fit the recipient site loosely, avoiding contact with adjacent bone and pro-

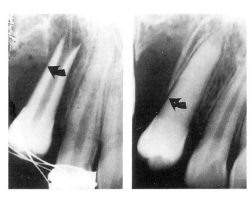

Fig. 19.1. Alveolar bone induction by a premolar transplant to the canine region

Due to a severe trauma considerable bone has been lost in the region (arrow). The auto-transplanted premolar has induced formation of alveolar bone distal to the transplant (arrow).

viding an approximately 1-mm space to the adjacent roots. Many potential grafts will exceed the existing labiolingual dimension, especially if atrophy of the alveolar process has taken place. However, special surgical techniques, such as intentional fracture of the labial bone plate or a composite tooth-labial bone plate graft can solve this problem (see p. 678). An important aspect is the dimension at the cervical part of the graft. This must be in reasonable harmony with its antimere. Such harmony can often be obtained if the graft is rotated 45° or 90°.

Fig. 19.2. Central incisor loss, possible donor teeth
Except for mandibular first premolars, all premolars can serve as donor teeth. In rare cases, diminutive maxillary third molars can also be used.

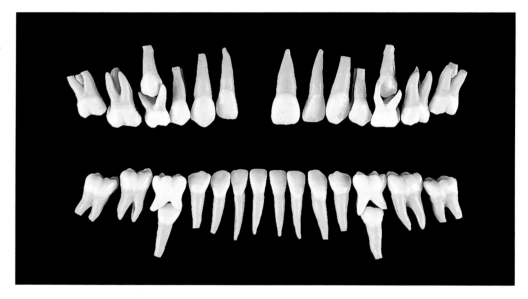

CHAPTER 19

With these limitations in mind, the following grafts (in order of preference) appear to be suitable for the *maxillary central incisor region* (Fig. 19.2): Second mandibular premolars, canines, first mandibular premolars, second maxillary premolars and diminutive third molars (Figs. 19.3 and 19.4). Maxillary first premolars should generally not be used because of their bifid roots, which present surgical obstacles to atraumatic graft removal.

Fig. 19.3. Central incisor region, transplantation of a mandibular second premolar
The double exposure illustrates where crown substance should be added or reduced.

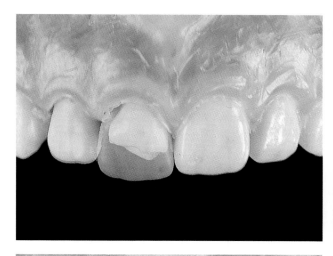
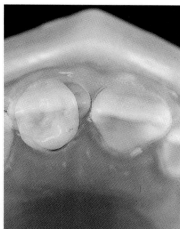

Fig. 19.4. Central incisor region, transplantation of a maxillary second premolar
The double exposure illustrates where crown substance should be added or reduced when the transplant is positioned without or with rotation.

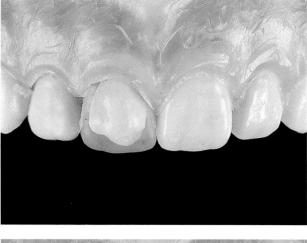
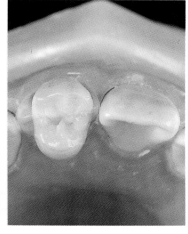

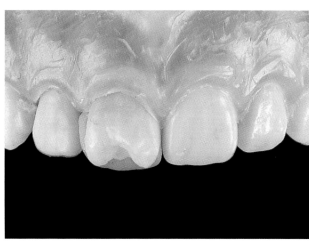
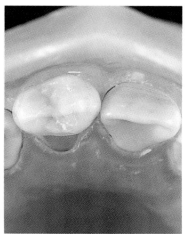

Fig. 19.5. Lateral incisor loss, possible donor teeth
Mandibular first premolars are optimal donor teeth.

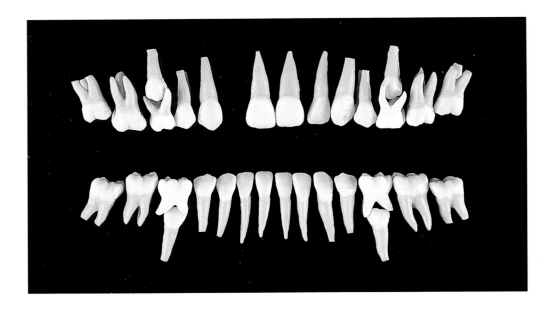

In the *lateral incisor region* the mandibular first premolar is, because of its size, the only good candidate for transplantation (Figs. 19.5 and 19.6).

In the *canine region*, all premolars, except the maxillary first, can be used (Figs. 19.7 and 19.8).

In general, grafts should be selected with 3/4 to full root formation with a wide open apex. At this stage of development, the graft is easy to remove and both periodontal and pulpal healing are very predictable (see p. 680).

Fig.19.6. Lateral incisor region, transplantation of a mandibular first premolar
The double exposure illustrates where crown substance should be added or reduced.

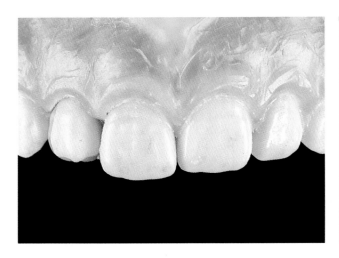 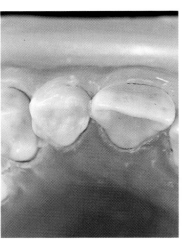

**Fig. 19.7. Canine loss,
possible donor teeth**
*Mandibular premolars are opti-
mal donor teeth.*

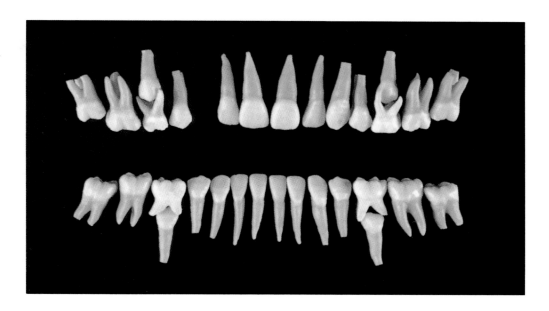

Analysis of the Recipient Site

A radiographic examination is necessary to analyze the vertical bone level and the space available between adjacent teeth. As a rule, the crown of the potential graft should fit into the space available mesio-distally above bone level. Furthermore, dimensions of the root of the graft should ensure 1 mm of bone between itself and the roots of adjacent teeth.

The labio-palatal dimension of the alveolar process can be estimated by inspection clinically. In case of doubt as to whether a potential graft can fit into the recipient site, an open surgical procedure should be chosen (see p. 678).

Surgical Procedure

In this context only certain principles of graft removal and recipient site preparation will be presented. Readers interested in details about the surgical procedures are referred to a recent textbook covering this subject (21).

**Fig. 19.8. Canine region,
transplantation of a man-
dibular first or second
premolar**
*The double exposure illustrates
where crown substance should be
added or reduced.*

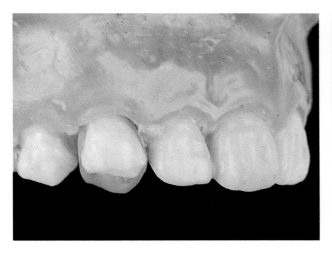
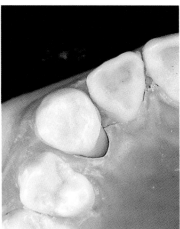

Preparation of the Recipient Site

Based on the radiographic and clinical examination, and depending on the fit of the graft in the existing alveolar process, a closed or open procedure is selected. As a rule, the recipient site is prepared prior to graft removal in order to shorten the extra-alveolar period for the graft. Before the surgical procedure, antibiotic coverage is achieved (e.g. penicillin, 1 million IU) 1 hour before surgery and maintained for a period of 4 days (2-4 million IU/day).

Closed Procedure

If a tooth is present at the recipient site, it is extracted and the socket enlarged so that the future graft will be surrounded by a 1-2 mm coagulum (Fig. 19.9). This will optimize periodontal and pulpal healing. The socket preparation should be performed atraumatically with a bur with internal saline cooling. Thereafter the entrance to the socket is covered with a gauze sponge while awaiting the graft.

Fig. 19.9. Autotransplantation of a premolar to the central incisor region using a closed procedure
The treatment plan is to transplant a maxillary second premolar to the central incisor region. The incisor is to be removed due to root resorption subsequent to replantation.

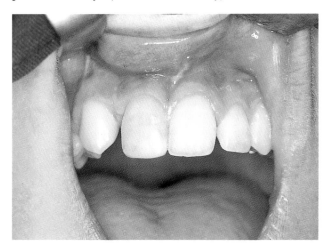 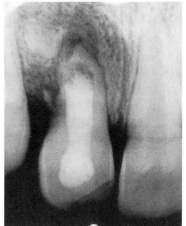

Extracting the incisor
The incisor is extracted. Note the extensive root resorption.

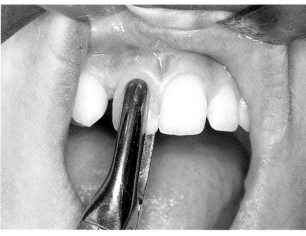 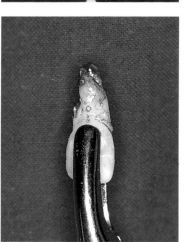

Preparing the socket
The socket is enlarged with a surgical bur with internal saline cooling. The socket is expanded palatally. The socket is then rinsed with saline.

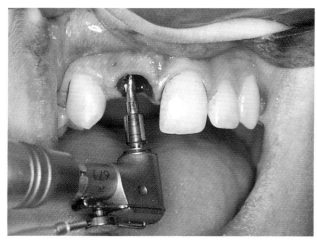 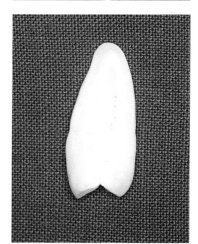

Testing the size of the socket

Using a glass replica of a premolar, the size of the socket is tested. Thereafter the socket is washed with saline.

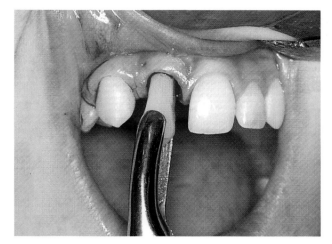 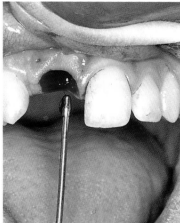

Removing the maxillary second premolar

After making a gingival incision and incising the cervical part of the PDL, the tooth is extracted using gentle luxation movements.

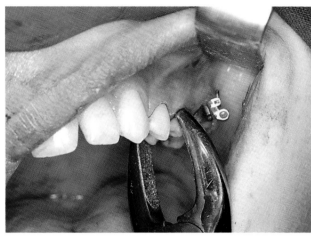 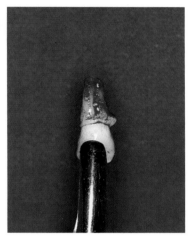

Repositioning the graft

The graft is placed 45° rotated in order to achieve sufficient cervical width.

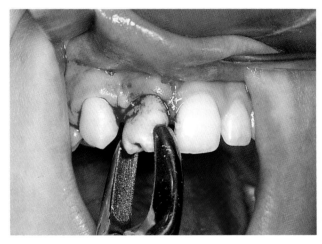 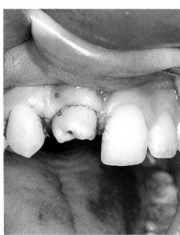

Splinting the graft

The tooth is splinted with an 0.2 mm stainless steel wire placed around the necks of the adjacent teeth. The position for the wire is ensured by etching the labial enamel of the adjacent teeth and incorporating the wire in composite.

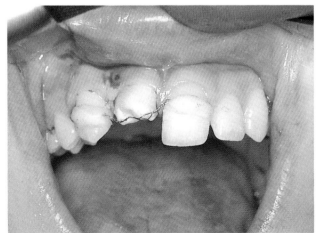 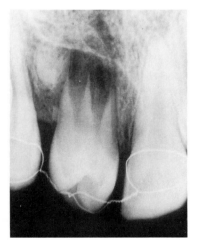

Open Procedure

A trapezoid incision is made in the attached labial gingival mucosa. A candidate tooth is extracted (Fig. 19.10) and an osteotomy cut is made with a thin bur at the site of the future alveolus. The labial bone plate is then removed with a chisel and stored in saline. Thereafter the socket is prepared with a bur with internal saline cooling. Finally, the socket is covered with a gauze sponge in order to prevent saliva contamination during graft removal.

Graft Removal and Insertion

The donor tooth is removed atraumatically, usually implying a flap procedure and removal of marginal bone labially in the case of mandibular premolars or palatally in the case of maxillary premolars. The graft is placed in a semi-erupted position in the new socket and stabilized with a suture cervically.

In case of an open procedure, the dissected labial bone plate is cut lengthwise with a heavy scissors into 2-3 pieces. These grafts are placed so that they cover the labial part of the root with the cortical surface facing the root. Thereafter the labial flap is elongated using periosteal incisions and then sutured tightly around the neck of the transplant. As experimental studies have shown that rigid splinting is detrimental to both pulpal and periodontal healing, this procedure should be avoided. To prevent vertical displacement during healing, a suture is placed over the occlusal surface of the graft. Alternatively, a figure-of-eight stainless steel wire (diameter 0.2 mm) inserted between adjacent teeth may serve the same purpose. The stabilizing sutures or wires are removed after 1 week.

Follow-up Period

Clinical and radiographic controls should be made after 4 and 8 weeks where healing complications, such as pulp necrosis or external root resorption (i.e. inflammatory or replacement resorption) can be diagnosed. After 4 months, the graft can be restored. Further clinical and radiographic controls should be performed at the following intervals: 6 months, 1 year, 2 years and 5 years after grafting in order to assess pulpal and periodontal healing.

Fig. 19.10. Autotransplantation of a premolar to the central incisor region using an open procedure

The treatment plan is to transplant a right maxillary premolar to the central incisor region where there is marked vertical and horizontal bone atrophy.

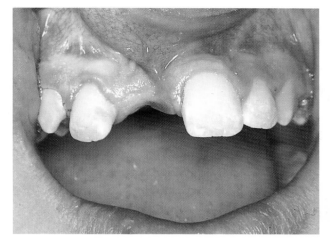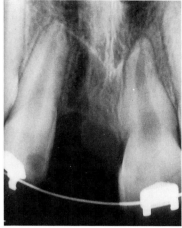

Flap procedure and socket preparation

A trapezoidal incision is made and the atrophied alveolar ridge exposed. Osteotomy cuts through the labial bone plates and subsequent removal of bone plate with a chisel will expose the future socket. The socket is prepared with a bur with internal saline cooling.

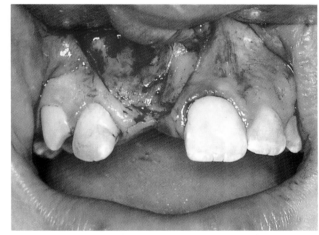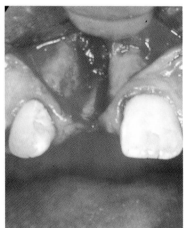

Transplanting the premolar

The premolar is seated in the socket and fixed in its new position with a suture placed cervically. Thereafter, the labial bone plate is cut lengthwise in 2-mm wide strips with heavy scissors and placed over the transplant, with the concave cortical surface against the periodontal ligament.

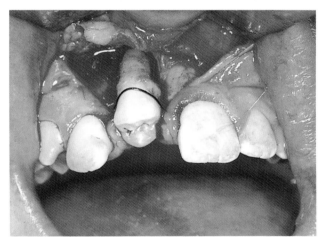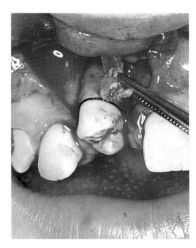

Flap repositioning and splinting

The flap is lengthened via periosteal incisions at its base and then sutured. A thin (0.2 mm) stainless steel wire anchored between the right lateral incisor and the left central incisor stabilizes the tooth during initial healing.

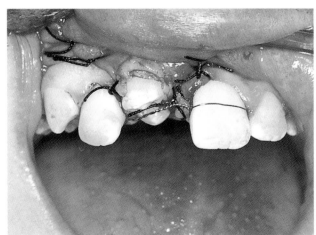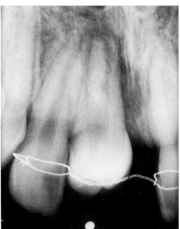

AUTOTRANSPLANTATION OF TEETH TO THE ANTERIOR REGION 679

Fig.19.11. Tooth survival of
autotransplanted teeth used
in the treatment of anterior
tooth loss
A life table analysis of two clinical studies representing 50 and 130 transplants to the anterior region. From KRISTERSON & LAGERSTRÖM (20) *1991 and* ANDREASEN ET AL. (22) *1992.*

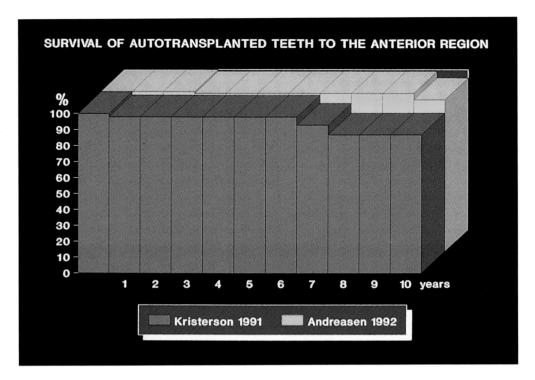

Tooth Survival

In two long-term studies of autotransplanted teeth to the anterior region 5-year survival ranged from 98% to 99% and 10-year survival from 87% to 95% (20-22) (Fig. 19.11). It appears that long-term survival can be found with an intact PDL and pulp vitality (Fig. 19.12).

Pulpal Healing

Three to 6 months after transplantation, pulpal healing can be diagnosed clinically by a positive sensibility response as well as radiographically by pulp canal obliteration, which is a sign of reinnervation and revascularization of the traumatized pulp (14). Pulp necrosis due to infection can usually be diagnosed after 4 to 8 weeks. Treatment of pulp necrosis is outlined in Chapter 14, p. 593. Secondary pulp necrosis may occur following pulp canal obliteration. This complication was found in 5% of transplanted cases and was usually related to a new trauma or dentin exposure during crown preparation.

Periodontal Healing

The earliest radiographic signs of healing (i.e. reformation of the periodontal ligament space) can be seen after 4 weeks and are usually manifest after 8 weeks. Inflam-

matory and replacement resorption are usually evident after 4 to 8 weeks. These complications were found with a frequency of 7% in the authors' material (22). The treatment of both resorption types follow the principles outlined for avulsed and replanted teeth (see Chapter 14, p.557).

Orthodontic Treatment of Transplanted Teeth

In many trauma cases, where autotransplantation to the anterior region has been performed, it is often necessary to reduce a maxillary overjet orthodontically.

Recent clinical studies indicate that orthodontic treatment is possible in the period 3-6 months after autotransplantation without a significant risk of progressive resorption (15, 20, 22).

Restoration of Transplanted Teeth

The general principles for restoration of transplanted teeth imply a minimum interference with the health of the pulp and the gingiva. In a tooth transplanted with an incompletely formed root, revascularization of the pulp normally occurs, but usually with pulp canal obliteration to follow. Pulp canal obliteration can usually be

Fig.19.12. Long-term survival of a grafted premolar
*A maxillary second premolar
transplanted to the lateral incisor
region.*

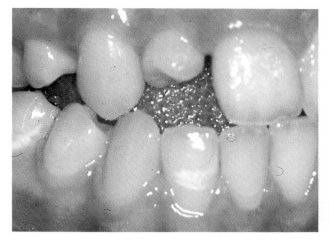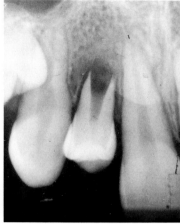

10- year control
*Stable periodontal and pulpal
healing is evident 10 years after
transplantation.*

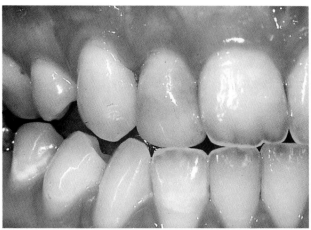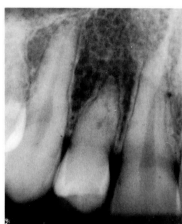

diagnosed 3 to 6 months after transplantation. This newly formed dentin differs from normal dentin by virtue of its cellular content and many vascular inclusions (21). Thus, any exposure of dentin, as during crown preparation or caries, may permit progressive bacterial invasion. As an adequate secondary dentin response in the pulp is not possible due to the constricted root canal, an infected pulp necrosis may occur (Fig. 19.13). For this reason, it is suggested that restorative procedures are performed prior to total canal obliteration, i.e. 3-9 months after transplantation.

Before restoration, the contour of the gingival margin should also be considered. If a gingivectomy is to be performed, coronal regrowth of approximately 1 mm in the anterior region should be anticipated (24).

Safe restoration of transplanted teeth implies the following considerations: (1) Pulpal status should be determined prior to restoration, i.e., a positive sensibility response should be elicited. (2) The restoration should be made so that no or only a minimum of dentin is exposed. At least no postransplantation dentin must be exposed. (3) The restorative procedure used should prevent or limit microleakage, which leads to bacterial invasion, hypersensibility and discoloration of the restoration. The use of the new dentin-bonding agents may help to eliminate these problems following tooth reduction.

If the tooth has been endodontically treated, the first two considerations can be ignored.

The restorative procedures are presently confined to two types: composite resin restoration or ceramic laminate veneers, both employed after adequate enamel reduction.

Composite Restoration

These restorations can be performed very soon after transplantation. After necessary enamel reduction, the crowns are built up according to the principles described for the use of composite resin in the treatment

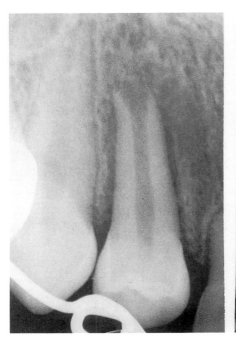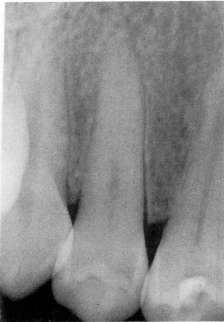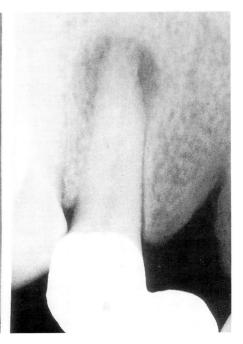

Fig.19.13.
Pulpal complications subsequent to crown preparation. One year after crown preparation, a periapical radiolucency is seen. From KRISTERSON (10) 1985.

of crown fractured teeth (see Chapter 16, p. 636) (Fig. 19.14).

An important aspect in the restoration of the traumatized dentition is the restoration of symmetry in the dental arch. A decisive factor is the cervical dimension of the graft, which can be adjusted during the surgical phase of treatment by graft rotation at the recipient site. However, in the case of anterior asymmetry, either due to deviation of graft dimension with its antimere, or where adjacent teeth have migrated into the site of tooth loss or infraocclusion in the case of protracted ankylosis, and where for various reasons orthodontic realignment is not possible, the problem arises as to how to reestablish lost symmetry.

Slight reduction of the proximal surface of the adjacent incisor may compensate for some space loss. There should be maximal length of the restored transplanted tooth to enhance the illusion of symmetry. The facial surface should be flattened, with maximum separation between mamelons, and acute proximal angles to allude to a broader tooth. Finally, the mesial and distal corners of the incisal edge should be squared (21).

Another situation can arise when the mesiodistal dimension of the transplant is greater than its antimere, as when a maxillary premolar has been transplanted and rotated 90°. In this situation, the opposite optical effect can be used to achieve optimal symmetry (21). The transplant should be restored to maximum length, with the facial surface as well as the mesial and distal corners rounded and minimal distance between mamelons. This technique will deflect light and suggest smaller dimensions. Moreover, the size of the contralateral can also be enhanced to improve symmetry (21).

Finally, in teeth with diminutive cervical dimensions, cervical build-up in ceramic, similar to that done in the case of single tooth implants can provide another solution to anterior asymmetry (25).

Ceramic Laminate Veneers

The conservative preparation necessary for veneer restoration makes this treatment procedure suitable for restoring the esthetics to the anterior region following premolar autotransplantation while preserving pulpal vitality following post-trans-

Fig.19.14. Maxillary central incisor replacement using *autotransplantation*
Right central incisor replaced with a left mandibular second premolar. *The tooth has been restored with composite.*

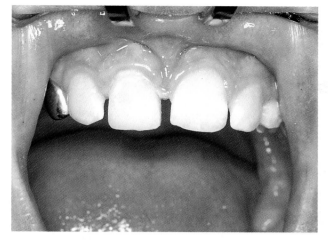
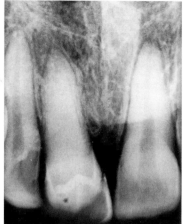

Right central incisor replacement
The incisor was replaced with a left mandibular second premolar. *The tooth has been restored with composite.*

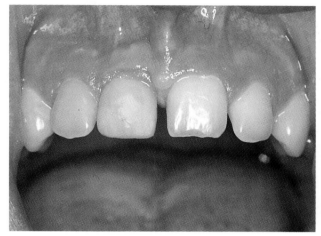
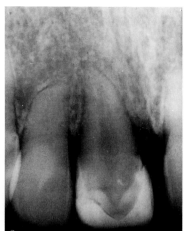

Right central incisor replacement
The incisor was replaced with a right maxillary second premolar. *The tooth has been restored with composite.*

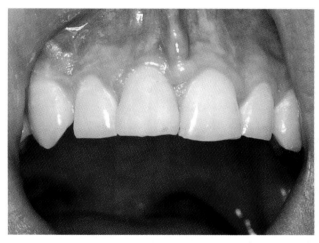
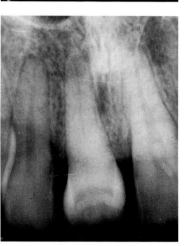

Left central incisor replacement
The incisor was replaced with a left maxillary third molar. *The tooth has been restored with composite.*

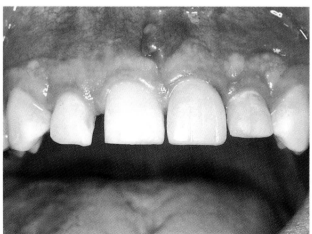
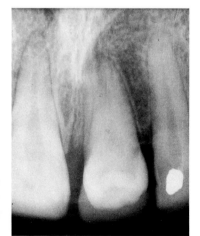

AUTOTRANSPLANTATION OF TEETH TO THE ANTERIOR REGION

Fig.19.15. Autotransplanted premolars restored with a porcelain laminate veneer
Two restored central incisors were replaced with 2 second maxillary premolars. The transplants were later restored with porcelain laminates.

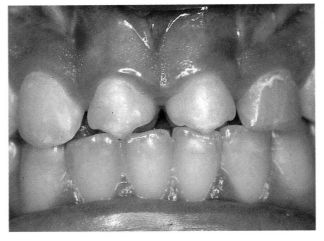 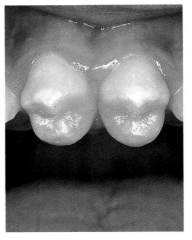

Completed treatment
The transplants, after grinding were restored with porcelain laminates.

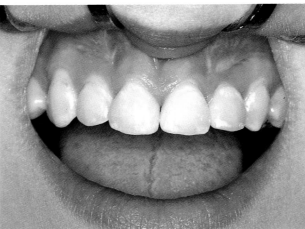 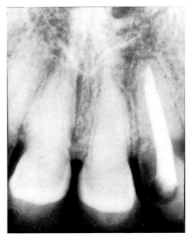

plantation canal obliteration (25) (Fig. 19.15). Although the crown height in younger individuals is very likely to undergo changes, the gingival margin of ceramic veneers cemented with a composite luting agent is esthetically acceptable despite its eventual visibility. Patient satisfaction with these restorations, including the prospect of revision at a later date due to maxillary skeletal growth, is more than adequate.

Special problems arise with respect to preparation of premolars for anterior restorations. Often orthodontic adjustment of the transplant is necessary prior to definitive restoration. In such cases, the period of retention must be complete before preparation for veneers. Otherwise, there is a risk of tooth migration. Alternatively, a retention wire should be applied palatally to assure transplant orientation even after restoration.

Other problems that also present in these cases concern the proximal extension of the preparation to ensure adequate ceramic bulk to withstand occlusal loading during function, as well as the extent of reduction of the palatal cusp to ensure

occlusal stability. It is still a matter of debate whether a bulky palatal cusp invites lingual pressure that could force the transplant facially or whether occlusion in the central fossa stabilizes the tooth. Esthetic demands might well dictate cusp reduction. Whatever decision is made with regard to tooth preparation, caution must exercised if dentin is exposed during tissue reduction. In such cases, it is advisable that the exposed dentin be treated with a dentin-bonding agent and a thin layer of unfilled composite resin immediately after preparation and prior to impression taking in order to seal dentinal tubules until veneer cementation.

The following procedures have been suggested for detecting exposed dentin: search under magnification or with an explorer, where dentin feels and looks smooth compared to a roughened, prepared enamel or by a 5-second etch, where enamel looks frosty and dentin dull. Provisional restoration would seem appropriate in such situations; also in the case of palatal-occlusal reduction (i.e. a reverse 3/4 crown) in order to maintain interdental and intermaxillary relationships. When

CHAPTER 19

Fig.19.16. Maxillary lateral and central incisor replacement with combined orthodontic space closure and premolar transplantation
Two incisors have been avulsed in a 9-year-old girl. The treatment plan is to orthodontically move the canine into the lateral incisor position, the first premolar into the canine position, and finally to transplant the mandibular second premolar into the central incisor position.

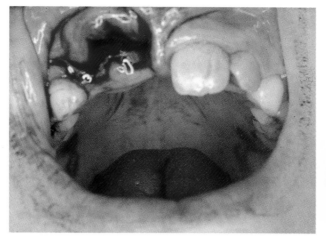
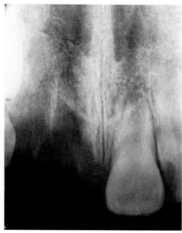

Restoration of the anterior segment
The premolar has been moved into the canine position, rotated 45° and the oral cusp reduced. The canine has been moved into the lateral incisor position and its cusp and proximal surfaces reduced. The transplanted premolar has been restored with composite. From ANDREASEN ET AL. (11) 1989.

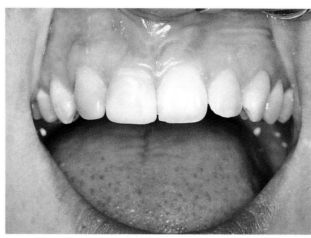
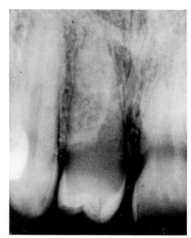

provisional restorations are indicated, they can be retained either as a resin splint by spot-etching the prepared and adjacent teeth or as a provisional veneer with a eugenol-free luting agent (27-29).

Figs. 19.16 and 19.17 demonstrate examples of final treatment results of autotransplantation in the treatment of anterior tooth loss.

Autotransplantation of Teeth with Completed Root Formation

Recently a technique for autotransplantation of teeth with completed root formation has been used in the initial or late treatment of acute dental trauma TSUKIBOSHI (30, 31) (Fig. 19.18 and 19.19)

In this technique, the socket is prepared atraumatically with surgical burs to a size which is slightly larger than the donor tooth. The graft tooth is luxated and extracted after incision of the periodontal

ligament with a thin scalpel blade and immediately transferred to the new socket and placed slightly out of occlusion. The graft is splinted for 8 weeks with a flexible wired splint and an acid-etch/composite technique.

After 3 to 4 weeks, endodontic treatment can be performed using an interim dressing of calcium hydroxide followed by a gutta-percha root filling (see Chapter 15, p. 554).

In cases of acute trauma, this technique can also be used to place the tooth in a site of less injury (Fig. 19.19). A tooth (usually an ectopically placed premolar) can be moved to the anterior region (Fig. 19.18).

In a follow-up study of 130 transplants over a period of 7 years, 97% tooth survival was recorded. Moreover, periodontal ligament healing without progressive root resorption (inflammatory resorption and replacement resorption) was observed in 97% of the cases (30,31).

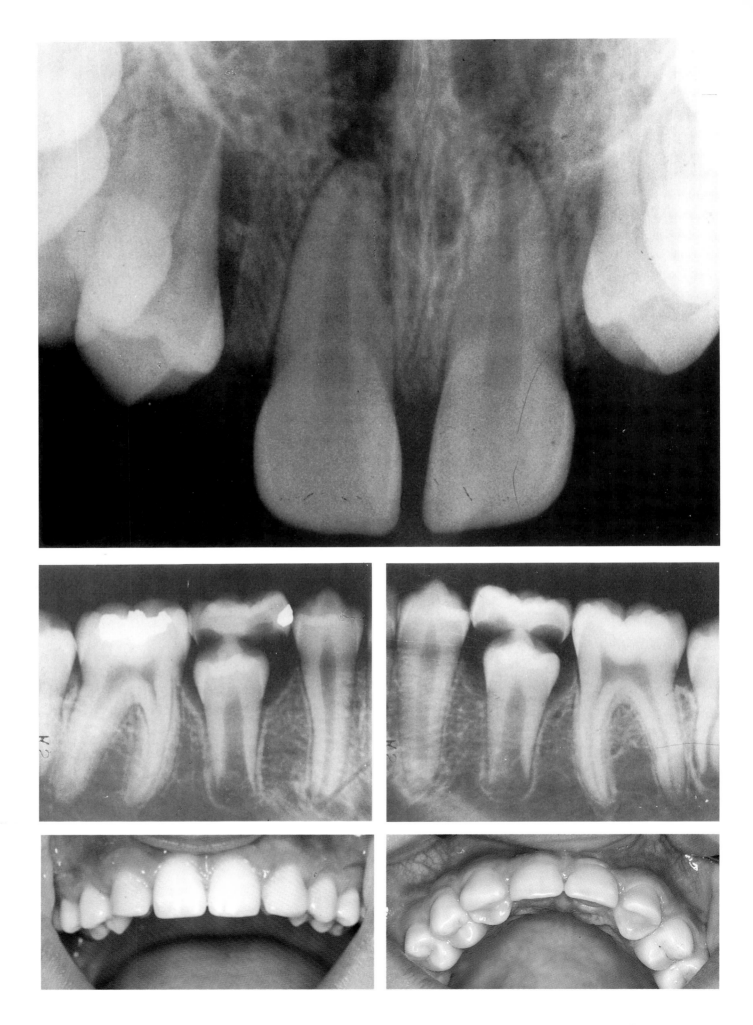

Fig.19.17. Maxillary lateral incisors replaced by a mandibular second premolar transplants
This patient suffered lateral incisor and canine aplasia. Orthodontic evaluation showed that mandibular second premolar transplantation to the lateral incisor position together with anterior orthodontic movement of the distally placed teeth was indicated in order to compensate for the missing teeth. The two mandibular premolars are at optimal stage of root development, with 3/4 of the anticipated root length. The clinical condition is shown 5 years after transplantation and after completion of orthodontic treatment.

Prognosis

In two long-term studies of autotransplanted teeth with immature root development, where data allow life table analysis of the prognosis there appears to be almost identical survival. Five-year survival ranges from 98 to 99%; and 10-year survival from 87 to 95% and 80% (20, 22, 23). This survival rate thus appears to be equal or superior to alternative treatment approaches, such as implants and fixed prosthetic appliances (see Chapters 17, 18 and 20).

With respect to pulpal and periodontal healing, it should be mentioned that 10%-20% of the cases may show complications, such as primary or secondary pulp necrosis as well as root resorption, which may require additional treatment.

With respect to the restorative procedures presently available, little is known about long-term success when applied to autotransplanted teeth.

In summary, autotransplantation of premolars in properly selected cases offers a unique treatment possibility with a high success rate, with esthetic reconstruction of both tooth and alveolar process and functional qualities (i.e. functional and adjustable PDL) which cannot be equalled or surpassed by present treatment alternatives.

Fig 19.18. Autotransplantation of 2 premolars with complete root formation to the central incisor region
This 14-year-old girl had lost her two central incisors due to progressive root resorption subsequent to replantation after avulsion. In conjunction with orthodontic reduction of a maxillary overjet, two second mandibular premolars were extracted and transplanted to the central incisor region.

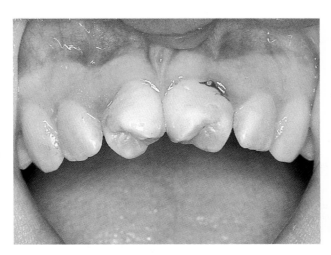
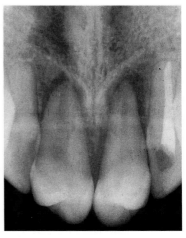

10-year follow-up
The clinical and radiographic condition is shown 10 years after transplantation. The transplanted teeth have been treated endodontically and later restored with post retained crowns.

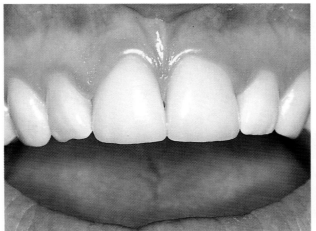
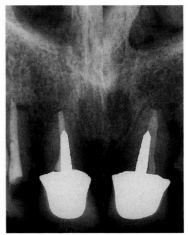

Fig. 19.19. Autotransplantation of an intruded central incisor with completed root formation
Radiographic and clinical condition at the time of injury in a 32-year-old woman. There is extrusion of the right maxillary lateral incisor with associated gingival laceration. The right central and left lateral incisors have been avulsed and the left central incisor intruded with severe crushing of the associated alveolar process.

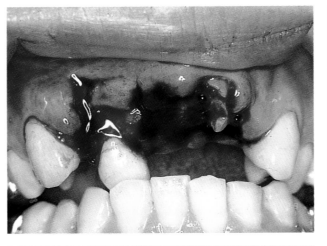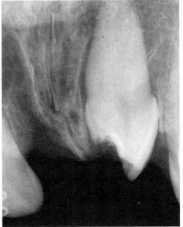

Treatment plan
Treatment includes autotransplantation of the left central incisor to a site with least bony injury in order to avoid later bone loss (i.e. the right central incisor socket) and repositioning of the extruded right lateral incisor.

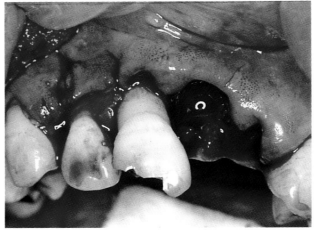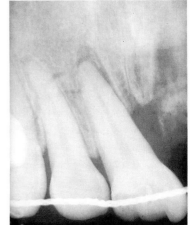

Clinical and radiographic condition after treatment
The teeth are repositioned and the gingiva sutured. The teeth are splinted with flexible wire and an acid-etch/composite resin technique for 3 months. The root canals were initially treated with a calcium hydroxide dressing for 3 months prior to final root filling with gutta percha and sealer.

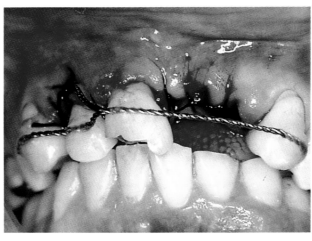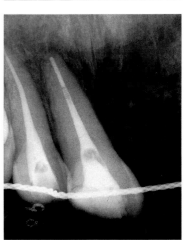

Follow-up
The clinical condition is shown 4 years after completed prosthetic treatment. Radiographic condition 6 years after completed treatment shows slight apical surface resorption of the transplanted central incisor.

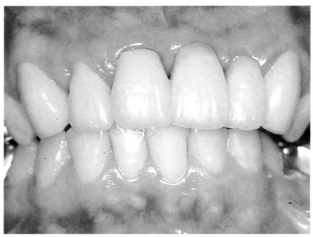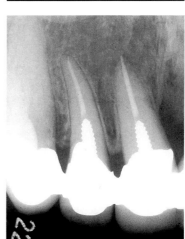

688

Essentials

Indications

All cases where an early loss of permanent incisors occurs - in that case a panoramic radiograph should be taken in order to detect possible tooth grafts.

The advantage of tooth autotransplantation in comparison to alternative treatment procedures is the establishment of a functional tooth unit, which allows tooth eruption and development of the alveolar process.

Graft Selection

Central maxillary incisor region
All premolars except maxillary first premolars, sometimes canines or maxillary third molars of small size.

Lateral maxillary incisor region
Only mandibular first premolars.

Canine region
All premolars except maxillary first premolars.

Stage of Graft Removal

3/4 or full root development with wide open apex.

Surgical Procedures

Closed procedure
In cases with adequate bone support (Fig. 19.9).

Open procedure
In cases with composite bone tooth grafting (Fig. 19.10).

Atraumatic graft removal and graft insertion is essential for successful long-term results.

Orthodontic Treatment

If orthodontic treatment is necessary, it can be performed when revascularization of the pulp has been completed, i.e. after 4 months.

Prosthetic Restoration:

Autotransplanted teeth can be restored by a composite technique after 3 months or after 6 months with a porcelain laminate technique.

Minimal or no dentin exposure during crown preparation is essential.

Prognosis

5-year *graft survival:* 98%-99%
10-year *graft survival:* 87%-95%

Bibliography

1. SLAGSVOLD O. Autotransplantation of premolars in cases of missing anterior teeth. *Trans Eur Orthod Soc* 1970;**66:**473-85.

2. KRISTERSON L. Unusual case of tooth transplantation: Report of case. *J Oral Surg* 1970;**28:**841-4.

3. DIXON DA. Autogenous transplantation of tooth germs into the upper incisor region. *Br Dent J* 1971;131:260-65.

4. KVAM E, BJERCKE B. Dentes confuse - en kasusrapport og et behandlingsalternativ. *Nor Tandlægeforen Tid* 1976;**86:**305-8.

5. SLAGSVOLD O, BJERCKE B. Applicability of autotransplantation in cases of missing upper anterior teeth. *Am J Orthod* 1978;**74:**410-21.

6. BRADY J. Transplantation of a premolar to replace a central incisor with advanced resorption. *J Dent* 1978;**6:**259-60.

7. BJERCKE B. Autotransplantasjon av tenner på børn. In: HJØRTING-HANSEN E, ed. *Odontologi*. Copenhagen: Munksgaard, 1979:1-25.

8. SHULMAN LB. Impacted and unerupted teeth: Donors for transplant tooth replacement. *Dent Clin North Am* 1979;**23:**369-83.

9. KRAGH MADSEN I. Autotransplantation i privat praksis. *Tandlægebladet* 1984:**88:**373-4.

10. KRISTERSON L. Autotransplantation of human premolars. A clinical and radiographic study of 100 teeth. *Int J Oral Surg* 1985;**14:**200-13.

11. DERMAUT L, DE-PAUW G. L'autogreffe de dents: une dimension supplémentaire dans la practique dentaire. *Rev Belge Med Dent* 1989;**44:**85-98.

12. ANDREASEN JO, PAULSEN HU, FJELLVANG H, BARFOD K. Autotransplantation af præmolarer til behandling af tandtab i overkæbefronten. *Tandlægebladet* 1989;**93:**435-40.

13. ANDREASEN JO, PAULSEN HU, YU Z, AHLQUIST R, BAYER T, SCHWARTZ O. A long-term study of 370 autotransplanted premolars. Part I. Surgical procedures and standardized techniques for monitoring healing. *Eur J Orthod* 1990;**12:**3-13.

14. ANDREASEN JO, PAULSEN HU, YU Z, BAYER T, SCHWARTZ O. A long-term study of 370 autotransplanted premolars. Part II. Tooth survival and pulp healing subsequent to transplantation. *Eur J Orthod* 1990;**12:**14-24.

15. ANDREASEN JO, PAULSEN HU, YU Z, SCHWARTZ O. A long-term study of 370 autotransplanted premolars. Part III. Periodontal healing subsequent to transplantation. *Eur J Orthod* 1990;**12:**25-37.

16. ANDREASEN JO, PAULSEN HU, YU Z, BAYER T. A long-term study of 370 autotransplanted premolars. Part IV. Root development subsequent to transplantation. *Eur J Orthod* 1990;**12:**38-50.

17. PAULSEN HU, ANDREASEN JO, SCHWARTZ O. Behandling af tab i fronten med autotransplantation of præmolarer. *Tandlægernes nye Tidsskrift* 1990;**5:**70-5.

18. BOWDEN DEJ, PATEL HA. Autotransplantation of premolar teeth to replace missing maxillary central incisors. *Br J Orthod* 1990;**17:**21-8.

19. OIKARINEN K. Replacing resorbed maxillary central incisors with mandibular premolars. *Endod Dent Traumatol* 1990;**6:**43-6.

20. KRISTERSON L, LAGERSTRÖM L. Autotransplantation of teeth in cases with agenesis or traumatic loss of maxillary incisors. *Eur J Orthod* 1991;**13:**486-92

21. ANDREASEN JO. *Atlas of replantation and transplantation of teeth*. Fribourg: Mediglobe, 1991.

22. ANDREASEN JO, ANDREASEN FM. Autotransplantation of premolars, canines and third molars to the anterior region. In preparation1993.

23. LAGERSTRÖM L, KRISTERSON L. Influence of orthodontic treatment on root development of autotransplantated premolars. *Am J Orthodont* 1986;**89:**146-9.

24. MONEFELDT I, ZACHRISSON BU. Adjustment of clinical crown height by gingivectomy following orthodontic space closure. *Angle Orthod* 1977;**47:**256-64.

25. ANDREASEN JO, DAUGAARD J, ANDREASEN FM. Autotransplantation of teeth to the anterior region. II. Restorative procedures. In preparation

26. GOLDSTEIN RE. *Esthetics in Dentistry*. Philadelphia: JB Lippincott Company, 1976.

27. BROOKS L. The porcelain bonded to tooth restoration. *J Pedod* 1987;**11:**269-80.

28. WILIS P. Temporization of porcelain laminate veneers. *Compendium of Continuing Education in Dentistry* 1987;**IX:**352-8.

29. GARBER DA, GOLDSTEIN RE, FEINMAN RA. *Porcelain laminate veneers*. Chicago: Quintessence Publishing Co., Inc 1988. 136 pp.

30. TSUKIBOSHI M. Autogenous tooth transplantation-Reevaluation. *Int J Periodontol Rest Dent.* 1993;**2:** (in press).

31. TSUKIBOSHI M. The efficacy of autogenous tooth transplantation. Abstract, AAP 79th annual meeting. Chicago, 1993.

CHAPTER 20

Implants in the Anterior Region

J. O. ANDREASEN, L. KRISTERSON, H. NILSON,
K. DAHLIN, O. SCHWARTZ, P. PALACCI & J. JENSEN

A new procedure has recently been developed for the treatment of anterior tooth loss, namely insertion of single standing implants (1-30).

This treatment modality offers patients with completed jaw growth a unique treatment possibility whereby biologically compatible materials such as titanium and aluminum oxide serve as an osseointegrated root which is subsequently united with a porcelain crown (suprastructure)(Figs. 20.1 and 20.2).

Fig. 20.1. Treatment of central incisor loss with an implant
The condition is shown before implant installation.

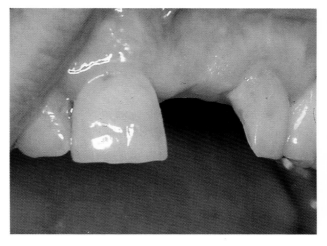 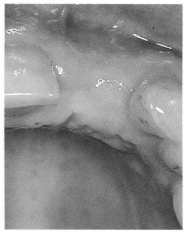

Condition after restoration
A good esthetic result has been obtained by the use of a ceramic crown restoration (Cera One®). Prosthetics performed by Dr. B. HOLM, Copenhagen.

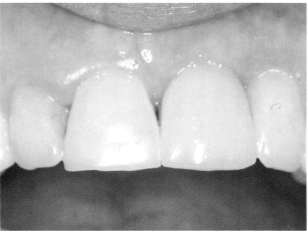 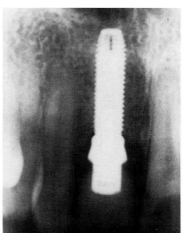

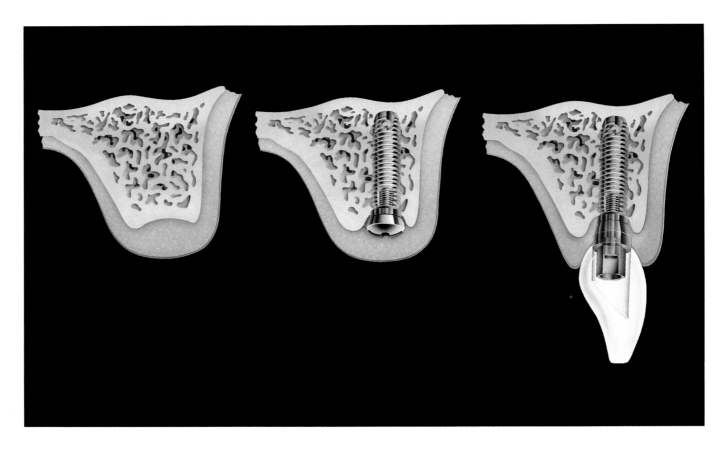

Fig. 20.2.
Treatment of maxillary incisor tooth loss with intact alveolar bone using an implant

In this context only those aspects of implantology which are related to the treatment of tooth loss after acute dental trauma will be presented. For a complete description of dental implantology the reader is referred to recent textbooks (31-34).

Treatment Planning

When anterior tooth loss has occurred or is anticipated (e.g. due to progressive root resorption) the most important factors to consider with respect to treatment planning are: age of the patient, anticipated vertical growth of the alveolar process, space available between crowns and roots adjacent to the recipient site, occlusal relations and condition of the alveolar process.

These factors usually determine the treat-

ment of choice, whether orthodontic space closure, resin-retained or conventional fixed prosthetics, autotransplantation or implantation (see Appendix 5, p. 751). To aid in the choice between these treatment possibilities, study models and panoramic radiographs, as well as a radiographic survey are essential (36).

Age of the Patient

In individuals where maxillary or mandibular vertical growth is not yet complete (36, 37) (Fig. 20.3), the use of implants is contraindicated as the osseointegrated implant will be maintained in its original position and progressive infraocclusion can be anticipated (38, 39). This process is identical to that seen with progressive replacement resorption in growing individuals (see Chapter 15, p. 621). However, if

Average path of eruption of maxillary central incisors

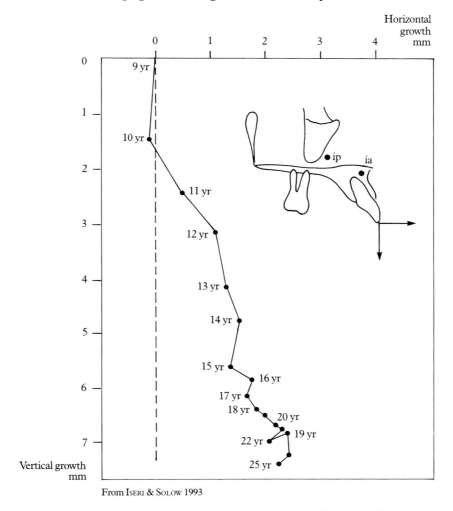

From ISERI & SOLOW 1993

Fig. 20.3. Estimate of expected infraposition for anterior dental implants inserted in children and young adults.
Based on data from a longitudinal growth study of 14 girls from 8-25 years, the expected residual vertical and horizontal component of continued eruption of the upper central incisors can be estimated in relation to age for girls. This measure is also an estimate of the amount of infraposition to be expected in the adult for a dental implant inserted at the age in question. The graph is consulted according to the subject's age; the expected infraposition can be determined from the vertical scale. Somewhat larger values can be expected for boys. Modifed from ISERI & SOLOW (37) 1991.

only 1 mm vertical growth of the alveolar process is expected (i.e. at the age of 18 years), implant treatment can be considered (Fig. 20.3).

The choice between implantation and autotransplantation is thus influenced by the age of the patient. As autotransplants are generally indicated only in cases where teeth with incomplete root formation can be transplanted, this naturally limits the use of autotransplantation to young individuals with a suitable tooth to transplant. Also the morphology of the alveolar process at the recipient region - i.e. reduced height and sharp ridge - is of significance when the choice between implants and autotransplants has to be made, because

bony reconstruction of the alveolar ridge is a necessary part of the treatment. An analysis of advantages and disadvantages of the two treatment modalities is presented in Appendix 5, p. 751.

Patient Selection - Prosthetic Aspects

The prosthetic aspects of implant selection for restoring lost anterior teeth depend upon various situations. These include:

-The condition of the adjacent teeth.
Thus, if the adjacent teeth are crowned or have large restorations, a conventional bridge could be considered.

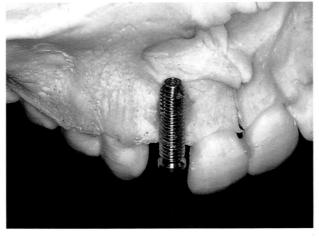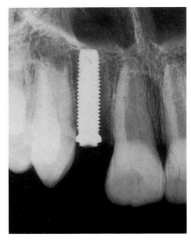

Fig. 20.4. Preoperative radiographic evaluation, angulated **exposure**
The space needed cervically amounts to the cervical diameter of the abutment plus adequate space to adjacent teeth, i.e. 1 mm mesially and 1 mm distally. The length of the implant cannot be accurately determined radiographically due to the oblique projection in the maxillary anterior region.

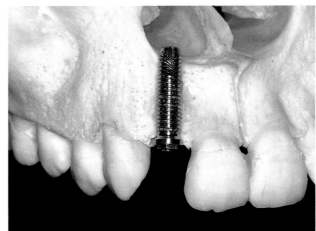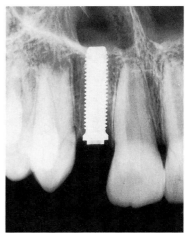

Preoperative radiographic evaluation, horizontal **exposure**
It appears that the actual distance between the crest of marginal bone and the nasal floor is approximately 1 mm shorter than the radiographic distance shown with an angulated exposure.

-Occlusal relationships and/or habits. Patients with deep overbite and/or severe parafunctional habits present contraindications.

-Interdental space relationships. The minimum space required between adjacent teeth is 6-7 mm for implant placement, as well as to permit adequate crown form and size (see later).

-Cuspid guidance. In restoring a cuspid, one should be aware of the occlusion. A cuspid-protected occlusion on an implant should be avoided due to the great forces a cuspid can exert in extreme excursions.

-Esthetic limits of an implant-borne crown, due to lack of bone or alignment of the fixture. These problems have become less significant, as the latest implant techniques imply surgical reconstruction of the alveolar process (see later).

The restorative dentist should guide the surgeon in placing the implant in the correct horizontal and axial orientation. This can be done in several ways, either indirectly by the use of surgical stents or directly by the restorative dentist being present during fixture insertion. A good general rule is that the axis of the implant should ideally be placed identically to the long axis of the tooth to be replaced.

There are several different types of surgical stent that can be used. All are aimed at aiding in the orientation of the labial surface of the future restoration.

Patient Selection - Surgical Aspects

Vertical and horizontal alveolar bone atrophy is a common problem following anterior tooth loss. This can be extreme following early tooth loss or in cases where the labial bone plate has been lost in connection with tooth avulsion. In order to evaluate the osseous condition at the proposed implant site, periapical orthoradial radiographs should be taken. With respect to the recipient site, there should be at least a distance of 1 mm between the potential position of the implant and adjacent teeth. This distance is especially important in the cervical region where the

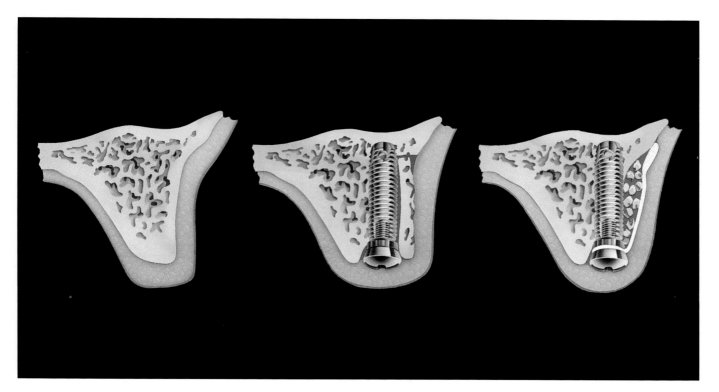

Fig. 20.5.
Methods for treatment of horizontal alveolar bone loss (A) in the maxillary incisor region include labial bone repositioning (B) and bone augmentation using guided tissue repair (C).

width of the cervical part of the fixture and the abutment should be considered (Fig. 20.4). If the distance appears critical, orthodontic expansion should be considered or a smaller implant size chosen.

The use of implants was previously contraindicated in cases of alveolar atrophy, as full bony coverage of the implant could not be obtained. However, recently developed surgical techniques have generally solved this problem. Thus, in case of labial alveolar atrophy the following techniques are available to augment the *width* of the alveolar process (Fig. 20.5):

1. Labial bone repositioning (40).
2. Maxillary bone transplants or free mandibular bone transplants (41).
3. Bone augmentation using guided tissue repair (42-59,96, 97).

All three techniques have been shown clinically to allow insertion of implants in the correct position in the alveolar process. However, long-term studies are needed to demonstrate whether a stable osseointegration is created under these conditions.

In case of combined *labial* and *vertical* bone atrophy, a free bone graft harvested from the mental region of the mandible or from the iliac crest can be used (Fig. 20.6) (41, 60-65).

To estimate the extent of labial bone atrophy, several methods have been advocated, such as CT- scanning, tomography (35) and direct probing under local anesthesia, using a measuring instrument which penetrates the gingival and alveolar mucosa (Fig. 20.7). If a very precise registration of alveolar atrophy is required, a plaster model is cast and sectioned at the implant site. The soft tissue depth is then marked after direct probing through the mucosa (Fig. 20.7). It is not unusual that a soft tissue thickness of 5-6 mm is present, whereby existing bone volume can be seriously overestimated. These techniques can determine whether there is sufficient horizontal bone support for the implant.

In conclusion, apart from the age factor (i.e. completion of vertical maxillary or mandibular growth), there are presently few contraindications to the use of single standing implants. It should, however, be mentioned that the implant solution in most countries represents one of the most expensive alternatives to the treatment of anterior tooth loss. However, in view of good long-term prognosis and low frequency of complications related to this form of treatment, as well as non-interference with adjacent teeth the implant solution would seem to be economically com-

Fig. 20.6. Method of treatment of vertical alveolar bone loss
A bone graft from the mental region augments the alveolar process in both vertical and in labial direction.

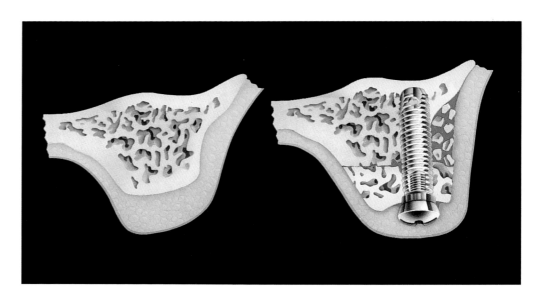

petitive with other treatment modalities in the long run (see Appendix 5 p. 751.).

Surgical Procedure

Present knowledge of the biology of osseous integration of implants has shown that the following features should be considered:

1. Use of an implant system which allows a *predictable* and *stable* osseous integration. Apart from type of material and surface texture, the length and the width of the implant appear to be of importance. In general, longer implants show a higher rate of success than shorter ones. Furthermore, wider fixtures, irrespective of length, are more stable than standard fixtures [66]. For predictable single tooth replacement the shortest fixture length is 10 mm [30].

2. Placement of the implant in a bony environment and with minimal or no contamination from the oral cavity during osseous integration. However, this requirement has been questioned by recent clinical and experimental studies, where implants inserted into fresh extraction sites healed similarly to implants inserted into healed sockets [69-74].

Fig. 20.7. Estimating the bony dimensions of the reduced alveolar process
An impression is taken and the model sectioned at the potential implant site. After administration of a local anesthetic, the mucosa is penetrated with a periodontal probe. These measurements are then transferred to the sectioned plaster model. In this way the sagittal extension of the alveolar process is accurately determined.

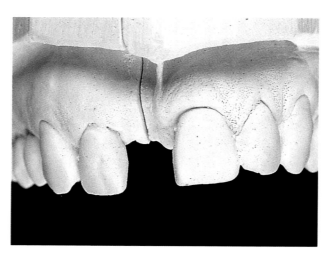 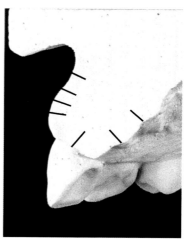

Fig. 20.8. Use of an implant to treat anterior tooth loss
A 24-year-old man has suffered anterior tooth loss due to trauma. As the alveolar process was intact, conventional implant insertion was planned.

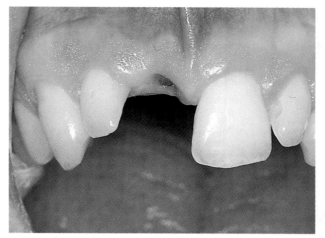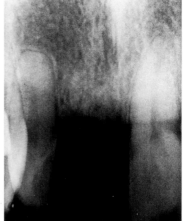

Raising a flap
A trapezoidal labial flap is raised which respects the interdental papillae. The flap is extended palatally so that sutures are not placed directly over the implant.

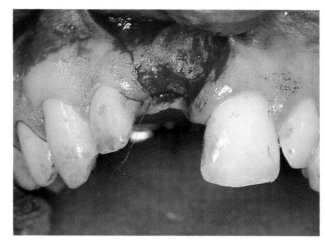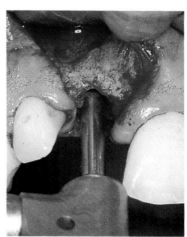

Insertion of the implant
The level of the implant before insertion of the healing cap should be 3 mm below the labial gingival margin of the homologous tooth.

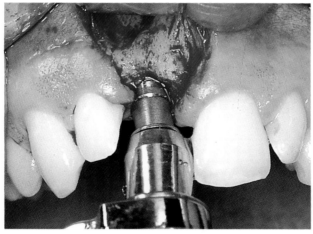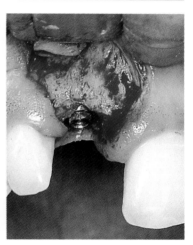

Completed restoration
After a healing period of 6 months and installation of an abutment, a porcelain crown is fabricated.

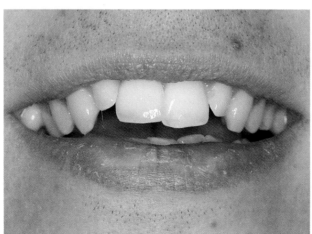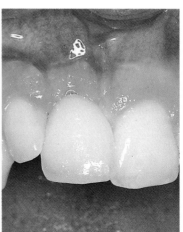

3. Appropriate timing with respect to the placement of the suprastructure.
4. Finally, esthetics dictate placement of the implant in such a position that the combined implant and suprastructure can mimic the tooth to be replaced.

The surgical procedure is entirely determined by the status of the alveolar process. In the following, different treatment solutions will be presented according to the condition of the alveolar bone.

Intact Alveolar Bone

In this situation, the tooth to be replaced can be present or extracted. In the former case it is an advantage to extract the tooth in question and allow a healing period of 2-3 months.

Atraumatic tooth removal is of the utmost importance with respect to the maintenance of an intact labial bone plate. Special instruments have been designed to facilitate tooth removal by severing cervical periodontal ligament fibers [75]. In the healing period a resin-retained temporary bridge or a spoon denture can be used.

Although the value of antibiotics has not yet been proven it seems advisable to administer penicillin for 2-4 days in connection with fixture installation.

To install the fixture, a trapezoidal flap is raised which avoids the marginal gingiva of adjacent teeth. The implant site is then prepared according to the implant system used (Fig. 20.8). The axis of the implant should ideally follow the axis of the tooth to be replaced and be directed at the proposed incisal edge. If a system is used where the suprastructure is cemented to the abutment (e.g. Brånemark® system) the axis of the implant is not as crucial as with systems where the crown is retrievably fixed with a screw. The ideal position and alignment of the implant is a situation in which the fixture resembles that of the natural tooth. If compromise is necessary, the axis of the implant can be deviated to some extent in most implant systems.

In some cases a large incisal canal may prevent optimal placement of the implant. In these cases it has been shown that elimination of the canal content and replacement with an autogenous bone graft (see later) can solve this problem [76].

The cervical level of the implant is important in ensuring an optimal esthetic suprastructure. Thus, in the central inci-

sor region, this level should be 2-4 mm below the level of the labial gingival margin of the adjacent central incisor. In the lateral incisor region the same position is chosen in relation to the contralateral incisor. After implant insertion, the flap is repositioned and sutured.

Horizontal Atrophy of the Alveolar Process

In these cases there are three different treatment options: namely, labial bone repositioning, bone grafting or bone augmentation using guided tissue repair.

LABIAL BONE REPOSITIONING
A trapezoidal flap is raised in which the marginal gingiva of adjacent teeth is avoided (Fig. 20.9). The labial outline of the socket for the implant in the atrophic part of the bone is defined using a narrow fissure bur penetrating the cortical bone. The bone plate is then removed with a narrow chisel and stored in saline or some drops of blood from the surgical area. The fibrin in the blood makes the bone fragments sticky and thereby easier to apply. The labial bone plate is cut lengthwise in 2-mm wide strips with heavy scissors and placed over the implant. It is especially important that the cervical aspect of the implant is covered with bone. The labial flap is then repositioned. If there is any tension during flap repositioning, the flap should be elongated at its base using periosteal incisions.

MANDIBULAR OR MAXILLARY FREE BONE GRAFTS
A trapezoidal flap is raised whereafter the implant is installed (Fig. 20.10). This will result in labial exposure of the implant which is then covered with free bone grafts harvested from the mental region of the mandible. After administration of a bilateral mandibular regional block anesthetic supplemented locally in the central incisor region, a flap is raised which includes separation of the mentalis muscle. A circular or ellipsoid osteotomy cut is made 5 mm apical to the incisors. The osteotomy is carried to a depth of 8 mm, whereafter a cone of bone is loosened with an elevator. The graft is then sectioned into small fragments using a bone cutter. The exposed part of the implant is then covered with the bone chips and the flap repositioned and

Fig. 20.9. Horizontal bone loss treated by labial bone repositioning and an implant
This 19-year-old man suffered anterior tooth loss 10 years previously. Note extensive horizontal bone atrophy.

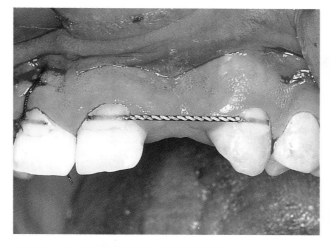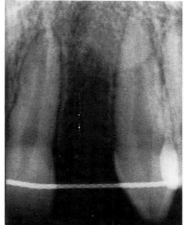

Raising a flap and removing the labial bone plate
A trapezoidal flap is raised which respects the interdental papillae. An osteomy cut is made through the labial bone plate corresponding to the future site of the implant.

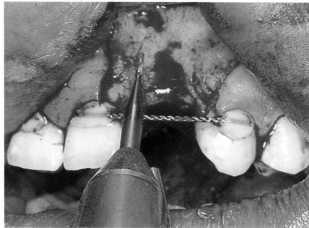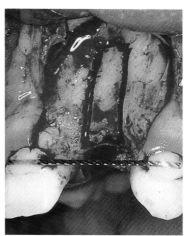

Removing the bone plate
The bone plate is then removed with a thin chisel and the graft stored in saline or a drop of blood. Thereafter preparation is made for the implant.

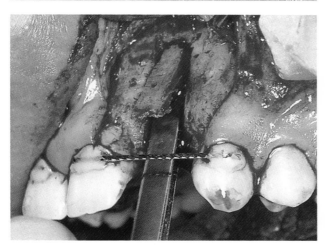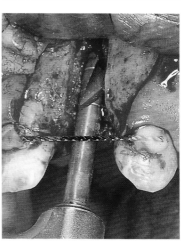

Inserting the implant and repositioning the bone plate
The implant is inserted and the bone plate is reversed so that the concave labial surface faces the implant.

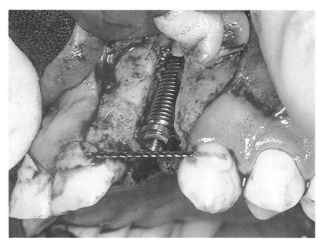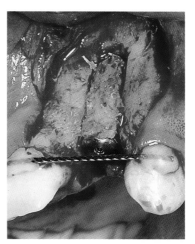

IMPLANTS IN THE ANTERIOR REGION

Repositioning and suturing the flap

If there is any tension along the flap during repositioning, a periosteal incision is made at the base of the flap to facilitate suturing without tension.

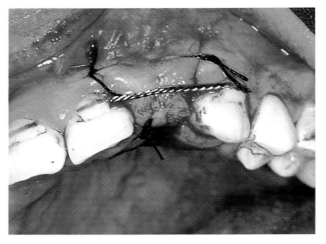

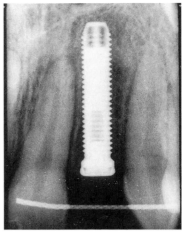

Condition after abutment insertion

At the time of insertion, it is apparent that the implant is completely osseous integrated.

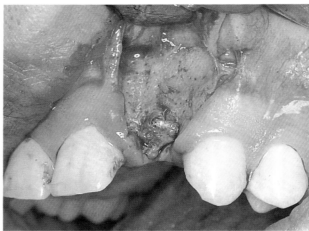

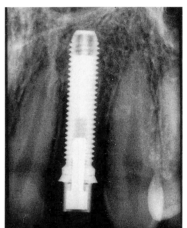

Final restoration

A porcelain crown has been inserted. Note the restoration of the alveolar ridge as well as the gingival anatomy. Prosthetics by Dr. B. HOLM, Copenhagen.

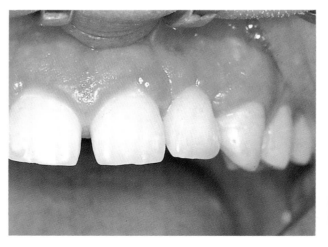

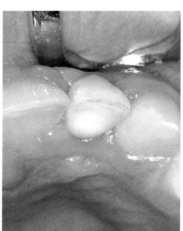

sutured. Alternatively bone can be harvested from the retromolar areas. After 6 months, abutments are installed and restorations inserted (Fig. 20.9).

BONE AUGMENTATION USING GUIDED TISSUE REPAIR

A substantial amount of data exists that support the use of guided tissue regeneration as an osteopromotive technique in conjunction with implant therapy. Basically the treatment can be performed in two separate ways, either as a pure ridge augmentation procedure which after 9-10 months of healing is followed by conventional fixture installation in the actual region (49), or the technique is used to create new bone cover over parts of the implants that have been exposed during the installation procedure (42-44, 46, 51-54).

The technique implies that a membrane barrier is placed in such a way that a secluded space is created. The occlusive membrane prevents ingrowth of the surrounding soft connective tissue. Thus cells with osteogenic potential from the sur-

Fig. 20.10. Atrophy of the alveolar bone, treated by augmentation using guided tissue repair and implants

Two Brånemark® implants have been inserted in the central incisor region of the maxilla. Note the buccal fenestration and the narrow buccal rim of bone adjacent to the right implant.

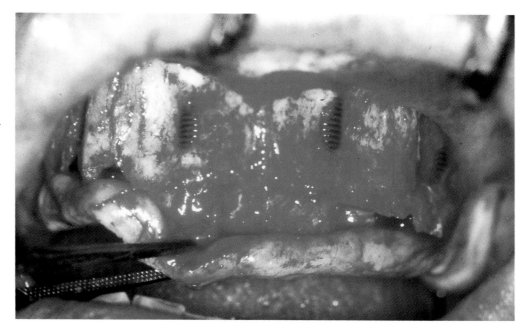

Placing a GTAM® membrane

The fenestration defect and the thin crest are covered by a GTAM® membrane which is kept in place by means of the cover screw.

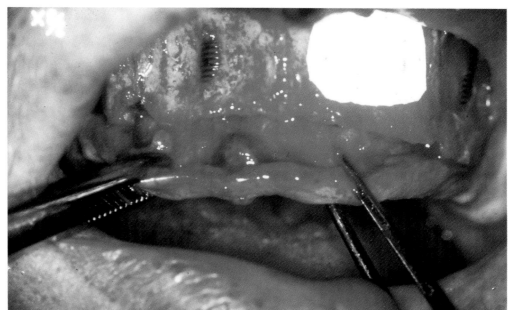

Clinical situation at the time of abutment connection

After 7 months of healing the membrane is found in proper position. No clinical signs of any adverse reaction towards the material is seen. A thin translucent layer of soft connective tissue (arrow) is found beneath the membrane which has been partly lifted away. Complete healing of the buccal fenestration is seen. Also note the increased width of the bucco-palatal bone at the top of the crest. From DAHLIN (52) 1991.

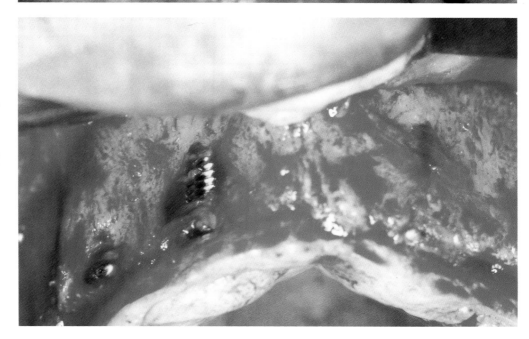

Fig. 20.11. Treatment of bone dehiscence with a GTAM® membrane
At second stage operation a dehiscence of the labial and cervical bone is found.

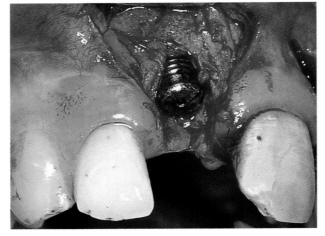

Harvesting cortical bone
Small fragments of bone are removed mesial to the implant with a chisel.

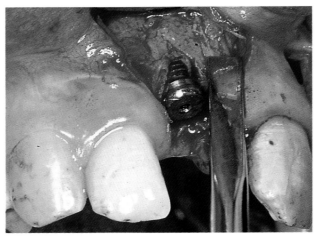
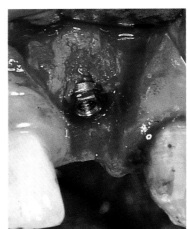

Trimming of a GTAM® membrane
The membrane is contoured so that it ends short of the incision of the flap. The membrane is anchored with the cover screw. Before placing the membrane, bone fragments are placed on top of the exposed part of implant.

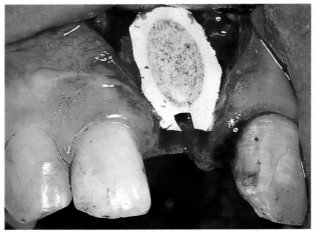
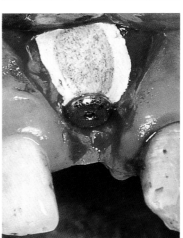

Sutured flap
The flap is repositioned and sutured with GTAM® sutures.

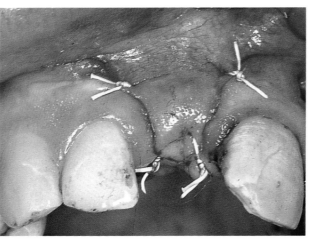
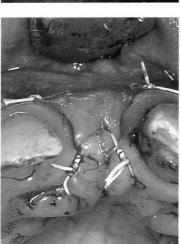

Fig. 20.12. Atrophy of the alveolar bone treated by augmentation using guided tissue repair and an implant.

Fixtures installed in the anterior region of the maxilla. Primary stability is achieved, but several threads are exposed at the mid-buccal portion. The exposed threads and the surrounding bone are covered with a GTAM® membrane placed in direct contact with the bone surface and tucked beneath the periosteal flap for stabilization. The contralateral fenestration defect served as a control. From DAHLIN ET AL. (52) 1991.

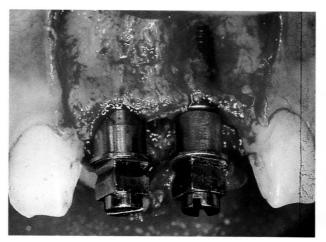
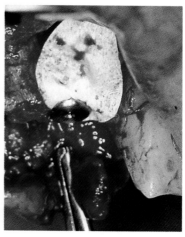

Condition at reentry

Membrane-treated fenestration after 6 months of healing. Complete regeneration of the bone is evident, covering the previously exposed titanium surface. An increased dimension of the bone in buccolingual direction is seen. Note the amount of visible threads at the untreated fenestration at the contralateral site.

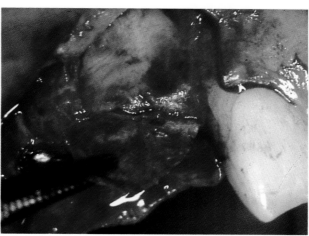
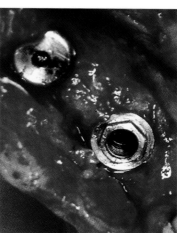

rounding bone margins can migrate into the defect relatively unimpeded and permit osteogenesis (42,43).

The choice between ridge augmentation or the use of membranes in conjunction with installed implants is very much dependent upon the extent and shape of the osseous defect in the actual region. If the rim of the alveolar crest is too narrow for fixture installation, initial ridge augmentation is recommended (49). If the labial defect is in the form of a concavity due to the atrophy of the crest after trauma, but with a normal width of the alveolar crest, there is a good chance for primary stability of the implant. However, exposure of threads at the buccal mid-portion is a common finding and has been reported to compromise long-term prognosis of the implant (82). Recent studies have shown promising results in the treatment of such defects with guided tissue regenerative techniques (51-52,54,96,97) (Figs. 20.10 to 20.12).

Presently the most commonly used mechanical barrier is the GTAM® (Guided Tissue Augmentation Material) made of expanded-Polytetra-fluoroethylene (e-PFTE, i.e. Teflon).

The flap procedure and implant insertion are identical to those described for labial bone or a mandibular free graft procedure. The importance of space making has been documented experimentally as well as clinically (51-53). In case of ridge augmentation in conjunction with implant therapy, a few autogenous bone chips beneath the membrane are recommended as a space maintainer in order to prevent collapse of the material. If the bone is very compact in the recipient site, perforation of the buccal bone plate with a small round bur is suggested in order to ensure bleeding and blood clot formation in the defect. Rigid fixation of the membrane to the bone surface also seems to be of importance for successful treatment (49). This can be achieved by anchoring the membrane to the cover screw (47, 54) (Figs. 20.5 and 20.11). Additional fixation could also be performed with miniscrews (Memfix®) which are placed along the periphery of the membrane. Finally the membrane could also be tucked beneath the periosteal flaps for stabilization (51, 52).

Tight suturing preferably with horizontal mattress sutures is essential for successful treatment. If there is any tension during flap repositioning, releasing incisions at the base through the periosteum are needed.

The membrane should be kept in place for the entire recommended healing period to achieve osseointegration of the implants. Therefore it is both logical and practical to remove the material at the time of abutment operation (i.e. 3-4 months in the mandible and 6-8 months in the maxilla). This has also been confirmed in a recent experimental study (96).

In case of exposure of the membrane through the oral mucosa, special attention is required. The patient is placed on a chlorhexidine rinse (0.2% solution) twice daily for 6-7 weeks, until the membrane is removed. In case of pain, swelling or pus, the membrane must be removed immediately. In these cases significantly less bone augmentation can be expected (97).

In summary, guided bone regeneration has a sound scientific basis and has been proven to be successful both experimentally and clinically. It is a practical treatment tool when atrophy of the alveolar bone is localized and sufficient vertical bone height is still present. The biologic rationale behind this concept is well understood today, but a number of changes can be anticipated in the nature of material and surgical technique.

Vertical Atrophy of the Alveolar Process

The extent and shape of bone atrophy is evaluated with the help of periapical radiographs and by probing the mucosal thickness, whereafter these measurements are transferred to a sectioned plaster model. The most likely donor sites appear to be the mandibular symphysis or iliac crest when a large amount of bone is needed. Often, only a minimum of bone is necessary for the reconstruction procedure. In contrast to reconstruction procedures using the iliac crest, hospitalization can be avoided by using mandibular bone as the grafting ma-

terial (41). Furthermore, mandibular bone is easier to harvest, has a shorter storage period, and seems to have less tendency towards resorption (41). The surgical description will therefore be based on the use of mandibular bone as the grafting material, which is then anchored by osseointegrated implants (Figs. 20.13 and 20.14).

After administration of sedation, antibiotics and local anesthesia, the alveolar crest is exposed surgically through a vestibular incision appoximately 1 to 2 cm from the mucogingival margin, with relieving incisions towards the alveolar crest. Depending on the number of implants to be installed, different types of preformed templates are available to prepare the recipient site for bone graft and implant installation (Fig. 20.13). The donor site at the mandibular symphysis is exposed through an incision in the vestibule. Using the template of choice, holes for implant placement are drilled and tapped prior to harvesting of the graft (Fig. 20.13). The edges of the template act as a guide for preparing the bone block and as a guide in preparing the implant bed, to ensure proper inter-implant distance. The bone block is loosened from the lingual cortex with specially designed chisels and transferred directly to the recipient site for fixation with implants (Fig. 20.13). After implant installation and fixation of the bone graft, final adjustments are made with burs or a bone cutter. The mucosal flap is sutured tightly with horizontal mattress sutures. Due to mobilization of lip tissue at the closure, one should be aware that a minor vestibuloplasty might be necessary at the abutment procedure.

Postoperative Follow-up

After implant insertion, a radiograph can be taken using a standardized technique for future reference. After suture removal, a healing period of 6-12 months is recommended.

The normal healing period after fixture installation is 3 to 6 months: 3 months in the mandible and 6 months in the maxilla. During this healing period it is important to construct an adequate temporary restoration. There are several temporary restorations that can be used during the healing phase: acid-etch retained bridge, an acrylic tooth bonded to the neighboring

Fig. 20.13. Horizontal and vertical bone loss treated by a mental bone graft and 2 implants

This 25-year-old male suffered avulsion of 2 incisors 2 years previously. Despite extensive horizontal and vertical atrophy, fixed prosthetics was the initial treatment of choice. The fixed bridge has been removed. Note extensive vertical and horizontal reduction of the alveolar ridge. The extent and type of bone loss indicated autogenous bone transplantation from the mental region.

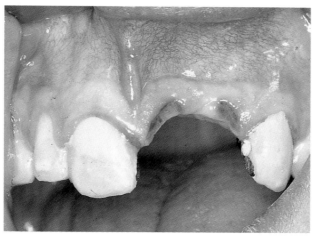

Raising a flap

The alveolar crest is exposed surgically by a vestibular incision 1 to 2 cm from the mucogingival margin, with relieving incisions towards the alveolar crest. These incisions should not be less than 1 mm from the gingival sulcus, in order to safeguard the integrity of this area.

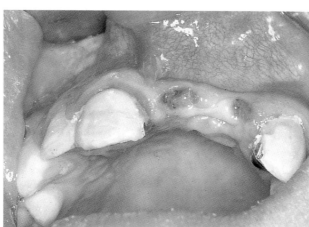 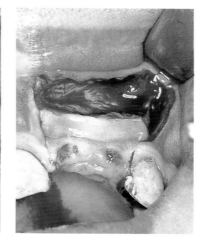

Dissection of the flap

The flap is loosened both labially and palatally. Sharp bone edges are reduced. Thereafter the mucosal flap is temporarily anchored in a palatal position with a horizontal mattress suture.

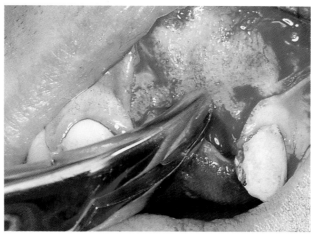 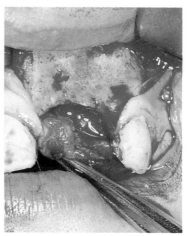

Assessing proper implant location

From a set of preformed templates, a template is selected which fits the available mesio-distal space (Leibinger® implant system). While this is held with a pincet, the two entrance holes for the implants are marked with round burs.

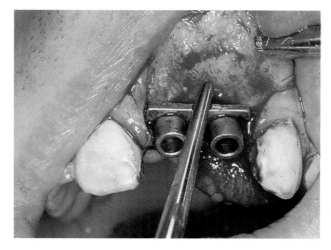 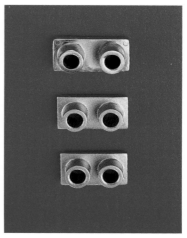

IMPLANTS IN THE ANTERIOR REGION

Preparing the site for the implants

The entire length of the implant canal is prepared with surgical burs. Due to the extent of labial bone atrophy, only the palatal aspect of the canal is fully supported by bone. The apical boundary is defined by the cortical bone of the nasal cavity. The use of the template ensures that the implants are parallel.

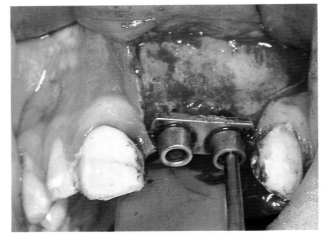 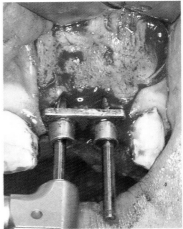

Harvesting the mental bone graft

A vestibular incision is made for exposure of bone apical to the incisors in the mandibular symphyseal region. To ensure parallelism and correct interimplant distance, the template is placed in contact with the bony surface and a round bur is used to mark the entrance sites for the implant channels, which are prepared to the depth of the lingual cortical bone.

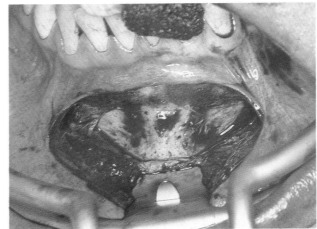 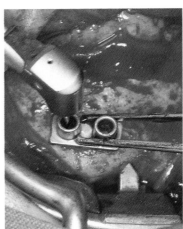

Final preparation of the mental graft

Before tapping, it is important to countersink approximately 2 mm in the graft due to the anticipated marginal resorption during the healing period. The edges of the template act as a guide for preparing the size of the bone block with a thin bur.

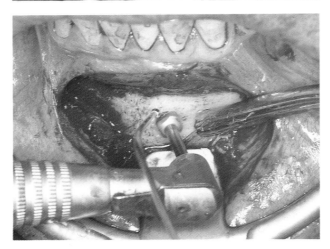 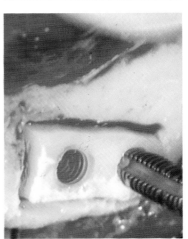

Removing the bone graft

The graft is loosened and removed with the help of thin chisels working to the extent of the lingual cortical bone and finishing up with curved chisels in the corners.

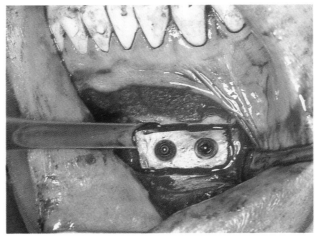 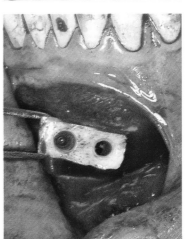

Testing the graft in the recipient region
The harvested graft is tested for fit in the recipient region.

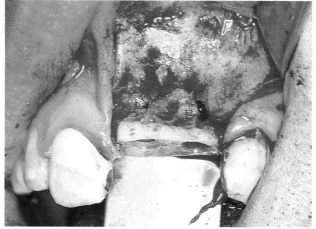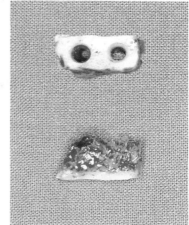

Adapting the graft and inserting the fixtures
The width of the graft is adjusted so that it fits into the site without pressure on the adjacent gingiva. The two fixtures are then inserted.

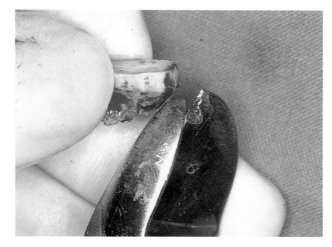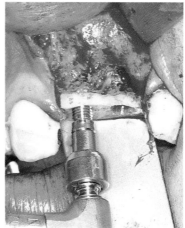

Implant installation and contouring
It is important that the top of the implants lie approximately 1 mm below bone in order to compensate for anticipated marginal bone resorption during the healing period. With a bur, sharp labial and palatal edges of the graft are reduced to simulate the normal contour of the alveolar ridge.

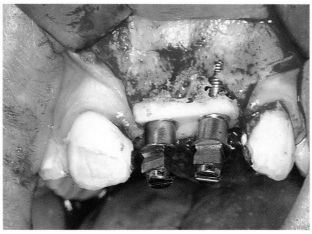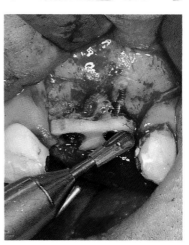

Additional grafting
Cancellous bone chips taken from the donor site in the mental region are placed along the facial aspect of the alveolar ridge to cover exposed implant surfaces and optimize facial contour.

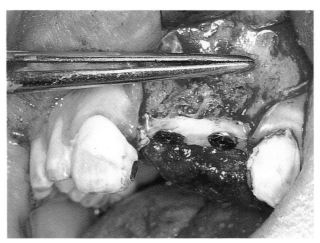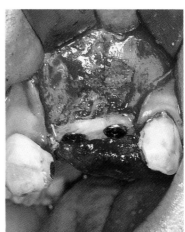

Closing the surgical site

The alveolar flap is repositioned and sutured to the labial mucosa using horizontal mattress sutures. To prevent hematoma in the region, it is an advantage to use a splint for coverage in the 1st post-operative week.

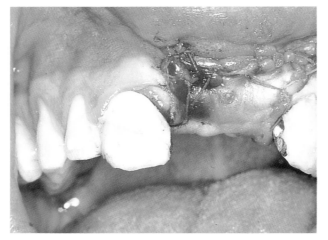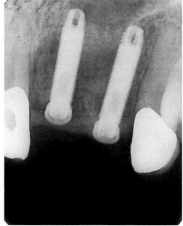

Abutment procedure

Six months later, abutments are connected. Note the integrity of the alveolar bone. There is almost complete bone coverage of the implants.

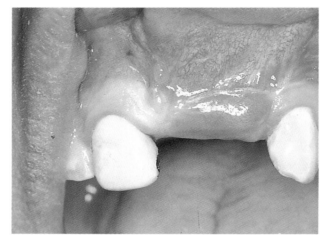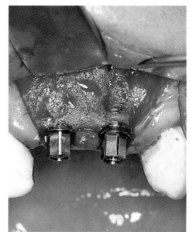

Temporary restoration

The flap is repositioned and sutured and a temporary restoration inserted.

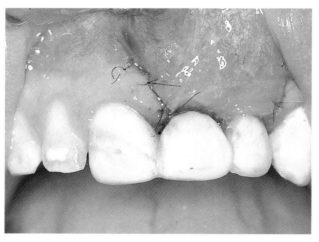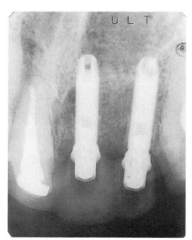

Final restoration

At the prosthetic procedure the restoration is completed by firing porcelain onto ceramic caps specially designed for use with Cera-One ® abutments. Prosthetics by Dr. C. FÆRCH, Copenhagen.

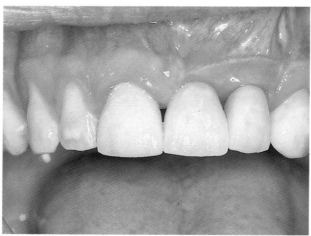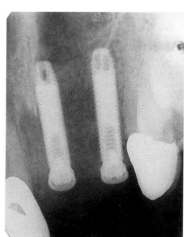

Fig. 20.14. Loss of several teeth and alveolar ridge reconstructed by mental bone grafts and implants
This 18-year-old man suffered avulsion of most of the right pre-maxilla including first premolar, canine, second and first incisor in a traffic accident. Only the bony floor of the nasal cavity remains. From JENSEN & SINDET - PEDERSEN (41) 1991

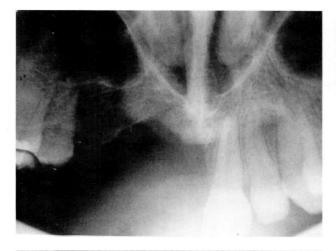 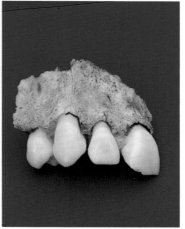

Immediate treatment and later reconstruction
Due to an associated jaw fracture an intermaxillary splint was applied. The alveolar ridge was reconstructed using bone harvested from the mental region fixed to residual bone by 4 implants. At the time of abutment implantation a vestibuloplasty with a palatal mucosal graft was performed to improve lip contour and width of attached gingiva.

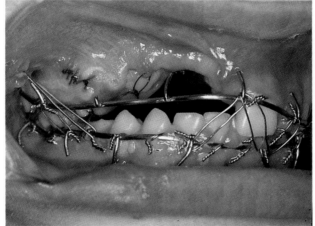 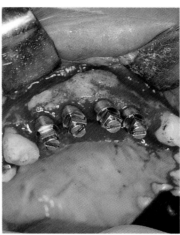

Follow-up 4 years after surgery
The implants have been restored with porcelain crowns. Note the very limited resorption of the bone graft.

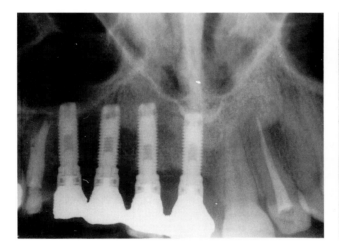 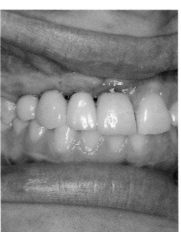

teeth, or a removable partial denture. If a removable partial denture is used as a temporary restoration, great care must be taken so that the load from the denture does not threaten the bone graft.

Abutment Installation and Prosthetic Procedure

It is usually an advantage to raise a labial flap in order to verify that the implant is properly osseointegrated and that there is no soft or hard tissue interposition between the fixture and the implant.

Before designing the flap for abutment installation the need for correction of the labial contour and the interdental gingival level should be considered.

The shape of an interdental papilla is determined primarily by the proximal position of the cemento-enamel junction in relation to the corresponding labio-lingual position (98-101). Due to the marked curvature of this border in the anterior region the interdental papilla has a markedly pointed appearance (Fig. 20.15).

In case of single tooth loss the interdental papillae are usually intact at the time of abutment installation unless the initial injury has resulted in tissue loss. If more than one tooth has been lost, the interdental gingival tissue will atrophy between the 2 extraction sockets and fixture installation with or without bone augmentation will not recreate the original form of the interdental papillae in these sites (Fig. 20.15).

A special flap design has recently been developed whereby the soft tissue overlying the buried implant is transposed to the proximal region(s) instead of being removed (102). Using this type of pedicled gingival graft, the interdental papilla can be recreated to the desired form. The surgical procedure of interdental papilla creation is shown in Fig. 20.15.

This procedure can be used to create interdental papillae between implants as well as between natural teeth and implants. A follow-up study of 130 procedures has demonstrated 95% successful results; complications being loss of the transposed papilla or dehiscence around the releasing incisions due to soft tissue tension.

At the abutment connection it is preferable to use a special healing abutment for the first weeks after the abutment operation, to allow the gingiva to heal properly. This normally takes 4 to 6 weeks and is especially important in the anterior region, where esthetics is of greatest concern. By the use of the healing abutment, the surgeon can leave the final selection of the correct abutment height to the restorative dentist.

After a sufficient healing period, the healing abutment is removed and the appropriate single tooth abutment chosen. Different abutment heights are available depending upon the height of the abutment collar. The abutment is placed 2 to 3 mm under the gingival margin in order to optimize esthetics. If there is inadequate space for a titanium abutment (i.e. superficial placement of the fixture) a UCLA abutment can be chosen whereby the crown is fitted directly to the fixture.

The abutment is attached to the fixture with a gold paladium screw with an electric torque controller at a torque of 30-32 N/cm. The use of the torque controller ensures that the gold screw will not loosen during function (77). Another benefit of the torque controller is that, in combination with a special countertorque device, the risk of transferring forces to the bone/implant interface is eliminated.

Radiographic control of the fit between the fixture head and the abutment is mandatory. If this is ignored prosthodontic and periodontal healing problems will occur. An impression coping is selected and an impression is taken using an elastic impression material. An index is then made.

The technician can use a special prefabricated ceramic cap or a conventional wax-up in order to create the final ceramic crown. With the use of the ceramic cap, porcelain is sintered to the ceramic cap, after which the necessary adjustments in form and height of the cap are made. The use of the prefabricated ceramic cap is recommended in those situations when the fixtures are positioned in a favorable site and axial orientation. If this is not possible, a conventional wax-up is made in order to permit uniform thickness of porcelain to cover the metal framework.

After try-in and adjustments, the crown can be cemented to the abutment. It is of utmost importance that all cement is removed from the gingiva in order to avoid severe gingival inflammation.

If there is a need to combine fixtures with natural teeth this can be done without complication (78-80).

Follow-up

After crown insertion, the status of the implant should be monitored clinically and radiographically on an annual basis. Following an initial marginal bone loss of approximately 1 mm, the process appears to level out at 0.1 mm bone loss annually (81-85). If marginal bone loss extends to the

Fig. 20.15. Anatomy of the interdental papillae

The shape of interdental papillae appears from this model where 2 incisors have been removed. The marked curvature of the cemento-enamel junction results in a markedly pointed interdental papilla. This papilla will atrophy after removal of the incisors.

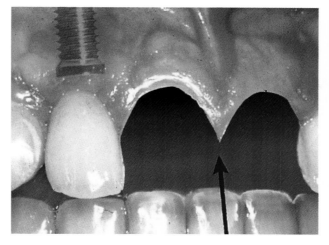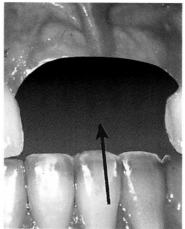

Interdental papilla creation associated with abutment installation

This patient has lost 2 central incisors and 1 lateral incisor. Fixtures have been installed 6 months earlier. There is a need to create interdental papillae and to augment the ridge labially. A trapezoidal paramarginal incision is made whereby the cover screws are exposed.

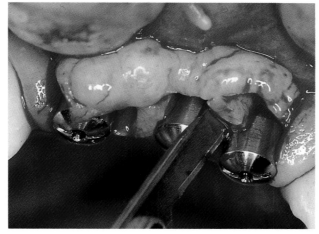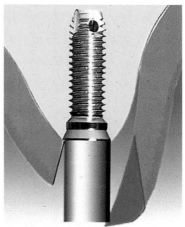

Creating the new papillae

With a no. 15 surgical blade, two oblique incisions are made in the palatal aspect of the flap. The length and width of these incisions determine the dimensions of the new interdental papilla. The flap is repositioned and trimmed so that there is tight adaptation between the flaps and the healing abutments. It is important that titanium healing abutments are used, to favor healing of the grafts.

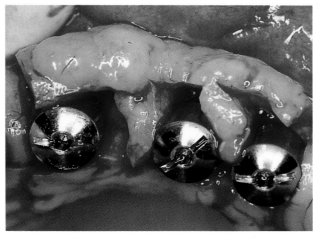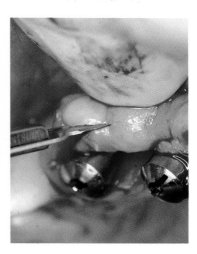

Suturing the flap

Horizontal mattress sutures are used to stabilize the position of the gingival pedicle grafts. It is important not to place a suture inside the interproximal wound. Furthermore gingival packing should be avoided as it may displace the newly created papillae. To the right is shown the condition after 3 weeks. The gingival tissue including the interdental papillae has healed around the healing abutments.

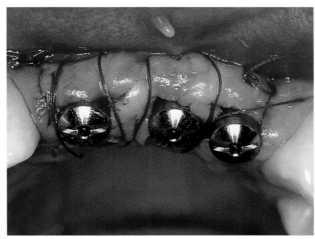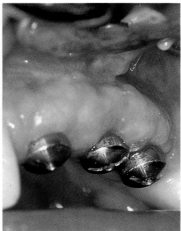

IMPLANTS IN THE ANTERIOR REGION

Table 20.1. Long-term prognosis of single standing implants

Authors	Implant type	Observation period	Age	No. inserted	Failures	Successes
Wagner et al.[4] 1981	Tübingen® (Al₂O₃)	1 year		35	8	77%
Wörle [5] 1981	Tübingen® (Al₂O₃)	2½ years	11-66	25	4	84%
Heners & Wörle [6] 1983	Heinrich-Schraube® Titanium	0-6 years ($\bar{x}$=3 years)		48	3	94%
	Schulte-Sofort(Al₂O₃)	0-4 years ($\bar{x}$=1.5 years)		27	5	82%
Tetsch [7] 1983	Pfeilstift®, TPS® and Bladevent®	5.2 years		288	36	87%
Scholz & d'Hoedt[11] 1984	Tübingen® (Al₂O₃)	1-5 years	8-17	134	31	77%
d'Hoedt [13] 1986	Tübingen® (Al₂O₃)	1-10 years		347	26	93%
Nordenram et al.[12]1986	Tübingen® (Al₂O₃)	0-2 years	14-56	70		93%
Schram-Scherer et al. [14] 1987	Tübingen® (Al₂O₃)	2 years		116	21	82%
Albrektsson et al. [15]1988	Brånemark® (Titanium)	0-5 years		152[1] 45[2]	7 2	95% 96%
Patrich et al. [16] 1992	Corevent® (Titanium)	1-5 years $\bar{x}$=2 years	15-48	94	0	100%
Jemt et al. [23] 1990	Brånemark® (Titanium)	3 years		23	2	91%
Jemt et al. [26] 1991	Brånemark® (Titanium)	1 year	<20-70	107	3	97%
Åstrand & Engquist [25] 1991	Brånemark® (Titanium)	1-4 years	20-50	35	2	94%

[1] Maxilla
[2] Mandible

threads of the implant, this may result in recurrent gingival irritation [86].

Prognosis

The criteria for implant success have been discussed in a number of articles [87-92]. The following criteria have recently been suggested for single standing implants [91]:
Criteria for success:
1. The individual unattached implant is immobile when tested clinically.
2. No evidence of peri-implant radiolucency is present as assessed on an undistorted radiograph.
3. The mean vertical bone loss is less than 0.2 mm annually after the 1st year of service.
4. No persistent pain, discomfort, or infection is attributable to the implant.
5. The implant design does not preclude placement of a crown or prosthesis with an appearance that is satisfactory to the patient and dentist.
6. By these criteria, a success rate of 85% at the end of a 5-year observation period and 80% at the end of a 10-year period are minimum levels for success.

Results from the few studies on long-term prognosis of single standing implants are presented in Table 20.1. It appears that two implant systems (Tübingen® Alu-

Fig. 20.16. Comparison between healing of titanium and aluminum oxide implants
A material of 48 titanium implants was compared with 27 aluminum oxide single standing implants. From HENERS & WÖRLE (10) 1983.

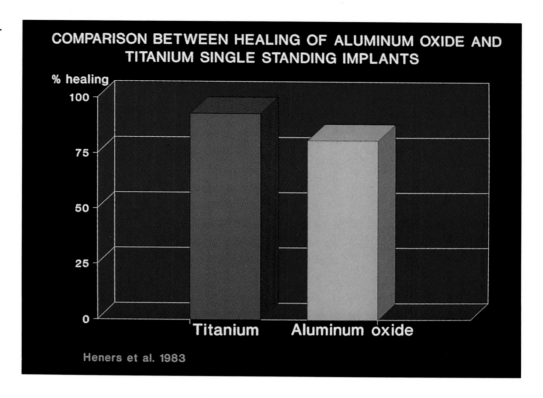

Fig. 20.17. Long-term survival of single standing Brånemark® implants inserted in two implant centers
The material consists of 149 and 131 single standing Brånemark® implants inserted in the period 1984-1992. All implants were installed by specially trained oral surgeons and subsequently restored by prosthodontists. From LINDEN & KISCH (93) 1992 and NILSON ET AL. (94) 1992 .

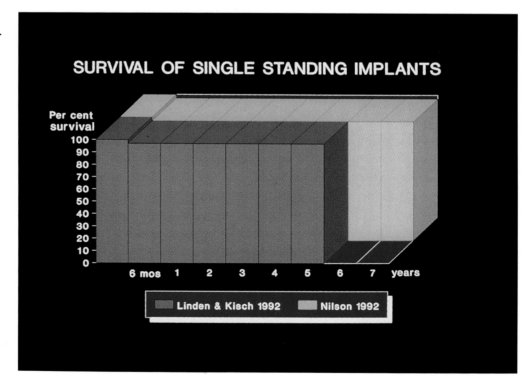

IMPLANTS IN THE ANTERIOR REGION

minum oxide implants (Tübingen® and Brånemark® titanium implants) have been extensively documented scientifically. Moreover, the reported studies reveal that the titanium implants generally perform better than aluminum oxide implants (10) (Fig. 20.16).

Presently only two studies, from Malmø and Umeå, Sweden, reveal data whereby a life-table analysis of implants can be calculated (93, 94) (Fig. 20.17). In both studies 97% survival was found after 5 years.

In the future, it can be anticipated that better documentation of various marketed implant systems will be seen. Thus, in the USA, a 5-year documentation of implant will be required in the future by the Food and Drug Administration (95). The authors of this chapter are in full agreement with this demand.

In summary, single standing implants appear to be a very promising treatment solution for anterior tooth loss. However, further studies are needed to analyze the effect of open or closed insertion as well as the long-term prognosis of the various bone augmentation techniques. Furthermore, it should be borne in mind that only a few implant systems have so far been tested in such long-term clinical studies as must be considered a prerequisite for their clinical use (95).

Essentials

Indications

All cases where jaw growth is completed

Implant Site Analysis

A clinical and radiographic examination should reveal the osseous dimensions horizontally and vertically. A minimum of 1 mm bone should be present between the potential implant and adjacent teeth. In case of labial or vertical bone atrophy, direct probing through the mucosa or tomography should disclose the extent of atrophy.

Surgical Procedure

No bone atrophy
Standard implant procedure

Labial bone atrophy
Labial bone repositioning
Mandibular free bone transplantation
Bone augmentation using guided tissue repair

Vertical bone atrophy
Mandibular free bone transplantation

Healing Phase before Abutment Installation

4-6 months.

Prosthetic Restoration

Preferably full porcelain crowns.

Prognosis

5-year implant survival: 97%

Bibliography

1. SCHULTE W, KLEINEIKENSCHEIDT H, LINDNER K, SCHA-REYKA R. Das Tübinger Sofortimplantat in der klinischen Prüfung. *Dtsch Zahnärztl Z* 1978;**33**:348-59.

2. SCHWARZ G, KÜMMERLE U. Erfahrungen bei der klinichen Erprobung des Tübinger Implantat. *Dtsch Zahnärztl Z* 1981;**36**:607-8.

3. SCHULTE W. Das enossale Tübinger Implantat aus Al₂O₃ (Frialit). Der Entwicklungsstand nach 6 Jahren. *Zahnärztl Mitt* 1981;**71**:1-20.

4. WAGNER W, TETSCH P, BOSSLER L. Bisherige klinische Erfahrungen mit dem Frialit-Implantat Typ Tübingen. *Dtsch Zahnärztl Z* 1981;**36**:585-90.

5. WÖRLE M. Klinische Erfahrungen mit enossalen Aluminiumoxidkeramik-Implantaten. *Dtsch Zahnärztl Z* 1981;**36**:591-5.

6. HENERS M, WÖRLE M. Indikation verschiedener Implantationsverfahren - Ergebnisse einer klinischen Langzeitstudie. *Dtsch Zahnärzl Z* 1983;**38**:115-8.

7. TETSCH P. Indikation und Erfolgsaussichten von enossalen Implantaten. *Dtsch Zahnärztl Z* 1983;**38**:111-4.

8. WAHL G. Das Tübinger-Sofort-Implantat im Frontzahnbereich. *Dtsch Zahnärztl Z* 1981;**36**:596-8.

9. TETSCH P. Indikation und Erfolgsaussichten von enossalen Implantaten. *Dtsch Zahnärztl Z* 1983;**38**:111-4.

10. HENERS M, WÖRLE M. Indikation verschiedener Implantationsverfahren - Ergebnisse einer klinischen Langzeitstudie. *Dtsch Zahnärtzl Z* 1983;**38**:115-8.

11. SCHOLZ F, D'HOEDT B. Der Frontzahnverlust im jugendlichen Gebiss - Therapiemöglighkeiten durch Implantate. *Dtsch Zahnärztl Z* 1984;**39**:416-24.

12. NORDENRAM Å, ZETTERQVIST L, LANDT H, EKENBÄCK J. Keramikimplantat Frialit. Ersättning vid förlust av enstaka tänder. *Tandläkartidningen* 1986;**78**:721-9.

13. D'HOEDT B. 10 Jahre Tübinger implantat aus Frialit. *Zahnärztl Implantol* 1986;**6**: Band II:6-12.

14. SCHRAM SCHERER B, REICH W, TETSCH P. Zweijährige Erfahrungen mit der Implantatdokumentation. *Z Zahnärztl Implantol* 1987;**3**:3-12.

15. ALBREKTSSON T, DAHL E, ENBOM L, et al. Osseointegrated oral implants. A Swedish multicenter study of 8139 consecutively inserted Nobelpharma implants. *J Periodontol* 1988;**59**:287-96.

16. PATRICK D, ZOSKY R, LUBAR R, BUCHS A. The longitudinal clinical efficacy of core-vent dental implants in partially edentulous patients: a 5-year report. In: LANEY WR, TOLMAN DE, eds. *Tissue Integration in Oral, Orthopedic & Maxillofacial Reconstruction*. Chicago: Quintessence Books, 1990:341-9.

17. ÖDMAN J, LEKHOLM U, JEMT T, BRÅNEMARK P-I, THILANDER B. Osseointegrated titanium implants - a new approach in orthodontic treatment. *Eur J Orthod* 1988;**10**:98-105.

18. NENTWIG H. Die Implantation im Frontzahnbereich bei reduziertem Alveolarfortsatz. *Z Zahnärztl Implantol* 1988;**4**:120-4.

19. LEWIS SG, BEUMER J III, PERRI GR. Single tooth implant supported restorations. *Int J Oral Maxillofac Implants* 1988;**3**:25-30.

20. ÖHRNELL L-O, HIRSCH JM, ERICSSON I, BRÅNEMARK P-I. Single-tooth rehabilitation using osseointegration. A modified surgical and prosthodontic approach. *Quintessence Int* 1988;**19**:871-6.

21. STEVEN G, LEWIS S, BEUMER J, PERRI G, HORNBURG W. Single tooth implant-supported restorations. *Int J Oral Maxillofac Implants* 1988;**3**:25-30.

22. PERRI G, LEWIS S, BEUMER J, AVERA S, NUNOKAWA G. Single tooth implants. A comparison of UCLA and Nobelpharma single tooth implant supported restoration systems. *Systems Update* 1989;**17**:30.

23. JEMT T, LEKHOLM U, GRÖNDAHL K. A 3-year follow-up study of early single implant restorations ad modum Brånemark. *Int J Periodontics Restorative Dent* 1990;**10**:341-9.

24. SCHER ELC. An osseointegrated implant to replace a missing incisor following orthodontic treatment. *Br J Orthod* 1990;**17**:146-54.

25. ÅSTRAND P, ENGQUIST B. Singeltandsersättning med implantat. *Tandläkartidningen* 1991;**83**:1008-1021.

26. JEMT T, LANEY WR, HARRIS D, et al. Osseointegrated implants for single tooth replacement. A one year report from a multicenter prospective study. *Int J Oral Maxillofac Implants* 1991;**6**:29-36.

27. SHERWOOD JR RI, SULLIVAN DY. Concepts and techniques of single-tooth implant restoration. *Esthet Dent Update* 1991;**2**:16-22.

28. SHERWOOD JR RL, SULLIVAN DY. Concepts and techniques of single-tooth implant resorations. *Esthet Dent Update* 1991;**2**:16-22.

29. HÜLSMANN M, ENGELKE W. Delayed endodontic and prosthetic treatment of two traumatized incisors. *Endod Dent Traumatol* 1991;**7**:90-5.

30. ÖHRNELL L-O, PALMQUIST J, BRÅNEMARK P-I. Single tooth replacement. In: WORTHINGTON P, BRÅNEMARK P-I, eds. *Advanced Osseointegration Surgery Applications in the Maxillofacial Region*. Chicago: Quintessence Books, 1992.

31. BRÅNEMARK P-I, ZARB GA, ALBREKTSSON T, eds. *Tissue-integrated prostheses: Osseointegration in clinical dentistry*. Chicago, Illinois: Quintessence Publishing Co, Inc; 1985.350pp.

32. HOBO S, ICHIDA E, GARCIA LT. *Osseointegration and occlusal rehabilitation*. Tokyo: Quintessence Publishing Co Ltd,1989.

33. PAREL S, SULLIVAN D. *Esthetics and osseointegration*. San Antonio: OSI publication, 1989.

34. BEUMER J, LEWIS S. *The Brånemark Implant System - Clinical and Laboratory Procedures*. St. Louis: Ishiyaku EuroAmerica, Inc;1990.

35. SCHWARZ MS, ROTHMAN SLG, CHAFETZ N, STAUTS B. Preoperative diagnostic radiology for the tissue-integrated prosthesis. In: LANEY WR, TOLMAN DE, eds. *Tissue Integration in Oral, Orthopedic & Maxillofacial Reconstruction*. Chicago: Quintessence Books, 1990:68-79.

36. SIERSBÆK-NIELSEN S. Rate of eruption of central incisors at puberty: an implant study on eight boys. *Tandlægebladet* 1971;**75**:1288-95.

37. ISERI H, SOLOW B. Growth displacement of the maxilla in girls studied by the implant method. *Tandlægebladet* 1991;**95**:839-46.

38. ÖDMAN J, GRÖNDAHL K, LEKHOLM U, THILANDER B. The effect of osseointegrated implants on the dento-alveolar development. A clinical and radiographical study in growing pigs. *Eur J Orthod* 1991;**13**:279-86.

39. THILANDER B, ÖDMAN J, GRÖNDAHL K, LEKHOLM U. Aspects on osseointegrated implants inserted in growing jaws. A biometric and radiographic study in the young pig. *Eur J Orthod* 1992;**14**:99-109.

40. ANDREASEN JO, SCHWARTZ O, FÆRCH C, HOLM B. The use of single standing Brånemark implants with and without bone autotransplantation. A prospective study of 60 cases. Unpublished study.

41. JENSEN J, SINDET-PEDERSEN S. Autogenous mandibular bone grafts and osseointegrated implants for reconstruction of the severely atrophied maxilla: a preliminary report. *J Oral Maxillofac Surg* 1991;**49**:1277-87.

42. DAHLIN C, LINDE A, GOTTLOW J, NYMAN S. Healing of bone defects by guided tissue regeneration. *Plast Reconstr Surg* 1989;**81**:672-6.

43. DAHLIN C, SENNERBY L, LEKHOLM U, LINDE A, NYMAN S. Generation of new bone around titanium implants using a membrane technique: an experimental study in rabbits. *Int J Oral Maxillofac Implants* 1989;**4**:19-25.

44. DAHLIN C, GOTTLOW J, LINDE A, NYMAN S. Healing of

maxillary and mandibular bone defects using a membrane technique. *Scand J Plast Reconstr Hand Surg* 1990;**24**:13-9.

45. NYMAN S, LANG N, BUSER D, BRAGGER U. Bone regeneration adjacent to titanium dental implants using guided tissue regeneration: a report of two cases. *Int J Oral Maxillofac Implants* 1990;**5**:9-14.

46. BECKER W, BECKER B, HANDELSMAN M, et al. Bone formation at dehisced dental implant sites treated with implant augmentation material: a pilot study in dogs. *Int J Periodontics Restorative Dent* 1990;**10**:93-102.

47. BECKER W, BECKER B. Guided tissue regeneration for implants placed into extraction sockets and for implant dehiscenses: surgical techniques and case reports. *Int J Periodontics Restorative Dent* 1990;**10**:377-91.

48. SEIBERT J, NYMAN S. Localized ridge augmentation in dogs: a pilot study using membranes and hydroxyapatite. *J Periodontol* 1990;**61**:157-65.

49. BUSER D, BRÄGGER U, LANG NP, NYMAN S. Regeneration and enlargement of jaw bone using guided tissue regeneration. *Clin Oral Impl Res* 1990;**1**:22-32.

50. JOVANOVIC SA, SPIEKERMANN H, RICHTE R E-J, KOSEOGLU M. Guided tissue regenration around titanium dental implants. In: LANEY WR, TOLMAN DE, eds. *Tissue Integration in Orthopedic & Maxillofacial Reconstruction.* Chicago: Quintessence Books, 1990:208-15.

51. DAHLIN C, LEKHOLM U, LINDE A. Induced bone augmentation at titanium implants using a membrane technique. A report on 10 fixtures followed 1 to 3 years after loading. *J Periodont Rest Dent* 1991;**11**:273-8.

52. DAHLIN C, LEKHOLM U, LINDE A. Bone augmentation at fenestrated implants by an ostopromotive membrane technique. A controlled clinical study. *Clin Oral Impl Res* 1991;**2**:159-65.

53. DAHLIN C, ALBERIUS P, LINDE A. Osteopromotion for cranioplasty. An experimental study in rats using a membrane technique. *J Neurosurg* 1991;**74**:487-91.

54. DAHLIN C, LEKHOLM U, LINDE A. Membraninduzierte Knochenaugmentation an Titanimplantaten. Ein Bericht über 10 Implantate nach 1- bis 3 jähriger Belastung. *Int J Parodontologie Rest Zahnheilk* 1991;**11**:291-9.

55. WACHTEL HC, LANGFORD A, BERNIMOULIN J-P, REICHART P. Guided bone regeration next to osseointegrated implants in humans. *Int J Oral Maxillofac Impl* 1991;**6**:127-35.

56. NEVINS M, MELLONIG JT. Enhancement of the damaged edentulous ridge to receive dental implants: a combination of allograft and the GORE-TEX membrane. *Int J Periodont Rest Dent* 1992;**12**:97-110.

57. ALBERIUS P, DAHLIN C, LINDE A. Role of osteopromotion in experimental bone grafting to the skull: a study in adult rats using a membrane technique. *J Oral Maxillofac Surg* 1992;**50**:829-34

58. LEHMANN B, BRÄGGER U, HÄMMERLE CHF, FOURMOUSIS I, LANG NP. Treatment of an early implant failure according to the principles of guided tissue regeneration (GTR). *Clin Oral Impl Res* 1992;**3**:42-8.

59. WEINGART D, BIGGEL A. Lokal periimplantäre Augmentation des anterioren Unterkiefer-Alveolarfortsatzes nach dem Prinzip der gesteuerten Geweberegeneration. *Quintessenz Int* 1992;**43**:403-16.

60. BRÅNEMARK P-I, BREINE U, HALLÉN O, HANSSON B-O, LINDSTRÖM J. Repair of defects in mandible. *Scand J Plast Reconstr Surg* 1975;**9**:100-8.

61. BRÅNEMARK P-I, LINDSTRÖM J, HALLÉN O, BREINE U, JEPPSON P-H, ÖHMANN A. Reconstruction of the defective mandible. *Scand J Plast Reconstr Surg* 1975;**9**:116-28.

62. BREINE U, BRÅNEMARK P-I. Reconstruction of alveolar jaw bone: An experimental and clinical study of immediate and preformed autologous bone grafts in combination with osseointegrated implants. *Scand J Plast Reconstr Surg* 1980;**14**:23-48.

63. KELLER EE, VAN ROEKEL NB, DESJARDINS RP, TOLMAN DE. Prosthetic-surgical reconstruction of the severely resorbed maxilla with iliac bone grafting and tissue-intergrated prosthese. *Int J Oral Maxillofac Implants* 1987;**2**:155-65.

64. KELLER EE, DESJARDINS RP, ECKERT SE, TOLMAN DE. Composite bone grafts and titanium implants in mandibular discontinuity reconstruction. *Int J Oral Maxillofac Implants* 1988;**3**:261-7.

65. ADELL R, LEKHOLM U, GRÖNDAHL K, BRÅNEMARK P-I. LINDSTRÖM J, JACOBSSON M. Reconstruction of severely resorbed edentulous maxillae using osseointegrated fixtures in immediate autogenous bone grafts. *Int J Oral Maxillofac Implants* 1990;**5**:233-46.

66. LEKHOLM U. The Brånemark implant technique: a standardized procedure under continuous development. In: LANEY WR, TOLMAN DE, eds. *Tissue Integration in Oral, Orthopedic & Maxillofacial Reconstruction.* Chicago: Quintessence Books, 1990:194-9.

67. LAZZARA F. Immediate implant placement into extraction sites: surgical and restorative advantages. *Int J Periodont Rest Dent* 1989;**9**:333-43.

68. LAZZARA RJ. Immediate implant placement into extraction sites: surgical and restorative advantages. In: LANEY WR, TOLMAN DE, eds. *Tissue Integration in Oral, Orthopedic & Maxillofacial Reconstruction.* Chicago: Quintessence Books, 1990:203-7.

69. YUKNA RA. Clinical comparison of hydroxyapatite-coated titanium dental imlants placed in fresh extraction sockets and healed sites. *J Periodontol* 1991;**62**:468-76.

70. GOTFREDSEN K, ROSTRUP E, HJØRTING-HANSEN E, STOLTZE K, BUDTZ-JØRGENSEN E. Histological and histomorphometrical evaluation of tissue reactions adjacent to endosteal implants in monkeys. *Clin Oral Impl Res* 1991;**2**:30-7.

71. GOTFREDSEN K, HJØRTING-HANSEN E, BUDTZ-JØRGENSEN E. Clinical and radiographic evaluation of submerged and nonsubmerged implants in monkeys. *Int J Prosthodontics* 1990;**3**:463-9.

72. GOTFREDSEN K, HJØRTING-HANSEN E. Histological and histomorphometric evaluation submerged and nonsubmerged titanium implants. In: LANEY WR, TOLMAN DE, eds. *Tissue Integration in Oral, Orthopedic & Maxillofacial Reconstruction.* Chicago: Quintessence Books, 1990:37-40.

73. BECKER W, BECKER BE, OCHSENBEIN C, HANDELSMAN M, ALBREKTSSON T, CELLETE R. The use of guided tissue regeneration for implants placed in immediate extraction sockets. In: LANEY WR, TOLMAN DE, eds. *Tissue Integration in Oral, Orthopedic & Maxillofacial Reconstruction.* Chicago: Quintessence Books, 1990:200-2.

74. WARRER K, GOTFREDSEN K, HJØRTING-HANSEN E, KARRING T. Guided tissue regeneration ensures osseointegration of dental implants placed into extraction sockets. An experimental study in monkey. *Clin Oral Impl Res* 1991;**2**:166-71.

75. QUALE AA. A traumatic removal of teeth and root fragments in dental implantology. *Int J Oral Maxillofac Implants* 1990;**5**:293-6.

76. ROSENQUIST JB, NYSTRÖM E. Occlusion of the incisal canal with bone chips. A procedure to facilitate insertion of implants in the anterior maxilla. *Int J Oral Maxillofac Surg* 1992;**21**:210-1.

77. RANGERT B, JEMT T, JÖRNEUS L. Forces and moments on Brånemark Implants. *Int J Oral Maxillofac Implants* 1989;**4**:241-7.

78. ERICSSON I, LEKHOLM U, BRÅNEMARK P-I, et al. A clinical evaluation of fixed bridge restorations supported by the combination of teeth and osseointegrated titanium implants. *J Clin Periodontol* 1986;**13**:307-12.

79. ERICSSON I, GLANTZ P-O, BRÅNEMARK P-I. Use of implants in restorative therapy in patients with reduced periodontal tissue support. *Quintessence Int* 1988;**19**:801-7.

80. ÅSTRAND P, BORG K, GUNNE J, OLSSON M. Combination of natural teeth and osseointegrated implants as prosthesis abutments: a 2-year longitudinal study. *Int J Oral Maxillofac Implants* 1991;**6**:305-12.

81. ADELL R, LEKHOLM U, ROCKLER B, BRÅNEMARK PI, LINDHE J. Marginal tissue reactions at osseointegrated titanium fixtures (I). A 3-year longitudinal prospective study. *Int J Oral Maxillofac Surg* 1986;**15**:39-52.

82. LEKHOLM U, ADELL R, LINDHE J, et al. Marginal tissue reactions at osseointegrated titanium fixtures (II) A cross-sectional retrospective study. *Int J Oral Maxillofac Surg* 1986;**15**:53-61.

83. COX CF, ZARB GA. The longitudinal clinical efficacy of osseointegrated dental implants. A 3 year report. *Int J Oral Maxillofac Implants* 1987;**2**:91-100.

84. CHAYTOR DV, ZARB GA, SCHMITT A, LEWIS DW. Der Langzeiterfolg osseointegrierter Implantate. II. Die Toronto-Studie: Veränderungen in der Knochenhöhe. *Int J Paradontologie Rest Zahnheilk* 1991;**11**:111-23.

85. QUIRYNEN M, NAERT I, VAN STEENBERGHE D, TEERLINCK J, KEKEYSER C, THEUNIERS G. Periodontal aspects of osseointegrated fixtures supporting an overdenture. A 4 year retrospective study. *J Clin Periodontol* 1991;**18**:719-28.

86. SENNERBY L, ERICSON LE, THOMSEN P, LEKHOLM U, ÅSTRAND P. Structure of the bone-titanium interface in retrieved clinical oral implants. *Clin Oral Impl Res* 1991;**2**:103-11.

87. SCHNITMAN PA, SHULMAN LB. Recommendations of the consensus development conference on dental implants. *J Am Dent Assoc* 1989;**98**:373-7.

88. CRANIN AN, SILVERBRAND H, SALTER N. The requirements and clinical performance of dental implants. In: SMITH DC, WILLIAMS DF, eds. *Biocompatibility of dental materials,* Vol 4. Boca Raton, FL: CRC Press, 1982:198.

89. MCKINNEY R, KOTH DL, STEFLIK DE. Clinical standards for dental implants. In: CLARK JE, ed. *Clinical dentistry.* Harperstown: Harper & Row, 1984:1-11.

90. ALBREKTSSON T, ZARB GA, WORTHINGTON P, ERIKSSON AR. The long-term efficacy of currently used dental implants: a review and proposed criteria of success. *J Oral Maxillofac Implants* 1986;**1**:11-25.

91. SMITH DE, ZARB A. Criteria for success of osseointegrated endosseous implants. *J Prosthet Dent* 1989;**62**:567-72.

92. VAN STEENBERGHE D, KELLER EE, SHULMAN LB. Intraoral consensus panel. In: LANEY WR, TOLMAN DE, eds. *Tissue Integration in Oral, Orthopedic & Maxillofacial Reconstruction.* Chicago: Quintessence Books, 1990:392-3.

93. LINDEN U, KISCH J, KRISTERSON L. Long term prognosis of single standing implants. An analysis of 149 cases. 1993 Unpublished data.

94. NILSON H. Long term prognosis of single standing implants. An analysis of 130 cases. 1993 Unpublished data.

95. ALBREKTSSON T, SENNERBY L. State of the art in oral implants. *J Clin Periodontol* 1991;**18**:474-81.

96. BECKER W, DAHLIN C, LEKHOLM U, BECKER B, DONATH K, SANCHEZ R. Role of early versus late removal of GTAM material on bone formation around dental implants. An experimental study in dogs. *Clin Oral Impl Res* 1993. Submitted.

97. SIMION M, BALDONI M, ZAFFE D. Guided tissue regeneration in osseointegrated implant II: extraction sockets. *Ital Osseointegration* 1991;**1**:40-54.

98. HOLMES CH. Morphology of the interdental papillae. *J Periodontol* 1965;**36**:455-60.

99. KOHL JT, ZANDER HA. Morphology of interdental ginginal tissues. *Oral Surg* 1961;**14**:287-95.

100. COHEN B. Morphological factors in the pathogenesis of periodontal disease. *Br Dent J* 1959;**107**:31-39.

101. MCHUGH WD. The interdental gingivae. *J Periodont Res* 1971;**6**:227-236.

102. PALACCI P. Amenagement des tissues periimplantaires interét de la regeneration des papilles. *Réalités Clinique* 1992;**3**:381-87.

Chapter 21

Prevention of Dental and Oral Injuries

B. SCHEER

Use of Mouthguards

Although the caries rate in children has fallen considerably in the last decade there has been a significant rise in the number of dental injuries (1) (Fig. 21.1). The major causes of these injuries vary considerably and include accidents in and around the home, playground injuries and injuries that result from violence(2) (Fig. 21.2). A significant number result from the participation in contact sports such as American football, rugby, soccer, boxing, wrestling, diving or "stick sports"(3-7). Other sport activities which are not necessarily associated with player contact may also place the participant at risk. These include horse riding, cycling and skiing. Injury may also occur during surgical procedures, from excessive pressure on the incisors while using a laryngoscope to pass anesthetic tubes or endoscopy instruments. This is particularly true in young patients where the anterior teeth are only partly erupted and root length is not complete, when the teeth may easily be displaced or fractured and cases have been reported of inhalation of teeth displaced during general anesthesia (8).

The appearance of a dentition mutilated by the fracture or loss of teeth may no longer be socially acceptable and although great advances have been made in the treatment of injuries, relatively little attention has been paid to ways in which they may be prevented.

The Federation Dentaire International (FDI) has recommended that an investigation into the effectiveness of mouthguards should be carried out, and has classified organized sport into two categories: *High risk sports* that include American football, hockey, ice hockey, lacrosse, martial sports, rugby and skating. The *medium risk sports* include basketball, diving, squash, gymnastics, parachuting and waterpolo (9).

In addition to dental injuries an important factor is the neurological effect of direct blows to the head or the indirect effect of rapid acceleration or deceleration following such impacts. When discussing oro-facial protectors, their possible value in preventing concussion or more severe neurological damage is an important consideration.

As the etiology of dental injuries is multifactorial, effective preventive measures are difficult to institute and assess. Attempts have been made to assess the factors which make some individuals more prone to injury than others and it has been shown that there is a significant difference between the sexes, and that individuals who take part in contact sports also have an increased prevalence of injuries(4-6).

Fig. 21.1. The prevalence of dental caries and dental injuries

The prevalence of dental injuries and caries was examined in the U.K. in 15-year old children in 1973 and 1983. From TODD (1) 1985.

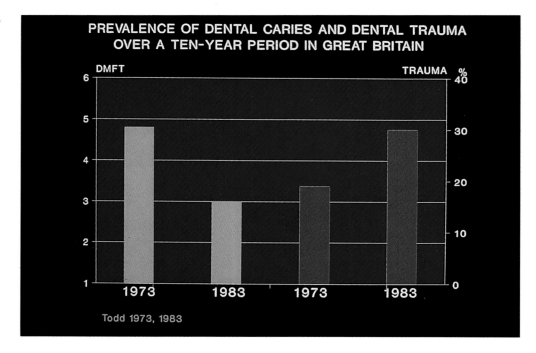

Injuries to the teeth are twice as frequent in children who have an increased overjet and inadequate lip coverage (10-12), and tend to be more severe (12). It has been suggested that women may be more susceptible than men to injury, as it has not been traditional for them to wear any form of mouth protection. OLVERA in a study of over 5000 female basketball players reported that they suffered an injury rate of 7.5%. This was greater than that reported for mens's football, and the dental injuries of 2% exceeded the prevalence of 0.5% reported for the football players (13).

Preventive measures, which include the wearing of seat belts in automobiles and the use of protective clothing when taking part in contact sports, have gained considerably in popularity during the last decade reflecting an attempt to reduce the number of injuries to the head, face and oral tissues (Fig. 21.3).

The use of mouth protectors and face masks has been made mandatory by the

Fig. 21.2. The cause of trauma related to sex
The etiology of dental trauma was examined in a clinical study from Sweden. From CRONA LARSON (2) 1989.

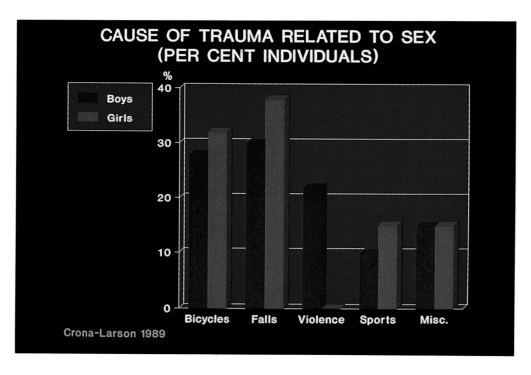

CHAPTER 21

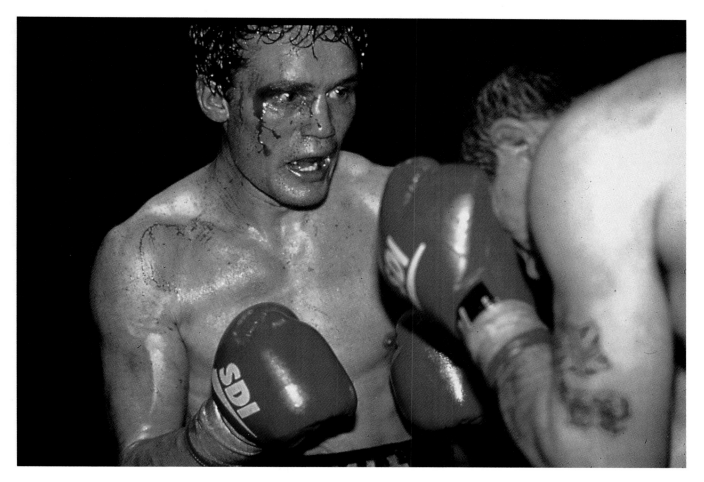

Fig. 21.3.
Despite severe facial injuries, and injuries including brain damage, boxing does not usually result in tooth damage, due to the use of mouth guards.

controlling bodies of some sports in different countries. While a certain uniformity has been established by the international governing bodies of many contact sports, there is no global consistency. Although in the United States, amateur boxers are required to wear head protectors (Figs. 21.3 and 21.4), in many other countries this is not a requirement.

Football

In the United States, early attempts to protect sports players from injury to the dento-facial tissues included the use of face masks which were attached to the helmets in American football (Fig. 21.4). These were recommended by the regulating authority of the sport and made compulsory in 1959 by the National Alliance of Athletic Associations (NAAA) (14). In 1962 it was made compulsory for football players to wear mouthguards in high

schools and junior colleges and it was made mandatory for university teams by the National Collegiate Athletic Association (NCAA) in 1973.

In 1990 the rules committee of NCAA adopted a rule that made it mandatory for all players to wear yellow mouthguards so that it could easily be seen if they were being worn. Ice hockey, men's lacrosse, women's field hockey and boxing are also strictly regulated by the appropriate sports authority. Investigations carried out in 1968 showed that 2.26% of all American football wounds involved injury to the dental or facial tissues.

When mandatory face masks and mouth protectors were introduced for college football players in the USA, the prevalence was reduced to 0.3% (15). Studies carried out more recently suggest that the prevalence of dento-facial injuries to football players is greater than previously recorded (16).

Fig. 21.4.
Head protectors as worn by amateur boxers and football helmet and face mask with full coverage to the face including chin support and mouthguard.

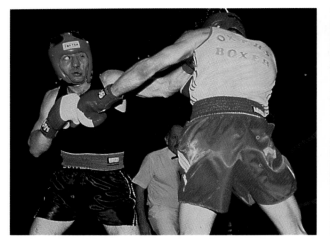 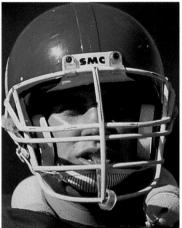

Thus it was shown in 1986 that 3.9% of adolescent football players sustained oral trauma even when wearing a mouthguard (16).

In several studies it has been confirmed that there was a considerable reduction in football and other sports injuries when a mouthguard was worn (5,16). While data demonstrates an increased susceptibility to injury in individuals not wearing mouthguards, it should be noted that in several sports it is not customary to wear mouthguards. The studies suggest that although football players who wear mouthguards still have a relatively high prevalence of soft tissue injury, the numbers of tooth injuries, hematomas fractures and brain concussions are reduced dramatically (5, 16).

In other countries, apart from regulatory bodies in boxing, the policy regarding the use of mouth protectors is less well defined.

Rugby

The injuries suffered by rugby players have been described in a several studies. DAVIES ET AL. (17) in 1977 showed that 45% of the players examined had injured front teeth, although the full extent of the injuries was probably underestimated, since soft tissue injuries and maxillo-facial injuries were not included and vitality testing of the teeth was not carried out. NICHOLAS in a study carried out in New Zealand found that 62% of rugby players had suffered injuries to the oral structures (18).

Hockey and Ice Hockey

In 1975 mouthguards were made mandatory for ice hockey players in the USA and 2 years later a rule enforcing full face protection was introduced. In the following 7 years the prevalence of dental injuries fell from 13% to 5% of all injuries (19). In Finland between 1984 and 1985 it was shown that while 5.8% of all ice hockey players suffered injury, 8.9% of those still received dental injuries even though full cage face masks had been introduced in 1979 (7). Other studies carried out with hockey and ice hockey players, showed a comparable prevalence of injuries (20,21). LEES ET AL. have reported that among university students in England, 32% had experienced dental injuries, approximately half of them sustained while participating in contact sports (22).

Soccer

A study of soccer players of all ages in Norway (23) reported that between 1979 and 1983, of 7319 injuries sustained, approximately 20% were dental injuries. The majority of injuries occurred among male players, the relative frequencies of dental injuries were also higher among men (13.5 injuries for each 10,000 male players compared to 3.5 per 10,000 female players). It was also noted that the prevalence of injuries was higher in players in the senior divisions.

When considering the soft tissue injuries, wearing mouth protectors appeared to reduce the potential for such an injury by a factor of 7.6 (5).

Fig. 21.5.
*The total number of sports in-
juries and the number of dental
injuries per 10,000 players for
the period 1981, 1982, 1983 in
Norway. From* NYSETHER (23)
1987.

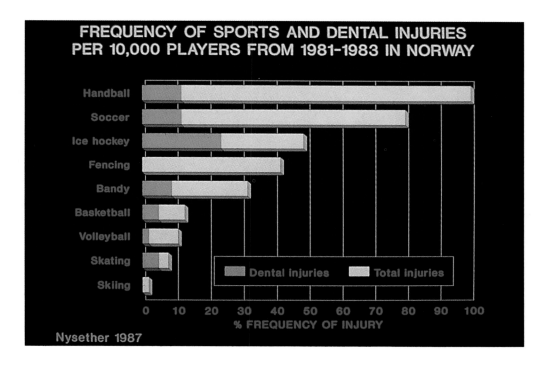

Cost Benefit of Mouthguard Protection

Although a number of studies have shown a dramatic reduction in the number of dental injuries (24-26), the direct effect of wearing a mouthguard is not without controversy.

Thus in rugby football, BLIGNAULT ET AL. reported that dental injuries did not appear to be associated with the use or non-use of mouthguards (7). They were also critical of the findings in a number of other studies and came to the conclusion that in rugby football failure to wear a mouthguard had no significant effect on the prevalence of dental injuries. Similar opinions were expressed by BOLHUIS ET AL. 1987 concerning field hockey (21).

The economic cost of treating dental sports injuries has not been studied in any depth. The cost of carrying out emergency treatment and subsequent treatment is high. It has been shown that a high number of endodontic and prosthetic treatments are responsible for a greater part of the cost and it has been suggested that with longer follow-up periods the costs would increase still further (28). It is possible that wearing a mouthguard might reduce the severity of the injury thus reducing the number of complex treatments necessary. However, since the way in which wearing a mouthguard affects the type of injury sustained is still not known, further information is required.

In an analysis of insurance records of reported injuries, NYSETHER showed that for the sports studied the proportion of dental injuries in relation to the overall number of injuries was fairly small and questioned the cost effectiveness of fitting mouthguards to all participant (23) (Fig. 21.5). SANE ET AL. 1988, however, in a study of contact sports injuries, concluded that dental protection for all players was justified to prevent unnecessary dental injuries and lifelong discomfort, as well as reducing the high costs involved in treatment of injuries (7).

It seems that although the protection of the oral and dental tissues is to be encouraged for all participants in contact sports, the precise value of mouthguards for individual sports has not yet been determined

Mechanism of Function of Mouthguards

The protection of the oral tissues during contact sports was first recorded by a boxer in 1913 who wore a mouthguard made of guttapercha in order to reduce "the jarring pain of jaws being smashed together, shattering teeth, severely lacerating lips, and transmitting spine-chilling chin blows to the base of the brain" (30). Since that time, the wearing of mouthguards and, in some countries, helmets has become mandatory in boxing.

Several papers have drawn attention to head injuries, including brain concussion resulting from impact blows to the mandible sustained during contact sports (31-35). Two types of acceleration have been described which result following an impact to the head (32). These are angular acceleration, caused by rapid rotation of the head and linear acceleration in a postero-anterior direction. Evidence suggests that their effects differ considerably; thus, angular acceleration is believed to be more damaging to the brain than linear acceleration because of the high shear strain it causes. The mechanism of injury is therefore not only related to the magnitude of the force but also to the resulting acceleration.

Impact to the the mandible during sport is usually direct, that is a blow from a fist, knee or elbow. The distribution of these forces has, together with the injury pattern to the oral soft tissues and teeth, led to the development of mouthguards (33,36,38), protective helmets and faceguards (37).

The different functions of mouthguards have been described by STEVENS (39).

1. They hold the soft tissues of the lips and cheeks away from the teeth, preventing laceration or bruising of the lips and cheeks against the hard and irregular teeth during impact.
2. They cushion the teeth from direct frontal blows and redistribute the forces that would otherwise cause fracture or dislocation of anterior teeth.
3. They prevent opposing teeth from coming into violent contact, reducing the risk of tooth fracture or damage to supporting structures.
4. They provide the mandible with resilient support which absorbs impacts that might fracture the unsupported angle or condyle of the mandible.
5. They help prevent neurological injury by holding the jaws apart and act as shock absorbers to prevent upward and backward displacement of the mandibular condyles against the base of the skull. Under experimental conditions, it has been shown that the use of mouth protectors may reduce intracranial pressure and bone deformation due to impacts (35).
6. They provide protection against neck injuries. It has been demonstrated on cephalometric radiographs that repositioning of the mandibular condyle, cervical vertebrae, and other cervical anatomic structures takes place when a mouthguard is in place. Comparative tracings, with and without a mouthguard, suggests a partial explanation for protection against traumatic shock to the head and neck (32).
7. They are psychological assets to contact sport athletes. Hockey players and football players feel more confident and aggressive if they believe that they are less likely to receive injuries to the head and mouth (24, 36, 40).
8. They fill the space and support adjacent teeth, so that removable prostheses can be taken out during contact sports. This prevents possible fracture of the denture and accidental swallowing or inhaling of fragments.

These criteria are frequently not adequately fulfilled in many of the types of mouthguards worn by athletes, a number of those readily available may in fact increase the likelihood of injury occurring. This is discussed later in this chapter.

Design of Mouth Protectors

Criteria for Construction

The principles for the construction of effective mouthguards have been suggested to be the following by TURNER and others (33, 41-45).

1. The mouthguard should fit the mouth accurately, and preferably be processed on models of the teeth.
2. It should have sufficient retention to prevent its displacement while being worn.
3. It must be comfortable.
4. It should not interfere with the soft tissues.
5. It should allow normal breathing and speech.
6. It should be formed from a material that:
   a. is easily manipulated,
   b. is sufficiently flexible to absorb impact,
   c. is sufficiently durable to prevent

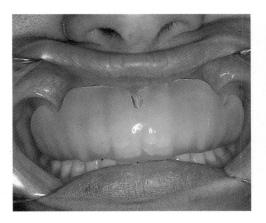

Fig. 21.6.
A correctly fitted mouthguard showing adequate extension and contouring.

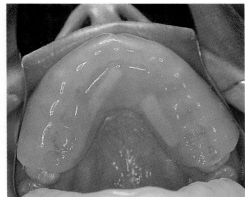

either breakage of the mouthguard or penetration by a tooth cusp.

d. will remain stable for at least 2 years,
e. can be sterilized,
f. has no odor or taste,
g. is approved alone or in combination with other materials and presents no risk to health from the longterm release of trace impurities as a result of the action of oral fluids and bacteria.

The FDI has listed the following criteria for constructing an effective mouthguard (9).

1. The mouthguard should be made of a resilient material which can be easily washed, cleaned and readily disinfected.
2. It should have adequate retention to remain in position during sporting activity, and allow for a normal occlusal relationship to give maximum protection.
3. It should absorb and disperse the energy of a shock by:
   a. Covering the maxillary dental arch.
   b. Excluding interferences.
   c. Reproducing the occlusal relationship.
   d. Allowing mouth breathing.
   e. Protecting the soft tissues.

The FDI also recommends that mouthguards should, preferably, be made by dentists from an impression of the athlete's teeth.

The U.S. Joint Committee on Mouth Protectors has recommended similar criteria (45).

Mouthguard Design

The accepted design for mouthguards is based on that suggested by TURNER in 1977 (3). The mouthguard should normally be fitted to the maxillary arch, al-

though in an Angles Class III malocclusion, the appliance should be placed over the mandibular arch.

The mouthguard should be close fitting (Fg. 21.6). It should cover the occlusal surfaces of the teeth except where it is anticipated that the exfoliation of primary teeth or further eruption of teeth will occur during the lifetime of the appliance. It should extend at least as far back as the distal surface of the first permanent molar. Although STEVENS suggests that it should extend to the tuberosity (39), there is no evidence that this improves protection; and it may reduce comfort.

The flanges of the mouthguard should extend beyond the gingival attachment, but short of the mucobuccal fold. There is no evidence that constructing a thick labial flange is of any advantage. It should be not more than 2 mm thick over the labial mucosa, to avoid stretching the lips which could lead to them splitting on impact. The buccal edge of the flange should be smooth and rounded and carefully relieved around the frena and muscle attachments.

The palatal aspect of the mouthguard should extend approximately 5 mm on to the palate and should be tapered to a smooth, thin, rounded edge to avoid interference with speech and breathing or stimulation of the "gagging" reflex.

The occlusal thickness of the mouthguard should not exceed the width of the freeway space and should occlude evenly and comfortably with the opposing arch.

Assessment of the Criteria

The design criteria described above have never been evaluated clinically, but appear to have gained wide acceptance. Different types of sports activity expose the partici-

Fig. 21.7
*A. Bimaxillary mouthguard as
suggested by* CHAPMAN (47) *1985
B. Design of mouthguard as recommended by* CHANDLER (48)
*1987 showing airway space ante-
riorly to facilitate breathing.*

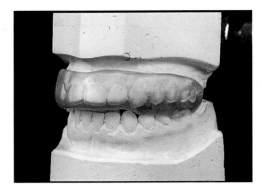

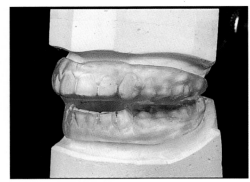

pants to different types of injury (45). It has been suggested that the design of the mouthguard should be modified to allow for these differences.

In a study carried out on Australian Rules Football, it was recorded that half of all blows were to the front of the face; and one-third were received under the mandible, necessitating particular protection of the occlusion (41). In the absence of more substantial evidence it is suggested that a mouthguard should give maximum protection of both hard and soft tissues irrespective of the sport and type of injury that is anticipated, so that modification of the basic design is not necessary.

CHAPMAN ET AL. describes a bimaxillary mouthguard (Fig. 21.7 A) that covers both arches and holds the mandible in a position that allows maximum oral air flow (7). It is claimed that this design offers several advantages by allowing complete protection of the teeth, as well as the intra- and extraoral tissues, from injury. It is also suggested that the bimaxillary mouthguard significantly increases mandibular protection by giving it rigid support, reducing the likelihood of concussion by preventing the transmission of forces through the temporomandibular joint to the base of the skull. CHANDLER ET AL. (48) describe thickening the occlusal surfaces over the molar teeth so as to disengage the incisors and suggests that this provides protection that is equal to the bimaxillary type described by CHAPMAN (47) (Fig. 21.7 B). It is clear that further studies are necessary to evaluate the design of mouthguards.

Mouthguard Materials

Mouthguards have been made of a large number of plastic materials. The earliest appliances were made by boxers who moulded a ball of softened guttapercha in their mouths. Since that time a number of materials have been developed and are in current use. These are:

Polyvinyl acetate-polyethelene co-
polymer (PVAc-PF)
Polyurethane (PU)
Polyvinyl chloride (PVC)
Soft acrylics
Natural rubber

Physical Properties of Mouthguard Materials

The most commonly used material is Polyvinyl Acetate-Polyethelene copolymer (PVAc-PE). Polyurethane is becoming less frequently used (49-51).

A number of studies have been carried out to examine the physical and mechanical properties of these materials and to test their ability to protect the oral tissues (49-53). It has been shown that the physical and mechanical properties vary with their chemical composition and this itself varies with different brands of the same material (50-55) (Table 21.1). The resilience of PVAc-PE materials appears to vary inversely with the magnitude of the impact energy at which they are tested (54). A number of factors may be responsible for this variation including the degree of crosslinking between polymer chains, the proportion of plasticizer present and the volume of filler particles (50-55). It has been suggested that laminated thermoplastic mouthguards are dimensionally more stable in use (50).

The clinical significance of these vari-

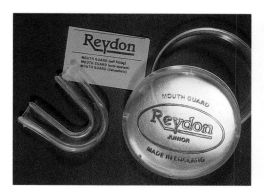

Fig. 21.8.
A stock mouthguard.

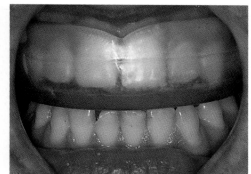

Types of Mouth Protector

ations has not been determined; but it has been suggested that high energy absorption does not necessarily indicate that the material will give maximum protection, since some of the absorbed energy may be transmitted directly to the underlying dental structures (49).

Mouthguards may be classified into three types:

A) *Stock*
B) *Mouth formed*
C) *Custom made.*

A). *Stock* mouthguards may be made either from rubber or one of the plastic materials (Fig. 21.8). They are generally made in three sizes and are supposed to be universal fitting. Modification is limited to trimming the margins to relieve the frena. The loose fit means that the wearer has to keep the teeth in contact to prevent the guard from being displaced. They also impede speech and respiration. Their only advantage is that they are inexpensive and may be obtained by the public from sports shops. There is no evidence that they are effective in redistributing forces of impact, and they may result in soft tissue injury from rough or sharp edges. The need to hold the teeth together may reduce the risk of mandibular fracture or neurological injury resulting from the sudden forced closure of the lower jaw. TURNER (43) has recommended that "on present evidence the stock type of mouthguard should be withdrawn from sale" and cites a case when a rugby player suffered a serious injury when a stock mouthguard blocked his airway.

B). There are two types of *Mouth Formed protectors* that may be made from a manufactured kit. The first consists of a hard and fairly rigid outer shell that provides a smooth, durable surface and a soft, resilient lining that is adapted to the teeth

Table 21.1. *The range of properties of polyvinyl acetate-polyethylene, polyvinyl chloride and soft liners used in mouthguards. After* CHACONAS ET AL. (50) *1985.*

Property	PVAc-PE	PVC	Liners
Tensile Strength (psi)	460-2860	1230-2480	140-530
Elongation (%)	700-1150	200-450	150-500
Tear Strength (lb/in)	120-210	150-420	30-85
Hardness(Rex A, 1sec.)	68-86	79-85	37-75
Hardness(Rex A, 15 sec.)	63-84	73-78	21.24
Water absorption (%)	0.13-2.07	0.38-0.88	0.54-1.27
Rebound (%)	45.0-53.9	11.6-26.1	7.7-56.9
Penetration (ins)	0.14-0.23	0.13-0.19	0.17-0.44

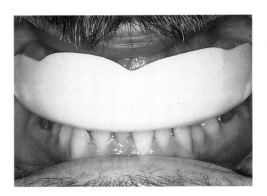

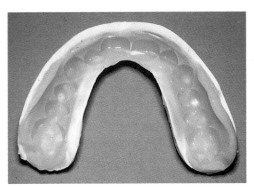

Fig. 21.9.
A mouth formed mouthguard consisting of a vinyl chloride outer shell lined with self-curing soft acrylic. It appears that the outer shell stands away from the teeth and may increase the distortion of the soft tissue during an impact.

(Fig. 21.9). The outer shell of vinyl-chloride may be lined with a layer of self-curing methyl-methacrylate or silicone rubber. The outer shell is fitted and trimmed, if necessary, around the sulci and frenal attachments. It is filled with the soft lining and seated in the mouth. Care must be taken to ensure that it is centrally placed. The lining is allowed to polymerize for 3-5 minutes. Excess material is trimmed with a sharp knife and the margins smoothed with dental stones. This type of mouthguard tends to be bulky and the margins of the outer shell may be sharp unless protected by an adequate thickness of the lining material.

The most commonly used type of mouth formed protector is constructed from a preformed thermoplastic shell of PVAc-PE copolymer or PVC (49) that is softened in warm water and then moulded in the mouth by the user (Fig. 21.10). These mouthguards have several distinct advantages over the stock mouthguard. If carefully adapted, they give a closer fit and are more easily retained than stock protectors. If care is not taken during the moulding process, however, the mouthguard may not fit accurately. The temperature

necessary to allow adequate adaptation to the teeth is fairly high, so that there is also a risk of burning the mouth.

In a study of mouthguards worn by boxers (56), it has been shown that only 31% fulfilled the criteria recommended for protection described earlier. It was shown that 72% were loose and 17% had sharp edges that could cause soft tissue injury (Fig. 21.11). The majority of mouthguards examined were only retained in the mouth by being held in place by the lower teeth.

KUEBKER ET AL. showed that 85% of the mouth formed guards were not large enough to meet the NCAA rules and recommended that a wider choice of sizes should be developed to meet the rules (7).

C) *Custom* mouthguards are individually made in a laboratory, on plaster of paris models poured from impressions of the player's mouth. Many studies have shown that these mouthguards are more acceptable and comfortable to athletes than the other types (18, 30, 58-60). There is no evidence, however, that custom made protectors are more effective in preventing injuries. STOKES ET AL. compared mouth formed and custom made mouthguards (57). They showed that although there were no dental injuries in either group, the users preferred laboratory formed mouthguards. This confirms the views of other workers (18, 59-61).

Historically, three groups of materials were used to fabricate custom made mouth protectors: these were moulded velum rubber (18, 58), latex rubber (18, 18) and resilient acrylic resins. They have been largely replaced by thermoplastic vinyl plastics that are available in sheets 3

Fig. 21.10.
Thermoplastic PVAc-PE copolymer mouthguard.

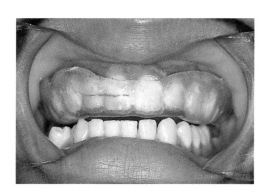

Fig. 21.11.
Mouthguards showing poor adaptation and sharp margins.

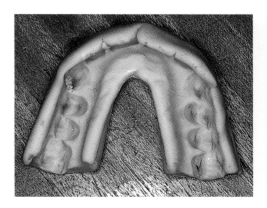 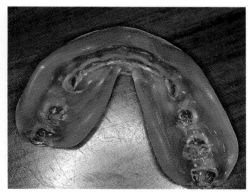

to 6 mm thick (Fig. 21.12). They can be moulded by vacuum or direct pressure on to a plaster model either singly or laminated when they are softened by heat (62). CHACONAS ET AL. have described a laminated thermoplasic mouthguard in use in the United States (49).

Alginate impressions are taken of both arches together with a wax bite taken with the patients's mandible in a physiological rest position. The mouthguard is constructed with an even occlusal imprint (Fig. 21.13) which enables the athlete to brace the muscles of the head and neck as the teeth come into uniform contact with the mouthguard (40). This increases the separation between the cranial base and the condyle and reduces the risk of brain concussion (47). If the occlusal thickness is greater than the "freeway space," clenching the teeth could result in temporomandibular discomfort and may result in the athlete chewing through the appliance (64). CHANDLER ET AL. recommend 4.5mm as the optimum thickness for the occusal surface and suggested that an airway space should be left anteriorly to facilitate breathing (47). CHAPMAN (46) describes the design for a bimaxillary mouthguard and suggests that the increased area of coverage results in improved protection against the risk of orofacial and head injury particularly in contact sports. No evidence is offered for this view and the involved technique inevitably increases the cost.

It has been suggested that a "standard" mouthguard should be worn by players until the age of 16 years because changes in the dentition and jaw development would necessitate a new mouthguard every year until then (65). A bimaxillary mouthguard made then should remain effective for at least 2 to 3 years. The mouthguard may need to be more robust at this age, as competition is often keener and the probability of severe injury greater (60).

Special Considerations in Fitting Mouthprotectors

Edentulous and partly dentate athletes should not wear removable prostheses while participating in sports, to prevent injury or aspiration of the fragments if the appliance were to be accidentally displaced or fractured. Vinyl occlusal rims may be constructed on a thermoplastic

Fig. 21.12.
A custom made thermoplastic mouthguard showing the correct extension and thickness to give maximum protection from injury.

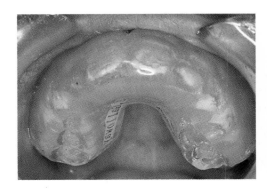 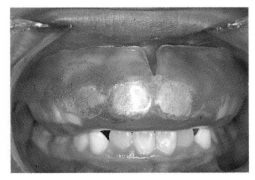

Fig. 21.13. Construction of custom made PVAc-PE thermoplastic mouthguard

The inner layer is vacuum moulded to a plaster model. Thereafter a second layer is moulded over the inner layer once it has been trimmed. An identifying label and a piece of radio-opaque foil may be inserted between the two layers.

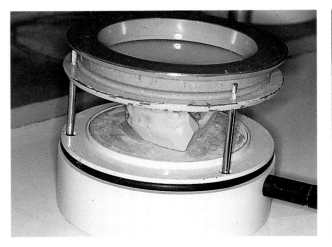
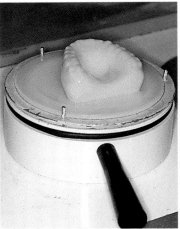

Trimming the mouthguards

The mouthguard is then again trimmed and placed on an articulator so that after softening the occlusal surface of the lower teeth can be imprinted into the surface.

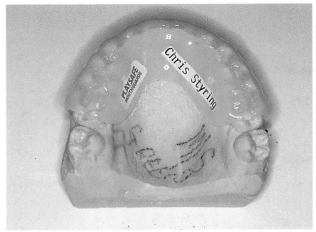
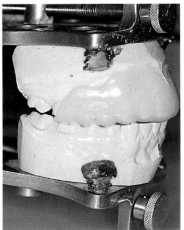

vinyl base to replace the missing teeth. If the user is edentulous, a space should be left anteriorly to facilitate breathing (64).

For patients undergoing orthodontic treatment involving the wearing of fixed appliances, the brackets and arch wires may be covered with boxing wax before the impressions are taken. The mouthguard may be made of a less elastic material, to protect the teeth, but care should be taken not to increase the thickness sufficiently to place the lips or other soft tissues under tension. Stock mouthguards that are specifically sold to athletes who are wearing orthodontic appliances appear to offer little protection (Fig. 21.14).

Care of Mouthguards

When fitted, instructions should be given for the care of the mouthguard. It has been reported that only half of athletes clean their mouthguards after use. Eight percent even lent them to other athletes (67). Bacteriological studies have led to the recommendation that mouthguards should a) be washed with soap and water immediately after use; b) they should be dried thoroughly and stored in a perforated box; and c) they should be rinsed in mouthwash or mild antiseptic (e.g. 0.2% Chlorhexidene) immediately before being used again (68).

The mouthguard should be inspected regularly to check its fit, especially in children who are still growing. During use it may become distorted or torn through chewing. Athletes should be warned that chewing the mouthguard will shorten its life. It was recommended by STEVENS that when not being worn, mouth protectors should be stored in a specially constructed case designed to carry all the mouth protector boxes of the team (38).

The Acceptability of Mouthguards

Considerable effort has been made in recent years to make mouthguards more acceptable to athletes. Although they have been made mandatory in a number of sports, where rules do not specify their use there is still often a resistance to their use

Fig. 21.14.
Stock mouthguard designed for individuals wearing orthodontic appliances.

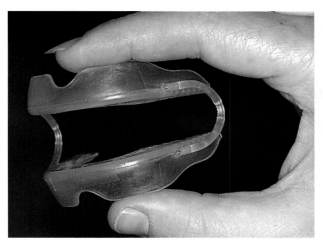 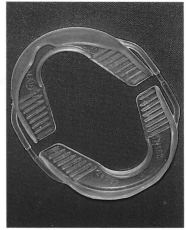

due to discomfort (21, 69-73). A number of authorities have suggested that custom formed latex mouth protectors provide the best protection (58, 63) and appear to be most acceptable. However, they have largely fallen into disuse due to cost of production and the low tear resistance of the material (24, 74).

The acceptability of different types of mouthguard by athletes has been examined by several investigators. Although it is generally accepted that custom made protectors give better protection and are more comfortable than stock mouthguards (5, 24, 42, 61, 72), it has been shown that only 13.2% of a sample of 16,000 athletes wore a mouthguard fitted by a dentist (71). These findings may be compared with a smaller study carried out by the author (55), in which it was shown that only 18% of young boxers wore a custom made mouthguard. Similar figures were suggested by JENSEN (75). Work published by CHAPMAN (76) states that among Australian rugby club players, the usage rate was 96%; although for the national team it was only 79% and over 80% were custom made. Although it has been recommended that stock protectors and self-made mouth formed guards should be withdrawn from sale (42) and athletes admit that they are less comfortable and restrict breathing, they are still used because of their cheapness compared with custom made guards (57, 71).

The athletes' view of mouthguards and the objections to wearing them have been studied by a number of workers (21, 57, 69, 71, 73). Reasons given include discomfort, nausea, interference with breathing or speech, expense and appearance.

In a study carried out among football players in 1963 each player wore the three types of mouth guard (stock, mouth formed and custom) in turn for 2 weeks. A comparative evaluation was made at the end of the period. The custom made protector was judged to have the best rating in all qualities, taste, lack of odour, comfort, speech, cleanliness and retention. The mouth formed protectors were rated next and the stock mouth guards rated the poorest (41). This preference for custom protectors has also been reported among ice hockey players (77). It has been recommended by a number of authorities that dentists should be appointed to sports teams with responsibility for diagnosing problems related to poorly fitting mouthguards, arranging for custom made protectors to be fitted and carrying out emergency treatment when necessary (15, 43, 52).

BLUM describes a project where a program to provide custom made mouthguards at minimal cost to the population was started in 1972. It is reported that the demand has increased steadily each year; although no data is published of any change in the prevalence of injuries (78).

Conclusion

In summary, while the evidence for the wearing of mouthguards for all contact sports is incomplete, there is strong data to suggest that they reduce the susceptibility to dental injury in many instances. While the design of mouthguards and the materials from which they are made need further investigation, in order to produce protectors that are not only effective but also inexpensive, there is sufficient evidence to suggest that a correctly made mouthguard at least reduces the severity of oral injuries considerably.

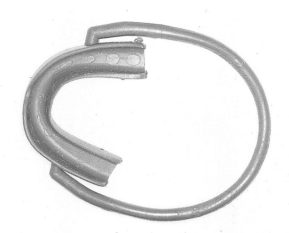

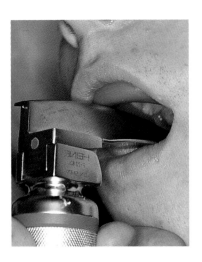

Other Applications for the Use of Mouthguards

Protection of the Dental Tissues during General Anesthesia

The use of laryngoscopes and surgical instruments has been associated with dental injuries 79-84. Oral endoscopy and orotracheal intubation may result in fracture or displacement of the teeth (79, 80, 84, 85). The damage may be inflicted by using the incisal edges of the anterior teeth as a fulcrum when inserting a laryngoscope, retractors or endoscopes. The fracture of prosthetic crowns has also been reported and injuries to the teeth are one of the most frequent complications during the delivery of general anesthesia (79, 86). Furthermore the most frequent of all anesthesia-related medico-legal claims was for dental injuries (87). It was suggested that some form of tooth damage occurs once in each 1000 inductions. Concern for dental injuries of this type has increased due to an awareness of the medico-legal responsibility of the surgeon or anesthetist for iatrogenic injury (86, 87).

A number of methods have been recommended to prevent injuries in these circumstances. These include mouth formed and custom made guards (83, 90, 91) (Fig. 21.15). EVERS (82) has described the use of an adhesive oral bandage(Orahesive®) to protect the tissues. Recently the use of an orthopedic bandage has been suggested. Ther-mo-plastic impregnated gauze mesh (Hexalite®) may be quickly adapted directly to the teeth and trimmed by the anesthetist before induction (92).

Injury to the soft tissues and in neonatal infants including the inducement of cleft palates due to the prolonged application of endotracheal tubes have been reported (84,88). Dilaceration of a primary incisor has been described following neonatal laryngoscopy (89). Evidence suggests that preterm infants who need prolonged intubation (93) may suffer long-term damage to their palates. SULLIVAN (94) has described an appliance that may be used to protect the palatal tissues of these children. A similar appliance was described by ASH & MOSS (93) (Fig. 21.16).

Protection of Neurological Patients from Self-Inflicted Injury

Self-inflicted injuries have frequently been reported in individuals who suffer from mental retardation, neurological damage due to anoxia or congenital syndromes e.g. *Lesch-Nyhan* syndrome (95-99). A number of methods have been described for the treatment of self-induced oral injury. These include the construction of processed hard acrylic splints, wire and acrylic splints (98) and tongue stents (97). FINGER & DUPERON (98) describe the construction of mouthguards for the mandibular and maxillary arches from a double thickness of soft vinyl. Holes were placed in each

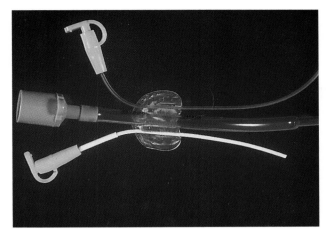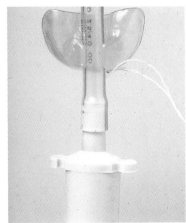

Fig. 21.16.
A. A neonatal protective plate supporting an endotracheal tube. B. A combined feeding and protective plate. Courtesy of Dr. S. P. ASH.

guard through which floss was threaded to provide a means of removal.

The protection of comatose patients from intra-oral injury may necessitate fitting a tongue stent that is wired to the mandible with brass ligatures (97).

Mouthguards have also been recommended for patients who traumatize their soft tissues due to the involuntary movements in *Parkinson's disease* (100).

Essentials

Preventive Measures in Sports

HIGH RISK SPORTS:
    American football
    Ice hockey
    Lacrosse
    Martial sports
    Rugby
    Skating

HIGH RISK INDIVIDUALS
    Maxillary overjet
    Inadequate lip coverage

COST BENEFIT OF MOUTHGUARD PROTECTION

TYPE OF PROTECTION
    Face masks
    Mouth Protectors
    a. Stock variety
    b. Mouth-formed
    c. Custom-made

Preventive Measures during Anesthetic Procedures

Preventive Measures of Oral Trauma in Intubated or Neonates

Bibliography

1. TODD JE, DODD T. *Childrens Dental Health in the UK* 1983. Office of Population Censuses and Surveys, Social Survey Div. London: HMSO 1985.

2. CRONA-LARSON G, NOREN JG. Luxation injuries to permanent teeth- A retrospective study of aetiological factors. *Endod Dent Traumatol* 1989; **5:** 176-79.

3. O'MULLANE DM. Injured permanent incisors of permanent incisors in school children. *Br Dent J* 1973; **134:** 328-32.

4. HEDEGARD B, STÅLHANE I. A study of traumatised permanent teeth in children aged 7-15 years. Part 1. *Swed Dent J* 1973; **66:** 431-50.

5. MCNUTT T, SHANNON SW, WRIGHT JT, FEINSTEIN RA. Oral trauma in adolescent athletes. *Paed Dent* 1989; **11:** 209-13.

6. GELBIER S. Injured anterior teeth in children. A preliminary discussion. *Br Dent J* 1967; **123:** 331-35.

7. SANE J, YLIPAAVALNIEMI P. Dental trauma in contact team sports. *Endod Dent Traumatol* 1988; **4:** 164-69.

8. POWELL JB, KEOWN KK. Endobronchial aspiration of a tooth. An unusual anaesthetic complication. *Anaesth Analg Curr Res* 1965; **44:** 355-57.

9. Federation Dentaire International *(FDI),* Commision on dental products, Working Party No. 7: 1990.

10. MCEWEN JD, MCHUGH WD, HITCHIN AD. Fractured maxillary incisors and incisal relationships. *J Dent Res* 1967; **46:** 1290. Abstract no. 87.

11. LEWIS TE. Incidence of fractured anterior teeth as related to their protrusion. *Angle Orthodont* 1959; **29:** 128-31.

12. EICHENBAUM IW. A correlation of traumatised anterior teeth to occlusion. *ASDC J Dent Child* 1963; **30:** 229-236.

13. OLVERA N. *8th Symposium on sports dentistry,* US Olympic Training Center, Colorado Springs, Co, USA

14. RANALLI DN. Prevention of craniofacial injuries in football. *Dental Clin of North Am* ed. 1991;**35:**627-45.

15. HEINTZ WD. Mouth Protectors: A progress report. *J Am Dent Assoc* 1968; **77:** 632-36.

16. GARON MW, MERKLE A, WRIGHT JT. Mouth protectors and oral trauma: A study of adolescent football players. *J Am Dent Assoc* 1986; **112:** 663-65.

17. DAVIES RM, BRADLEY D, HALE RW, LAIRD WRE, THOMAS PD. The prevalence of dental injuries in rugby players and their attitude to mouthguards. *Br J Sports Med* 1977; **11:** 72-74.

18. NICHOLAS NK. Mouth protection in contact sports. *N Z Dent J* 1969; **65:** 14-24.

19. CASTALDI CR. Sports related oral and facial injuries in the young athlete; a new challenge for the paediatric dentist. *Paed Dent* 1986; **8:** 311-15.

20. NADEAU J. Special prosthesis. *J Pros Dent* 1978; **20:** 62-76.

21. BOLHUIS JHA, LEURS JMM, FOGEL GE. Dental and facial injuries in international Field Hockey. *Br J Sports Med* 1987; **21:** 174-77.

22. LEES GH, GASKELL PHF. Injuries to the mouth and teeth in an undergraduate population. *Br Dent J* 1976; **140:** 107-08.

23. NYSETHER S. Dental injuries among Norwegian soccer players. *Community Dent Oral Epidemiol* 1987; **15:** 141-43.

24. STEVENS OO. Mouth protectors: Evaluation of twelve types-second year. *ASDC J Dent Child* 1965; **32:** 137-43.

25. WATTS G, WOOLARD A, SINGER CE. Functional mouth protectors for contact sports. *J Am Dent Assoc* 1954; **49:** 7-11.

26. BUREAU OF DENTAL EDUCATION, COUNCIL ON DENTAL MATERIALS AND DEVICES. Mouth Protectors. 11 years later. *J Am Dent Assoc* 1973; **86:** 1365-67.

27. BLIGNAULT JB, CARSTENS IL, LOMBARD CJ. Injuries sustained by wearers and non-wearers of mouthguards. *Br J Sports Med* 1987; **21:** 5-7.

28. SANE J. Maxillo-facial and dental injuries in contact team sports. *Proc Finnish Dent Soc* 1988;**84,** Suppl. Vl.

29. NYSETHER S. Tannskader i norsk idrett. *Norske Tannlegefor Tid* 1987; **97:** 512-14.

30. DUKES HH. Latex football mouthpieces. *J Am Dent Assoc* 1954; **49:** 445-48.

31. HUGENHOLTZ H, RICHARD MT. Return to athletic competition following following concussion. *Can Med Assoc J* 1982; **127:** 827-29.

32. STENGER JM. Mouthguards: protection against shock to the head, neck and teeth. *J Am Dent Assoc* 1964; 69: 273-81.

33. CHAPMAN PJ. Concussion in contact sports and importance of mouthguards in protection. *Aust J Sci Med Sport* 1985; **17:** 25-28.

34. GENNARELLI TA. In: TORG JS, ed. *Athletic injuries to the Head, Neck and Face.* Philadelphia: Lea & Febiger, 1982.

35. HICKEY JC, MORRIS AL, CARLSON LD, et al. The relation of mouth protectors to cranial pressure and deformation. *J Am Dent Assoc* 1965; **74:** 735-40.

36. UNTERHARNSCHEIT F. About boxing: a review of the historical and medical aspects. *Texas Rep Biol Med* 1970; **28:** 421-95.

37. HEINTZ WD. The case for mandatory protectors. *Phys Sports Med* 1975; **3:** 60-63.

38. JOSELL SD, ABRAMS RG. Traumatic injuries to the dentition and its supporting structures. *Paed Clin N Am* 1982; **29:** 717-43.

39. STEVENS OO. In: ANDREASEN JO, ed. *Traumatic Injuries to the Teeth.* Copenhagen: Munksgaard 1981:p.442.

40. WALKDEN L. The medical hazards of rugby football. *Practitioner* 1975; **215:** 201-07.

41. DENNIS CG, PARKER DAS. Mouthguards in Australian sport. *Aust Dent J* 1972; **17:** 228-35.

42. BUREAU OF DENTAL HEALTH EDUCATION AND BUREAU OF ECONOMIC RESEARCH AND STATISTICS. Evaluation of mouth protectors used by high school football players. *J Am Dent Assoc* 1964; **68:** 430-42.

43. TURNER CH, Mouth Protectors. *Br Dent J* 1977; **143:** 82-86.

44. MOON DG, MITCHELL DF. An evaluation of a commercial protective mouthpiece for football players. *J Am Dent Assoc* 1961; **62:** 568-72.

45. Report of the Joint Committee of the American Association for Health, Physical Education and Recreation and American Dent Assoc 1962.

46. OIKARINEN K. Pathogenesis and mechanism of traumatic injuries to teeth. *Endod Dent Traumatol* 1987; **3:** 220-23.

47. CHAPMAN PJ. The bimaxillary mouthguard: Increased protection against orofacial and head injuries in sport. *Aust J Sci Med Sport* 1985; **17:** 25-29.

48. CHANDLER NP, WILSON NHF, DABER BS. A modified maxillary mouthguard. *Br J Sports Med* 1987; **21:** 27-28.

49. GOING RE, LOEHMAN RE, CHAN MS. Mouthguard materials: Their physical and mechanical properties. *J Am Dent Assoc* 1974; **89:** 132-38.

50. CHACONAS SJ, CAPUTO AA, BAKKE N K. A comparison of mouth guard materials. *Am J Sports Medicine* 1985; **13:** 193-97.

51. CRAIG RG, GODWIN WC. Physical properties of materials for custom made mouthguards. *J Mich Dent Assoc* 1967; **49:** 34-40.

52. GODWIN WC, CRAIG RG. Stress transmitted through mouth protectors. *J Am Dent Assoc* 1970; **77:** 1316-20.

53. Bureau of Health Education and Audiovisual Services Council on Dental Materials, Mouth protectors and sports team dentists. *J Am Dent Assoc* 1984; **109:** 84-87.

54. YOUNG MR. *Mouthguard materials: A comparative study of resilience and chemical composition.* Master of Science thesis, Univ. of London, 1990.

55. BISHOP BM, DAVIES EH, VON FRAUENHOFER JA, et al. Materials for mouth protectors. *J Prosthet Dent* 1985; 53: 256-60.

56. SCHEER B. Unpublished data, 1993

57. KUEBKER WA, MORROW RM, COHEN PA. Do mouth-formed mouthguards meet the NCAA rules? *Phys Sports Medicine* 1986; 14: 69-74.

58. STOKES ANS, CROFT GC, GEE D. Comparison of laboratory and intraorally formed mouth protectors. *Endod Dent Traumatol* 1987, 3: 255-58.

59. CHAPMAN PJ. Mouthguards in sport. *Sport Health* 1983; 1: 13-15.

60. CHAPMAN PJ. The prevalence of oro-facial injuries and use of mouthguards in rugby union. *Aust Dent J* 1985, 30: 364-67.

61. UPSON N. Mouthguards, an evaluation of two types for rugby players. *Br J Sports Med* 1985; 19: 89-92.

62. GODWIN WC. Simplified mouth protector technique. *J Mich Dent Assoc* 1962; 44: 132-34.

63. CATHCART JF. Mouthprotectors for contact sports. *Dent Digest* 1951; 57: 346-48.

64. CASTALDI CR. Mouthguards in contact sports. *J Conn State Dent Assoc* 1974; 48: 233-41.

65. NICHOLAS NK. Mouth protection for children. *N Z Dent J* 1982; 78: 62-64.

66. BARANKOVICH GJ. Mouth protector for an edentulous patient. *J Prosth Dent* 1975; 34: 588-90.

67. NACHMAN BM, SMITH JF, RICHARDSON FS. Football players opinions of mouthguards. *J Am Dent Assoc* 1965; 70: 62-69.

68. RENDER TP. Mouth protector sanitation. *J Am Dent Assoc* 1963; 66: 709.

69. GODWIN WC, CRAIG RG, KORAN A, et al. Mouthprotectors in junior football players. *Phys Sports Medicine* 1982; 10: 42-48.

70. UPSON N. Dental injuries and the attitudes to mouthguards. *Br J Sports Med* 1982; 16: 241-44.

71. SEALS RS, KUEBKER WA, MORROW RM, FARNEY WD. An evaluation of mouth guard programs in Texas high school football. *J Am Dent Assoc* 1985; 110: 904-09.

72. DE WET FA. The prevention of orofacial sports injuries in the adolescent. *Int Dent J* 1981; 31: 313-19.

73. MAESTRELLO-DEMOYA MG, PRIMOSCH RE. Orofacial trauma & mouthprotector wear among high school varsity players. *ASDC J Dent Child* 1989; 56: 36-39

74. WILKINSON EE, POWERS JM. Properties of mouthprotector materials. *Phys Sports Med* 1986; 14: 77-84.

75. JENSEN J. Intra oral mouth guards in a group of athletes (Boxers). *Tandlægebladet* 1984; 88: 681-86.

76. CHAPMAN PJ. The prevalence of orofacial injuries and the use of mouth guards in Rugby Union. *Aust Dent J* 1985; 30: 364-67.

77. BLACKBURN MM. One year evaluation of twelve mouth protectors for Edmonton hockey players. *J Can Dent Assoc* 1964; 30: 560-64.

78. BLUM J, KRANZ S. Operation mouth guard: A model program designed to prevent dental trauma. *ASDC J Dent Child* 1982; 49: 22-24.

79. SEALS RR, DORROUGH BC. Custom mouth protectors: A review of their applications. *J Prosthet Dent* 1984; 51: 238-42.

80. BAMFORTH BJ. Complications during endotracheal anaesthesia. *Anesth Analges* 1963; 42: 727-32.

81. McCARTHY G, CARLSON O. A dental splint for use during peroral endoscopy. *Acta Otolaryngol* 1977; 84: 450-52.

82. EVERS W, RACZ GB, GLAZER J, DOBKIN AB. Orahesive as a protection for the teeth during general anaesthesia and endoscopy. *Canad Anaesthes Soc J* 1967; 14: 123-28.

83. NAYEK AM, WINNICK AM. An acrylic dental protector in oral endoscopy. *J Otolaryngol* 1976; 5: 86-88.

84. BLANC VF, TREMBLAY NAG. The complications of tracheal intubation: a new classification with review of the literature. *Anesth Analges* 1974; 53: 202.

85. WRIGHT RB, MANFIELD FFV. Damage to the teeth during the administration of general anaesthesia. *Anesth Analges* 1974; 53: 405-08.

86. LOCKHART PB, FELDBAU EV, GABEL RA, et al. Dental complications during and after tracheal intubation. *J Am Dent Assoc* 1986; 112: 480-83.

87. RISK MANAGEMENT FOUNDATION. Anaesthesia claims analysis show frequency low, losses high. *Risk Management Foundation* 1983; 4: 1-2.

88. DUKE PM, COULSON JD, SANTOS JI, JOHNSON JD. Cleft palate associated with prolonged orotracheal intubation in infancy. *J Pediatr* 1976; 89: 990-91.

89. SEOW WK, PERHAM S, YOUNG WG, DALEY T. Dilaceration of a primary incisor associated with neonatal laryngoscopy. *Paed Dent* 1990; 12: 321-24.

90. HENRY PJ, BARB RE. Mouth protectors for use in general anaesthesia. *J Am Dent Assoc* 1964; 68: 569-70.

91. DAVIS FO, DEFREECE AB, SHROFF PF. Custom made plastic guards for tooth protection during endoscopy and endotracheal intubation. *Anesth Analg* 1971; 50: 203-06.

92. ANDREASEN JO. Personal communication. 1993.

93. ASH SP, MOSS JP. An investigation of the features of the preterm infant palate and the effect of prolonged orotracheal intubation with and without protective appliances. *Br J Orthod* 1987; 14: 253-61.

94. SULLIVAN PG. An appliance to support oral intubation in the premature infant. *Br Dent J* 1982; 103: 191-95.

95. FENTON SJ. Management of oral self mutilation in neurologically impared children. *Spec Care Dentist* 1982; 2: 70-73.

96. FREEDMAN A, SEXTON T, REICH D, et al. Neuropathologic chewing in comatose children: a case report. *Paediatr Dent* 1981; 3: 334-36.

97. HANSON GE, OGLE RG, GIRON L. A tongue stent for the prevention of oral trauma in the comatose patient. *Crit Care Med* 1975; 3: 200-203.

98. FINGER S, DUPERON DF. The management of oral trauma secondary to encephalitis: a clinical report. *ASDC J Dent Child* 1991; 58: 60-63.

99. TURLEY PK, HENSON JL. Self injurous lip biting; etiology and management. *J Pedod* 1983; 7: 209-20.

100. HUSSEIN SB. Use of a gum shield for Parkinsons disease patients. *Br Dent J* 1989; 166: 320.

CHAPTER 22

Prognosis of Traumatic Dental Injuries

P. K. ANDERSEN, F. M. ANDREASEN &
J. O. ANDREASEN

Expressing Prognosis Quantitatively

In the dental literature, the most frequently used method for expressing prognosis is as proportion survival, where **n** treatments are followed for time intervals of varying length and x/n x 100% of these procedures develop a given complication. Prognosis then relates to an average or median interval (1,2).

When analyzing the occurrence of events such as pulp necrosis (PN), pulp canal obliteration (PCO) and root resorption (RR) after dental trauma, **time**

becomes very important. First, from a clinical point of view, the time after injury at which complications are likely to occur and the order in which different complications can be anticipated play an important role for clinical decision making.

As healing complications usually appear with some time variation, the length of observation period of patients followed is decisive (Fig. 22.1). If, for example, the observation period for an overwhelming majority of patients in a trauma study is so long that most complications will have appeared (period C), conventional frequency calculations will provide a reliable picture of the likelihood of a given event.

Fig. 22.1.
Typical time relation between occurrence of healing complications after dental trauma. After AN-DREASEN (1) *1987.*

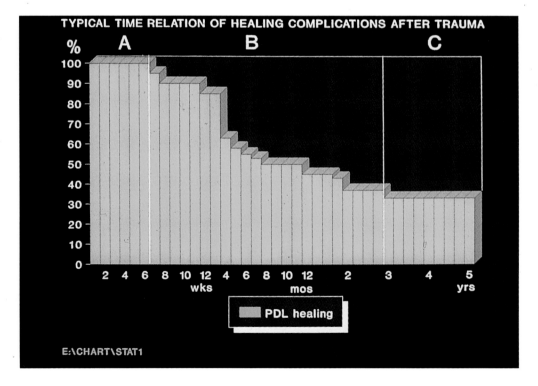

Fig. 22.2.
Observation time and probability of diagnosis of <u>pulp necrosis</u> *of extrusion of mature permanent teeth. After* ANDREASEN & PETERSEN (3) *1985.*

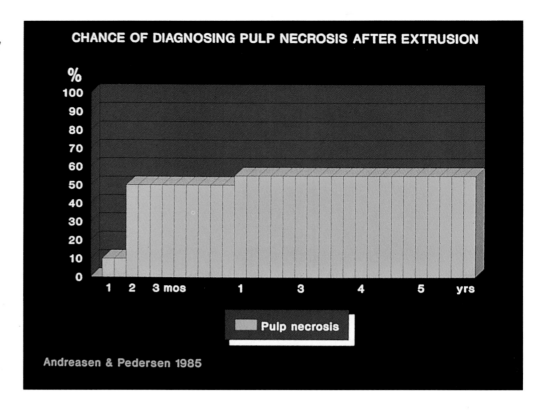

However, if prognosis is calculated from a material with a very short observation period (period A), an unrealistically optimistic picture of complication events will be presented. In period B, a varied picture of the appearance of complications will be seen due to variation in length of observation periods and their relation to the chance of detecting a given complication (1).

It can be seen from Figs. 22.2 to 22.4 that *pulp necrosis*, *pulp canal obliteration* and *root resorption* after luxation or avulsion with subsequent replantation of permanent teeth appear with relatively large variations in time (3-8). Thus, expression of prognosis for these complications will show great variation from one investigation to another, making comparison of results difficult, if not impossible. However, using the method of **meta-analysis** (see later), it is possible to summarize the results from similar investigations in a quantitative manner.

Also, from a statistical point of view, the *time* factor is important because teeth are observed at varying time intervals due to staggered entry and a fixed closing date, implying different probabilities of experiencing a given complication within the

period of observation. This fact must be taken into account in statistical analyses of clinical data on dental trauma. This problem can be overcome by focusing on events during a time interval of fixed length and expressing prognosis as proportion survival as explained above, but such a procedure may involve a serious loss of information.

An informative expression of prognosis is achieved by means of *life table*, or *actuarial statistics*, by which variation in prognosis with variation in observation period can be described. Such an analysis permits full utilization of all "survival" information accumulated up to the closing date of the study, including information from patients with partial follow-ups (i.e. patients not followed through to the occurrence of a given complication or terminal event). This form of analysis is well known and widely applied in studies of life expectancy with cancer (9-12); and more recently it has been applied to long-term dental investigations, such as the longevity of dental filling materials (13-16), pulp capping procedures (17), tooth transplantation (18, 19), and long-term prognosis of various dental trauma entities (3-8, 20, 21).

A crucial difference in survival data

Fig. 22.3.
Observation time and probability of <u>pulp canal obliteration</u> *subsequent to lateral or extrusive luxation of mature permanent teeth. After* ANDREASEN ET AL. (5) *1987.*

Fig. 22.3.
Observation time and probability of <u>pulp canal obliteration</u> *subsequent to lateral or extrusive luxation of mature permanent teeth. After* ANDREASEN ET AL. (5) *1987.*

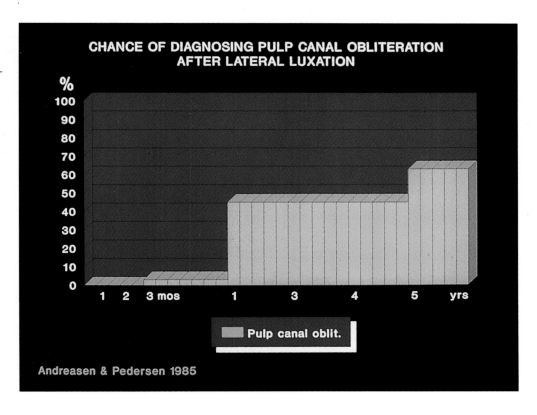

from, e.g., cancer trials and data on occurrence of complications after dental trauma results from the non-fatal nature of the latter complications. Typically, the occurrence of a dental complication must be diagnosed in a clinical investigation, and this means that only at some predetermined observation periods can it be seen whether a given complication has arisen since the previous follow-up examination; but the precise time of occurrence in the time interval cannot be determined. Thus, the relevant statistical analysis of occurrences of complications is an analysis of *grouped survival data* (3).

A calculation illustrating the principles of life-table analysis is presented in the following example of patients suffering

Fig. 22.4.
Observation time and probability of diagnosis of <u>external root resorption</u> *after replantation of avulsed permanent teeth. After* ANDREASEN ET AL. (7) *1992.*

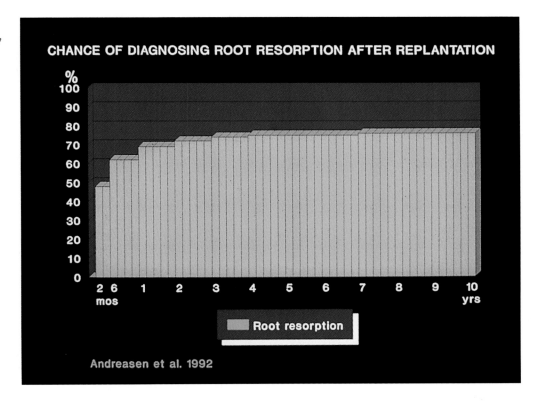

Fig. 22.5.
Calculation of periodontal liga-ment survival in a theoretical clinical dental trauma study. After ANDREASEN (1) 1987.

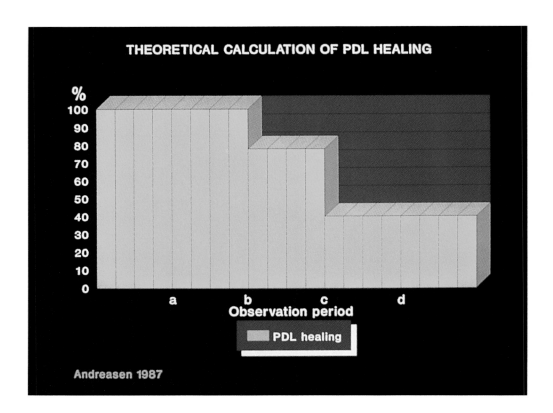

dental trauma (e.g. replantation of avulsed teeth) (Fig. 22.5). Each patient will repre-sent one of the following three outcomes:

Failed - if the replanted tooth has de-veloped one of the complications under study.

Withdrawn - if the tooth (patient) is lost from the trial for any reason other than healing complications from the injury. For example, if a patient stopped attending recall examinations and was lost to follow-up, or if a tooth was lost due to causes unrelated to the initial trauma, e.g. a new acute injury.

Censored - if the tooth is still in function at the end of the investigation and does not show the complications being stu-died.

The following example will show the principles of the calculations behind a tooth survival analysis: Ten patients with a total of 10 replanted incisors participate in a prospective investigation. There are no teeth showing failure at the end of the first observation period (a). Tooth survival at the end of the first interval is therefore 100%. At the end of the next interval (b), failure is seen in 2 teeth. Tooth survival is now:

$$\frac{10-2}{10} \times 100\% = 80\%$$

In the third observation period (c), there are now only 8 teeth at risk. Of these 8

teeth, 4 fail; that is, 4/8 of 80% have survived, yielding 40% survival. No com-plications are registered in the fourth in-terval (d), but 2 patients have such short observation periods that they are with-drawn from the study. There are now only 2 teeth left. Tooth survival is therefore 2/2 of 40% = 40%. It can be seen from Fig. 22.5 that the risk for a given complication can now be calculated for a given observa-tion period (3).

Life table statistics are very sensitive to a number of factors, such as definitions of failed, withdrawn and censored patients, as well as recall procedures and sample size. The significance of these factors will therefore be discussed.

Importance of Definition of Failures

Failures can be defined according to the type of dental trauma analyzed, such as loss of tooth, root resorption, devel-opment of pulp necrosis, pulp canal obliteration or loss of marginal bone sup-port. Each of these conditions (apart from tooth loss) represents unique diagnostic difficulties. Thus, *pulp necrosis* is depend-ent upon a number of diagnostic proce-dures, where none is conclusive (see Chapter 9, p. 352). *Pulp canal obliteration, root resorption* and *loss of marginal bone sup-*

port are primarily dependent upon radiographic examination procedures. This implies that a variation in technique could influence the sensibility of the analysis. Concerning *tooth loss*, it should be established whether the tooth in question was otherwise intact and in function, and that the extraction was *not* related to the previous trauma (e.g. a traffic accident, extraction for orthodontic or prosthetic purposes). Otherwise serious bias might arise.

Importance of Censored Patients

The definition of a censored event (i.e. tooth survival or tooth presence without pathology) is, like failures, entirely dependent upon the established criteria for pathology. Furthermore, it is important that the majority of censored data represent adequate observation periods for the complication to have had a chance to appear. Otherwise problems may arise regarding the reliability of the survival analysis.

Importance of Withdrawn Patients

The usual reason for withdrawal of patients from continuing examination appears to be one of the following:
-The patient cannot be traced (moved without a forwarding address, emigration, death).
-The patient has received a recall notice and chosen not to respond
-The tooth in question is lost.
-The tooth in question has survived and the patient does not feel the need for a follow-up examination.
-The patient ignores the recall notice for other reasons (e.g. inconvenience or lack of interest).

If the reasons for no-show at a scheduled follow-up are centered around the first two, the analysis may be seriously jeopardized. The relevance of no-shows has only been studied in a few dental investigations (20-26). Thus, it was shown in a long-term study of healing after surgical endodontics that patients not initially responding to recall notices, when later examined after extensive recall efforts demonstrated the same healing pattern as the rest of the material (24). This illustrates that, at least

in the cited study, the no-shows were usually related to inconvenience for the patient of the scheduled examination.

Importance of the Length of the Investigation Period

This is a crucial factor and should be related to the mean or median observation period for the occurrence of the event under investigation. Thus, root resorption requires extended observation periods for the material before any meaningful survival statistics can be established (7, 8).

Importance of Sample Size

The sample size becomes very important especially when the pathological event under investigation occurs infrequently.

Effect of Recall Schedule

As mentioned above, it can usually only be established at some prescheduled follow-up examinations whether a given complication has arisen since the previous examination, whereas the precise time of occurrence within that period cannot be determined. The recall schedule is therefore important. Short time intervals between successive follow-up examinations are recommended when the rate of failure is high, whereas longer time intervals may be chosen when few failures are likely to occur.

Comparing Life Tables

The Logrank Test for Comparison of Life Tables

Life table estimates for the survival probability in two groups, e.g. two randomized treatment groups, may be compared at a single point in time, **t**, using the variance estimate based on Greenwood's formula (12). It would be more efficient, however, to compare survival of the two groups on the entire survival functions and not only on their value at a single point in time. This may be done using the *logrank test statistic* for the case of continuously observed i.e. *non-grouped survival data* (9, 10). For *grouped survival data*, a similar test has been developed (12).

Further Treatment Comparisons, Multivariate Analysis

In almost all clinical investigations, the identification of clinical factors which have an effect on the occurrence of healing complications after trauma has been achieved using univariate statistical analysis where it is assumed that all teeth in the group for which the estimate is calculated have the same survival probability. In this type of analysis, each potential causative factor is considered individually, usually with the result that numerous clinical factors can be identified that are significantly related to the given healing complication. In many cases, however, the groups are heterogeneous and the relationships found may have little biological relevance, as they may be due to associations between registered clinical parameters. As an example, assume that the stage of root development is the only clinical parameter related to a given complication, and a given type of treatment (e.g. repositioning and splinting) is chosen according to stage of root development. In such a case, in a univariate analysis, there may be a significant relationship between treatment procedure and complication due to this association.

In order to identify and eliminate such associations, various multivariate analyses have been developed whereby the effect of several factors is studied simultaneously. For the case of continuously observed data the *Cox regression model* is frequently used (12, 27). It is also possible to use such a model for grouped survival data when, e.g., treatment comparisons are to be made in the presence of other prognostic factors (3, 28). In this way, associations can be disclosed and/or eliminated and this has been shown to significantly reduce the number of predictors for healing complications after dental traumas (3,6-8,29).

The Use of Predictors and Confidence Limits

From a regression model it is possible to estimate the probability that a given complication will arise during a given interval for a patient having a tooth with the given characteristics. Confidence limits for such a predictor may also be estimated.

Comparing Tooth Survival or Healing Results from various Studies

In the evaluation of the effect of various treatment modalities, the usual approach is to report the individual findings from clinical studies, the so-called narrative review (31). Such an analysis usually results in a range of treatment effects from which it is difficult to summarize the effect of a given treatment. To overcome this difficulty, **meta-analysis** can be used. This method uses statistical techniques to summarize estimates from a series of studies with common underlying characteristics (31) and thus allows estimation of the magnitude of a treatment effect. The principle is that when the effect of the same treatment has been estimated in a number of similar studies (together with confidence limits), a quantitative overview can be obtained as a weighted average of the individual estimates using as weights the precision of the individual estimates.

Essentials

Expressing Prognosis Quantitatively
> Percent calculation (i.e. disregarding relationship to observation period)
> Life table statistics (i.e incorporating relationship to observation period)

Factors of Importance for Life Table Analysis
> Definition of healing and non-healing
> Censored patients
> Withdrawn patients
> Length of period under consideration

> Sample size
> Recall schedule

Comparing Life Tables
> Log rank test for treatment comparisons
> Multivariate analysis

Predictors and Confidence Intervals

Comparing Healing Results
> Meta-analysis

Bibliography

1. ANDREASEN FM. Prognoser ved tandskader i det permanente tandsæt. *Odontologi '87.* Copenhagen: Munksgaards Forlag, 1987:149-64.

2. DAVIES JA. Dental restoration longevity: a critique of the life table method of analysis. *Community Dent Oral Epidemiol* 1987;**15**:202-4.

3. ANDREASEN FM, PEDERSEN BV. Prognosis of luxated permanent teeth - the development of pulp necrosis. *Endod Dent Traumatol* 1985;**1**:207-20.

4. ANDREASEN F, YU Z, THOMSEN BL. The relationship between pulpal dimensions and the development of pulp necrosis after luxation injuries in the permanent dentition. *Endod Dent Traumatol* 1986;**2**:90-8.

5. ANDREASEN FM, YU Z, THOMSEN BL, ANDERSEN PK. The occurrence of pulp canal obliteration after luxation injuries in the permanent dentition. *Endod Dent Traumatol* 1987;**3**:103-15.

6. ANDREASEN JO, BORUM M, JACOBSEN HL, ANDREASEN FM. Replantation of 400 avulsed permanent incisors. II. Factors related to root growth after replantation. 1993: To be submitted.

7. ANDREASEN JO, BORUM M, JACOBSEN HL, ANDREASEN FM. Replantation of 400 avulsed permanent incisors. IV. Factors related to periodontal ligament healing. 1993: To be submitted.

8. ANDREASEN JO, BORUM M, JACOBSEN HL, ANDREASEN FM. Replantation of 400 avulsed permanent incisors. V. Factors related to the progression of root resorption. 1993: To be submitted.

9. PETO R, PIKE MC, ARMITAGE P, et al. Design and analysis of randomized clinical trials requiring prolonged observation of each patient. II. Analysis and examples. *Br J Cancer* 1977;**35**:1-39.

10. PETO R, PIKE MC, ARMITAGE P, et al. Design and analysis of randomized clinical trials requiring prolonged observation of each patient. I. Introduction and design. *Br J Cancer* 1976;**34**:585-612.

11. LEE ET. *Statistical methods for survival data analysis.* Belmont, California: Lifetime learning publications, 1980.

12. ANDERSEN PK, VÆTH M. *Statistisk analyse af overlevelsesdata ved lægevidenskabelige undersøgelser.* Copenhagen: FADL's Forlag 1984.

13. THYLSTRUP A, RÖLLING I. The life table method in clinical dental research. *Commun Dent Oral Epidemiol* 1975;**3**:5-10.

14. WALLS AWG, WALLWORK MA, HOLLAND IS, MURRAY JJ. The longevity of occlusal amalgam restorations in first permanent molars of child patients. *Br Dent J* 1985;**158**:133-6.

15. SMALES RJ. Effects of enamel-bonding, type of restoration, patient age and operator on the longevity of an anterior composite resin. *Am J Dent* 1991;**4**:130-3.

16. SMALES RJ, WEBSTER DA, LEPPARD PI. Survival predictions of four types of dental restorative materials. *J Dent* 1991;**19**:278-82.

17. HØRSTED P, SØNDERGAARD B, THYLSTRUP A, EL ATTAR K, FEJERSKOV O. A retrospective study of direct pulp capping with calcium hydroxide compounds. *Endod Dent Traumatol* 1985;**1**:29-34.

18. SCHWARZ O, BERGMANN P, KLAUSEN B. Autotransplantation of human teeth. A life-table analysis of prognostic factors. *Int J Oral Surg* 1985;**14**:245-58.

19. ANDREASEN JO, PAULSEN HU, YU Z, BAYER T, SCHWARTZ O. A long-term study of 370 autotransplanted premolars. Part II. Tooth survival and pulp healing subsequent to transplantation. *Eur J Orthod* 1990;**12**:14-24.

20. ANDREASEN FM, ANDREASEN JO, BAYER T. Prognosis of root fractured permanent incisors - prediction of healing modalities. *Endod Dent Traumatol* 1989;**5**:11-22.

21. MITCHELL L, WALLS AWG. Survival analysis in practice. *Dental Update* 1990;April:125-8.

22. STRINDBERG LZ. The dependence of the results of pulp therapy on certain factors. An analytic study based on radiographic and clinical follow-up examinations. *Acta Odontol Scand* 1956;**14**:Suppl 21.

23. MÜHLEMANN HR. Zur statistischen Beurteilung von Wurzelbehandlungserfolgen. *Schweiz Monatschr Zahnheilk* 1965;**75**:1135-42.

24. RUD J, ANDREASEN JO, MØLLER JENSEN JE. A follow-up study of 1000 cases treated by endodontic surgery. *Int J Oral Surg* 1972;**1**:215-28.

25. FAZIO RC, BOFFA J. A study of "Broken Appointment" patients in Children's Hospital Dental Clinic. *J Dent Res* 1977;**56**:1071-6.

26. APT H, DYRNA G, NITZSCHE W, VÖLKER J. Mathematisch-statistische Aussagekraft klinisch-röntgenologischer Nachuntersuchungen von Wurzelbehandlungen. *Zahn Mund Kieferheilk* 1975;**63**:819-22.

27. COX DR. Regression models and life tables. *J Royal Stat Soc* 1972;**34**:187-220.

28. PRENTICE RL, GLOECKLER LA. Regression analysis of grouped survival data with applicaton to breast cancer data. *Biometrics* 1978;**34**:57-67.

29. ANDREASEN FM. Pulpal healing after luxation injuries and root fracture in the permanent dentition. *Endod Dent Traumatol* 1989;**5**:111-31.

30. EARLY BREAST CANCER TRIALISTS' COLLABORATIVE GROUP. Effects of adjuvant tamoxifen and of cytotoxic therapy on mortality in early breast cancer: an overview of 61 randomized trials among 28,896 women. *New Engl J Med* 1988;**319**:1681-92.

31. COHEN PA. Meta-analysis: application to clinical dentistry and dental education. *J Dent Education* 1992;**56**:172-5.

Appendix 1

Emergency record for acute dental trauma

Patient's name	
Birth date	

Date of examination:	Referred by:
Time of examination:	Referring diagnosis:

General medical history: any serious illness?　　　　　yes　no
If yes, explain.
Any allergy?　　　　　yes　no
If yes, explain.
Have you been vaccinated against tetanus?　　　　　yes　no
If yes, when.

Previous dental injuries:　　　　　yes　no
If yes,
　　When?
　　Which teeth were injured?
　　Treatment given and by whom?

Present dental injury:
　　Date:　　　　　　　Time:
　　Where?
　　How?

Have you had or have now *headache?*　　　　　yes　no

Have you had or have now *nausea?*　　　　　yes　no

Have you had or have now *vomiting?*　　　　　yes　no

Were you *unconscious* at the time of injury?　　　　　yes　no
If yes, for how long (minutes)?
Can you *remember* what happened before,　　　　　yes　no
during or after the accident?

The emergency record is constructed so that wherever a question is answered by *yes,* more details must be provided. Finally, the last question in the record is whether the examiner has re-read the chart. This is a reminder to check that all relevant points have been registered.

Emergency record for acute dental trauma

Diagnoses (check appropriate boxes and designate tooth no. or indicate correct anatomical region)

☐ Infraction

☐ Complicated crown fracture

☐ Uncomplicated crown fracture

☐ Complicated crown-root fracture

☐ Uncomplicated crown-root fracture

☐ Root Fracture

☐ Alveolar fracture

☐ Mandibular fracture

☐ Maxillary fracture

☐ Concussion

☐ Subluxation

☐ Extrusion

☐ Lateral luxation

☐ Intrusion

☐ Exarticulation

☐ Skin abrasion

☐ Skin laceration

☐ Skin contusion

☐ Mucosal abrasion

☐ Mucosal laceration

☐ Mucosal contusion

☐ Gingival abrasion

☐ Gingival laceration

☐ Gingival contusion

Supplementary remarks:

Treatment plan
At time of injury: *Final therapy:*
Repositioning (time finished)
Fixation (time finished)
Pulpal therapy (time finished)
Dentinal coverage (time finished)

Chart re-read by examining dentist   ☐ yes ☐ no

Appendix 2

Clinical examination form for the time of injury and follow-up examinations

	Tooth no.	12		11		21		22	
TIME OF INJURY	Date								
TIME OF INJURY	Tooth color normal yellow red grey crown restoration								
TIME OF INJURY	Displacement (mm) intruded extruded protruded retruded								
TIME OF INJURY	Loosening (0-3)								
TIME OF INJURY	Tenderness to percussion (+/−)								
TIME OF INJURY	Pulp test (value)								
TIME OF INJURY	Ankylosis tone (+/−)								
TIME OF INJURY	Occlusal contact (+/−)								
CONTROL	Fistula (+/−)								
CONTROL	Gingivitis (+/−)								
CONTROL	Gingival retraction (mm)								
CONTROL	Abnormal pocketing (+/−)								

Each column represents an examination of a given tooth. The first column for each tooth gives the values from the time of injury. *Only* the parameters listed in the top half of the form ("Time of injury") are to be recorded at the time of injury. The information from this examination as well as the information collected on the emergency record are used to determine the final diagnoses for the injured teeth. Those parameters *and* the last four (fistula, gingivitis, gingival retraction, abnormal pocketing) are to be registered at all follow-up controls.

Emergency record for acute dental trauma

Objective examination – Extraoral findings (contd.)

Bleeding from nose, or rhinitis	yes	no
Bleeding from ext. auditory canal	yes	no
Double vision or limited eye movement	yes	no
Palpable signs of fracture of facial skeleton	yes	no

If yes, *location of fracture*

Objective examination – Intraoral findings

Lesions of the *oral mucosa*	yes	no
If yes, *type* and *location*		
Gingival lesion	yes	no
If yes, *type* and *location*		
Tooth fracture	yes	no
If yes, *type* and *location*		
Alveolar fracture	yes	no
If yes, *type* and *location*		

Supplemental information:

General condition of the dentition

Caries	poor	fair	good
Periodontal status	poor	fair	good
Horizontal occlusal relationship	undr bite	over jet	norm
Vertical occlusal relationship	deep	open	norm

Radiographic findings

Tooth dislocation

Root fracture

Bone fracture

Pulp canal obliteration

Root resorption

Photographic registration yes no

Appendix 3

Clinical and radiographic findings with the various luxation types

Findings	Concussion	Subluxation	Extrusion	Lateral Luxation	Intrusion
Clinical					
Abnormal mobility	−	+	+	−(+)	−(+)
Tenderness to percussion	+	+(−)*	+/−	−(+)	−(+)
Percussion sound**	normal	dull	dull	metallic	metallic
Response to pulp testing	+/−	+/−	−(+)	−(+)	−(+)
Clinical dislocation	−	−	+	+	+
Radiographic dislocation	−	−	+	+	+

* A sign in parentheses indicates a finding of rare occurrence.

** Teeth with incomplete root formation and teeth with marginal or periapical inflammatory lesions will also elicit a dull percussion sound.

Appendix 4

Summary of treatment and follow-up procedures and recall schedule following the various trauma types

Post-traumatic interval*	Radiographic exposure for various trauma types		
	Luxation of 21**	Replantation of 21	Root fracture of 21
Time of injury	OI 11,21*** BI 12,11,21,22	OI 11,21 BI 12,11,21,22	OI 11,21 BI 12,11,21,22
1 week		BI 21,22£$	
2-3 weeks	OI 11,21£$	BI 21,22	OI 11,21
6-8 weeks	BI 12,11,21,22£	BI 12,11,21,22	BI 12,11,21,22
3 months		BI 21,22	BI 12,11,21,22£
6 months		BI 21,22	
1 year	BI 12,11,21,22	BI 12,11,21,22	BI 12,11,21,22
2, 3, 4 years		BI 21,22	
5, 10, 15 years	BI 12,11,21,22	BI 12,11,21,22	BI 12,11,21,22

   * All examinations include radiographs as well as information from the clinical examination form (see Appendix 2).

  ** Tooth designation is according to the FDI two-digit system.

 *** Regarding radiographic exposure, OI implies "Occlusal Identical", or occlusal exposures; BI implies "bisecting identical". Both designations imply the use of standardized techniques and filmholder.

  £ Removal of fixation. The following fixation periods are suggested. The reader is referred to the respective chapters for details: Replantation, 1 week; Extrusion, 2-3 weeks; Lateral luxation, 3-8 weeks (depending on radiographic findings); Intrusion, see text for discussion of repositioning and fixation; Root fracture, 3 months.

  $ Begin endodontic therapy: Replantation, after 1 week, Intrusion, after 2 weeks.

Emergency record for acute dental trauma

Is there pain from *cold air?*   yes | no
If yes, *which teeth?*

Is there pain or tenderness from *occlusion?*   yes | no
If yes, *which teeth?*

Constant pain?   yes | no
If yes, *which teeth?*

Treatment elsewhere?   yes | no
If yes, *what treatment?*

After *exarticulation,* the following information is needed:
Where were the teeth found (dirt, asphalt, floor, etc.)?
When were the teeth found?
Were the teeth *dirty?*
How were the teeth *stored?*
Were the teeth *rinsed* and *with what* prior to replantation?
When were the teeth replanted?
Was *tetanus antitoxoid* given?
Were *antibiotics* given?
  Antibiotic?
  Dosage?

Objective examination
Is the patient's general condition affected?   yes | no
If yes, *pulse*
      blood pressure
      pupillary reflex
      cerebral condition
Objective findings beyond the head and neck?   yes | no
If yes, *type* and *location*
Objective findings within the head and neck?   yes | no
If yes, *type* and *location*

Appendix 5

Comparison between cost/effectiveness of different treatment solutions for anterior tooth loss

	Ortho-dontics	Implants	Resin-retained bridges	Conventional bridges	Auto-transplants
Cost	+++	+++	+	+++	+
Long-term service	+++	+++	+	+	+++
Use in growing individuals	+++	0	+	0	+++
Bone-inducing potential	+	0	0	0	+++

Scale used: 0 = not to be used or non-existent
+ = minimum (low)
++ = medium (moderate)
+++ = maximum (high)

Subject Index

Root resorption, internal
  after luxation injuries, 366
  after pulpotomy, 525
  after root fractures, 309
  treatment of, 563

S

Scutane® (see Epimine material)
Schulte-Sofort® implant (see Implants)
Seasonal variations in frequency of injuries, 175
Self-curing resin for splinting, 348
Semi-permanent restorations
  in crown fractures, 229
Sequestration of permanent tooth
    germs, 483
  bibliography, 491
  classification of, 459
  clinical findings of, 483
  essentials, 490
  etiology of, 483
  frequency of, 459
  radiographic findings of, 483
  terminology of, 459
  treatment of, 488
Serotonin in wound healing, 26, 120
Sevriton® (see Cast silver cap splint)
Sex distribution of dental injuries, 172
Shape of the impacting object (see Impact and dental injury)
Silver cap splint (see Cast silver cap splint)
Sodium hypochlorite solution, use in
    endodontics, 549
Sodium perborate for bleaching, 571
Space closure in orthodontic
    treatment, 608
Space maintainers in orthodontic treatment, 608
Space maintenance after loss of anterior
    teeth, 608
Splinting
  acid-etch/resin splint, 348
  acrylic splint, 348
  after crown fractures, 231
  after injuries to supporting bone, 438
  after luxation injuries, 348
  after replantation, 400
  after root fractures,
  arch bar, 174
  cast silver cap splint, 348
  interdental, 442
  intermaxillary, 442
  orthodontic band/brackets and resin
  splint, 348
  resin full arch splint
  self-curing resin used for
    splinting, 348

Spontaneous root fractures in osteogenesis and dentinogenesis imperfecta, 161
Sports injuries (see Athletics)
Stainless steel crowns
  in treatment of crown fractures, 229
Steel crowns (see Stainless steel crowns)
Statistical analysis, 737
Stock variety of mouth guards, 726
Storage media for avulsed
    teeth, 399, 408
Subluxation, 315
  bibliography, 378
  classification of, 155, 315
  clinical findings of, 317
  color changes of crown, 355
  endodontic treatment of, 543, 554
  essentials, 376
  etiology of, 315
  frequency of, 315
  laser Doppler flowmetry, 206, 355
  loss of marginal bone support, 373
  orthodontic treatment of, 608
  pathology of, 323
  prognosis of, 350
  pulp canal obliteration, 362
  pulp healing, 351
  pulp necrosis, 351
  pulp testing, 353
  radiographic findings of, 320
  root resorption, external, 366
  root resorption, internal, 370
  splinting, 347
  terminology of, 155, 315
  transient apical breakdown, 359
  transient marginal breakdown, 373
  treatment of, 332
Substance P in wound healing, 116
Superoxide in wound healing, 57, 58
Surface resorption
  after luxation injuries, 366
  after replantations, 410
  after root fractures, 287
Surgical exposure in crown-root
    fractures, 266
Surgical extrusion
  in crown-root fractures, 269
Surgicel® in wound healing, 62
Surgical treatment
  in crown dilacerated teeth, 485
  in crown-root fractures, 266, 269
  in disturbances in eruption, 488
  in lateral root angulation or dilacerations, 488
  in odontoma-like malformations, 488
  in replacement resorption, 621
  in root duplication, 488
  in root fractures, 306